AMYLOID AND AMYLOIDOSIS
1990

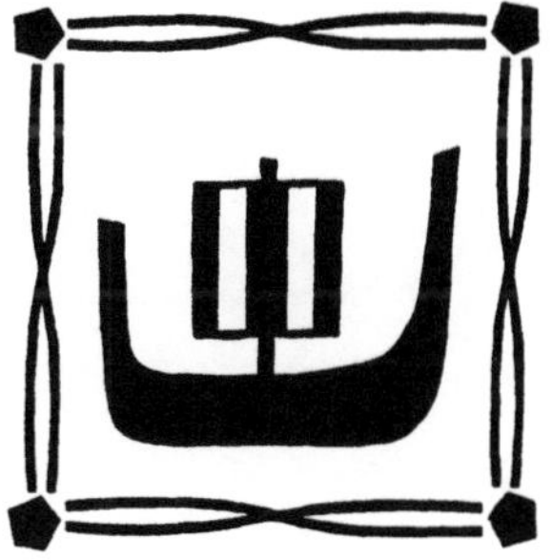

AMYLOID AND AMYLOIDOSIS 1990

VIth International Symposium on Amyloidosis,
August 5–8, 1990, Oslo, Norway

edited by

JACOB B. NATVIG

Institute of Immunology and Rheumatology,
University of Oslo, Oslo, Norway

ØYSTEIN FØRRE

Oslo Sanitetsforenings, Rheumatism Hospital,
University of Oslo, Oslo, Norway

GUNNAR HUSBY

Department of Rheumatology,
University of Tromsø, Tromsø, Norway

ANNE HUSEBEKK

Department of Immunology and Bloodbank,
University of Tromsø, Tromsø, Norway

BJØRN SKOGEN

Department of Immunology and Bloodbank,
University of Tromsø, Tromsø, Norway

KNUT SLETTEN

Department of Biochemistry,
University of Oslo, Oslo, Norway

PER WESTERMARK

Department of Pathology,
University of Linköping, Linköping, Sweden

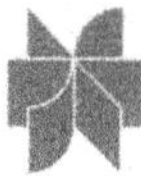

KLUWER ACADEMIC PUBLISHERS

DORDRECHT / BOSTON / LONDON

Library of Congress Cataloging-in-Publication Data

International Symposium on Amyloidosis (6th : 1990 : Oslo, Norway)
Amyloid and amyloidosis 1990 / VIth International Symposium on Amyloidosis, August 5-8, 1990, Oslo, Norway ; edited by Jacob B. Natvig.
p. cm.
Includes bibliographical references and index.

1. Amyloidosis--Congresses. I. Natvig, Jacob B. II. Title.
RC632.A5I57 1990
616.3'995--dc20 90-25031

Published by Kluwer Academic Publishers,
P.O. Box 17, 3300 AA Dordrecht, The Netherlands.

Kluwer Academic Publishers incorporates
the publishing programmes of
D. Reidel, Martinus Nijhoff, Dr W. Junk and MTP Press.

Sold and distributed in the U.S.A. and Canada
by Kluwer Academic Publishers,
101 Philip Drive, Norwell, MA 02061, U.S.A.

In all other countries, sold and distributed
by Kluwer Academic Publishers Group,
P.O. Box 322, 3300 AH Dordrecht, The Netherlands.

Printed on acid-free paper

PREFACE

Both scientifically and socially the VIth International Symposium on Amyloidosis, August 5 - 8, 1990 in Oslo was a great success. There were three and a half intensive days.

It started with the Opening Ceremony, particularly highlighted with the Norway-Norway multi media show by David Cochron, and ended with a visit to the Edvard Munch museum and the Farewell Salmon-Dinner on the evening of August 8 (not to forget the "happy birthday" song for Dorothea Zucker-Franklin at the breakfast table the following morning).

In between was the intellectual penetration into the science of amyloidosis and amyloid proteins, and a deepening of many friendships among young and old "amyloidologists", together with some of the cultural and historical features of Oslo and Norway. Among the numerous letters of thanks and gratitude that we have received, the senior organizer of the previous meeting, Takashi Isobe said it briefly and eloquently:

"You have overwhelmed us,
you have performed a drama with joy and cheer,
you have hosted so nicely with lovely secretariat,
you have arranged impressive hospitality in every respect,
you certainly did for all of us"

Now we are left with the proceedings book for the three coming years until the next symposium in Kingston, Canada, which will be organized by Drs. Robert Kisilevsky and Thomas Muckle from the Department of Pathology at Queens University in 1993.

The scientific contributions herein cover all the sessions of the meeting. In order to keep the structure of the book within the framework of about 900 pages, we have had to limit the size of each contribution in the following way. For each abstract submitted, we have allotted four pages of printed report to the proceedings, and for the introductory and summing up speakers, six pages. In a few instances we have accepted that contributors who submitted a shorter manuscript than required could add another, slightly longer manuscript, as long as the total was within the number of pages allotted. Some people have put in several abstracts and therefore had a greater amount of space available. In a couple of exceptional cases, for people who had only submitted one abstract and were session chairmen etc., we have accepted the same number of pages as for an introductory speaker.

The contributions have come in very rapidly. The best service to the scientific community is a speedy publication. Therefore, we decided to make the deadline for accepting more papers the end of August 1990, and left all the manuscripts to the efficient "camera-ready" publication of the book. We thank Kluwer Academic Publishers for all their efforts in making this publication of the proceedings a success. In addition, we would also like to particularly thank our two secretaries at the Institute of Immunology and Rheumatology in Oslo, Ms. Bente Brenna and Ms. Suzanne Garman-Vik for their conscientious help throughout the symposium and in organizing the scientific papers for the book. We also thank Ms. Hanne Haugen at the Winge Travel Bureau, Drammen, who did so much to see that everything went well. In addition, a group of students from the Department of Biochemistry, University of Oslo, contributed a great deal to the scientific success of the meeting. Finally, we will again thank our advertisers, exhibitors and sponsors who made the conducting of the symposium possible as well as the publication of this symposium book.

Linköping, Oslo, Tromsø, September 1990

Jacob B. Natvig
Øystein Førre Gunnar Husby
Anne Husebekk Bjørn Skogen
Knut Sletten Per Westermark

CONTENTS

III AMYLOID ENHANCING FACTOR (AEF), AMYLOID P-COMPONENT AND PROTEOGLYCANS IN AMYLOIDOSIS

We will hereby thank our advertisers, Applied Biosystems page 12, ABK Tek page 124, Nycomed Pharma page 248, Ciba Geigy page 328, Blackwell Scientific Publications page 422, Scandinavian Journal of Rheumatology page 564, Pfizer page 626, MSD page 732 and Sandoz page 850.

WELCOME!

Jacob B. Natvig
Chairman of the Organizing Committee.

Welcome to the Soria Moria Conference Center, to Oslo and Norway for the VIth International Symposium on Amyloidosis.

At the very pleasant and active meeting in Hakone, Japan three years ago, it was decided to hold the next meeting in Oslo. An organizing committee was established with Knut Sletten, Øystein Førre and myself from the Oslo group, Gunnar Husby, Anne Husebekk and Bjørn Skogen from the Tromsø group, and our close friend and collaborator through many years, Per Westermark from Linköping, Sweden. We have worked hard to try and organize a good meeting.

The best guarantee for a successful meeting, however, is all of you, the participating scientists from 18 different countries all over the world. We are very happy that so many came, altogether 235 registered participants and 70 accompanying persons bringing the total to just over 300. We are very pleased that all the senior scientists who are still in the field came to participate. There were also many young researchers, and several are here for the first time attending an International Symposium on Amyloidosis.

Perhaps most impressively, 226 abstracts have been submitted. They have been selected for oral presentations or for posters. This means that there is virtually a 1:1 ratio between scientific contributions and active participants. This should make the foundation for a most dynamic and vibrant scientific meeting.

The field of amyloidosis research is presently growing, and the numbers of participants and abstracts are the highest to date in the series of international symposia.

Who and what are we? We are not a society. Maybe we are a club? However, that is not an adequate expression either. A club is often a closed circle, but here we are a very open, outgoing group that would still like to have many more participants to help us solve all the problems and questions about amyloidosis and amyloid proteins.

And what should we name ourselves? Perhaps you would like to be named an "amyloidologist"? One of our problems is that the name of our group of scientists is as well as the name of the disease and these terms are very unfamiliar to most people.

This reminds me of the "diagnosis law" by Professor Gudmund Hernes, Oslo; "Even if the doctor has a name for your disease, it does not mean that he knows what you are suffering from" (1). This notion that we doctors in a deeper sense do not know what our patients are suffering from is certainly true in many ways of amyloidosis. We have had a name for this condition for about 150 years. However, only in the last 20 years have we been able to identify and classify a number of proteins that can give rise to amyloidosis. We certainly expect there to be even new reports of such proteins at this symposium. However, the true nature of amyloidosis and how we can prevent it, or cure it, is still only in the initial stages of research. Therefore, although we have had great success in classifying, describing and diagnosing amyloid proteins and amyloidosis, a curative therapy or an effective prophylaxis is still pending.

When the first Nobel Prize in medicine was awarded in 1901 to Emil von Behring it was for; "his work on serum therapy, especially its application against diphtheria by which he has opened a new road in the domain of medical science and thereby placed in the hands of the physicians a victorious weapon against illness and death". This is our aim as scientists in the amyloidosis field also: To find a victorious weapon against illness and death from amyloidosis.

Now, why are we scientists and why are we struggling for these goals? Many different forces may drive us. In my experience, curiosity is perhaps the most central factor. Let me tell you a small episode about curiosity. As a young boy I walked hand in hand along the road with my father on a nice, nordic summer evening like this one here in Oslo. As usual I asked some questions. What the questions were is long forgotten, but not the answer to one of them; "this is something you will learn when you get older". I felt uncomfortable with the answer. That is probably why I still remember it so vividly almost 50 years later. Perhaps that was the moment that out of curiosity something was born inside that made me want to become a scientist, dissatisfaction with unanswered questions.

That is what science is all about, we strive to know the unknown and to penetrate the dark areas of the map of knowledge. In this way, science becomes not only a work, but a life style. A famous professor, Otto Lous Mohr, gave many excellent talks when he was the dean of the University of Oslo after the second world war. Several times he cited his teacher and friend, the Nobel Laureate T.H. Morgan, who once said; "A scientist is a man who loves science more than himself" (2). Morgan also, according to Professor Mohr, once divided his experiments into "fool experiments, damned fool experiments and those that are still worse". "No matter what the circumstances, you want to do those tiresome and sometimes silly experiments in order to know and to answer the unanswered questions". These quotations from a great scientist of this century tell a lot about science and scientists.

So I welcome you again to this international group of "amyloidologists" and this symposium of "amyloidology" where we will put together all our experiments, fool, damned fool and those that are still worse, as well as all our knowledge and efforts to try what Emil von Behring achieved, namely to place in the hands of the physician a victorious weapon against illness and death.

REFERENCES

1. Hernes, Gudmund. Hvorfor mer går galt (Why more things go wrong - More laws for modern man). Universitetsforlaget Bergen - Oslo - Tromsø 1981, pp. 144.
2. Mohr, Otto Lous. Taler (Speeches). Gyldendal Norsk Forlag, Oslo 1952, pp. 145.

and to answer the unanswered questions". These questions [illegible]

[illegible]

" Truth exists for the wise,
beauty for a sensitive heart.
The two are destined for each other."
(Beethoven's own words by P. Kruseman)

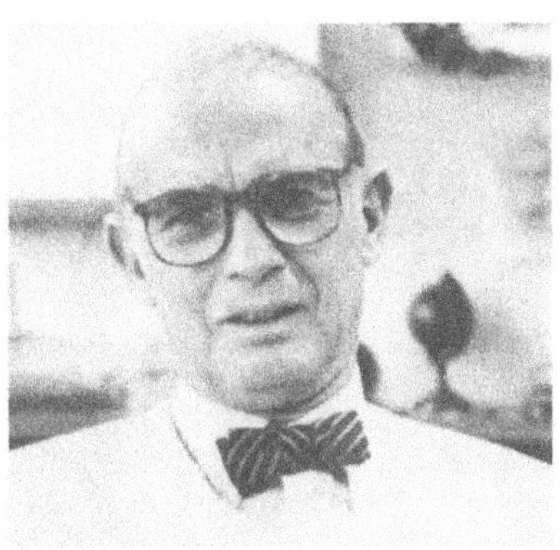

Dr. Elliott F. Osserman died on April 13, 1989. He was an active participant in amyloidosis symposia. In 1974 at the 2nd International Symposium, he delivered a closing remarks, summarizing the great wealth of information. In 1984, he organized the 4th International symposium at Arden House, New York. Elliott spent his entire career in Columbia University, College of Physicians & Surgeons, New York. He became a physician in 1947 and was promoted to Professor of Medicine in 1971. He also received a life time Professorship of American Cancer Society at the age of 43.

Without question, Elliott was a major contributor to amyloidosis research starting with the publication of "Amyloidosis: Tissue proteinosis: Gammaloidosis (editorial)", appeared in Annals of Internal Medicine in 1961. He continued to insist that certain Bence Jones proteins could be responsible to the antibody to certain tissue components and in-situ deposition of Ig-light chains or their fragments by means of his immunochemical method. Later in 1971, "Ig light chain origin of amyloid" was clearly established on the basis of amino-acid sequence study of the purified amyloid-fibril-proteins from patients with primary amyloidosis. He had a rare quality of combining the important biological observation with the laboratory study of molecular basis of the clinical manifestations derived from amyloidosis, myeloma, heavy chain disease and lysozyme-related disorders. He was the man who was passionate to provide essential knowledge on the general concept of plasma cell dyscrasia, including AL amyloidosis.

Most of us know that Elliott was very bright and charming. Beyond and above Elliott's scientific achievements, there are the international friendships he made. These are not only professional acquaintances, but warm relationships that continued across countries, oceans, and time.

Takashi Isobe, M.D.

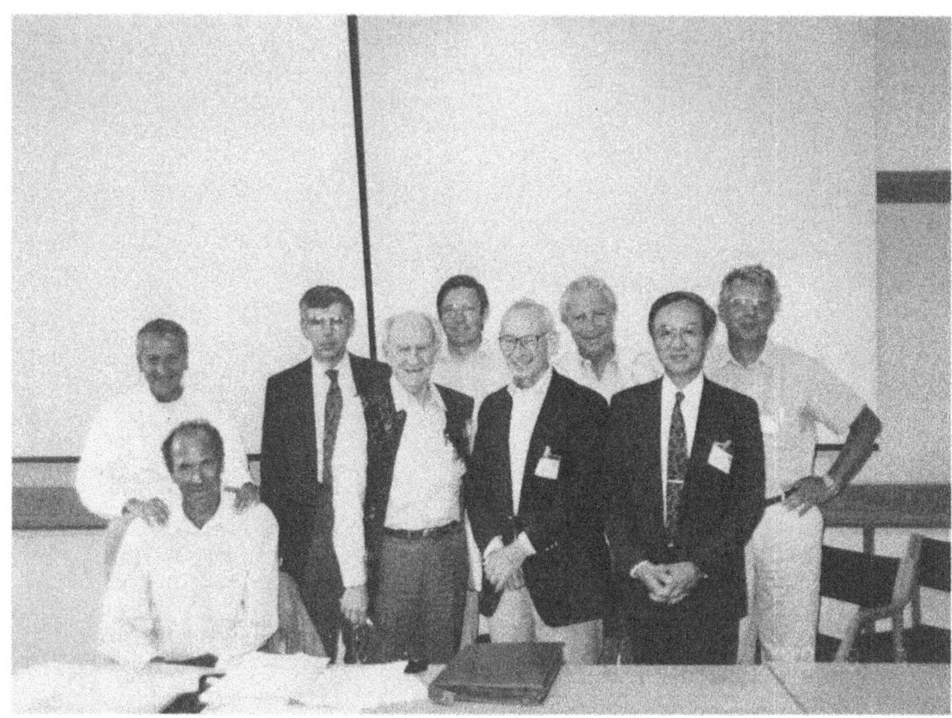

Members of The International Nomenclature Committee for Amyloidosis. The committee was appointed at the Vth International Symposium on Amyloidosis in Hakone, Japan in October 1987 and finished it's work during the VIth International Symposium on Amyloidosis in Oslo, Norway in August 1990. The members are front row from left to right Gunnar Husby (chairman), Earl P. Benditt, Alan S. Cohen, Shukuro Araki. Back row from left to right Blas Frangione, Merrill D. Benson, Jacob B. Natvig, George G. Glenner, Per Westermark.

THE 1990 GUIDELINES FOR NOMENCLATURE AND CLASSIFICATION OF AMYLOID AND AMYLOIDOSIS

Gunnar Husby[a], Shukuro Araki[b], Earl P. Benditt[c], Merrill D. Benson[d],Alan S. Cohen[e], Blas Frangione[f], George G. Glenner[g], Jacob B. Natvig[h] and Per Westermark[i]

a Department of Rheumatology, University of Tromsø, Norway
b Department of Neurology, Kumamoto University Medical School, Japan
c Department of Pathology, University of Washington, Seattle, USA
d Department of Rheumatology, Indiana University, Indianapolis, USA
e Thorndike Memorial Laboratory, Boston City Hospital, Boston, USA
f New York University Medical Center, New York, USA
g School of Medicine, University of California, San Diego, USA
h Institute of Immunology and Rheumatology, Rikshospitalet, Oslo, Norway
i Department of Pathology, University of Uppsala, Sweeden

Introduction

A group of experts in amyloidosis met during the Second International Symposium on Amyloidosis held in Helsinki in 1974 to discuss nomenclature for amyloid and amyloidosis. The results of this discussion provided the basis for the first nomenclature in this field of medicine which was published in the Proceedings of that symposium (1). Most of it showed to be useful for both research and clinical practice. The scientific developments regarding amyloid and amyloidosis have been very rapid, and already at the 3rd International Symposium on Amyloidosis in Povoa de Varzim, Portugal, in 1979, the nomenclature was again the subject of discussion among a group of researchers including those who had agreed upon the first nomenclature 5 years earlier. A chapter called "Guidelines for nomenclature" was published in the Proceedings of the symposium (2). This nomenclature was very similar to that agreed upon in 1974, but with some revisions.

The 1979 revision of the nomenclature has been widely accepted, however, not consistently used. Since a steadily increasing number of amyloid proteins characterized by amino acid sequencing and their clinical correlates have been disclosed, the need for an updated nomenclature for amyloid and amyloidosis is clear. During the 5th International Symposium on Amyloidosis in Hakone, Japan, 1987, an International Nomenclature Committee for Amyloidosis was established and includes the members who are co-authors of these Guidelines, with Gunnar Husby as chairman.

The main points agreed upon by the Committee members are outlined in the following.

Main Principles

When possible, the basis for nomenclature and classification should be the fibril protein making up the amyloid deposits in the case of amyloidosis under examination.

---

[1]This nomenclature has been submitted to the WHO/IUIS Nomenclature Committee in order to become an official nomenclature for amyloid proteins.

Nomenclature and Classification of Amyloid and Amyloidosis

Amyloid protein[a]	Protein precursor	Protein type or variant	Clinical	Ref.no.
AA[b]	apoSAA		Reactive(secondary)	4,5,6,7
			Familial Mediterranean Fever	8
			Familial amyloid nephropathy with urticaria and deafness (Muckle-Wells' syndrome)	9
AL	κ, λ e.g. κ III	Aκ, Aλ, e.g. AκIII	Idiopathic (primary), myeloma- or macroglobulinemia-associated	10,11
AH	IgG 1 (γ1)	Aγ1		3
ATTR	Transthyretin	e.g. Met 30[c]	Familial amyloid polyneuropathy, Portuguese	12,13,14,15
		e.g. Met 111	Familial amyloid cardiomyopathy, Danish	16
		TTR or Ile 122	Systemic senile amyloidosis	17,18
AApoAI	apoAI	Arg 26	Familial amyloid polyneuropathy, Iowa	19
AGel	Gelsolin	Asn 187[d] (15)	Familial amyloidosis, Finnish	20,21,22
ACys	Cystatin C	Gln 68	Hereditary cerebral hemorrhage with amyloidosis, Icelandic	23
Aß	ß protein precursor e.g. ßPP 695[e]		Alzheimer's disease	24,25
			Down's syndrome	
		Gln 618 (22)	Hereditary cerebral hemorrhage with amyloidosis, Dutch	26
Aß2M	ß2-microglobulin		Associated with chronic dialysis	27,28
AScr	Scrapie protein precursor 33-35[f], cellular form	Scrapie protein 27-30	Creutzfeldt-Jakob disease etc.	29
		e.g. Leu 102	Gerstmann-Straüssler-Scheinker syndrome	30
ACal	(Pro)calcitonin	(Pro)calcitonin	In medullary carcinomas of the thyroid	31
AANF	Atrial natriuretic factor		Isolated atrial amyloid	32
AIAPP	Islet amyloid polypeptide		In islets of Langerhans Diabetes type II, insulinoma	33
AIns[g]	Insulin		Islet amyloid in the degu (a rodent)	34
AApoAII[g]	apoAII (murine)	Gln 5	Amyloidosis in senescence accelerated mice	35

a Non-fibrillar proteins e.g. protein AP (amyloid P-component) excluded.

b Abbreviations not explained in the table:
AA: amyloid A protein; SAA: serum amyloid A protein; apo: apolipoprotein;
L: immunoglobulin light chain; H: immunoglobulin heavy chain.

c ATTR Met 30 when used in text.

d Amino acid position in the mature precursor protein. The position in the amyloid fibril protein is given in parentheses.

e Number of amino acid residues.

f Molecular mass (Kilodaltons).

g Not found in humans.

In many instances, the amyloid fibril proteins are identical to/or derived from intact or fragments of proteins present in serum. Such fibril protein precursors should be listed as a second set of data.
In cases where the given amyloid protein exists in the form of different types or variants, this should be given as additional information when necessary.

A fourth type of information is a description of the disease process affecting the patient. These 4 sets of information are given in the form of a table made up by 5 columns (Table):
1. Amyloid protein. 2. Protein precursor. 3. Protein type or variant. 4. Clinical description.
5. Relevant references.

Amyloid Proteins

When possible, amyloid and amyloidosis should be classified by the fibril protein.
Only proteins which have been characterized by their amino acid sequence and are known to be integrated in the amyloid fibrils should be listed (Table). Extrafibrillar proteins, like protein AP (the amyloid P-component), although regularly present in amyloid deposits are thus excluded.

The protein designations and abbreviations are chosen in order to use those accepted in the relevant fields of medicine and basic sciences. They should also be recognized and understood by people in clinical practice, students etc.

The capital letter A (for Amyloid) should be used as a first letter of all designations for amyloid proteins. The protein designation in abbreviated form should then follow without any open space after the first capital A. When a given term is abbreviated to one single letter, this letter should be a capital, Roman letter or a Greek lower case letter, e.g. AA, Aß. When a term is abbreviated into an acronym, e.g. transthyretin to TTR, all letters are capitalized. When the spelling of the term is maintained, but the word abbreviated; the first letter is capitalized and the remaining are in lower case (e.g. cystatin to Cys).

Regarding numbers, both Arabic and Roman numbers are used in order to meet abbreviations/designations widely and traditionally accepted in the scientific world. Subscripts or superscripts are not used in order to simplify typing and use of word processing.

Aß and ß protein precursor (ßPP) are designations for the fibril protein and its precursor in Alzheimer's disease etc. (Table).

The recently discovered amyloid fibril protein of immunoglobulin heavy chain nature (3) has been given the designation AH.

Protein Precursor

The term protein precursor (Table) refers to the protein from which the actual amyloid fibril protein (normal or variant) is thought to be derived. With the exception of ß protein precursor these amyloid related proteins can be demonstrated in serum, and in many cases the amyloid protein is a fragment i.e. an incomplete degration product of its precursor.

Protein Type or Variant

These represent a variety of classes and variable subgroups of immunoglobulins, molecular variants related to inherited amyloidoses, and a prohormone (i.e. procalcitonin). Class designati- on of immunoglobulin chains are given in Greek, lower case letter, γ-chain subclass in Arabic number and variable subgroups in Roman numbers.

The (single) amino acid substitutions in transthyretin and other proteins that account for the inherited amyloid protein variants are indicated by the amino acid that substitutes for the normal one using the 3 letter code, following one open space after the protein designation. This is followed by a single open space, again followed by the position in the protein (i.e. residue number from the N-terminal) in the respective intact, normal protein where the substitution occurs, e.g. ATTR Met 30. The number of the variant amino acid, relates to that in the mature (native) precursor protein, whereas the position in the corresponding amyloid protein which is a fragment of the precursor, is given in parentheses.

The Table shows only one example of protein type or variant for each amyloid protein. The only exception is TTR, where 3 different variants are related to different clinical forms of inherited amyloid disease. In the cases of multiple protein types or variants (i.e. immunoglobulins, TTR, Scrapie protein) "sub-tables" should be designed to include all those known at the present time.

Clinical Descriptions

The clinical descriptions used in the Table are those traditionally used in clinical practice up to now. No attempt has thus been made to revise them except that the Roman numbers used to classify various familial amyloid polyneuropathies have been omitted, and replaced by the geographic origin of the actual families.

Because the fibril protein in many forms of amyloidosis is not known, and because only few examples of amyloid protein variants or subtypes are given in the Table, some clinical forms of amyloidosis are not listed.

Finally, it should be noted that the distinction between systemic and localized (organ or tissue-limited) amyloidoses has been avoided. This is because some amyloid deposits thought to be localized, may represent a predilection site of systemic amyloidosis.

References

1.Cohen, A.S., Franklin, E.C., Glenner, G.G., Natvig, J.B. Ossermann, E.F. and Wegelius, O. (1975) P. IX in O. Wegelius and A. Pasternack (eds.) Amyloidosis. Academic Press, London, New York and San Francisco.
2.Benditt, E.P., Cohen, A.S, Costa, P.P., Franklin, E.C., Glenner, G.G., Husby, G., Mandema, E., Natvig, J.B.,Ossermann, E.F., Sohar, E., Wegelius, O. and Westermark, P. (1980) Pp. XI - XII in G.G. Glenner, P.P. Costa and A.F. deFreitas (eds.), Amyloid and Amyloidosis. Exerpta Medica, Amsterdam, Oxford, Princeton.
3.Eulitz, M., Weiss. D.T. and Solomon, A. (1990) In J.B. Natvig, Ø. Førre, G. Husby, A. Husebekk, B. Skogen, K . Sletten and P. Westermark (eds.), Amyloid and Amyloidosis, Kluwer Academic Publishers, Dordrecht
4.Benditt, E.P., Eriksen, M., Hermodsen, M.A., and Ericsson, L.H. (1971) FEBS Lett 19, 169-173.
5.Levin, M., Pras, M., Franklin, E.C. (1973) J. Exp. Med. 138, 373-380.
6.Husby, G., Natvig, J.B., Michaelsen, T.E., Sletten, K.and Høst, H. (1973) Nature 244, 362-364.
7.Parmelee, D.C., Titani, K., Ericsson, L.H., Eriksen, N. Benditt, E.P. and Walsh, K.A. (1982) Biochemistry 21, 3298-3303.
8.Levin, M., Franklin, E.C., Frangione, B. and Pras, M. (1972) J. Clin. Invest. 51, 2773-2776.

9.Linke, R.P., Heilmann, K.L., Nathrath, W.B.J., Eulitz,M. (1983) Lab. Invest. 48, 698-704.
10.Glenner, G.G., Harbaugh, J., Ohms, J.E., Harada, M. and Cuatrecasas, P. (1970) Biochem. Biophys. Res. Comm. 41, 1287-1289.
11.Glenner, G.G., Terry, W., Harada, M., Isersky, C. and Page, D. (1971) Science 172, 1150-1151.
12.Costa, P.P., Figueira, A.S. and Bravo, F.R. (1978) Proc. Natl. Acad. Sci. USA 75, 4499-4503.
13.Tawara, S., Nakarato, M., Kengawa, K., Matsuo, K. and Araki, S. (1983) Biochem. Biophys. Res. Commun. 116, 880-888.
14.Francis, E., Dwulet and Benson, M.D. (1983) Biochem. Biophys. Res. Comm. 114, 657-662.
15.Saraiva, M.J.M., Birken, S., Costa, P.P. and Goodman, D.S. (1984) J. Clin. Invest 74, 104-119.
16.Nordlie, M., Sletten, K., Husby, G. and Ranløv, P.J.(1988) Scand. J. Immunol. 27, 119-122.
17.Gorevic, P.D., Prelli, F.C., Wright, J., Pras, M. and Frangione, B. (1989) J. Clin. Invest. 83, 836-843.
18.Westermark, P., Sletten, K., Johansson, B. and Cornwell, G.G. (1990) Proc. Natl. Acad. Sci. USA 87, 2843-2845.
19.Nichols, W.C., Dwulet, F.E., Liepnieks, J. and Benson,M.D. (1988) Biochem. Biophys. Res. Comm. 156, 762- 768.
20.Maury, C.P.J., Alli, K. and Baumann, M. (1990) FEBS Lett. 260, 85-87.
21.Haltia, M., Prelli, F., Ghiso, J., Kiuru, S., Somer, H., Palo, J. and Frangione, B. (1990) Biochem. Biophys. Res. Commun. 167, 927-932.
22.Maury, P. (1990) in J.B. Natvig, Ø. Førre, G. Husby,A. Husebekk, B. Skogen K. SLetten and P. Westermark (eds.) Amyloid and Amyloidosis, Kluwer Academic Publishers,Dordrecht
23.Ghiso, J., Jensson, O., Frangione, B. (1986) Proc.Natl. Acad. Sci. USA 83, 2974-2978.
24.Glenner, G.G. and Wong, C.W. (1984) Biochem. Biophys. Res. Comm. 120, 885-890.
25.Glenner, G.G. (1988) Cell 82, 307-308.
26.Levy, E., Carman, M.D., Fernandez-Madrid, I.J., Power,M.D., Lieberburg, I., van Duinen, S.G., Bots,G.T.A.M., Luyendijk, W. and Frangione, B. (1990) Science 248, 1124-1126.
27.Gejyo, F., Yamada, T., Odani, S., Nakagawa, Y., Arakawa, M., Kunitomo, T., Kataoka, H., Suzuki, M.,Hirasawa, Y., Shirahama, T., Cohen, A.S. and Schmid, K. (1985) Biochem. Biophys. Res. Comm. 129, 701-706.
28.Gorevic, P.D., Casey, T.T., Stone, W.J., DiRaimondo, R., Prelli, F.C. and Frangione, B. (1985) J. Clin. Invest. 76, 2425-2429.
29.Prusiner, S.B., Groth, D.F., Bolton, D.C., Kent, S.B.and Hood, L.E. (1984) Cell 38, 127-134.
30.Hsiao, K., Baker, H.F., Crow, T.J., Poulter, M., Owen, F., Terwilliger, J.D., Westaway, D., Ott, J.Prusiner, S.B. (1989) Nature, 3338, 342-345.
31.Sletten, K., Westermark, P. and Natvig, J.B. (1976) J. Exp. Med. 143, 993-998.
32.Johansson, B., Wernstedt, C. and Westermark, P. (1987) Biochem. Biophys. Res. Commun. 148, 1087-1092.
33.Westermark, P., Wernstedt, C., Wilander, E. and Sletten, K. (1986) Biochem. Biophys. Res. Commun.140, 827-831.
34.Hellman, U., Wernstedt, C., Westermark, P., O'Brien T.and Johnson, K.H. (1990) Biochem. Biophys. Res.Commun. In press.
35.Higuchi, K., Yonezu, T., Tsunasawa, S., Sakiyama, F. and Takeda, T. (1986) FEBS Lett. 207, 23-27.

THE HUMAN SERUM AMYLOID A GENES AND THEIR REGULATION BY INFLAMMATORY CYTOKINES

P. Woo, J. Betts, M. Edbrooke
Section of Molecular Rheumatology, Clinical Research Centre, Northwick Park Hospital, Watford Road, Harrow, HA1 3UJ, UK.

INTRODUCTION.

Serum amyloid A or apoSAA comprise a family of amphipathic proteins with the approximate size of 12k daltons. These proteins have been described in rodents and a large number of mammals in addition to man. ApoSAA from plasma is found mainly as part of the high density lipoprotein (HDL) fraction, but can also associate with other lipoprotein fractions. HDL associated apoSAA has been shown to be a mixture of the products of two genes, SAA1 and SAA2 (1). The HDL SAA proteins are acute phase reactants and serum levels can rise to over 1,000 fold during an inflammatory response.

ApoSAA was first discovered because of its reactivity with antibodies made against protein A obtained from amyloid fibres in tissues of man and mouse. Subsequent amino acid sequence analysis of both AA protein and SAA showed amino acid identity from the N-terminal ends, with the AA protein being shorter at the C-terminal end. These observations suggest that serum amyloid A is the precursor for amyloid A protein, and indeed the transfer of human acute phase HDL into amyloidotic mice has resulted in human SAA being incorporated into mouse amyloid tissue (2).

The fact that only one of the mouse SAA gene products SAA2, is deposited as murine amyloid fibres, raises the possibility of there being one species of amyloidogenic SAA. In humans however, the situation is a little more complicated. There are two types of AA amyloidosis: (1) those associated with chronic inflammatory conditions, ie. reactive amyloidosis and (2) those associated with familial mediteranean fever (FMF)in specific ethnic groups, eg. North African Jews and Turks, but rarely in Ashkenazi Jews, and Armenians. From the published amino acid sequences of amyloid proteins, it appears that there is only one type of SAA deposited in reactive amyloidosis (ie. SAA1). In FMF however, both SAA1 and SAA2 have been found in amyloid deposits from FMF patients (Pras pers.comm). Therefore there is unlikely to be one particular amyloidogenic form of human SAA.

SAA Genes.

Studies of HDL SAA have revealed many isoforms. Therefore it is important to define the entire gene family of SAA and analyse their pattern of expression. There are 3 murine genes and 1 pseudogene, only the products of 2 are found in HDL. At the previous international amyloidosis meeting, it was suggested that there were at least 3 human gene loci. We present data here for 4 gene loci, which account for the

Southern analysis patterns seen in population and family studies. Combined data available from our lab and those of Sack (Ref 3) and Kluve-Beckerman (4) are represented in the diagram below (Fig 1). Overlapping genomic clones from two lambda phage libraries were used to define SAA1 and SAA2 genes in our laboratory. SAA3 was described by Sack *et al* (3). In addition, a clone containing both SAA2 and a 4th SAA gene, SAA4, has been obtained from a cosmid library in our laboratory. All of these genes are contained within Fig No: 1.

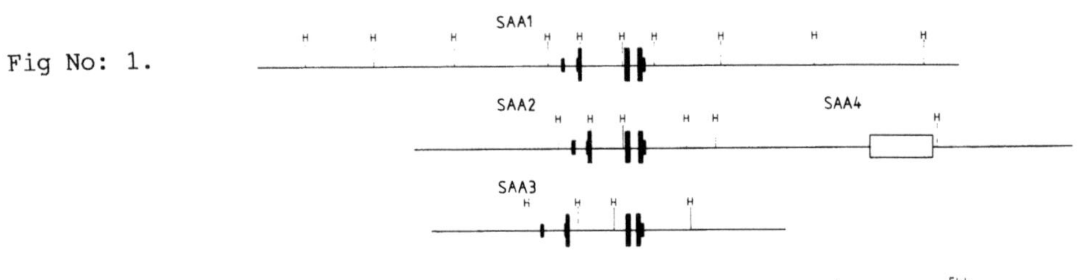

Fig No: 1.

a 350 kb Not I fragment in the genome using pulse-field gel electrophoretic analysis. SAA1-3 have the same highly conserved region (from amino acid residues 33 to 45, as originally described in the cDNA clones for SAA1 (5)). This conserved region is present in all SAA protein in all species except in the rat, where it is deleted. Interestingly, rat SAA-like protein is an acute phase protein, but is not associated with HDL. Moreover, rats do not develop reactive amyloidosis.

So far cDNA from hepatic libraries have shown gene products of SAA1 and SAA2, but not SAA3 and SAA4. In addition, SAA3 may be a pseudogene from the data of Dr. Kluve-Beckerman (see her chapter in this volume). Further work obviously is necessary to clarify the situation. Our restriction map of SAA4 shows that this is a distinct gene loci, but the sequence is not yet complete. A comparison between human and mouse SAA genes shows 71.2% homology between human SAA1α and mouse SAA1 and SAA2, 72.1% between human SAA1α and mouse SAA3, and 73% homology between human and mouse SAA3.

Detailed restriction maps of the human genes have allowed us to assign the bands seen on Southern blots in population and family studies. Five families with 82 members and 53 unrelated subjects were analysed for SAA1 alleles and 3 different alleles with the restriction enzyme Bgl I were defined. Two alleles for SAA2 were found using 54 unrelated members and 3 families containing 68 members. There is one individual with an extra RFLP band. This could represent a private polymorphism, but could indicate a duplicated gene. Table 1 shows the number of genes with their corresponding cDNAs. The recent data from Linke's cDNA library (6) suggest that there maybe gene duplication of SAA1. Unfortunately it was not possible to do Southern analysis on the original donor. Table 2 shows the isoforms of SAA in human HDL.

Regulation of SAA2β by Interleukin 1.

Chronically elevated levels of HDL SAA seems to be a prerequisite factor in reactive amyloidosis. Even so, only a small percentage of patients with an inflammatory disease appear to develop amyloidosis. Therefore there are likely to be genetically determined factors interacting with high levels of SAA. In order to examine whether the gene specific deposition of SAA is related to the control of synthesis of different types of SAA in the process of amyloidogenesis, we have examined the transcriptional control of the SAA1 and SAA2 genes by the inflammatory cytokines interleukin 1 (IL-1) and interleukin 6 (IL-6).

Tables 1 and 2.

Genomic clones and their corresponding cDNA's

	Genomic clones	cDNA clones
SAA1α	-	pA1, pAS1
SAA1β	1.1	-
SAA2α	2.2, GSAA3	pA10, pSAA82, pAS8
SAA2β	2.1 (SAAg9)	pAS2
SAA3	GSAA1	-
SAA4	cos361	

HUMAN SERUM AMYLOID A PROTEIN

MAJOR ISOFORMS

pH

8.0

7.5

7.4

7.0

6.4

6.0

1 2 3

Interleukin 1 has been shown by Osbourn *et al* (7) to induce a nuclear factor, NF_kB, first described by Sen and Baltimore in B cells (8). NF_kB is responsible for the transcription of the immunoglobulin κ light chain, and binds to the sequence (GGGACTTTCC) in the enhancer region of the gene. DNA from the HIV genome containing 2 recognition sites of this transcription factor was used in transfection studies to show NF_kB binding inducible by IL-1 (7). Previous analysis in our laboratory has shown that the SAA promoter contains a recognition sequence for NF_kB. Furthermore, this region is responsible for induction by phorbol esters (9). To see whether interleukin 1 has a similar effect on SAA via the transcription factor NF_kB, transfection experiments were performed. We were able to obtain consistently 6 fold induction of the reporter gene in this system, and IL-1 induction appears to be entirely via this region since mutating the recognition sequence from GGGACTTTCC to CTCACTTTCC abolish this effect. Further analysis of upstream regions of the SAA promoter has revealed that the control of SAA gene expression is more complex. The diagram below illustrates our present hypothesis.

Fig No: 2.

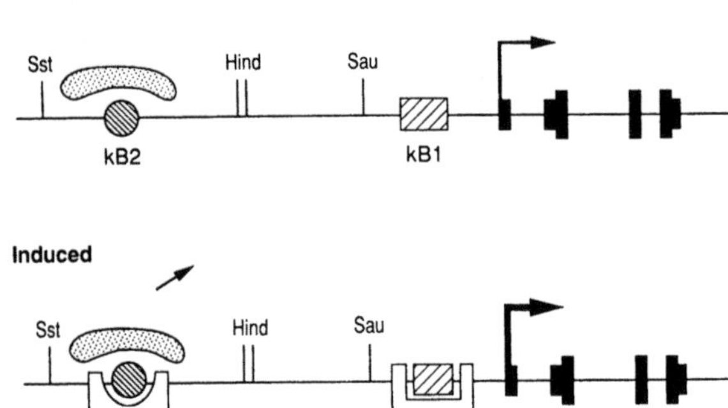

kB1 is the NF_kB recognition site which responds to IL-1 and it is situated at nucleotide -82 to -91. Further upstream, there is a second NF_kB recognition site designated kB2 (nucleotide -635 to -626). This is in the opposite orientation and appears to be able to bind nuclear factors from IL-1 stimulated HepG2 nuclear extracts. We have data now to suggest that a constitutive protein factor binding to the region near the kB2 site has the effect of switching off the SAA gene. The induction of SAA requires a new protein binding to the kB2 region which interfere with the negative factor and allows transcription to proceed.

Induction of SAA1 and SAA2 by Interleukin 6.

There is 88% nucleotide identity between the SAA1 and SAA2 promoter as far as -450. Within this region is the kB1 site as described above, and also region that has been suggested as the interleukin 6 responsive element based on nucleotide homology between different acute phase genes. The activity of the SAA promoter has been studied with transient transfection experiments in HepG2 cell lines as before. Our results show that the mechanism by which IL-6 induces gene activation is different than that of IL-1. We were able to demonstrate binding of SAA promoter DNA fragments by nuclear extracts from IL-6 induced HepG2 cells using gel retardation assays. The noticeable difference between IL-1 and IL-6 extracts is that the binding of the transcription factor(s) have different time courses

(Fig. 3).

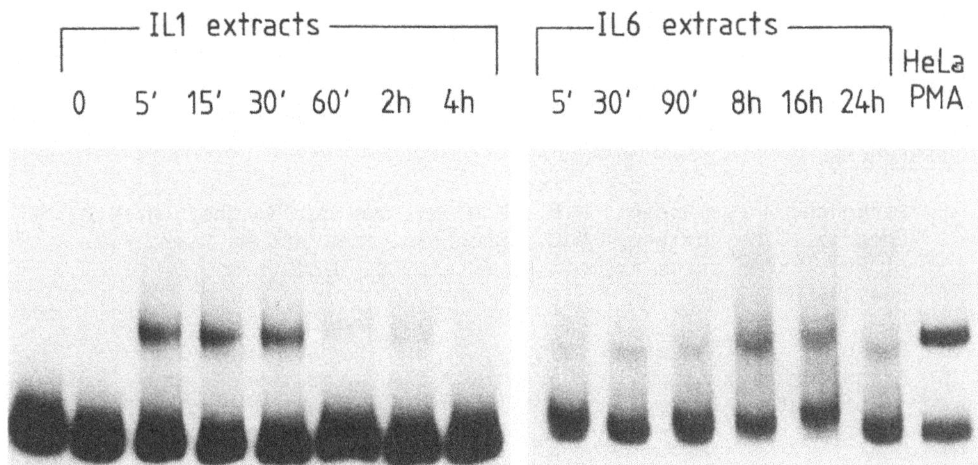

Subsequent footprint analysis show different nuclear protein binding sites. In the case of IL-1 it is kB1, in the case of IL-6 we were able to obtain a footprint in the IL-6 responsive element identical to the sequence recognised by a newly described nuclear factor, NFIL-6. This is the factor shown by Kishimoto & colleagues (11), to be induced by IL-1 to bind to the promoter region of IL-6 in glioblastoma cells. It is interesting that in our system we do not see a NFIL-6-like factor induced by interleukin 1, but by interleukin 6. Transfection studies reveal in addition, that IL-6 requires both NF_kB site and the NFIL-6 site for full inductive activity.

Synergism between IL-1 and IL-6 in the induction of SAA.

In the physiological state during acute inflammation, activated monocytes produce a cocktail of inflammatory cytokines which include interleukin 1, interleukin 6 and tumour necrosis factor as well as other growth factors. Therefore combinations of these cytokines may produce different levels of each SAA isotype. In the case of IL-1 and IL-6 they seem to be synergistic rather than just simply additive for SAA1 and SAA2. In transient transfections experiments, our results showed that IL-1 alone will induce an approximately 6 fold increase in transcription, approximately 3 fold increase by IL-6, but greater than 20 fold by the same quantity of IL-1 and IL-6 added simultaneously in tissue culture.

Conclusions and Perspectives.

The mechanisms of AA amyloidogenesis still alludes us. However, the application of molecular genetics has defined the polymorphic nature of the precursor proteins, apoSAA. Furthermore, the mechanisms of their differential synthesis under inflammatory stimuli are able to be dissected. SAA isotype expression and their tissue distribution are important questions that need to be explored and hopefully answered by the next international amyloidosis meeting.

REFERENCES.

1. Strachan, A.F., Brandt, W.F., Woo, P., van der Westhuyzen, D.R., Coetzee, G.A., de Beer, M.C., Shephard, E.C. and de Beer, F.C. (1989). Human serum amyloid A protein, J. Biol Chem 264,18368-18373.

2. Husebekk, A., Skogen, B., Husby, G. and Marhaug, G. (1985). Transformation of amyloid precursor SAA to protein AA and incorporation in amyloid fibrils *in vivo*, Scand J Immunol 21, 283-287.

3. Sack, G.H. and Talbot, C.C. (1989). The human serum amyloid (SAA) encoding gene GSAA1: nucleotide sequence and possible autocrine - collagenase-inducer function, Gene 84, 509-515.

4. Kluve-Beckerman, B: see later in this volume.

5. Sipe J.D., Colten, H.R., Goldberger, G., Edge, M.D., Tack, B.F., Cohen, A.S. and Whitehead, A.S. (1985). Human serum amyloid A (SAA): biosynthesis and postsynthetic processing of pre SAA and structural variants defined by complementary DNA, Biochemistry 24, 2931-2936.

6. Steinkasserer, A., Weiss, E.H., Schwaeble, W. and Linke, R.P. (1990). Heterogeneity of human serum amyloid A protein, Biochem J 268, 187-193.

7. Osborn, L., Kunkel, S. and Nabel, G.J. (1989). Tumor necrosis factorα and interleukin 1 stimulate human immunodeficiency virus enhancer by activation of the nuclear factor kB, Proc Natl Acad Sci USA 86, 2336-2340.

8. Sen, R. and Baltimore, D. (1986). Multiple nuclear factors interact with the immunoglobulin enhancer sequences, Cell 46, 705-716.

9. Edbrooke, M.R., Burt, D.W., Cheshire, J.K. and Woo, P. (1989). Identification of cis-acting sequences responsible for phorbol ester induction of human serum amyloid A gene expression via a nuclear factor kB-like transcription factor, Mol Cell Biol 9, 1908-1916.

10. Fey, G.H., Hattori, M., Northemann, W., Abraham, L.J., Baumann, M., Braciak, T.A., Fletcher, R.G., Gauldie, J., Lee, F. and Reymond, M.F. (1989). Regulation of rat liver acute phase genes by interleukin-6 and production of hepatocyte stimulating factors by rat hepatoma cells, Ann N Y Acad Sci 557, 317-329.

11. Akira, S., Isshiki, H., Sugita, T., Tanabe, O., Kinoshita, S., Nichio, Y., Nakajima, T., Hirano, T. and Kishimoto, T. (1990). A nuclear factor for IL6 expression (NF-IL6) is a member of a C/EBP family, EMBO J 9, 1897-1906.

GENETIC ISOFOCUSING VARIANT OF HUMAN SERUM AMYLOID A

A. Steinmetz, H. Vitt#, S. Motzny, H. Kaffarnik
Zentrum Innere Medizin, Endokrinologie und Stoffwechsel,
Philipps-Universität Baldingerstrasse D-3550 Marburg, F.R.G.
#DRK Kinderkrankenhaus D-5900 Siegen, F.R.G.

ABSTRACT. The acute phase reactant serum Amyloid A (SAA) is the putative precursor of the tissue amyloid deposits in AA-amyloidosis. As point mutations in the precursor protein may be a possible underlying cause of the development of amyloidosis we looked for variants of SAA using isofocusing (IEF) combined with immunoblotting employing sheep anti human SAA antibody. In this system SAA1 and SAA2 (now called SAA1 and SAA1 des Arg) can directly be visualized from serum. In a family of Turkish origin we detected an isofocusing genetic variant of SAA1 and SAA2. The mutant forms show a charge shift of about one charge unit towards the anode (IP of 6.1 and 5.7, respectively) and immunoblotting experiments with anti SAA-peptide antibodies indicated that the two mutant proteins are most likely to be derived from SAA1 and SAA1 des Arg. The mutant proteins have the same apparent MW as the normal SAA proteins. They could be shown in a three month old girl, her brother and her mother. All carriers of the mutant were apparent heterozygotes expressing both the normal SAA1 and SAA1 des Arg forms and the described variants. Although the propositus and her brother were seen repeatedly for fever of unknown origin we do not know at present if this is linked to the SAA mutant. We also do not yet know if carriers of the mutant protein are prone to develop amyloidosis. This is the first mutant protein of SAA described so far.
INDEX WORDS: SAA genetic variant, isoelectric focusing, family study.

INTRODUCTION

Protein amyloid A (AA), characteristic of amyloid deposits in tissues of patients with e.g.chronic inflammatory diseases has an immunologically and structurally (sequence homology in its first 76 amino acids) related plasma protein, serum amyloid A (SAA). SAA was found in plasma associated with high density lipoprotein (HDL) and is thought to be the putative precursor of amyloid fibril protein AA. An amphiphilic character was demonstrated for AA and SAA and apoprotein (apo) SAA isolated from human high density lipoprotein revealed two major components upon isofocusing, named SAA_1 and SAA_2 differing in their NH_2

terminal amino acid arginine, which was missing in SAA_2 (for a review see ref. 1). Upon isofocusing of serum and subsequent immunoblotting these two major and several minor forms are detectable (2,3). Sequencing analysis of one of the major forms of human SAA from pooled human serum revealed a 104 amino acid protein homogeneous in charge but polymorphic by reverse phase HPLC (4). The primary structures of six SAA forms from the plasma of an individual donor were then determined (5). Three different patterns of human apo SAA isoforms were reported to be identified by electrofocusing of apo HDL. The authors found one pattern showing six major SAA isoforms, the other two patterns missing two of these isoforms at a time, respectively (6). Also N-terminal sequence and amino acid analysis was performed of these six isoforms from HDL of pooled plasma (7). According to these results three different SAA proteins are present in plasma, each with and without the aminoterminal arginine (and some also without arg and ser) residue, giving rise to six isoforms. One of the proteins sequenced matched the primary structure determined by Parmelee et al. (4) which was also derived from a cDNA (8) except for the alanine/ valine polymorphism at positions 52/57. The other proteins, SAA2Á and SAA2ß, differed from this major plasma peptide in seven amino acid positions, with an additional arginine for histidine exchange at position 71 in the latter, matching cDNA derived amino acid sequence of Kluve-Beckerman et al. (9,10).

In order to identify isofocusing variants of SAA from human plasma as possible amyloidogenic proteins (11) we (3) and others (2) developed immunoblotting procedures for SAA isoforms from human plasma and applied them to clinical screening studies. The paper reports the first isofocusing variant of human SAA found and described so far.

MATERIALS AND METHODS

Subjects. Blood was obtained from patients with rheumatoid arthritis, systemic lupus erythematosus (SLE) or apparently healthy volunteers. Blood was also collected from the members of a Turkish family identified as carriers of the SAA variant.

Materials. Antibodies to apo SAA were raised in sheep as reported be fore (12). Blood samples were drawn into tubes containing Na_2 EDTA-2 H_2O, 1.5 g/l (final concentration) and plasma was obtained by immediate low speed centrifugation and kept at 4°C for a maximum of one day before use. Thawing and refreezing up to three times in several samples with or without the variant SAA did not change the isofocusing pattern of SAA originally obtained with the same sample when fresh.

Isoelectric focusing (IEF) and protein blotting. Plasma was subjected to IEF as described by Menzel et al. (13) with an ampholite pH-range of 3-9. After IEF proteins were electrophoretically blotted onto nitrocellulose sheets and SAA was detected by peroxidase labeled anti sheep antibodies in the presence of 4-chloro-1-naphthol.

RESULTS AND DISCUSSION

As amyloid fibrillar deposits in reactive amyloidosis occur only in a few cases with elevated SAA plasma levels, it seems likely that additional factors are necessary for the development of the disease. One of these factors might be that some of the SAA plasma proteins may be more amyloidogenic than others (11). Thus genetic variants of the SAA proteins may be responsible for their abnormal processing and subsequent deposition as was demonstrated for genetic variants of transthyretin and apo AI (1,14). By using the described procedure we were able to detect a genetic isofocusing variant in a family of Turkish origin. The variant could be shown in apparently heterozygous form in the propositus, her brother and in the mother of the children.

The mutant protein underwent a charge shift of about one charge unit toward the anode. Both, the normal SAA_1 and SAA_2 (IP 6.4 and 6.0) and the variant SAA_1* and SAA_2* (IP 6.1 and 5.7) were present in each affected individual. The likelyhood of the variant form to be a mutant form of SAA_1 and SAA_2 (SAA1 and SAA1-des Arg) is supported by several observations: i) the variants show similar apparent intensity upon isofocusing and blotting as SAA_1 and SAA_2; ii) it is, as are SAA_1 and SAA_2, also recognized by the antipeptide 58-69 antibody (15) and iii) the PH difference between the two variant forms is identical to that between SAA_1 and SAA_2. We therefor hypothesize a mutation having taken place in the gene corresponding to the cDNA pA1 (8). Fig. 1 shows an isofocusing pattern of a normal control (A) and of the plasma of the propositus (B).

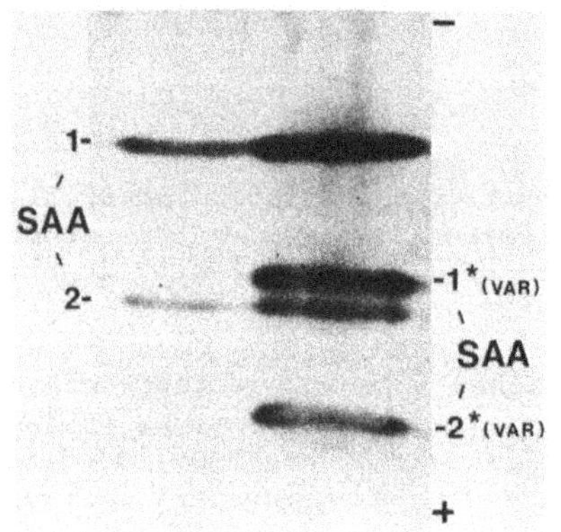

Fig. 1
Immunoblotting analysis of plasma from a normal control person (A) and from a carrier of the SAA (Marburg) variant (B). Only the SAA_1 and $_2$-region of the nitrocellulose is shown. The two mutant bands are labelled SAA_1* and SAA_2* (or SAA1-des Arg)* as they most likely arouse from SAA_1 and SAA_2. All carriers of the mutant identified so far are heterozygotes expressing both SAA isoforms in the usual focusing position and variant isoforms.

Two dimensional gel electrophoresis revealed similar apparent molecular weights both for the normal and the variant isoforms (data not shown). The propositus, a three month old girl, was repeatedly hospitalized for recurrent fever, the origin of which could not be determined so far. Family history revealed that also the brother of the propositus has been seen for several years repeatedly in children's hospitals for fever of unknown origin, possibly familial Mediterranean fever. No such history of fever could be remembered during the child-

hood of the parents. Two older sisters of the propositus were not available for study. Unfortunately the family has not yet given consent to investigate the possible presence of amyloidosis.
As this is to our knowledge the first genetic isofocusing variant of SAA we propose to name the mutant $SAA_{Marburg}$.

References

1 Benson, M.D. and Wallace, M.R., (1989) in: Scriver, C.R., Beaudet, A.L., Sly, W.S. and Valle, D. ed. The Metabolic Basis of Inherited Disease. Mc Graw Hill, New York, 6th ed. 2439-2460.
2 Maury, C.P.J., Ehnholm, C. and Lukka, M., (1985), Ann. Rheum. Dis., 44, 711-715.
3 Hocke, G. and Steinmetz, A., (1985), Elektrophorese Forum 85, München, 449-453.
4 Parmelee, D.C., Titani, K., Ericsson, L.H., Eriksen, N., Benditt, E.P. and Walsh, K.A., (1982), Biochemistry, 21, 3298-3303.
5 Dwulet, F.E., Wallace, D.K. and Benson, M.D., (1988), Biochemistry, 77, 1677-1682.
6 Strachan, A.F., de Beer, F.C., van der Westhuyzen, D.R. and Coetzee, G.A., (1988), Biochem. J., 250, 203-207.
7 Strachan, A.F., Brandt, W.F., Woo, P., van der Westhuysen, D.R., Coetzee, G.A., de Beer, M., Shephard, E.G. and de Beer,F.C. (1989), J. Biol. Chem. 264, 18368-18373.
8 Sipe, J.D., Colten, H.R., Goldberger, G., Edge, M.D., Track, B.F., Cohen, A.S. and Whitehead, A.S., (1985), Biochemistry, 24, 2931-2936.
9 Kluve-Beckerman, B., Long, G.L. and Benson, M.D., (1986), Biochem. Genet., 24, 795-803.
10 Kluve-Beckermann, B., Dwulet, F.E. and Benson, M.D., (1988), J. Clin. Invest., 82, 1670-1675.
11 Gorevic, P.C., Levo, Y., Frangione, B. and Franklin, E.C., (1978), J Immunol., 121, 138-140.
12 Hocke, G., Ebel, H., Bittner, K., Müller, T., Kaffarnik, H. and Steinmetz, A., (1989), Klin. Wochenschr., 67, 447-451.
13 Menzel, H.J., Kladetzky, R.G. and Assmann, G., (1982), J. Lipid Res., 23, 915-922.
14 Nichols, W.C., Dwulet, F.E., Liepnieks, J. and Benson, M.D., (1988), Biochem. Biophys. Res. Commun., 156, 762-768.
15 Saïle, R., Hocke, G., Tartar, A., Fruchart, J.C. and Steinmetz, A., (1989), Biochim. Biophys. Acta, 992, 407-408.

SEQUENCE ANALYSIS OF A THIRD HUMAN SAA GENE

Kluve-Beckerman, B., Brinckerhoff, C., and Benson, M.D.
Indiana University School of Medicine, Department of Medicine, Rheumatology Division, Clinical Building 492, 541 Clinical Drive, Indianapolis, IN 46223; and Veterans Affairs Medical Center (583/111RH), 1481 West 10th Street, Room #A772, Indianapolis, IN 46202; Dartmouth Medical School, Department of Medicine, Connective Tissue Disease Section, Hanover, NH 03756; USA.

ABSTRACT. A candidate for the human SAA3 gene has been cloned and characterized. The sequence derived from this clone (HDgl-1) for amino acids 1-12 most closely resembles that of rabbit SAA3 with which it has 75% identity, compared to 25% identity with the corresponding sequences in human SAA1 and SAA2. In the region spanning exon 3 - exon 4, however, HDgl-1 and the human SAA1 and SAA2 genes are 87% homologous. The exon 3 sequence of HDgl-1, as well as the exon 3 sequence of this gene in four unrelated individuals, was found to have an "extra" base which would distrupt the appropriate reading frame for SAA and generate a premature stop codon. In addition, no mRNA corresponding to the HDgl-1 sequence has been detected. These data point to the possibility that the SAA3 gene may not be expressed in humans.

INTRODUCTION

Serum amyloid A (SAA), a prominent acute phase reactant in humans and other species, is a polymorphic protein encoded by a family of genes. The well-characterized murine SAA gene family consists of four genes [1,2]; two (SAA1 and SAA2) are very similar and encode proteins synthesized by the liver and released into the general circulation where they travel in association with HDL particles. The third gene (SAA3) differs from SAA1 and SAA2 not only in sequence, but also in terms of its extrahepatic transcription. Although murine SAA3 mRNA has been demonstrated in a variety of tissues [3,4], the protein product has yet to be identified. The corresponding rabbit protein, however, has been characterized [5]. The fourth murine SAA sequence represents a pseudogene due to its apparent lack of exon 1 and exon 2 and a deletion in exon 3.

Although less is known about human SAA genes, it is apparent that there are at least three. As in the mouse, two of the genes encode very homologous plasma proteins synthesized by the liver. The mRNAs for these proteins have been cloned [6,7] and the complete structure of one of the corresponding genes determined [8]. The hybridization pattern of SAA fragments in Southern analyses has suggested a third gene somewhat divergent from the other two [7]. We contribute here the sequence of a human SAA gene significantly different from those encoding either of the two major plasma isoforms.

MATERIALS AND METHODS

Library Construction and Screening. DNA was purified from a human lymphoblastoid cell line designated HD-1 and then partially digested with MboI. Human genomic fragments 15-20 kb in length were ligated to λFIX vector arms following a partial fill-in reaction (Stratagene, LaJolla, CA). DNA was packaged using the Gigapack II Gold packaging extract (Stratagene). Titration at the library on E.coli TAP 90 cells revealed approximately 10^6 independent clones. Initially 2.3 X 10^5 plaques were screened using an SAA cDNA probe. Clone HDg1-1 was isolated and DNA prepared.

Sequencing. Various regions of HDg1-1 DNA were amplified by the polymerase chain reaction (PCR). The primers used for amplification represented sequences previously determined for clone SAAg5-1-1 [9] or clone SAAg9 [8]. Amplification mixtures contained 1 ng HDg1-1 or genomic DNA, primers (0.3 μM each), 1-2 units Amplitaq DNA polymerase (Perkin-Elmer Cetus, Norwalk, CT), 10 mM Tris, pH 8.3, 1.5 mM $MgCl_2$, 50 mM KCl, and 0.01% gelatin in 100 μl. Thirty cycles of 1 minute at 94°C, 1 minute at a temperature several degrees above the Tm of the primers, and 1 minute at 72°C were carried out. Fragments resulting from amplification were either reamplified asymmetrically to generate single-stranded templates for direct sequencing or cloned into M13 via restriction sites built into the primers. DNA was prepared for asymmetric amplification and purified after amplification as described by Nichols [10]. All templates were sequenced by the dideoxy method using Sequenase Version 2.0 (U.S. Biologicals, Cleveland, OH).

RESULTS AND DISCUSSION

Sequencing and restriction enzyme mapping indicates that clone HDg1-1 contains an entire SAA gene. Within the clone is a 3.6 kb HindIII fragment corresponding to the SAA fragment seen in Southern analyses of HindIII-digested total genomic DNA [7]. The sequence of HDg1-1 from intron 1 through exon 4 is shown in Figure 1. Of special note is the sequence of nucleotides 1299-1308 in exon 3 corresponding to codons 30-32. This sequence is AAA AAAT TCA. The bases must be grouped as indicated to maintain the appropriate reading frame for SAA. According to this grouping, codon 31 would have four bases suggesting that there has been a single base insertion (A or T) at this position. Regrouping the bases into triplets causes the sequence 3' to the insertion to be out-of-frame and generates a premature TGA termination signal at the position corresponding to codon 43. The same exon 3 sequence was previously determined for clone SAAg5-1-1 isolated from a chromosome 11 library and sequenced by traditional methods not employing PCR [9]. An SAA gene with the AAA AAAT TCA sequence was also identified in four unrelated individuals by means of amplification and direct sequencing of genomic DNA. The primers used for these amplifications were designed to equally recognize the HDg1-1 sequence and the sequence of a closely related clone, GSAA1, which does not contain an extra base [11]. No sequences matching that of GSAA1 were detected.

```
   1  CCACCTTTTC CAATGAATGG AAGTTGTGTA GGGAATATTC AAATGTTGCT TAGCATTGCC TTAGATAAGA ACCAAAGGGA CAGGGAAATC CTCTGACAGC  100
 101  TATCTGCCTT ATAACTTTCA TTTTACTGTG CCTAAAATAT GCTCAGAACC CAGAAAGAGG CATAATTCCT AATTTTGGCA GGCTCTAATC TAAAATAATG  200
 201  ATTCTCAAAC ATGGTGTGAC TTTTGTCTAT TTTGCTTTAT CCTGGGTCAC TGCTCCTCTT CTGTCAGATA CTGGGATTCC AATGAGACAA AATGGAAATG  300
 301  AGACGTAGAC CCTCTGACCT TCTATCTTTA TCTATCACAT ACACATGTGT GTGTGTGTGT GTGTGTGTGC GTGTGTAAAA CCGAGTGGGT TTTTTTCTTG  400
                                                                                                            Met
 401  GAATGAAAGA ATGGACTAAC ATTACAAAAA ATAAAAACTT GAAACAGAAT GTGTATTATC CTTGGTTGTG TTTCCTTGGC CCTGCAGCAG GATGAAGCTC  500
                                                       1                     13
 501  TCCACTGGCA TCATTTTCTG CTCCCTGGTC CTGGGTGTCA GCAGCCAAGG ATGGTTAACA TTCCTCAAGG CAGCTGGCCA AGGTGAGGTC CACAGGATAG  600
 601  GGGGCAGGAG GCTGCTTCTG GCTGCCCCCA GGATGCAGCT GAGCAGAGGC CACATCCCCC ACTGGGCAAA GGTGCTAGTG ATGCCACAGA TGGATAGAGA  700
                         ******
 701  AGGGG<—— ~ 2 kb ——> AAGCTTTCTT AGGTAACTCA CCTTTATCAC TTGCTGACTG AATTCTGACA GATGTCAGTT TCTAATTATA GCCTGGACAT  785
 786  TCAGATGTAT TCAGGACCAA GTTGTCCTCA CTCTACCTAC AGGCATGAAT TTCTCTCATT GACTAGGTTA GGAGCGCCAT ATGTCTGCAG CCTCCCTCAG  885
 886  AATCCCCTGT GTTCTCACAC AGGAACTGAG GGTTCCCTGG GTCTTCCAGG TAGAAGTTCA TTGTACAATG AAACATCCCT TAAGGACCAT TTCATCTCTT  985
 986  CTTTAGGTGC ATCACACATG GTTAAAACAA AGTAATAACA GAACTTAGAA TGGAATCAAA CAGAATGAAA CTTACACCAA GTACAATTCT CATTACATTA  1085
1086  ACCCAGAGAA GTGAAAAGTA GAAGAATATT TATTTCAAGC CAATATAATT TCCAAGGGCT TTGTTGAAGG CTGAAATCTT CGGGAGGAAA GTAGTGAGAA  1185
                                                                  13
1186  GAAAACTGTT CATTCCTCTA TTTCCAGTAT ATAATTGTTT TGATCATTTT CTTTCCTTTC CAGGGACTAA AGACATGTGG AAAGCCTACT CTGACATGAA  1285
1286  AGAAGCCAAT TACAAAAAAT TCAGACAAAT ACTTCCATGC TTGGGGGAAC TATGATGCTG TACAAAGGGG GCTTGGGGCT GTCTGGGCTA CAGAAGTGAT  1385
      59
1386  CAGGTAATGC ACATTCCTGA TGTTGCCAGG AATGAGTGAG CAGAGCTTGA CTGCCTTGGA CAGTCAGGAG AGAGGTAAGC TCCTTGCAGA GAAGTTAGAG  1485
1486  GCTGCAGCCC CTCCTCCTCT TGCCCTCTCT CTGCCTGTGT GCTTAGTGCG AGGGTCTGAG TGGATGGTAG AAGTGAGTGA TTCCTCACCC TCCCTCTCTG  1585
1586  GGTGCTGTTC ATCCAGCCTA GGGGTGCCCA GCCTGGCTGA GTGGGGCAGT GCCAGGCAGG GTCATTGTTT TCACCCCTCC TTCCTTGGCC TTCCTGGGCT  1685
                                                                                                          59
1686  TCTCCCAGAG TCCTCCCTTG GAAAGCAGAG AATGGGAAGG TGGGCTGTTG CTCACTGGCC TGGTGATTAA TCTCCTTGCT TGCCTGGACT ACAGCGATGC  1785
1786  CAGAGAGAAC GTCCAGAGAC TCACAGGAGA CCATGCAGAG GATTCGCTGG CTGGCCAGGC TACCAACAAA TGGGGCCAGA GTGGCAAAGA CCCCAATCAC  1885
                            104
1886  TTCCGACCTG CTGGCCTGCC AGAGAAATAC TGAGCTTCCT TTTCAATCTG CTCTCAGGAG ACCTGGCTGT GAGCCCCTGA GGGCAGGGAC ATTTGTTGAC  1985
1986  CTACAGTTAC TGAATTCTAT ATCCCTAGTA CTTGATATAG AACACATAAA AATGCTTAAT AAA  2048
```

Figure 1. Nucleotide sequence of the SAA portion of human genomic clone HDgl-1. The underlined sequences represent exons 2, 3, and 4. Nucleotides at the beginning and end of exons are overlined and the codons to which they correspond indicated. Also overlined are nucleotides corresponding to the AUG start codon in exon 2 (Met), codon 1 in exon 2, and codon 104 in exon 4.

A comparison of the nuclotide and derived amino acid sequences of HDg1-1 with those of human SAA1 and SAA2 shows: (1) no homology in introns 1 and 2, but nearly 90% homology in intron 3, (2) 83% identity in the exon 2 encoded signal peptide, but only 25% identity over the first 12 amino acids of the mature protein which are also encoded in exon 2, (3) 86% nucleotide and 72% amino acid identity in exon 3, and (4) 86% nucleotide and 81% amino acid identity in the coding region of exon 4. For these calculations the extra base in exon 3 was not considered.

While the NH_2-terminal region derived from HDg1-1 was most divergent from human SAA1 and SAA2, its sequence matched that of rabbit SAA3 at 9 of the first 12 positions. Based on its collagenase-inducing capabilities, the rabbit protein has been implicated as a mediator of connective tissue breakdown [5]; presumably the corresponding protein in humans could have an important role in the pathogenesis of rheumatoid arthritis. However, no mRNA for human SAA3 was detected in liver, lung, or synovium either by enzymatic amplification of RNA or by Northern analysis. The presence of the extra base in exon 3, together with the absence of detectable mRNA, suggests that this SAA3 gene in human is not expressed.

ACKNOWLEDGEMENTS

This work was supported by VA Medical Research, the United States Public Health Service (RR-00750, NIDDK-34881, NIAMS-AR20582, AR7448), The Arthritis Foundation, The Grace M. Showalter Trust and The Marion E. Jacobson Fund.

REFERENCES

1. Lowell, C.A., Potter, D.A., Stearman, R.S., and Morrow, J.F. (1986), J. Biol. Chem. 261, 8442-8452.
2. Yamamoto, K.-I., Goto, N., Kosaka, J., Shiroo, M., Yeul, Y.D., and Migita, S. (1987), J. Immunol. 139, 1683-1688.
3. Ramadori, G., Sipe, J.D., and Colten, H.R. (1985), J. Immunol. 135, 3645-3647.
4. Meek, R.L. and Benditt, E.P. (1986), J. Exp. Med. 164, 2006-2017.
5. Brinckerhoff, C.E., Mitchell, T.I., Karmilowicz, M.J., Kluve-Beckerman, B., and Benson, M.D. (1989), Science 243, 655-657.
6. Sipe, J.D., Colten, H.R., Goldberger, G., Edge, M.D., Tack, B.F., Cohen, A.S., and Whitehead, A.S. (1985), Biochemistry 24, 2931-2936.
7. Kluve-Beckerman, B., Dwulet, F.E., and Benson, M.D. (1988), J. Clin. Invest. 82, 1670-1675.
8. Woo, P., Sipe, J., Dinarello, C.A., and Colten, H.R. (1987), J. Biol. Chem. 262, 15790-15795.
9. Kluve-Beckerman, B., Benson, M.D., and Benson, M.D. (1989), Arthritis Rheum. 32, D109.
10. Nichols, W.C., Liepnieks, J.J., McKusick, V.A., and Benson, M.D. (1989), Genomics 5, 535-540.
11. Sack, G.S. and Talbot Jr., C.C. (1989), Gene 84, 509-515.

HUMAN SERUM AMYLOID-A PROTEIN: VARIABILITY DEMONSTRATED BY CDNA SEQUENCING AND EXPRESSION STUDIES

A. Steinkasserer*, E. Weiss, V. Bock, and R.P. Linke
Institute of Immunology, Goethestr. 31, D-8000 München 2,
*present address: MRC Immunochemistry Unit, Dept. of Biochemistry, South Parks Road, Oxfors OX1 3QU UK

ABSTRACT. To investigate the variability of the SAA gene family in one individual an acute phase liver cDNA library was screened and the sequence of all SAA cDNA clones was determined resulting in at least five variants. Based on sequence homology in the coding region and identical 3' untranslated segments our cloned sequences fall into two groups. By Northern blot analysis three distinct mRNA species were distinguished. No correlation was observed between the SAA cDNA groups and individual mRNA bands, as variant specific oligonucleotides hybridized to all three mRNA molecules suggesting that the three SAA mRNA species are due to variations in the poly(A) tail. We propose that the variant 3' untranslated regions and the poly(A) tail have a function in the differential expression of the SAA polypeptide family.

1. INTRODUCTION.

The serum amyloid proteins are chemically heterogeneous, and in man six isoforms have been characterized (1), pointing to the presence of a family of SAA genes. This concept is supported by the description of individual genomic or cDNA sequences (2, 3, 4, 5, 6, 7) demonstrating the existence of three different genes in the human genome. We took the approach to determine the complexity of SAA by the isolation and sequencing of cDNA clones isolated from an acute phase human liver cDNA library and obtained evidence for a minimum of at least five distinct SAA transcripts. A more detailed account of this work is given elsewhere (8).

2. MATERIALS AND METHODS

Isolation of SAA specific cDNA clones and sequence determina tion of SAA cDNA clones in the procaryotic expression vector pEX2 has been described previously, as has been the high the high resolution RNA gel electrophoresis (8).

3. RESULTS AND DISCUSSION

The sequence determination of a large number of SAA cDNA clones led to the identification of a minimum of five distinct SAA transcripts, some of which differ only by few bases. The majority of the coding substitutions are present in the 3' portion. A comparison of known cloned sequences (Fig.1) demonstrates that the sequences fall into three classes of homologous clones. Members of one group differ only by few exchanges and are characterized by an identical, unique 3' untranslated region (group I: a,g h; group II: d, e, f; group III: b, c). Sequences of one group have a distinctive set of aminoacids in positions 60, 68, 69 and 90, whereas the two variations specific for α- and ß- forms of SAA polypeptides can be found within one group. A minimal number of three loci (isotypes) could explain the spectrum of our cloned SAA sequences; each locus then would show considerable polymorphism.
On high resolution polyacrylamide gels three SAA mRNA species were always detected. To test the possibility that each class of SAA transcripts might be presented by one size of mRNA, we used group specific oligonucleotides derived from the 3' untranslated regions to probe Northern blots obtained from RNA gels run for improved separation on 6 % acrylamide gels. Whereas with the group I/group II crossreactive cDNA probe, the two largest SAA mRNA species of 650n and 600n gave roughly the same hybridization signals, the oligomer probes specific for either the group I (Fig.2, lane 2) or group II (Fig.2, lane 1) sequences detected preferentially the 600n transcript. Thus, the three SAA mRNA species do not correspond with the classes of distinct SAA cDNA sequences, but might be explained by differences in the length of the poly (A) tail.
Considering the variation of SAA sequences, the results indicate that at least four genes are present in the human genome. Three genes have to be postulated to account for the group I/group II sequences and another one to code for group III SAA variants. The finding that SAA polypeptides are coded by a possibly polymorphic gene family stresses the necessity for continuing investigation on a possible differential function of the molecules. We used an eucaryotic expression system to start isolating pure recombinant SAA polypeptide. We took advantage of a full length cDNA clone isolated from the CDM8 cDNA library, the sequence of which is identical to pAP1 (see a) in Fig.1. Transient expression in COS7 cells resulted in the secretion of SAA polypeptides also present in human serum.
In view of increasing evidence that the 3' untranslated reg-

	-4	15	23	25	30	31	41	43	45	46	47	48	52	53	54	55	57	58	60	62	63	64	65	66	68	69	70	71	72	73	75	78	79	81	82	83	84	87	90	101
a	GGT	CGG	GAC	AGA	ATC	GGC	AAC	GAT	GCC	AAA	AGG	GGA	GTC	TGG	GCT	GCA	GCG	ATC	GAT	AGA	GAG	AAT	ATC	CAG	TTC	TTT	GGC	CAT	GGT	GCG	GAC	GCT	GAT	GCT	GCC	AAT	GAA	AGG	AAA	CCT
	G	R	D	R	I	G	N	D	A	K	R	G	V	W	A	A	A	I	D	R	E	N	I	Q	F	F	G	H	G	A	D	A	D	A	A	N	E	R	K	P
b		AAA	...	.A.	.AA	AAT	...	...	..A	.C.	..A	..G	.CT	...	...	A..	.TC	...	...	..G	..A	..C	G..	...	C..	ACA	..A	AGG	AC.	..A	..T	...	..C	...	A.G	..C	A..	CA.	...	..A
		K	.	K	K	N	.	.	.	T	.	.	A	.	.	T	V	.	.	.	.	.	V	.	L	T	.	R	T	.	.	.	.	.	T	.	K	Q	.	.
c		AAA	...	.A.	.AA	AAT	...	...	..A	.C.	..A	..C	...	...	...	A..	.T.	...																						
		K	.	K	K	N	.	.	.	T	.	.	.	.	.	T	V	.																						
d		...	...	...	...	...	...	...	...	...	...	...	.C.	...	..C	...	.T.	...																						
		.	.	.	.	.	.	.	.	.	.	.	A	.	.	.	V	.																						
e	...	...	...	...	...	...	...	...	...	...	...	...	.C.	...	...	...	.T.	...	A..	...	...	...	...	...	C..	ACA	...	.G.	...	...	...	...	...	...	...	...	A..	...	.G.	...
	.	.	.	.	.	.	.	.	.	.	.	.	A	.	.	.	V	.	N	.	.	.	.	.	L	T	.	R	.	.	.	.	.	.	.	.	K	.	R	.
f	A..	...	...	...	...	...	...	...	...	...	...	...	.C.	...	..C	...	.T.	...	A..	...	...	...	...	...	C..	ACA	...	...	...	...	...	..C	...	...	...	...	A..	...	.G.	...
	S	.	.	.	.	.	.	.	.	.	.	.	A	.	.	.	V	.	N	.	.	.	.	.	L	T	.	.	.	.	.	.	.	.	.	.	K	.	R	.
g															...	...	...	...	A..	...	...	...	...	...	...	...	...	...	...	...	...	..C	...	...	...	...	...	...	...	...
															.	.	.	.	N	.	.	.	.	.	.	.	.	.	.	.	.	.	.	.	.	.	.	.	.	.
h															...	...	.T.	...	A..	...	...	...	...	...	...	...	...	...	...	...	...	..C	...	...	...	...	...	...	...	...
															.	.	V	.	N	.	.	.	.	.	.	.	.	.	.	.	.	.	.	.	.	.	.	.	.	.

Fig.1: Comparison of the nucleotide and deduced amino acid sequences of distinct SAA cDNA: a: pAP1 (2); b: pGS14/1 (3); c: GSAA2 and d: GSAA3 (3); e: SAA_g9 (6); f: pAS_8 (8); g: $pAS_{3\alpha}$, and h: $pAS_{3\beta}$ (8).

Fig.2: Northern blot analysis of total RNA isolated from acute phase liver and electrophoresed on a 6 % acrylamide-/7M urea gel (8). Hybridized: Lane 1: with oligomer oAS_8 GTGAGGTCTATGTCCAGG derived from the 3' untranslated segment specific for group II SAA cDNA;
2: oligomer oAS_1 GGGGAGGGTACACAATGGG from the 3' untranslated region of the group I transcripts.

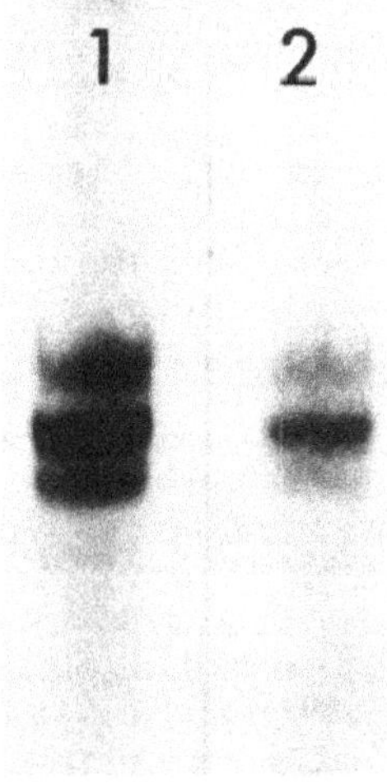

ion and the poly (A) tail not only control mRNA stability, but also have a role in the control of translation, an intriguing possibility is that the similar but distinct 3' untranslated sequences and the different poly (A) tails of SAA transcripts might influence, possibly independently, the translation efficiency of SAA mRNA. It is conceivable that some SAA variants are synthesized in the very early stage of acute phase reaction whereas another group of SAA transcripts is translated more efficiently during later stages. Thus, the production of variant SAA polypeptides during the acute phase reaction is not only differentially regulated at the level of transcription but might also modulated by the translation efficiency.

4. ACKNOWLEDGEMENTS

This study was supported by the DFG, SFB 207, Projekt G8.For technical assistance we thank Mrs. A. Reil and A. Kerling

5. REFERENCES

1) Strachan, A.F., Brandt, W.F., van der Westhuyzen, D.R., Coetzee, G.A., de Beer, M.C., Shepardt, E.G., de Beer F.C. (1989) Human serum amyloid A protein. J. Biol. Chem. 264 18368-18373.
2) Sipe, J.D., Colten, H.R., Goldberger , G., Edge, M.D., Tack, B.F., Cohen, A.S., Whitehead, A.S. (1985) Human serum amyloid A (SAA): Biosynthesis and postsynthetic processing of preSAA and structural variants defined by complementary DNA. Biochemistry 24, 2931-2936.
3) Sack, G.H. and Lease, J.J. (1986) Human serum amyloid genes - molecular characterization. Amyloidosis, Plenum press, New York and London, pp. 61-68.
4) Kluve-Beckerman, B., Lang, G.L., Benson, M.D. (1986) DNA sequence evidence for polymorphic forms of human serum amyloid a (SAA). Biochem. Genet. 24, 795-803.
5) Kluve-Beckerman, B., Dwulet, F.E., Benson, M.D. (1988) Human serum Amyloid A. Three hepatic mRNAs and the corresponding proteins in one person. J. Clin. Invest. 82, 1670-1675.
6) Woo, P., Sipe, J.D., Dinarello, C.A., Colten, H.R. (1987) Structure of a human serum amyloid A gene and modulation of its expression in transfected L cells. J. Biol. Chem. 261, 15790-15795.
7) Sack, G.H. and Talbot, C.C. (1989) The human serum amyloid A (SAA)-encoding gene GSAA1: nucleotide sequence and possible autocrine-collagenase-inducer function. Gene 84, 509-515.
8) Steinkasserer, A., Weiss, E.H., Schwaeble, W., Linke, R.P. (1990) Heterogeneity of human serum amyloid A protein. Five different variants from one individual demonstrated by cDNA sequence analysis. Biochem. J. 268, 187-193.

ABYSSINIAN CAT MODEL OF AA AMYLOIDOSIS: SAA GENE ANALYSIS

Harats, N., DiBartola, S.P., Benson, M.D., and Kluve-Beckerman, B., Indiana University School of Medicine, Department of Medicine, Rheumatology Division, Clinical Building 492, 541 Clinical Drive, Indianapolis, IN 46223; USA.

ABSTRACT. Amyloidosis of the amyloid A (AA)-type develops fairly frequently in Abyssinian cats and is similar in many respects to the amyloidosis associated with FMF in humans. To reveal clues about the pathogenetic mechanism of amyloid formation, we have studied the SAA genes in these cats. The study was approached by amplifying SAA exon 4 sequences from genomic DNA, cloning the amplification products into M13, and determining the exon 4 sequences of 7-9 clones from each of 4 cats. The 12 different sequences that were present among 32 clones could be grouped into 3 sequence motifs. All 4 cats had sequences belonging to each of the three motifs, but no cat had more than 2 sequences of any one motif, suggesting that the slightly different sequences within a motif were allelic. These sequence data, along with the results of Southern analyses, provide evidence that there are a minimum of three genes and multiple alleles for SAA in the cat.

INTRODUCTION

Amyloidosis is a common disease in the Abyssinian breed of cat, but quite rare in the general cat population. Abyssinian cats are affected with the disease in a familial fashion underscoring a genetic contribution to its pathogenesis. The fibrillar amyloid deposits are composed of SAA-derived AA protein as they are in human reactive amyloidosis, although the cats usually have no obvious chronic infection or inflammation [1]. Similar to human amyloidosis of the AA-type, the feline disease is systemic with the kidneys a predominant target organ and renal failure the most common cause of death [2]. While reactive amyloidosis develops in only a small percentage of individuals with predisposing diseases, it is relatively common in patients with familial Mediterranean fever (FMF), an autosomal recessive disease affecting people of Mediterranean descent [3,4]. In light of the similarities between FMF-associated amyloidosis and amyloidosis in Abyssinian cats, we have studied feline SAA genes with the hope that they might provide clues about the pathogenetic mechanism of amyloid formation.

MATERIALS AND METHODS

An SAA gene was cloned from a cat genomic library [5] and partially sequenced. Based on the sequence of this clone (cSAAg2-1-1), 20-mer oligonucleotides were synthesized to use as linker-primers in the enzymatic amplification of cat SAA gene sequences and subsequent M13 cloning of the amplification products. The sequences of the linker-primers (LP) were as follows. LP1: 5'-TGACCTGCAGGCGACGCCAGAGAGAATT-3'; LP2: 5'-TGACCTGCAGGCAGAGCAAAGAGGAAGC-3'. LP1 corresponded to SAA codons 59-64 and LP2 to the sequence immediately 3' to the stop codon. At the 5'-end both oligonucleotides contained a PstI recognition sequence plus four additional bases. Amplification reactions contained 1 ug of genomic DNA, LP1 and LP2 (500 nM each), dGTP, dATP, dTTP, and dCTP (200 uM each), and 1 unit of Amplitaq DNA polymerase (Perkin-Elmer Cetus) in a 100 ul solution of 10 mM Tris, pH 8.3, 1.5 mM $MgCl_2$, 50 mM KCl, and 0.01% gelatin. Amplification was accomplished by 30 reaction cycles, each consisting of denaturing at 94°C for 2 minutes, annealing at 60°C for 2 minutes and elongating at 72°C for 3 minutes. The 150 bp amplification product was digested with PstI, purified by spin dialysis using Centricon 100 membranes (Amicon), and then cloned into M13 mp19. M13 clones were selected and the exon 4 sequences in each clone determined by the dideoxy method using Sequenase Version 2.0 (U.S. Biochemicals).

RESULTS AND DISCUSSION

A total of 32 clones containing SAA exon 4 sequences were analyzed (7-9 from each of 4 cats; cats D and S had amyloidosis, cats W and F were healthy). Twelve different sequences were present among the 32 clones. These 12 sequences could be grouped into three sequence motifs (Figure 1). The nucleotide sequence shown as Motif 1 encoded the amino acid sequence previously determined for protein AA isolated from an Abyssinian cat (6), and nucleotide sequence designated as Motif 2 matched that of an SAA gene (cSAA2-1-1) cloned in this laboratory.

All three motifs were represented in the 5 sequences found for each cat, i.e. none of the cats had more than two sequences of any one motif, suggesting that the slightly different sequences within a motif were allelic. Intra-motif variations consisted of the following: Motif 1 - both AGG and AGC were found to specify Arg 67; Motif 2 - sequences had either AGA specifying Arg 102 or AGC specifying Ser 102; Motif 3 - sequences had either AGA or AGG specifying Arg 67, AGT or AGC specifying Ser h, and GAA or GAG specifying Glu 84. Two of the 12 sequences contained an exception from the motif into which they were grouped. One clone isolated from cat D had a motif 3 sequence except that it had GAG specifying Glu 98 as in motif 1, and a clone isolated from cat S had a motif 2 sequence except for GAG specifying Glu 74 as in motif 3. Although amyloid-affected cats D and S each contained a sequence not found in healthy cats W and F, any statement regarding the amyloidogenicity of these sequences would require analyses of a much greater number of cats. The isolation of 5 sequences from each of the 4 cats does indicate that the cat, like other species, has multiple genes for SAA. There appear to be a minimum of 3 genes with 2 or more alleles for each.

Data corroborating SAA gene multiplicity was provided by Southern analyses of cat genomic DNA digested with a variety of enzymes (BamHI,

	64	65	66	67	68	69	a	b	c	d	e	f	g	h	70	71	72
Motif 1	AAT	TCT	CAG	AGA	GTC	ACA	GAC	TTT	TTC	AGG	CAC	GGA	AAC	AGC	GGC	CAC	GGA
	N	S	Q	R	V	T	D	F	F	R	H	G	N	S	G	H	G
2	·	·	·	·	·	·	·	·	·	AGC	·	AGA	AGC	·	·	·	·
										S		R	S				
3	·	·	·	·	·	·	·	·	·	AGG	·	GGA	AAC	AG(C/T)	·	·	·
										R		G	N	S			

	73	74	75	76	77	78	79	80	81	82	83	84	85	86	87	88	89
Motif 1	GCA	GAG	GAC	TCG	AAG	GCT	GAC	CAG	GAA	GCC	AAT	GAA	TGG	GGC	CGG	AG(C/T)	GGC
	A	E	D	S	K	A	D	Q	E	A	N	E	W	G	R	S	G
2	·	CAG	·	·	·	·	·	·	GCC	·	·	·	·	·	·	AGC	·
		Q							A							S	
3	·	GAG	·	·	·	·	·	·	GCC	·	·	·	·	·	·	AGC	·
		E							A							S	

	90	91	92	93	94	95	96	97	98	99	100	101	102	103	104
Motif 1	AAA	GAC	CCC	AAC	CAC	TAT	CGA	CCT	GAG	GGC	CTG	CCT	GAC	AAG	TAC
	K	D	P	N	H	Y	R	P	E	G	L	P	D	K	Y
2	·	·	·	·	·	TTT	·	·	GCT	·	·	·	AG(A/C)	·	·
						F			A				R / S		
3	·	·	·	·	·	TTT	·	·	GCT	·	·	·	AGC	·	·
						F			A				S		

Figure 1. Three sequence motifs into which the 12 different sequences determined for exon 4 could be grouped. All three sequences, or some minor variation thereof, were found in each cat.

Motif 1: Corresponds to the sequence previously determined for an isolated feline AA protein.

Motif 2: Matches that determined for a cloned feline SAA gene (cSAAg 2-1-1) cloned from a non-Abyssinian cat.

BglI, BglII, BstEII, EcoRI, EcoRV, HincII, HindIII, NsiI, PstI, PvuII, ScaI, SstI, StuI, StyI, and XbaI) and probed with a 610 bp SAA gene fragment restricted to exon 3-exon 4 sequences. Regardless of the enzyme used for digestion, hybridization to a minimum of three fragments was seen, suggesting that there are at least three SAA genes (data not shown).

In addition to gene multiplicity, the sequences presented here also show the nucleotide basis for the stretch of 8 amino acids (a-h, Figure 1) identified in cat AA protein between residues 69 and 70 based on alignment with the human SAA sequence [6]. The nucleotide sequence specifying this "insertion" was present in all 32 clones.

ACKNOWLEDGEMENTS

This work was supported by VA Medical Research, the United States Public Health Service (RR-00750, NIDDK-34881, NIAMS-AR20582, AR74480), The Arthritis Foundation, The Grace M. Showalter Trust and The Marion E. Jacobson Fund.

REFERENCES

1. DiBartola, S.P., Benson, M.D., Dwulet, F.E., and Cornacoff, J.B. (1985), 'Isolation and characterization of amyloid protein AA in the Abyssinian cat', Lab. Invest. 52, 485-489.
2. DiBartola, S.P., Tarr, M.J., and Benson, M.D. (1986), 'Tissue distribution of amyloid deposits in Abyssinian cats with familial amyloidosis', J. Comp. Pathol. 96, 387-398.
3. Gafni, J., Ravid, M., and Sohar, E. (1968), 'The role of amyloidosis in familial Mediterranean fever. A population study', Israel J. Med. Sci. 4, 995-999.
4. Meyerhoff, J. (1980), 'Familial Mediterranean fever: Report of a large family, review of the literature, and discussion of the frequency of amyloidosis', Medicine 59, 66-77.
5. Soe, L.H., Devi, B.G., Mullins, J.I., and Roy-Burman, P. (1983), 'Molecular cloning and characterization of endogenous feline leukemia virus sequences from a cat genomic library', 46, 829-840.
6. Kluve-Beckerman, B., Dwulet, F.E., DiBartola, S.P., and Benson, M.D. (1989), 'Primary structures of dog and cat amyloid A proteins: Comparison to human AA', Comp. Biochem. Physiol. 94B, 175-183.

MINK SERUM AMYLOID A PROTEIN - EXPRESSION AND PRIMARY STRUCTURE OF AMYLOIDOGENIC AND NON-AMYLOIDOGENIC ISOTYPES

G.MARHAUG*, G.HUSBY*, K.NORDSTOGA$ and S.B.DOWTON #

Institute of Clinical Medicine, University of Tromsø and $ Norwegian College of Veterinary Medicine, Oslo, Norway, #Division of Medical Genetics, Edward Mallinckrodt Department of Pediatrics and the James S. McDonnell Department of Genetics, Washington University School of Medicine, St. Louis, Missouri, U.S.A.

ABSTRACT. When Northern blot analysis of LPS stimulated mink liver RNA was performed using a SAA specific probe, several signals were found. Nucleotide sequence analysis of two clones from a cDNA library was performed. Deduced amino acid sequence of the longer one, SAA1 (776 bp), indicates that it represents a SAA isotype found only in serum, while the shorter one, SAA2 (552 bp), corresponds to an isotype found both in serum and degraded to protein AA in secondary amyloid. These results show that the situation in mink is the same as in mice, where only one out of at least two SAA isotypes has been shown to be amyloidogenic. Northern blot analysis also showed that almost all SAA mRNA was found in the liver, while only minor amounts of SAA1 and SAA2 mRNA was found in the brain and the lungs. No signals could be detected in amyloid prone organs like intestine and spleen. In the liver a SAA specific signal was found corresponding to 2.2 kb, and after in vitro translation a protein SAA band corresponding to 28,000 Daltons was detected, indicating that a SAA isotype with high molecular weight exists in this animal.

Introduction

Serum amyloid A (SAA) is a sensitive acute phase protein, which was first recognized in serum because of its cross-reactivity with antisera to protein AA from secondary amyloid [1]. IL-1, IL-6 and TNF released during inflammation stimulate hepatic SAA production [2]. Administration of LPS to mice produces a 2000-fold increase in the level of hepatic SAA mRNA [3]. Heterogeneity of amino acid sequences in SAA proteins may confer properties which result in deposition of some SAA isotypes as AA protein in amyloid. Only SAA2 has been demonstrated in murine amyloidosis, suggesting that various murine SAA isotypes may have different amyloidogenic potential [4]. In man, several SAA genes have been characterized by nucleotide sequence analysis [5], but, in contrast to murine models, no obvious difference in amyloidogenicity among human SAA isotypes has been detected. Mink are susceptible to the development of AA amyloidosis, and the observation that only valine occurs in amino acid position 10 of mink AA [6] while mink apoSAA contains isoleucine or valine at that position [7] has supported the postulate that certain SAA isotypes may be more amyloidogenic than others.

Materials and methods

Isolation and Analysis of SAA mRNA. Two mink (Mustela vision) were injected with LPS (E. coli 026:B6) 1 mg/kg, while saline was administrated to one control animal. After 18 hrs brain, lungs, heart, liver, spleen and intestine were frozen in liquid nitrogen. Total cellular RNA from organs was prepared by extraction in guanidinum isothiocyanate and centrifugation over a CsCl cushion. The polyadenylated (poly A^{+}) fraction was purified by affinity chromatography on oligo(dT) cellulose. RNA from different organs was fractionated by agarose-formaldehyde electrophoresis, and transfered to nylon membranes. RNA blots were hybridized with either labeled mink SAA cDNA inserts or sequence specific oligonucleotides.

Analysis of Primary Translation Products. RNA aliquots were translated in a rabbit reticulocyte lysate cell free system in the presence of (^{35}S)methionine. The radiolabeled translation products were precipitated with rabbit anti mink SAA antiserum, and analyzed by SDS-PAGE.

cDNA Library Construction and Screening. Analysis of Mink SAA Clones. An acute phase mink liver cDNA library was constructed from poly A^{+} RNA isolated from LPS stimulated mink using M-MTV reverse transcriptase for first strand cDNA synthesis. The second strand DNA was synthesized using a modification of the method of Gubler and Hoffman. cDNA were ligated into lambda ZAPII arms. Transformant plaques ($4.4x10^{5}$) were screened with a Syrian hamster SAA cDNA insert. Selected clones were plaque purified, and in vivo excision of pBS SK(-) phagemids was achieved by addition of R408 helper phage. Nucleotide sequencing was performed using the dideoxy-chain termination method.

Results

The nucleotide sequences and the corresponding amino acid sequences of two mink SAA cDNA clones, one (SAA1) 776 bp long, the other (SAA2) 552 bp long, are shown in Fig.1. The amino acid sequences of apoSAA and protein AA are shown for comparison. Previous studies of mink protein SAA and AA suggest that only one SAA isotype is amyloidogenic. The cDNA clone for SAA2 defines the amyloidogenic isotype, while SAA1 is found only in serum. Mink SAA1 has alanine in position 10, isoleucine in position 24, 67 and 71, lysine in position 27 and proline in position 105. Residue 10 in mink SAA2 is valine while arginine and asparagine are at positions 24 and 27 respectively, characteristics of protein AA isolated from mink amyloid fibrils. Mink SAA2 also has valine in position 67, phenylalanine in position 71, and amino acid 105 is serine. After LPS stimulation mink SAA mRNA of three different sizes, 0.6, 0.8 and 2.2 kb, are found in the liver (Fig.2), while no signal could be detected in the control animal. SAA mRNA is abundant in liver with relatively minor accumulations in brain and lung (Fig.2). Radiolabeled synthetic 18-mer oligonucleotides specific for mink SAA1 and SAA2 mRNA species (Fig.1) identify the 0.8 kb mRNA as SAA1 and the 0.6 kb signal as corresponding to SAA2. Genes encoding both SAA isotypes are expressed in all three organs, while no SAA mRNA was detectable in amyloid prone organs including spleen and intestine, indicating that deposition of AA from locally synthesized SAA is unlikely. A third mRNA species (2.2 kb) is identified only in the liver, and hybridizes with cDNA probes for mink SAA1

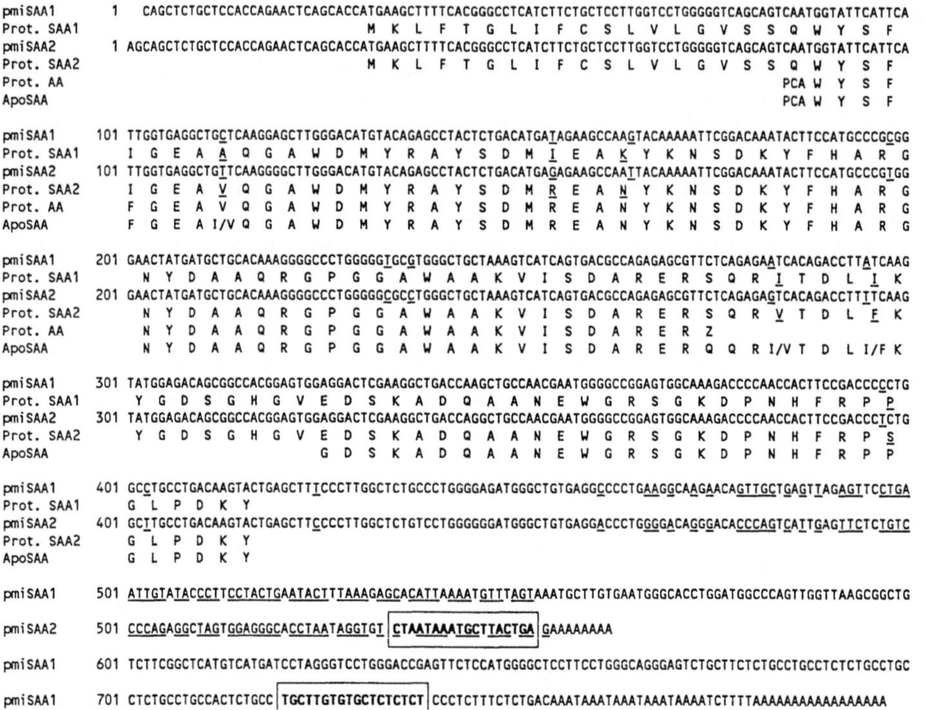

Fig.1. Nucleotide sequences of two mink SAA clones and their deduced amino acid sequences. Differences between the two are underlined. Synthetic 18-mer oligonucleotides specific for the two cDNAs and used for mRNA studies are showed in open boxes. Mink apoSAA and mink protein AA are shown for comparison.

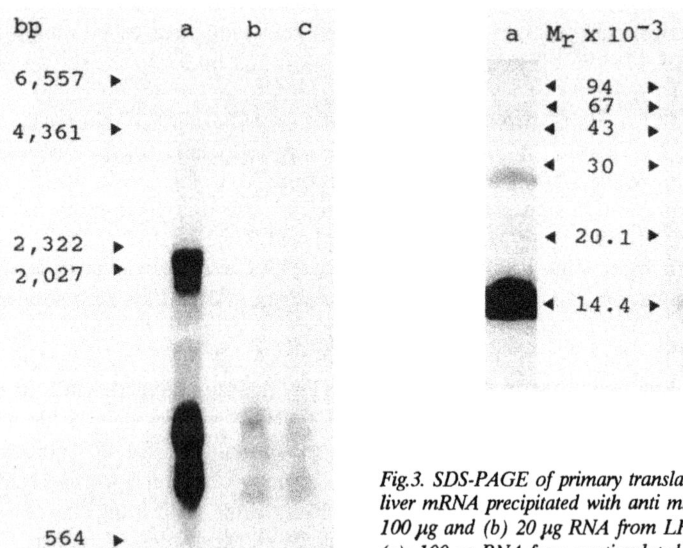

Fig.3. SDS-PAGE of primary translation products from mink liver mRNA precipitated with anti mink SAA. Lane (a) 100 μg and (b) 20 μg RNA from LPS-stimulated mink liver, (c): 100 μg RNA from unstimulated mink liver.

Fig.2. Northern blot of RNA from LPS-stimulated mink hybridized with a RNA-probe transcribed from pmiSAA1. Lane (a):liver; (b):brain; (c) lung. (a) exposed for 15 min, (b) and (c) for 24 hrs.

and SAA2 (Fig.2). In addition to a major primary translation product (molecular mass 14,400 Da) an additional product with molecular mass 28,000 Da is immunoprecipitable (Fig.3)

DISCUSSION

The derivation of isoleucine at positions 67 and 71 from one cDNA clone, and valine and phenylalanine at these respective positions in the other, has defined SAA1 and the amyloidogenic SAA2 primary structure for mink. The six amino acid substitutions, including three in the NH_2-terminal portion of the SAA molecule found in protein AA, indicate that SAA2 is the amyloidogenic isotype. Prediction of secondary structure based upon amino acid sequence of mink SAA1 and SAA2 did not reveal any major differences in helical content or hydrophilicity of these two polypeptides. Although the hepatic mRNA species for mink SAA1 and SAA2 are equally abundant 18 hrs after LPS stimulation, SAA2 account for only 20% of apoSAA isolated from mink serum after 36 hrs [7]. This may be due to selective removal of SAA2 from the circulation, as has been shown in the murine model [8]. Anti SAA antiserum immunoprecipitates a 28,000 Da primary translation product in addition to a major 14,400 Da species, suggesting that the 2.2 kb SAA mRNA may be the transcription product of a third SAA gene. Anti AA reactivity in HDL at high molecular weights has been observed in Western blotting experiments [9]. Mink SAA mRNA was not identified in amyloid-prone organs such as spleen and intestine. This data support the observation that amyloid deposition does not arise from locally produced SAA isotypes, but rather from hepatically derived SAA.

References

1. Husby, G., Sletten, K., Michaelsen, T.E. and Natvig, J.B. (1972) 'An alternative non immunoglobulin origin of amyloid fibrils', Nature (London) 238, 187
2. Ramadori, G., Van Damme, J., Rieder, H. and Meyer zum Buschenfelde, K.-H. (1988) 'Interleukin 6, the third mediator of acute phase proteins. Comparison with interleukin 1ß and tumor necrosis factor-α', Eur. J. Immunol. 18, 1259-1264
3. Lowell, C.A., Stearman, R.S. and Morrow, J.F. (1986) 'Transcriptional regulation of serum amyloid A gene expression', J. Biol. Chem. 261, 8453-8461
4. Hoffman, J.S., Ericsson, L.H., Eriksen, E., Walsh, K.A. and Benditt, E.P. (1984) 'Murine tissue amyloid protein AA. NH_2-terminal sequence identity with only one of two serum protein (ApoSAA) gene products', J. Exp. Med. 159, 641-646
5. Kluve-Beckerman, B., Long, G.L. and Benson, M.D. (1986) 'DNA-sequence evidence for polymorphic forms of human serum amyloid A(SAA)', Biochemical Genetics 24, 795-803
6. Waalen, K., Sletten, K., Husby, G. and Nordstoga, K. (1980) 'The primary structure of amyloid fibril protein AA in endotoxin-induced amyloidosis of the mink', Eur. J. Biochem. 104, 407-417
7. Syversen, V., Sletten, K., Marhaug, G., Husby, G. and Lium, B. (1987) 'The amino acid sequence of serum amyloid A (SAA) protein in mink', Scand. J. Immunol. 26, 763-767
8. Meek, R.L., Hoffman, J.S. and Benditt, E.P. (1986) 'One serum amyloid A isotype is selectively removed from circulation', Exp. Med. 163, 499-510
9. Husebekk, A., Skogen, B., Husby, G. and Marhaug, G. (1985) 'Transformation of amyloid precursor SAA to protein AA and incorporation in amyloid fibrils in vivo', Scand. J. Immunol. 21, 283-287

PRIMARY STRUCTURE OF TWO RABBIT SERUM AMYLOID A PROTEINS (SAA) BASED ON cDNA SEQUENCE

M. RYGG, G. HUSBY, B. DOWTON, G. MARHAUG*
Institute of Clinical Medicine, University of Tromsø, Norway
** Division of Medical Genetics, Edward Mallinckrodt Department of Pediatrics and the James S. McDonnell Department of Genetics, Washington University School of Medicine, St. Louis, Missouri, USA*

ABSTRACT. The aim of this study was to predict the complete amino acid sequence of rabbit serum amyloid protein A (SAA) and identify heterogenities and amyloidogenic isotypes. After stimulation with turpentine a SAA specific mRNA signal was detected in the rabbit liver, and a cDNA library was made. Selected clones were sequenced. The deduced amino acid sequences of two rabbit SAA proteins differ in five amino acid residues, four of which are located in the NH_2-terminal part. Only one of these two isotypes, SAA2, seems to be involved in amyloid formation.

Introduction

SAA is a sensitive acute phase protein reaching levels 1000-fold or more above normal concentration during inflammation (1). IL-1, IL-6 and TNF released during inflammation induce hepatic SAA mRNA, indicating a pretranslational regulation (2). In circulation SAA is bound to high density lipoprotein. During inflammation apoSAA accounts for as much as 50% of total apo-proteins in this lipoprotein fraction (3). The function of SAA still remains unclear. A precursor-product relationship between SAA and amyloid protein AA isolated from secondary amyloid has been established (4).

Amino acid sequence heterogenity of SAA has been demonstrated in all species studied, while protein AA from most species is more homogeneous. Murine protein AA shears amino acid sequence with the SAA2 isotype, but differs from SAA1 in several residues (5), suggesting that various murine SAA isotypes may have different amyloidogenic potential. The same phenomenon has recently been seen in mink (6). Several human SAA isotypes have been characterized, but no obvious difference in amyloidogenicity has so far been detected (7).

In contrast to in mice and mink, experimental amyloidosis has been difficult to induce in rabbits (8). A previous report has indicated two forms of rabbit SAA based on differences in isoelectric focusing (9). The two forms have very similar amino acid composition and molecular weight. Amino acid sequence of rabbit protein AA has been described (10) and demonstrated several heterogenities. The present study was undertaken to establish the nucleotide and deduced amino acid sequence of rabbit SAA, look for heterogenities and if possible identify amyloidogenic isotypes.

Methods

Induction of SAA mRNA. One rabbit (New Zealand White) was injected intramuscularly with turpentine, and another with saline as control. Both were sacrifized after 18 hrs. Liver tissue was frozen in liquid nitrogen.

cDNA library construction and screening. Total liver RNA was prepared (11) and the polyadenylated (poly A^+) fraction was purified using oligo(dT) cellulose. An acute phase rabbit liver cDNA library was constructed from poly A^+RNA using M-MTV reverse transcriptase for first strand cDNA synthesis. The second strand cDNA was synthesized using a modification of the method of Gubler and Hoffman (12). cDNAs were ligated into Lambda ZAPII arms, packed and plated. Transformant plaques were screened with a radiolabeled mink SAA cDNA insert. Selected clones were plaque purified and in vivo excision of pBS SK(-) phagemids was achieved by addition of R408 helper phage.

Analysis of rabbit SAA clones. Nucleotide sequencing was performed using the dideoxy-chain termination method (13).

Results

So far two complete nucleotide sequences have been determined from two rabbit SAA cDNA clones. The deduced amino acid sequences for rabbit SAA1 and SAA2 are shown in Fig 1. The nomenclature was adopted according to the convention established in the murine system where SAA2 is amyloidogenic and SAA1 is not.

The deduced polypeptide sequences for rabbit SAA both have a total of 104 residues, as human apoSAA. SAA1 differs from SAA2 by five amino acid substitutions, four of which are located in the NH_2-terminal part sheared with protein AA. The nucleotide sequence of SAA1 predicts arginine in position 2, threonine in position 11, glutamine in position 12 and glycine in position 15, while the nucleotide sequence of SAA2 predicts glycine, valine, arginine and glycine in the corresponding positions. In addition there is a substitution of alanine for valine in position 61, outside the described rabbit protein AA sequence.

Discussion

The described amino acid composition of rabbit SAA (9) is in good agreement with our prediction based on cDNA sequences. Tobias and co-workers (9) demonstrated that one of the two SAA isotypes probably had a threonine residue and the other had not, which corresponds with our deduced sequences.

Amyloidogenic SAA isotypes have been demonstrated both in mouse (5) and mink (6) and suspected in several other species because of amino acid sequence heterogenities in SAA with no or far less polymorphism in the corresponding AA protein (6). Amino acid sequence study of rabbit protein AA (10) has demonstrated two heterogenities, one in position 4 (of rabbit SAA) and another in position 12. This rabbit protein AA correspond to one of our two predicted SAA isotypes, designated SAA2. This agreement goes for the glycine residue in position 2, valine in position 11, arginine in position 12 and glycine in position 15 and indicates that SAA2 is an amyloidogenic isotype. Threonine in position 22 as found in protein AA (10), was found in none of the SAA isotypes.

The heterogenities in position 4 and 12 in rabbit protein AA and the discrepancy between the amino acid analysis (9) and the cDNA sequences may reflect the prescence of an additional amyloidogenic SAA isotype.

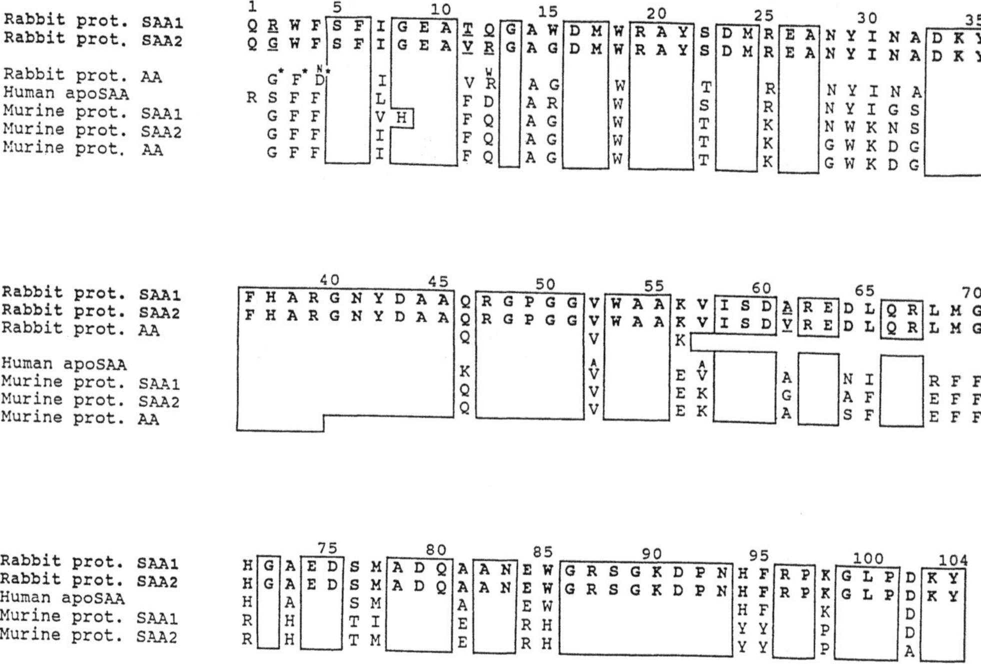

Fig 1. Deduced amino acid sequences of two rabbit SAA isotypes, protein SAA1 and SAA2, based on cDNA sequences. Differences in amino acid sequence between the two are underlined. Rabbit protein AA (10), human apoSAA (14), murine SAA1 and SAA2 (15) and murine protein AA (5) are shown for comparison. Identical residues are enclosed in boxes.

** The sequence of the three NH_2-terminal amino acids was not determined.*

References

1. Kushner, I. (1982) 'The phenomenon of the acute phase response', Ann. NY Acad. Sci. 389, 39-48.
2. Ramadori, G., Van Damme, J., Rieder, H. and Meyer zum Buschenfelde K.-H. (1988) 'Interleukin 6, the third mediator of acute phase reaction, modulates hepatic protein synthesis in human and mouse. Comparison with interleukin 1ß and tumor necrosis factor-α', Eur. J. Immunol. 18, 1259-1264.
3. Marhaug, G., Sletten, K. and Husby, G. (1982) 'Characterization of amyloid related protein SAA complexed with serum lipoproteins (apoSAA)', Clin. Exp. Immunol. 50, 382-389.
4. Husebekk, A., Skogen, B., Husby, G. and Marhaug, G. (1985) 'Transformation of amyloid precursor SAA to protein AA and incorporation in amyloid fibrils in vivo', Scand. J. Immunol. 21, 283-287.
5. Hoffman, J.S., Ericsson, L.H., Eriksen, N., Walsh, K.A. and Benditt, E.P. (1984) 'Murine tissue amyloid AA', J. Exp. Med. 159, 641-646.
6. Marhaug, G., Husby, G. and Dowton, S.B. (1990) 'Mink serum amyloid A protein - expression and primary structure based on cDNA sequences', J. Biol. Chem. 265, 10049-10054.
7. Sletten, K., Marhaug, G. and Husby, G. (1983) 'The covalent structure of amyloid-related serum protein SAA from two patients with inflammatory disease', Hoppe-Zeylers Z. Physiol. Chem. 364, 1039-1046.
8. Wagner, T., Swierezynska, Z., Stankiewicz, C., Bujalska, H. and Kosowska, E. (1981) 'A new model of experimental amyloidosis?', Z. Rheumatol. 40, 234-235.
9. Tobias, P.S., McAdam, K.P.W.J. and Ulevitch, R.J. (1982) 'Interaction of bacterial lipopolysaccaride with acute-phase rabbit serum and isolation of two forms of rabbit serum amyloid A', J. Immunol. 128, 1420-1427.
10. Sano, K. (1988) 'Experimental amyloidosis induced by saponin', Acta Pathol. Jpn. 38, 1241-1253.
11. Chirgwin, J.M., Przybyla, A.E., MacDonald, R.J. and Rutter, W.J. (1979) 'Isolation of biologically active ribonucleic acid from sources enriched in ribonuclease', Biochemistry 18, 5294-5299.
12. Gubler, U. and Hoffman, B.J. (1983) 'A simple and very efficient method for generating cDNA libraries', Gene 25, 263-269.
13. Sanger, F., Nicklen, S. and Coulsen, A.R. (1977) 'DNA sequencing with chain-terminating inhibitors', Proc. Natl. Acad. Sci. USA 74, 5463-5476.
14. Parmelee, D.C., Titzni, K., Ericsson, L.H., Eriksen, N., Benditt, E.P. and Walsh, K.A. (1982) 'Amino acid sequence of amyloid-related apoprotein (apoSAA) from human high-density lipoprotein', Biochemistry 21, 3298-3303.
15. Yamamoto, K.-I., Migita, S. (1985) 'Complete primary structures of two major murine serum amyloid A proteins deduced from cDNA sequences', Proc. Natl. Acad. Sci. USA 82, 2915-2919.

BIOSYNTHESIS AND PROCESSING OF SAA BY MOUSE L-CELLS TRANSFECTED WITH THE HUMAN SAAg9 GENE

I.P. FRASER,* D.R. VAN DER WESTHUYZEN,* G.A. COETZEE,* F.C. DE BEER,+ E.G. SHEPHARD°, and A.F. STRACHAN°

U.C.T./M.R.C. Unit for the Cell Biology of Atherosclerosis, University of Cape Town, Observatory 7925, +Department of Rheumatology, University of Kentucky Medical Center, and °Department of Internal Medicine, University of Stellenbosch Medical School, P.O. Box 63, Tygerberg 7505, South Africa.

ABSTRACT

Pulse-chase studies of SAA biosynthesis and processing in mouse L-cells transfected with the SAAg9 gene have shown that, over a 2h time period, intracellular SAA does not show amino-terminal trimming. Extracellular SAA, although principally composed of the pI=8.0 isoform, shows limited conversion from the pI=8.0 to pI=7.4 isoform over a 2h period.

INTRODUCTION

During the acute phase response cytokines mediate greatly increased transcription of SAA genes with a resultant elevation in plasma SAA levels. In the human, three genes (pA1, pSAA82 and SAAg9) give rise to three unique primary 104-amino acid SAA peptides [1]. It has been established that each of these peptides is subsequently trimmed at the amino terminus to yield 103 and 102 residue peptides [2]. As the enzymatic breakdown of SAA has relevance to the process of amyloidogenesis, we have initiated studies of the process of amino terminus trimming of SAA. In this report we describe the results of our studies of the biosynthesis, secretion and processing of SAA by mouse L-cells.

MATERIALS AND METHODS

Mouse L-cells transfected with the human SAA genomic clone SAAg9 [3] were incubated with monocyte-conditioned medium, as previously described [2]. Cells were pulse-labelled with ^{35}S-methionine for varying times. ^{35}S-SAA was recovered by immunoprecipitation using preformed immune complexes and intra- and extracellular SAA analyzed by SDS/PAGE and isoelectric focusing (IEF) [2].

For intracellular SAA, cells were washed with 1ml trypsin (0.1% (w/v) in PBS) at 37°C before being incubated for 5 minutes at 37°C in the presence of 1ml/dish of this trypsin solution. At the end of this period, 1ml MEM-HEPES, 5% (v/v) LPDS, 0.7mg/ml soybean trypsin inhibitor (activity : 1mg inhibits 1.4mg trypsin) at 4°C was added to each dish. Cells were removed from the dish by repeated aspiration through a plastic transfer pipette. The resulting cell suspension was spun for 1 min in a microfuge and the supernatant discarded. Cells were resuspended in 1ml PBS and transferred to a clean microfuge tube prior to being spun for a further minute. The supernatant was again discarded and the remaining cells lysed by the addition of 400ul cell lysis buffer (10mM HEPES, 200mM NaCl, 2mM $CaCl_2$, 2.5mM $MgCl_2$, 1mM PMSF (0.5% (v/v) in DMSO), 0.1mM leupeptin, 1% (v/v) Triton X-100, pH7.4) accompanied by repeated aspiration through a plastic pipette tip. Lysates were spun in a microfuge prior to immunoprecipitation.

Efficacy of trypsinization of cell surface protein was assessed as follows : L-cells were grown in medium containing ^{35}S-SAA (in the presence of 100uM cycloheximide and 200uM L-methionine) for 2h at 37°C. The cells were then trypsinized, lysed, SAA immunoprecipitated and the samples analyzed by SDS/PAGE.

RESULTS

Trypsinization of cell-surface SAA

In order to determine the nature of the newly synthesized isoforms present within the secretory pathway in L-cells, it was necessary to remove any SAA that may have become associated with the cell surface following secretion of SAA into the medium. When cells were offered ^{35}S-SAA, subsequent trypsinization resulted in no ^{35}S-SAA being detectable on SDS/PAGE (Fig. 1).

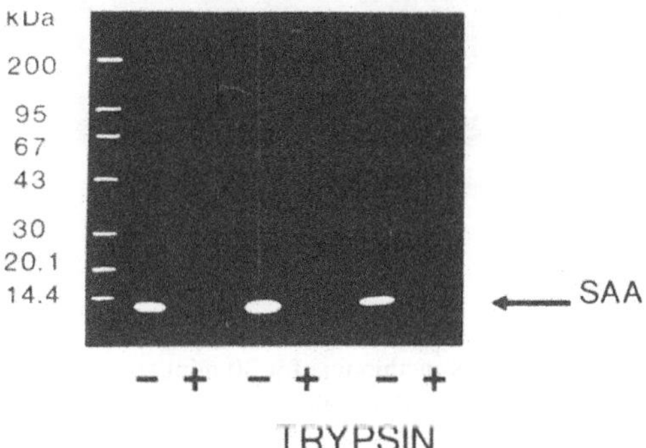

Figure 1. Cells were incubated with ^{35}S-SAA (see Materials and Methods) and subsequently treated with (+) or without (-) trypsin at 37°C for 5 minutes. The figure shows a fluorogram of immunoprecipitated cell lysate material.

Pulse-chase kinetics

When L-cells were subjected to a continuous pulse of ^{35}S-methionine, intracellular ^{35}S-SAA reached a maximum after 30 minutes. ^{35}S-SAA in the medium was not identified until after 30 minutes after initiation of pulse (data not shown). When cells were pulsed for 30 minutes and chased in medium containing L-methionine a gradual disappearance of ^{35}S-SAA was noted over a 2h period (Fig. 2) with a corresponding appearance in the medium (data not shown). An increase in cell-surface bound ^{35}S-SAA was noted with respect to time and can be seen by the increasing difference in the SAA band intensity between cells treated or not treated with trypsin (Fig. 2).

SAA isoforms

Duplicate samples from the abovementioned experiment were subjected to electrofocusing. Intracellular ^{35}S-SAA existed as the pI=8.0 isoform at all time points up to 2h. In the medium ^{35}S-SAA existed principally as the pI=8.0 isoform with an increasing proportion of the pI=7.4 isoform developing over the time period (Fig. 3).

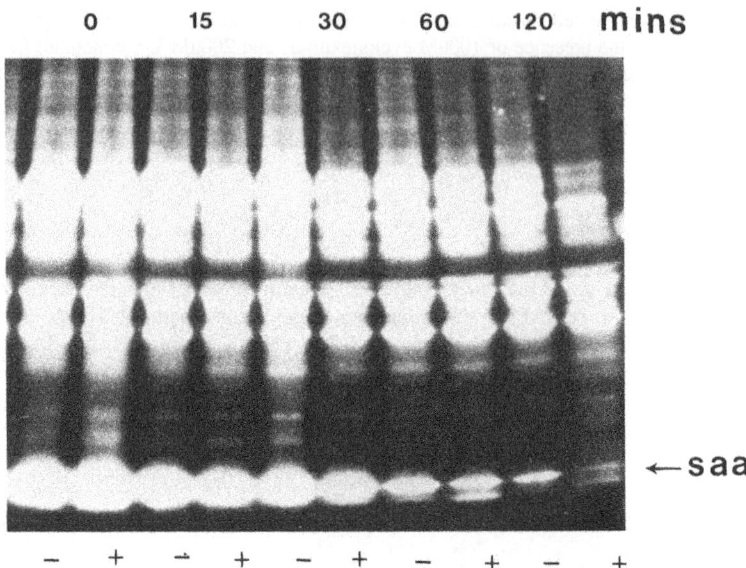

Figure 2. Cells were pulse-labelled with ^{35}S-methionine for 30 minutes and chased for the times shown. At each time point one dish was trypsinized (+) and the other not (-) prior to SDS/PAGE and fluorography.

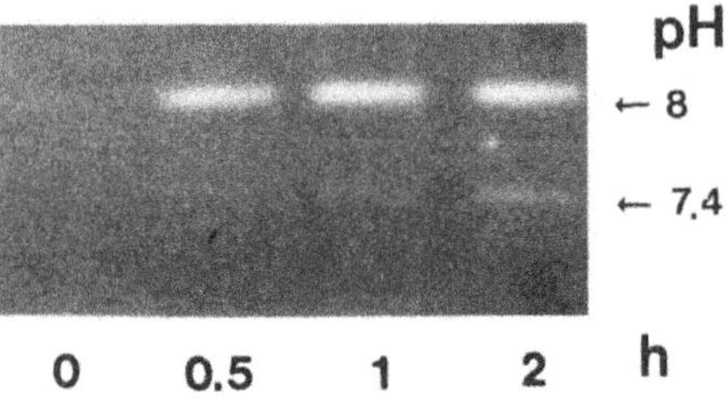

Figure 3. IEF gel of SAA isoforms present in medium following a 30 minute ^{35}S-methionine pulse and chases for the times indicated. Note the very faint pI=7.4 band on the fluorogram.

DISCUSSION

In these studies we have established a protocol for the study of SAA synthesized by L-cells stimulated by monocyte-conditioned medium. Use of this protocol has revealed the existence of only one of the two SAAg9-derived SAA isoforms intracellularly over a two hour time period following pulse labelling. Over the same period however, extracellular SAA, although principally composed of the pI=8.0 isoform, showed a time-related increase in the relative amount of the pI=7.4 isoform. Further studies over an extended time period are therefore necessary to fully characterize intracellular and extracellular SAA processing.

ACKNOWLEDGEMENTS

The financial assistance of the University of Cape Town, the S.A. Medical Research Council and the S.A. Arthritis and Rheumatism Association is acknowledged. Mrs B. Henstock is thanked for manuscript preparation. The transfected L-cells were a gift from Dr P. Woo, Division of Molecular Rheumatology, Clinical Research Centre, Northwick Park Hospital, London.

REFERENCES

Strachan A.F., de Beer, F.C., van der Westhuyzen D.R. and Coetzee G.A. (1988) "Identification of three isoform patterns of human serum amyloid A protein", Biochem. J. 250, 203-207.

Strachan A.F., Brandt W.F., Woo P., van der Westhuyzen D.R., Coetzee G.A. and de Beer M.C. et al (1989) "Human serum amyloid A protein : the assignment of the six major isoforms to three published gene sequences and evidence for two genetic loci." J. Biol. Chem. 264, 18368-18373.

Woo P., Sipe J., Dinarello C.A. and Colten H.R. (1987) "Structure of a human serum amyloid A gene and modulation of its expression in transfected L-cells", J. Biol. Chem. 262, 15790-15795.

Regulation of serum amyloid A (SAA) synthesis in Hep 3B cells by cytokines and corticosteroids.

I Kushner, MK Ganapathi, D Schultz, SL Jiang, D Samols
Case Western Reserve University at MetroHealth Medical Center, Department of Medicine, Cleveland, Ohio 44109

Abstract

In Hep 3B cells, in which the combination of IL-6 and IL-1 had previously been found to be required for SAA induction, checkerboard titration of these cytokines showed that each cytokine played an enabling role, permitting the effect of the other cytokine to be perceived at the level of synthesis in a dose-related manner. Dexamethasone (dex) markedly potentiated SAA induction by both monocyte conditioned medium and IL-6 plus IL-1α, although it had no effect when employed alone. SAA induction by these cytokine preparations in the presence of dex was inhibited by TGFß-1 at concentrations of 4-10 ng/ml. The combination of IL-6 and TNFα was capable of SAA induction at levels about 20-60% of those achieved by IL-6 and IL-1α. [TGFß-1 (4-10 ng/ml) inhibited SAA induction by cytokine.] These cytokine effects were detectable at the pretranslational level. These data suggest that SAA synthesis in human hepatocytes might be regulated by IL-6, IL-1, TNFα, and TGFß and corticosteroids in various combinations.

Introduction

Several different cytokines and corticosteroids have been reported to induce synthesis of SAA in various in vitro model systems derived from different species. (1-5) We have previously reported that SAA can be induced in serum free medium, in the presence of 1.0 μM dexamethasone (dex) and 0.02 U/ml of insulin, in the human hepatoma cell lines NPLC/PRF/5 and Hep 3B by conditioned medium (CM) from LPS-stimulated human monocytes (6). Comparable induction could be achieved in the former cells by recombinant interleukin 6 (IL-6), while SAA induction in Hep 3B cells required the combination of IL-6 and IL-1 (5).

It has become clear that different cytokines and corticosteroids can interact to influence production of a number of acute phase proteins (7-14). This study was undertaken to further explore the effects of combinations of corticosteroids, insulin and human cytokines on synthesis of SAA in the well-defined model system, Hep 3B cells.

Materials and Methods

Hep 3B cells were cultured in RPMI 1640 supplemented with dex and insulin, incubated with cytokines, and metabolically labelled with ^{35}S methionine as previously described (5,6). SAA synthesis was estimated by specific immunoprecipitation of radiolabelled protein from medium followed by SDS PAGE. Radioactivity in SAA bands was quantitated by liquid scintillation counting following digestion in 30% hydrogen peroxide. RNA was extracted from cells and Northern blot analysis carried out employing a cDNA probe PA10, generously provided by Dr. J. D. Sipe, Boston. Recombinant IL-6 from CHO cells and IL-1α from E. Coli were gifts of Drs. G. Wong, Boston and P. Lomedico, Nutley, NJ, respectively. Recombinant tumor necrosis factor α (TNF) and purified transforming growth factor ß-1 (TGFß) were purchased from Genzyme and R&D systems respectively.

Results

Checkerboard titration of different doses of IL-6 and IL-1α revealed that increases in concentration of either cytokine led to progressive increases in SAA synthesis as long as a minimal dose of the other cytokine was present. Thus, the effect of each cytokine was enabling, permitting the effect of the other cytokine to be perceived at the level of synthesis.

Dex alone had no effect on synthesis of SAA, while CM led to modest SAA induction in the absence of dex. Addition of dex to CM caused a concentration dependent, marked potentiation of SAA induction. Similarly, dex potentiated the SAA response to the combination of IL-6 and IL-1α. In contrast, SAA induction was unaffected by the presence or absence of insulin.

Since TGFß has been shown to alter production of some acute phase proteins (12), we studied the possible effect of this cytokine on SAA induction. TGFß-1 alone, in concentrations of 4-10 ng/ml, did not induce SAA synthesis. However, these concentrations of TGFß did inhibit induction of SAA by either CM or IL-6 plus IL-1α, with parallel decreases in SAA mRNA concentrations.

Because of the considerable overlap in functions of IL-1 and TNFα, we explored the possible role of the latter cytokine in SAA induction. TNFα alone, like IL-6, IL-1, or the combination of IL-1 and TNFα, caused minimal if any induction of SAA in Hep 3B cells. However, the combination of IL-6 and TNFα was capable of SAA induction to levels about 20 to 60% of those achieved with IL-6 plus IL-1α. Both combinations of cytokines, IL-6 plus IL-1α, and IL-6 plus TNFα, caused increased SAA mRNA accumulations which roughly paralleled increases in synthesis.

Discussion and Conclusions

These data demonstrate that SAA synthesis in Hep 3B cells can be influenced by IL-6, IL-1α, TNFα, TGFß-1 and dexamethasone, and that the cytokine effects are apparent at the pre-translational level. Delineation of these effects opens the door to more targeted studies of the precise steps in the sequence of signal transduction, transcriptional regulation and post-transcriptional regulation by which extracellular messengers, alone or in combination, may regulate gene expression and protein synthesis.

Our findings differ from those of Castell et al (3) in human primary hepatocyte cultures. They found that IL-6 alone and dex alone were each capable of SAA induction, and that IL-6 and dex were synergistic. In contrast, we found that detectable SAA induction in Hep 3B cells required both IL-6 plus IL-1 and could not be achieved by dex alone, but was potentiated by dex. These differences might reflect differences between primary cultures and the Hep 3B hepatoma cell line, although other explanations are possible.

Taylor et al have reported that TGFß may have either an up- or down-regulatory effect on induction of C-reactive protein in hepatoma cell lines, depending on the concentration employed (13). The studies of the effects of TGFß on SAA synthesis reported here were carried out in a narrow range of TGFß concentrations. We do not yet know what the effects of lower TGFß concentrations would be.

These data, derived from Hep 3B cells, indicate that SAA synthesis is not controlled by a single extracellular signal, and raise the possibility that SAA synthesis in human hepatocytes, in vivo, might be regulated by IL-6, IL-1, TNFα, TGFß and corticosteroids in various combinations. Different pathophysiologic conditions may lead to induction of different cytokines. Several different cytokines, either alone or in combination with one another or with corticosteroids, may influence SAA induction in different circumstances.

Acknowledgements

We are grateful for the secretarial assistance of Barbara Faber. These studies were supported by NIH grant AG02467.

References

1. Ramadori, G., Sipe, J.D., Dinarello, C.A., Mizel, S.B., Colten, H.R. (1985) 'Pretranslational modulation of acute phase hepatic protein synthesis by murine recombinant interleukin 1 (IL-1) and purified human IL-1.' J Exp Med 162:930-942.
2. Woo, P., Sipe, J., Dinarello, C.A., Colten, H.R. (1987) 'Structure of a human serum amyloid A gene and modulation of its expression in transfected L cells.' J Biol Chem 262:15790-15795.
3. Castell, J.V., Gomez-Lechon, M.J., David, M., Hirano, T., Kishimoto, T., Heinrich, P.C. (1988) 'Recombinant human interleukin-6 (IL-6/BSF-2/HSF) regulates the synthesis of acute phase proteins in human hepatocytes.' FEBS Lett 232:347-350, 1988.
4. Mackiewicz, A., Ganapathi, M., Schultz, D., Samols, D., Reese. J., Kushner, I. (1988) 'Regulation of rabbit acute phase proteins by monokines.' Biochemical J 253:851-857.
5. Ganapathi, M.K., May, L.T., Schultz, D., Samols, D., Reese, J., Kushner, I. (1988) 'Role of interleukin-6 in regulating synthesis of C-reactive protein and serum amyloid A in human hepatoma cell lines.' Biochem Biophys Res Commun 157:271-277.

6. Ganapathi, M.K., Schultz, D., Mackiewicz, A., Samols, D., Hu, S-I., Brabenec, A., Macintyre, S.S., Kushner, I. (1988) 'Heterogeneous nature of the acute phase response. Differential regulation of human serum amyloid A, C-reactive protein and other acute phase proteins by cytokines in Hep 3B cells.' J Immunol 141:564-569.
7. Magielska-Zero, D., Bereta, J., Czuba-Pelech, B., Pajdak, W., Gauldie, J., Koj, A. (1988) 'Inhibitory effect of human recombinant interferon gamma on synthesis of acute phase proteins in human hepatoma Hep G2 cells stimulated by leukocyte cytokines, TNFα and IFN-$ß_2$/BSF-2/IL-6.' Biochem Intl 17:17-23.
8. Rokita, H., Bereta, J., Koj, A., Gordon, A.H., Gauldie, J. (1990) 'Epidermal growth factor and transforming growth factor-ß differently modulate the acute phase response elicited by interleukin-6 in cultured liver cells from man, rat and mouse.' Comp Biochem Physiol 95A:41-45.
9. Baumann, H., Richards, C., Gauldie, J. (1987) 'Interaction among hepatocyte-stimulating factors, interleukin 1, and glucocorticoids for regulation of acute phase plasma proteins in human hepatoma (Hep G2) cells.' J Immunol 139:4122-4128.
10. Otto, J.M., Grenett, H.E., Fuller, G.M. (1987) 'The coordinated regulation of fibrinogen gene transcription by hepatocyte-stimulating factor and dexamethasone.' J Cell Biol 105:1067-1072.
11. Darlington, G.J., Wilson, D.R., Revel, M., Kelly, J.H. (1989) 'Response of liver genes to acute phase mediators.' Ann NY Acad Sci 557:310-316.
12. Mackiewicz, A., Ganapathi, M.K., Schultz, D., Brabenec, A., Weinstein, J., Kelley, M.F., Kushner, I. (1990) 'Transforming growth factor ß1 regulates production of acute phase proteins.' Proc Natl Acad Sci USA 87:1491-1495.
13. Taylor, A.W., Ku, N-O., Mortensen, R.F. (1990) 'Transforming growth factor ß regulates C-reactive protein synthesis by hepatocytes.' FASEB J 4:A1714.
14. Kushner I, Mackiewicz A, Ganapathi MK, Schultz D. (1990) 'Cytokine interaction in regulation of the acute phase response', in Oppenheim J, Dinarello CA, Kluger M, Powanda M (eds): Proc of the 2nd intl Workshop on Cytokines, Vol I, Molecular and cellular biology of cytokines, New York, Alan R. Liss.

REGULATION OF SAA SYNTHESIS BY CYTOKINES IN A HUMAN HEPATOMA CELL LINE.

J.G. Raynes, S. Eagling and K.P.W.J. McAdam
Department of Clinical Sciences,
London School of Hygiene and Tropical Medicine,
Keppel St.,
London WC1E 7HT

Abstract

In the search for an in vitro model of SAA synthesis we discovered that the human hepatoma cell line HuH-7 responded to recombinant IL-1 by increasing SAA synthesis by up to 100 fold. The dose response curve for IL-1 reached a maximum at about 1 ng/ml and half-maximal stimulation was at 100 pg/ml. The presence of IL-6 further stimulated levels by at least twofold. Leukaemia inhibitory factor (LIF;HSF III) had limited effect and TNF could stimulate SAA but less than IL-6. However the cells express IL-6 receptors since they have the ability to synthesise haptoglobin in response to IL-6 but poorly in response to IL-1. Neutralising monoclonal antibodies against IL-1α and IL-6 selectively neutralised the response due to the respective cytokine.

Introduction

Interleukin 6 has been demonstrated to be the major stimulator of many of the acute phase proteins synthesised in the liver during the acute phase response [1,2,3]. The overall response, however reflects contributions from other cytokines such as IL-1, TNF and LIF as well as modulation by hormonal influences such as the glucocorticoids [4,5,6]. Whilst IL-6 has been demonstrated to be the major cytokine for many proteins, there remain areas of uncertainty, as for example, in the case of SAA. There is no cell line that has been found to synthesise SAA in appreciable quantities until the HuH-7 cell line as described in this report. Also primary cell cultures suffer from the problems of contamination of the cultures with cytokine producing cells and the trauma of isolation may render the cells incapable of responding to further stimulation.

The HuH-7 cell line was developed as a well differentiated tumour cell line that produced many plasma proteins [7]. The HuH-7 cell line is becoming a popular cell model for research into hepatitis B, α-fetoprotein and lipoprotein metabolism. Since HuH-7 cells can be cultured in the absence of serum but presence of selenite it has proved to be of great use in examining the role of other serum components in secretion and in the effects of modulating hormones [8].

In this report we have looked at the SAA response of the cell line to various stimulating cytokines and confirmed the data by using neutralising monoclonal antibodies against IL-1 and IL-6.

Materials and Methods

CELL CULTURE

HuH-7 cells were grown in 24 well plates to confluence in RPMI containing 10% foetal calf serum, 1 mM pyruvate, 2mM glutamine, penicillin (100 ug/ml) and streptomycin (100ug/ml). In the experiment with neutralising monoclonal Ab to IL-6, serum was replaced with an equivalent concentration of HDL. Wells were then stimulated with various cytokines in medium containing 10^{-7} M dexamethasone and 10^{-8} M insulin. Supernatants were assayed for SAA, haptoglobin and albumin. Cells were counted after trypsinization. IL-1ß and TNF were kindly provided by Dr C Dinarello (Tuft's University, Boston) and Il-α was a gift from Dr Lomedico (Hoffman LaRoche, Nutley, N.J). Human IL-6 was from Dr S Clark (Genetics Institute, Cambridge, Mass.). Leukaemia inhibitory factor (LIF) was kindly provided by Dr G Wong (Genetics Institute, Cambridge, Mass.) and neutralising monoclonal to IL-1α (M3) was from Dr S Gillis (Immunex Corporation, Washington). Neutralising monoclonal antibody to human IL-6 was obtained from Dr N Ida (Toray industries, Inc, Japan).

ELISA ASSAYS

Immulon 2 plates (Dynatech) were coated with affinity purified anti-human SAA in 0.13M borate pH 9.6 overnight at 4^{0}C, and washed with PBS containing 0.05% Tween. The standards and samples were added to wells together with an SAA-alkaline phosphatase conjugate prepared by the one-step glutaraldehyde method. The ability of sample to inhibit SAA conjugate binding to the antibody coated plate was compared with that of standard. Substrate was p-nitrophenylphosphate in carbonate/bicarbonate buffer pH 9.6 containing 2 mM $MgCl_2$. Standards were high density lipoprotein with a known SAA concentration diluted in culture medium.

Haptoglobin assays were performed in a similar manner using a rabbit anti-human haptoglobin antibody coated onto the Immunol 2 plates. Haptoglobin conjugated to peroxidase by the periodate method was competed with the haptoglobin in the sample and compared with samples of purified haptoglobin added to culture medium. Albumin was also measured by a similar ELISA using alkaline phophatase conjugated human albumin. All assay results are expressed per 48h per 10^{6} cells.

Results

The SAA ELISA was sensitive to 2-8 ug/ml of SAA. The supernatants were removed at 48h from cells stimulated with IL-1ß, IL-6 or TNF. It was found that the major cytokine responsible for the stimulation of SAA was IL-1. This can be seen in Table I which shows the mean concentrations of SAA in culture supernatant at 48h. It was previously shown that the time course of SAA secretion from the cells showed a peak synthesis at about 24 h. By day 4 levels were back to control unstimulated concentrations. TNF stimulated only twofold and LIF (results not shown was only marginally stimulating.

The time taken for the secretion of SAA reflects that seen in vivo with levels returning to normal within several days of a defined stimulus. The dose of IL-1 required to produce a maximal response was 1-10 ng/ml; half maximal responses were seen at about 100 pg/ml, and some response could still be seen at only 1-10 pg/ml. The SAA response to increasing concentrations of IL-1α showed the same sensitivity and approximately the same response in SAA concentrations. The cells were capable of responding fully to IL-6 since the synthesis of haptoglobin was mainly induced by IL-6 as found previously for other cell lines. An increase of fourfold in response to IL-6 can be seen in Table II although this is lower in Table I, probably because of the baseline stimulation by serum cytokines.

Table I. Cytokine stimulation of HuH-7 cells (n=6)

Cytokine	SAA(ng/ml)	Hapt(ng/ml)	Alb(ug/ml)
Control	5 ± 2	265 ± 28	14.6 ± 1.1
IL-1 (10 ng/ml)	180 ± 80	400 ± 23	11.5 ± 0.7
IL-6 (200 U/ml)	40 ± 30	672 ± 50	15.8 ± 2.0
TNF (10 ng/ml)	15 ± 25	327 ± 28	12.9 ± 2.0
IL-1 /IL-6	375 ± 63	860 ± 108	10.1 ± 0.7
IL-1 /TNF	305 ± 50	565 ± 33	10.6 ± 0.9
IL-6 /TNF	60 ± 40	745 ± 35	12.2 + 1.6
IL-1 /IL-6 /TNF	450 ± 160	720 ± 43	8.5 + 0.6

Table II Neutralisation with α-IL-1α. (n=4)

Added cytokine	Neutralising McAb	SAA (ng/ml)
Control	Control	2 ± 2
Control	α-IL-1	4 ± 4
IL-1α(100 U/ml)	Control	100 ± 5
IL-1α+IL-6(10U)	Control	145 ± 23
IL-1α	α-IL-1α	10 ± 8
IL-1α + IL-6	α-IL-1	20 ± 6

Table III Neutralisation with α-IL-6 (n=6).

Added cytokine	Neutralising McAb	SAA (ng/ml)	Hapt(ng/ml)
Control	Control	25 ± 10	105 ± 33
Control	αIL-6 (1 ug/ml)	20 ± 10	78 ± 20
IL1ß (1 ng/ml)	Control	130 ± 13	208 ± 48
IL-6 (10 U/ml)	Control	45 ± 35	430 ± 100
IL-6 + IL-1ß	Control	233 ± 42	640 ± 170
IL-6	α-IL-6	15 ± 2	183 ± 23
IL-1ß	α-IL-6	118 ± 33	222 ± 43
IL-1ß + IL-6	α-IL-6	138 ± 13	240 ± 60

Monoclonal antibody to IL-1α (25 ug/ml) was capable of inhibiting the response to IL-1α (1 ng/ml) by 80% (Table II). Monoclonal antibody to IL-6 did not decrease the response to IL-ß, whilst it was capable of inhibiting the response to IL-6 as shown by decreases in both haptoglobin and SAA. A monoclonal to IL-1ß neutralised the stimulation by IL-1ß (results not shown). The use of monoclonals was required for inhibition of these responses because polyclonal antiserum often caused an increase in the synthesis rather than a decrease (results not shown).

Discussion

The results described here suggest that IL-1 is the major stimulating cytokine for SAA synthesis. One interesting possibility that arises from this finding, is that since CRP is mainly under the control of IL-6 [9], this may provide an explanation for observations of high CRP and low SAA or low CRP and high SAA in individual patients, due to high levels of IL-1 or IL-6. It has been observed before that the ratios of SAA to CRP can vary between different diseases, and this may well be due to differential stimulation of IL-1 and IL-6 reflected in the acute phase proteins.

It was clear that the neutralising monoclonal antibodies were capable of inhibiting the responses of HuH-7 cells to their respective stimulating cytokines. This fact together with the differential regulation of SAA and haptoglobin suggests that IL-1 is not acting through IL-6. It was found that polyclonal antisera did not inhibit the responses to their respective cytokine perhaps because of other cytokines in the antibody preparation. The difference between our results and those obtained with primary cultures which suggested that IL-6 was the main stimulator of SAA, may be due to stimulation of the cells during the hepatocyte isolation procedure, a possibility reinforced by consideration of the high SAA levels seen in unstimulated primary cultures. SAA stimulation by IL-1 has been shown in transfected cell lines [9,10].

This model of SAA synthesis and secretion will be valuable to elucidate the mechanisms of contol at the transcriptional and post-transcrpitional level as well as determining mechanisms that control secretion.

Acknowledgements

We would like to thank the Medical Research Council, the Wellcome Trust, and the Arthritis Research Council for support that funded this work.

References

1. Heinrich P.C. Castell J.V. and Andus T (1989) Interleukin-6 and the acute phase response Biochem J, 265, 621-636.
2. Gauldie J. Richards C., Harnish D., Lansdorf P., and Baumann H. 1987. Interferon ß-2/B-cell stimulatory factor type 2 shares identity with monocyte derived hepatocyte stimulating factor and regulates the

major acute phase response in liver cells. Proc. Natl. Acad Sci.,84, 7251-7256.
3. Castell J.V. Gomez-Lechon M.J. David M., Hirano T., Kishimoto T and Heinrich P.C. 1988. Recombinant human interleukin 6 (IL-6/BSF-2/HSF) regulates the synthesis of acute phase proteins in human hepatocytes. FEBS Lett, 232, 347-350.
4. Kushner I., Ganapathi M. Schultz D. 1989 The acute phase response is mediated by heterogeneous mechanisms. Ann. N. Y. Acad. Sci.,557, 19-30.
5. Baumann H., Richards C, Gauldie J. 1987. Interaction among hepatocyte stimulating factors, interleukin 1 and glucocorticoids for regulation of acute phase plasma proteins in human hepatoma (Hep G2) cells. J. Immunol, 139, 4122-4128.
6. Baumann H. and Wong G.G. 1989. Hepatocyte-stimulating factor III shares structural and functional identity with leukemia- inhibitory factor. J. Immunol., 143, 1163-1167.
7. Nakabayashi H. Taketa K., Miyano K. Yamne T and Sato J. 1982. Growth of human hepatoma cell lines with differentiated functions in chemically defined medium. J. Cancer Res. 42, 3858-3863.
8. Eagling S., McAdam K.P.W.J. & Raynes J.G. 1990 SAA secretion from cytokine stimulated hepatoma cells requires HDL. Proc VIth Int Symp on Amyloidosis, Oslo (eds Natvig JB, Forrw O. Husby G., Husebekk A, Skogen B Sletten K and Westermark P.) Kluwer Press, Dordrecht.
9. Ganter U., Arcone R., Toniatti C., Morrone G., Ciliberto G. 1989 Dual control of C-reactive protein gene expression by interleukin-1 and interleukin-6. EMBO J. 8,3773-3779
10 Woo P., Sipe J. Dinarello C.A, Colten R.A 1987. Structure of a human serum amyloid A gene and modulation of its expression in transfected L cells. J. Biol. Chem ,262, 15790-15795.
11 Edbrooke M.R. Burt D.W. Cheshire J.K. Woo P. 1989. Identificatiwn of cis-acting sequences responsible for phorbol ester induction of human serum amyloid A gene expression via a Nuclear Factor kB-like transcription factor. Mol. Cell. Biol., 9, 1908-1916 (1989).

SAA SECRETION FROM CYTOKINE-STIMULATED HUMAN HEPATOMA CELLS REQUIRES HDL

S. EAGLING, J. G. RAYNES and K. P. W. J. McADAM
Department of Clinical Sciences
London School of Hygiene and Tropical Medicine
Keppel Street
London WC1E 7HT
England

ABSTRACT. We have recently found that in the presence of fetal calf serum (FCS), the human hepatoma cell line, HuH-7, can increase SAA synthesis and secretion up to 100-fold after stimulation by a combination of cytokines. We required a serum-free model using HuH-7 cells to investigate further the control of SAA synthesis and secretion by cytokines and hormones. In serum-free medium, HuH-7 cells were found to increase only marginally the secretion of SAA after cytokine stimulation. Ultracentrifugally separated serum fractions were added to stimulated HuH-7 cultures to find the serum fraction that could fully restore SAA secretion. The high density lipoprotein (HDL) fraction was observed to restore SAA secretion and the amount of SAA secreted was dependent on HDL concentration in the culture medium. The dependency of protein secretion on the presence of HDL was found to be unique to SAA, as the secretion of haptoglobin, α_1-acid glycoprotein and albumin were unaffected by the adittion of HDL to cytokine stimulated cells. We have therefore established a good model for studying SAA synthesis and secretion and have observed a dependency of SAA secretion on the presence of HDL.

Introduction

The synthesis of SAA in the human hepatoma cell line, HuH-7, can be stimulated 100-fold by a combination of cytokines in 10% bovine serum (1). Other human hepatoma cell lines such as Hep 3B and NPLC/PRF/5 have been observed to synthesize SAA after cytokine stimulation in culture medium containing fetal bovine serum (2,3).

However, HuH-7 cells can be successfully cultured in serum-free medium containing sodium selenite (4). Therefore, the abilities of HuH-7 to grow in serum-free medium and to synthesize SAA in response to cytokines presented the cell line as a candidate for studying the cytokine and hormonal regulation of SAA synthesis and secretion under serum-free conditions. Here, we describe how high levels of SAA secretion are not obtained from stimulated HuH-7 cells cultured in serum-free medium.

As SAA exists as an apolipoprotein of high density lipoprotein (HDL) during inflammation (5,6), serum was fractionated by sequential ultracentrifugation to isolate lipoprotein fractions and analyse their influences on SAA secretion.

Materials and Methods

HDL and other fractions of fetal calf serum (FCS) were isolated by sequential ultracentrifugation (adaptation of (7)).

HuH-7 cells were seeded in medium containing 10% FCS. 24hrs after seeding the medium was replaced by serum-free medium containing $3x10^{-8}$M sodium selenite.

Recombinant human IL-1ß and IL-6 were used at 10ng IL-1ß + 10U IL-6/ml in culture medium containing 0.2% BSA, 10^{-7}M dexamethasone and 10^{-8}M insulin. FCS, HDL or other serum fractions were added to this medium. The defined media were added to cells when they had reached confluency. The cells were cultured for a further 48hrs. The media was then removed for protein assays.

Human SAA, albumin and haptoglobin were measured in the cell supernatants by competitive inhibition ELISAs. α_1-acid glycoprotein (AGP) was measured by rocket immunoelectrophoresis using concentrated supernatants.

Results

HuH-7 cells stimulated by cytokines in the absence of serum secreted only marginally higher levels of SAA than unstimulated cells. However, stimulation in 10% FCS medium greatly increased their secretion of SAA (table 1). Fractions of serum, separated by their densities, indicated that the HDL fraction of serum was the most potent serum fraction in restoring SAA secretion. The next most potent fraction was the LDL and VLDL containing fraction, F1 (table 2). The secretion of SAA increased with the HDL concentration in the surrounding medium in stimulated cells, but not in unstimulated cells. The secretion of haptoglobin and albumin did not increase with HDL concentration in stimulated cells, nor did albumin in unstimulated cells. However, haptoglobin secretion did increase with HDL in unstimulated cells (table 3). HDL did not increase AGP secretion in either stimulated or unstimulated cells (table 4).

TABLE 1. Secretion of SAA in the absence or presence of serum

Sample	Secretion of SAA (ng/10^6cells/48hrs) Mean ± SD (n = 6)
SFM no cytokines	45 ± 17
SFM IL-1 + IL-6	127 ± 25
10% FCS no cytokines	119 ± 47
10% FCS IL-1 + IL-6	708 ± 83

SFM denotes serum-free medium.

TABLE 2. Effect of serum fraction on SAA secretion

Serum fraction	Secretion of SAA (ng/10^6cells/48hrs) Mean ± SD (n = 6)
Whole serum (FCS)	220 ± 15
HDL (d = 1.063 - 1.21)	207 ± 18
F1 (d ≤ 1.063)	130 ± 20
F2 (d ≥ 1.21)	123 ± 23
Serum-free medium	53 ± 15

All samples were cytokine stimulated. FCS was used at 10% in the culture medium, HDL and all other serum fractions were at a concentration equivalent to 10% of whole serum.

TABLE 3. Effect of HDL concentration on protein secretion

HDL concentration (as a % of whole serum)	Protein secreted (weight/10^6cells/48hrs) Mean ± SD (n = 6)		
	SAA(ng)	Haptoglobin (ng)	Albumin (μg)
With cytokines:			
0	33 ± 18	883 ± 50	13 ± 3
4	40 ± 15	973 ± 93	10 ± 2
10	105 ± 33	1048 ± 43	11 ± 2
40	263 ± 45	775 ± 73	10 ± 1
60	470 ± 128	757 ± 40	10 ± 3
80	390 ± 90	845 ± 63	9 ± 2
100	467 ± 150	860 ± 30	8 ± 1
Without cytokines:			
0	31 ± 14	142 ± 25	20 ± 2
10	30 ± 11	230 ± 25	21 ± 2
100	29 ± 9	470 ± 80	18 ± 3

TABLE 4. Effect of HDL on AGP secretion

Sample	AGP secreted (μg/10^6cells/48hrs) Mean ± SD (n = 4)
Serum free, no cytokines	1.6 ± 0.2
2.5% HDL, no cytokines	1.6 ± 0.2
Serum-free + cytokines	5.5 ± 0.3
2.5% HDL + cytokines	4.9 ± 0.3

Discussion

We have shown that cytokine stimulated HuH-7 cells do not secrete high levels of SAA in the absence of serum. The requirement for serum was found to be associated mainly in the HDL fraction. The addition of HDL to cultures of stimulated HuH-7 cells can totally restore SAA secretion and increasing HDL concentrations cause increases in SAA secretion. However, SAA secretion reaches a maximum by 60% of the HDL levels found in serum, suggesting that in vivo variations in circulating HDL levels do not greatly influence SAA secretion. HDL itself does not stimulate SAA secretion, although it can marginally increase haptoglobin secretion, probably due to small amounts of cytokines in the HDL preparation. In stimulated cells, HDL is unable to increase further the secretion of haptoglobin, AGP or albumin. HDL therefore has a unique relationship with SAA secretion and is an essential component of the culture medium used in studying the in vitro secretion of SAA from HuH-7 cells.

This is probably one of the best available models for the in vitro study of cytokine and hormonal control of SAA synthesis and secretion as it allows large amounts of SAA to be secreted into the medium and reduces the confounding influence of ranging levels of hormones and cytokines in serum-containing medium.

Acknowledgements

We thank Steve Clark of The Genetics Institute, Cambridge, USA for his kind gift of recombinant human interleukin-6, and Dr Charles A. Dinarello of Tufts University School of Medicine and the New England Medical Center, Boston, USA for his kind gift of recombinant human interleukin-1ß. These studies were supported by grants from the Wellcome Trust and The Arthritis and Rheumatism Council.

References

(1) Raynes J.G., Eagling S., McAdam K.P.W.J. (1990), 'Regulation of SAA synthesis by cytokines in a human hepatoma cell line', in Natvig J.B. et al. (eds.), Amyloidosis, Kluwer Academic Publishers, Dordrecht.
(2) Ganapathi M.K., Schultz D., Mackiewicz A.J., Samols D., Hu S., Brabenec A., Macintyre S.S., Kushner I. (1988), 'Heterogenous nature of the acute phase response. Differential Regulation of Human Serum Amyloid A, C-Reactive Protein, and Other Acute Phase Proteins by Cytokines in Hep3B cells', J.Immunol., 141, 564-569.
(3) Ganapathi M.K., May L.T., Schultz D., Brabenec A., Weinstein J., Sehgal P.B., Kushner I. (1988), 'Role of interleukin-6 in regulating synthesis of C-reactive protein and serum amyloid A in human hepatoma cell lines', Biochem.Biophys.Res.Comm., 157, 271-277.
(4) Nakabayashi H., Taketa K., Miyano K., Yamane T., Sato J. (1982),'Growth of Human Hepatoma Cell Lines with Differential Functions in Chemically Defined Medium', Cancer Research, 42, 3858-3863.
(5) Benditt E.P. and Eriksen N. (1977),'Amyloid protein SAA is associated with high density lipoprotein from human serum', Proc.Natl.Acad.Sci.USA, 74, 4025-4028.
(6) Coetzee G.A., Strachan A.F., Van der Westhuyzen D.R., Hoppe H.C., Jeenah M.S., De Beer F.C. (1986),'Serum amyloid A-containing human high density lipoprotein 3. Density, size and apoprotein composition', J.Biol.Chem., 261, 9644-9651.
(7) Havel R.J., Eder H.A., Bragdon J.H. (1955),'The distribution and chemical composition of ulracentrifugally separated lipoproteins in human sera', J.Clin.Invest., 34, 1345-1353.

INTERFERON ALFA INDUCE TNF ELEVATIONS IN VIVO. CORRELATION WITH OTHER ACUTE PHASE REACTANTS.

Morton A. Scheinberg, Eliana Chapira, Marcia Gordon de Carvalho, Maria Isabel Mota, Merrill D. Benson, from the Department of Rheumatology/Immunology, Cancer Institute Arnaldo Vieira de Carvalho, São Paulo, Brazil, 01221 and Rheumatology Section Richard Roudebush Veterans Administration Medical Center, Indiana University School of Medicine, IN. 46223, USA.

ABSTRACT.

Patients with solid Neoplasms requiring therapy with interferon had serial measurements of IL-1, TNF, and SAA Evaluated before and after repeated injections. TNF elevations were observed in all patients while IL-1 and SAA showed no significant changes.

INTRODUCTION

Interferons are a unique set of proteins that possess potent antiviral, antiproliferative and immunoregulatory activities. From encouraging clinical trials in osteosarcoma and Hodgkin's disease interferon alpha of various origins are now being used in the treatment of certain viral diseases and cancer in general. (1). Many patients needing interferon therapy have shorter courses of treatment due to the presence of side effects. (2). In particular, constitutional symptoms "flu-like" after single injections are seen in the majority of patients.

In this study we have looked at serum levels of amyloid protein SAA and two lymphokines, interleukin 1 (IL-1) and Tumor Necrosis Factor (TNF) in a group of cancer patients undergoing interferon alpha therapy.

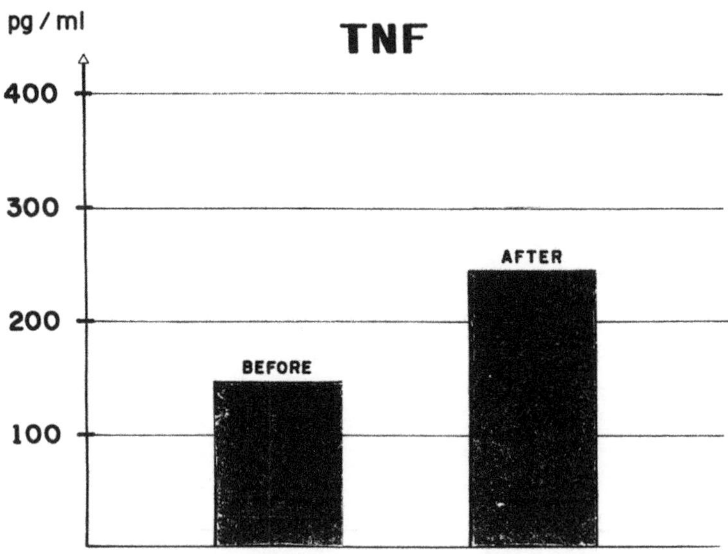

Fig 1 - Serum TNF levels in Cancer Patients on Chronic Interferon Therapy

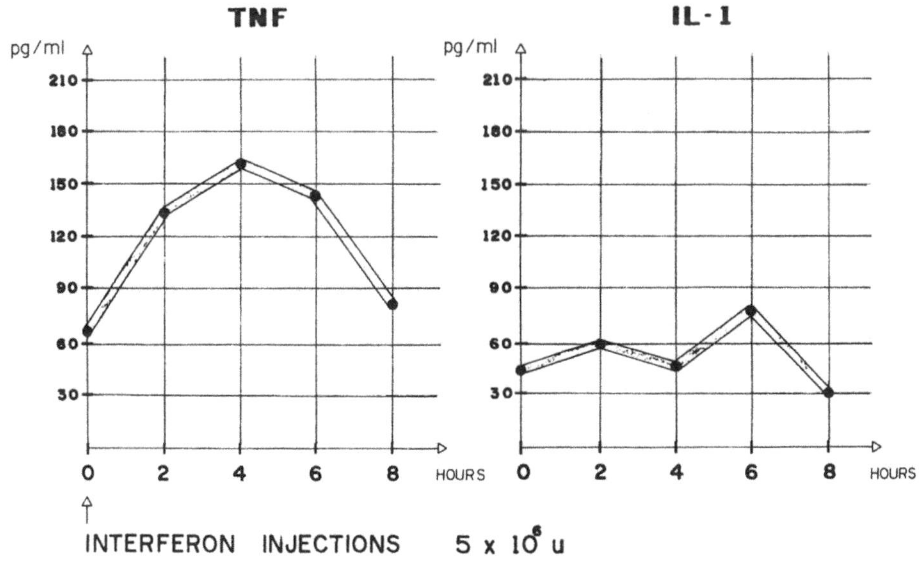

Fig 2 - Serial measurments of TNF and IL-1 before and after a single injection of interferon ($5x10^6U$)

TABLE 1. SAA serum levels in cancer patients after interferon injection (5 x 10^6 U)

	SAA (ug/ml)					
Patient	Before	Two	Four	Six	Eight	(hours)
1	4.1	4.3	4.2	4.2	4.1	
2	2.8	2.9	2.5	1.8	2.6	
3	2.5	2.7	3.2	- -	4.0	
4	2.9	2.8	2.5	2.6	1.8	
5	4.2	4.1	4.3	4.2	4.2	
6	9.0	9.0	6.5	9.0	9.1	

Control values - below 3.0 ug/ml

MATERIAL AND METHODS

Patients with solid neoplasms requiring therapy with alpha interferon had blood drawn before and various periods after interferon treatment. In six patients serial determinations were done every two hours for TNF, IL-1 and SAA levels. The Endogen TNF and IL-1 Elisa were used in this study. Both assays detect at least 50 pg/ml of biologically active TNF and IL-1. Serum SAA levels were performed also by an Elisa technique developed in our laboratory that detects between 0.5 to 3 ug/ml in normal controls.

RESULTS AND DISCUSSION

Patients on chronic interferon therapy had higher levels of serum TNF when compared to values before therapy when interferon was started. (Fig. 1). Six patients had serial measure-

ments done after a single injection of interferon by the intra muscular route. A progressive elevation was observed in serum TNF while IL-1 values remained essentially unchanged. SAA levels had patterns of fluctuation similar to those observed with IL-1 determinations. (Fig. 2 and Table 1).
These results taken together point to a persistent elevation of TNF levels in cancer patients on chronic interferon therapy and raises the possibility that TNF may be the lymphokine involved on the appearence of constitutional symptoms and not IL-1 which is also known to generate similar effects in experimental models. This notion is also supported by the lack of significant alterations on SAA levels which can be affected by changes inIL-1 concentrations.

REFERENCES

1. Fighen, R.A.: 'Biotherapy in clinical practice' (1989) Seminars in Hematology 26: 15-24, 1989.
2. Parkinson, DR.: 'Cytokines in Cancer Therapy' (1989) Urology 34: 87-96.

ACKOWLEDGEMENTS

This is publication nº 105 from the Division of Rheumatology/Immunology. Funds of these investigations were provided by CNPq/FAPESP. Address reprint requests to: Morton A. Scheinberg, Rua Dr. Cesario Mota Jr., 112 - Capital, São Paulo - 01221 - Brazil.

ACUTE PHASE PROTEIN, SERUM AMYLOID A, INHIBITS IL-1- AND TNF-INDUCED FEVER AND HYPOTHALAMIC PGE_2 IN MICE

Ruth Shainkin-Kestenbaum,[1] Geffry Berlyne,[2] Shulamit Zimlichman[1] and Abraham Danon.[3]
Departments of Nephrology,[1] and Clinical Pharmacology,[3]
Soroka Medical Center and Ben-Gurion University of the Negev,
P.O.Box 653.
Beer-Sheva, 84105 Israel.
Nephrology, [2] Brooklyn VA Medical Center and Health Science Center,SUNY, Brooklyn, NY, USA.

The effect of serum amyloid A (SAA) on fever, induced by recombinant interleukin-1β (rIL-1β) or recombinant tumor necrosis factor α (rTNFα), was studied in mice. Serum amyloid A is an acute phase protein whose rise in pathological events is induced by the cytokines IL-1 and TNF. The rise in SAA blood level, occurring during acute events, exhibits the most intense and rapid increase among all acute phase proteins (1). These cytokines mediate the many diverse events of the acute phase response, among which is the production of fever (2). It was recently shown that the endogenous pyrogens IL-1 and TNF initiated fever by increasing PGE_2 synthesis in the thermoregulatory center of the hypothalamus. PGE_2 is thus known to be a central mediator of fever and its release correlates directly with the magnitude of fever (3).

Serum amyloid A was isolated from human sera of patients, who had undergone severe musculoskeletal trauma, according to the method of Rosenthal et al. (4), as modified by Pras (personal communication). For the fever studies female RCNIH mice, 8-10 weeks old, were allowed free water, but deprived of food for 18 hours to avoid temperature changes due to food ingestion. The mice were kept at room temperature in plastic restrainers to prevent excessive motion and temperature was recorded continuously by a thermocouple. In the experiments designed to look at hypothalamic PGE_2, male MCR mice, 6-8 weeks old, were decapitated, the hypothalamic region was removed immediately and cut into 4 slices, 1-2 mm^3 each. Slices obtained from 4 animals were pooled in one vial containing 1 ml Dulbecco's Modified Eagle's Medium (DMEM) supplemented with 2 mM glutamine, 100 U/ml penicillin, 0.1 mg/ml streptomycin, and 12.5 U/ml nystatin. Vials were incubated in a shaking bath at 37^0C in an atmosphere of O_2/CO_2 (95%/5%). Media were changed at 30 min intervals and PGE_2 in the media was assayed by RIA.

25 U rIL-1β induced fever in all five mice, whereas simultaneous administration of 250 μg serum amyloid A with rIL-1β prevented the induction of fever, and even subnormal temperatures were observed ($p<0.001$). Likewise, when rTNFα was injected alone, 50 U induced an increase in

rectal temperature. Serum amyloid A injected simultaneously prevented the development of fever ($p<0.01$). Injection of 250 µg serum amyloid A alone to control mice had no effect on body temperature. These data suggest a role for serum amyloid A in modulating the pyrogenic activity of IL-1 and TNF in vivo. Likewise, in vitro , addition of 50 µg/ml serum amyloid A simultaneously with 5 U/ml rIL-1β inhibited the increase in PGE_2 output from mouse hypothalamic slices. A similar inhibitory effect of serum amyloid A (50 µg/ml) was observed on hypothalamic PGE_2 output that was induced by 25 ng/ml rTNFα. PGE_2 output was not affected by serum amyloid A alone. Since fever is a major symptom of inflammation, its possible regulation by an endogenously-produced acute phase protein may be of particular importance in the course of these events. As IL-1 and TNF are biochemically distinct proteins, acting through different receptors, a direct interaction of serum amyloid A with the cytokines or their receptors is not likely. Serum amyloid A, however, may affect intracellular messages common to both cytokines. Since serum amyloid A did not affect body temperature or hypothalamic PGE_2 levels when administered alone, it may represent a specific servo-mechanism for fever regulation in acute events, and it suggests, for the first time, a possible feedback relationship between serum amyloid A and the immunoregulatory cytokines.

References

1. Kushner , I. (1982) The phenomenon of the acute phase response, Ann NY Acad Sci 389, 39-48.
2. Dinarello, CA. (1989) Interleukin-1 and its biologically related cytokines, Adv Immunol 44, 153-205.
3. Dinarello, CA. Cannon , GJ., and Wolfe SM. (1988) New concepts on the pathogenesis of fever. Rev Infect Dis 10, 168-189.
4. Rosenthal , CJ. Franklin , EC. , Frangione, B. and Greenspan , J. (1976) Isolation and partial characterization of SAA - an amyloid-related protein from human serum, J Immunol 116, 1415-1418.

HUMAN RECOMBINANT TNF-α AND POLY I.POLY C INDUCE SAA AND ENHANCE AMYLOIDOSIS IN HAMSTER.

Niewold ThA, Arakawa T[o], Kisilevsky R[*], Shirahama T[#], Gruys E.
Dept. of Vet. Pathol., Univ. of Utrecht, The Netherlands.
[o]Amgen, Thousand Oaks, Ca, USA, [*]Dept. of Pathol., Kingston School of Med., Kingston, Canada. [#]Arthritis Center, Boston School of Med., Boston, USA.

ABSTRACT

Interleukin 1 and 6 (IL1, IL6) and tumor necrosis factor (TNF) were described to stimulate SAA-production. In the present study, the role of TNF and IL6 in SAA-induction was examined, using human recombinant TNF-α (hrTNF-α) and the IL6 inducer polyI.polyC. The injection of both compounds gave rise to a SAA-response in a dose-dependent way. Furthermore, both substances enhanced amyloid deposition in hamster. The results obtained stress the importance of mediators in both the acute phase response and amyloidogenesis.

INTRODUCTION

The precursor of AA-amyloid is serum amyloid A (SAA), an acute phase protein that is produced by the liver upon stimulation with cytokines. Interleukin 1 and 6 (IL1, IL6) and tumor necrosis factor-α (TNF-α) were identified as SAA-stimulating factors and they were shown to act synergistically. The interrelationship between cytokines is very complex, IL1 and TNF-α stimulate the production of IL6, whereas IL6 inhibits LPS-induced TNF-α production (4,5). It was shown previously, that sustained high SAA-levels alone do not produce amyloid. Amyloid deposition requires the presence of amyloid enhancing factor (AEF) (3,6). However, IL1 induced SAA-levels in the presence of AEF did not lead to amyloid deposition (3).

In the present study, the role of TNF-α in amyloidogenesis is studied for the following reasons.

1. TNF-α stimulates the production of SAA.
2. The protein structure of TNF-α has a high content of β-pleated sheet (1), as is the case with fibril-derived AEF (FAEF) (6).

These properties of TNF-α led to the following questions:

1. are TNF-α-induced SAA-levels sufficient to produce amyloidosis?
2. does TNF-α possess AEF-activity?

MATERIALS AND METHODS

Young male hamsters (Mesocricetus auratus, 100g) were used in all the experiments. In a first experiment, TNF-α was tested intraperitoneally (i.p.) in hamster for its SAA-inducing activity, in comparison with the IL6 inducer polyI.polyC (pIpC)(7)(i.p.), and lipopolysaccharide (LPS) (subcutaneously). After 24 h the animals were bled and the serum SAA-levels determined. In the second experiment, one group of hamsters received 7 daily injections of TNF-α (i.p.), with a single i.p. injection of FAEF or PBS on day one. Another group received 7 daily subcutaneous LPS-injections, with on day one a single i.p. injection of PBS, FAEF, TNF-α or pIpC. Animals were killed on day 7, their spleens fixed in buffered formalin. Alkaline Congo red stained paraffin sections were screened for the presence of amyloid.

The injected materials were: human recombinant TNF-α (hrTNF-α) with a cytolytic activity of 2×10^6 U/mg (1), polyI.polyC (Sigma, Chemical Company, St.Louis MO), LPS (E.coli, 0.127:B8, Difco Labs, Detroit), hamster fibril derived AEF was prepared as described (6).

Serum SAA-levels were determined as described before (8), and expressed as a percentage of a known positive control serum (containing approximately 1 mg SAA/ml serum).

RESULTS

Table 1. Serum SAA-levels in hamster (n=2) 24 h after intraperitoneal injection of human recombinant TNF-α and polyI.polyC, in comparison with a subcutaneous injection of lipopolysaccharide.

substance	amount (μg)	% SAA ± sd
hrTNF-α	0.2	40 ± 3
	1.0	74 ± 2
	5.0	71 ± 1
pIpC	20	9 ± 1
	100	26 ± 6
	300	83 ± 1
LPS	40	83 ± 4

Both hrTNF-α and pIpC did induce serum SAA in a dose dependent way (Table 1).

Table 2. The effect of various treatments on splenic amyloid deposition after 7 days.

injected daily (7x)	injected on day one (1x)	splenic amyloid/n
hrTNF-α (1 μg)	+PBS	0/3
	+FAEF	0/3
LPS (40 μg)	+PBS	0/4
	+FAEF	4/4
	+hrTNF-α (25 μg)	4/4
	+pIpC (300 μg)	2/4

Daily injections of 1 μg hrTNF-α resulted in elevated SAA-levels at day

7 (not shown) but even in the presence of FAEF no amyloid was deposited. A single intraperitoneal injection of 25 μg of hrTNF-α followed by 7 daily subcutaneous LPS-injections resulted in enhanced amyloid deposition. The IL6 inducer pIpC also showed amyloid enhancing activity, albeit to a lesser extent (Table 2).

DISCUSSION

It was shown previously, that the induction of SAA in experimental animals is not mediated by IL1 alone (2,4,5). From the results obtained here it can be concluded that TNF-α and probably IL6 (induced by pIpC (7)) play an important role in SAA-induction in hamster.

Sustained high serum levels of SAA induced by daily injections of TNF-α were not sufficient to produce amyloid, even in the presence of FAEF. A similar result was obtained in the murine model, using IL1-rich macrophage supernatant and AEF (3).

In the standard hamster model of accelerated amyloid induction, both hrTNF-α and pIpC appeared to have AEF-activity. Given the complex nature of the interrelationship between mediators these results do not allow attributing AEF-activity to one specific mediator itself. Furthermore, differences in the known biological activities between AEF and TNF (and IL6), speak against complete identity. It is suggested that the injection of hrTNF-α (and pI.pC) disturbs the normal equilibrium between mediators, leading to endogenous AEF-production.

REFERENCES

1. Davis JM, Narachi MA, Alton NK, Arakawa T: Structure of human tumor necrosis factor α derived from recombinant DNA. Biochem. 26:1322, 1987
2. Hol PR, Snel FWJJ, Draayer M, Gruys E: The serum amyloid A stimulatory factor (SAASF) in the hamster. J.Comp.Pathol. 97:677, 1987
3. Kisilevsky R, Tan R, Subrahmanyan L, Snow A: Are elevated serum amyloid A levels and amyloid-enhancing factor sufficient to induce inflammation-associated amyloid deposition? Appl.Pathol. 2:308, 1984
4. Le J, Vilcek J: Tumor necrosis factor and interleukin 1: cytokines with multiple overlapping biological activities. Lab.Invest. 56:234, 1987
5. Le J, Vilcek J: Interleukin 6: a multifunctional cytokine regulating immune reactions and the acute phase protein response. Lab.Invest. 61:588, 1989
6. Niewold ThA, Hol PR, van Andel ACJ, Lutz ETG, Gruys E: Enhancement of amyloid induction by amyloid fibril fragments in hamster. Lab.Invest. 56:544, 1987
7. Sehgal PB, Sagar AD: Heterogeneity of poly(I).poly(C)-induced human fibroblast interferon mRNA species. Nature 288:95, 1980
8. Snel FWJJ, Niewold ThA, Baltz ML, Hol PR, van Ederen AM, Pepys MB, Gruys E: Experimental amyloidosis in the hamster: correlation between hamster female protein levels and amyloid deposition. Clin.Exp.Immunol. 76:296-300, 1989

THE PHYSIOLOGY OF THE ACUTE PHASE SERUM AMYLOID A (SAA) RESPONSE IN MICE

J. D. SIPE, R. NETA, P. GHEZZI AND R. NUMEROF
Boston Univ. Sch. Med., Boston, MA; Armed Forces Radbiol. Res. Inst., Bethesda, MD; Istituto "Mario Negri", Milan, Italy; and Div. Hem.-Onc., Tufts Univ. Sch. Med., Boston, MA.

ABSTRACT. LPS stimulates the mononuclear phagocyte system to produce interleukin 1 (IL-1) and tumor necrosis factor (TNF) which in turn activate the murine serum amyloid A gene family to result in synthesis of apo-SAA isoforms. The molecular mechanism by which purified recombinant IL-1 regulates the quantity of apo-SAA production was investigated in CD2F1, C3H/HeJ and CD1 mice. Three observations support a physiological role for IL-1 in regulation of SAA gene expression: 1) Monoclonal antibodies to the EL-4 IL-1 receptor significantly inhibited IL-1 induced SAA production; 2) The recombinant IL-1 receptor antagonist (IL-1ra) completely blocked IL-1 induced SAA mRNA transcription; and 3) The calcium antagonist chlorpromazine inhibited LPS, IL-1 and TNF induced SAA synthesis. Phorbol myristate acetate (PMA) stimulated SAA production maximally at 6 rather than 24 hours, a time course more similar to IL-1 and TNF than to LPS. Repeated administration of PMA resulted in tolerance (reduced capacity for SAA production) to further stimulation with either PMA or LPS suggesting the two agents share a pathway of signal transduction to the transcriptional machinery of the SAA gene family.

INTRODUCTION. Inbred strains of mice have been used to decipher the pathway leading to expression of the serum amyloid A (SAA) gene family [1]. The amount of SAA synthesized during disturbances of homeostasis is proportional to the extent of injury or the amount of inciting stimulus [1,2]. While interleukin-1 (IL-1) and tumor necrosis factor (TNF) have been implicated as modulators of lipopolysaccharide (LPS)-stimulated hepatic SAA mRNA and/or protein synthesis in mice [3-5], the precise temporal order of signaling pathways regulating the prompt and large variations in the magnitude of transcription and translation of SAA mRNA is still largely unknown. In this study, the capacity of both monoclonal antibodies to the p80 (EL-4) receptor for IL-1 alpha and beta [6] and the naturally occurring IL-1 receptor antagonist (IL-1ra) (which bind to the same receptor) [7] to block IL-1 induced SAA synthesis was investigated. The ability of the calcium antagonist and phospholipase A2 inhibitor chlorpromazine (CPZ), known to protect against endotoxic shock in mice [8], to inhibit LPS, TNF and IL-1 stimulated SAA production was measured. Phorbol myristate acetate (PMA), known to alter expression of genes such as collagenase through activation of protein kinase C [9], appears to stimulate SAA gene expression through a pathway shared with LPS.

MATERIAL AND METHODS. Recombinant human IL-1 alpha and anti IL-1 (EL4) receptor antibody (35F5) were prepared at Hoffman-La Roche, Nutley, NJ. IL-1 receptor antagonist (IL-1ra) was obtained from Synergen, Inc., Boulder CO. Chlorpromazine was obtained from Farmitalia Carlo Erba, s.p.a. Milan, Italy; phorbol 12-myristate 13-acetate (PMA) and LPS (E. coli) serotype 055:B5) were purchased from Sigma Chemical Co., St. Louis, MO. The oligonucleotide probe corresponding to residues 33-38 of apo-SAA1, apo-SAA2 and SAA3 was synthesized in the Department of Biochemistry core facility, Boston University School of Medicine. Northern blot analysis of liver RNA was carried out as described [3,4] and serum SAA concentrations were measured by ELISA [10].

RESULTS. Intraperitoneal (ip) administration of rat monoclonal antibodies to the murine IL-1 receptor 6 hours prior to ip injection of IL-1 reduced the SAA response of CD2F1 male mice (Table 1).

TABLE 1. **Inhibition of apo-SAA Response by Anti-IL-1 Receptor Ab**

Treatment	SAA (ug/ml)
None	6
Saline	28
Saline + 500ng IL-1	219
30ug Ab + 500ng IL-1	74
150ug Ab + 500ng IL-1	79
Saline + 100ng IL-1	103
30ug Ab + 100ng IL-1	52
150ug + 100ng IL-1	9

Administration of 30 ug of human IL-1 receptor antagonist completely abolished SAA mRNA expression (unpublished observations). CPZ inhibited LPS, IL-1 and TNF stimulated SAA production (Table 2). PMA was a potent stimulus of SAA production (Control mice, SAA = 2.2 (1.4) ug/ml, mice 6 hours after 5 ug PMA, SAA = 99 (15) ug/ml and mice 24 hours after 5 ug PMAS = 44 (34) ug/ml. The maximum at 6 hours

TABLE 2. Chlorpromazine inhibition of murine SAA synthesis

Treatment	SAA (ug/ml)
Saline	<1
LPS	71 (20)
LPS + CPZ	16 (8) *
TNF	68 (18)
TNF + CPZ	18 (6) *
IL-1	40 (9)
IL-1 + CPZ	15 (4) *

CD-1 mice were treated with LPS (2.5 ug), TNF (1 ug) or IL-1 (1ug) with or without CPZ pretreatment (4mg/kg, 30 min before LPS, TNF or IL-1). SAA concentration was measured by ELISA in serum obtained 24 hours after LPS and 8 hours after TNF and IL-1. Data are mean $\pm$ standard deviation in parentheses(5 mice per group). * = $p < 0.05$ versus respective treatment group (LPS, TNF or IL-1 without CPZ) by Fisher´s exact test.

for PMA is unlike LPS which is maximal at 16-24 hours [1]. In tolerance experiments (Table 3) either PMA or LPS was administered for 4 days, then after one day CD-1 mice were given either a PMA or LPS challenge and SAA was measured 6 hours later. Repeated administration of PMA or LPS resulted in cross-resistance to SAA induction.

TABLE 3. LPS/PMA cross tolerance to SAA induction

Treatment	Experiment 1	2	3	4
	SAA (ug/ml)			
PMA	51(5)	48(44)	74(7)	126(32)
LPSx4/PMA	14(9)	3(3)	20(13)	26(15)
LPS	29(5)	18(4)	42(8)	55(14)
PMAx4/LPS	20(16)	14(7)	28(23)	31(6)

LPSx4/LPS and saline were always less than 2 ug/ml SAA. PMA tolerance: Exp 1, PMA, 59 (27), PMAx4/PMA, 3(3); Exp 2, PMA 114 (11), PMAx4/PMA, 19(5). In tolerance experiments, the agent was administered for 4 days, then 1 day later mice were given challenge and SAA measured 6 hours later for PMA, 24 hours later for LPS. Values are mean $\pm$ standard deviation in parenthesis, 5 mice/group.

DISCUSSION. Anti-IL-1 receptor antibody (35F5) given to mice prior to IL-1 reduces SAA production, providing direct evidence that IL-1 regulates SAA gene expression. Consistent with these findings presented in Table I is the fact that the IL-1 receptor antagonist totally blocks IL-1 induced IL-1 induced mRNA transcription in murine liver (unpublished observations). Chlorpromazine inhibits the SAA inducing activity of LPS, TNF and IL-1 (Table 2). CPZ can bind calmodulin and inhibit calcium activated enzymes and the synthesis of diacylglycerol and phosphatidylcholine [reviewed in reference 8]. This suggests that the CPZ sensitive pathway represents a non-receptor mediated mechanism of stimulus-response coupling. PMA regulates gene expression through inducible transcriptional enhancers [9]. The demonstration of PMA and LPS cross-tolerance suggests the exxistence of long-lived negative regulatory elements and that the PMA and LPS pathways share common regulatory features.

ACKNOWLEDGMENT. The authors thank Dr. Manuela Mengozzi for valuable contributions to this study.

REFERENCES.

1. McAdam, K.P.W.J. and Sipe, J.D. (1976) ´Murine model for human secondary amyloidosis: Genetic variability of the acute-phase serum protein SAA response to endotoxins and casein.´, J. Exp. Med., 144,1121-1127.
2. Sipe, J.D., Vogel, S.N., Ryan, J.L., McAdam, K.P.W.J. and Rosenstreich, D.L. (1979) ´Detection of a macrophage-derived mediator for induction of the acute phase SAA response in mice by endotoxin´, J. Exp. Med. 150,597-606.
3. Ramadori, G., Sipe, J.D., Dinarello, C.A., Mizel, S.B. and Colten, H.R. (1985) ´Pretranslational modulation of acute phase hepatic protein synthesis by murine recombinant interleukin 1(IL-1) and purified human Il-1´, J. Exp. Med. 162, 930-942.
4. Woo, P., Sipe, J.D., Dinarello, C.A. and Colten, H.R. (1988) ´Structure of a human SAA gene and modulation of its expression in transfected L cells´ J. Biol. Chem. 262, 15790-15797.
5. Sipe, J.D., Vogel, S.N., Douches, S. and Neta, R. (1987) ´Tumor necrosis factor/cachectin is a less potent inducer of SAA synthesis than interleukin 1´ Lymphokine Res., 6, 93-101.
6. Chizzonite, R., Truitt, T., Kilian, P.L., Stern, A.S., Nunes, P., Parker, K.P., Kaffka, K.L., Chua, A.O., Lugg, D.K., Gubler, U. (1989) ´Two high affinity interleukin 1 receptors represent separate gene products´ Proc. Natl., Acad. Sci. USA, 86, 8029-8034.
7. Eisenberg, S.P., Evans, R.J., Arend, W.P., Verderber, E., Brewer, M.T., Hannum, C.H. and Thompson, R.C. (1990) ´Primary structure and functional expression from complementary DNA of a human interleukin-1 receptor antagonist´, Nature 343:341-346.
8. Bertini, R., Bianchi, M., Mengozzi, M. and Ghezzi, P. (1989) ´Protective effects of chlorpromazine against lethality of IL-1 in adrenalectomized or actinomycin D sensitized mice", Biochem. Biophys. Res. Comm., 65, 942-946.
9. Angel, P., Imagawa, M., Chiu, R., Stein, B., Imbra, R.J., Rahmsdorf, HJ.J., Jonat, C., Herrlich, P. and Karin, M. (1987) ´Phorbol ester-inducible genes contain a common cis element recognized by a TPA-modulated trans-acting factor´ Cell, 49,729 -739.
10. Sipe, J.D., Gonnerman, W.A., Loose, L.D., Knapschaefer, G., Xie, W -J. and Franzblau, C. (1989) ´Direct binding enzyme-linked immunosorbent assay (ELISA) for SAA´ J. Immunol. Methods, 1225, 125-135.

MOUSE SAA_3: DETECTION IN MOUSE TISSUES WITH SPECIFIC ANTIBODY

R. MEEK, N. ERIKSEN, AND E.P. BENDITT
Dept. of Pathology (SJ-60), University of Washington
Seattle, Washington 98195, U.S.A.

ABSTRACT. Antibodies to a protein A-SAA_3 fusion protein were generated in rabbits. Immunochemical studies using SAA_3 antiserum were performed on tissues from LPS treated mice and revealed positive reactions to liver hepatocytes and other tissues.

Introduction

Serum amyloid A (SAA) is a family of acute phase proteins found circulating mainly associated with high density lipoproteins (HDL) [1-4]. Usually at trace levels, the concentrations are elevated several hundred fold [1,5-7] in response to a variety of injuries. In the mouse, SAA is encoded by a family of three active genes [8,9]. SAA_1 and SAA_2 are HDL apoproteins but the SAA_3 protein has not been identified. The major site of SAA_1, SAA_2, and SAA_3 synthesis is the liver, where mRNA for each of the three genes is elevated approximately 1,000-fold in mice challenged with lipopolysaccharide (LPS) [10]. SAA genes are also expressed in extrahepatic tissues in response to LPS injection [11, 12]; however, this expression is almost exclusively limited to the SAA_3 mRNA [11]. In situ hybridization studies showed that adipocytes are a major extrahepatic tissue of SAA_3 mRNA transcription in mice challenged with LPS and may account for much of the extrahepatic SAA_3 mRNA expressed [13]. Here we report immunocytochemical studies on tissues from LPS challenged mice with antibodies against an SAA_3 protein construct expressed in bacteria.

Materials and Methods

The plasmid RS48 (Dr. John Morrow) containing an SAA_3 cDNA was cleaved with Ava-II, blunt ended with the Klenow fragment of DNA polymerase alpha and cleaved with Pst-I. The SAA_3 cDNA fragment was subcloned into pRIT2T (Pharmacia), prepared by double digestion with Sma-I and Pst-I. The resultant chimeric plasmid (pRIT2T-SAA_3) encoded a fusion product of truncated bacterial protein A (residues #1-263) and SAA_3 (residues #48-103). Expression of protein A-SAA_3 in E. coli N4830-1 was induced by temperature elevation and the fusion protein was isolated by affinity chromatography on IgG-Sepharose. Antibodies were raised in rabbits immunized with acrylamide gel slices containing the fusion protein.

Western blotting. Bacterial extracts, separated by electrophoresis through SDS-acrylamide gels [14] and blotted onto nitrocellulose, were exposed to antisera at 1:100-1:400 dilutions; bound antibodies were detected by peroxidase-conjugated goat anti-rabbit IgG and visualized with 4-chloro-1-napthol [15].

Immunocytochemistry. Tissues of Balb/c mice given 50 μg of LPS W (Difco) i.p. were removed 20 hours later, fixed in methyl-Carnoy's fixative and embedded in paraffin. Sections were treated with SAA_3 antisera and detected with biotinylated goat anti-rabbit antibody with a Vectastain kit (Vector Laboratories).

Identification of Antibody to SAA3. Because the protein A - SAA_3 antigen contains 4 domains capable of binding the Fc portion of IgG, another bacterial fusion product protein was raised for Western blotting with the anti-SAA_3 antisera. The plasmid vector (Dr. H. Rienhoff) coded for a fusion product, bacterial Tryp E (residues #1-323) and SAA_3 (residues #14-103). Antiserum from one rabbit was positive (Fig. 1) and specific for SAA_3 as shown by the lack of reaction with

SAA_1 or SAA_2 in Western blots of SAA-rich HDL or with tissues from casein challenged mice expressing high levels of SAA_1 and SAA_2.

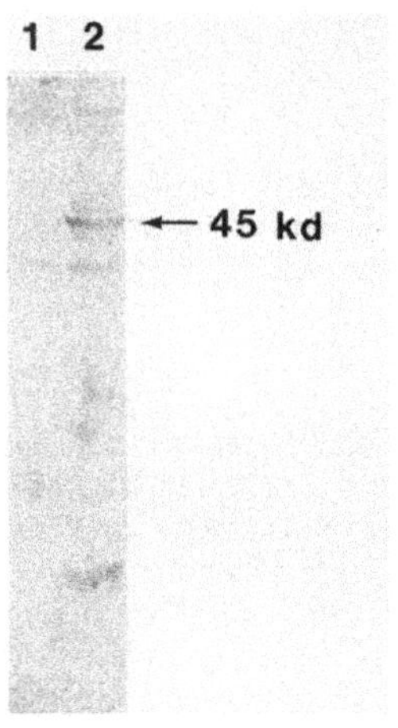

Fig. 1 E. coli harboring the Tryp-E - SAA_3 plasmid were induced by adding 3-ß-indole-acrylic acid (IAA) to a final concentration of 20 ng/ml. After 3 hrs the cells were harvested, lysed in 1x sample buffer, separated by SDS-PAGE and blotted onto nitrocellulose. Western blotting was performed with rabbit antibodies to protein A-SAA_3. Lane 1, control uninduced; lane 2, IAA induced bacterial extracts.

Results

Examination of liver shows that, compared to pre-immune serum, SAA_3 antiserum stains all hepatocytes; some cells stain more intensely than others (Fig. 2). This observation is consistent with _in situ_ hybridization studies which revealed SAA_3 mRNA in all hepatocytes.

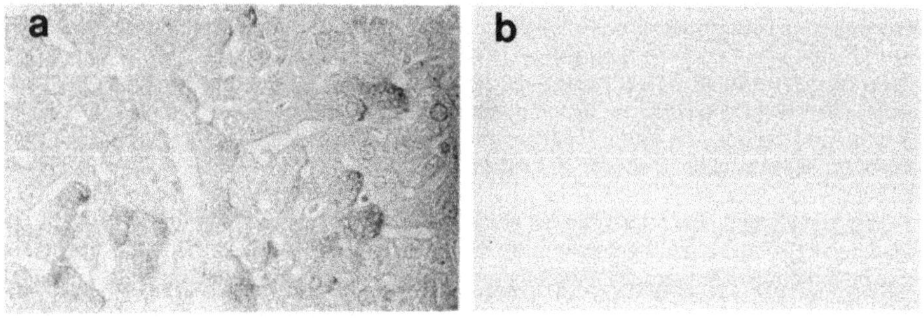

Fig. 2 Immunocytochemistry of liver from LPS challenged mouse. Panel a, antiserum to mouse SAA_3. Panel b, pre-immune antiserum.

Spleen shows a general perifollicluar staining pattern (Table 1). Megakaryocytes appear positive. Other cells, perhaps macrophages, known to have high levels of SAA_3 mRNA [11], stain with the antibody. In addition, the matrix appears to be stained.

Intense anti-SAA_3 staining is observed in the epithelial cells of the thin loops of Henle (Table 1). General overall staining of tubules with anti-SAA_3 compared with pre-immune serum was also observed. This generalized pattern of SAA_3 protein levels is consistent with the presence of SAA_3 mRNA throughout the kidney (unpublished observations).

Cytoplasmic staining of fat cells is seen with anti-SAA_3 compared to pre-immune serum. Adipocytes adherent to the adrenal glands, lymph node and kidney all stain with anti-SAA_3 (Table 1). Other locations have not yet been examined. This finding is consistent with our observations that SAA_3 mRNA is expressed by adipocytes from LPS challenged mice [12].

Lymph nodes revealed specific staining of mononuclear cells (Table 1). Two patterns are evident: very light staining in large cells with abundant cytoplasm and very dark staining in some cells which contain little cytoplasm; only a few cells of these types are positive.

Table 1: SAA_3 Immunoreactivity of Various Tissues from Mice Challenged with LPS

Tissue	SAA_3 Antibody
Liver: hepatocytes	+ + +
Kidney: loop of Henle	+ +
tubules	+
Fat: adipocytes	+ + +
Spleen: perifollicular sites	+ +
megakaryocytes	+ +
Lymph node: macrophages?	+, + + +
lymphocytes?	

Discussion

The conservation and the dramatic elevation of the message levels of the SAA gene family members in response to injury suggest an important functional role for them but their function(s) is still elusive.

This paper is the first report identifying the SAA_3 protein. In these initial studies, identification of SAA_3 in hepatocytes, adipocytes and kidney parallels our observation by _in situ_ hybridization that these cells transcribe SAA_3 mRNA (13, unpublished observation). This correlation is not seen in other sites. SAA_3 mRNA is transcribed by some cells found in splenic perifollicular regions [13], but SAA_3 protein appears to be present in most perifollicular cells. Thus far we have not investigated whether SAA_3 circulates. SAA_3 protein appears extracellularly in perifollicular regions of spleen, where we previously found $SAA_{1\&2}$, which circulate [16]; however, as indicated, cells in these regions also react with anti-SAA_3 antibody and have SAA_3 mRNA.

Acknowledgments

We express our appreciation to Jeanette Carlson for dedicated service in preparation of the manuscript.

This work was supported by United States Public Health Service Grants HL-03174 and HL-40079.

References

1. Hoffman, J.S., Benditt, E.P. (1982) `Changes in high density lipoprotein content following endotoxin administration in the mouse', J. Biol. Chem. 257, 10510-10517.
2. Bausserman, L.L., Herbert, P.N., McAdam, K.P.W.J. (1980) `Heterogeneity of human serum amyloid A proteins', J. Exp. Med. 152, 641-656.

3. Benditt, E.P., Eriksen, N. (1977) `Amyloid protein SAA is associated with high density lipoprotein from human serum', Proc. Natl. Acad. Sci. USA 74, 4025-4028.
4. Benditt, E.P., Eriksen, N., Hanson, R.H. (1979) `Amyloid protein SAA is an apoprotein of mouse plasma high density lipoprotein', Proc. Natl. Acad. Sci. USA 76, 4092-4096.
5. Kushner, I. (1982) `The phenomenon of the acute phase response', Ann. NY Acad. Sci. 389, 39-48.
6. McAdam, K.P.W.J., Sipe, J.D. (1976) `Murine model for human secondary amyloidosis: genetic variability of the acute-phase serum protein SAA response to endotoxins and casein', J. Exp. Med. 144, 1121-1127.
7. Benson, M.D., Schneider, M.S., Shirahama, T., Cathcart, L.S., Skinner, M. (1977) `Kinetics of serum amyloid protein A in casein-induced murine amyloidosis', J. Clin. Invest. 59, 412-417.
8. Lowell, C.A., Potter, D.A., Stearman, R.S., Morrow, J.F. (1986) `Structure of the murine serum amyloid A gene family', J. Biol. Chem. 261, 8442-8452.
9. Yamamoto, K.-I., Shiroo, M., Migita, S. (1986) `Diverse gene expression for isotypes of murine serum amyloid A protein during acute phase reaction' Science, 232, 227-229.
10. Lowell, C.A., Potter, D.A., Stearman, R.S., Morrow, J.F. (1986) `Transcriptional regulation of serum amyloid A gene expression', J. Biol. Chem. 261, 8453-8461.
11. Meek, R.L., Benditt, E.P. (1986) `Amyloid A gene family expression in different mouse tissues', J. Exp. Med. 164, 2006-2017.
12. Ramadori, G., Sipe, J.D., Colten, H. (1985) `Expression and regulation of the murine serum amyloid A (SAA) gene in extrahepatic sites', J. Immunol. 135, 3645-3647.
13. Benditt, E.P., Meek, R.L. (1989) `Expression of the third member of the serum amyloid A gene family in mouse adipocytes', J. Exp. Med. 169, 1841-1846.
14. Laemmli, U.K. (1970) `Cleavage of structural proteins during the assembly of the head of bacteriophage T4', Nature 227, 680-685.
15. Monroe, D. (1985) `The solid-phase enzyme linked immunospot assay: current and potential applications', BioTechniques May/June, 222-229.
16. Meek, R.L., Eriksen, N., Benditt, E.P. (1989) `Serum amyloid A in the mouse: sites of uptake and mRNA expression', Am. J. Pathol. 135, 411-419.

GENERATION AND USE OF SITE-SPECIFIC ANTIBODIES AGAINST SAA.

S-T. JU, T. SHIRAHAMA, K. MIURA, AND A. S. COHEN.
The Arthritis Center,
Boston University School of Medicine,
Boston, MA. 02118. USA.

Abstract

Polyclonal antibodies against purified mouse AA and a synthetic peptide of the SAA2 C-terminal 20 amino acids were made in rabbits. The anti-AA serum reacted with both AA and SAA, but the anti-peptide serum reacted with SAA only. Interestingly, anti -peptide serum stained AA deposits, indicating the presence of either intact SAA or partially degraded SAA. Moreover, it stained predominantly the rims of AA deposits. In contrast, homogeneous stainings of AA deposits were obtained with anti-AA serum. Our results provided visual evidence that AA deposits contain both SAA and AA and that these SAA molecules are processed, in situ, into AA as the maturation of AA fibril progresses.

1. Introduction

Murine serum amyloid A2 (SAA2) protein has 103 amino acids while the major sequence of AA amyloid contains 75 amino acids [1]. It is generally believed that cleaving the C-terminal portion of SAA2 is an important process for AA amyloid formation. To be able to visualize this process during amyloid formation, specific antisera were generated to AA protein lacking the C-terminal peptide and to a synthetic peptide corresponding to the 20 amino acid residues of the C-terminal peptide (SAA2 -C20) of SAA2. These antisera were successfully used to demonstrate the transitional process from SAA2 to AA within an individual amyloid deposit.

2. Materials and Methods

2.1. REAGENTS: Mouse (CBA/J) AA protein was extracted and purified as described previously [2]. The C-terminal (84-103) 20 amino acid peptide bearing the sequence, His-Gly-Arg-Ser-Gly-Lys-Asp-Pro-Asn-Tyr-Tyr-Arg-Pro-Pro-Gly-Leu-Pro-Ala-Lys-Tyr, was synthesized according to the method of Merrifield [3] and coupled onto human albumin with 0.05% glutaraldehyde. Antisera were prepared in rabbits by repeated immunizations with antigens emulsified in complete Freund's adjuvant.

2.2. RADIOIMMUNOASSAYS: AA protein and SAA2-C20 peptide were labeled with ^{125}I by chloramine T [4] and free iodine was removed by Sephadex G25 chromatograph. Various amounts of antisera were incubated with 10 ng of labeled ligands in a total mixture of 50 ul at 37°C for 30 minutes. Bound ligands were precipitated with an excess amount (50 ul) of goat anti-rabbit Ig serum. After centrifugation, 50 ul of supernatants were removed and counted. The % binding was determined by the formula: 100 - (Sample cpm - background cpm)/(Total cpm

- background cpm) x 100. Background cpm was obtained with normal rabbit serum.

2.3. WESTERN BLOT ANALYSIS: The specificity of antisera was examined by Western immunoblotting according to the method of Towbin [5]. One ul of inflammed serum containing approximately 0.3 ug SAA and 30 ug of purified AA protein were electrophresed through a 15% SDS-PAGE, blotted onto nitrocellulose paper, and developed with immune sera.

2.4. IMMUNOHISTOCHEMISTRY: Formalin-fixed, paraffin-embedded sections of amyloidotic liver of CBA/J mice were stained with the antisera using Vectastain ABC kits (Vector, Burlington, CA) [6]

3. Results and Discussion

Because SAA2-C20 peptide contains many charged and aromatic amino acids, it is expected to be an excellent antigenic peptide. Indeed, upon coupling onto human serum albumin, it becomes strongly immunogenic and induced high titered anti-peptide antibodies. As shown in Table 1, this antiserum exhibits strong and specific binding activity toward radiolabeled SAA2-C20 without detectable binding activity to AA. Conversely, anti-AA antiserum expresses potent binding activity to AA but shows no binding activity toward SAA2-C20 peptide. The data demonstrate the specificity of these antisera. It also indicate that the AA preparation is free of C-terminal 20 amino acids.

Table 1. Specificity of antisera to AA protein and SAA2-C20.

Antiserum (ul)	% AA binding	%SAA2-C20 binding
Anti-SAA2-C20 (5 ul)	4	100
Anti-SAA2-C20 (1 ul)	3	70
Anti-SAA2-C20 (0.2 ul)	2	36
Anti-AA (5 ul)	100	3
Anti-AA (1 ul)	88	1
Anti-AA (0.2 ul)	59	3

Western immunoblotting was used to determine whether the anti-SAA2-C20 and anti -AA antisera react with SAA in a site-specific fashion. As shown in Figure 1, both antisera reacted positively with a protein of 12 kDa in the inflammed serum (lane 2). This protein corresponded to SAA and was undetectable in normal serum. In addition, anti-AA, but not anti-SAA2-C20 antiserum specifically reacted with purified AA protein (lane 3). The result demonstrates that these two antisera behave as site-specific antibodies toward SAA subregions.

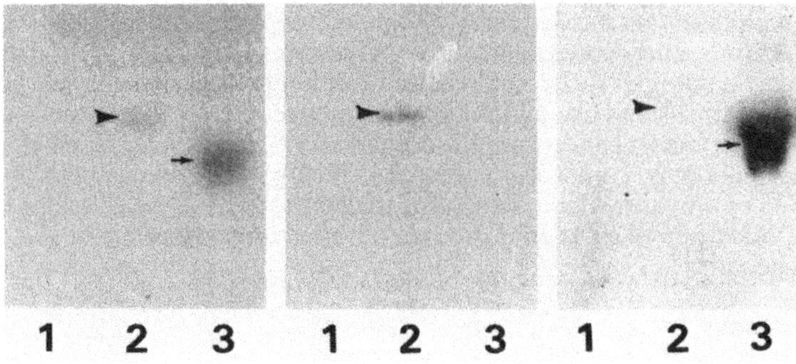

Figure 1. Western blot analyses of antisera to SAA2-C20 and AA protein. Samples were electrophoresed through a 15% SDS-PAGE, followed by Coomasie blue staining (left) immunoblotting with anti-SAA2-C20 serum (middle panel) and anti-AA serum (right panel). Samples were normal mouse serum (lane 1), LPS-inflammed mouse serum (lane 2), and purified mouse AA protein (lane 3). Arrow heads indicate the position of SAA and arrows point to the position of AA.

These antisera were used to visualized the location of SAA and AA in the livers of normal, inflammed, and amyloidotic hosts. The hepatocytes of inflammed and amyloidotic livers, but none of the normal liver were positively stained with these antisera (not shown). Although amyloid deposits were stained with both antisera, distinct patterns of stainings were observed. While anti-AA stained the overall area of amyloid deposits (Figure 2a), anti-SAA2-C20 selectively stained the rims of amyloid deposits (Figure 2b). This distinction is particularly evident on small(early) amyloid deposits. Anti-SAA2-C20 antiserum also preferentially stained the contour area of larger amyloid deposits, leaving central area translucent, whereas anti-AA stained overall deposits homogeneously (not shown).

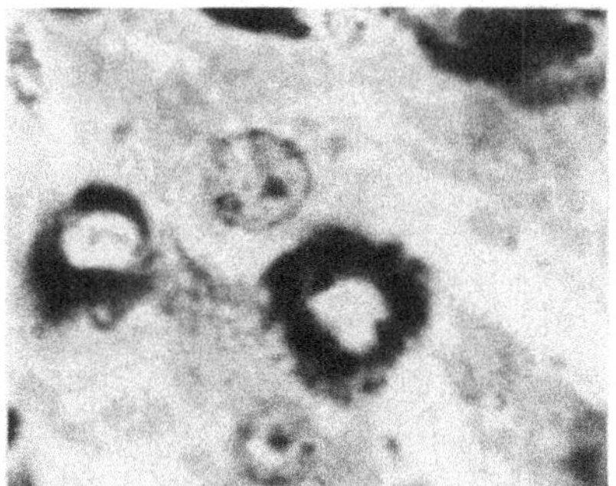

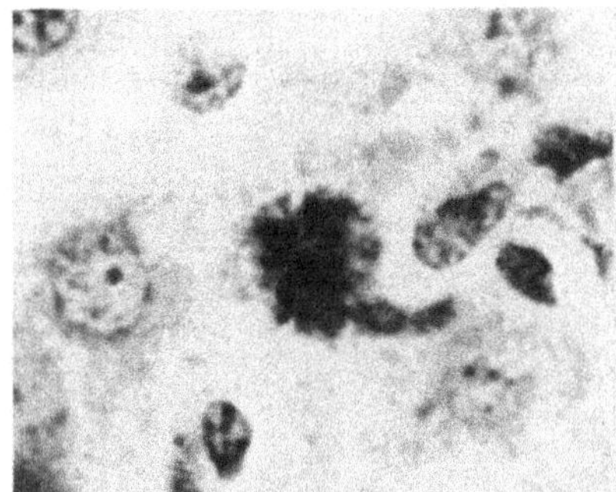

Figure 2. Amyloid-laden mouse liver sections were immunohistochemically stained with anti-SAA2-C20 antiserum (left panel), and anti-AA antiserum (right panel). Anti-SAA2-C20 stains predominantly the marginal portion of early (small) amyloid deposits . In contrast, anti-AA serum stains the overall deposits almost uniformly. 900x.

These observations provided firm evidence that either intact or partially degraded SAA proteins are present on the periphery of amyloid deposits and degraded or processed AA products are concentrated in the center of the amyloid mass. We speculate that SAA concentrated on the cell surface of localized Kupffer cells or hepatocytes, polymerizes into amyloid fibrils and as amyloidogenesis progresses, local enzymes continues to cleave the C-terminal peptide from fibril-bound SAA, forming larger amyloid deposits and larger inner mass composed of pure AA. Finally, this approach can be applied to other types of amyloid which involve degraded products as constituents of amyloid deposits. Such approach should provide a better understanding of the process of amyloidogenesis.

4. References

1. Yamamoto, K. and Migita, S. (1985) 'Complete primary structures of two major murine serum amyloid A proteins deduced from cDNA sequences', Proc. Natl. Acad. Sci. USA. 82, 2915.
2. Skinner, M. Shirahama, T. Benson, M. D. and Cohen, A. S. (1977) 'Murine amyloid protein AA in casein-induced experimental amyloidosis', Lab. Invest. 36, 420.
3. Merryfield, R. B. (1963) 'Solid phase peptide synthesis. I. The synthesis of a tetrapeptide' J. Am. Chem. Soc. 85, 2149.
4. Hunter, W. M. and Greenwood, F. C. (1962) 'Preparation of iodine-131 labeled human growth hormone of high specific activity', Nature. 194, 495.
5. Towbin, H. Slaehelin, T. and Gordon J. (1979) 'Electrophoretic transfer of proteins from polyacrylamide gels to nitrocellulose sheets: procedure an some applications',Proc. Natl. Acad. Sci. USA. 76, 4350.
6. Shirahama, T. Skinner, M. Cohen, A. S. Gejyo, G. Arakawa, M. Suzuki, M. and Hirasawa, Y. (1985) ' Histochemical and immunohistochemical characterization of amyloid associated with chronic hemodialysis as beta-2 microglobulin', Lab. Invest. 53, 705.

THE N-TERMINUS IS THE LIPID-BINDING SITE OF SAA: SUPPORTING EVIDENCE BY MoAbs

YIFAT ZIQ-BACHAR[1], DAVID LEVARTOWSKY[1,2], MORDECHAI PRAS[1], ALISTAIR F. STRACHAN[3], MATI FRIDKIN[2] AND NECHAMA I. SMORODINSKY[4]

[1]Heller Institute for Medical Research, Sheba Medical Center 52621, Israel. [2]Department of Organic Chemistry, The Weizmann Institute of Science, Rehovot 76100, Israel. [3]Department of Internal Medicine, Faculty of Medicine, University of Stellenbosch, Tygerberg 7505, Republic of South Africa. [4]George S. Wise, Faculty of Life Sciences, Tel Aviv University, Ramat Aviv 69978, Israel.

ABSTRACT. SAA is a major acute-phase protein comprising of 104 amino acids ciruclating in the plasma, assembled to subfraction of high density lipoproteins (HDL_3). Two amyloid A proteins, NOR1 and NOR2, corresponding to residues 2-82 and 2-45, respectively, were extracted from an amyloidotic goiter of an FMF patient's NOR. Three MoAbs against NOR2 were raised in mice. Two MoAbs recognize AA and SAA in addition to NOR2 and the third one recognizes NOR2 only. The binding of these MoAbs to NOR2 was inhibited by SAA-related peptides 2-82, 2-45, 2-15, 1-6. Almost no inhibition was observed with peptide 29-41. Two MoAbs recognize purified SAA dissolved in normal human sera. These MoAbs could not detect SAA in various acute-phase sera. Nevertheless, subjecting acute-phase HDL to denaturing conditions (SDS, urea) enables recognition of six SAA isoforms by these MoAbs. Supposing that denatured SAA is detached from HDL, these findings support the theory that the N-terminus of SAA functions as an anchor to the lipid layer of HDL.

Introduction

SAA is a notable acute-phase protein, its circulating concentration increases rapidly and extensively in response to most forms of tissue injury, infection and inflammation. During acute-phase response, SAA associates with pre-exisiting HDL particles in the circulation, displacing Apo-AI and perhaps Apo-AII from the HDL, and may comprise of up to 90% of the total apolipoproteins of HDL, resulting in remodelling the surface of such particles to yield particles which have greater size, higher hydrated density and relatively less Apo-AI [1,2,3]. This association is consistent with its primary structure, which resembles other apolipoproteins as it contains amphipathic helical sequences capable of lipid-binding [4,5]. It is not yet clear whether the binding of SAA to HDL involves displacement of some phospholipid or if these changes, that occur with the acute phase response, take place independently. The lipid binding site of SAA has not yet been characterized, though it has been predicted to lie within sequences 2-25 [4] or, a part of it, in sequence 1-11 [5] of the N-terminus of the SAA molecule according to its hydrophobicity and amphipathic α-helical content. Although the NH_2-terminal sequence of SAA is not identical in different species, it is homologous and, most importantly, the linear pattern of hydrophilicity is conserved [5]. Another presumptive lipid-binding site -

residues 47 to 58 - lies within the predicted calcium binding site, but calcium-mediated attachment cannot be the sole bond to lipid because SAA is not eluted from HDL by EDTA [5].

Materials and Methods

Peptides: *a.* Naturally occurring fragments NOR1 and NOR2, corresponding to residues 2–82 and 2-45, were purified from amyloidotic goiter of FMF patient NOR [6]. *b.* Synthetic peptides, corresponding to residues 1-6, 2-15, 6-11, 7-15, 7-19, 11-19, 12-19, 15-19 and 29-41, were synthesized by solid phase peptide synthesis according to Merrifield [7] (Fig. 1). *Production of monoclonal antibodies*: AA peptide corresponding to residues 2-45 (NOR2) was covalently linked to a carrier protein (KLH, BSA) via a bifunctional reagent [1-ethyl-3-(3'-dimethylaminopropyl)carbodiimide hydrochloride] [8]. Two-month old BALB/c mice were immunized with NOR2-KLH conjugate. Spleen cells were hybridized with NSo myeloma cells. Hybridoma supernatants were screened for antibody production on NOR2-BSA conjugate using ELISA. Three MoAbs were chosen for the following studies. *Direct binding of anti-NOR2 MoAbs to SAA and related fragments*. Microtiter plates were coated with SAA and related fragments. Serial dilutions of MoAbs 450/1, 485/11 and 872/18 were added to the plates and the binding to the antigen was quantitated by adding goat anti-mouse IgG conjugated to alkaline phosphatase, following by p-nitrophenyl phosphate. The results were monitored with an automatic ELISA reader (405 nm). *Inhibition of binding of anti-NOR2 MoAbs to NOR2 by SAA-related peptides*. The MoAbs [in dilutions of 1/600 (450/1), 1/120 (485/11) and 1/3000 (872/18)], preincubated with serial dilutions (0.1-5000 μg/ml) of the SAA-related peptides (0.1-5,000 μg/ml) were added to NOR2 coated plates. Inhibition of the binding was monitored by ELISA. *Electrofocusing and immunoblotting*. Acute-phase HDL was electrofocused in denaturing conditions and immunoblotted using the MoAbs [9].

Results and Discussion

Three MoAbs of the IgG1 isotype were prepared from mice immunized with NOR2-KLH. Two of these MoAbs (450/1 and 872/18) bind to SAA and AA, in addition to NOR2, while a third one (485/11) binds to NOR2 only (Fig. 2). In order to locate the antigenic determinant SAA-related peptides (Fig. 1) were used in competition assays. The results of these assays are summarized in Fig. 3. The binding of all three MoAbs to NOR2 was inhibited by free NOR1 and NOR2, though considerably lower concentrations were needed to inhibit MoAb 485/11. Significant inhibition of MoAbs binding was obtained with peptide 2-15 only. Poor inhibition was obtained for MoAb 485/11 with peptides 1-6 and 29-41, while for MoAbs 450/1 and 872/18 with 29-41 only. No inhibition was noticed with peptides 1-6 (for MoAbs 450/1 and 872/18), 6-11, 7-15, 7-19, 11-19, 12-19 and 15-19. The amount of peptides needed for 50% inhibition is summarized in Table 1. The results indicate that all three MoAbs are directed against the N-terminal region of the SAA molecule.

Despite the fact that MoAbs 450/1 and 872/18 recognize purified SAA (Fig. 2), as well as SAA dissolved in normal human sera, they do not recognize SAA in acute-phase sera (results not shown). When SAA-enriched acute-phase HDL was electrofocused in denaturing conditons (8M urea) and immunoblotted (Fig. 4), all SAA isoforms were recognized by the MoAbs. It should be emphasized that these MoAbs recognize SAA in its delipidated form. In the case of MoAb 485/11, a complete denaturation of SAA is required for recognition (recognizes SAA after IEF in denaturing conditions but not after purification procedures - Fig. 2). Another MoAb derived from rat immunized with NOR2-KLH recognizes SAA in the SAA-HDL complex of acute-phase sera. This MoAb was significantly inhibited by peptide 29-41. These findings denote that the antigenic determinant of the mouse MoAbs, which lies within the N-terminal of SAA, contrary to the rat MoAb determinant, which lies within the 29-41 residues of SAA, is not exposed in the SAA-HDL complex. It also implies that the N-terminus of SAA is its lipid binding site. The conclusion reached from all our results supports the computer-based predictions that sequences 2-25 [4] or a part of it, sequence 1-11 [5], due to their hydrophobicity and amphipathic helical regions, are suitable for lipid-associated domain.

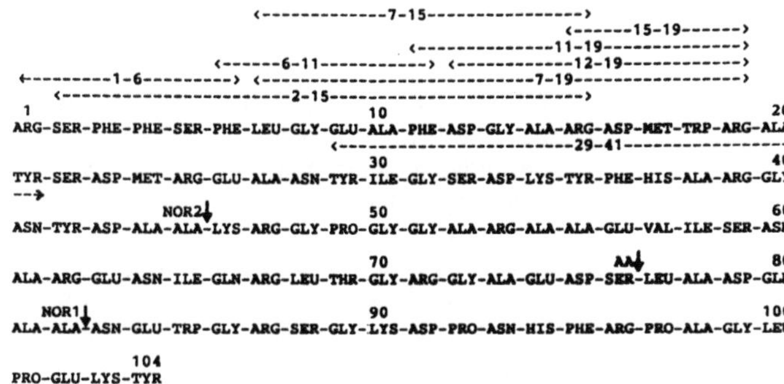

Fig. 1. SAA and related peptides

Fig. 2. Binding of MoAbs 450/1, 485/11, 872/18, respectively, to SAA (⊞), AA (■) NOR2-BSA (◆) as determined by ELISA. Second antibody (BSA ▲)

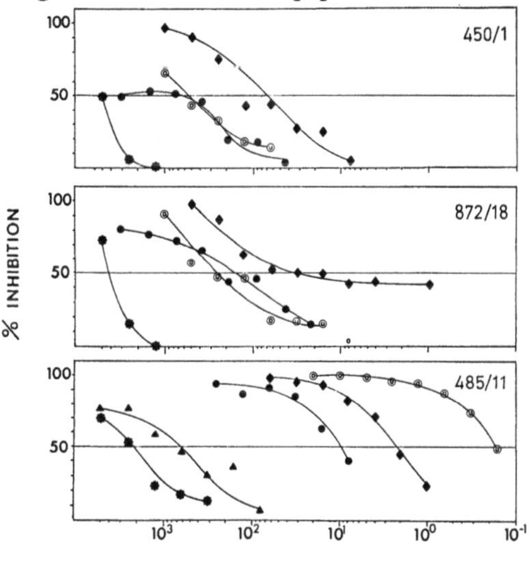

Fig. 3. Competition assay in which the binding of MoAb to NOR2-coated plates was inhibited by prior incubation of the the MoAbs NOR1 (●), NOR2 (◆), 2-15 (◎), 1-6 (▲) 29-41 (✱). No inhibition was obtained with the other peptides.

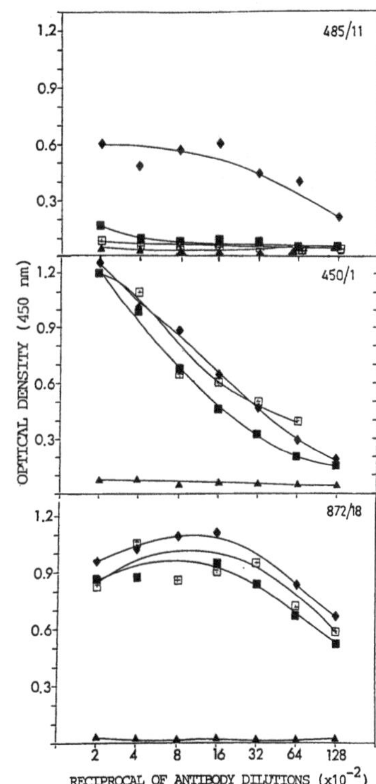

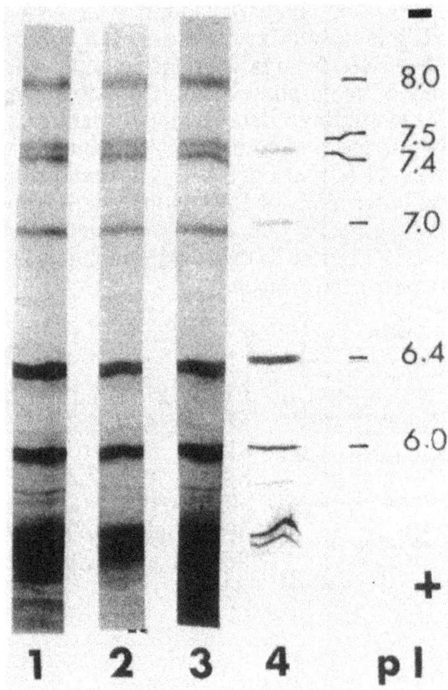

Table 1. Peptide concentration μg/ml

MoAbs	1-6	2-15	6-11	29-41	NOR2	NOR1
450/1	*	530	*	5000	620	73
485/11	640	0.17	*	2300	2.2	10
872/18	*	270	*	4200	45	160

*No inhibition was observed with 5000 μg/m

Fig. 4. Immunogold silver staining of nitrocellulose blots of electrofocused, delipidated, acute-phase-HDL, with MoAbs (αNOR2) showing 6 isoforms of SAA. LANES 1-3: MoAbs 872/18, 485/11, 450/1, respectively. LANE 4: Coomasie blue staining of electrofocusing gel of SAA, which was performed on acrylamine gel containing ampholytes 20%, pH 3.0-10.0, 40% pH 4.0-6.5, 40% pH 7.0-9.0 in the presence of 8 M urea.

References

1. Benditt, E.P. and Erikson, N. (1977) 'Amyloid protein SAA is associated with high density lipoprotein from human serum', Proc. Natl. Acad. Sci. USA 74, 4025-4028.
2. Coetzee, G.A., Strachan, A.F., van der Westhuyzen, D.R., Hoppe, H.C., Jeenah, M.S. and de Beer, F.C. (1986) 'Serum amyloid A - containing human high density lipoproteins', J. Biol. Chem. 261, 9644-9651.
3. Clifton, P.M., Mackinnon, A.M. and Barter, P.J. (1985) 'Effects of serum amyloid A protein (SAA) on composition, size and density of high density lipoproteins in subjects with myocardial infarction', J. Lipid Res. 26, 1389-1398.
4. Segrest, J.P. and Feldman, R.J. (1977) 'Amphipathic helixes and plasma lipoproteins: a computer study', Biopolymers 16, 2053-2065.
5. Turnell, W., Sarra, R., Glover, I.D., Baum, J.O., Caspi, D., Blatz, M. and Pepys, M.B. (1981) 'Secondary structure prediction of human SAA_1. Presumptive identification of calcium and lipid binding sites', Mol. Biol. Med. 3, 387-407.
6. Prelli, F., Pras, M. and Frangione, B. (1987) 'Degradation and deposition of amyloid AA fibrils are tissue-specific', Biochemistry 26, 8251-8256.
7. Merrifield, R.B. (1963) 'Solid phase synthesis. I. The synthesis of a tetrapeptide', J. Am. Soc. Chem. 85, 2149-2154.
8. Müller, G.M., Shapira, M., Arnon, R. (1982) 'Anti-influenza response achieved by immunization with a synthetic conjugate', Proc. Natl. Acad. Sci. USA 79, 569-573.
9. Strachan, A.F., Shephard, E.G., Bellstedt, D.U., Coetzee, G.A., van der Westhuyzen, D.R. and de Beer, F.C. (1989) 'Human serum amyloid A protein. Behaviour in aqueous and urea-containing solutions and antibody production', Biochem. J. 263, 365-370.

EPITOPE MAPPING OF AMYLOID-A PROTEIN USING MONOCLONAL ANTIBODIES

B. Frankenberger, S. Modrow, R.P. Linke

Institute for Immunology, Goethestr.31, D-8000 Munich
Pettenkofer-Department of Microbiology, D-8000 Munich

ABSTRACT. In order to identify the fine-specificity of monoclonal antibodies (mc8, mc12, mc20, mc29) against amyloid A, which were shown before to bind to both, the isolated AA and the AA-type amyloid fibrils in tissue sections, we employed synthetic peptides covering the entire length of AA as well as CNBr polypeptides. The results show, that the monoclonals bind to different epitopes.
Out of four anti-AA antibodies two could be assigned to distinct regions of the AA_9 molecule: mc20 recognizes AA 60-75 and mc29 recognizes AA 28-40, while mc8 and mc12 did only bind to the intact protein and the largest CNBr-peptide, but not to any of the tested AA-peptides.

1. INTRODUCTION

The deposition of amyloid-A (AA) in degradation-resistant fibrillar form is characteristic for the life-threatening disease AA-amyloidosis, which often follows long lasting inflammations (1).
AA-amyloidosis is best diagnosted in tissue sections by AA-type antibodies using immunohistochemistry (2). For diagnostic purposes we have produced murine monoclonal antibodies against human AA (3).
In order to better define the target-specificities of our monoclonals we employed different antigenic probes together with a high sensitive micro-ELISA.
The tested probes were the following:
1) isolated AA protein as well as the serum precursor SAA_{12}
2) a series of 7 different partially overlapping, synthetic peptides of AA
3) cyanogen bromide generated AA-polypeptides

2. MATERIAL AND METHODS

2.1 Monoclonal antibodies

Monoclonal antibodies against amyloid fibril protein AA were produced by cell fusion of murine P3x63-Ag8.653 myeloma cells with spleen cells of immunized BALB/c mice (3).

The specificity of these monoclonals, prepared in our laboratory, was demonstrated by non-reactivity to serum proteins and other non-AA amyloid fibril proteins, i.e. Aλ (LOH). Only protein AA and its precursor-molecule SAA_{12} showed strong reaction employing an micro-ELISA . Furthermore, monoclonality was demonstrated by the presence of only one single isotype. Additional characteristics such as reactivity-strength in the immunoperoxidase-technique (IP) or in electronmicroscopy (EM) are described in Table 1.

2.2 Peptides

Besides the insoluble AA protein and its serum precursor SAA_{12}, a series of various synthetic peptides have been used for the epitope mapping. These peptides represent partially overlapping streches corresponding to human AA protein according to the sequence of SAA_{12} by Parmelee et al.(5). All these peptides corresponding to their respective residues are summarized in Table 2. They have been synthesized by an automatic peptide synthesizer (430-A, Applied Biosystem. Inc., USA). Moreover, additional peptides of AA were prepared by CNBr-digestion and separation on Sephadex G-100 in 6M guanidine-HCl.

2.3 Micro-ELISA

The above-mentioned antigenic probes have been employed (at 2µg/ml) for the epitope mapping of our monoclonals using the high sensitive micro-ELISA detection system.
Antigens were coupled to micro-ELISA plates (Dynatech M129B, Plochingen) in 0,1M NH_4HCO_3. The monoclonal antibody was used as culture supernatant at serial dilutions. The detection system consisted of anti-murine IgG from sheep (1/200) and a monoclonal (mc100) antiperoxidase peroxidase complex; the substrate-chromogen solution was ABTS (3). The oxidized chromogen was measured at 420nm using a micro-ELISA reader (Flow Laboratories, Munich). The reaction was considered positive when the signal was more than 20 times over background.

3. RESULTS AND DISCUSSION

Out of four monoclonal AA-antibodies tested two, mc20 and mc29, could be assigned to distinct regions of the intact proteins AA and SAA_{12}. So, peptide 5 corresponding to positions 60-75 reacted with mc20, while peptide 7 (residues 28-40) showed reaction with mc29. All monoclonal antibodies recognized not only the intact proteins AA and SAA_{12}, but also the largest CNBr-peptide 10, while fetal calf serum or non-AA amyloid fibril proteins have been negative in the micro-ELISA (negative control).
Most of the peptides did not react at all, despite covering the entire molecule. The reasons may be as follows: it is possible that short peptides consisting of about 10-15 amino acids are showing a different conformation as compared to the equivalent region within the intact protein. Therefore,

Table 1. Characteristics of monoclonal anti-AA antibodies

No.	Clon-No.	Isotype (3)*	IP (3)	EM (4)
1	mc8	IgG3 k	++	o
2	mc12	IgG2bk	++	o
3	mc20	IgG2ak	++	++
4	mc29	IgG1 k	+++	+

* References in brackets

Table 2. Reactivity of antigenic probes with our four monoclonal antibodies by micro-ELISA

Peptide	Residues	Monoclonal antibodies mc8	mc12	mc20	mc29
SAA_{12}(KEL)*	AA 1-104	+	+	+	+
AA_9(KIR)	AA 1- 76	+	+	+	+
FCS		-	-	-	-
Aλ(LOH)		-	-	-	-
1	AA 7- 22	-	-	-	-
2	AA23- 32	-	-	-	-
3	AA33- 44	-	-	-	-
4	AA45- 59	-	-	-	-
5	AA60- 75	-	-	+	-
6	AA76- 91	-	-	-	-
7	AA28- 40	-	-	-	+
8	AA 1- 17	-	-	-	-
9	AA18- 24	-	-	-	-
10	AA25- 76	+	+	+	+

A = proteins, isolated from serum and organs
B = synthetic peptides
C = CNBr-fragments of AA_9
* = abbreviation of patient's name

monoclonal antibodies raised against native proteins often fail to recognize peptides of the corresponding area. Another possible reason could be conformational changes of the peptides by adsorption to the ELISA plate or low affinity of short peptides to the antibody caused by missing stability from flanking streches. Furthermore, the full heterogeneity of the AA molecule is not reflected by the choice of synthetic peptides, which were chosen according to the sequence reported by Parmelee (5).
By contrast, distinct regions of a peptide frequently constitute a stable threedimensional conformation, thus forming an epitope which is very similar to that in the intact protein. We can assume that the two epitopes described here belong to these peptides.
Interestingly, peptide 9 (comprising by residues 28–40), which forms the epitope for mc29 is evolutionary conserved within the AA proteins. So it is conceivable that this anti-AA antibody mc29 could be a useful tool in identifying the amyloid fibrils of AA-type on paraffin-embedded sections and their precursor proteins from various animal species.
Epitope mapping may be important for revealing functionally important epitopes as well as different iso- and allotypes of AA and SAA_{12}.

4. REFERENCES

1. Benditt, E.P., Eriksen, N.: Chemical classes of amyloid substance.
   Am. J. Pathol. 65, 231, 1971
2. Glenner, G.G.: Amyloid deposits and amyloidosis. The β-fibrilloses.
   New Engl. J. Med. 302, 1283, 1333, 1980
3. Linke, R.P.: Monoclonal antibodies against amyloid fibril protein AA.
   J. Histochem. Cytochem. 32, 322, 1984
4. Linke, R.P., Huhn, D., Casanova, S., Donini, U.: Immuno-electron microscopic identification of human AA-type amyloid.
   Lab. Invest., 61, 691, 1989
5. Parmelee, D.C., Titani, K., Ericsson, L.H., Eriksen, N., Benditt, E.P., Walsh, K.A.: Amino acid sequence of amyloid-related apoprotein ($apoSAA_1$) from human high-density lipoprotein.
   Biochemistry, 21, 3298, 1982

5. ACKNOWLEDGMENTS

This study was supported by the Deutsche Forschungsgemeinschaft, SFB 207, project G8. We thank Mss. A. Kerling and A. Rail for technical assistance.

REACTIVE (AA) AMYLOIDOSIS IN A 14 YEAR OLD WITH NO PREDISPOSING DISEASE

Quinn, L., Shafer, E., Liepnieks, J.J., and Benson, M.D.
Indiana University School of Medicine, Department of Medicine
Rheumatology Division, Clinical Building 492, 541 Clinical Drive
Indianapolis, IN 46223; VA Medical Center (583/111RH), 1481 West
10th Street, Indianapolis, IN 46202, USA.

ABSTRACT. Reactive (AA) amyloidosis usually occurs in relation to chronic inflammation or infection. It also occurs in individuals with familial Mediterranean fever (FMF) and occasionally in asymptomatic individuals within FMF kindreds. Infrequently, adults present with AA amyloidosis without predisposing disease, but such cases are extremely rare in children. We report the case of a 13 year old Caucasian male who presented with weakness, lethargy, and an abdominal mass. Resection of the mass revealed mesenteric lymph nodes heavily infiltrated with amyloid. Liver, gastric, duodenal, and rectal biopsies were positive for amyloid. Immunohistochemistry of the resected lymph nodes with monoclonal antibody to human AA was positive. Amyloid fibrils isolated from the nodes were solubilized, fractionated, and digested with trypsin. Amino acid sequence analysis of tryptic peptides confirmed the AA structure with predominance of SAA1-derived AA. Complete patient history and physical exam elicited no evidence of infection, inflammation, or family history of FMF type illness. We report this as a case of spontaneous reactive (AA) amyloidosis in the pediatric age group.

INTRODUCTION

Reactive (AA) amyloidosis involves the deposition of amyloid fibrils composed of protein AA, a degradation product of the polymorphic serum amyloid A (SAA) protein. It is usually associated with chronic infections or inflammatory diseases such as rheumatoid arthritis, granulomatous bowel disease, or osteomyelitis. It also occurs in individuals with FMF or occasionally in asymptomatic individuals within FMF kindreds. Infrequently, there are reports of adults diagnosed with AA amyloidosis by immunohistochemistry, but with no evidence of underlying disease [1,2,3]. Similar instances in the pediatric age group are extremely rare. We are reporting the case of an otherwise healthy Caucasian male initially diagnosed with AA amyloidosis by immunohistochemistry at 13 years of age; we have sequenced his isolated amyloid fibrils to verify the AA structure.

CASE REPORT

A 13 year old previously healthy Caucasian male presented to his local physician with a history of lethargy, weakness, decreased appetite,and increased fluid intake of several months duration. Urinalysis showed

4+ protein, so he was referred to the University of Kentucky for further evaluation. On physical exam he was noted to have hepatosplenomegaly and an abdominal mass. Laboratory tests indicated anemia and proteinuria. Bone marrow aspirate was normal. As the patient's mass was thought to be cancer, he underwent exploratory laparotomy. During surgery, the mass was found to consist of enlarged mesenteric and periaortic lymph nodes. Pathology of the resected mass revealed no evidence of cancer, but extensive amyloid deposition within lymph nodes. The patient was referred to the Indiana University Amyloid Research Center.

Immunohistochemistry of pathology specimens showed positive staining with monoclonal antibody to human AA, consistent with a diagnosis of reactive (AA) amyloidosis. For this reason the patient was carefully evaluated for any predisposing conditions. History and physical exam were negative for chronic infection, inflammatory disease, neoplasia, or family history of FMF type illnesses. He did have one episode of anemia at six years of age that resolved with a three month course of vitamins and iron. He was otherwise a healthy and active child. Laboratory evaluation was significant for a hemoglobin of 12.4 g/dl, with a mean corpuscular volume of 62.9 fl. Serum liver enzyme levels were mildly elevated. Blood urea nitrogen and creatinine were within normal limits, but urinalysis showed 2+ protein and 5-10 red blood cells per high power field. A 24 hour urine collection contained 432 mg protein. Creatinine clearance was 108 ml/min. Further evaluation included a ^{99}Technetium pyrophosphate bone scan which revealed hepatosplenomegaly with marked uptake of tracer by liver and spleen, and bilateral renal enlargement. Cardiac evaluation was normal. Chest X-ray was normal, and roentgenograms of the lumbar spine and sacroiliac joints showed no evidence of ankylosing spondylitis. Upper and lower endoscopies as well as upper GI series with small bowel follow through were normal, but biopsies of the stomach, duodenum, colon, rectum, and liver were all strongly positive for amyloid.

The patient was felt to have reactive (AA) amyloidosis, although no predisposing conditions were detected. He was discharged on ferrous sulfate and 0.6 mg colchicine a day. Reevaluation one year later showed a continuing negative history and physical exam for infection, inflammation, neoplasia, or other predisposing condition. The patient had gained considerable weight and was active again. His anemia had completely resolved, and repeat pyrophosphate bone scans revealed absence of hepatomegaly with remarkably reduced uptake by the liver and spleen.

MATERIALS AND METHODS

Amyloid fibrils were isolated from formaldehyde fixed lymph nodes by homogenization and centrifugation. The isolated fibrils were reduced and alkylated, then fractionated on a Sepharose CL6B column (2.5 X 90 cm). The subunit protein was digested with TPCK-treated trypsin at pH

8.0. Tryptic peptides were fractionated on an Altex Ultrasphere C-18 column eluted with an acetonitrile gradient in 0.1% TFA. Peptides were sequentially degraded on a Beckman 890C sequenator and PTH-amino acids were identified by HPLC.

RESULTS AND DISCUSSION

Biochemical studies were undertaken to confirm the AA sequence of the amyloid fibrils and to identify any abnormalities in protein structure. Reduction and alkylation of amyloid fibrils extracted from mesenteric lymph nodes gave a subunit protein of approximately 8,000 daltons. Amino acid sequence analysis of peptides after trypsin digestion revealed typical AA structure.

SAA, the serum precursor of AA, is polymorphic; the three forms identified are SAA1, SAA2α, and SAA2β. We evaluated the yields on sequence analysis of tryptic peptides T9 and T8-9, which are unique in SAA1 and SAA2 as shown in the figure below, to determine the percentage of SAA1- to SAA2-derived AA in the amyloid deposits.

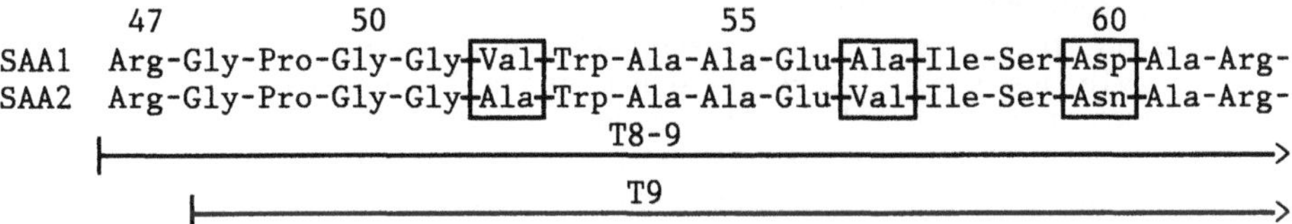

The results indicated a predominance of SAA1-derived AA, with a ratio of 89% SAA1 to 11% SAA2α and 2β. This ratio is similar to that found in other patients with reactive (AA) amyloidosis [4]. Interestingly, the ratio of SAA1 to SAA2 in the serum of patients with reactive amyloidosis is approximately 2:1 [5]. The reason for this disparity in serum as well as the further enhanced presence of SAA1-derived AA in amyloid fibrils, is unclear. Possible explanations could include increased turnover of SAA2α and 2β or differences in gene expression.

The distribution of amyloid deposits in the patient, his clinical course, and the results of the biochemical analysis of his amyloid fibrils are all consistent with reactive (AA) amyloidosis. This disease, when seen in children, is frequently associated with juvenile rheumatoid arthritis (JRA). To date, however, there is no evidence of any predisposing disease in our patient. There is also no evidence of any abnormality in the AA structure of his amyloid fibrils. The etiology of this patient's amyloidosis remains uncertain, but may involve abnormal gene expression or SAA protein processing.

There is no known specific therapy for reactive amyloidosis. There are several well-documented cases of spontaneous regression of amyloid deposits in children with JRA usually corresponding to remission of the underlying JRA. Our patient's improvement on colchicine is remarkable in that he has no identifiable predisposing disease.

Colchicine has been shown to prevent the occurrence of amyloidosis in individuals with FMF, and may inhibit further deposition of fibrils in patients with amyloidosis. It is not known to cause regression of the disease. The disappearance of amyloid deposits in this patient is therefore highly unusual. Whether it is related to the colchicine therapy or to pathogenetic mechanisms involved in the initial disease process remains to be investigated.

ACKNOWLEDGEMENTS

This work was supported by VA Medical Research, the United States Public Health Service (RR-00750, NIDDK-34881, NIAMS-AR20582, AR7448), The Arthritis Foundation, The Grace M. Showalter Trust and The Marion E. Jacobson Fund.

REFERENCES

1. Pras, M., Zaretzky, J., Frangione, B., Franklin, E.C. (1980) 'AA protein in a case of "primary" or "idiopathic" amyloidosis,' Am. J. Med. 68, 291-294.
2. Picken, M.M., Pelton, K., Frangione, B., Gallo, G. (1987) 'Primary amyloidosis A. Immunohistochemical and biochemical characterization,' Am. J. Pathol. 129, 536-542.
3. Glantz, L.K., Miller, F., Gorevic, P.D. (1989) 'Idiopathic amyloidosis due to AA protein: a report of 2 cases,' J. Histotechnol. 12, 137-140.
4. Liepnieks, J.J., Leagre, C., Kluve-Beckerman, B., Benson, M.D. (1990) 'Predominance of one SAA isotype (SAA1) in human reactive amyloid,' VIth International Symposium on Amyloidosis, Oslo, Norway.
5. Kluve-Beckerman, B., Liepnieks, J., Benson, M.D. (1990) 'Differential regulation of human serum amyloid A isoforms,' VIth International Symposium on Amyloidosis, Oslo, Norway.

INDUCTION OF AMYLOIDOSIS IN MICE: PREPARATION OF ACTIVE AZOCASEIN (AZO) AND EFFECT OF ENDOTOXIN (LPS).

Louise M. Greene, Wayne A. Gonnerman, Edgar S. Cathcart
Departments of Medicine and Biochemistry
Boston University School of Medicine, Boston, MA and
E.N. Rogers Memorial VA Hospital, Bedford, MA.

ABSTRACT. Frequent failure to induce amyloidosis in mice with multiple injections of casein prompted this study to compare the effectiveness of AZO prepared and sterilized by various methods. The direct effect of LPS contamination of AZO was determined by comparing four protocols all including daily subcutaneous (s.c.) injections of AZO for 20 days; a) no other injections; b) daily intraperitoneal (i.p.) injections of 1 μg LPS; c) a single initial i.p. injection of 10 μg LPS; and d) daily i.p. injections of 10 μg LPS. Daily i.p. injections of 1 μg LPS had no additional effect on amyloid induction when compared to AZO alone. With both C57Bl and CBA/J mice, daily 10 μg LPS injections protected against amyloid deposition. With C57Bl mice, both severity and incidence of amyloid were reduced. With CBA/J mice, the severity of amyloid deposition was reduced, but not the incidence. The three types of casein derivatized to prepare AZO (purified grade, or technical grade with one or with two precipitations) resulted in a progressively increasing incidence of amyloidosis. After derivatization of casein to AZO and concentration by ultrafiltration, sterilization by autoclaving or filtration produced a less-effective material than sterilization by exposure to diethyl pyrocarbonate (DEP).

INTRODUCTION

Murine amyloidosis has been shown to be a useful model of human secondary amyloidosis (1). We have examined the effect of LPS on the incidence and severity of amyloid induction by AZO in two strains of mice. The AZO was prepared by improved methods, sterilized by autoclaving, filtration, or DEP treatment, and evaluated for efficacy in inducing amyloid.

MATERIALS AND METHODS.

Mice: Male CBA/J mice, 2 months old, were obtained from Jackson Laboratory, Bar Harbor, Maine. Male C57Bl/6N mice, 4 months old, were obtained from Charles River Laboratories, Wilmington, MA.

Azocasein: Azocasein was prepared by modifications of the method of Janigan and Druet (2) from Casein, purified grade (Sigma), or Casein, technical grade (Sigma) with either 1 or 2 precipitations. After dialysis, the azocasein was concentrated 2-fold by Omegacell 30 K (Pharmacia) ultrafiltration and sterilized by autoclaving for 20 minutes, filter-sterilizing with a disposable 0.45 μm filter unit (Nalgene), or treatment with diethyl pyrocarbonate (DEP) (3) (0.5 ml per 50 ml AZO solution for 2 hours with mixing). The protein concentration was measured by the method of Lowry, *et al.* (4).

Amyloid Induction: Mice were given daily (five times per week), subcutaneous injections of sterile 10% (w/v) AZO in 0.3 ml doses for 20 days. Some mice were also injected intraperitoneally (i.p.) with LPS from *S. typhimurium* (RIBI Immunochem), either 1 µg/day, 10 µg/day, or a single initial injection of 10 µg LPS. After the mice were sacrificed by CO_2 asphyxiation, sections of spleen were removed from identical central locations, squashed and stained with Congo Red (5). Green birefringent material when viewed by polarized light microscopy was considered a positive test for amyloid. The degree of amyloid formation was scored blindly on a scale from 1+ to 4+ (6).

RESULTS

At 10 µg daily, injections of LPS protected C57Bl mice against amyloid induction in both incidence and severity (Fig. 1). AZO solutions prepared from purified grade casein, technical grade casein precipitated only once, and technical grade casein precipitated twice were compared for efficacy in inducing amyloid. Commercial purification of casein reduced its ability to stimulate amyloid production when it was used as the starting material for AZO preparation. Precipitating the technical grade casein only once during AZO preparation resulted in AZO which produced only a 20% incidence of amyloid (data not shown) compared to 80% incidence when two precipitations were done (Fig. 1).

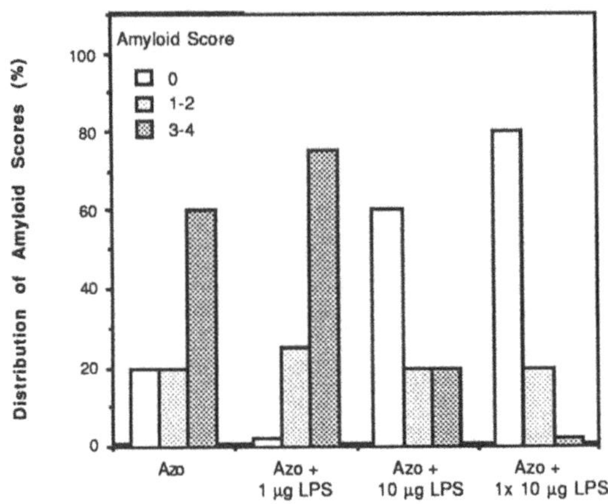

Figure 1. Effect of LPS on Induction of Amyloidosis in C57Bl Mice. Mice were injected daily (0.3 ml s.c., 5 times per week) with AZO and i.p. with 0, 1 µg LPS, or 10 µg LPS, or once on day 1 with 10 µg LPS. After 20 injections, mice were sacrificed and the severity of amyloid in the spleen was assessed.

It appears that since CBA/J mice are more susceptible to the induction of amyloidosis than C57Bl mice (7), the protective effect of LPS is more easily overcome in these mice. While LPS does not influence the incidence of amyloidosis in CBA/J mice, it does reduce the severity of the amyloid deposited (Table 1). While all AZO-injected mice got amyloidosis, those also injected with 10 μg LPS daily had much less amyloid deposited in their spleens.

Table 1. Effect of LPS on Induction of Amyloid in CBA/J Mice

	AZO	AZO + 1 μg LPS	AZO + 1x 10 μg LPS	AZO+Daily 10 μg LPS	Control
Number	8	4	4	4	4
Score (Mean±S.D.)	3.3 ± 0.5	2.75 ± 0.5	3.25 ± 0.9	1.5 ± 0.6	0
Incidence(%)	100	100	100	100	0

AZO was injected daily (0.3 ml s.c., 5 days per week). LPS was injected i.p. at the same time in the dose indicated. After 20 injections, mice were sacrificed and the severity of amyloid in the spleens was assessed.

AZO solutions sterilized by different methods induced amyloidosis at different times and at different rates (Fig. 2). AZO sterilized by treatment with DEP induced amyloid earliest, after only 12 injections. Autoclaved AZO and filtered AZO required 20 injections to achieve the same level of amyloid scores as the DEP-treated AZO achieved with 12 injections. All three preparations had comparable levels of protein (data not shown).

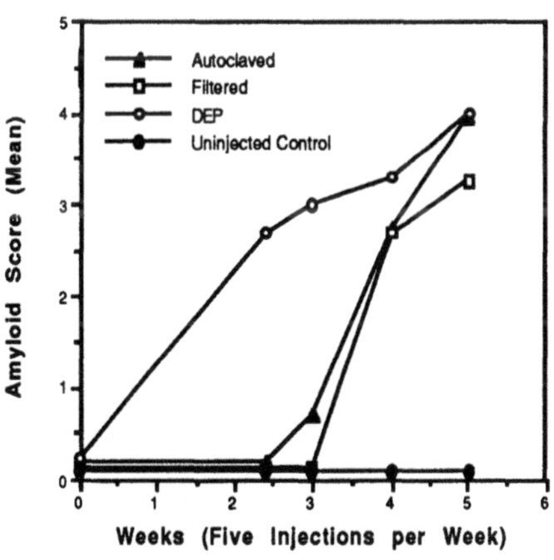

Figure 2. Induction of Amyloid in CBA/J Mice by Azocasein Sterilized by Various Means. Azocasein solutions were sterlizedby different methods. CBA/J mice were injected with AZO daily (0.3 ml s.c., five times per week). At the indicated times 3 mice were sacrificed and the severity of amylolid in the spleen was assessed.

DISCUSSION

LPS is known to be a potent inducer of acute-phase reactants such as serum amyloid A (SAA)(8). SAA is thought to give rise to amyloid A (AA), the fibril protein, by proteolytic cleavage (9). Since AZO induces deposition of amyloid, it was expected that LPS, which independently causes an increase in SAA, would enhance amyloidosis, not diminish it. This unexpected protective effect of LPS may be a reflection of the complex nature of the immunological events involved in amyloidosis.

By rendering AZO solutions sterile, the variation in amyloid induction due to possible bacterial growth and consequent LPS contamination is eliminated. Sterilization with DEP avoids the protein denaturation which occurs on autoclaving and the lengthy sterile filtration method. After derivatization of casein to AZO and concentration by ultrafiltration, sterilization by DEP treatment produced an effective inducer of amyloid.

ACKNOWLEDGEMENT.

We thank Dr. Richard A. Greene for his excellent technical assistance in the preparation of this manuscript.

REFERENCES.

1. Skinner, M., Shirahama, T., Benson, M.D. and Cohen, A.S. (1977) Murine amyloid protein AA in casein-induced experimental amyloidosis. Lab. Invest. 36, 420-427.
2. Janigan, D.T. and Druet, R.L. (1966) Experimental Amyloidosis. Am. J. of Pathol. 48,1013-25.
3. Huvos, P., Gaal, O., Vereczkey, L. and Solymosy, F. (1971) Dissociation of rat liver polyribosomes upon treatment with diethyl pyrocarbonate. Acta Biochim. et Biophys. Acad. Sci. Hung. 6, 317-325.
4. Lowry, O.H., Rosebrough, N.J., Farr, A.L. and Randall, R.J. (1951) Protein measurement with the Folin phenol reagent. J. Biol. Chem. 193, 265-275.
5. Puchtler, H., Sweat, F. and Levine, M. (1962) On the binding of Congo red by amyloid. J. Histochem. Cytochem 10, 355-363.
6. Cathcart, E.S., Leslie, C.A., Meydani, S. and Hayes, K.C. (1987) A fish oil diet retards experimental amyloidosis, modulates lymphocyte function, and decreases macrophage arachidonate metabolism in mice. J. Immunol. 139, 1850-1854.
7. Wohlgethan, J.R. and Cathcart, E.S. (1981) Amyloidosis in (CBA/J x A/J) F_2 mice: Correlation of amyloid resistance and low mitogenic response to Concanavalin A. J. Immunol. 127, 1003-1007.
8. Morrison, D.C. and Ulevitch, R.J. (1978) The effects of bacterial endotoxins on host mediation systems. Am. J. Pathol. 93, 526-617.
9. Husebekk, A., Skogen, B., Husby, G.and Marhaug, G. (1985) Transformation of amyloid precursor SAA to protein AA and incorporation in amyloid fibrils in vivo. Scand. J. Immunol. 21, 282-287.

SERUM AMYLOID A (SAA) INDUCTION IN THE SERUM HIGH DENSITY LIPOPROTEINS OF THE SYRIAN HAMSTER

N. ERIKSEN, R. L. MEEK, AND E. P. BENDITT
Dept. of Pathology (SJ-60), University of Washington
Seattle, Washington 98195, U.S.A.

ABSTRACT. SAA elevations in the serum lipoproteins of hamsters were induced by injection of lipopolysaccharide intraperitoneally or turpentine subcutaneously. Lipoprotein fractions isolated by sequential density centrifugation of serum samples obtained 20-hours post-stimulus were examined by SDS-PAGE followed by electroimmunoblotting. We observed a marked enhancement of a ~12-kDa doublet in the electrophoretic pattern of the acute-phase HDL_3. Antibodies to human or monkey AA reacted preferentially with the leading member of the doublet, whereas antibodies to mouse AA reacted preferentially with the trailing member. Antibodies to human and mouse SAA and to duck AA reacted with both members. The different reactions displayed by the members of the hamster SAA doublet against the several antibody preparations suggest that at least two of the three proteins predicted by a study of SAA-gene expression in the hamster may circulate in the HDL.

Introduction

Serum amyloid A (SAA) levels in hamsters that had been injected with casein or with amyloid enhancing factor followed by casein have been measured by use of rabbit antibodies to hamster AA [1]; more recently an association between SAA and the plasma lipoproteins of hamsters has been reported [2]. In this paper we describe the induction of SAA apoproteins in the high density fraction of the serum lipoproteins of hamsters by injection of turpentine or bacterial lipopolysaccharide (LPS), and immunoreactions of these apoproteins with antibodies made against AA and SAA proteins derived from three mammalian and one avian species.

Materials and Methods

Acute-Phase Induction. A group of eight female golden Syrian hamsters (age 7-8 weeks) was divided into sets of two. One pair was untreated. A second pair was injected intraperitoneally, per animal, with 50 μg E. coli LPS W in 100 μl PBS; a third pair, with 250 μg LPS in 500 μl PBS. The fourth pair was injected subcutaneously, per animal, with 0.5 ml gum turpentine; the dose was divided among three sites. Serum samples were obtained 20 hours later; paired serums were pooled and stored at -18° C for two weeks before separation of lipoprotein fractions.

Preparation of Serum Lipoprotein Fractions. Lipoprotein fractions were separated by sequential density centrifugation [3] of 3.0-ml serum samples initially diluted to fill tubes of ~6-ml capacity. Flotation layers (top 1.5 ml) were removed by aspiration at each density, dialyzed in 3.5-kDa-cutoff tubing against PBS, made up to 2.0 ml with PBS, and stored at -18° C until analyzed.

Molecular-Sizing Electrophoresis. The lipoprotein fractions were analyzed by SDS-PAGE [4] modified by the inclusion of urea: 6.4 M in the separating gel, 4.3 M in the stacking gel, and 5M in the sample buffer. Before application to the gel, samples were heated for 3 minutes at 100° C with sufficient sample buffer (5% 2-mercaptoethanol added) to provide a several-fold excess of SDS over protein. Molecular mass standards were commercially available proteins, duck AA protein [5], and human $apoSAA_1$ and $apoSAA_2$, purified by ion-exchange chromatography [6]. The calculated molecular mass of duck AA, a 106-residue protein, is 11,587 Da [7]; of human $apoSAA_1$, a 104-residue protein, 11,685 Da [8]; of human $apoSAA_2$, which is identical to human $apoSAA_1$

except that it lacks the N-terminal arginine, 11,529 Da. These two human apoSAA proteins correspond respectively to the human apolipoproteins SAA_1 and SAA_1 des Arg described by Dwulet et al. [9].

Antibody Preparation. Antibodies were raised in rabbits against human, monkey, mouse, and duck AA proteins, and against human $apoSAA_2$. A sodium sulfate precipate of rabbit antiserum to mouse apoSAA, absorbed with normal mouse serum, was a gift from Dr. Mark B. Pepys. The antisera to monkey and duck AA were prepared in our laboratory by Dr. Stanley Fowler.

Electroimmunoblotting. Samples resolved by SDS-PAGE were transferred in 25 mM Tris/192 mM glycine/0.01% SDS/10% (v/v) CH_3OH to nitrocellulose, which, after blocking with Tris-buffered 5% BSA, pH 7.4, was exposed to antibody diluted in BSA/TBS and developed with peroxidase-conjugated goat anti-rabbit IgG followed by 4-chloro-1-naphthol/H_2O_2 [10].

Results

A prominent doublet in the 12-kDa region was revealed by SDS-PAGE of the HDL_3 fraction (d 1.125-1.21 g/ml) from the turpentine-injected hamsters; the leading member of the doublet, the more intense of the two bands, had a mobility slightly greater than that of duck AA (11.6 kDa), which comigrated with the trailing member (Fig. 1). The doublet was present but less intense in the HDL_2 fraction (d 1.063-1.125 g/ml), fainter in the lower density lipoprotein fractions (d<1.063 g/ml), and hardly detectable in any of the lipoprotein fractions derived from the control hamsters. The subcutaneous injection of 0.5 ml turpentine evoked a greater SAA response than the intraperitoneal injection of 50 μg LPS; a more toxic dose of LPS (250 μg) diminished the response (Fig. 2).

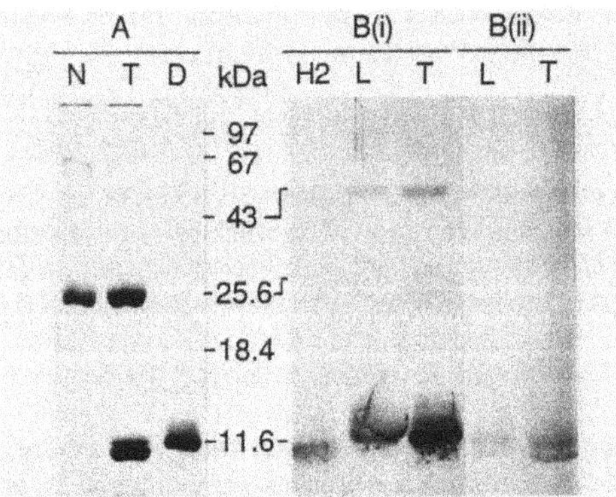

Fig. 1. A) SDS-PAGE of duck AA (D) and HDL_3 from untreated (N) and turpentine (T)-injected hamsters; 10.8% total acrylamide (17:1 acrylamide:bis); stain, 0.25% Coomassie Blue R-250. B) Electroimmunoblots of human $apoSAA_2$ (H_2) and HDL_3 from 50-μg-LPS(L)- and turpentine (T)-injected hamsters vs. anti-mouse AA (i) and anti-mouse SAA (ii). Sample volumes, initial-serum equivalent: A) 5 μl (N,T); B) 15 μl (L), 8 μl (T).

Antibodies to mouse SAA reacted with both members of the doublet, whereas antibodies to mouse AA reacted preferentially with the trailing member; in addition to their reactions in the 12-

kDa region, antibodies to mouse AA and SAA revealed a band (also a doublet) in the 40-kDa region of the acute-phase electrophoretic pattern (Fig. 1). Antibodies to human SAA and duck AA, which is very similar to known SAA proteins in size and sequence, reacted with both members of the doublet; antibodies to human and monkey AA reacted preferentially with the leading member. Weak reactions in the 25-kDa region observed with several antibody preparations are believed to be mainly nonspecific interactions involving the major apolipoprotein apoA-I.

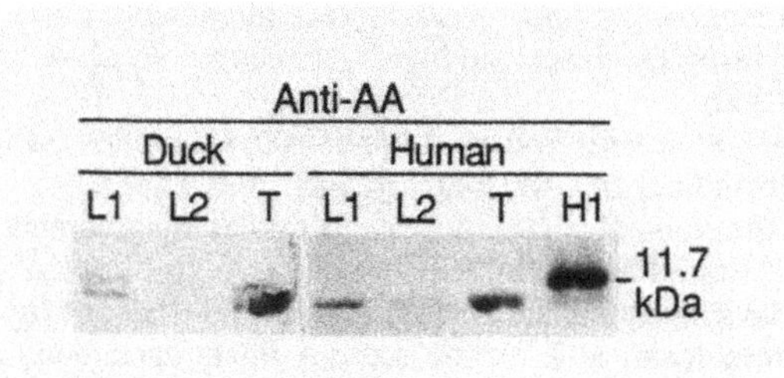

Fig. 2. Electroimmunoblots of human apoSAA_1 (H1) and HDL_3 from 50–μg-LPS (L1)-, 250–μg-LPS (L2)-, and turpentine (T)-injected hamsters vs. antibodies to duck and to human AA. Sample volumes, initial-serum equivalent: 6 μl (L1, L2, T).

Discussion

The 12-kDa doublet that became evident on SDS-PAGE of the serum HDL from the treated hamsters could represent separate gene products or post-translational modifications of a single gene product. The differences among the immunoreactions of members of the doublet with antibodies to human, monkey, mouse and duck AA and/or SAA must depend upon reactions with different epitopes and are compatible with the existence of more than one gene product. A recent study of SAA-gene structure and expression in the Syrian hamster indicates three SAA genes; the corresponding derived amino-acid sequences have been designated $hSAA_1$, $hSAA_2$, and $hSAA_3$ [11]. There is a 96.7% similarity between $hSAA_1$ and $hSAA_2$ and an 88.5% similarity between $hSAA_1$ and $hSAA_3$. The three sequences are very similar (84.5-88.3%) to the derived sequence of mouse SAA_3, for which the mRNA exists [12] but a corresponding protein has not yet been reported. In mice injected with an inflammatory agent such as LPS, SAA_1 and SAA_2 temporarily become major HDL apoproteins [13]. Our results suggest a similar situation in the Syrian hamster, but a strict parallelism between the mouse and the hamster seems unlikely because of the close similarity between the three hamster SAA genes and the mouse SAA_3 gene, which according to available evidence does not encode a protein that associates with HDL. Four SAA isotypes have been recognized by isoelectric focusing of acute-phase hamster HDL [2]. These isotypes were characterized only by second-dimension SDS-PAGE, so their genetic individuality remains in question.

Acknowledgments

We express our appreciation to Jeanette Carlson for dedicated service in preparation of the manuscript.

This work was supported by United States Public Health Service Grants HL-03174 and HL-40079.

References

1. Snel, F.W.J.J., Niewold, Th.A., Baltz, M.L., Hol, P.R., van Ederen, A.M., Pepys, M.B. and Gruys, E. (1989) `Experimental amyloidosis in the hamster: correlation between hamster female protein levels and amyloid deposition', Clin. Exp. Immunol, 76, 296-300.
2. Niewold, Th.A. and Tooten, P.C.J. (1990) `Purification and characterization of hamster serum amyloid-A protein (SAA) by cholesteryl hemisuccinate affinity chromatography', Scand. J. Immunol. 31, 389-396.
3. Eriksen, N. and Benditt, E.P. (1984) `Trauma, high density lipoproteins, and serum amyloid protein A', Clin. Chim. Acta 140, 139-149.
4. Laemmli, U.K. (1970) `Cleavage of structural proteins during the assembly of the head of bacteriophage T4', Nature 227, 680-685.
5. Benditt, E.P. (1976) `The structure of amyloid protein AA and evidence for a transmissible factor in the origin of amyloidosis', in O. Wegelius and A. Pasternack (eds.), Amyloidosis, Academic Press, London, pp. 323-332.
6. Eriksen, N. and Benditt, E.P. (1980) `Isolation and characterization of the amyloid-related apoprotein (SAA) from human high density lipoprotein', Proc. Natl. Acad. Sci. USA 77, 6860-6864.
7. Ericsson, L.H., Eriksen, N., Walsh, K.A. and Benditt, E.P. (1987) `Primary structure of duck amyloid protein A', FEBS Lett. 218, 11-16.
8. Parmelee, D.C., Titani, K., Ericsson, L.H., Eriksen, N., Benditt, E.P. and Walsh, K.A. (1982) `Amino acid sequence of amyloid-related apoprotein (apoSAA_1) from human high-density lipoprotein', Biochemistry 21, 3298-3303.
9. Dwulet, F.E., Wallace, D.K. and Benson, M.D. (1988) `Amino acid structures of multiple forms of amyloid-related serum protein SAA from a single individual', Biochemistry 27, 1677-1682.
10. Monroe, D. (1985) `The solid-phase enzyme-linked immunospot assay: current and potential applications', BioTechniques May/June, 222-229.
11. Webb, C.F., Tucker, P.W. and Dowton, S.B. (1989) `Expression and sequence analysis of serum amyloid A in the Syrian hamster', Biochemistry 28, 4785-4790.
12. Stearman, R.S., Lowell, C.A., Peltzman, C.G. and Morrow, J.F. (1986) `The sequence and structure of a new serum amyloid A gene', Nucleic Acids Res. 14, 797-809.
13. Hoffman, J.S. and Benditt, E.P. (1982) `Changes in high density lipoprotein content following endotoxin administration in the mouse', J. Biol. Chem. 257, 10510-10517.

THE COMPLETE PRIMARY STRUCTURE OF BOVINE SERUM AMYLOID PROTEIN A (SAA) AND OF TISSUE AMYLOID FIBRIL PROTEIN A (AA) SUBSPECIES

K. ROSSEVATN*, P.K. ANDRESEN*, K. SLETTEN*,
G. HUSBY**, K. NORDSTOGA***, K.H. JOHNSON****
& P. WESTERMARK*****.
**Department of Biochemistry, University of Oslo P.O.Box 1041, Blindern, N-0361 OSLO 3, Norway*
***Department of Rheumatology, University Hospital of Tromsø, Norway*
****National Veterinary Institute, Oslo, Norway*
*****College of Veterinary Medicine, University of Minnesota, St.Paul, USA*
******Department of Pathology, University of Linkøping, Sweden*

ABSTRACT. The goal of this work was to determine the complete covalent structures of the bovine proteins SAA and AA. Protein AA was isolated from the amyloid fibrils extracted from the kidneys. Three molecular species of protein AA was characterised and were found to consist of 68, 81 and about 112 amino acid residues, respectively. The protein SAA isolated from acute phase HDL was composed of 112 amino acid residues. The amino acid sequence elucidated for the protein AA subspecies was identical to that determined for protein SAA. No microheterogeneity could be detected in the amino acid sequence of protein SAA or of protein AA subspecies. The data thus suggest the existence of only one molecular species of protein SAA and that this species is amyloidogenic. As shown for the equine protein SAA, an insertion of several amino acid residues between positions 68 and 69 could be established.

1. Introduction

In our laboratories, we are performing comparative and structural studies of SAA and AA from man and different animal species, in order to disclose common characteristics and differences which may be related to their physiological function and their role in the formation of amyloid.

The domestic cow develops AA type amyloidosis quite frequently with particular affection to the kidneys (4). In previous reports (3,9), we have characterised bovine SAA and AA by immunologic chemical studies including partial amino acid sequencing. The covalent structure of a bovine protein AA has recently been reported by others (1). We here report the complete primary structures of bovine SAA and AA.

2. Materials and Methods

Isolation and purification of protein SAA. Acute-phase serum was obtained from a cow suffering from septicemia. The high density lipoprotein fraction was isolated by ultracentrifugation, delipidised with methanol and diethylether and subjected to gel filtration. Apo-SAA was further purified by reverse phase high performance liquid chromatography.

Preparation of amyloid fibrils and purification of the protein AA. The amyloid fibrils were extracted from the kidney of a Norwegian cow suffering from chronic infection (7). Purified protein AA was obtained by gel-filtering the fibrils. Protein AA was also purified from renal cortical tissue of an American cow (9).

Amino acid composition and sequence determination. Polypeptides were hydrolysed in 6M HCl and amino acid analysis was performed. Opening of the pyrrolidone ring of the amino-terminal pyroglutamic acid was performed by methanolysis (5). N-terminal analysis was performed using an automatic sequence analyser of the micro-type (8). The proteins were cleaved by BNPS-skatole and cyanogen bromide and digested with trypsin and Staphylococcus aureus V8 proteinase. The generated peptides were purified by HPLC using neutral and acidic elution system, TLC and gel filtration (8).

3. Results and Discussion

Bovine protein SAA was found to consist of 112 amino acid residues (Fig.1). Two main molecular species of protein AA was found in the fibrils from the Norwegian cow, and these consisted of 68 and 81 amino acid residues, respectively (Fig.1). Renal cortical tissue from the American cow contained the shortest of these two species, in addition to a molecular form corresponding to a SAA-like or an intact protein SAA (Fig.1). This support earlier data that intact protein SAA is being incorporated in the fibrils.

Both protein SAA and all molecular forms of protein AA were found to have pyroglutamic acid as the N-terminal residue.

No microheterogeneity could be detected in the amino acid sequence of protein SAA or in the protein AA subspecies, and the amino acid sequence of the protein AA subspecies were identical to that of protein SAA. Furthermore, the amino acid sequence agrees with the protein AA, studied by Benson et al. (1). The data thus suggest the existence of only one molecular species of protein SAA and that this species is amyloidogenic.

Compared to human SAA both the equine (8) and bovine SAA has an insertion of several amino acid residues between positions 68 and 69 (Fig.2). This insertion has been allocated in order to maximize the homology.

The bovine amyloid fibrils were found to consist of the following protein AA subspecies: position 1 to 68, position 1 to 81 and position 1 to about 112 (Fig.1). Only the two largest contain the inserted region, which suggest that this region has no primary effect on the fibrillogenesis.

Preliminary results of protein SAA from sheep shows also this insertion (6). It is interesting to note that in most of the protein AA so far studied, the C-terminal region including the insertion is more or less degraded (2).

```
                  5                   10                  15
PCA-Trp-Met-Ser-Phe-Phe-Gly-Glu-Ala-Tyr-Glu-Gly-Ala-Lys-Asp-

                  20                  25                  30
Met-Trp-Arg-Ala-Tyr-Ser-Asp-Met-Arg-Glu-Ala-Asn-Tyr-Lys-Gly-

                  35                  40                  45
Ala-Asp-Lys-Tyr-Phe-His-Ala-Arg-Gly-Asn-Tyr-Asp-Ala-Ala-Gln-

                  50                  55                  60
Arg-Gly-Pro-Gly-Gly-Ala-Trp-Ala-Ala-Lys-Val-Ile-Ser-Asp-Ala-

                  65             ↓    70                  75
Arg-Glu-Asn-Ile-Gln-Arg-Phe-Thr-Asp-Pro-Leu-Phe-Lys-Gly-Thr-

                  80     ↓            85                  90
Thr-Ser-Gly-Gln-Gly-Gln-Glu-Asp-Ser-Arg-Ala-Asp-Gln-Ala-Ala-

                  95                  100                 105
Asn-Glu-Trp-Gly-Arg-Ser-Gly-Lys-Asp-Pro-Asn-His-Phe-Arg-Pro-

                110         ↓
Ala-Gly-Leu-Pro-Asp-Lys-Tyr
```

Fig.1. The complete amino acid sequence of bovine amyloid fibril proteins and of the corresponding protein SAA. C-terminii of AA subspecies are marked with an arrow.

```
       67    a   b   c   d   e   f   g   h   i   70
Cow    Phe-Thr-Asp-Pro-Leu-Phe-Lys-Gly-Thr-Thr-Ser-Gln-Gln
Horse  ------------Arg-Phe-Ser-Phe-----    Gly---------Arg
Human  Phe-Phe-                                   ----His
       Leu Thr                                        Arg
```

Fig.2. A comparison of the amino acid residues in position 67 to position 70 in protein SAA.

4. Acknowledgements

The work was supported by the Norwegian Council for Science and the Humanities. The technical assistance of Jessie Juul is gratefully acknowledged.

5. References

1. Benson, M.D., Dibartola, S.P. and Dwulet, F.E. (1989) 'A unique insertion in the primary structure of bovine amyloid AA protein', J. Lab. Clin. Med. 113, 67.
2. Husby, G. and Sletten, K. (1986) 'Chemical and clinical classification of amyloidosis', Scand. J. Immunol. 23, 253.
3. Husebekk, A., Husby, G., Sletten, K. Skogen, B. and Nordstoga, K. (1988) 'Characterization of bovine amyloid proteins SAA and AA', Scand. J. Immunol. 27, 739.
4. Jakob, W. (1971) 'Spontaneous amyloidosis of mammals', Vet. Path. 8, 292.
5. Kawasaki, I. and Itano, H.A. (1972) 'Methanolysis of the pyrrolidone ring of amino terminal pyroglutamic acid in model peptides', Anal. Biochem. 48, 546.
6. Marhaug, G., Sletten, K. and Husby, G. (1987) 'Charac terization of serum amyloid A (SAA) protein in the sheep', in T. Isobe et al. (eds.), Amyloid and Amyloidosis, Plenum press, New York and London, pp. 217-222.
7. Pras, M. Schubert, M., Zucker-Franklin, D. Rimon, A. and Franklin, E.C. (1968) 'The characterization of soluble amyloid prepared in water', J. Clin. Invest. 47, 923.
8. Sletten, K. and Husby, G. (1989) 'The primary structure of equine serum amyloid A (SAA) protein', Scand. J. Immunol. 30, 117.
9. Westermark, P., Johnson, K.H., Westermark, G.T., Sletten, K. and Hayden, D.W. (1986) 'Bovine amyloid protein AA: Isolation and amino acid sequence analysis' Comp. Biochem. Physiol. 85B, 609.

DEGRADATION OF SAA IN AMYLOID FIBRILS BY ELASTASE.

Anne Husebekk & Bjørn Skogen
Department of Immunology and Bloodbank
University Hospital of Tromsø, Norway.

Amyloid fibrils were isolated from the kidneys of two different cows by standard washing procedure (fibril preparation I and II). Both fibril preparations were subjected to enzymatic degradation by incubation with elastase (37°C, 2 and 4 hours). The main protein in fibril preparation I (9-10 kD;AA) was not significantly degraded by elastase, whereas a 14 kD protein (SAA) in fibril preparation II was totally degraded. A 9-10 kD (AA) protein in this preparation, was unchanged after incubation with elastase. Bovine serum SAA was isolated by ultracentrifugation and this SAA protein was totally degraded after 2 hour incubation with elastase. These results indicate that fibril SAA is more susceptible to enzymatic degradation by elastase than fibril AA, but more stable than serum SAA. The fibril SAA may thus be in an intermediate form between serum SAA and fibril AA. This finding may have therapeutical consequences for secondary amyloidosis.

Introduction

Amyloid fibrils are relatively resistant to enzymatic degradation and resolution of amyloid fibrils in patients with secondary amyloidosis has hardly been observed. Purified serum SAA and dissociated AA protein from the fibrils are easily degraded by different serine proteases (1).
It is shown that amyloid fibrils may consist of either undegraded SAA (2), the partly degraded SAA, namely AA molecule (3,4), or a mixture of the two proteins (5,6,7). We have described a bovine preparation with a mixture of SAA and AA (8).
The aim of the present study was to investigate the effect of elastase on SAA and AA in an aqueous solution of bovine amyloid fibrils.

Materials and Methods

Amyloid fibril preparation. Amyloid fibrils were isolated by the standard washing procedure with destilled water. (Tissues were kindly provided by K. Nordstoga).
Serum SAA. Bovine serum SAA was prepared by gel filtration of delipidized and dissociated acute phase HDL apolipoproteins.
Antiserum. Antiserum to bovine SAA/AA was made by immunization of a rabbit with purified bovine AA in Complete Freunds adjuvans.
Enzymatic degradation. Enzymatic degradation was performed by incubating protein and enzym (Elastase E 1250, Sigma Chemical Company, St. Louis, USA) at a ratio of 80 to 1 for 2 and 4 hours and at 37°C.
SDS-PAGE. SDS-PAGE was performed with Pharmacia Phast Gel System using homogeneous 20% gels stained with Coomassie Brilliant Blue.
Double immuno diffusion. Double immuno diffusion was performed in 1% agarose gels in barbital buffer, pH 8,6.
Congo Red staining. A 1% Congo Red solution was used. Destaining with KOH was performed.

Results

Amyloid fibril preparation I contained mainly a 9-10 kD protein which was not degraded after 4 hours incubation with elastase (Fig. 1).
Amyloid fibril preparation II contained a 9-10 kD protein and a 14 kD protein. The 14 kD protein was partly degraded after 2 hours incubation with elastase and totally degraded after 4 hours. The 9-10 kD protein band was almost unchanged (Fig.2).

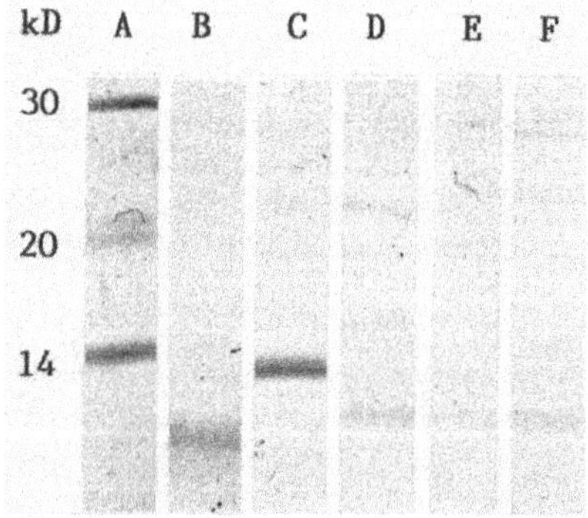

Fig.1. SDS-PAGE (20%) showing that the main protein (9-10 kD) in bovine fibril preparation I was not degraded by elastase. Lane A: MW standards. Lane B: human AA. Lane C: human SAA. Lane D: bovine fibril prep. I. Lane E: fibril prep. I + elastase incub. for 2 h. Lane F: fibril prep. I + elastase incub. for 4 h.

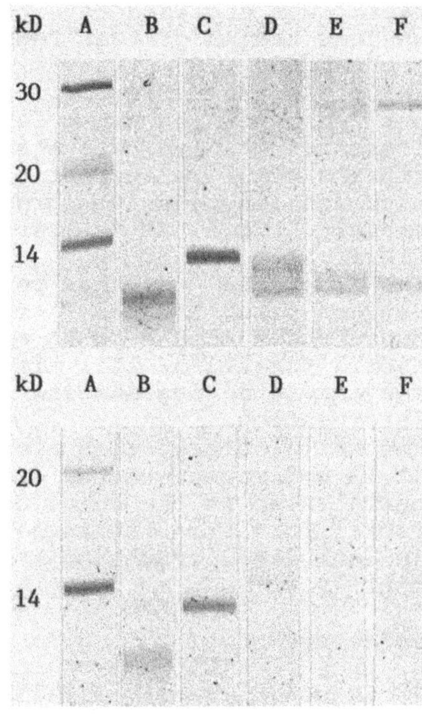

Fig.2. SDS-PAGE (20%) showing that the 14 kD protein in bovine fibril prep. II was degraded by elastase. Lane A: standards. Lane B: human AA. Lane C: human SAA. Lane D: bovine fibril prep. II. Lane E: fibril prep. II + elastase incub. for 2 h. Lane F: fibril prep. II + elastase incub. for 4 h.

Fig.3. SDS-PAGE (20%) showing that purified bovine serum SAA was degraded by elastase after 2 h incubation. Lane A: standards. Lane B: human AA. Lane C: human SAA. Lane D: bovine serum SAA. Lane E: bovine serum SAA + elastase incub. for 2 h. Lane F: bovine serum SAA + elastase incub. for 4 h.

Purified cow SAA was totally degraded after 2 hours incubation with elastase (Fig.3).
In double immunodiffusion there were precipitation lines between an antiserum to bovine (SAA/AA) and both amyloid fibril preparations as well as the fibrillar proteins subjected to elastase.

Discussion

Elastase has been shown to degrade isolated SAA and AA proteins very efficiently (1). Although different serine proteases are present in most tissues, amyloid fibrils consisting of SAA and AA proteins, seem to be relatively resistant to enzymatic degradation.
Aquous solutions of bovine amyloid fibrils were subjected to elastase in order to follow the degradation of the fibrillar proteins.
In fibril preparation I, containing mainly AA proteins, no significant degradation after incubation with elastase occured. This strongly indicates that protein AA is protected from enzymatic attack and fit with the in vivo observation of hardly any resolution of the fibrils. In fibril preparation II, the SAA like constituent of the

fibril was degraded after 4 hours incubation with enzyme whereas the AA protein remained electrophoretically unchanhged.
Serum SAA was easily degraded, in accordance with an earlier report on human SAA (1).
These results indicate that SAA incorporated in amyloid fibrils still is susceptible for enzymatic degradation, although less easily degradable than the serum SAA protein. Fibril AA is more resistant to degradation than fibril SAA.
The fibril SAA may thus be in an intermediate form between serum SAA and fibril AA. Predicting that the degradation of SAA to AA mainly take place at the site of fibril formation, this tissue SAA still is susceptible for enzymatic degradation and possibly for therapeutic intervention.
The normal degradation procedure for SAA is unclear, and it is not known whether degradation to AA represent a normal step in the total degradation of SAA. In amyloid fibril formation the total degradation of SAA in any way is inhibited, resulting in the deposition of amyloid fibrils.

References

1. Skogen,B.,Natvig,J.B.(1981) Degradation of Amyloid Proteins by Different Serine Proteases. Scand J Immunol, 14,389.
2. Westermark,P.,Johnson,K.H.,Westermark,G.T.,Sletten,K.,Hayden,D.W.(1986) Bovine amyloid protein AA:Isolation and amino acid sequence analysis. Comp Biochem Physiol,85B, 609.
3. Levin,M.,Franklin,E.C.,Frangione,B.,Pras,M. (1972) The amino acid sequence of a major non-immunoglobulin protein of amyloid. J Clin Invest,51,2773.
4. Sletten,K.,Husby,G.(1974) The complete amino acid sequence of non-immunoglobulin amyloid fibril AS in rheumatoid arthritis. Eur J Biochem,41,117.
5. Isobe,T.,Husby,G.,Sletten,K. (1980) Characterization of an amyloid protein AA similar to SAA.Pp.331-336 in Glenner,G.G.,Costa,P.& Freitas,F.(eds) Amyloid and Amyloidosis.Excerpta Medica, Amsterdam.
6. Shiroo,M,Kawahara,E.,Nakanishi,I,Migita,S. (1987) Specific deposition of serum amyloid A protein 2 in the mouse. Scand J Immunol, 26,709.
7. Tape,C.,Tan,R.,Nesheim,N.,Kisilevsky,R.(1988) Direct evidence for circulating SAA as the precursor of tissue AA deposits. Scand J Immunol,42,139.
8. Husebekk,A.,Husby,G.,Sletten,K.,Skogen,B.,Nordstoga,K. (1988) Characterization of bovine amyloid proteins SAA and AA.Scand J Immunol,27,739.

EVOLUTIONARY ASPECTS OF PROTEIN SAA

SYVERSEN, P.V.*, SLETTEN, K.* and HUSBY, G.**
*Department of Biochemistry, University of Oslo, Norway. **Department of Rheumatology, University of Tromsø, Norway.

ABSTRACT. By comparing the so far known protein SAA sequences, it appears to be two separate branches in the evolutionary pattern of SAA. One branch includes those species in which protein SAA has an insertion in position 72-81. This region is a very heterogeneous area. Three regions with invariability has been observed for those species with the described insertion. In addition to the inserted area, protein SAA consists of two other variable regions. For all species putative sites for phosphorylation has been elucidated.

1. Introduction

In a variety of species the serum amyloid protein A (SAA) has been isolated and characterized and found to be an apolipoprotein mainly associated with high density lipoprotein (HDL). Protein SAA behaves like an acute phase protein in man and in various animals (1), and is the precursor for amyloid protein A (AA), which is the main amyloid fibril protein in secondary amyloidosis.
The physiological function of protein SAA is not clear, but the results so far suggest a multifunctional protein.
The aim is to elucidate structural similarities and differences of importance in the formation of amyloid and function of the protein.

2. Results and discussion

The complete primary structure of the SAA proteins, is shown in Fig.1. The mouse SAA1 and SAA2 are from gene sequences. Cat and dog protein AA have been included because of their extended C-terminal region. By comparing the sequences in this way a clear delineation of the conserved and divergent regions is obtained (Fig.1).
It appears to be two separate branches in the evolutionary pattern of protein SAA. One branch includes the species of mink#, cat, dog, cow and horse, in which protein SAA has an insertion in position 72-81. Preliminary studies of sheep SAA also indicate an insertion in the same region.

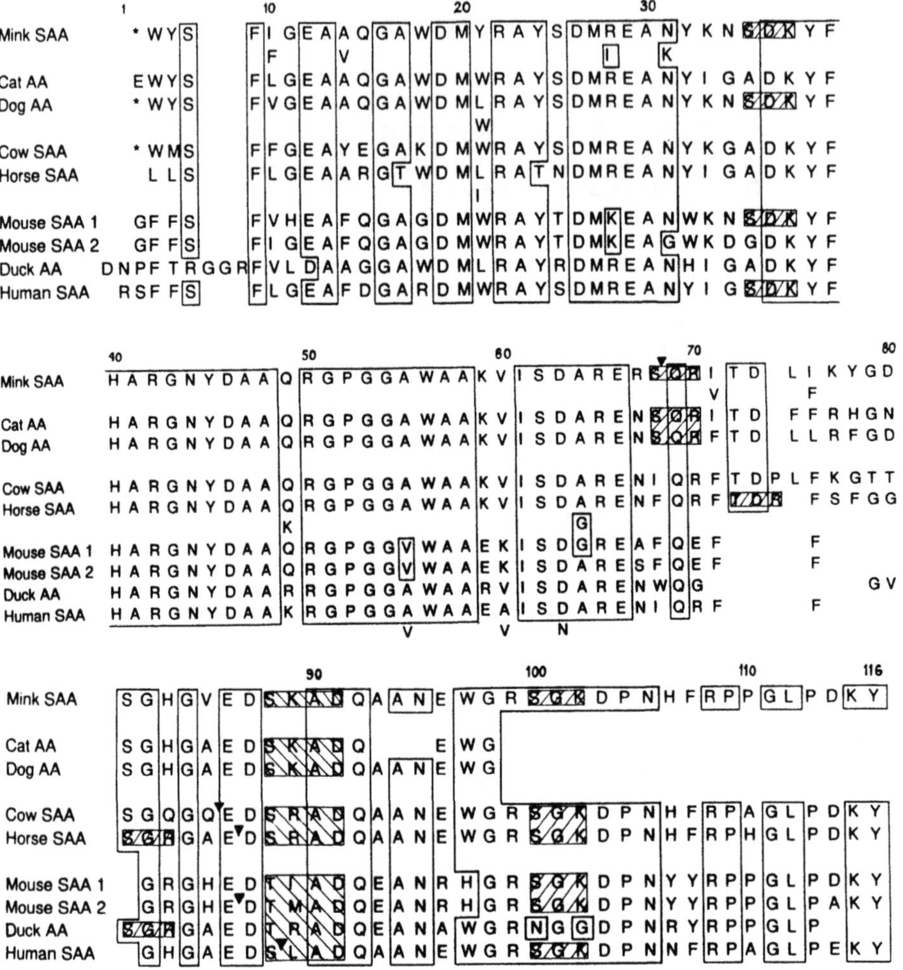

* Pyroglutamic acid

Fig.1. Comparison of protein SAA and AA from different species. Alignment is done to maximize homology. Boxed regions are areas with invariable residues. The sequences used for comparison are from Refs. 9 (cat AA, dog AA), 10 (horse SAA, mouse SAA 1,2, human SAA), 11 (duck AA), (cow SAA/AA in prep. 1990).
The C-terminal of the corresponding protein AA is indicated by: ▼
Phosphorylation site Protein kinase C :
Phosphorylation site Casein kinase II :

The inserted region, position 72-81, is a very heterogeneous area in the protein, indicating a high tendency of mutation.
An interesting observation is the invariability in positions 59-60(KV), 70,72-73(R,TD) and 96-98(EWG) for those species with the described insertion. In addition, position 71 constitutes an hydrophobic amino acid, and the question is whether there exists a specific association between the insertion and the consistent amino acid residues.
In addition to the inserted area in positions 72-81, there are two other variable regions, namely in positions 1-4 and 32-35. However, these species show a stronger homology in the two variable areas than those lacking this insertion (mouse,duck,human).
All the SAA proteins are strongly hydrophobic in the 11 N-terminal residues, and this part of the molecule is probably responsible for the binding to HDL (2).
Another question is the importance of the insertion for the degradation of the SAA in the amyloidogenesis. The human and mouse protein AA often terminate in the inserted area. These sites of cleavage are just C-terminal to an amphipathic helical region predicted to end at position 86 (3).
As indicated in Fig.1, the protein AA from cat, dog, cow and horse all constitute an extention in the C-terminal region compared to the protein AA from mouse and man. In the case of mink AA the protein ends in position 68.
Computer analyses have revealed putative sites for phosphorylation as marked in Fig.1.
It remains to be seen whether the constant and the variable regions in protein SAA have functional implication, for example that they may be involved in inflammatory and immunological reactions (4) and in the regulation of the enzyme lecithin-cholesterol acetyltransferase(L-CAT) (5).
In addition, the capability to protein SAA phosphorylation may indicate an involvement in the Protein kinase C system (6).
A recent observation that SAA may possess collagenase-like activity (7) should also be studied in a comparative manner.

#The amino acid sequence for protein SAA mink differ in some positions from previous published sequence (8). Data to be published.

3. References

1. Pepys, M.B. & Baltz, M.L.(1983). 'Acute phase proteins with special reference to C-reactive protein and related proteins (pentraxins) and serum amyloid A protein.' Adv. Immunol. **34**, 141.
2. Turnell, W.G., Sarra, R., Glover, I.D. & Baum, J.O.(1986). 'Secondary structure prediction of human SAA 1. Presumptive identification of calcium and lipid binding sites.' Mol. Biol. Med. **3**, 387.
3. Parmelee, D.C., Titani, K., Ericsson, L.H., Eriksen, N., Benditt, E.P. & Walsh, K.A.(1982). 'Amino acid sequence of amyloid-related apo-protein (apo SAA) from human high density lipoprotein.' Biochemistry **21**, 3298.
4. Ramadori, G., Damme, J.V., Rieder, H. & Meyer zum Buscenfeld, K.-H. (1988). 'Interleukin 6, the mediator of the acute phase reaction, modulates hepatic protein synthesis in human and mouse. Comparison with interleukin 1b and tumor necrosis factor-A.' Eur. J. Immunol. **18**, 1259.
5. Steinmetz, A., Hocke, G., Saile, R., Puchois, P. & Fruchart, J.-C.(1989). 'Influence of serum amyloid A on cholesterol esterification in human plasma.' Biochim. Biophys. Acta **1006**, 173.
6. Nel, A.E., De Beer, M.C., Shepard, E.G., Strachan, A.F., Vandenplas, M.L. & De Beer, F.C.(1988). 'Phosphorylation of human serum amyloid A protein by protein kinase C.' Biochem. J. **255**, 29.
7. Sack Jr., G.H. & Talbot Jr., C.C.(1989). 'The human serum amyloid A (SAA)-encoding gene GSAA1: nucleotide sequence and possible autocrine-collagenase-inducer function.' Gene **84**, 509.
8. Syversen, V., Sletten, K., Marhaug, G., Husby, G. & Lium, B.(1987). 'The amino acid sequence of serum amyloid A (SAA) protein in mink.' Scand. J. Immunol. **26**, 763.
9. Kluve-Beckerman, B., Dwulet, F.E. DiBartola, S.P. & Benson, M.D.(1989). 'Primary structures of dog and cat amyloid A proteins: comparison to human AA.' Comp. Biochem. Physiol. **94B**, 175.
10. Sletten, K., Husebekk, A. & Husby, G.(1989). 'The primary structure of Equine serum amyloid A (SAA) protein.' Scand. J. Immunol. **30**, 117.
11. Ericsson, L.H., Eriksen, N., Walsh, K.A. & Benditt, E.P.(1987). 'Primary structure of duck amyloid protein A.' FEBS Lett. **218**, 11.

STRAIN SPECIFIC VARIATION IN EXPRESSION OF NOVEL MOUSE APO-SAA ISOFORMS

J. D. SIPE, M. C. DE BEER AND F. C. DE BEER
Boston University School of Medicine, Boston, MA 02118 and
University of Kentucky School of Medicine, Lexington, KY
40506

ABSTRACT. In addition to apo-SAA 1 (pI 6.45) and apoSAA 2 (pI 6.3), three novel minor apo-SAA isoforms (pI 6.15, 6.0 and 5.9) have been identified by isoelectric focusing analysis of plasma from lipopolysaccharide treated BALB/c mice and other haplotype A strains. SJL/J mice (SAA gene family haplotype B), previously thought to be defective in SAA2 expression, were found to produce apo-SAA 2 as a minor isoform and the novel pI 5.9 isoform as the second quantitatively major apo-SAA species. The results suggest that the novel apo-SAA isoforms are products of genes distinct from, but closely related to, SAA1 and SAA2, and that the haplotype specificity of quantitative expression of the individual SAA genes reflects genomic differences in the control regions of the genes.

INTRODUCTION. Inbred strains of mice are powerful tools with which to analyze the cellular and molecular events in apo-SAA synthesis, catabolism and amyloidosis. The genomic structure of the murine SAA gene family has been studied extensively in BALB/c mice [1]. Cloning, sequencing and mapping studies have identified three active genes and a pseudogene with deletion of exons 1 and 2 and a portion of exon 3 resulting in an inframe stop codon. The SAA1 and SAA2 genes, 3200 bp long, are 96% identical; their mature products apo-SAA 1 and apo-SAA 2, differing in 9 of 103 amino acids, both associate with the HDL3 subclass of lipoproteins and are rapidly transported from the plasma compartment to peripheral tissues [2]. The third active gene, SAA3, is transcribed in liver coordinately with SAA1 and SAA2, but the corresponding protein has not been found on HDL [3].

Taylor and Rowe [4] surveyed 48 inbred murine strains and substrains for restriction fragment length polymorphisms (RFLPs) associated with the SAA gene family. A group of 33 strains, including BALB/c, CBA/J, C57BL/6, C3H, and A/J, which exhibited common restriction fragment patterns, was designated haplotype type A. Eight of the remaining 15 strains, one of which was SJL/J, which exhibited a common set of RFLP variants distinct from group A were designated haplotype B. SJL/J mice, originally thought to be resistant to

AA amyloidosis due to a defect in apo-SAA 2 production, were recently found to develop amyloidosis of the AA type using amyloid enhancing factor [5]. This study addressed the question of from which isoform precursor are AA fibrils produced in SJL/J mice by comparative isoelectric focusing analysis of SJL/J and BALB/c apo-SAA isoforms. The results suggest that, among inbred strains of mice, more than one SAA gene product has the potential to be converted to amyloid fibrils.

MATERIALS AND METHODS. BALB/c and SJL/J mice, female or male, were obtained at 5-8 weeks of age from Jackson Laboratories, Bar Harbor, ME. Plasma was isolated from EDTA-anti-coagulated blood obtained 16-20 hours after the intraperitoneal injection of 100 ug of lipopolysaccharide (W) from Salmonella typhosa from Difco Laboratories, Detroit, MI. High density lipoprotein (HDL) was prepared by sequential ultracentrifugation of the plasma [6]. Delipidated HDL was electrofocused on 0.3mm acrylamide gels containing 7M urea and 20% (v/v) ampholines pH 3-10, 40% (v/v) ampholines pH 4-6.5 and 40% (v/v) ampholines pH 7-9 [7]. Coomassie-stained proteins were excised from electrofocusing gels and analyzed in a second dimension in a 5-20% (w/v) acrylamide SDS-gel [7]. In order to optimize protein staining, several bands of a particular pI were pooled.

RESULTS. The apo-SAA isoforms of SJL/J mice were compared with that of BALB/C and several other type A murine strains (Fig. 1, Table 1) In addition to the major isoforms apo-SAA 1 (pI 6.45) and apo-SAA 2 (pI 6.3), 3 novel isoforms were identified in BALB/c mice by immunochemical staining. Phosphorylation [7] and glycosylation (Glycan detection kit, Boehringer Mannheim, Indianapolis, IN) of these novel apo-SAA isoforms were excluded. All have a molecular weight identical to apo-SAA when analyzed by two dimensional gel electrophoresis (Fig. 1a,b).

TABLE 1. Genetic variation in mouse serum amyloid A (SAA)

Strain	Genotype	Phenotype
Type A		
BALB/c	SAA1, SAA2	Major: apo-SAA 1, apo-SAA 2
(prototype)	SAA3, pseudo	Minor: pI 6.15, pI 6.0, pI 5.9
A/J		" " "
		" " "
Type B		
129/J		
(prototype)		
SJL/J		Major: apo-SAA 1, pI 5.9
		Minor: apo-SAA 2, pI 6.15

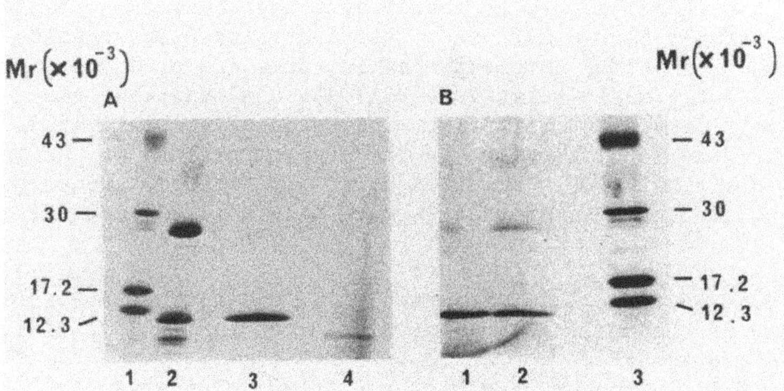

Figure 1. Molecular weight analysis of BALB/c and SJL/J apo-SAA isoforms. A: Lane 1, molecular weight markers ovalbumin (43,000), carbonic anhydrase (30,000), myoglobin (17,200) and cytochrome c (12,300); Lane 2, murine type A acute phase HDL containing apo-A-I (28,000), apo-SAA (11,500) and apo-A-II (9,000); Lane 3 SJL/J protein pI 5.9 with molecular weight similar to apo-SAA (11,500); and Lane 4, SJL/J protein with pI 6.0 with molecular weight similar to apo-A-II (9,000). B: Lanes 1 and 2, BALB/c proteins with respective pI´s 6.0 and 5.9 showing size homogeneity to apo-SAA (11,500); Lane 3, molecular weight markers as in Figure 3A. The pI 6.15 isoform present in LPS treated BALB/c and SJL/J mice has the molecular weight of apo-SAA. SJL/J mice lack the pI 6.0 isoform, the Coomassie Blue stained band present at that position does not stain with rabbit anti-mouse AA and has a molecular weight corresponding to apo-A-II. The identification as SAA of three novel isoforms present in HDL during the acute phase response was also established by immunoblotting with anti-murine AA antiserum (unpublished observations).

DISCUSSION. Taylor and Rowe´s RFLP based classification of murine SAA gene structure could have a range of implications for apo-SAA phenotypes. If the RFLPs identify mutation only in silent portions of the genes, then there would be no change in apo-SAA isoforms. If the RFLPs identify differences in the coding regions, then one would expect to find strain-specific isoforms. If the RFLPs identify differences in control regions, then one would expect to find an identical spectrum of isoforms in both type A and type B haplotypes with quantitative differences in expression. One or more combinations of these three possibilities might occur.

Our data show that BALB/c mice (Type A) produce, in addition to apo-SAA 1 and apo-SAA 2, quantitatively minor novel apo-SAA isoforms and that SJL/J mice (Type B) produce the same spectrum of isoforms qualitatively with quantitative differences. As the pI 6.0 isoform was not detected in SJL/J mice, it is conceivable that this is a strain-specific isoform for BALB/c anf other Type A strains. The results of our study suggest that the novel apo-SAA isoforms are products of genes distinct from, but closely related to SAA1 and SAA2 and that the haplotype specificity of quantitative expression of the individual genes reflects genomic differences in the control regions of the genes. Furthermore, our finding of a novel major pI 5.9 isoform, the amino-terminal of which resembles apo-SAA 2, make this a likely candidate.

REFERENCES.

1. Lowell, C.A., Potter, D.A., Stearman, R.S. and Morrow, J.F. (1986) ´Structure of the murine serum amyloid A gene family´, J. Biol. Chem., 261, 8442-8452.
2. Yamamoto, K-I, Shiroo, M. and Migita S. (1986) ´Diverse gene expression for isotypes of murine serum amyloid A during acute phase reaction´, Science, 232, 227-229.
3. Hoffman, J.S. and Benditt, E.P. (1982) ´Changes in high density lipoprotein content following endotoxin administration in the mouse. Formation of serum amyloid protein rich subfractions. J. Biol. Chem. 257, 10510-10517.
4. Taylor, B.A. and Rowe, L. (1984) ´Genes for serum amyloid A proteins map to chromosome 7 in the mouse´, Mol Gen Genetics 195, 491-499.
5. Rokita, H., Shirahame, T., Cohen, A.S., Meek, R.L., Benditt, E.P. and Sipe J.D. (1987) ´Differential expression of the amyloid SAA3 gene in liver and peritoneal macrophages of mice undergoing dissimilar inflammatory episodes´, J. Immunol. 139, 3848-3853.
6. Godenir, N.I., Jeenah, M.S., Coetzee, G.A., van dr Westhuyzen, D.R., Strachan, A.F., de Beer, F.C. (1985) ´Standardization of the quantitation of serum amyloid A protein (SAA) in human serum´, J. Immunol. Methods, 83, 217-225.
7. Strachan, A.F., Brandt, W.F., Woo, P., van der Westhuyzen, D.R., Coetzee, G.A., De Beer, M.C., Shepard, E.G., De Beer, F.C. (1989) ´Evidence that the six major isoforms of human serum amyloid A protein are coded for by three genes at two genetic loci´, J. Biol. Chem., 264,18368-18373.

SAA ISOTYPES IN PATIENTS WITH SECONDARY AMYLOIDOSIS

J. G. Raynes[1], Hultquist R.[2], Molyneux M[3], Griffin G[4] and McAdam K.P.W.J.[1]

1.Department of Clinical Sciences,
London School of Hygiene and Tropical Medicine,
Keppel St., London WC1E 7HT.
2.Department of Rheumatology,
University Hospital of Lund,
S-221 85 Lund, Sweden
3.Liverpool School of Tropical Medicine,
Pembroke Place, Liverpool L3 5QA
4.Department of Communicable Diseases
St George's Hospital Medical School,
Tooting, London SW17 ORE

Abstract

SAA isotypes were examined in a group of patients from Papua New Guinea where there is a very high incidence of amyloidosis. The expression of SAA2ß was more common than observed in patients from Europe/USA but similar to that observed in a group of patients from Malawi with malaria. After examination of matched pairs of patients with and without amyloidosis we could find no evidence for qualitative differences in isotypes present in patients with or without amyloidosis. We have also looked at the isotypes in a group of patients from Lund with rheumatoid disease, with or without amyloidosis, matched for age, sex and duration of disease. There was no qualitative difference in SAA isotype expression in individuals who develop amyloidosis and those who do not. There was no evidence for quantitative differences in SAA1 and SAA2α in patients who had amyloidosis and those who did not. Further studies are in progress on the quantitation of isotypes with arginine at the N-terminal.

Introduction

Serum amyloid A (SAA) is synthesised by the liver and concentrations increase following inflammation by a factor of up to 1000 [1]. Isotypes of SAA have been described before using a variety of methods of separation and detection. In most cases six isotypes have been described, including two major isotypes and 4 minor components [2-4]. The two major isotypes of SAA correspond to the sequences derived from clones pA1 [5] and SAA1 [6] with or without the N-terminal arginine [7]. Other sequences that have been obtained for human SAA include pSAA82 [8] and SAAg9 [9] which code for more basic SAA proteins. Recent reports have identified 3 hepatic mRNA species that code for the main isotypes purified from serum [7,10].

Using the octyl-Sepharose method for extracting SAA and other apolipoproteins we were able to demonstrate a sufficiently high recovery for us to attempt to quantitate the isotypes of SAA from small samples of acute phase sera [11]. In this study we have examined the isotypes present in sera from several groups of patients in order to evaluate the possibility that differences in isotypes present in the acute phase sera might be associated with the propensity to form AA amyloid deposits.

Materials and Methods

Octyl-Sepharose and ampholines were obtained from Pharmacia, Milton Keynes and other chemicals were obtained from BDH Chemicals, Poole, Dorset. Serum samples were collected from patients with malaria (Dr M.Molyneux, Liverpool, U.K.) and suffering from inflammatory bowel disease and infective gastroenteritis (Dr G Griffin, St George's, Tooting, London). Matched pairs of patients with and without amyloidosis were obtained from leprosy patients in Papua New Guinea (Dr K.P.W.J. McAdam). Acute phase sera was also obtained from individuals from Papua New Guinea 36 h after TAB vaccination. Sera was collected from rheumatoid arthritis patients with or without amyloidosis matched for age, sex and duration of disease in Lund (Dr R. Hultquist).

Thawed sera (0.5 ml) were added to Octyl-Sepharose beads (1 ml, 50% settled bed volume) equilibrated in phosphate buffered saline (PBS). The beads were washed with PBS (5 x 5 ml) and protein was eluted with 4M Guanidine hydrochloride, 30 % ethanediol, 10 mM NaOH. The supernatants were dialysed agianst distilled water and concentrated to 0.5 ml.
IEF was performed according to published methods [12] in vertical mini-gel apparatus using ampholines pH range 5-8. Quantitative measurements were obtained by scanning protein stained bands at 595 nm. Peak height was used to calculate the percentage SAA in each isotype and values for each isotype calculated from the total SAA in the sample measured by ELISA.

The SAA ELISA was a competitive inhibition method [11] using affinity purified antibody to human SAA bound to the solid phase and alkaline phosphatase conjugated SAA. Electroblotting was performed using semi-dry apparatus and PVDF membranes. SAA isotypes were visualised with goat anti-human SAA and alkaline-phosphatase conjugated anti-goat immunoglobulin.

Results

Extracted apolipoproteins from acute phase and normal sera were electrofocused and stained with Coomassie blue or electroblotted onto PVDF and stained immunoenzymatically. SAA isotypes pI 5.9 and 6.1 were always detectable by immunoblotting in acute phase and in most normal sera regardless of the origin of the sera. Protein staining detected these SAA isotypes in acute phase samples and some but not all normal sera. Recovery of SAA using this method has been shown to be 82 $\pm$ 20% after analysis of 8 sera. Presence of the isotypes was determined by electroblotting and quantitation performed by densitometric scanning of Coomassie blue stained gels. Isotypes with pI 6.6 and 6.9 were present in all European and North American samples. Isotypes with pI 6.8 and 7.1 were present in only 10 out of 53 samples from Europe and North America (Table 1). SAA2α isotypes were present in all 53 sera studied. In samples from Papua New Guinea there was a much higher incidence of SAA2ß although most of the individuals also expressed SAA2α (Table 2). Comparison with the European/USA sample was significant (chi square, $p= 0.0032$). There was no qualitative difference between the isotypes of patients from Papua New Guinea with or without amyloidosis (Table 2). The high frequency of SAA2ß was also seen in 22 patients from Malawi, where there is no evidence for high incidence of amyloidosis (chi square test against European/USA samples $p= 0.0047$). A series of samples from rheumatoid arthritis with or without amyloidosis matched for age, sex and duration of illness from Lund, Sweden showed no difference in type of isotype expressed. The SAA2ß isotypes were present in only 5 patients, 3 with amyloidosis and 2 without amyloidosis (Table 3). It was found that the SAA2α isotypes were present in all patients as expected from the distributions found previously (Table 1). The presence of amyloidosis was not associated with higher SAA concentrations, or increased percentage of either gene product (SAA1 or SAA2α) (Table 3).

Table 1
Frequency of SAA isotypes

Location	Stimulus	SAA1	SAA2α	SAA2ß
Europe	Gastroenteritis	23(100%)	23(100%)	2(9%)
USA	Etiocholanolone	7(100%)	7(100%)	1(14%)
Europe/USA	Various	23(100%)	23(100%)	7(30%)
Total		53(100%)	53(100%)	10(19%)
Malawi	Malaria	22(100%)	20(91%)	15(68%)
Papua New	Vaccination	20(100%)	19(95%)	14(70%)
Guinea	Leprosy	14(100%)	12(86%)	12(86%)
Total		34(100%)	31(91%)	26(76%)

Table 2
Isotypes in Papua New Guinea patients

Patients	Amyloidosis	SAA1	SAA2α	SAA2ß
Vaccination	+	10	10	7
	-	10	9	7
Leprosy	+	7	6	6
	-	7	6	6

Table 3
Isotypes in rheumatoid arthritis

		Amyloidosis	No amyloidosis
No. of patients		16	14
Total SAA		34 ± 35	65 ± 43
Frequency	SAA1	13	13
	SAA2α	13	13
	SAA2ß	3	2
% total	SAA1	80 ± 10	77 ± 9
	SAA2	17 ± 11	21 ± 10

Discussion

We investigated the frequency and concentration of SAA1, SAA2α and SAA2ß isotypes in populations from several countries. It was found that the frequency of SAA2ß was much higher in Papua New Guinea and Malawi than in Europe or North America. However there was no association of increased expression of any gene product with the presence of SAA2ß to presence of amyloidosis. This was confirmed in the group of samples from Sweden with rheumatoid arthritis. There was no difference in these samples between the quantity of SAA1 and SAA2α expressed as a ratio of total SAA. It would thus appear unlikely that high expression of a particular isotype might lead to an increased likelyhood of forming AA amyloid deposits.

Further studies are continuing on the quantitation of SAA isotypes with and without an N-terminal arginine and on the changes in their concentration during inflammation. The isotype patterns were the same to those described previously [13] although the pI values of SAA2α and SAA2ß were reported to be different (not shown in this report).

References

1. Fey GH., and G.M. Fuller. 1987. Regulation of acute phase gene expression by inflammatory mediators. Mol Biol Med. 4:323- 338.
2. Bausserman, L.1., P.N. Herbert, and K.P.W.J. McAdam. 1980. Heterogeneity of human serum amyloid A proteins. J. Exp. Med. 152:641-656.
3. Eriksen, N., and E.P. Benditt. 1980 Isolation and characterisation of the amyloid related apoprotein (SAA) from human high density lipoprotein. Proc. Acad. Natl. Sci. U.S.A. 77:6860-6864.
4. Martin M.E., C.J. Rosenthal, and A. Huq. 1986. The physico-chemical, antigenic, and functional heterogeneity of human serum amyloid A. in Amyloidosis Proc IVth Symp on amyloidosis, Plenum Press, New York. 27-38.
5. Sipe J.D., H.R. Colten, D. Goldberg, M.D. Edge, B.F. Tack, A.S. Cohen, and A.S. Whitehead. 1985. Biosynthesis and postsynthetic processing of preSAA and structural variants defined by complementary DNA. Biochemistry. 24:2931-2936.

6. Parmalee, D.C., K. Kitani, L.H. Ericsson, N. Eriksen, E.P. Benditt and K.A. Walsh. 1982. Aminoacid sequence of amyloid- related apoprotein (apoSAA) from human high density lipoprotein. Biochemistry. 21:3298-3303.
7. Dwulet F.E., D.K. Wallace and M.D. Benson. 1988. Amino acid structures of multiple forms of amyloid related serum protein SAA from a single individual. Biochemistry. 27:1677-1682.
8. Kluve-Beckerman B., G.L. Long & M.D. Benson 1986. DNA sequence evidence for polymorphic forms of human serum amyloid A. Biochem Genet. 24:795-803.
9. Woo, P. 1986 Gene structure of human serum amyloid A protein and comparison with amyloid A. In amyloidosis. (Marrink J., & Van Rijswijk, W.H, Eds.), Martinus Nijhoff, Dordrecht, 135- 139.
10. Kluve-Beckerman B., F.E. Dwulet, and M.D. Benson. 1988. Human serum amyloid A. Three hepatic mRNAs and the corresponding proteins in one person. J. Clin Invest. 82:1670-1675.
11. Raynes J.G. and K.P.W.J. McAdam. 1988. Purification of serum amyloid A and other high density apolipoproteins by hydrophobic interaction chromatography. Anal. Biochem. 173,116-124
12. Robertson E.F., H.K. Dannelly, P.J. Malloy and H.C. Reeves. 1987. Rapid isoelectric focusing in a vertical polyacrylamide minigel system. Anal. Biochem. 167:290-294.
13. Strachan AF., F.C. de Beer, D.R. van der Westerhuyzen and G.A. Coetzee. 1988. Identification of three isoform patterns of human serum amyloid A protein. Biochem J. 250:203-207 (1988).

DIFFERENTIAL REGULATION OF HUMAN SERUM AMYLOID A ISOFORMS

Kluve-Beckerman, B., Liepnieks, J. and Benson, M.D.
Indiana University School of Medicine, Department of Medicine, Rheumatology Division, Clinical Building 492, 541 Clinical Drive, Indianapolis, IN 46223 and Veterans Affairs Medical Center (583/111RH), 1481 West 10th Street, Room #A772, Indianapolis, IN 46202, USA.

ABSTRACT. Significantly more SAA1 than SAA2 is routinely purified from the plasma of patients studied by this laboratory. Investigating the reason for this disparity, we have compared mRNA levels for SAA1 and SAA2 in a patient whose ratio of purified SAA1/SAA2 was approximately six. Relative levels of SAA1 and SAA2 mRNA were determined by Northern analysis using isotype-specific oligonucleotide probes. Scanning densitometry of the resulting autoradiographs revealed a 2-fold predominance of SAA1 over SAA2 mRNA. Thus, a higher steady state level of SAA1 mRNA explains in part the predominance of the SAA1 isotype.

INTRODUCTION

There are two major forms of serum amyloid A (SAA) in both mouse and human plasma. In the mouse only one form, SAA2, is deposited as amyloid A (AA) protein [1,2]. Over a 20-day course of murine amyloid induction, the ratio of plasma SAA2/SAA1 drops dramatically from 1.28 to 0.15, while the ratio of SAA2/SAA1 mRNA as measured by immunoprecipitation of cell-free translation products remains fairly constant (day 1=1.36; day 20=1.23) [3]. These data have been explained by the selective and rapid removal of SAA2 from the circulating pool of SAA1 and SAA2.

Similar to the monotypy of murine amyloid deposits, a single human isotype, SAA1, accounts for the vast majority (80-100%) of the AA protein isolated from any one individual [4]. In contrast to the murine model, however, SAA1 is also the predominant isotype purified from plasma. Although the ratio of human SAA1/SAA2 has not been followed during the amyloidogenic period, significantly more SAA1 than SAA2 has been isolated from the plasma of patients experiencing an acute phase response as well as from those with end-stage reactive amyloidosis. We have initiated a study to determine if the increased level of purified human SAA1 versus SAA2 reflects the physiologic state or is due to selective loss of SAA2 during purification. Relative levels of mRNA for the two isotypes have been measured in a patient from whom approximately six times more SAA1 than SAA2 was purified.

MATERIALS AND METHODS

Northern Blot Analysis. Total RNA was isolated from human liver tissue [5] and poly A+ RNA selected by chromatography on oligo(dT) cellulose. Poly A+ RNA (900, 450, and 225 ng) was fractionated in a 1% agarose gel containing 1.1 M formaldehyde and 10 mM sodium phosphate, pH 7.4 by electrophoresis at 50 volts for 3.5 hours. Transfer of the RNA to nitrocellulose was in 20X SSPE. Nitrocellulose filters were prehybridized in 6X SSPE, 5X Denhardt's, and 0.1% SDS for 2.5 hours at 47°C and hybridized with SAA1 and SAA2 specific probes overnight in 6X SSPE, 1X Denhardt's, 0.1% SDS, and 150 ug/ml tRNA at 47°C. Both probes were 17mer oligonucleotides with Tm's of 52°C and designed to specifically recognize sequences in the 3'-untranslated region of either SAA1 mRNA or SAA2 mRNA. The SAA1 probe consisted of: 5'-CCATTGTGTACCCTCTC-3' and the SAA2 probe: 5'CTCAGCTTCTCTGGACA-3'. Following hybridization the filters were subjected to three 20 minute washes in 6X SSPE, 0.1% SDS at room temperature and one 5 minute wash in 6X SSPE, 0.1% SDS at 47°C. Autoradiography was carried out with Kodak AR film and intensifying screens. Autoradiographs were scanned on a Hoefer GS365 P5 densitometer and the scans integrated with the complementary Hoefer/IBM software package.

Southern Blot Analysis. Cloned SAA1 and SAA2 cDNAs in pBR322 [6] were linearized by digestion with EcoRI and then aliquots of each (80, 40, and 20 ng) electrophoresed in a 1% agarose gel in Tris-borate-EDTA buffer, pH 8.3. Before transfer to nitrocellulose, the DNA was stained with ethidium bromide and visualized under UV light to confirm that appropriate amounts of DNA were present in each lane. Strips of nitrocellulose containing both SAA1 cDNA and SAA2 cDNA were prehybridized, hybridized, washed, and autoradiographed together with each of the RNA filters to evaluate the specificity and hybridizability of the SAA1 and SAA2 oligonucleotide probes.

RESULTS AND DISCUSSION

The autoradiographic signal produced by hybridizing acute phase liver RNA with an SAA1-specific oligonucleotide probe was approximately twice as intense as that produced with an SAA2-specific probe (Figure 1). Hybridization to filters containing SAA1 and SAA2 cDNAs included with the RNA blots demonstrated the specificity of each probe (Figure 1). The SAA1 probe showed virtually no hybridization to SAA2 cDNA and strong hybridization to the complementary SAA1 cDNA, while the SAA2 probe barely detected SAA1 cDNA and gave an intense signal with SAA2 cDNA. The lack of cross-hybridization allowed the intensity of the signal produced by each probe on the RNA blots to be considered a relative measure of the amount of mRNA for that particular isotype. Thus, the 2-fold stronger signal generated by the SAA1 probe indicates that the steady state level of SAA1 mRNA was approximately 2 times that of SAA2 mRNA in the liver under investigation. The donor of this liver was known to have elevated serum SAA due to traumatic injury.

The yield of SAA purified from 100 ml of plasma obtained from this patient at the time of organ donation was 5.3 mg SAA1 versus 0.8 mg SAA2 after fractionation of the two isotypes by reverse phase HPLC. Such a predominance of SAA1 over SAA2 also has been noted for three other individuals from whom SAA has been purified in this laboratory.

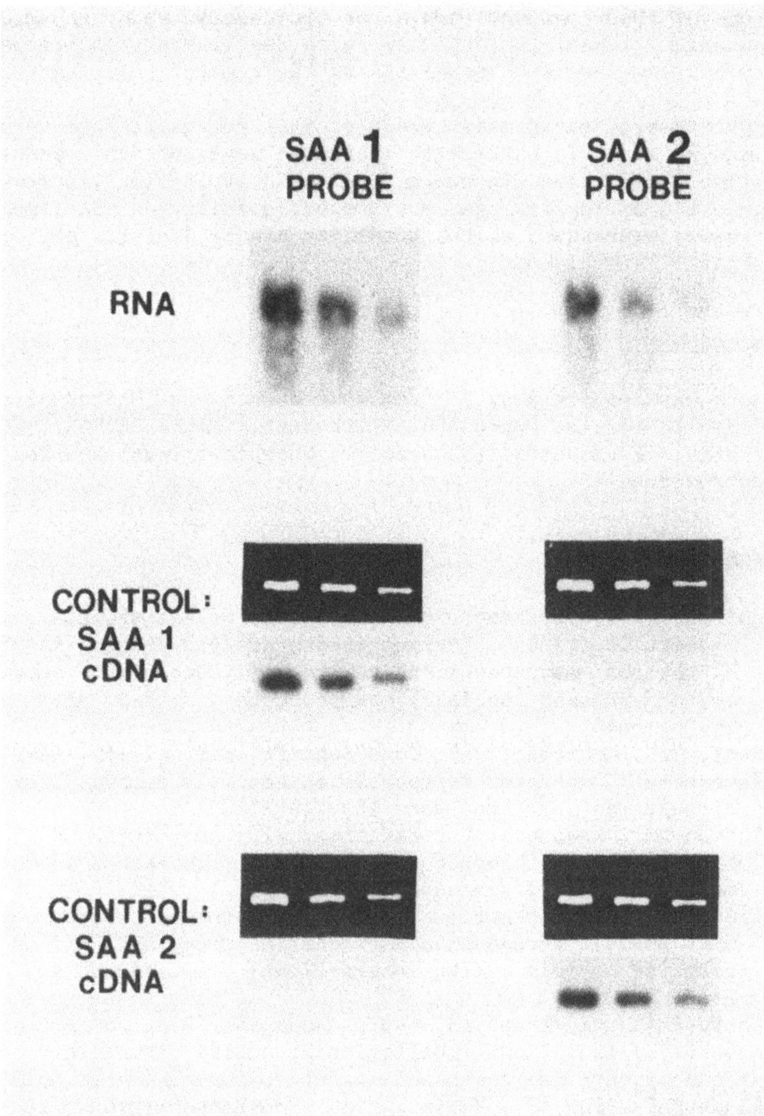

Figure 1. Northern analyses of human liver polyA+ RNA and Southern analyses of cloned SAA1 and SAA2 cDNAs using isotype-specific of oligonucleotide probes. RNA (left to right: 900, 450, and 225 ng) was electrophoresed in a 1% agarose gel containing 1.1 M formaldehyde, transferred to nitrocellulose, and hybridized with SAA1 and SAA2 specific oligonucleotides. As controls, SAA1 and SAA2 cDNAs in pBR322 (left to right: 80, 40, and 20 ng) were also electrophoresed in a 1% agarose gel, transferred to nitrocellulose, and included in the hybridizations with each probe. Ethidium bromide-stained cDNA before transfer is shown above the autoradiographs of hybridization.

While one of these patients had a chronic disease and high serum concentration of SAA, the other two were reactive amyloid patients who notably had low levels of total SAA at the time of their deaths.

As reported here, the greater yield of SAA1 versus SAA2 protein can be explained at least in part by an increased level of SAA1 versus SAA2 mRNA. The 2-fold predominance of SAA1 mRNA may reflect increased transcription of the SAA1 gene or greater stability of SAA1 mRNA. In either case, expression of the two major plasma isoforms appears to be differentially regulated.

ACKNOWLEDGEMENTS

This work was supported by VA Medical Research, the United States Public Health Service (RR-00750, NIDDK-34881, NIAMS-AR20582, AR7448), The Arthritis Foundation, The Grace M. Showalter Trust and The Marion E. Jacobson Fund.

REFERENCES

1. Hoffman, J.S., Ericsson, L.H., Eriksen, N., Walsh, K.A., and Benditt, P. (1984), 'Murine tissue amyloid protein AA. NH-terminal sequence identity with only one of two serum amyloid protein (ApoSAA) gene products', J. Exp. Med. 159,641-646.
2. Meek, R.L., Hoffman, J.S., and Benditt, E.P. (1986), 'Amyloidogenesis: One serum isotype is selectively removed from the circulation', J. Exp. Med. 163, 499-510.
3. Shiroo, M., Kawahara, E., Nakanishi, I., and Migita, S. (1987), 'Specific deposition of serum amyloid A protein 2 in the mouse', Scand. J. Immunol. 26, 709-716.
4. Liepnieks, J.J., Leagre, C., Kluve-Beckerman, B., and Benson, M.D. (1990), 'Predominance of one SAA isotype (SAAI) in human reactive amyloid', VIth International Symposium on Amyloidosis, Oslo, Norway.
5. Chirgwin, J.M., Przybyla, A.E., MacDonald, R.J. and Rutter, W.J. (1979), 'Isolation of biologically active ribonucleic acid from sources enriched in ribonuclease', Biochemistry 18, 5294-5299.
6. Kluve-Beckerman, B., Dwulet, F.E., and Benson, M.D. (1988), 'Human serum amyloid A: Three hepatic mRNAs and the corresponding proteins in one person', J. Clin. Invest. 82, 1670-1675.

THE EFFECT OF SAA-DERIVED FRAGMENT - SAA_{2-82} - ON PLATELET AGGREGATION

DAVID LEVARTOWSKY[1,2], MORDECHAI PRAS[1]
[1]Heller Institute for Medical Research, Sheba Medical Center 52621, Israel.
[2]Department of Organic Chemistry, The Weizmann Institute of Science, Rehovot 76100, Israel.

ABSTRACT. SAA is a highly conserved acute phase protein among animals. Various inflammatory stimuli induce vigorous synthesis of SAA, which comprises up to 2.5% of the hepatic protein synthesis capacity. Despite the ubiquity of SAA and the existance of such elaborate synthetic mechanism, the biological functions of SAA remain obscure. FMF patients are subjected to recurrent inflammatory attacks, which impose physiological and biochemical changes, that are associated with propensity to cardiovascular morbidity. However, this anticipation is being challenged by the clinical observation of significantly reduced prevalence of myocardial infarctions and thromboembolic phenomena among these patients. We evaluated the potential cardioprotective effect of SAA via a tentative platelet anti-aggregatory effect. Platelet-rich plasma was pre-incubated for 20 minutes with SAA fragment, corresponding to residues 2–82, and thereafter were treated with four different aggregating agents, namely Epinephrine, Ristocetine, Collagen, and ADP. SAA-fragment, especially in its higher concentrations, was found to inhibit signficantly the normal pattern of platelet aggregation with all these four aggregants. SAA, by its platelet inhibitory property, particularly in an acute-phase response like concentration, may regulate various clinical expressions of cardiovascular morbidity. This cffect should not be limited to FMF patients.

Introduction

Despite the fact that SAA is a highly conserved protein among animals, and its elaborate synthetic mechanisms during acute-phase response, its physiological functions remain obscure, though immunomodulation was suggested. Platelet activity and platelet-derived mediators of inflammation are accessory elements of the acute-phase response. We studied the potential modulatory effect of SAA on platelet aggregation. Our results suggest attenuation of platelet aggregation in a dose-dependent manner. The tentative importance of this effect will be discussed.

Materials and Methods

SAA related peptide: Peptide SAA 2-82, corresponding to residues was extracted from amyloidotic goiter of FMF patient as previously described [1]. *SAA_{2-82} solutions* were prepared by dissolving SAA_{2-82} in normal human sera which were previously subjected to complement deactivation (60 min x 56°C). *Platelets preparation*: Citrated venous blood was centrifuged at 250 x g for 10 min. to obtain platelet-rich plasma (PRP). The remaining blood was recentrifuged to obtain platelet-poor plasms (PPP), which was used as a blank. *Aggregating agents:* (Sigma) Epinephrine - 5μM, calf skin collagen - 0.1 mg/ml, ADP - 10 μM, and ristocetin - 0.75 mg/ml. *Platelet aggregation:* Measurements were carried out in a four channel aggregometer (PAF-4, Bio-data). Platelets, at final concentration of 2 x 10^8 cells/ml were stirred at 1200 rpm at 37°C in the presence of SAA_{2-82}, 0.6-600 μg/ml and was allowed to equilibrate for 20 min. Then one of the aggregating agents were added into a total volume of 0.250 ml, and the light transmittance was recorded for 4 min [2,3]. The signficance of the results was evaluated by students t-test.

Results and Discussion

The effect of SAA-related peptide-SAA_{2-28} on platelet aggregation induced by ADP, collagen, epinephrine and ristocetin is summarized in Table 1, and shown in Figure 1.

Table 1: Inhibition of aggregating agent induced platelet aggregation by SAA_{2-82}

	PLATELET AGGREGRATION (%)			
	Aggregation agent			
SAA_{2-82} μg/ml concentration	ADP	Collagen	Epinephrine	Ristocetin
0.6	78±10	75±12	71±6	78±8
6	77±4	71±5	71±9	76±9
60	73±10	66±10	69±1	*65±10
120	*64±4	--	--	--
600	**45±7	**40±7	**38±4	**35±6

The results are expressed as means ± SD of 9 experiments. *P <0.05, **P <0.0005 (students t-test).

The results imply that platelet aggregation that was induced by either ADP, collagen, epinephrine or ristocetin was attenuated in a dose-dependent fashion by SAA-related peptide SAA_{2-82}. Significant inhibition was observed only in concentrations that simulate full-blown acute-phase response (60-600 μg/ml). It should be emphasized that these aggregating agents are chemically distinct and also vary in their receptors and modes of action. However, they are all capable of platelet activation and facilitation of clot formation [4].

The results of this study fall into line with the not yet described clinical observations regarding FMF patients - i.e. significantly reduced prevalence of myocardial infarctions (about 1.5% out of 450 patients beyond 40y of age) and thrombo-embolic phenomena. This anti-aggregative effect of SAA upon platelets should be further stressed in view of the fact that FMF patients recurrently sustain inflammatory attacks, which introduce physiological and biochemical changes that are well known for their association with hypercoagulability, thromboembolic phenomena, and cardiovascular morbidity and mortality [5], e.g. presence of cryofibrinogen [6], circulating fibrin [7], procoagulant activity [8], leukoagglutinins [9], circulating immune complexes [5,10,11] and the increased levels of fibrinogen [12] and alpha-2 macroglobulin [10,13]. Uncontrolled complement system due to C_{5a} inhibitor deficiency may further induce pro-coagulability [10]. Additional impacts on aggregation and hemostasis in these patients should be referred to the presence of C-reactive protein (CRP), serum amyloid P (SAP), glycosaminoglycans (especially heparan sulfate), colchicine therapy and amyloidosis (Nephrotic syndrome and renal failure). Involvement of the prostaglandin system is implied by the presence of hydroxy fatty acids in patients' sera, which could be related to

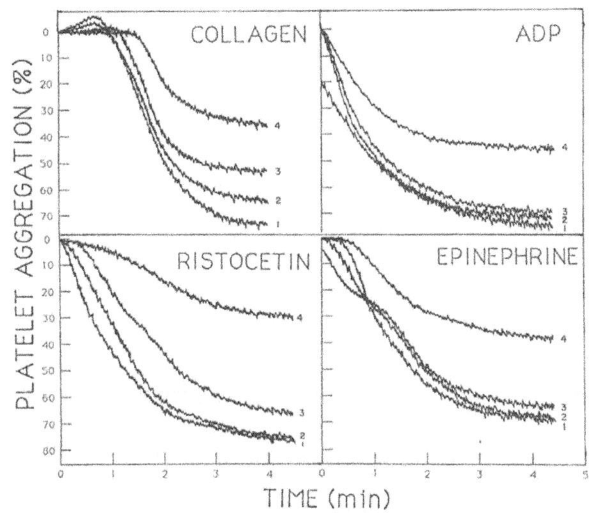

Figure 1. Characteristics effect of SAA_{2-82} on platelet aggregation that was induced by ADP, collagen, epimephrine and ristocetin. SAA_{2-82} concentration (μg/ml): (1) 0.6, (2) 6, (3) 60, (4) 600

an aspirin-like effect of a serum factor (possibly SAA) that interferes with the cyclooxygenase pathway and prefers the synthetic products of the lipooxygenase route [14]. Furthermore, reduced prostacyclin (PG-I_2) production was observed in macrophages obtained from mice with AA-amyloidosis, compared to the amyloid resistant strain [15]. It is of interest that in Behcet's disease and systemic lupus erythematosus (SLE), which are reputed for being associated with thromboembolism, the SAA level is considerably low compared to similar diseases. The interaction of SAA and HDL is intriguing, since cardio-protective effect is attributed to HDL. The effect of SAA on platelets is suggested to be mediated by the sequence corresponding to residues 39-41 of SAA, i.e. Arg-Gly-Asn (RGN). This sequence closely resembles that of Arg-Gly-Asp (RGD) that mediates the binding of certain proteins (fibrinogen, fibronectin, VWF, vitronectin) to platelet membranal receptor - GP IIb-IIIa (a member if the integrin family of receptors) that play a fundamental role in platelet adhesion. RGD-related peptides are capable of inhibiting platelet adhesion and aggregation [16].

This effect can take place during the acute-phase response by the SAA, as a whole, or by inflammatory cell-mediated degradative related peptides that contain this sequence Further evaluation of this theory is warranted. Alternatively, SAA as a superoxide production inhibitor may regulate platelet aggregation [17,18], possibly concomitantly to other mechanisms. This effect, in fact, potentially involves any situation that is associated with acute-phase response.

References

1. Prelli, F., Pras, M., Frangione, B. (1987) 'Degradation and deposition of amyloid A fibrils are tissue specific', Biochemistry 26, 8251-8256.
2. Weiss, H.J. (1983) 'Platelet aggregation', in W.J. Willliams, E. Beutler, A.J. Erslev and M.A. Lichtman (eds.), Hematology, McGraw-Hill Publishers, New York, pp. 1673-1675.
3. Yardumian, D.A., Mackie, I.J., Machin, S.J. (1986) 'Laboratory investigation of platelet function. A review of methodology', J. Clin. Pathol. 39, 701-712.
4. Kroll, M.H. and Schafer, A.I. (1989) 'Biochemical mechanisms of platelet activation', Blood 74, 1181-1195.
5. Schafer, A.I. (1985) 'The hypercoagulable state', Ann. Intern. Med. 102, 814-828.
6. Shamir, H., Pras, M., Sohar, E. and Gafni, J. (1974) 'Cryofibrinogen in familial Mediterranean fever', 134, 125-126.
7. Mosesson, M.W., Wautier, J.L., Amrani, D.L., Dervichian, M. and Catan, D. (1982) 'Evidence for circulating fibrin in familial Mediterranean fever', J. Lab. Clin. Med. 99, 559-567.
8. Courillon-Mallet, A., Bevilacqua, M., Wautier, J.L., Dervichian, M., Cattan, D. and Caen, J. (1986) 'Increased procoagulant response of monocytes from patients with familial Mediterranean fever', Thromb. Haemostas. 56, 211-213.
9. Eliakim, M., Levy, M. and Ehrenfeld, M. (1981) Recurrent polyserositis (familial Mediterranean fever, periodic disease), Elsvier, North-holland, Amsterdam.
10. Blajchman, M.A. and Ozge-Anwar, A.H. (1986) 'The role of complement system in hemostasis', Progress in Hematology 14, 149-182.
11. Levy, M., Ehrenfeld, M., Levo, Y., Fischel, R., Zlotnick, A. and Eliakim, M. (1980) 'Circulating immune complexes in recurrent poly serositis (familial Mediterranean fever, periodic disease),' J. Rheumatol. 7, 886-890.
12. Frensdorff, A., Sohar, E. and Heller, H. (1961) 'Plasma fibrinogen in familial Mediterranean fever', Ann. Intern. Med. 55(3), 448-455.
13. Frensdorff, A., Shibolet, S., Lamprecht, S. and Sohar, E. (1964) 'Plasma proteins in familial Mediterranean fever', Clin. Chim. Acta 10, 106-113.
14. Aisen, P.S., Haines, K.A., Given, W. et al. (1985) 'Circulating hydroxy fatty acids in familial Mediterranean fever', Proc. Natl. Acad. Sci. U.S.A. 82, 1232-1236.
15. Leslie, C.A., Lazzari, A. and Cathcart, E.S. (1986) 'Prostacyclin and thromboxane production from macrophages of amyloid resistent and sensitive mice', in G.G. Glenner, E.F. Osserman, E.P. Benditt, E. Clakins, A.S. Cohen and D. Zucker-Franklin (eds.) , Amyloidosis, Plenum Press, New York, pp.175-185.
16. Plow, E.F., Pierschbacher, M.D., Rouslahti, E., Marguerie, G.A. and Ginsberg, M.H. (1985) 'The effects of Arg-Gly-Asp containing peptides on fibrinogen and von Willebrand factor binding to platelets', Proc. Natl. Acad. Sci. U.S.A. 82, 8057-8061.
17. Del Principe, D., Menichelli, A., De Matteis, W., Di Corpo, M.L., Di Giulio, S. and Finazzi-Agro, A. (1985) 'Hydrogen peroxide has a role in the aggregation of human platelets', FEBS Lett. 185, 142-146.
18. Levartowsky, D., Pras, M., Shephard, E., Rosen, O. and Fridkin, M. (1990) 'Serum amyloid A (SAA)-related peptide isolated from synovial fluid modulates superoxide production by human neutrophils', This Symposium.

SERUM AMYLOID A, AN ACUTE PHASE PROTEIN, INHIBITS PLATELET ACTIVATION

Shulamit Zimlichman,[1] Abraham Danon,[2] Ilana Nathan,[3] Gabriel Mozes[4] and Ruth Shainkin-Kestenbaum[1]
Departments of Nephrology,[1] Clinical Pharmacology,[2]
Hematology,[3] and Orthopedic Surgery[4]
Soroka Medical Center and Ben-Gurion University of the Negev,
P.O.Box 653
Beer-Sheva, Israel.

Serum amyloid A is an acute phase protein known to circulate in blood as a component of high density lipoprotein. Platelets and mediators released from activated platelets are involved in various inflammatory reactions (1). It was, therfore, of interest to investigate whether this protein could play a role in modulating platelet function.

Serum amyloid A was purified from sera of patients who had undergone severe musculoskeletal trauma, according to Rosenthal et al.(2) as modified by Pras (personal communication). Gel filtered platelets were separated using a Sepharose 2B-CL column.

Serum amyloid A (50 μg/ml) inhibited the platelet aggregation that was induced by thrombin (0.05 u/ml) ($p<0.005$). Serum amyloid A also inhibited TxB_2 generation and serotonin release by thrombin-activated gel filtered platelets The time-course of inhibition by serum amyloid A reveals attenuation with time of this effect. Thus, TxB_2 generation in the presence of serum amyloid A was only 14.2±7.1% of control at 2 min, compared to 46.0±15.5% at 6 min following stimulation with 0.05 u/ml thrombin. In the presence of 25 and 50 μg/ml serum amyloid A, the cytosolic $[Ca^{2+}]$ rose 2 min following thrombin induction by only 46.0 and 25.0 nM, respectively, compared with 90 nM in the control system. The mean inhibition over time by 50 μg/ml serum amyloid A of cytosolic $[Ca^{2+}]$ increase was 45.0±16.0%. We also studied the effect of human amyloid A, purified from amyloidotic spleen of a Familial Mediterranean Fever patient, on the aggregation of thrombin-induced gel filtered platelets. 25 μg/ml of this protein also markedly suppressed aggregation. In order to find out whether serum amyloid A interacts directly with thrombin, its effect on clotting and amidolytic activities of the enzyme were studied. Serum amyloid A (50 μg/ml) did not affect the clotting or amidolytic activities of thrombin. To further investigate the possibility of direct interaction between serum amyloid A and thrombin, serum amyloid A was labeled with ^{125}I and chromatographed . The elution pattern and retention time of serum amyloid A were similar in the presence and absence of thrombin, excluding any possible interaction between these two proteins.

The results indicate that serum amyloid A, an acute phase protein, specifically inhibits thrombin-induced platelet aggregation, reduces TxB_2 production and serotonin release, and attenuates the increase in cytosolic [Ca^{+2}]. This inhibitory effect of serum amyloid A was most pronounced during the initial stage of aggregation and exhibited an inverse relationship with thrombin concentration, thus suggesting a competitive type antagonism. It is intriguing to hypothesize that serum amyloid A, the concentration of which increases many-fold following acute myocardial infarction, could serve to modulate the thrombin-induced platelet aggregation that may be associated with this event. The results presented here, and the possible involvement of serum amyloid A in immunoregulation (3), may suggest a putative role of this acute phase protein in the modulation of some of the processes occurring in acute phase events.

References

1. Oxholm, P. and Winther, K. (1986) Thrombocyte involvement in immune inflammatory reactions, Allergy 41, 1-10.
2. Rosenthal, CJ., Franklin, EC. Frangione, B. and Greenspan, J. (1976) Isolation and partial characterization of SAA - an amyloid-related protein from human serum, J Immunol 116, 1415-1418.
3 Benson, MD. and Aldo-Benson, M. (1979) Effect of purified SAA on immune response *in vitro*: Mechanisms of suppression, J Immunol 122, 2077-2082.

SERUM AMYLOID A (SAA)-RELATED PEPTIDE ISOLATED FROM SYNOVIAL FLUID MODULATES SUPEROXIDE PRODUCTION BY HUMAN NEUTROPHILS.

DAVID LEVARTOWSKY[1,3], MORDECHAI PRAS[1], ENID SHEPHARD[2], OREN ROSEN[3] AND MATI FRIDKIN[3]

[1]Heller Institute for Medical Research, Sheba Medical Center, Israel 52621. [2]Clinical Science and Immunlogy, University of Cape Town Medical School, Cape Town, R.S.A. [3]Department of Organic Chemistry, The Weizmann Institute of Science, Rehovot 76100, Israel

ABSTRACT. A mixture of low-molecular weight peptides was isolated from an inflammatory synovial fluid and fractionated by high performance liquid chromatography (HPLC). One fraction, capable of inhibiting lucigenin-enhanced chemiluminescence of activated neutrophils, was found to be the peptide H-Ala-Gly-Leu-Pro-Glu-Lys-Tyr-OH corresponding to amino acid residues 98-104 of SAA. Respective synthetic peptide, coeluted on HPLC with the natural fraction, was found to modulate superoxide anion production by activated human neutrophils. Related synthetic peptides were found to have modulatory effects. Taking together the fact that toxic free-radicals have been implicated as important pathological mediators of organ injury in a wide range of human diseases, and the fact that these diseases are usually associated with induction of acute phase response, modulatory effect of SAA-related peptides on superoxide release from PMNs, shed new light on the potential functional importance of SAA in a broad spectrum of clinical situations.

Introduction

Various diseases involving the joints result in accumulation of inflammatory synovial fluid. The inflammatory changes include, among other elements, the presence of highly increased levels of the acute-phase proteins (CRP) and SAA [1], as well as elevated numbers of white blood cells.

Recently, CRP and SAA were shown to be degraded by inflammatory cells into smaller peptides [2,3]. The CRP-derived peptides are bioactive and display anti-inflammatory properties [3]. These findings have prompted us to explore the possibility that peptides related to acute-phase proteins are present in inflammatory, synovial, and perhaps other, fluids and play a defensive role in these loci.

Materials and Methods

Synovial fluids were collected at the time of diagnostic arthrocentesis of inflamed knee joints. After immediate centrifugation at 1500 xg for 10 min, the cell-free supernatant was aliquoted and stored at -20°C. *Isolation of crude low molecular weight peptide mixtures* was affected by: (1) removal of hyaluronic acid and of protein content by ethanol (75%) precipitation; (2) TCA-precipitation of remaining high molecular weight material and (3) lyophilization. *Fractionation of peptide mixtures* was achieved by HPLC on C_8 and C_{18} silica columns, employing linear acetonitrile: water (containing 0.1% trifluoroacetic acid) gradients. *Structural determination of fractions* was achieved by amino acid analysis, following automatic amino acid sequence determination. *Peptide synthesis* was accomplished through the solid-phase strategy of Merrifield [4]. *Neutrophils* were isolated from healthy volunteers using Ficoll-Hypaque gradient. *Generation of oxygen radicals from fMLP-stimulated human PMN-leukocytes* was measured by lucigenin-enhanced chemiluminescence (LECL) [3]. *Generation of superoxide anions from stimulated human PMN-leukocytes* was assessed by cytochrome C reduction [5]. Cells were stimulated by the chemotactic peptide fMLP, PMA, or by histone-opsonized [6] *streptococci.*

Results and Discussion

HPLC-fractionations of various inflammatory synovial fluids reveal similar, though not identical, elution patterns. As illustrated in Table 1, several fractions obtained from one of the synovial fluids (49y diabetic woman, suffering from monoarthritis of the knee) inhibited LECL of fMLP and PMA-stimulated neutrophils. The fraction eluted at 25.77 min was found to contain the peptide H-Ala-Gly-Leu-Pro-Glu-Lys-Tyr-OH corresponding to amino acid residues 98-104 of SAA. A respective synthetic peptide was coeluted with a section of the natural fraction (Fig. 1). Synthetic 98-104 peptide and related synthetic analogs (sequences corresponding to residues 77-104, 99-104 and 100-104 of SAA) were found to modulate superoxide generation from activated human PMNs (Fig. 2).

Toxic free-radicals have been implicated as important pathologic mediators of organ injury in a wide spectrum of human diseases. Oxygen radicals are capable of reversibly or irreversibly damaging compounds of all biochemical classes, including nucleic acids, connective tissue macromolecules, carbohydrates, lipids and lipoproteins, proteins and free amino acids. These species may have an impact on such cell activities as membrane function, metabolism and gene expression. Oxygen free-radicals have a putative role as agents of tissue damage in a vast number of diseases and pathologic mechanisms ranging from carcinogenesis and cancer to aging, autoimmune conditions, acute and chronic inflammatory diseases, atherosclerosis, ischemia-induced diseases and, particularly, myocardial infarcation.

Table 1. Inhibition of superoxide production (LECL) by fractions from synovial fluid

Fraction number	retention times (min)	% superoxide inhibition
1	5.17	14±0.28
2	10.10	34±0.68
3	20.39	16±0.32
4	25.77	75±1.5
5	36.20	27±0.54

Many defense mechanisms within the organism have evolved to limiting the level of reactive oxygen species and the damage they induce. Tissue insult invovles free-radical release and induction of acute phase response. This includes synthesis of proteins known to be scavengers of free-radicals, i.e. haptoglobin and ceruloplasmin, but especially synthesis of two major acute phase proteins - CRP and SAA - the level of which may increase up to 1000-fold [7]. These proteins were found to be degraded by proteolytic enzymes derived from inflammatory cells into peptides. Several CRP-related peptides are potent modulators of superoxide release from PMNs.

The present findings suggest that proteolysis of SAA may give rise to bioactive peptides that modulate the inflammatory response within the synovial fluid, and probably other extracellular fluids.

Special consideration should be referred to certain conditions, i.e. reperfusion injury of myocardial infarction [8], cancer [9], aging [9] and inflammatory artritides [1], in which the toxic effect of free-radicals is essential to its pathogenesis and SAA level is significantly increased.

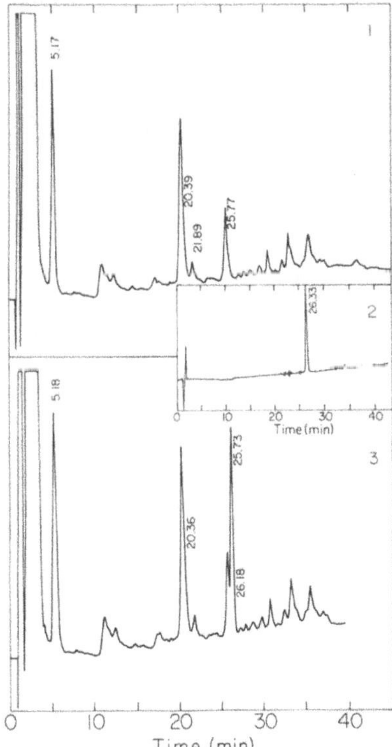

Figure 1. HPLC profiles of (1)synovial fluid derived low molecular weight peptides; (2) synthetic SAA 98-104 peptide; (3) co-injection 1 and 2.

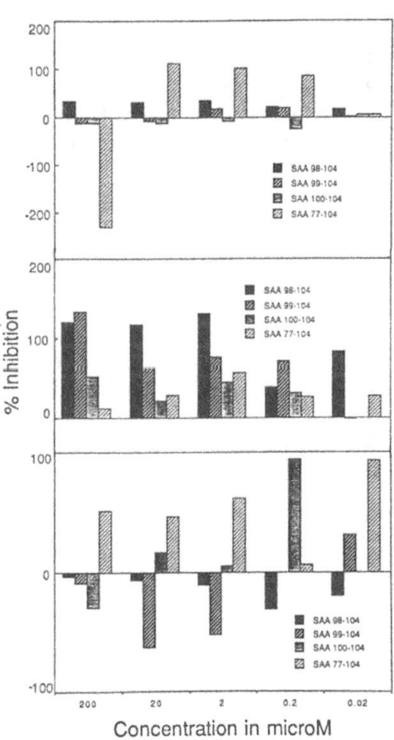

Figure 2. The effect of SAA related peptide on superoxide production by stimulated PMNs: (1) fMLP, (2) PMA, (3) *sterptococci*-opsonized with histone.

References

1. Sukenik, S., Henkin, J., Zimlichman, S., Skibin, A., Neuman, L., Pras, M., Horowitz, J. and Shainkin-Kestenbaum, R. (1988) 'Serum and synovvial fluid levels of SAA protein and CRP in inflammatory and non-inflammatory arthritis', J. Rheumatol. 15, 942-945.

2. Lavie, G., Zucker-Franklin, D. and Franklin, E.C. (1978) 'Degradation of SAA protein by surface-associated enzymes of human blood monocytes', J. Exp. Med. 148, 1020-1031.

3. Shephard, E.G., Beer, S.M., Anderson, R., Strachan, A.F., Nel, A.E. and De Beer, F.C. (1989) 'Generation of biologically active C-reactive protein peptides by a neutral protease on the membrane of phorbol myristate acetate-stimulated neutrophils', J. Immunol. 143, 2974-2981.

4. Merrifield, R.B. (1963) 'Solid phase synthesis. (I). The synthesis of a tetrapeptide', J. Am. Chem. Soc. 85, 2149-2154.

5. Bellavite, P., Dri, P., Della Bianca, V. and Serra, M.C. (1983) 'The measurement of superoxide anion production by granulocytes in whole blood. A clinical test for the evaluation of phagocyte function and serum opsonic capacity', Eur. J. Clin. Invest. 13, 363-368.

6. Ginsburg, I., Borinski, R., Malamud, D., Struckmeier, F. and Klimetzek, V. (1985) 'Chemiluminescence and superoxide generation by leukocytes stimulated by polyelectrolyte-opsonized bacteria', Inflammation 9, 245-271.

7. Kushner, I. (1989) 'Erythrocyte sedimentation rate and the acute phase reactants', in W.N. Kelley, E.D. Harris Jr., S. Ruddy and L.B. Sledge (eds.), Textbook of Rheumatology, W.B. Sanders Company, Philadelphia, pp. 719-727.

8. Shainkin-Kestenbaum, R., Winikoff, Y., Cristal, N. (1986) 'SAA concentrations during the course of actute ischemaemic heart disease', J.Clin. Pathol. 39, 635-637.

9. Rosenthal, C.J., Franklin, E.C. (1975) 'Variation with age and disease of an amyloid A protein-related serum component', J. Clin. Invest. 55, 746-753.

ANTIPLATELET AGGREGATION ACTIVITY OF SERUM AMYLOID A (SAA) RELATED PEPTIDES

R. SHAINKIN-KESTENBAUM[a], D. LEVARTOWSKY[b,c], S. ZIMLICHMAN[a], M. FRIDKIN[c] AND M. PRAS[b]

[a]Soroka Medical Center and Ben Gurion University of the Negev, Beer-Sheva, Israel. [b]Heller Institute for Medical Research, Sheba Medical Center, Israel 52621. [c]Department of Organic Chemistry, The Weizmann Institute of Science, Rehovot 76100, Israel

ABSTRACT. The effect of Serum Amyloid A (SAA), Amyloid A (AA) and related peptides on thrombin-induced platelet activation was studied, in order to locate the site of the SAA molecule, in which the inhibitory effect, previously been reported by us, resides. The results suggest that the N-terminal hydrophobic region between amino acid residues 2-15 is responsible for most of the inhibitory activity of the SAA molecule. 6.5 μg/ml of this peptide inhibits aggregation. Other regions, including C-terminal related peptides exhibit milder inhibitory activity. Although this main active site is also the lipid binding site of the SAA molecule to HDL, the small amount of lipid-free SAA required for biological activity, in comparison to the high serum level in acute event, like acute myocardial infarction, possibly enables SAA to exert its activity in the presence of serum. This activity may contribute to the relatively low incidence of thromboembolic phenomena in FMF patients and in acute septic diseases in which SAA levels are highly increased.

Introduction

In a previous study, we described specific inhibition of thrombin- induced platelet activation by the acute phase protein SAA. This inhibition, however, was not observed in platelet-rich plasma [1]. One could speculate that as most of the SAA in plasma is bound to HDL [2], and as we were limited in our in vitro studies to small amounts of SAA, due to its poor solubility, the inhibitory effect could not be detected. Since the pathogenesis of thromboembolic phenomena are of special importance in many acute events, e.g. myocardial infarction, it was of interest to locate the biologically active site of thrombin-induced platelet activation in the SAA molecule.

Materials and Methods

Isolation of Serum Amyloid A from serum of patients was performed as described previously [1].

Amyloid A 1-76 and 2-46 amino acids were extracted from amyloidotic tissue of FMF patients as described previously [3].

Polypeptides from various regions of SAA were synthesized by the solid phase peptide synthesis method according to Merrifield [4]. The following peptides were prepared: 2-15 amino acids corresponding to the N-terminal region: H-Ser-Phe-Phe-Ser-Phe-Leu-Gly-Glu-Ala-Phe-Asp-Gly-Ala-Arg-OH; sequence 76-104 from the C-terminal region: H-Leu-Ala-Asp-Gln-Ala-Ala-Asn-Glu-Trp-Gly-Arg-Ser-Gly-Lys-Asp-Pro-Asn-His-Phe-Arg-Pro-Ala-Gly-Leu-Pro-Glu-Lys-Tyr-OH.

Platelet separation and aggregation was performed as previously described [1].

DATA EVALUATION

The effect of SAA, AA and related peptides on thrombin- induced aggregation was calculated for 2 to 6 min. and expressed in percent of inhibition of control system. The significance of the effect was evaluated by student's T-test.

Results

Attenuation of thrombin-induced platelet aggregation by 50 μg/ml SAA or AA is summarized in Table 1. As shown, AA (1-76 amino acids) has a stronger inhibitory effect on aggregation than the entire molecule of SAA (1-104 amino acids). The inhibition by both proteins was more pronounced during the initial stage of aggregation (2 min) and decreased with time. Table 2 demonstrates the inhibition by peptides from various regions of SAA, as compared to the inhibition by AA. As shown, the N-terminal hydrophobic region, 2-15, exerts the most pronounced effect of all the tested polypeptides and was also highly significant in the presence of 6.5 μg/ml. This higher effect became more stable with time as well. The C-terminal region of SAA, which is absent in AA and in the smaller peptides, also represent inhibitory activity, but milder than that of the hydrophobic N-terminal region.

Discussion

This study indicates that the specific inhibition of thrombin-induced platelet activation [1] is located mainly in the N-terminal hydrophobic region of SAA. This region was previously described as the lipid binding site of SAA through which the association of SAA with plasma HDL occurs [5-7]. This finding may explain our failure to detect the inhibitory effect by 50 μg/ml SAA on platelet-rich plasma. Due to the poor solubility of SAA in the in-vitro system, we were limited to the above amount of SAA. However, in the acute event as myocardial infarction, the plasma concentration may reach levels up to a few thousand μg/ml [8,9]. In these situations, despite the dramatic increase in SAA concentrations, its association with HDL may represent available storage of SAA, of which only small amounts of free protein is needed to exert its biological activity. Therefore, physiological importance in modulating thromboembolic events is suggested for SAA. It may contribute to the relatively lower incidence of thromboembolic phenomena in FMF patients and in acute septic diseases, in which SAA levels are greatly increased.

Table 1. Inhibition of thrombin-induced platelet aggregation by serum amyloid A (SAA) and amyloid A (AA).

	Control	SAA	control	AA
INITIAL SLOPE (cm/0.5 min)	2.3±0.3	1.6±0.2 (31.3)*	1.9±0.3	0.1±0.1 (96.0)**
AGGREGATION EXTENT (cm)				
at 2 min.	4.1±0.3	3.3±0.4 (22.1)*	5.7±0.6	0.4±0.4 (95.0)**
at 6 min.	7.9±0.6	7.2±0.6 (10.6)++	11.1±0.7	1.3±1.3 (89.0)**

Described are means±SEM of 14 experiments with SAA, and means±SEM of 3 experiments with AA. Numbers in parenthesis are % inhibition. Thrombin; 0.05-0.1 U/ml; serum amyloid A - 50 μg/ml AA equivalent; amyloid A - 50 μg/ml.
*$p < 0.02$, **$p < 0.0025$, ++$p < 0.05$, paired Student's t test.

Table 2. Inhibition of thrombin-induced platelet aggregation by AA and SAA-related peptides.

Amino Acid region	% INHIBITION 6.5 μg/ml		13 μg/ml		25 μg/ml	
	2 min	6 min	2 min	6 min	2 min	6 min
1-76, tissue	0	0	23	8	42*	5
2-46, tissue	0	0	0	0	16	8
2-15, synthetic	37*	5	48**	16**	64**	32**
76-104, synthetic	0	0	12	4	19*	4

The extent of aggregation was measured at 2 and 6 minutes, following stimulation with thrombin (0.05-0.1 U/ml); *significant, **highly significant in Student's t test.

References

1. Zimlichman, S., Danon, A., Nathan, I., Mozes, J. and Shainkin-Kestenbaum, R. (1990) 'Serum, amyloid A, an acute phase protein, inhibits platelet activation', J. Lab. Clin. Med. in press.

2. Skogen, B., Borresen, A.L., Natvig, J.B., Berg, K. and Michaelsen, T.E. (1979) 'High density lipoprotein as carrier for amyloid-related protein SAA in rabbit serum', Scand. J. Immunol. 10, 39-45.

3. Pras, M., Schubert, M., Zucker-Franklin, D., Rimon, A. and Franklin, E.C. (1968) 'The characterization of soluble amyloid prepared in water', J. Clin. Invest. 47, 924-933.

4. Merrifield, R.B. (1963) 'Solid phase peptide synthesis, I. The synthesis of a tetrapeptide', J. Am. Chem. Soc. 85, 2149-2154.

5. Segrest, J.P., Pownall, H.J., Jackson, R.L., Glenner, G.G. and Pollock, P.S. (1976) 'Amyloid A: amphipatic helixes and lipid binding', Biochemistry 15, 3187-3191.

6. Clifton, P.M., Mackinnon, A.M. and Barter, P.J. (1985) 'Effect of serum amyloid A protein (SAA) on composition, size and density of HDL in subjects with myocardial infarction', J. Lipid Res. 26, 1389-1398.

7. Turnell, W., Sarra, R., Glover, I.D., Baum, J.O., Caspi, D., Baltz, M.L. and Pepys, M.B. (1986) 'Secondary structure prediction of human SAA_1 presumptive identification of calcium and lipid binding sites', Mol. Biol. Med. 3, 387-407.

8. Kushner, I. (1982) 'The phenomenon of the acute phase response', Ann. N.Y. Acad. Sci. 389, 39-48.

9. Shainkin-Kestenbaum, R., Winikoff, Y. and Cristal, N. (1986) 'Serum amyloid A concentrations during the course of acute ischaemic heart disease', J. Clin. Pathol. 39, 635-637.

EFFECT OF PURIFIED SERUM AMYLOID A ON GROWTH AND DIFFERENTIATION OF TRANSFORMED CELLS

I. Nathan [1] D. Goldfarb[2], A. Dvilansky[1], Z. Zolotov[1]. and R. Shainkin-Kestenbaum[3].
Departments of [1]Hematology, [2]Pediatrics, and [3]Nephrology.
Soroka Medical Center and Ben-Gurion University of the Negev
P.O.Box 653 Beer-Sheva Israel.

ABSTRACT. The potential effect of the acute phase protein serum amyloid A (SAA) on the myeloid leukemia cell-line HL-60 was studied. Inhibition of cell proliferation was observed following 5 days incubation with 50 μg/ml of purified SAA. This inhibitory level of SAA is within the range of SAA levels in cancer patients, *in vivo*. Purified SAA by itself affected differentiation of HL-60 cells. Concomitant addition of sodium butyrate (0.5mM) or TPA (10^{-8}M) with purified SAA markedly potentiated the inhibitory effect on cell growth and enhanced the differentiation of these cells. These results suggest that SAA may play a role in modulation of cancer cells.

Introduction

Serum amyloid A (SAA) is an acute-phase apolipoprotein (1) associated with active malignant diseases. Previous studies have demonstrated a direct correlation between serum levels of SAA and disease activity (2-4). Recently, we also demonstrated the prognostic value of SAA in malignancy, whereby SAA levels correlate to the clinical course of the disease, and inversely correlate to survival time (5). The overall role of SAA in acute-phase response and in malignancy is far from being clear. HL-60 cells serve as a model for studies of tumor cell proliferation and differentiation. In the present study we investigated whether purified SAA affects the proliferation and differentiation of HL-60 promyelocyte leukemic cells into monocyte macrophage-like cells.

Materials and Methods

SAA was purified from sera of patients who had undergone severe musculoskeletal trauma, according to the method of Rosenthal *et al.* (6), as modified by Pras (personal communication). HL-60, promyelocytic leukemia cells (7) were grown in culture as previously described (8). HL-60 cells were seeded at $2\text{-}4 \times 10^5$/ml and incubated with TPA (10^{-8} M) for two days. Incubation with 0.5mM butyrate was carried out for five days. Cell number and adherent cells were determined using trypan blue exclusion method. Mac-1 positive cells were identified using the indirect immunofluorescent method (8). Statistical analysis was done by means of Student's t test.

Results

The effect of purified SAA on the proliferation of HL-60 cells was studied in the presence and absence of TPA, following two days of incubation. Purified SAA, at a concentration of 75 μg/ml, had a mild inhibitory effect on HL-60 cell proliferation, which was not statistically significant Higher concentrations of SAA could not be used due to insolubility of the purified material. TPA, at a concentration of 10^{-8} M, caused inhibition of HL-60 cell proliferation. However, when 75 μg/ml.SAA was added concomitantly with TPA, total cell number was reduced from 3.5±0.6 $x10^5$/ml to 1.5±0.4$x10^5$/ml ($p<0.05$).

Purified SAA by itself induced differentaion in 4 out of 7 experiments. (In four experiments, SAA induced 13.5±1.7% Mac 1 positive cells. In two experiments increased adhesiveness was also observed). In the presence of 10^{-8} M TPA, SAA affected differentiation in all performed experiments . Mean percent of adhesive cells of TPA treated cells was 55.5±0.7, as compared to 85.3±2.9 percent in the presence of both TPA and SAA (75 μg/ml) (p=0.001). There was no parallel increase in Mac-1 expression (75 μg/ml SAA even reduced the percentage of Mac-1 positive cells).

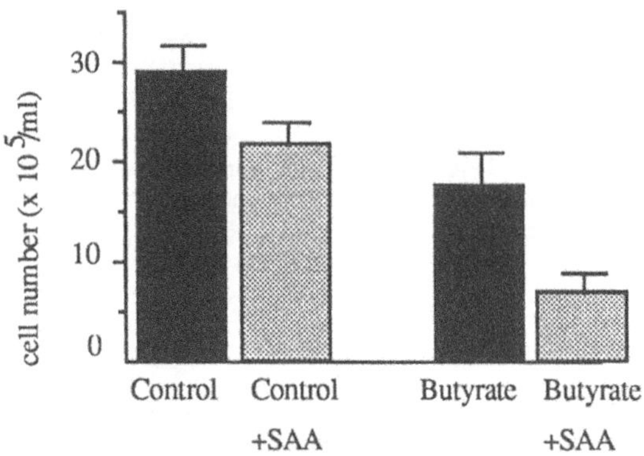

Figure 1. Effect of purified SAA (50μg/ml) on HL-60 cell growth following five days treatment in the presence and absence of 0.5 mM butyrate

Incubation of HL-60 cells for five days with SAA increased the inhibition of cell growth as depicted in Figure 1. Butyrate (0.5mM) attenuated the proliferation of HL-60 cells more pronouncely than SAA. The concomitant addition of both SAA and butyrate synergisticaly decreased the growth of HL-60 cells in comparison to butyrate itself (p=0.026). In two experiments in which NBT reduction was studied in parallel to cell growth, SAA increased the differentiation that was induced by butyrate.

Discussion

Our study suggests the potential role of SAA in modulating cancer cell proliferation and differentiation. These results demonstrate inhibition of proliferation of cells by SAA which is already observed after two days of incubation and further augmented after five days (Figure 1). The concentrations used in our experiments are lower than the levels observed by us in cancer patients (5). Higher levels of SAA could not be used because of SAA insolubility. Purified SAA markedly potentiated the inhibitory effect of TPA and butyrate on the growth of HL-60 cells which are well known leukemic cells. The ability of SAA to promote HL-60 differentiation is of special interest. This effect was more prominent in the presence of TPA where inhibition of proliferation was accompanied by increased adhesivenesss.

It is worth noting that the purified SAA used in this study yields many heterogeneous fractions. The polymorphysm of SAA was already described previously (9). Since we used a mixture of isomers which were isolated from different patients, the variation in the purified SAA effect in causing self-differentaion could be due to the variation in the relative content of specific isomers. Alternatively, it could be attributed to another material copurified with SAA .

The phenomenon of the inhibitory effect of purified SAA on proliferation and its interaction with other differantiation inducers suggests a potential role for SAA in the modulation of cancer cell growth in vivo.

References

1. Benditt, E.P. and Erikson, N.(1977) . Amyloid protein SAA is associated with high density lipoprotein from human serum. *Proc. Natl. Acad. Sci. USA.* ;74:4025-4028.
2. Rosenthal, C.J. and Sullivan, L.M. (1979). Serum amyloid A to monitor cancer dissemination. *Ann. Intern. Med.* 91:383-390.
3. Raynes, J.G. and Cooper, E.H. (1983) Comparison of serum amyloid A protein and C-reactive protein concentration in cancer and nonmalignant disease. *J. Clin. Pathol.* 36:798-803.
4. Kaneti, J., Winikoff, Y., Zimlichman, S. and Shainkin-Kestenbaum, R. (1984). Importance of serum amyloid A (SAA) level in monitoring disease activity and response to therapy in patients with prostate cancer. *Urol. Res.* 12:239-241.
5. Biran, H., Friedman, N., Neumann, L., Pras, M. and Shainkin-Kestenbaum, R. (1986.) Serum amyloid A variations in patients with cancer. Correlation with disease activity stage, primary site and prognosis. *J. Clin. Pathol.* 39:794-797.
6. Rosenthal, C.J. and Franklin, E.C. (1975.) Variation with age and disease of an amyloid A protein related serum component. *J. Clin. Invest.* 55:746-753.
7. Collins, S.J., Gallo, R.C. and Gallagher, R.E. (1977). Continuous growth and differentiation of human myeloid leukemic cells in suspension culture. *Nature (Lond.).* 270:347-349.
8. Kafka, M., Dvilansky, A. and Nathan, I.(1990.) Mechanism of interaction between interferon-γ and antineoplastic agent on the differentiation of HL-60 promyelocytic cells. *Exp. Hematol.* 18:153-158.
9. McAdam K., Bausserman I., Herbert P.N. and Green K.(1980). Polymorphism of SAA within high density lipoproteins in amyloid and amyloidosis. In: Glenner, G., *et al.* eds.), *Excerpta Medica.* Amsterdam, pp. 302-312.

PRIMARY SYSTEMIC AMYLOIDOSIS (AL) IN 1990.

Robert A. Kyle, M.D., Mayo Clinic, Rochester, Minnesota 55905 USA

Amyloidosis was described over 300 years ago, but it was not until 1856 that Wilks described a 51-year-old man with "lardaceous viscera" in whom the changes were unrelated to syphilis, osteomyelitis, other osseous disease, or tuberculosis. The patient had dropsy and albumin in his urine. At autopsy the heart was enlarged and the spleen was hard and lardaceous. Similar changes were found in the kidney. This patient probably had primary amyloidosis (AL).

Amyloid appears to be homogeneous and amorphous under the light microscope and when stained with Congo red produces an apple-green birefringence under polarized light. The amorphous, hyalin-like appearance of amyloid is misleading because it is a fibrous protein. Electron microscopy reveals that amyloid consists of rigid, linear, nonbranching, aggregated fibrils. The fibrils consist of the variable portion of a monoclonal light chain (Glenner, et al., 1971). The light-chain class is more frequently of λ than κ (2:1). There is a predominance of the λ_{VI} subgroup.

From 1977 to 1989, 1,150 patients with amyloidosis were diagnosed at the Mayo Clinic. Seven hundred seventy-six patients (68%) had primary amyloidosis (AL). Two hundred fifty-two (22%) had localized amyloidosis. The majority had amyloid localized to the carpal ligament. Secondary amyloidosis (AA) was found in only 45 patients (4%) while familial amyloidosis was recognized in 39 patients (3%). The remainder had senile amyloidosis.

AL is a disease of older male patients. The incidence of AL in Olmsted County, Minnesota is 8.5/million/year. Five hundred seventy patients with AL were recognized at the Mayo Clinic from 1982 to 1989. The median age was 62 years with a range from 32 to 90 years. Two-thirds were male. Weakness or fatigue and weight loss are the most frequent symptoms and are seen in more than half the patients. Loss of weight may be striking and amounted for 45 kg in three of our patients. The median loss of weight was 10 kg. Dyspnea and pedal edema are frequently noted by patients with congestive heart failure. Paresthesias, lightheadedness, and syncope are seen in those with peripheral neuropathy or autonomic neuropathy. Hoarseness or change of voice to a weak, high pitched, or a deep, husky tone should alert the physician to the possibility of amyloidosis.

The liver was palpable in slightly less than one-fifth of our patients while splenomegaly was recognized in only 4%. Macroglossia was found in 11%. Purpura is common and often involves the neck and face, particularly the upper eyelids. Orbital purpura may be striking after proctoscopy. The skin is fragile and may be easily traumatized during physical examination.

Approximately one-third of patients have the nephrotic syndrome at the time of diagnosis of AL. Congestive heart failure is present at diagnosis in about one-fourth of patients while one-six of patients present with orthostatic hypotension or peripheral neuropathy. Congestive heart failure or orthostatic hypotension often develops during the course of the disease. The presence of one of these syndromes and an M-protein in the serum or urine raises a strong suspicion of amyloidosis.

Anemia is not a prominent feature of AL and when present is due usually to renal insufficiency, multiple myeloma, or gastrointestinal bleeding. Thrombocytosis occurs in 5% to 10% of patients and may be an important clue to the diagnosis. Functional hyposplenism is one cause of thrombocytosis. The presence of Howell-Jolly bodies in the peripheral blood smear is an indicator of hyposplenism. Proteinuria is present in approximately 80% of patients. Some degree of renal insufficiency is seen in almost half of the patients at the time of diagnosis. In almost one-fourth of patients, the serum creatinine is 2 mg/dL or more at diagnosis. Levels of serum alkaline phosphatase are increased in approximately one-fourth of patients. Hyperbilirubinemia is an infrequent finding and when present is an ominous sign. The prothrombin time is increased in about 15% of patients and the thrombin time is prolonged in 60% of patients. The factor X level is decreased in less than 5% of patients and is rarely the cause of bleeding. Serum carotene and vitamin B_{12} levels are each reduced in approximately 5% of patients.

The serum protein electrophoretic pattern shows a localized band or M-spike in one-half of patients; even when present, the spike is usually of modest size and often is not easily recognized in the densitometer tracing. Hypogammaglobulinemia is seen in about one-fifth of patients and the remainder have a normal-appearing pattern. Serum IgG levels are reduced in approximately one-half of patients whereas IgA and IgM values are often normal. Immunoelectrophoresis or immunofixation of the serum reveals a monoclonal protein in two-thirds of patients. About 45% have a monoclonal heavy chain in the serum while almost 20% have a free monoclonal light chain. Of our patients with a monoclonal protein, almost three-fourths have λ light chains in their sera in contrast to patients with multiple myeloma in whom two-thirds have κ light chains.

Immunoelectrophoresis and immunofixation of an adequately concentrated urine specimen reveals a monoclonal light chain in almost two-thirds of patients. A monoclonal protein was found in the serum or urine in 83% of our 553 patients who were studied between 1982 and 1989. An M-protein is most common in the nephrotic syndrome and is least common in peripheral neuropathy.

Almost three-fourths of patients have 10% or fewer plasma cells in the bone marrow. We find that only 15% of patients have more than 20% plasma cells in the bone marrow. These patients generally do not have symptomatic myeloma despite the significant plasmacytosis. The median percentage of plasma cells in our patients was 6%.

The heart is frequently involved in AL. The electrocardiogram frequently shows either low voltage in the limb leads or characteristics consistent with anterior septal infarction (loss of anterior forces), but there is no evidence of myocardial infarction at autopsy (Smith, et al., 1984). Arrhythmias, including atrial fibrillation, atrial or junctional tachycardia, ventricular premature complexes, or heart block, are common electrocardiographic features. Amyloid may infiltrate the sinus node and produce the sick sinus syndrome. Echocardiography is a valuable technique for the evaluation of amyloid heart disease. In a series of 132 patients with AL (Cueto-Garcia, et al., 1985), found a relationship between an increasing incidence of congestive heart failure and increasing thickness of the ventricular wall and septum. Patients with greater wall thickness also had a higher frequency of associated echocardiographic abnormalities such as left atrial enlargement, granular sparkling, and reduced systolic function. The median survival was 2.4 years for patients with ventricular and septal thickness of ≤12 mm, while it was only 0.4 years for patients with thickness ≥15 mm. Serial echocardiography is also useful in documenting the progression of disease. Congestive heart failure or arrhythmias (or both) developed or worsened in 14 of 27 patients with cardiac AL who had serial echocardiographic studies. These 14 patients had significant increases in left ventricular wall thickness and in left atrial size and a decrease in fractional ventricular shortening. The 13 patients without clinical progression showed no significant echocardiographic changes (Cueto-Garcia, et al., 1984).

Comprehensive Doppler echocardiographic assessment of diastolic function in AL demonstrates impressive abnormalities (Klein, et al., 1989). Early cardiac amyloidosis is characterized by abnormal relaxation, whereas advanced involvement (mean wall thickness of 15 mm or more) is characterized by restrictive hemodynamics. Right ventricular diastolic function is also abnormal in most patients with AL. A major abnormality is a short deceleration time which is consistent with restriction in the advanced stages of the disease (Klein, et al., 1990). All patients with biopsy-proven AL should have an echocardiographic study.

Involvement of the kidneys is extremely common in AL and is one of the major clinical problems. At the time of diagnosis of AL, the nephrotic syndrome was present in one-third of our patients. Amyloid is first deposited in the mesangium of the glomerulus and later extends along the basement membrane. The degree of proteinuria in the nephrotic syndrome does not correlate well with the extent of amyloid deposition in the kidneys. The severity of proteinuria correlates better with the presence of spicules and podocyte destruction. Because minimal deposits of amyloid may be associated with the nephrotic syndrome, kidney biopsy specimens that have the appearance of minimal change, glomerulopathy must be carefully stained for amyloid when the nephrotic syndrome is recognized in older patients.

Histologic involvement of the gastrointestinal tract occurs in most cases of AL. The involvement is often asymptomatic but widespread dysfunction may occur. Malabsorption occurs in approximately 5% of patients. Decreased motor activity of the small bowel is not uncommon. In some instances, apparent mechanical obstruction may actually be pseudo-obstruction for which surgical treatment is ineffectual and actually dangerous. Although amyloid deposits may be extensive, severe diarrhea is more often due to neurologic (autonomic) dysfunction than to the deposition of amyloid. Gastrointestinal bleeding may be a prominent feature. Ascites is not uncommon.

The liver is involved frequently by amyloidosis. Elevation of serum alkaline phosphatase is common, but hyperbilirubinemia is unusual. The presence of jaundice is associated with short survival. Patients with portal hypertension and bleeding esophageal varices have been observed. Hepatomegaly may be striking, but other physical findings of primary liver disease are uncommon. Spontaneous rupture of the spleen followed by hemorrhagic shock has been noted.

Peripheral neuropathy occurs in about one-sixth of our patients with AL. The neuropathy is usually distal, symmetric, and progressive. Initial manifestations are due to sensory rather than motor nerve dysfunction. Dysesthetic numbness is more frequent than paresthesias and is extremely troublesome to some patients. Pain and temperature sensations are reduced earlier and to a greater degree than are sensations of vibration and position. The lower extremities usually are more involved than the upper. Autonomic dysfunction may be a prominent feature and is often manifested by lightheadedness or syncope from orthostatic hypotension, by gastrointestinal disturbance and bladder dysfunction, and by impotence in men. Carpal tunnel syndrome is seen in approximately one-fourth of patients.

The possibility of AL must be considered in every patient who has an M-protein in the serum or urine and who also has nephrotic syndrome, congestive heart failure, sensorimotor peripheral neuropathy, carpal tunnel syndrome, hepatomegaly, or idiopathic malabsorption. The diagnosis depends on the demonstration of amyloid deposits in tissue. Congo red produces an apple-green birefringence under polarizing light, and is the most commonly used stain. Antiserum to amyloid P component reacts with virtually all types of amyloid deposits and is useful in demonstrating the presence of amyloid. Hawkins, et al. (1988) subsequently used ^{123}I-labeled purified human serum amyloid P component and found uptake in AL, AA, and β_2-microglobulin (β_2-M) amyloid patients in contrast to the complete absence of tissue localization in control subjects. Minor deposits of amyloid (such as in the carpal tunnel) were seen in high-resolution scintigraphic images. Using the direct or the unlabeled immunoperoxidase method, Linke, et al. (1986) correctly identified 112 (98%) of 114 patients with systemic amyloidosis using antisera to AA, Aλ, Aκ, AF, and AS_{C1}.

The initial diagnostic procedure should be an abdominal fat aspirate because this test is positive in 70% to 80% of patients. If this is negative, a bone marrow aspirate and biopsy specimen may be helpful because marrow contains amyloid in about one-half of the patients. If the bone marrow and abdominal fat are negative, a rectal biopsy specimen should be taken. This procedure is reasonably free of complications and produces positive findings in approximately 80% of patients. If these sites are negative, tissue should be obtained from a suspected involved organ such as the kidney, liver, heart, or peripheral nerve.

The median survival of the 570 patients with AL that we have seen from 1982 to 1989 was 1.8 years. The median survival from onset of congestive heart failure until death was 0.6 years. The 170 patients with nephrotic syndrome had a median survival of 2.4 years while those with peripheral neuropathy had a median survival of 4.4 years. In a multivariate analysis of 168 AL patients at the Mayo Clinic, four variables--congestive heart failure, presence of monoclonal urinary light chain, hepatomegaly, and amount of weight loss--all had a highly significant influence on survival during the first year. Elevation of creatinine, diagnosis of multiple myeloma, presence of orthostatic hypotension, and the presence of a monoclonal serum protein all had a highly significant adverse influence on survival in those who lived for 1 year after diagnosis. In a group of 131 patients at the Mayo Clinic with AL without myeloma, the median survival was 10.8 months for those with an elevated β_2-M level (2.7 μg/μL or more) compared with 32.9 months for those with a normal β_2-M level. The impact of β_2-M on survival was independent of the serum creatinine level. A plasma cell labeling index >0% predicted a survival disadvantage (14.1 months vs. 30.9 months; P = <0.05) in 103 AL patients. The 1-year survival of patients with an initial deceleration time of 150 msec or less in the echocardiogram was 55%, whereas 90% lived for more than 1 year when the deceleration was more than 150 msec (P <0.01).

Treatment for AL is unsatisfactory. The amyloid fibrils consist of the variable portion of monoclonal immunoglobulin light chains and are synthesized by plasma cells. Increased numbers of monoclonal plasma cells are commonly found in the bone marrow of patients with AL. It is therefore reasonable to attempt treatment with alkylating agents which are known to be affective against plasma cell proliferative processes such as multiple myeloma. In a prospective randomized study of melphalan (0.15 mg/kg/day for 7 days) plus prednisone (0.8 mg/kg/day for the same 7 days) every 6 weeks versus daily colchicine therapy, 101 patients were stratified according to their dominant clinical manifestation. If the disease progressed, the other regimen was added. There was no statistically significant difference in survival when the two groups were compared in total (melphalan-prednisone, 25 months; colchicine, 18 months; P = 0.23). When the survival of patients who received only one regimen was analyzed or when survival was analyzed from the time of entry into the study to the time of death or progression of disease, significant differences (P <0.001 and P <0.0001, respectively) favoring melphalan-prednisone were evident. Four patients died of acute nonlymphocytic leukemia and two patients had a myelodysplastic syndrome.

We are currently engaged in a prospective study in which patients with AL are stratified according to their dominant clinical manifestation--nephrotic syndrome or renal failure, congestive heart failure, peripheral neuropathy, or other. Patients were randomized to regimen I (colchicine, 0.6 mg b.i.d. which was increased gradually to the point of toxicity), regimen II (melphalan, 0.15 mg/kg daily plus prednisone, 0.8 mg/kg daily, both for 7 days every 6 weeks), or regimen III (melphalan, prednisone, and colchicine as in regimens I and II). One hundred sixty-three patients have been entered. Fifty-three were assigned to regimen I, 57 to regimen II, and 53 to regimen III. The nephrotic syndrome was the most common followed by congestive heart failure and peripheral neuropathy. Forty-four of the 53 patients in regimen I have died while 40 of the 57 patients in regimen II have expired. Nineteen of the 53 patients in regimen III are alive. The median survival of those receiving colchicine was 9 months; melphalan and prednisone, 16 months; and melphalan, prednisone, and colchicine, 18 months. The study is continuing.

REFERENCES

Glenner, G.G., Terry, W., Harada, M., et al. (1971) Amyloid fibril proteins: proof of homology with immunoglobulin light chains by sequence analyses. Science, 172:1150-1151.

Smith, T.J., Kyle, R.A., Lie, J.T. (1984) Clinical significance of histopathologic patterns of cardiac amyloidosis, Mayo Clin Proc, 59,547-555.

Cueto-Garcia, L., Reeder, G.S., Kyle, R.A., et al. (1985) Echocardiographic findings in systemic amyloidosis: spectrum of cardiac involvement and relation to survival, J Am Coll Cardiol, 6:737-743.

Cueto-Garcia, L., Tajik, A.J., Kyle, R.A., et al. (1984) Serial echocardiographic observations in patients with primary systemic amyloidosis: an introduction to the concept of early (asymptomatic) amyloid infiltration of the heart, Mayo Clin Proc, 59:589-597.

Klein, A.L., Hatle, L.K., Burstow, D.J., et al. (1989) Doppler characterization of left ventricular diastolic function in cardiac amyloidosis, J Am Coll Cardiol, 13:1017-1026.

Klein, A.L., Hatle, L.K., Burstow, D.J., et al. (1990) Comprehensive Doppler assessment of right ventricular diastolic function in cardiac amyloidosis, J Am Coll Cardiol, 15:99-108.

Hawkins, P.N., Myers, M.J., Lavender, J.P., Pepys, M.B. (1988) Diagnostic radionuclide imaging of amyloid: biological targeting by circulating human serum amyloid P component, Lancet, 1:1413-1418.

Linke, R.P., Nathrath, W.B.J., Eulitz, M. (1986) Classification of amyloid syndromes from tissue sections using antibodies against various amyloid fibril proteins: report of 142 cases. in G.G. Glenner, E.F. Osserman, E.P. Benditt, et al (eds), Amyloidosis, Plenum Press, New York, p. 599-606.

COMPARISON OF THE AMINO ACID SEQUENCES OF TEN KAPPA I AMYLOID PROTEINS FOR AMYLOIDOGENIC SEQUENCES

Liepnieks, J.J., Benson, M.D., and Dwulet, F.E.
Veterans Affairs Medical Center (583/ 111RH), 1481 West 10th Street, Room #A772, Indianapolis, IN 46202; Indiana University School of Medicine, Department of Medicine, Rheumatology Division, Clinical Building 492, 541 Clinical Drive, Indianapolis, IN 46223, USA

ABSTRACT. It has been proposed that amyloid forming immunoglobulin light chains contain specific amino acid sequences in their variable region which predispose them to form amyloid. To elucidate whether such sequences exist and can be identified, we have investigated the amino acid sequence of the variable region of ten kappa I immunoglobulin light chains associated with amyloid. Comparison of the ten kappa I amyloid proteins to nonamyloid kappa I light chains identifies a number of amino acid substitutions which are presumed to be on the outside surface of the light chain dimer and which may participate in fibril formation by promoting dimer aggregation. Changes to more hydrophobic residues or from neutral to charged residues are present in the inner beta sheet which forms some of the contact regions for monomer-monomer interaction. These changes may increase dimer stability which then could form the amyloid aggregating subunit. In two proteins, the usual Arg at position 61 is replaced by an Asn with carbohydrate attached. It is possible that the presence of carbohydrate at the outer edge of this beta turn may promote fibril formation.

INTRODUCTION

Immunoglobulin light chains present in amyloid have been proposed to possess secondary and tertiary structures which predispose them to selfaggregate and form amyloid [1]. Thus, specific alterations in the primary sequence which determines the secondary and tertiary structure of the light chains may be a controlling factor for amyloid formation. However, the limited number of complete immunoglobulin amyloid sequences in the literature has hampered the analysis for such amyloidogenic sequences. To test this hypothesis, we have investigated the sequence of the variable region of kappa I immunoglobulin light chains associated with amyloid. This subgroup was chosen for study for several reasons. The kappa I subgroup accounts for approximately 20% of all AL amyloid deposits [2]. There are a large number of sequenced myeloma kappa I proteins to use as non-amyloid controls for evaluation of amino acid substitution patterns [3]. Finally, the 3-dimensional structure of a kappa I variable region protein is known from X-ray diffraction studies [4] which will assist in evaluating the effects of amino acid substitutions. We report here our results on the studies on the primary structure of 10 kappa I immunoglobulin light chains associated with amyloid.

MATERIALS AND METHODS

Amyloid fibrils were isolated from amyloid laden tissues by the procedure of Pras et al. [5] using repeated washings with first saline and then water [6,7]. The isolated fibrils were treated with guanidine hydrochloride, reduced, alkylated, and fractionated on Sepharose CL6B [6,7]. Immunoglobulin light chains were isolated from urine by chromatography on DEAE Sephadex and Ultragel ACA 34 [8]. The protein was treated with guanidine hydrochloride, reduced, alkylated, and recovered by lyophilization after dialysis against water [6-8]. Reduced and alkylated amyloid subunit proteins and light chain proteins were digested with TPCK-treated trypsin or Staphylococcus protease [6-9]. Peptides were fractionated by HPLC on a Beckman Ultrasphere C-18 or Synchrom Synchropax RPP or RP8 columns using an acetonitrile gradient in 0.1% TFA [6-9]. When necessary, peptides were subdigested with TLCK-treated chymotrypsin or Staphylococous protease [6-9]. Peptides were sequentially degraded on Beckman 890C sequenator, and PTH-amino acids were identified by HPLC [6-9].

RESULTS AND DISCUSSION

Four of the kappa I variable region sequences were determined from light chains isolated from urine (NIE, BRE, COL, and EPP). The amyloid subunit protein isolated from the spleen of NIE was subsequently sequenced and had residues 1 to 20 identical to the urinary protein. The other six sequences were from the amyloid subunit protein isolated from spleen (BAN, AND, and HAC), liver (COZ and MUM), or heart (CRU).

The outer surface of a typical kappa I light chain REI as determined by X-ray crystallography consists of a beta sheet containing 4 polypeptide strands from residues 5-7, 19-24, 63-65, and 71-75 [4]. In residues 5-7, EPP has a hydrophobic Ile at residue 5 compared to the usual Thr (Figure 1). Also, BAN and MUM have a Leu and EPP a Val at position 4, both more hydrophobic than the usual Met. While several residues removed from the beta sheet, the Pro at position 9 in HAC is unique for kappa I proteins. In the 19-24 region, NIE and MEV contain a hydrophobic Ile at residue 20 in place of Thr. In the 63-65 region, EPP and MEV contain a Gly at position 65 in place of the usual Ser. Also, MEV is unique with Arg at position 66 in place of Gly. In the 71-75 area, BAN contains the hydrophobic Ile at residue 72 in place of the usual Thr. Also, MUM and CRU have Arg and Ile respectively at position 76 instead of the usual Ser. Thus, six of the kappa I proteins contain hydrophobic for hydrophilic substitutions on the outer beta sheet of the dimer which may promote hydrophobic interactions and aggregation.

The inner beta sheet consisting of polypeptide strands 34-38, 43-50, 51-61, and 85-89 forms some of the contact regions for monomer-monomer interaction in the dimer [4]. Substitutions in these regions

PROTEIN	RESIDUES			
	4-9	19-24	62-66	71-76
ROY	-M-T-Q-S-P-S-	-V-T-I-T-C-Q-	-F-S-G-T-G-	-F-T-T-T-I-S-
BAN	-L-T-Q-S-P-S-	-V-T-I-T-C-R-	-F-T-G-S-G-	-F-I-L-T-I-S-
AND	-M-T-Q-S-P-S-	-V-T-I-T-C-R-	-F-S-G-S-G-	-F-T-L-T-I-T-
NIE	-M-T-Q-S-P-S-	-V-I-I-T-C-R-	-F-S-G-S-G-	-F-T-L-T-I-S-
COZ	-M-T-Q-S-P-S-	-V-T-I-T-C-R-	-F-S-G-S-G-	-F-T-L-T-I-T-
MUM	-L-T-Q-S-P-S-	-V-T-I-T-C-R-	-F-S-G-S-G-	-F-T-L-T-I-R-
CRU	-M-T-Q-S-P-S-	-V-T-I-T-C-Q-	-F-S-G-S-A-	-F-T-F-T-I-I-
BRE	-M-T-Q-S-P-S-	-V-T-I-T-C-Q-	-F-S-G-S-G-	-Y-T-F-T-I-S-
EPP	-V-I-Q-S-P-S-	-V-T-I-T-C-Q-	-F-S-G-G-G-	-F-T-F-T-I-S-
HAC	-M-T-Q-S-P-P-	-V-T-I-T-C-R-	-F-S-G-S-G-	-F-T-L-T-I-S-
COL	-M-T-Q-S-P-S-	-V-T-I-T-C-R-	-F-S-G-S-G-	-F-T-L-T-I-S-
MEV	-M-T-Q-S-P-S-	-V-I-I-T-C-R-	-F-S-G-G-R-	-F-T-L-T-I-S-

PROTEIN	34-38	42-50	51-61
ROY	-N-W-Y-Q-Q-	-K-A-P-K-L-L-I-Y-D-	-A-S-K-L-E-A-G-V-P-S-R-
BAN	-A-W-F-Q-Q-	-K-A-P-K-S-L-I-Y-D-	-A-S-T-L-Q-S-G-V-P-S-N-
AND	-N-W-Y-H-Q-	-K-A-P-S-L-L-I-F-G-	-A-S-S-L-R-S-G-V-P-S-R-
NIE	-A-W-F-Q-Q-	-K-A-P-K-S-L-I-Y-A-	-A-S-N-L-Q-S-G-V-S-S-K-
COZ	-N-W-Y-Q-H-	-K-A-P-N-V-L-I-Y-A-	-A-S-N-L-Q-S-G-V-P-S-G-
MUM	-N-W-Y-Q-Q-	-K-A-P-N-L-L-I-Y-D-	-A-S-S-L-Q-S-G-V-P-S-N-
CRU	-N-W-Y-Q-Q-	-K-A-P-K-L-L-I-Y-D-	-A-S-N-L-E-T-G-F-P-S-R-
BRE	-I-W-Y-Q-Q-	-K-A-P-N-L-L-I-Y-D-	-A-S-T-L-E-T-G-V-P-S-R-
EPP	-N-W-F-Q-Q-	-K-A-P-K-L-L I Y D	-A-S-N-L-E-R-G-V-P-S-R-
HAC	-A-W-F-Q-Q-	-K-A-P-K-S-L-I-Y-A-	-A-S-S-L-Q-S-G-V-P-S-K-
COL	-A-W-Y-Q-Q-	-E-A-P-K-L-L-I-Y-K-	-A-S-T-L-Q-S-G-V-P-S-R-
MEV	-N-W-Y-Q-Q-	-K-A-P-K-L-L-I-F-D-	-T-S-N-L-Q-S-G-V-P-S-R-

Figure 1. Amino acid sequence of polypeptide strands involved in outer and inner beta sheets of kappa I proteins. Sequences for ROY, BAN, AND, and MEV are from references 3, 6, 7, and 10 respectively. MEV is an amyloid Bence-Jones Kappa I protein and ROY is a non-amyloid myeloma kappa I protein. Residues possibly involved in amyloid formation are boxed.

may increase the stability of the dimer which then could form the amyloid aggregating subunit. BRE has Ile at residue 34 in place of the usual Ala or Asn (Figure 1). BAN, NIE, EPP, and HAC have Phe at position 36 in place of the usual Tyr. AND and COZ have His at residues 37 and 38 respectively in place of the usual Gln. COL has Glu at residue 42 instead of the usual Lys. COZ, MUM, and BRE have Asn and AND Ser at position 45 instead of Lys. BAN, NIE, and HAC have Ser at position 46 instead of the usual hydrophobic Leu. AND and MEV have Phe at position 49 instead of Tyr. AND and EPP have the basic Arg at positions 55 and 56 respectively in place of the usual acidic or neutral amino acid. CRU has Phe at position 58 instead of Val. In place of the usual Arg at residue 61, NIE and HAC have Lys, COZ has Gly, and BAN and MUM have Asn with carbohydrate attached. Position 61 is on the outer edge of a beta turn and faces toward the C-region away from the antigen binding site [4]. These changes from hydrophilic to hydrophobic residues or from neutral to charged residues may affect monomer-monomer interaction possibly increasing dimer stability.

No single unique amyloidogenic sequence or feature common to all the amyloid kappa I proteins is apparent. Possibly, an alteration in one of several regions could each lead to self aggregation and fibril formation. In some cases, this could involve changes to more hydrophobic residues in the outer beta sheet of the dimer leading to dimer aggregation. In others, changes in residues involved in monomer-monomer contact could alter dimer stability and formation. Possibly the change to an Asn at residue 61 and subsequent carbohydrate attachment somehow results in aggregation. Further studies on the 3 dimensional structure of amyloid proteins are needed to clarify how their structures are different from non-amyloid forming proteins and the factors which lead to aggregation and fibril formation.

ACKNOWLEDGEMENTS

This work was supported by VA Medical Research, The United States Public Health Service (RR-00750, NIDDK-34881, NIAMS-AR20582, AR7448), The Arthritis Foundation, The Grace M. Showalter Trust and The Marion E. Jacobson Fund.

REFERENCES

1. Solomon, A., Frangione, B., and Franklin, E.C. (1982), J. Clin. Invest. 70, 453-460.
2. Glenner, G.G. (1980), New Engl. J. Med. 302, 1283-1292 and 1333-1343
3. Kabat, E.A., Wu, T.T., Reid-Miller, M., Perry, H.M. and Gottesman, K.S. (1987) 'Sequences of Proteins of Immunological Interest', NIH, Bethesda, MD, pp. 41-49.
4. Epp, O., Tattman, E.E., Schiffer, M., Huber, R., and Palm, W. (1975), Biochemistry 14, 4943-4952.
5. Pras, M., Schubert, M., Zucker-Franklin, D., Rimon, A., and Franklin, E.C. (1968), J. Clin. Invest. 47, 924-933.
6. Dwulet, F.E., O'Conner, T.P., and Benson, M.D. (1986), Mol. Immunol. 23, 73-78.
7. Liepnieks, J.J., Dwulet, F.E., and Benson, M.D. (1990), Mol. Immunol. 27, 481-485.
8. Glueck, H.I., Coots, M.C., Benson, M., Dwulet, F.E., and Hurtubise, P.E. (1989), J. Lab. Clin. Med. 113, 269-277.
9. Kluve-Beckerman, B., Dwulet, F.E., DiBartola, S.P., and Benson, M. D. (1989), Comp. Biochem. Physiol. 94B, 175-183.
10. Eulitz, M. and Linke, R.P. (1982), Hoppe-Seyler's Z. Physiol. Chem. 363, 1347-1358.

CHARACTERIZATION OF A kAL PROTEIN AND TWO AMYLOIDOGENIC kBJP IN THREE CASES OF IMMUNOGLOBULIN AMYLOIDOSIS

T. SHINODA, T. TAKENAWA, A. HOSHI AND T. ISOBE
Department of Chemistry, Tokyo Metropolitan University,
Setagaya-ku, Tokyo 158 ; School of Alied Medical Science,
Kobe University, Kobe 650, Japan

ABSTRACT. Characterization of an amyloid fibril protein kAL(Am 81) and two amyloidogenic Bence Jones proteins(Am107, 113) were made in three cases of immunoglobulin amyloidosis. On SDS-disc electrophoresis, Am81 extract showed four distinct bands, all of which reacted only with anti k antiserum, with molecular weights of 26k, 18k, 14k and 12k, respectively. Sequence analysis was mainely done on 12k component with conventional techniques. It consisted of 126 residues and had a sequence characteristic of VkI subgroup. Sequence studies made on two amyloidogenic kBJPs, Am107 and 113, revealed that both of them also had the sequence characteristic of VkI subgroup. Although three specimens studied in the present cases had sequence characteristics of VkI, they also have individual characteristics especially in FR3-CDR3-FR4 regions, which may in some correlations with the fibril formation in the amyloid process.

1. INTRODUCTION

Current studies on the primary structure of amyloid fibril proteins(AL), in primary and in myeloma-associated amyloidosis, have reveiled that they are derived from monoclonal immunoglobulin light(L) chains and/or their fragments which vary in size ranging from 6k to 24k daltons[1,2]. Although sequence data are still limited, it is assumed that AL proteins consist of the V region of the L chains, the V region flanked by a portion of the C region, the intact L chain , or a combination of various intermediate molecular forms. These data strongly suggest that the V domain plays more role than does the C domain in the formation of such pathological fibrils. If this is the case, question may be raised as to whether there is any association between the primary structure of the V region(i.e.subgroups) and amyloidogenicity, and whether or not there is any difference in this regard between two types, amyloidogenic and non-amyloidogenic, of the L chains.

We have previously reported sequences of several L chains,including three amyloidogenic BJPs and two AL proteins, and have proposed that these proteins could further be classified into distinct "subsubgroups"

1 10 20 30
Am107 D I Q M T Q S P S S L S A S V G D R V T I T C R A S Q T S L
AM113 D I Q M T Q S P S S L S A S V G N R V T I T C R A S Q S S V
40 50 60
D Y L N W Y Q Q K P G K A P K L L I Y D A S S - L Q T G V P
D Y V A W Y Q Q K P G K A P K L L I F D A S N S L Q S G V P
70 80 90
S R F S G S G S G T D F T L T I S G L Q P E D F A T Y F C Q
S R F S G T G S G T D F T L T I S S L Q P E D F A T Y Y C Q
100
Q Y D T G P V T F G G G T K V D I K R T
Q F D N L P K T F G G G T K I D I K R T

Figure 2. Amino acid sequence of the V region of two amyloidogenic BJPs in myeloma associated amyloidosis. Amino acids underlined indicate those differ to each other.

3.2. Amino acid sequence of two amyloidogenic BJPs

Tentative sequence of the V region of two amyloidogenic kBJPs, Am107 and Am113 are shown in Figure 2. Peptides obtained from the C region were analyzed only for partial N-terminal sequnce and their amino acid compositions, since no sequence difference was seen as compared with that of the C region of k light chain.

4. DISCUSSION

A 12k component of AL protein Am81 composed of 126 residues with a flushed C-terminal sequence. This probably be resulted from partial processing during the couse of fibrilogenesis. Similar cases have also been reported by others[6] as well as by ourselves[5]. Thus, the total number of residues found would be a mean value. As illustrated in Figure 1, the sequence is most homologous with that of the corresponding region of the reported VkI chains[7]. In addition to this common feature, it has individual characteristics: whereas all the reported VkI specimens have Ile at position 76, Am81 lacks one residue at this position. It has several rare replacements along the sequence: these are Thr-31,Ile-47, Thr-52, Leu-55, Lys-62, Ser-69, Ser-75, and Ser-100. These uncommon replacements might cause some local distortion in their conformation, some of which might lead the protein being more prone to association with the amyloid processes.

As to the V region sequences of two amyloidogenic BJPs, Am107 and Am113, they are homologous to each other and have the characteristics of VkI subgroup. Inspite of their homology in sequence, there are also individual characteristics: for Am107, such residues are Thr-28, Phe-88, Tyr-92, Val-96, and Val-104, and for Am113, beside having unique replacements, it has novel insertion of Ser-54 in the CDR2 region(Fig.2). Such

on the basis of chemical characteristics of their V region sequences[3,4]. By such classification, though sequence data are still limited, amyloidogenic BLPs and AL proteins seemed to fall into common subsubgroups within any given subgroup. The present paper describes the sequences of two amyloidogenic BJPs and a kAL protein.

2. MATERIALS AND METHODS

2.1. Isolation and Purification of AL and BJPs

Crude AL fraction extracted from amyloid-laiden liver(Am81) and amyloidogenic BJPs(Am107 and 113) from urine were purified by reverse phase HPLC on a colomn of Toso phenyl 5PWRP(0.45 x 10cm) under the conditions reported elsewhere[5].

2.2. Enzyme Digestion and Peptide Separation

Purified AL protein and BJPs, following the complete reduction and carboxymethylation, were digested either with lysyl endopeptidase(E/S: 1/50, 0.1M DMAA-TFA, pH9.2) or with trypsin(E/S: 1/80, 0.2M NH_4CO_3, pH8.1) at 37 C for 3h. The digests were chromatographed by HPLC with C18 resin as described[5]. The peptides were further purified , if nessary, by HPLC under similar conditions as reported.

2.3. Sequence Analysis

Sequence analyses of the purified proteins and peptides(0.4-1.5nmole) were performed by Edman degradation with an automatic sequenator(ABI470A) under the standard conditions recommended. Carboxy terminal sequence of some peptides was determined after digestions with carboxypeptidase Y followed by amino acid analysis.

3. RESULTS

3.1. Amino Acid Sequence of Am81

Amino acid sequence of the V region of Am81, obtained from 12k component was shown in Fig.1. It has 109 residues in total and shows VkI subgroup characteristic as will be discussed later.

```
1                 10                        20                  30
D I Q M T Q S P S T L S A S V G D R V I I T C R A S Q S V L T Y L
            40                      50                    60
N W Y Q Q K P G K A P K L I I Y D A T L L L T G V P S K F S G S G
      70                    80                    90
S G S D F N I S S G L Q P E D F A T Y Y C Q Q F D A G P K T F G S
100
G T K L E I K R T
```

Figure.1. Amino acid sequence of the V region of Am81 AL protein

event wil more or less cause certain conformational modification at this region. In many cases, novel replacements of amino acids can be found in the sequences of Als and amyloidogenic BJPs when compared with those of non-amyloidogenic light chains. Some of such residues might positive ly participate in the fibril formation in the amyloid processes.

Although our data presented here also suggest that there are some preferences for amyloidogenicity in relation to V region sequences of AL proteins as described by others[8], it is not yet possible to identify definitely any specific residue(s) or sequence(s) which is essential to such proteins being endowed with amyloidogenicity. Appalently further sequence study is needed before clarifying the problems.

5. ACKNOWLEDGEMENTS

This work was supported in part by grants-in-aid from the Primary Amyloidosis Research Committee of the Ministry of Health and Welfare, and by the Human Science Foundation.

6. REFERENCES

[1] Glenner, G. G.(1980) 'Amyloid deposit and amyloidosis', N. Engl. J. Med. 306, 1283-1342.
[2] Glenner, G. G.(1980) 'Amyloid and amyloidosis', in G. G. Glenner, P. P. Costa et al (eds.), Amyloid and Amyloidosis, Excepta Medica, Amsterdam, pp. 3-13.
[3] Tonoike, H., Kametani, F., Hoshi, A. and Shinoda, T.(1985) 'Primary structure of an amyloidogenic Bence Jones protein NIG77', Biochem. Biophys. Res. Comm. 126, 1228-1234.
[4] Tonoike, H., Kametani, F., Shinoda, T. and Isobe, T.(1985) 'Amino acid sequence of an amyloidogenic Bence Jones protein in myeloma associated amyloidosis', FEBS Lett. 185, 139-141.
[5] Shinoda, T., Kametani, F., Takenawa, T. and Isobe, T.(1988), 'Molecular heterogeneity of amyloid fibril proteins in primary amyloidosis', in T. Isobe, S. Araki, F. Uchino et al(eds.), Amyloid and Amyloidosis, Plenum, New York, pp. 151-156.
[6] Sletten. K., Natvig, J. B. and Husby, G.(1981), 'The complete amino acid sequence of a prototype immunoglobulin L chain type amyloid fibril protein AR', Biochem. J. 195, 561-572.
[7] Shinoda, T.(1989) 'Biochemistry of amyloids', J. Med. Technol. 33, 993-1006.
[8] Eulitz, M. and Linke, P.(1982) 'Primary structure of variable region of an amyloidogenic Bence Jones protein(MEV)', Hoppe-Seyler's Physiol. Chem. 363, 1347-1358.

BICLONALITY IN AMYLOIDOSIS PATIENT MAL: ONE CLONE PRODUNCING AN AMYLOIDOGENIC, THE OTHER A NON-AMYLOIDOGENIC KAPPA L-CHAIN

- AL Amyloidosis -

Rodilla Sala, E., Kratzin, H. D., Pick, A. I.*, and Hilschmann, N.
*Max-Planck-Institute for Experimental Medicine, Hermann-Rein-Str. 3, D-3400 Göttingen, FRG and *Beilinson Med. Center, Petah Tikva, Tel Aviv University, Tel Aviv, Israel*

1. Abstract

Investigation of liver, urine, and serum of amyloidosis patient MAL established the presence of two idiotypically different kappa L-chains. The liver kappa-chain was isolated as an intact fibril precursor from the sodium chloride extracts of the liver and as a kappa L-chain fragment (pos.1-113) from the water extracts representing the fibril. The missing C-part was found in the urine. Kappa L-chain fragments were isolated from the urine consisting of V- and glycosylated J-C fragments reported in the previous paper. Inspite of 20 amino acid substitutions no V-region sequences characteristic of the liver fragment could be detected in the urine and vice versa. The MAL serum contained an intact monoclonal IgG1(kappa) protein whose L-chain was structurally identical to the urinary L-chain fragments.

2. Introduction

In the previous paper [1] we have described the amino-acid sequence of the urinary kappa Bence-Jones fragment MAL consisting of a glycosylated N-terminally truncated J-segment and the complete constant part. The C-region represents the Km3 allotype, the V-region was missing. Since mostly N-terminal fragments of light chains are deposited as fibrils we isolated the fibril and elucidated its primary structure. Unexpected findings prompted us to further characterize the monoclonal components in the sodium chloride extracts of the liver, the urine, and the serum.

3. Material and Methods

Amyloid fibrils were isolated from the MAL liver according to Pras et al. [2]. For N-terminal gas-phase sequencing aliquots were separated by SDS-PAGE and electroblotted to Immobilon membranes. Primary structure analyses were performed after isolation, reduction, caboxymethylation or succinylation followed by reduction and aminoethylation and either cleavage with trypsin, SV8-protease or endo-Lys protease. The peptides were separated by RP-HPLC and subjected to gasphase sequencing.

4.Results

4.1. Partial characterization of the monoclonal AL-kappa I light chain from the water supernatants (MAL-H_2O)

Five fragments were identified ranging from 14kD to 31kD. N-terminal gas-phase sequencing revealed in all except the 31kD band (blocked) kappa I sequences. For the major 14 kD band amino acids 1 - 77 were established by gas-phase sequencing. The J-segment sequence V-E-I-K and the putative C-terminus T-V-A-A-P (109-113) were also identified. The J-segment sequence differed from the corresponding urinary J-segment indicating heterogeneity. The sequence is designated MAL-H_2O (Fig. 1).

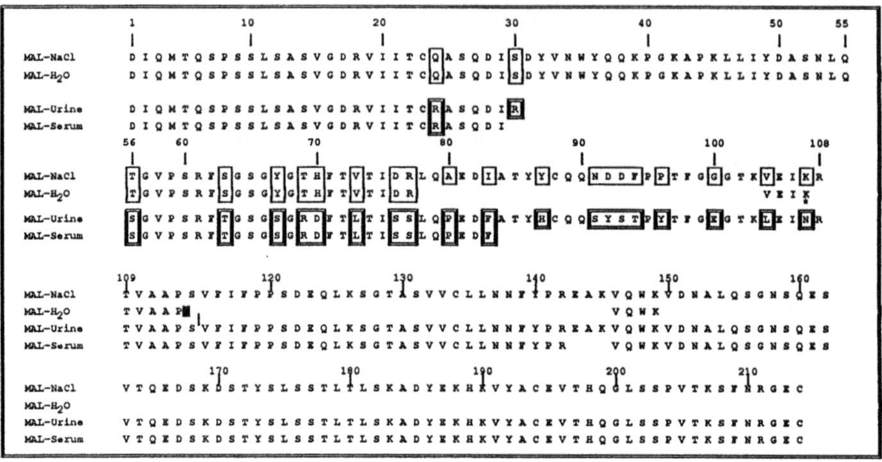

Fig. 1

4.2. Complete amino-acid sequence of a monoclonal kappa I light chain from sodium chloride extracts (MAL-NaCl)

The unexpected finding of different kappa J segements prompted us to look for the AL-precursor molecule. The anti-kappa positive Mr 29 kD fraction was isolated from MAL-NaCl, after reduction and carboxymethylation, by ion exchange chromatography employing a Mono Q column followed by gel filtration employing Sephacryl S200. After tryptic digestion the peptides were isolated by RP-HPLC chromatography and subjected to gas-phase sequencing. The results, designated MAL-NaCl, are depicted in Fig.1. The V-region sequence characterizes this polypeptide as a member of the kappa I subgroup and indicates that it is the intact precursor L-chain of the AL-fibril fragment described above. No consensus sequence for carbohydrate attachment was detected.

We have isolated from patient MAL two idiotypic monoclonal kappa light chains, both representing the Km3 allotype but joined to different J-segments. These derive from either the human kappa J2 (urine) or J4 (liver) amino-acid sequences.

4.3. Partial characterization of monoclonal urinary kappa V-region sequences (MAL-Urine)

From gas-phase sequencing of urine samples separated by SDS-PAGE and electrophoretically transferred to Immobilon membranes the following results were obtained: (1) The MAL urine contains numerous kappa V-fragments starting at positions 1, 13, 56, 61, 97, 104 and 115 of kappa I light chains. In contrast to this finding all fragments isolated from the liver start at the N-terminus. In the search for fragments complementary to the urinary J-C fragments (previous paper) a fraction of the urine was succinylated prior to reduction and aminoethylation. This material was digested with endoproteinase Lys-C, generating fragments starting after the cysteine residues of the starting peptide. To generate smaller fragments a portion of the urinary succinylated and aminoethylated material was subjected to tryptic digestion resulting in cleavage after arginine and aminoethyl cysteine residues. The following amino-acid sequences were determined from peptides isolated by RP-HPLC: (1) R-A-S-Q-D-I-R, (2) Q-Q-S-Y-S-T-P-Y-T, (3) Q-Q-S-Y-S-T-P-Y-T-F-G-E-G-T-Ksucc, (4) L-L-N-N-F-Y-P-R, and (5) E-V-T-H-Q-G-L-S-S-P-V-T-K-S-F-N-R. Peptides 1, 4 and 5 derive from cleavage after the first, third and fourth cysteines of kappa L-chains. Peptides 2 and 3, starting with amino-acid sequences following the second cysteine of kappa L-chains, represent the C-termini of the urinary kappa variable regions and end one amino acid away from the identified N-termini of the urinary J-C fragments. We assume that these represent the carboxy termini of the variable region fragments which have been cleaved from the urinary J-C fragments reported in the preceeding paper.

All gas-phase sequencing results obtained from urinary L-chain fragments are designated MAL-Urine (Fig. 1). In comparison to the amino-acid sequences found in the liver twenty amino-acid substitutions were detected. Therefore, this amino-acid sequence derives from a different kappa I idiotype than the one determined from the liver material. Patient MAL produced two different kappa I chains: the first one exclusively found in the liver and the second detected exclusively in the urine.

According to gas-phase sequencing of urine samples blotted to Immobilon membranes the Mr 14 kD band commences with V-F-I-F-P-P-S-D-Q-K. This sequence starts two amino acids after the carboxy terminus determined for the liver AL fragment (T-V-A-A-P) and therefore represents presumably the C-terminus of the liver kappa L-chain.

4.4. Partial sequence of a monoclonal kappa I light chain isolated from the serum (MAL-Serum)

We investigated the serum of patient MAL in search for both kappa I light chains. Under non-reducing conditions SDS-PAGE of MAL-Serum showed a band with Mr 155 kD along with two others of Mr 140 kD and 120 kD. These reacted positively with anti-kappa and anti-gamma antisera. On SDS-PAGE in the presence of reducing agents three bands with molecular weights of 25kD, 29kD and 31kD reacted positively with an anti-kappa antiserum whereas two bands with molecular weights of 32 kD and 55kD reacted with an anti-gamma antiserum. These data indicated the presence of at least one intact IgG immunoglobulin (155 kD = IgG, 55 kD = H-chain, 31 kd = glycosylated L-chain). N-terminal sequencing of the three lower bands identified these as kappa light chains or fragments thereof. To elucidate whether these light chains are related to the tissue light chain, the urine light chain or both, reduction and carboxymethylation was performed, followed by SDS-PAGE, transfer to Immobilon membranes and elution of the excised bands with the aid of Triton X-100. The proteins were then precipitated with acetone and digested with trypsin.

Tryptic digestion of the Mr 29 kD and 31 kD bands resulted in almost identical elution profiles after RP-HPLC. N-terminal as well as C-terminal peptides, up to position 214, were isolated in both cases, indicating the presence of intact light chains. The difference of approximately 2 kD in Mr may be due to the lack of carbohydrate in the band with a slightly smaller molecular weight. The results obtained from the serum were designated MAL-Serum (Fig. 1).

These data show that the serum contains a monoclonal kappa I light chain of the same idiotype as the urinary L-chain probably deriving from an intact IgG molecule.

5. Discussion

To summarize the main points of the above findings a schematic drawing is depicted in Fig.2. From the liver sodium chloride extracts the complete amino-acid sequence of a kappa I (allotype Km3) L-chain was established. It is marked with the number 1 in Fig.2. This is the precursor of the AL-fibril fragment (number 2) which comprises positions 1 - 113 of the precursor. The tryptic peptide TVAAP characterizes its carboxyl terminus.

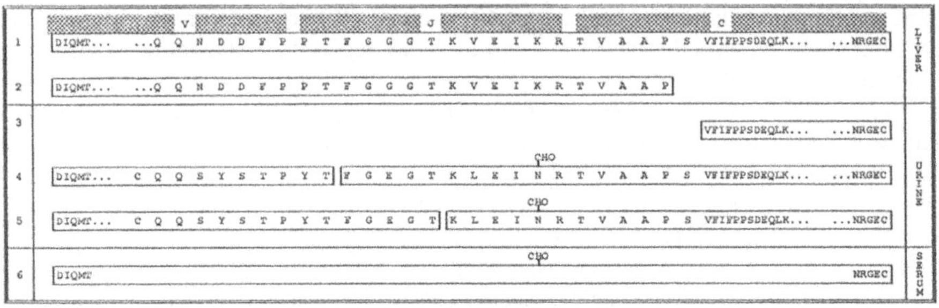

Fig. 2

Fragments 3, 4, and 5 were isolated from the urine. Fragment 3 starts at the termination of AL-fragment 2 with one serine residue missing at the N-terminus. We have good reason to assume that fragment 2 represents the N-terminal half and fragment 3 the C-terminal half of the amyloidogenic L-chain 1 identified in the liver. After cleavage of precursor molecule 1 the N-terminal moiety is deposited as the main fibril component in the liver while the soluble C-terminal half is secreted into the urine. Fragments 4 and 5 are polypeptides derived from the second kappa I chain (also of the Km3 allotype). This is distinguished from the precursor molecule 1 since a variable part characterized by at least 20 amino-acid substitutions was found. Hence, it represents the other L-chain-idiotype. Furthermore, the detected J-segment amino-acid sequence is different, it derives from the human kappa J2 germline sequence and due to a carbohydrate recognition signal is glycosylated in position 107. In the urine the V- and C-region fragments (numbers 4 and 5) have been isolated and their sequences were found to be complementary. No amino acid degradations due to aminopeptidase or carboxypeptidase activities were observed.

From V-region peptides isolated from a glycosylated and anti kappa positive serum 31 kD band we conclude that the uncleaved precursor of the urinary kappa L-chain fragments is present in the serum (Fig.2, number 6). Work is in progress to elucidate whether small amounts of the liver kappa L-chain or fragments thereof are also detectable in the serum.

Acknowledgments
We thank Mrs. R. Fröhlichmann, Mrs. D. Hesse, R. Merker, Mrs. E. Nyakatura, N. Otte, Mrs. M. Praetor, W. Sinn, and Mrs. H. Weiss for their expert technical assistance.

6. References

[1] Kratzin, H. D., Pick, A. I., and Hilschmann, N. (1990) 'Complete amino-acid sequence of a kappa light chain fragment isolated from the urine of amyloidosis patient MAL', in Amyloidosis, Natvig, J. B., Oystein, O., Husby, G., Husebekk, A., Skogen, B., Sletten, K., Westermark, P., (eds), Kluwer academic publishers, Dordrecht, Netherlands, in press.

[2] Pras, M., Schubert, M., Zucker-Franklin, D., Rimon, A., and Franklin, E. C. (1968) 'The characterization of soluble amyloid prepared in water', J. Clin. Invest. 47, 924-933.

COMPLETE AMINO-ACID SEQUENCE OF A KAPPA LIGHT CHAIN FRAGMENT ISOLATED FROM THE URINE OF AMYLOIDOSIS PATIENT MAL

-AL Amyloidosis-

Kratzin, H. D., Pick, A. I.*, and Hilschmann, N.
*Max-Planck-Institute for Experimental Medicine, Hermann-Rein-Str 3., D-3400 Göttingen, F.R.G., and * Beilinson Medical Center, Petah Tikva, Tel Aviv University, Tel Aviv, Israel*

1. Abstract

A kappa light chain fragment comprising the J-piece and the complete C-part was isolated from AL patient MAL. Amino-acid sequencing of this main urinary monoclonal component revealed a protein including residues 98 - 214 of a human kappa light chain. The J-piece sequence starts at three different positions (98, 104, and 105) indicating either unspecific or specific cleavage followed by degradation by aminopeptidases. Due to an amino-acid substitution which replaces lysine 107 with asparagine, a consensus glycosylation recognition site is generated (N-X-T/S) and accordingly a carbohydrate moiety N-glycosidically attached to Asn in position 107 was identified.

2. Introduction

The major protein in primary and myeloma associated amyloidosis deposited as fibrils in various organs is an immunoglobulin light chain or fragments thereof. The kappa/lambda ratio is reversed when compared to that determined for non amyloid Bence-Jones proteins [1,2], a finding which suggested that structural peculiarities make certain L-chains more amyloidogenic than others. A similar conclusion is drawn from enzymatic digestions of Bence-Jones proteins which have shown that proteolytic cleavage of some, but not all, Bence-Jones proteins results in congophilic peptide mixtures with ultrastructural features of amyloid fibrils [3].

The unusual molecular weight of a 20 kD monoclonal anti- kappa positive component isolated from the urine of amyloidosis patient MAL promted us to elucidate its primary structure.

3. Material and Methods

The source of the material was the urine of a 56 year old woman (patient MAL) who died from congestive heart failure. She had been hospitalized because of severe weight loss. Serum protein electrophoresis and immunoelectrophoresis showed a monoclonal Ig kappa protein. Hepatomegaly developed during hospitalization, the liver increased rapidly in size, and filled the whole abdomen after a two month period. The rectal biopsy was positive for amyloid but osteolytic lesions were not observed. She was not treated with alkylating agents or steroids.

The main protein from the MAL urine was isolated by ammonium sulfate precipitation and DEAE Sephadex chromatography resulting in a high degree of purity as shown by SDS-polyacrylamide gel electrophoresis. The molecular weight as calculated from comparison with commercially available molecular weight standards (LMW marker proteins, Pharmacia, Uppsala, Sweden) was 20kD. After electrophoretic transfer to Immobilon membranes (Millipore Corporation,Bradford,U.S.A.) according to Hirano [4] this protein was characterized as a kappa

L-chain fragment. The protein was reduced, carboxymethylated and digested with either TPCK treated trypsin (Merck, Darmstadt, F.R.G.) or staphylococcal protease (Boehringer Mannheim GmbH, F.R.G.). The generated peptides were separated by reverse-phase high-performance liquid chromatography and characterized by amino-acid analysis and automated sequencing using a gas-phase sequencer (Applied Biosystems, Foster City, U.S.A.).

4. Results and Discussion

The complete amino-acid sequence was deduced from tryptic peptides and fragments generated by digestion with staphylococcal protease (Fig.1). The results obtained after conventional ninhydrin amino-acid analyses from aliquots of the RP-HPLC purified tryptic and SV8 peptides will be reported elsewhere.

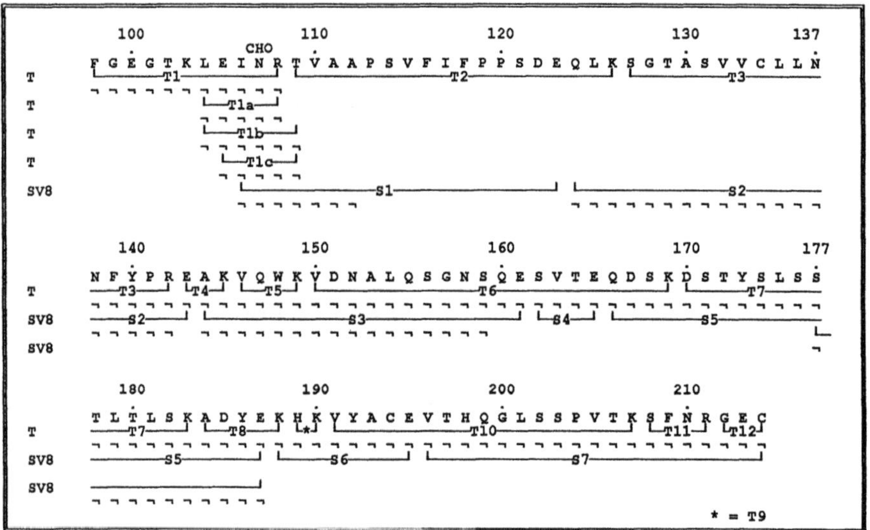

Fig. 1

The data show that in amyloidosis patient MAL a urinary monoclonal immunoglobulin kappa L-chain fragment, comprising residues 98 - 214 (nomenclature according to Kabat et al.) [5] and consisting of nearly the complete J-segment and the constant part, was isolated. With alanine in position 153 and valine in position 191 the polypeptide has the amino acids characteristic for the Km3 allotype. The molecular weight for the unmodified kappa J-C fragment, calculated according to its amino-acid sequence, is 12851.2 D. As this is not in agreement with the apparent molecular weight determined by SDS-PAGE (20kD), further investigation has revealed the replacement of the lysine, usually found in the J-segment position 107, by asparagine due to a pointmutation. This substitution has generated the signal sequence Asn-Arg-Thr for the attachment of carbohydrate to asparagine. After Edman degradation no PTH derivative could be detected for the Asn position. Presumably this residue is modified by a N-glycosidically linked carbohydrate moiety. This was demonstrated by staining with dansylhydrazine on Immobilon membranes. This glycosylation explains the unusually high molecular weight observed in SDS-PAGE. The carbohydrate side chain attached to asparagine residues of immunoglobulins are mostly of the triantennary type accounting for a molecular mass of about 3 kD. This shifts the molecular mass for the modified polypeptide chain to 15.9 kD. Since the carbohydrate side chain represents about 18.9% of the total molecular mass it accounts for the difference between calculated and observed molecular weight after SDS-PAGE.

An unusual splitting after threonine in position 109 occurred after tryptic digestion generating peptides T1b and T1c (Fig.1). Presumably, this is due to the steric effect of the carbohydrate moiety identified in position 107. The structure of this region is remarkable since glycosylation of myeloma proteins is rare. It is observed in only 4-15% of the investigated proteins. Among AL proteins it has been observed in the lambda as well as the kappa subgroup. AL-lambda II protein Es492 is glycosylated in positions 28 and 93, AL-lambda III protein MOL is glycosylated in position 92, AL-lambda protein EPS in position 103 and the AL kappa I chain BAN [6] is glycosylated in position 61. The numbering of the lambda chains has been corrected and is according to Kabat et al.[5]. The carbohydrate side chains of Es492, MOL, and EPS are located in hypervariable regions CDR1 and CDR3. If these L-chains derive from complete immunoglobuline molecules the glycosylation must influence the tertiary structure of the antibody combining sites rendering these more hydrophilic and hindering bulky antigens from getting into close contact with the antibody combining sites. In protein BAN position 61 is located at a β-turn of the five segment layer which is outside the CDR regions. This position, therefore, might well accept the bulky carbohydrate moiety without disruption of the tertiary structure. The carbohydrate of the MAL fragment is attached to Asn 107 of the J-segment, a region located in the intact precursor L-chain between the V- and the C-regions. Similar to position 61 in the BAN protein, position 107 in the J-segment of MAL does not participate in the combining site. However, it is sterically predisposed to allow the covalent attachment of hydrophilic and bulky posttranslational modifications. Interestingly, the identical replacement of Lys 107 by Asn and its glycosylation has been reported for kappa I light chain HOM [7]. In AL polypeptides the glycosylation is located at the edges of the β-pleated sheet structure. Since β-pleated sheet conformation seems to be a prerequisite for all protein components of amyloid fibrils we deduce that glycosylations which do not disturb the β-pleated sheet do not interfere with fibril formation. To evaluate the influence of carbohydrate upon amyloidogenicity however, more sequence data are necessary.

The N-terminus of the MAL polypeptide starts with phenylalanine at position 98. This is the third amino acid of the J segment as deduced from kappa J-segment DNA sequences [8]. Additionally, the tryptic peptides T1a, T1b, and T1c characterize a ragged N-terminus which might be generated by either cleavage after positions 97, 103, and 104 or specific cleavage after position 97 followed by degradation with an aminopeptidase. To answer this question additional investigation was necessary (See the following paper).

The truncated J-segment sequence Phe-Gly-Glu-Gly-Thr-Lys-Leu-Glu-Ile-Asn-Arg besides its amino-acid substitution and glycosylation in position 107 includes another replacement. The glutamine usually observed in position 100 is replaced by glutamic acid. At the amino acid level it remains unclear whether this is the result of a pointmutation, derives from deamidation after protein biosynthesis, or is the result of the purification procedure. Nevertheless, its amino-acid sequence derives from the sequence of the human kappa J2-segment [8]. Such a J-segment was identified in AL protein BAN [6] in germline configuration [8] while proteins MEV and TEW have kappa J3- and kappa J5-segments, respectively. For conclusions concerning the preferential usage of certain J-segments in AL proteins more sequence data have to be obtained.

As mentioned above AL fibril components usually consist of N-terminal fragments of immunoglobulin L-chains. The isolation of a kappa L-chain J-C fragment from the urine of amyloidosis patient MAL deserves special attention. The missing variable part may be deposited in the form of fibrils in the liver and other organs while after cleavage the reported constant part is secreted into the urine. Preliminary results of the elucidation of the amino-acid sequence of the AL polypeptide are reported in the paper communicated by Rodilla et al [9].

Acknowledgments
We thank Mrs. R. Fröhlichmann, Mrs. D. Hesse, R. Merker, Mrs. E. Nyakatura, N. Otte, Mrs. M. Praetor, W. Sinn, and Mrs. H. Weiss for their expert technical assistance.

5. References

[1] Solomon, A., Kyle, R.A., and Frangione, B. (1986) Amyloidosis, Glenner, G.G., Osserman, E.F., Benditt, E.P., Calkins, E., Cohen, A.S. and Zucker-Franklin, D., (eds.), Plenum Press, New York, 449-462.

[2] Glenner, G. G. (1980) 'Amyloid Deposits and Amyloidosis, The β-Fibrilloses' (First of two parts), N. Engl. J. Med. Vol. 302, No. 23, 1283-1292.

[3] Cohen, A. S., (1986) in Amyloidosis : Marrink, J. and Van Rijswijk, M. H., (eds.) Martinus Nijhoff Publishers , Dordrecht-Boston-Lancaster , 2-22.

[4] Hirano, H. (1989) ' Microsequence analysis of winged bean seed proteins electroblotted from two-dimensonal gel', J. Prot. Chem. 8 , 115-130.

[5] Kabat, E. A., Wu, T. T. (1987) ,'Sequences of proteins of immunological interest', Fourth Edition, Ed. Reid- Miller, M., U.S. Dep. of Health and Human Services.

[6] Dwulet, F. E., O'Connor, T. P., Benson, M. D. (1986), ' Polymorphism in a kappa I primary (AL) amyloid protein (BAN)', Mol. Immunol., Vol. 23, No. 1, 73-78.

[7] Savvidou, G., Klein, M., Horne, C., Hofmann, T., Dorrington, K. J. (1981), 'A monoclonal immunoglobulin G1 in which some molecules possess glycosylated light chains I. Site of glycosylation', Mol. Immunol., Vol. 18, No. 9, 793-805.

[8] Hieter, P. A., Maizel, J. V. Jr., Leder, P. (1982), 'Evolution of human immunoglobulin kappa J region genes', J. Biol. Chem. Vol. 257 , No. 3, 1516-1522.

[9] Rodilla-Sala, E., Kratzin, H.D., Pick, A.I., and Hilschmann, N. (1990) ' Biclonality in amyloidosis patient MAL : One clone producing an amyloidogenic, the other a non-amyloidogenic kappa L-chain', in Amyloidosis, Natvig, J. B., Oystein, O., Husby, G., Husebekk, A., Skogen, B., Sletten, K., Westermark, P., (eds), Kluwer academic publishers, Dordrecht, The Netherlands, this volume.

COMPARATIVE STUDIES OF TWO AL CHAINS OF KAPPA-III LIGHT CHAIN ORIGIN WITH AND WITHOUT ATTACHED CARBOHYDRATE (AL So124 AND AL 700)

[1]Toft, K.G., [2]Olstad, O.K., [2]Sletten, K., [3]Westermark, P.
[1]*Dept. of Peptide & Protein Chem., Nycomed Imaging A/S, P.O.Box 4220 Torshov, N-0401 Oslo 4, Norway*
[2]*Dept. of Biochemistry, University of Oslo, P.O. Box 1041 Blindern, N-0316 Oslo 3, Norway*
[3]*Dept. of Path., University of Linköping, Sweden*

ABSTRACT. The primary structure of the two AL chains was established from N-terminal analyses of their fragments obtained after enzymatic digestion with trypsin, thermolysin and S. aureus V8 and chemical cleavage with BNPS-skatole. Both proteins showed a heterogeneous C-terminal. The longest polypeptide chains extended up to postition 145 for AL 700 and position 103 for AL So124. Several amino acid exchanges not previously observed in kappa-III chains were detected. AL So124 contained a carbohydrate moiety linked to an Asn-residue in postion 72. AL 700 did not contain any carbohydrate, nor any acceptor sequence. Comparative studies indicated a higher homology between the two AL chains, than between the AL chains and other kappa-III chains. It may be possible that the unique amino acid substitutions found in the two AL chains will render them more amyloidogenic, and that the carbohydrate moiety could have some stabilizing or receptor function with regard to the amyloid fibrils.

1. INTRODUCTION

Immunoglobulin light chain fragments (AL), or less commonly whole chains, constitute the major part of the amyloid fibrils from patients with plasma cell dyscrasia and systemic amyloidosis (1). Hitherto no common structural feature in AL chains giving them a more amyloidogenic property has been identified, although the following aspects regarding the structure has been given special attention; i) some subgroups occur more frequently as components of amyloid fibrils than others (2), ii) a higher rate of glycation has been detected in AL chains than in normal L chains (3,4), iii) several unique amino acid substitutions has been reported in AL chains (3,4,5). In order to decide whether some of these structural features of AL chains give them a more amyloid-forming potential than normal L chains, it is neccessary to have more sequence data on AL chains. The two AL chains described in this paper is? the first example showing a greater homology between AL chains than between an AL chain and a Bence Jones protein.

2. MATERIALS AND METHODS

The isolation, purification and structure determination of So124 has been described elsewere (6).

2.1. PREPARATION OF AMYLOID FIBRILS AND PURIFICATION OF AL 700.

Amyloid fibrils were extracted from the spleen of a 62 year old person (male), with primary amyloidosis with heavy involvement of liver and spleen. Preparation of the fibrils and purification of AL 700 was performed as described earlier (6). Estimation of the molecular mass was done by sodium dodecylsulphate (SDS) polyacrylamide gel electrophoresis (7).

2.2. STRUCTURAL ANALYSIS OF AL 700.

The amino acid sequence of AL 700 was elucidated after digestion with trypsin, thermolysin and S. aureus proteinase, and cleavage with BNPS-skatole. The resulting subfragments were isolated by TLC, gel-filtration, HPLC and electroblotted from PAGE, and characterized by amino acid analysis and Edman degradation as described in (6). In cases where no overlapping peptide fragments could be found, the alignment of the peptides was based on the homology with other kappa-III chains. Homology search was performed using the UWGCG program (8).

3. RESULTS AND DISCUSSION

The C-terminus of the two AL proteins were shown to be heterogenous, from the results obtained with SDS-PAGE together with the finding of several versions of the same peptide from the C-terminal part. This phenomenon is probably due to an incomplete proteolytic degradation, as has been observed earlier in AL chains (3,4). One possible implication of this incomplete proteolytic prosess, is that a conformational change leads to a more stable protein structure that eventually starts the polymerization and fibril formation.
Some groups have argued that especially hydrophobic for polar amino acid exchanges in certain regions of the polypeptide chain could promote these structural changes that leads to fibril formation (9). In AL 700, the exchanges Trp for Arg in pos. 24 and Phe for Tyr in pos. 86 are examples of such exchanges, and they have not previously been found in kappa-III chains (Fig.1). In AL So124 the exchange Val for Ser is found in pos. 29 and 31 (Fig.1). However, both AL chains also show hydrophilic for hydrophobic exchanges, notably in position 28, 51 and 96. This may also add to the structural changes that eventually leads to fibril formation.
An interesting observation is that there is a greater extent of homology between the two AL chains (84.6%) than between the AL chains and the most homologous Bence-Jones kappa-III protein POM (81.7% for So124 and 81.5% for AL 700). More sequence information is needed to decide whether this observation is significant in describing a group of kappa chains with increased amyloidogenic properties.
The role of the carbohydrate moiety is still obscure. It is obviously not a prerequisite for fibril formation since several AL proteins including AL 700, lacks carbohydrate.

```
                              FR I                              →|←     CDR I
             1       5        10        15        20        25    27A    30
AL 700      E I  V M T Q S  P  A T L S  V S  P G G R A T L S  C W A S  Q .  S V T
AL So124    - - - - - - - - - - - - - - - - - E - V - - - - R - - - . - - R
B-J POM     - - - - - - - - - V - - - - - - - - E - - - - - - - R - - - S I S N

                  →|←             FR II          →|←  CDR II  →|←
                   35        40        45        50        55        60
AL 700      S N L  A W Y Q Q H P G Q A P R L L I  Y A T S  T R A T G T P A
AL So124    V - - - - - - - - K - - - - - - N F - - - G S T - - - - - - I - -
B-J POM     - Y - - - - - - - K -  S G S - - - - - - - G A - - - - - - - I - -

                                    FR III                               →|←
                   65        70        75        80        85        90
AL 700      R F S  G S  G S  G T Q F T L T I  S S L Q S  E D F  A V F  Y C Q Q
AL So124    - - - - - - - - - - E - N F - - - - - - - - - - - - - - Y - - - -
B-J POM     - - - - - - - - - - E - - - - - - - - - - - - - - - - - Y - - - -

                CDR III  →|←     FR IV
                   95        100       105
AL 700      Y N N W P  Y T F  G Q G T  K L E I  K
AL So124    - - - - - - - - - - - - - -
B-J POM     - - - - - P - - - - - - - R V - - -
```

Fig 1. A comparison of the amino acid sequence of the variable regions of the AL proteins 700 and So124 with the most homologous Bence-Jones kappa-III protein, POM.

One cannot, however, exclude the possibility that the carbohydrate may have some stabilizing function in the fibril formation, or perhaps some kind of receptor function as to where the fibrils locate in the organism.

4. ACKNOWLEDGEMENTS

This work was supported by the Norwegian Council for Science and the Humanities, the Swedish Medical Research Council and the Research fund of King Gustaf V.
The assistance of Kari Christiansen, NYCOMED Imaging, in preparing the manuscript is greatly appreciated.

5. REFERENCES

1) Husby, G. & Sletten, K. (1986) 'Chemical and clincal classification of Amyloidosis 1985' Scand. J. Immunol. **23**, 253-265.
2) Solomon A., Frangione B. & Franklin E.C. (1982) 'Bence Jones proteins and light chains of immunoglobulins. Preferensial association of the VλVI subgroup of human light chains with amyloidosis Al (lambda)' J. Clin. Invest. **70**, 453
3) Toft, K.G., Sletten, K. & Husby, G. (1985) 'The Amino-Acid Sequence of the Variable Region of a Carbohydrate-Containing Amyloid Fibril Protein EPS (Immunoglobulin Light Chain, Type λ)' Biol. Chem. Hoppe-Seyler **366**, 617-625
4) Tveteraas, T., Sletten, K. & Westermark, P. (1985) 'The amino acid sequence of a carbohydrate-containing immunoglobulin-light-chain-type amyloid-fibril protein' Biochem. J. **232**, 183-190
5) Eulitz, M., Breuer, M. & Linke, R.P. (1987) 'Is the Formation of AL-Type Amyloid Promoted by structural Peculiarities of Immunoglobulin L-Chains?' Biol. Chem. Hoppe-Seyler **368**, 863-870
6) Olstad, O.K., Sletten, K., Toft, K.G. & Westermark, P. (1988) 'The amino acid sequence of a carbohydrate-containing immunoglobulin-light-chain-type amyloid fibril protein (AL)' in Isobe, T., Araki, S., Uchino, F., Kito, S. & Tsubura, E. (eds.), Amyloid and Amyloidosis, Plenum Press, New York, pp. 157-162.
7) Laemmli, U.K. & Favre, M. (1973) 'Maturation of the head of bacteriophage T-4' J. Mol. Biol. **80**, 575
8) Devereux, J., Haeberli, P. & Smithies, O. (1984) 'A comprehensive set of sequence analysis programs for the VAX' Nucleic Acids Res. **12**, 387.
9) Benson, M.D., Dwulet, F.E., Madura, D. & Wheeler, G. (1989) 'Amyloidosis Related to a λIV Immunoglobulin Light Chain Protein' Scand. J. Immunol. **29**, 175-179

STRUCTURAL STUDIES OF TWO CARBOHYDRATE-CONTAINING AL CHAINS (ΛII) AL NØV AND AL MC.

GULLAKSEN,N., IDSØ,H., NILSEN,R., SLETTEN,K.*, HUSBY,G.**, CORNWELL,G.G.***

*Department of Biochemistry, University of Oslo, Norway.

**Department of Rheumathology, University Hospital of Tromsø, Norway.

***Dartmouth Medical School, Hanover, NH. 03756, U.S.A.

ABSTRACT.

The amino acid sequence of the AL chains NØV and MC were elucidated from peptides derived from digestion of the proteins with trypsin, thermolysin,chymotrypsin,pyrroglutamate amino peptidase, Endoproteinase Asp-N and Staphylococcus aureus V8 protease, and from cleavage of the proteins with CNBr and BNPS-skatole.Analyses revealed that both AL chains contained carbohydrate attached at different regions. Distinct differences were observed in the amino acid sequence, however, both AL chains were shown to have the most extensive homology to subgroup VλII

1.Introduction

To elucidate any association between the primary structure of the variable region of immunoglobulin light chains and the amyloidogenicity, we have investigated the amino acid sequence of two lambda chains (subgroup II) associated with amyloidosis.

2.Materials and Methodes

Amyloid fibrils were extracted with distilled water (Pras et al., 1968) from the lymph nodes (NØV) and from the spleen (MC) of two patients with plasma cell dyscrasia. The AL chains were isolated by two successive gel-filtrations on a Sephadex G-100 column, of amyloid fibrils treated with 6M guanidine-HCl, pH 8.0, containing 0.1 M DTT. The fractions containing the main retarded peak were pooled, dialysed against water and freez-dried.SDS-polyacrylamide-gel electrophoresis (PAGE) was carried out using the Laemmli system (Laemmli,1970).

Tryptic digestion of carboxymethylated protein was performed in 0.2 M NH_4HCO_3 pH 8.5, containing 2M Urea (Sletten et al.,1981).

Digestion with thermolysin and chymotrypsin was performed as described previously (Sletten et al.,1981). Digestion with Staphylococcus aureus V8 protease was as described by Austen & Smith (1976). Digestion with Endoproteinase Asp-N was performed as described by Noreau and Drapeau (1979).

Deblocking was performed by removal of pyrroglutamic acid from the N-terminal peptid using calf liver pyrroglutamate amino peptidase (Podell et al., 1978).

In addition, the AL chains were cleaved by CNBr and BNPS-skatole, as described previously (Sletten et al.,1974.,Fontana,1972).The peptides resulting from the cleavage with CNBr were separated on a Sephadex G-50 column (0.5 cm x 108 cm) eluted with 10 % (v/v) formic acid. Revers phase HPLC was also used for separation of proteins and peptides.

The amino acid composition of the polypeptides was determined as described (Sletten et al.,1981). Approx.10-15 ug of material was applied to a Biotronic LC 5000 amino acid analyser. Edman degradation was performed with an automatic protein sequencer,477A, from Applied Biosystems.

Results

Gel-filtration of denatured, reduced and carboxymethylated amyloid fibril proteins from patients MC and NØV resulted in two characteristical elution profiles (Fig.1). The elution patteren for patient MC is quite unique in that the retarded peak is much larger than that of the void volum material. SDS-PAGE of the retarded fractions revealed several bands corresponding to molecular weights ranging from 15 to 33 kDa. The major band in AL NØV was at 15.8 kDa, whereas that in AL MC was at 17.6 kDa. N-terminal analyses of the retarded fractions, containing the AL chains, showed that the AL chains from both patients, had a blocked N-terminal residue. Digestions with pyrroglutamate aminopeptidase resulted in a free N-terminal residue in both fractions. Extensive use of automatic Edman degradation on different purified peptides, revealed a sequence of 165 amino acid residues for AL chain MC and 145 residues for AL chain NØV (Fig.2). In AL chain MC, a tryptic peptide corresponding to positions 191-213 was isolated and the structure elucidated. However, no peptides between positions 165 and 191 could be obtained. Determination of the amino acid composition of AL MC and AL NØV revealed 0.5-2.0 residues of glucosamine per molecule for both AL chains. The structural studies revealed that the AL chain NØV was N-glycosylated in position 94 (Fig.2). We were unable to isolate the glycopeptide from the AL chain MC, however, an acceptorsite for N-glycosylation was found in position 152-154 (Fig.2).

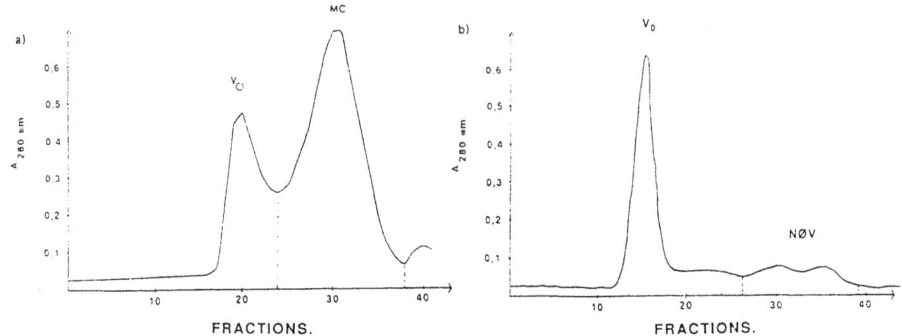

Fig.1. Elution profile from gel-filtration of a) AL MC and b) AL NØV.

```
          FR1                   CDR1               FR2               CDR2
          1    5    11   15   20   25  27 D E F 28  30    35     40    45   50    55
AL MC:    ZSALTQPAS_VSGSPGQSITISCTGTSSDVGGYNYVSWYQQHPGKAPQLMIYEVSNRPSG
AL NØV:          T                   D                    K   D  D
AL ES492:               ( , )A  H    NFTBA_ _     L    I  K    FD
VIL:      H             L                      F       T  K I S  R
```

```
              FR3                         CDR3            FR4
60   65   70   75   80   85  88  90    95 A B 96   100   106A107  110   115   120
VSNRFSGSKSGNSASLTISGLQAEDEADYYCS(S)YAIGS(R)_WVFGGGTKVTVLGQPKAAPSVTLFPPSS
 Y         T                     S  TSD  T  R    T                N  T
           T                     S FTDTT  QL V          L
 D       A T                     S  TSSN S  V           L
```

```
125  130  135  140  145  150  155  160                  191  195  200  205  210
EELQANKATLVCLISDFYPGAVTVAWKADSSPVKAGVET(               )STSCQVTHEGSTVEKTVAPTE
```

Fig.2. The amino acid sequnece of AL MC compared to the AL chains NØV and ES492, and an immunoglobulin light-chain from a person without amyloidosis. The amino acid residues are numbred according to the system used in 'Sequences of proteins of immunological interest', Kabat,E .et al.,(1987).

Discussion

The elucidated amino acid sequence for AL MC and AL NØV was compared with other human lambda immunoglobulin-light-chains and were shown to be of subgroup II.

The results obtained from SDS-PAGE and the primary structure determination gave evidence for a 'ragged' C-terminus in both AL chains and taht the AL MC was the largest of the two. The question may be raised whether or not the location of the carbohydrate had any influence on the degradation and deposition of amyloid fibrils.

A comparative study of AL MC, AL NØV, AL Es492 (Tveteraas et al.,1985), and the Bence Jones protein VIL (Kabat, E. et al.,1987) obtained from a person presumably without amyloidosis, shows a high degree of homology in the framework regions (Fig.2). However, distinct differences were observed in the complementarity determing regions (CDR), especially, in CDR 2 and CDR 3, which again support our earlier data.

References

Austen,B.M. and Smith,E.L.(1976) 'Action of Staphylococcal proteinase of varying chain length and composition'. Biochem.Biophys.Res.Commun.**7 2**,411-417

Doolittle,R.F.(1970).'Pyrrolidonecarboxylyl-Peptidase'.Meth.Enzymology.**1 9**.555-567.

Fontana,A.(1972)'Modification of tryptophan with BNPS-skatole'.Meth.Enzymol.**2 5**.419-423

Kabat,E.A.,Wu,T.T., Reider-Miller,M., Perry,H.M. and Gottesman,K.S. (1987) 'Sequences of proteins of immunological interest'. U.S: Department of immunological and human service.National Institutes of Health.

Laemmli,U.K.(1970)'Cleavage of structural proteins during the assembly of the head of bacteriophage T-4'.Nature.**2 2 7**.680-685.

Noreau,J. and Drapeau,G.R.(1979) 'Isolation and properities of the protease from the wild-type and mutant strains of Pseudomonas fragi' .J.Bacteriol.**1 4 0**.911.

Podell,D.N. and Abraham,G.N.(1978)'A Technique for the removal of pyrroglutamic acid from the amino terminus of proteins using calf liver pyrroglutamate amino peptidase' Biochem.Biophy.Res.Comm.**8 1** .176-185.

Pras,M.,Schubert,M.,Zucker-Franklin,D.,Rimon,A.&Franklin,E.C.(1968)'The characterization of soluble amyloid prepared in water.'J.Clin.Invest.**4 7**.924-933.

Sletten,K. and Husby,G.(1974).'The complete amino acid sequence of non-immunoglobulin amyloid fibril protein AS in rheumatoid arthritis'.Eur.J.Biochem.**4 1** .117-125.

Sletten,K.,Natvig,J.B.,Husby,G.&Juul,J.(1981).'The complete amino acid sequence of a prototype immunoglobulin λ-lightchain-type amyloid-fibril protein AR'.Biochem.J.**1 9 5**.561-572.

Tveteraas,T., Sletten,K.& Westermark,P.(1985).Biochem.J.,**2 3 2**,183-190.

COMPLETE AMINO-ACID SEQUENCE OF AL-BENCE-JONES PROTEIN POL OF THE LAMBDA I SUBCLASS

Pick, A. I.*, Kratzin, H. D., Barnikol-Watanabe, S., and Hilschmann, N.
*Max-Planck-Institute for Experimental Medicine, Hermann-Rein-Str 3., D-3400 Göttingen, FRG, and *Beilinson Med. Center, Petah Tikva, Tel Aviv University, Tel Aviv, Israel*

1. Introduction

Various types of amyloid fibril proteins were described but the mechanism of their formation, from "fragments" of Bence-Jones proteins (B.J.), remains unresolved. It is generally accepted that in AL-amyloidosis they represent degradation products of B.J.-proteins rather than independently synthesized polypeptides [1]. Amyloid fibrils are deposited in 6-15% of patients with "Plasma Cell Dyscrasias" (PCD) [2] and in 20 to 25% of patients with "Light Chain disease" [3]. The amino-acid sequences of amyloid fibril polypeptides and of monoclonal proteins, isolated from the serum and/or urine of PCD patients, were determined and found to be structurally closely related [3,4,5]. Certain types of light chains may be more "amyloidogenic" than others and such "amyloidogenic" proteins could be unusually susceptible to proteolysis, due to distinctive segments in their variable regions [6]. We have determined the complete amino-acid sequence of the urinary AL Bence-Jones protein POL and compared its primary structure to that of other B.J. proteins from patients with multiple myeloma with and without amyloidosis.

2. Materials and Methods

AL-B.J. protein POL was isolated from the urine of a patient who suffered from a PCD. The lyophylised protein was purified by ion exchange chromatography on a DE-52 column reduced and aminoethylated. The tryptic digestion was performed by TPCK treated trypsin (Merck Darmstadt), at an enzyme / substrate ratio of 1:35. Certain tryptic peptides were further cleaved by SV-8 protease (Miles Laboratories, Slough-England). Cleavage with alpha-chymotrypsin (Wortington Biochem. Corp., Freehold, N.J., U.S.A.), was performed at an enzyme / substrate ratio of 1:25. Isolation of tryptic peptides was performed on a Dowex 1x2 column (acetate form, 2000 mesh, 2 x 150 cm, Serva-Heidelberg). Each Dowex 1x2 peak was rechromatographed by RP-HPLC (Dupont, Model 850, Shandon ODS - Hypersil, 5 µm, 250 x 4.6 mm) and amino-acid analyses were performed with a Durrum amino acid analyser (Model D 500, Dionex Corpor. Palo Alto., Cal., U.S.A.). Amino-acid sequence analysis was performed with HPLC purified peptides using either the manual Edman degradation according to Chang [7] and Yang [8] or automatic gasphase sequencing with on-line PTH identification (Applied Biosystems, Foster City, U.S.A.). Amino-acid sequence homology analysis was carried out by a crosscorrelation program and is based on the Kabat classification [9], on the Protein Sequence Data Base [10] and the AL protein sequence data base compiled by us [11].

3. Results

Al Bence-Jones protein POL has 217 amino acids and due to its amino-acid sequence belongs to the lambda type L-chains. The complete sequence is shown in Fig. 1.

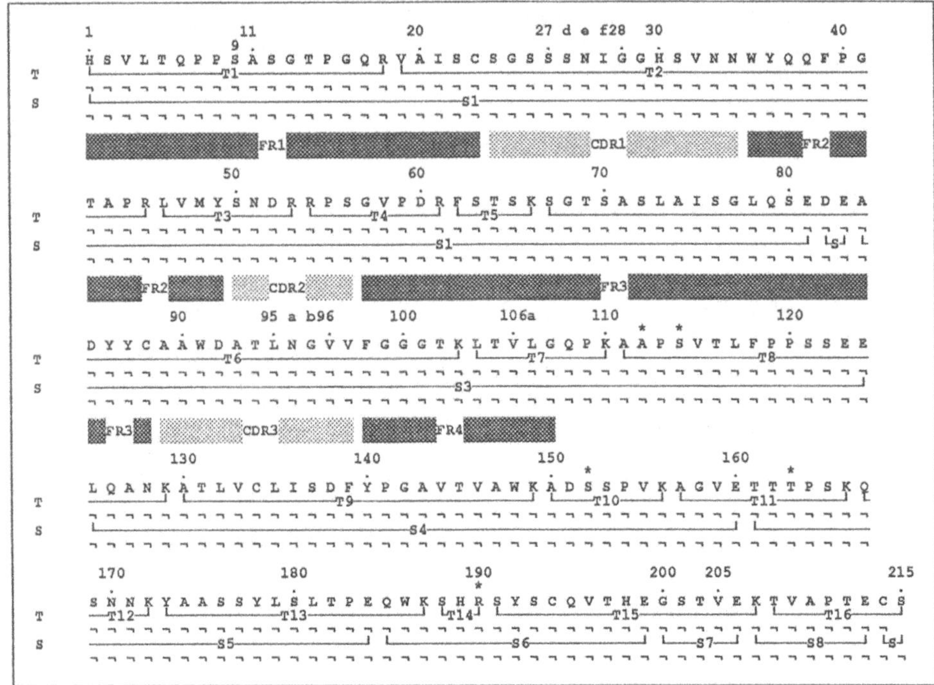

Fig. 1 Aminoacid sequence of the lambda I.2 AL Bence-Jones protein POL. ¬ = residue identified as PTH- or DABTH-amino acid; T = tryptic peptides; S = SV8-peptides; FR = framework regions; CDR = complementarity determining region; * = isotype specific residue.

The quantitative comparison of its V-region with polypeptides of the lambda I-VII subgroups classifies the Pol V-region as a member of the lambda I subgroup (Tab.1). According to Kametani et al. [12] the lambda I subgroup is split up into two subsubgroups, lambda I.1 and lambda I.2. The Pol sequence shows 68.91% to the lambda I.1 and 76.91% homology to the lambda I.2 subsubgroups, respectively. This results in a lambda I.2 assignment (Tab. 2) which is underlined by subsubgroup

	λ1	λ2	λ3	λ4	λ5	λ6	λ7
POL	73.71	60.79	59.26	58.95	57.41	57.12	52.29

Tab. 1

	λI.1	λI.2
POL	68.91	76.91

Tab. 2

specific amino acids A, G, T , N, S, V, S, A, S, S, E, A, and A in positions 11, 13, 14, 34, 50, 58, 72, 74, 76, 80, 81, 89, and 90. The C-region is Mcg(-), Kern(-), and Oz(-) with amino acids A,S,S,T, and R in positions 112, 114, 152, 163, and 190.

4. Discussion

The reason why some immunoglobulin light chains are preferentially involved in amyloidogenesis is still unknown, but reports on unusual amino-acid substitutions have been published for several AL proteins [13,14]. For example, certain V region subgroups, such as the V-lambda-VI, are apparently overrepresented in AL amyloid sequences and have a three to four times higher incidence than the one expected in the normal population [15]. Patient POL was a typical "primary" type amyloidosis patient with widespread organ involvement and excreted in her urine 1 to 2 gr of B.J.-protein per day. 28 amino acid substitutions as compared to lambda I.2 protein VOR [9] are scattered over Fr as well as CDR regions. From these no amyloidogenic pattern could be conceived. Computer assisted comparison of the POL AA sequence with B.J.-proteins isolated from patients with and without amyloidosis [11,12] revealed no apparent homology with AL associated polypeptides; its V-region has 77.7% homology to the amyloid BJ proteins NIG-77 [9] and NIG-51 [9] and 75% and 76.8% homology to non-amyloid B.J.-proteins VOR [9] and KOL [16], respectively. Due to the variability of immunoglobulin L-chains this characterizes only the subsubgroup assignment and no "amyloidspecific" identity is apparent. The N-terminal His, which is similar to the V-lambda-II subgroup B.J.-protein VIL [9], as well as Ala in position 20, are unusual findings. Ala 20 appears to be unique and has not been found in other human λ I L-chains. It remains to be shown that a single hydrohilic/hydrophobic substitution such as the Thr/Ala replacement in position 20 is sufficient to render a L-chain amyloidogenic.

Acknowledgments

We would like to thank Mr. R. Merker for help in the establishment of the amino acid sequence data base, Mrs. R. Fröhlichman, Mrs. H. Weiss and Mrs. D. Hesse for outstanding technical assistance and Mrs. M. Praetor for the performance of amino-acid analyses.

5. References

[1] Eulitz, M.(1985) 'Amyloid fibril derived from V -region together with C-region fragments from a lambda-II immunoglobulin light chain', Hoppe Seyler's Z. Physiol. Chem. 366, 907- 915.

[2] Isobe, T., Osserman, E.F.(1974) 'Patterns of amyloidosis and their association with Plasma Cell Dyscrasia', N. Engl. J. Med. 290, 473-477.

[3] Kyle, R.A.,(1982) Amyloidosis. Clinics in Hematology; 11, 151-179.

[4] Glenner, G.G., Terry, W., Harada, M., Iserski, C., Page, D., (1971) 'Amyloid fibril proteins: Proof of homology with immunoglobulin light chains by sequence analysis', Science 172, 1150 - 1151.

[5] Natvig, J. B., Westermark, P., Sletten, K., Husby, G., Michaelsen, (1980) 'Structure and antigenic analysis of light chain amyloid proteins' In: Amyloid and Amyloidosis - Glenner, G. (Editor) p.257-265 Excerpta Medica.

[6] Solomon, A., Kyle, R.A., Frangione, B. (1986) 'Light chain variable region subgroups of monoclonal immunoglobulins in amyloidosis-AL', in: Amyloidosis, Glenner et al. (Editor) Plenum Press, N.Y., p. 449-462.

[7] Chang, J.Y., Brauer, D., Wittmann-Liebold, B. (1978) 'Microsequence analysis of peptides and proteins', Febs Lett. 93, 205 -214.

[8] Yang, C.Y. (1979) 'Die Trennung der 4-(4-Dimethylamino) phenylazo) phenylthiohydantoin-Derivate des Leucins und Isoleucins über Polyamid-Dünnschichtplatten im Picomol-Bereich', Hoppe Seyler's Z. Physiol. Chem. 362, 1131-1146.

[9] Kabat, E.A., Wu, T.T.: Reid-Müller, M. (1987) Sequences of proteins of immunological interest. U.S. Department of Health and Human Services.

[10] Protein Sequence Data Base: Protein identification resource (PIR). National Biochem. Res. Fdn. 3900 Reservoir Rd., N.W. Washington D.C. 20009, U.S.A.

[11] Pick, A.I., Kratzin, H., Rodilla, E., Merker, R., Hilschmann, N. (1989) 'Computer data-base of 21 V-lambda region amino acid sequences from AL urinary Bence Jones and tissue fibrillar proteins, unpublished data.

[12] Kametani, F., Takayasu, T., Suzuki, S. Shinoda, T., Okuyama, T., and Shimizu, A.(1983) 'Comparative structures on the structure of light chains of human immunoglobulins. IV Assignment of a subgroup', J. Biochem. 93, 421 - 429.

[13] Tveteraas, T., Sletten, K., Westermark, P., (1985) 'The amino acid sequence of a carbohydrate-containing immunoglobulin-light chain-type amyloid fibril protein', Biochem. J. 232, 183-190.

[14] Toft, K.G., Sletten, K., Husby, G. (1985) 'The amino acid sequence of the variable region of a carbohydrate-containing amyloid fibril protein EPS (immunoglobulin light chain type lambda)', Biochem. Hoppe Seyler 366, 617-625.

[15] Frangione, B., Moloshok, T., Solomon., A. (1983) 'Primary structure of the variable region of a human lambda VI light chain, Bence Jones protein SUT', J. Immunol. 131, 2490-2493.

[16] Kratzin, H. D., Palm, W., Stangel, M., Schmidt, W.E., Friedrich, J., Hilschmann, N. (1989) 'Die Primärstruktur des kristalisierbaren-monoklonalen Immunoglobulins IgG-1 KOL', Biol. Chem. Hoppe Seyler 370, 263- 272 .

COMPLETE AMINO-ACID SEQUENCE OF AL-LAMBDA 1.1 BENCE-JONES PROTEIN EZI

-AL-Amyolidosis-

Kratzin, H. D., Pick, A. I.*, Stangel, M., and Hilschmann, N.
*Max-Planck-Institute for Experimental Medicine, Hermann-Rein-Str. 3, D-3400 Göttingen, FRG and *Beilinson Med. Center, Petah Tikva, Tel Aviv University, Tel Aviv, Israel*

1. Abstract

The complete amino-acid sequence of the AL Bence-Jones protein was determined from amyloidosis patient EZI. The protein was isolated from the urine by ammoniumsulfate precipitation, ion exchange chromatography, reduced, aminoethylated or carboxymethylated, and digested with either trypsin or staphylococcal protease. The peptides were separated using RP-HPLC and characterized by amino-acid sequence analysis and amino-acid analysis. The EZI polypeptide consists of 216 amino acids. It has a N-terminus blocked by PCA and amino-acid residues specific for the lambda 1.1 subgroup. Wit Ala, Ser, Ser, Thr, and Arg in pos. 112, 114, 163, and 190 the constant part belongs to the K(-), Oz(-), Mcg (-) isotype. An alanine was identified in position 90. This replaces the hydrophilic threonine or serine residues determined in the other lambda 1.1 L-chains and represents the only hydrophilic/hydrophobic substitution.

2. Introduction

Homogeneous polypeptide chains of immunoglobulin Bence-Jones proteins, especially their variable domain related fragments, are the major protein constituents of the amyloid fibrillar substance found in patients with primary or multiple myeloma associated amyloidosis [1]. Although a large body of amino-acid sequence data on Bence-Jones proteins as well as on light chains has been accumulated to date [2], only limited and mostly incomplete sequence data are available on AL proteins. It is known that lambda light chains are more "amyloidogenic" than kappa [3] and according to Sletten [4] there seems to be increasing evidence that uncommon subclasses, such as the V-lambda-VI subclass, are overrepresented among immunoglobulin light chain derived amyloid proteins. Whether amyloid-associated light chains, possess distinct structural features which render them "amyloidogenic" or alternatively, the light chain degradative process is abnormal in patients with amyloidosis AL, remains to be established [5]. To date no special amino-acid substitutions have been shown to be common or typical for amyloid proteins of most light chain subgroups and the existing sequence data seem to be insufficient to elucidate the relationship between their primary structure and pathogenic functions [6]. We have recently reported the complete amino-acid sequence of the V-lambda 1.2 AL Bence-Jones protein POL [7] and herewith report the complete amino-acid sequence of another AL V-lambda 1 subclass Bence-Jones protein.

3. Materials and Methods

AL BJ protein EZI was isolated from the urine by ammonium sulfate precipitation, followed by ion exchange chromatography. After reduction, alkylation, and cleavage with either trypsin or SV8-protease the generated peptides were separated by RP-HPLC. These were characterized by conventional amino-acid analysis (Fa. Dionex, Durrum D-500) and either automated (Applied Biosystems, model 479 A gas-phase sequencer and Beckman Instr., model B liquid-phase sequencer) or manual sequencing [8,9].

4. Results

Bence-Jones protein EZI consists of 216 amino acids. The N-terminus is blocked by pyroglutamate and with subgroup specific amio acids V, A, A, N, Y, S, D, K, I, T, G, T, T, G, G, and S in positions 11, 13, 14, 30, 32, 34, 50, 53, 58, 72, 74, 76, 80, 81, 89, and 93 it belongs to the lambda 1.1 subsubgroup [10]. The constant part represents the Kern(-), Oz(-), Mcg(-) isotype due to amino acids A, S, S, T, and R in positions 112, 114, 152, 163, and 190 (Fig.1). Compared to EPS [11], BL2 [12], NIG-64 [10], and NEW [13] only the replacement of T or S by A in position 90 (CDR3) represents a hydrophilic/hydrophobic substitution.

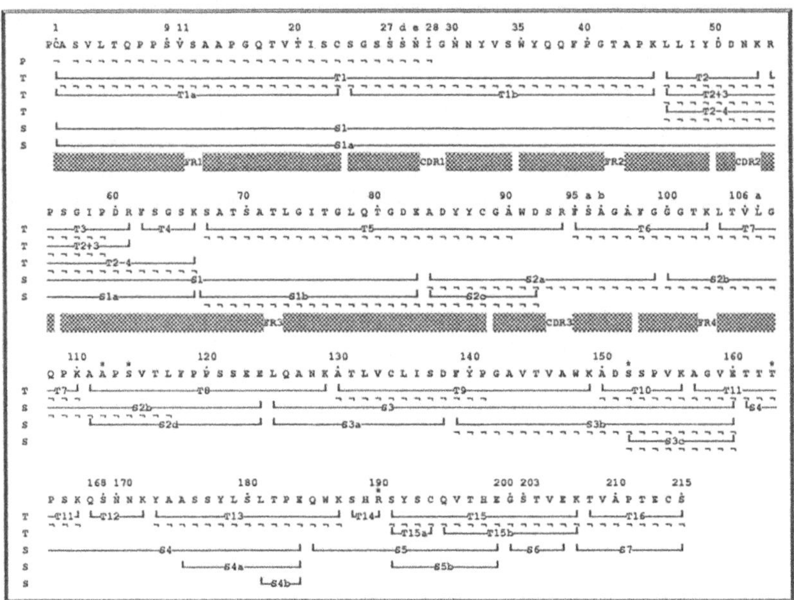

Fig. 1: Amino-acid sequence of AL Bence-Jones protein EZI
¬ = Amino acid identified by sequencing; P = Sequencing of the intact protein after treatment with pyroglutamate-aminopeptidase; T = Tryptic peptides; S = Peptides isolated after digestion with SV8-Protease ; * = isotype specific residues.

5. Discussion

Since Glenner has shown the homology of tissue AL fibril proteins with urinary Bence-Jones proteins [1], investigators are searching for structural features which could explain the mechanism of AL fibril formation from Bence-Jones proteins. Despite of the fact that, partial or complete, amino-acid sequences are available to date, for over 40 AL Bence-Jones proteins and amyloid fibril proteins [2], the physico-chemical conditions required for fibril formation are still unknown. It is well established that the AL amyloid fibril subunit can derive by enzymatic cleavage from a precursor, a Bence-Jones protein, and that lambda Bence-Jones proteins have a higher propensity for fibril formation, than light chains of the kappa type [3]. AL BJ-protein EZI is a typical representative of the V-lambda 1.1 subsubgroup. Its V-J part shows 67.8%, 80.4%, 88.4%, 88.4%, and 84.8% identity to proteins NEWM, EPS, BL2, NIG-64, and NEW which belong to the same subsubgroup. This demonstrates that EZI is more homologous to non-AL BJ-proteins BL2, NIG-64, and NEW than to the AL fibril polypeptide EPS. Therefore, by comparing identity values of complete VJ-parts no correlation with respect to amyloidogenicity could be deduced. To identify amyloid specific sequences shorter segments were compared revealing only the above mentioned substitution of the hydrophilic T or S residues of the other lambda 1.1 polypeptides for the hydrophobic A in position 90 of EZI. Although the fibril protein EPS has a hydrophilic T in this position and resembles the non-AL BJ proteins a similar hydrophilic/hydrophobic replacement is observed in EPS position 85. A hydrophobic I replaces the hydrophilic D. To decide whether single substitutions render polypeptides amyloidogenic more sequence data are necessary and most propably have to be combined with tertiary structure analysis. Presumably, this approach will show that hydrophilic to hydrophobic as well as hydrophobic to hydrophilic substitutions in framework regions inluencing the beta-pleated sheetare decisive for aggregation and fibril formation.

Acknowledgements.
We would like to thank Mrs. R. Fröhlichmann, Mrs. D. Hesse, Mrs. B. Wehle and Mrs. E. Nyakatura for excellent technical assistance, Mrs. M. Praetor and W. Sinn for performing the amino-acid analyses, and R. Merker for the computer-assisted sequence comparisons.

6. References

[1] Glenner, G., Terry, W., Harada, M., Iserski, C., Page, D. (1971) 'Amyloid fibril proteins: proof of homology with immunoglobulin light chains by sequence analysis', Science 172, 1150-1151.

[2] Kabat, E.A., Wu, T.T., Reid-Miller, M, Perry, H.M., Gottesman, K.S. (1987) 'Sequences of proteins of immunological interest', U.S. Department of Health and Human Services.

[3] Levo, Y., Pick, A.I., Fröhlichmann, R. (1976) 'Predominance of lambda type Bence-Jones proteins in patients with both amyloidosis and Plasma Cell Dyscrasias', in: Amyloidosis, Wegelius, O. (ed.), 291 - 297, Academic Press.

[4] Sletten, K., Husby, G., Natvig, J.B. (1974) 'N-terminal amino-acid sequence of amyloid fibril protein AR, prototype of a new lambda-variable subgroup V-lambda', Scand. J. Immunol. 3, 833-836

[5] Solomon, A., Kyle, R.A., Frangione, B. (1986) 'Light chain variableregion Subgroups of monoclonal immunoglobulins in amyloidosis - AL', in: Amyloidosis,

Glenner, G.G., Osserman, E.F., Benditt, E.P., Calkins, E., Cohen, A.S., Zucker-Franklin, D. (eds.), 449-462, Plenum Press, New York.

[6] Takahashi, N., Takayasu, T., Shinoda, T., Ito, S., Okuyama, T., Shimizu, A. (1980) 'Amino-acid sequence of a lambda Bence-Jones protein from a case of primary amyloidosis', Biochem. Res. 1, 321-333.

[7] Pick, A.I., Kratzin, H.D., Barnikol-Watanabe, S., Hilschmann, N. (1990) 'The complete amino-acid sequence of AL amyloidosis Bence-Jones protein POL of the lambda one subclass', in: Amyloidosis, Natvig, J.B., Oystein, O., Husby, G., Husebekk, A., Skogen, B., Sletten, K., Westermark, P. (eds.), Kluwer academic publishers, Dordrecht, in press.

[8] Chang, J.Y., Brauer, D., Whittmann-Liebold, B. (1978) 'Micro sequence analysis of peptides and proteins', FEBS Letters 93, 205-214.

[9] Yang, Ch.Y. (1979) 'Die Trennung der 4(4(dimethylamino) phenylazo) phenylthiohydantoin-derivate des leucins und isoleucins über Polyamid-Dünschichtplatten im Picomol - Bereich' Hoppe Seyler's Z. Physiol. Chem. 360, 1673-1675.

[10] Tonoike, H., Kametani, F., Hoshi, A., Shinoda, T., Isobe, T. (1985) 'Primary structure of the variable region of an amyloidogenic Bence-Jones protein NIG-77', Biochem. Biophys. Res. Commun. 126, 1228-1234.

[11] Toft, K.G., Sletten, K., Husby, G. (1985) 'The amino-acid sequence of the variable region of a carbohydrate-containing amyloid fibril protein EPS (immunoglobulin light chain type lambda)', Biol. Chem. Hoppe Seyler 366, 617-625.

[12] Tsujimoto, Y., Croce, C. M. (1984) 'Molecular cloning of a human immunoglobulin lambda chain variable sequence', Nuc. Acids. Res. 12, 8407-8414.

[13] Langer, B., Steinmetz-Kayne, M., Hilschmann, N. (1968) 'Die vollständige aminosäure sequenz des Bence-Jones-Proteins NEW (lambda typ)', Hoppe Seyler's Z. Physiol. Chem. 349, 945-951.

COMPLETE AMINO-ACID SEQUENCE OF A LAMBDA AMYLOID FIBRIL PROTEIN ISOLATED FROM THE LIVER OF AMYLOIDOSIS PATIENT DIA

Klafki, H.-W., Kratzin, H. D., Pick, A. I.*, Eckart, K., and Hilschmann, N.
*Max-Planck-Institute for Experimental Medicine, Hermann-Rein-Str. 3, D-3400 Göttingen, FRG, and *Beilinson Med. Center, Petah Tikva, Tel Aviv University, Tel Aviv, Israel*

1. Abstract

Amyloid fibrils were prepared from the liver of amyloidosis patient DIA by water extraction, reduced and carboxymethylated and purified by gel chromatography. SDS-PAGE revealed a major protein component with an apparent Mr of approx. 26 kD and two protein doublets of approx. 19 and 22 kD, respectively. All were positive with anti lambda L-chain antiserum on immunoblots. The most prominent protein component on SDS-PAGE with an apparent Mr of approximately 26 kD was digested with trypsin and the resulting peptides were separated by RP-HPLC. Amino-acid sequence determination was performed on an automatic gas phase sequencer and molecular weights of the tryptic peptides were confirmed by plasma desorption mass spectrometry.

Amyloid protein DIA is a lambda light chain belonging to subgroup 1.2. Preliminary results indicate the missing of two carboxy-terminal residues.

2. Introduction

Amyloidosis is a term describing a group of diseases characterized by extracellular deposition of fibrillar proteins. Under light microscopic investigation the amyloid substance appears to be homogeneous and amorphous and when stained with Congo Red it shows typical green birefringence when viewed under polarized light [1]. Ultrastructurally it consists of rigid, linear, nonbranching fibrils that are 7.5 to 10 nm wide [2]. Cross beta pleated sheet conformation of amyloid protein components [3] is believed to be responsible for the physicochemical properties of the fibrils [2,4]. In AL- amyloidosis intact monoclonal immunoglobulin light-chains, amino-terminal fragments, or both are the main protein components of the amyloid deposits [2].

In this paper we describe the determination of the complete amino-acid sequence of AL-protein DIA isolated from the liver of an amyloidosis patient.

3. Materials and Methods

Fibril preparation: Amyloid fibrils were isolated post mortem from the liver of amyloidosis patient DIA basically according to Pras et al. (1968) [5].

Subunit isolation: Reduction and carboxymethylation were performed as described by Dwulet et al. (1985) [6]. Insoluble material was removed by centrifugation and the sample was fractionated on a column of Sephacryl S 200 Superfine (180x1.5 cm), eluted with 6M guanidine HCl/0.1M Tris-HCl pH 8.5. Fractions were pooled according to UV-absorption at 280 nm, dialyzed against bidistilled water and lyophilized.

Sequence determination: The 26 kD protein was subjected to tryptic digestion (trypsin sequencing grade, Boehringer, Mannheim, FRG) for 4 h at 37°C at an enzyme to substrate ratio of 1:50. The peptide comprising residues 67-103 was digested with endoproteinase Asp-N (Boehringer, Mannheim, FRG) for 22 h at 37°C in 50 mM sodium-phospate buffer pH 8.0 at an enzyme to substrate ratio of 1: 40. Deblocking of the N-terminus was performed with pyroglutamate aminopeptidase (Sigma, Deisenhofen, FRG) [7].

The generated peptides were separated by RP-HPLC using Synchropak-RPP WP C18, Shandon ODS Hypersil and Spherisorb ODS II columns equilibrated in 0.1% TFA or 0.025M ammonium acetate using a gradient of CH_3CN. Amino-acid sequence determination was performed on an automatic gas phase sequencer (470 A, Applied Biosystems, Weiterstadt, FRG). Molecular masses of the tryptic peptides were confirmed by plasma desorption mass spectrometry using a Bio Ion mass spectrometer (Bio Ion 20, Applied Biosystems, Weiterstadt, FRG).
Gel electrophoresis on gradient and homogenous gels was performed according to Laemmli [8,9]. Separated proteins were electroblotted onto Immobilon PVDF membranes as described by Hirano [10]. *Immunostaining* was performed with rabbit-anti lambda antiserum (Behring-Werke, Marburg, FRG) 1:50 in TBS in combination with peroxidase conjugated swine anti-rabbit- Ig antibody (Nordic, Uppsala, Sweden) 1:500 in TBS/0.5% (w/v) SKIM as second antibody.

4. Results

The total yield of lyophilized fibrils was 300 mg from 10 g of wet tissue that had been stored at -20°C previously.

SDS-PAGE and subsequent immunoblotting of pooled fractions of isolated amyloid fibrils after reduction, carboxymethylation and gel-filtration revealed one major protein component, with an apparent Mr on SDS-PAGE of approx. 26 kD and two protein doublets of approx. 19 and 22 kD, respectively. All were positive with anti-lambda antiserum. The most prominent protein component on SDS-PAGE (Fig.1) with an apparent Mr of 26 kD was subjected to tryptic digestion and automatic gas phase sequencing. Amino-acid sequences and molecular masses of the identified tryptic peptides are listed in Table 1. Figure 2 shows the complete amino-acid sequence of amyloid fibril protein DIA.

Characterized by subsubgroup specific residues Ala, Gly, Thr, Gln, Val, Ser, Ala, Ser, Ser, Glu, Ala, Asp in positions 11, 13, 14, 53, 58, 72, 74, 76, 80, 81, 89, 93, respectively, amyloid protein DIA is a lambda immunoglobulin light chain, belonging to subgroup 1.2 (assignment of subsubgroup according to [14]). Preliminary results indicate the missing of two carboxy-terminal amino acids.

The protein has a blocked amino terminus but fragments lacking the first 4 residues have also been identified.

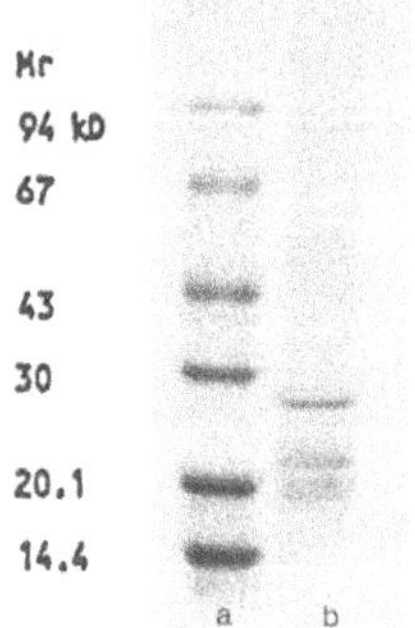

Fig. 1. Coomassie stained 5-17.5% gradient SDS-PAG. a: LMW-marker (Pharmacia, Uppsala, Sweden). b: reduced and carboxymethylated amyloid fibrils

Table 1: Amino-acid sequence and molecular weights of the tryptic peptides determined by gas phase sequencing and plasma desorption mass spectrometry, respectively. Z=pyrrolidone carboxylic acid.

Peptide	Sequence	PDMS Mr	calculated Mr	position
1	ZSVLTQPPSASGTPGQR	1694.6	1694.8	1- 18
1a	TQPPSASGTPGQR	1283.9	1283.6	5- 18
2	VTISCSGSSSNIGSNVVTW-YQQLPGTAPK	3041.6	3040.3	19- 45
3	LLIYTNNQRPSGVPGR	1784.4	1785.0	46- 61
4	FSGSK	525.2	524.6	62- 66
5	SGTSASLAVSGLQSEDEAD-YYCATWDDSVNGWVFGGGTK	4088.7	4089.4	67-103
6	LTVLGQPK	855.6	855.0	104-110
7	AAPSVTLFPPSSEELQANK	1987.0	1986.2	111-129
8	ATLVCLISDFYPGAVTVAWK	2213.2	2212.6	130-149
9	ADSSPVKAGVETTTPSK	1675.3	1674.8	150-166
9a	ADSSPVK	703.3	702.7	150-156
10	AGVETTTPSK	991.1	989.5	157-166
11	QSNNKYAASSYLSLTPEQWK	2317.3	2315.5	168-187
11a	YAASSYLSLTPEQWK	1744.1	1743.9	173-187
12	SHK	370.6	370.4	188-190
13	SYSCQVTHEGSTVEK	1712.9	1712.8	191-207
14	TVAPTE	616.7	616.4	208-213

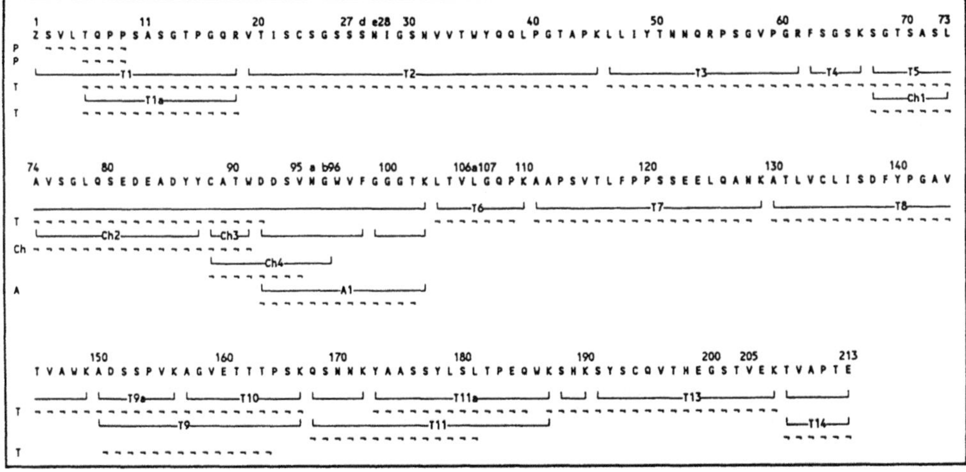

Fig 2: Amino acid sequence of amyloid protein DIA. Z= pyrrolidone carboxylic acid; P= sequenced after deblocking of the N-terminus with pyroglutamate aminopeptidase; T= peptides after tryptic digestion; Ch= peptides obtained after cleavage of the tryptic peptide T5 with α-chymotrypsin; A=peptides isolated after cleavage of the tryptic peptide T5 with endoproteinase Asp-N; = amino-acid identified as PTH-amino acid after gas phase sequencing. Amino-acid positions were numbered according to Kabat E. A., Wu T. T., Reid-Miller M., Perry M., Gottesman K. S.,: "Sequences of proteins of immunological interest", 4th. ed., US Department of Health and Human services 1987 [15].

5. Discussion

The lambda to kappa ratio of 2:1 in AL-amyloidosis [1], which is reverse of that seen in most cases of multiple myeloma and other monoclonal gammopathies [1], the finding that proteolytic digestion of some Bence-Jones Proteins results in amyloid like fibrils [11] and the observation that subgroup lambda VI appears to be especially "amyloidogenic" [6,12] supported the hypothesis that distinct structural properties are responsible for the "amyloidogeneity", but so far no primary structural feature common to all AL-proteins has been identified.

The amyloid fibril protein prepared from the liver of patient DIA represents an immunoglobulin light chain of the lambda 1.2 subsubgroup, presumably lacking two carboxy terminal amino-acids, Cys in pos. 214 and Ser in pos. 215. This observation might be of some importance since cysteine residues in this position are usually involved in the covalent attachment of immunoglobulin light chains to the H- chains in complete antibodies or to a second L-chain in Bence-Jones protein dimers [13]. Val in pos. 32 and Gly in pos. 60 represent hydrophilic/ hydrophobic exchanges. Considering the normal variability among V-parts of L-chains, tertiary structure data are necessary for evaluation of the significance of single amino-acid substitutions in AL-proteins .

In addition to the intact blocked N-terminus starting with pyroglutamate, amino-terminal fragments beginning at pos. 5 with threonine have been identified, indicating cleavage after Leu in pos. 4. Two smaller lambda light chain fragments with apparent Mr on reducing SDS-PAGE of approximately 19 and 22 kD, respectively, have been identified by immunoblotting.

The occurrence of different sized aminoterminal fragments as well as intact L-chains in the same amyloid preparation is not an unusual finding [2]. It seems that proteolytic cleavage makes L-chains more liable to fibril formation [11].

Further characterization of the two light chain fragments found in the amyloid deposits and of the BJP of the same patient are in progress.

References

[1] Kyle, R. A. (1982): "Amyloidosis", Clinics in Haematology 11 (1), 151-180

[2] Glenner G. G. (1980):"Amyloid deposits and amyloidosis. The ß-fibrilloses", N. Engl. J. Med. 302, 1283-1292, 1338-1343.

[3] Eanes, E. D., and Glenner G. G. (1968): "X-ray diffraction studies on amyloid filaments", J. Histochem. Cytochem. 16 (11), 673-677.

[4] Glenner G. G., Eanes E. D., and Page D. L. (1972): "The relation of the properties of congo red stained amyloid fibrils to the beta pleated sheet conformation", J. Histochem. Cytochem. 20, 821-826.

[5] Pras M., Schubert M., Zucker-Franklin D. Rimon A., and Franklin E. C. (1968): "The characterization of soluble amyloid prepared in water", J. Clin. Invest 47, 924-933

[6] Dwulet F. E., Strako K., and Benson M. D. (1985): "Amino acid sequence of a lambda VI primary (AL) amyloid protein (WLT)", Scand. J. Immunol. 22, 653-660.

[7] Podell D. N., and Abraham G. N. (1978): "A technique for the removal of pyroglutamic acid from the aminoterminus of proteins using calf liver pyroglutamate amino peptidase", Biochem. Biophys. Res. Comm. 81,176-185.

[8] Laemmli U. K. (1970): "Cleavage of structural proteins during the assembly of the head of bacteriophage T4", Nature 227, 680-685.

[9] Laemmli U. K. and Favre M. (1973): "Maturation of the head of bacteriophage T4", J. Mol. Biol. 80, 575-599.

[10] Hirano H. (1989): "Microsequence analysis of winged bean seed proteins electroblotted from two-dimensional gel", J. Prot. Chem. 8, 115-130.

[11] Glenner G. G., Eanes E. D., Bladen H. A., Terry W., and Page D. L. (1971): "Creation of "Amyloid" fibrils from Bence Jones Proteins in vitro", Science 174, 712-714.

[12] Solomon A., Frangione B., and Franklin E. S. (1982): "Bence Jones Proteins and light chains of immunoglobulins. Preferential association of the V lambda VI subgroup of human light chains with amyloidosis AL", J. Clin. Invest. 70, 453-460.

[13] Nisonoff A., Hopper J. E., and Spring S. B. (1975):"The antibody molecule", Acad. Press NY., San Francisco, London, 143-144.

[14] Kametani F., Takayasu T., Suzuki S., Shinoda T., Okuyama T., and Shimizu A. (1983): "Comparative studies on the structure of the light chains of human immunoglobulins. IV assignment of a subsubgroup", J. Biochem. 93: 421-429.

[15] Kabat E. A., Wu T. T., Reid-Miller M., Perry M., and Gottesman K. S. (1987): "Sequences of proteins of immunological interest", 4th. ed., US Department of Health and Human services.

Acknowledgements:

We thank D. Hesse, R. Merker, M. Praetor, D. Vana and H. Weiss for their expert technical assistance.

SYSTEMIC AL AMYLOIDOSIS IN A CAT

Liepnieks, J.J., Benson, M.D., and *DiBartola, S.P.
Veterans Affairs Medical Center (583/111RH), 1481 W.10th St., Room #A772, Indianapolis, IN 46202; Indiana University School of Medicine Department of Medicine, Rheumatology Division, Clinical Building 492, 541 Clinical Dr., Indianapolis, IN 46223; *Department of Veterinary Clinical Sciences, College of Veterinary Medicine, Ohio State University, Columbus, OH, 43210, USA

ABSTRACT. A tarsal mass removed from a 10 year old cat proved to be an extramedullary plasmacytoma which was largely composed of amyloid. Subsequent histological examination at necropsy indicated amyloid was also present in lymph nodes, spleen, and liver. Amyloid fibrils isolated from the tarsal mass were reduced, alkylated, and fractionated on Sepharose CL6B in 4M guanidine hydrochloride. The subunit protein was digested with trypsin or Staphylococcus protease, and the resulting peptides were fractionated by reverse phase HPLC. Sequence analysis of the tryptic peptides showed that the amyloid subunit protein was derived from an immunoglobulin lambda light chain. The variable region framework sequence resembled most closely the human lambda II subgroup. This represents the first structurally characterized immunoglobulin amyloid protein in a species other than human.

INTRODUCTION

Primary amyloidosis is associated with increased production of monoclonal immunolgobulin light chains in multiple myeloma and other plasma cell dyscrasias [1]. Approximately 15% of humans with multiple myeloma develop primary amyloidosis [1]. While other species develop multiple myeloma, no structurally characterized immunoglobulin amyloid protein has been reported in a species other than man. Recently we reported that a tarsal mass removed from a cat proved to be an extramedullary plasmacytoma largely composed of amyloid [2]. Subsequent histological examination indicated amyloid was also present in lymph nodes, spleen, and liver. Sequence analysis of fragments of the subunit protein isolated from the amyloid showed homology with human lambda light chain. Further structural analysis confirmes the immunoglobulin origin of this amyloid subunit protein

MATERIALS AND METHODS

Amyloid Fibril And Subunit Protein Isolation. Amyloid fibrils were isolated from the tarsal mass removed from a 10 year old cat by the procedure of Pras et al. [3] using repeated washes with first saline and then water [4]. The isolated fibrils were treated with 6M guanidine hydrochloride, reduced, alkylated, and fractionated on a Sepharose CL6B column [4].

Proteolytic Digestion And Peptide Separation. The subunit protein was digested with TPCK-treated trypsin (2%) for 7 hours or with Staphylococcus protease (5%) for 24 hours at 37°C and pH 8.0 as previously described [4]. Tryptic peptides were fractionated on a Beckman Ultrasphere C-18 column and Staphylococcus protease peptides on a Synchrom Synchropax RP8 column, both eluted with an acetonitrile gradient in 0.1% TFA [4].

Sequence Determination. Peptides were sequentially degraded on a Beckman 890C sequenator and PTH-amino acids were identified as previously described [4].

RESULTS AND DISCUSSION

Chromatography of the reduced and alkylated fibrils on Sepharose CL6B yielded a major subunit peak of approximately 20,000 daltons and a smaller peak of approximately 10,000 daltons. Fractionation of the lower molecular weight peak on a Beckman Ultrasphere C-18 column yielded over 10 peaks. Sequence analysis of three peaks yielded the sequences from residues 125 to 136, 130 to 141, and 178 to 192 in Figure 1. These peptides are highly homologous to the constant region of human immunoglobulin lambda light chains [5] suggesting that the amyloid protein was derived from immunoglobulin light chains.

The major subunit peak from Sepharose CL6B was proteolytically digested, the peptides separated by reverse phase HPLC, and the purified peptides subjected to sequence analysis. Figure 1 summarizes the sequence of the amyloid subunit protein to date and gives the peptides used for determining the sequence. The approximately 40 N-terminal residues and positions 167-172 have not been determined yet. Comparison of the cat sequence to that of the constant region of NIG 84, a human lambda light chain [5], shows that the two are highly homologous (Figure 1). Cat differs from NIG 84 in only 23 of 100 residues. Seven of these differences are the same as in other human lambda chains, residues 144, 152, 153, 155, 156, 163, and 212 [5]. Many of the other differences are conversative changes such as Ser versus Thr. Thus, the constant region in the cat is highly homologous to human lambda chain constant region.

The partial sequence of the variable regions, especially in the framework regions, resembles that of human lambda II light chains more than the other lambda subgroups [5]. The K-L-L-I-Y sequence at residues 45-49 resembles the lambda I and II sequences more than the other lambda subgroups. The sequence at residues 58-70 differs only at position 66 from that most common in lambda II and V. The sequence at residues 71 to 78 is identical to that in lambda II and VI while differing in at least one residue in the other subgroups. In resides 98 to 107, the cat differs only by a His in place of the Lys at position 103 from the usual sequences in human lambdas.

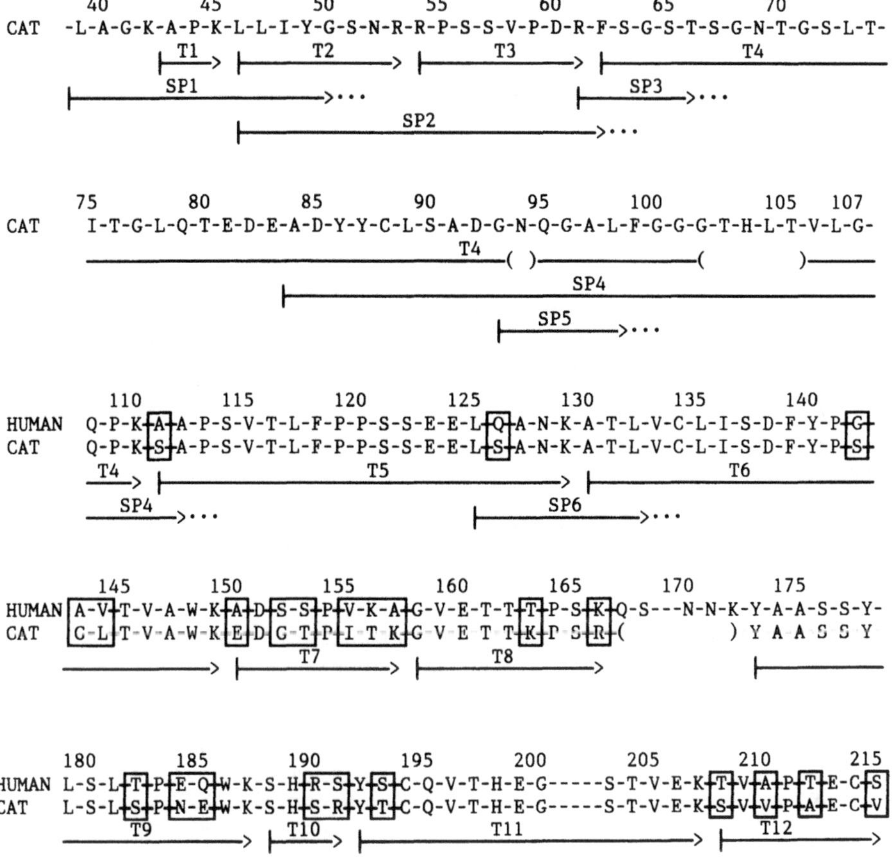

Figure 1. Amino acid sequence of the cat amyloid subunit protein. Numbering of residues is according to reference 5. Residues 1-38 and 167-172 have not been determined. The arrows indicate the tryptic (T) and Staphylococcus protease (SP) peptides used to determine the cat sequence. Parentheses indicate residues not identified in the peptide. Dots at the end of the arrows indicate that the peptide continues, but was not sequenced further. The constant region sequence of NIG 84, a human lambda light chain [5], is included for comparison. Boxed residues indicate residues different in the cat light chain and NIG 84.

Fractionation of the major CL6B peak on a Beckman Ultrasphere C18 reverse phase HPLC column resolved several peaks. Direct sequencing of one of these peaks yielded no sequence suggesting that the N-terminus is blocked. Human lambda I, II, and V contain N-termini blocked by pyroglutamic acid.

In summary, the amyloid in the tarsal mass of the cat contains an immunoglobulin light chain as the major subunit protein. The sequence of the protein is highly homologous to human lambda light chain. The variable region framework sequences resemble most closely the human lambda II light chain subgroup. This is the first structurally characterized immunoglobulin amyloid protein in a species other than man.

ACKNOWLEDGEMENTS

This work was supported by VA Medical Research, The United States Public Health Service (RR-00750, NIDDK-34881, NIAMS-AR20582, AR7448), The Arthritis Foundation, The Grace M. Showalter Trust and The Marion E. Jacobson Fund.

REFERENCES

1. Glenner, G.G. (1980) 'Amyloid deposits and amyloidosis: the beta-fibrilloses', N. Engl. J. Med., 302, 1283-1292 and 1333-1343.
2. Carothers, M.A., Johnson, G.C., DiBartola, S.P., Liepnieks, J., and Benson, M.D. (1989) 'Extramedullary plasmacytoma and immunoglobulin-associated amyloidosis in a cat', J. Am. Vet. Med. Assoc., 195, 1593-1597.
3. Pras, M., Schubert, M., Zucker-Franklin, D., Rimon, A., and Franklin, E.C. (1968) 'The characterization of soluble amyloid prepared in water', J. Clin. Invest. 47, 924-933.
4. Kluve-Beckerman, B., Dwulet, F.E., DiBartola, S.P., and Benson, M.D. (1989) 'Primary structures of dog and cat amyloid A proteins: Comparison to human AA', Comp. Biochem. Physiol. 94B, 175-183.
5. Kabat, E.A., Wu, T.T., Reid-Miller, M., Perry, H.M., and Gottesman, K.S. (1987) 'Sequences of proteins of immunological interest', NIH, p63-77 and 287-292.

EXPERIMENTAL PRODUCTION OF HUMAN AMYLOIDOSIS AL

ALAN SOLOMON and DEBORAH T. WEISS
Department of Medicine, University of Tennessee Medical Center
1924 Alcoa Highway
Knoxville, TN 37920

ABSTRACT. Amyloidosis AL is characterized by the deposition in tissue of monoclonal light chains or light-chain fragments. The lack of an *in vivo* model has limited acquisition of information regarding the pathogenesis of this disease. We now report that it has been possible, for the first time, to induce human light-chain-related amyloidosis through use of an experimental mouse model. The injection into mice of Bence Jones proteins obtained from patients with amyloidosis AL resulted in the deposition of the human proteins as amyloid. The deposits exhibited Congo red positivity, birefringence, and a fibrillar ultrastructure. They were located primarily within the blood vessel walls of the mouse kidneys but were also found in spleen, liver, and other organs. In control experiments, mice injected in identical fashion with non-amyloid-associated Bence Jones proteins did not develop amyloidosis. The experimental mouse model provides a means to study further protein and host factors responsible for the development of human amyloidosis AL.

Introduction

The prediction by Osserman and colleagues (1-2) that monoclonal Igs found in patients with plasma cell dyscrasias could be implicated in amyloid formation was subsequently established by Glenner (3), who demonstrated the seminal role of the light polypeptide chain in the pathogenesis of primary or multiple myeloma-associated amyloidosis, i.e., amyloidosis AL. The presence of a monoclonal Ig, however, does not invariably result in amyloid formation. The pathophysiological factors responsible for the development of amyloid in some but not all such patients are presently unknown.

The availability of an *in vivo* model for amyloidosis AL would provide a means to study further the pathogenic role of protein, as well as host factors, in this disease. Although it is possible to induce amyloidosis experimentally, e.g., through injection of mice with casein or endotoxin (4), the type of amyloid protein deposited is not Ig-related but rather is a totally different protein, namely, the degradation product of the acute-phase serum protein SAA (5).

In an effort to elucidate the protein and/or host factors essential to the development of amyloidosis AL, we have utilized an experimental model first described in 1976 by Koss, Pirani, and Osserman (6). These investigators found that the single injection into mice of certain human Bence Jones proteins produced the renal lesions characteristic of myeloma (cast) nephropathy. We now report that, using this model, we have been able to produce *in vivo* human light-chain-associated amyloid by injecting mice repeatedly with Bence Jones proteins obtained from patients with amyloidosis AL.

Material and Methods

Bence Jones proteins were isolated by zone (block) electrophoresis from urine specimens obtained from patients with multiple myeloma or amyloidosis AL (7): Their purity was determined by electrophoresis in agarose gels and by SDS/PAGE. The Bence Jones proteins were classified serologically using specific anti-κ and anti-λ light-chain antisera (7). Pairs of 6-wk-old C3H/HEJ mice were injected intraperitoneally with up to 200 mg twice weekly of purified Bence Jones protein dissolved in 2 ml of a physiological buffer. Forty-eight hrs after the period of protein injection specified, the mice were sacrificed and the organs processed appropriately for light microscopy (histochemistry and immunohistochemistry) and electron microscopy.

Results

Based on the finding that λVI light chains are invariably found in patients with amyloidosis AL (8), we first selected for injection into mice one such λVI amyloid-associated Bence Jones protein. Attempts to produce amyloid lesions in mice by single 300-mg injections according to the protocol described by Koss, et al (6) produced neither renal tubular casts nor Congo red-positive deposits. Negative results were also obtained when the protocol was changed so that mice received 200 mg of the λVI Bence Jones protein twice weekly for 4 consecutive wks or 100 mg of protein twice weekly for 8 wks. However, when the comparably scheduled 200-mg dose of protein was given to mice dehydrated for 24 hrs prior to each injection (in an attempt to accelerate light-chain nephrotoxicity [9]), Congo red-positive, birefringent material was detected in the mouse renal arterial walls after 8 wks (Fig. 1, left). These amyloid deposits contained the injected human light chain, as evidenced immunohistochemically by their reaction with a specific anti-human-$V_{\lambda VI}$ antiserum (Fig. 1, middle), as well as with a general anti-λ-chain antiserum (not illustrated). That the experimentally-induced amyloid deposits consisted of the injected human light chain and not mouse Ig or amyloid A protein was conclusively demonstrated using appropriate antisera. A similar pattern of reactivity was found in the renal vascular amyloid deposits in a patient with λVI-associated amyloidosis. Electron microscopic analyses demonstrated the characteristic fibrillar nature of the mouse amyloid deposits (Fig. 1, right) and their ultrastructural similarity to human amyloid. When the period of injections was extended to 12 wks, the renovascular deposition of amyloid was more pronounced and extended into the interstitial tissue. In contrast, no renal amyloid deposits were found in mice injected with a κ Bence Jones protein obtained from a patient who did not have amyloidosis.

Using this protocol, we injected mice with a κI Bence Jones protein obtained from a patient with widespread amyloidosis AL. These injections also resulted, after 8 wks, in the renovascular deposition of the human κ chain as amyloid. After 16 wks, Congo red-positive, birefringent deposits that reacted with specific anti-κ-chain and anti-idiotypic antisera were also found systemically in mouse heart, liver, adrenal gland, and spleen. The

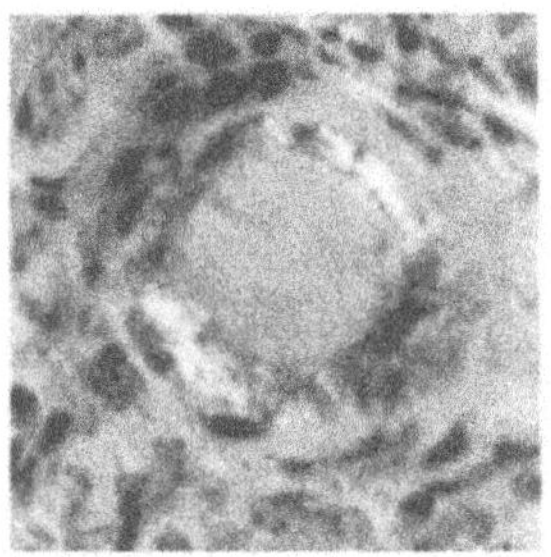
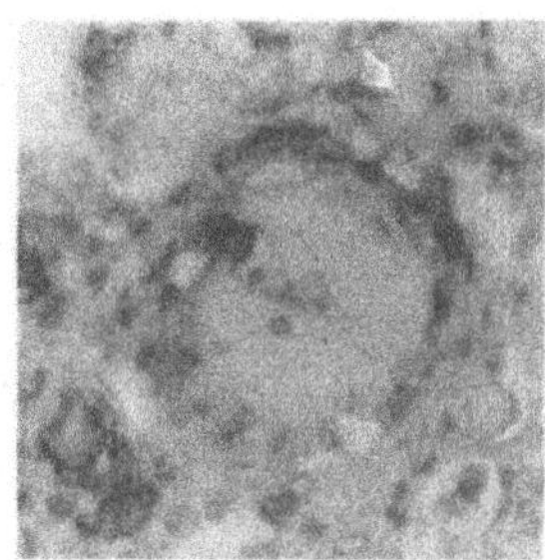
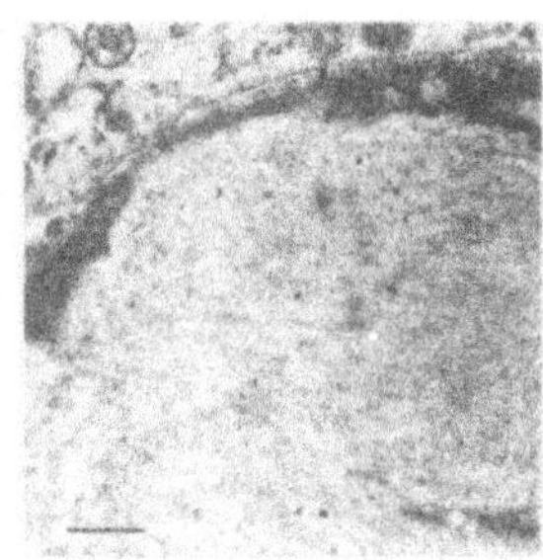

Figure 1. Experimental production of renovascular amyloidosis AL. *Left:* Birefringent Congo red-positive light chain deposits (polarizing microscopy; 2X enlargement/original 200X magnification). *Middle:* Human λVI light chain deposits (immunoperoxidase technique; anti-λVI primary antiserum; magnification 400X). *Right:* Fibrillar ultrastructure of light-chain deposits (electron photomicrograph; magnification 14,500X, bar = 500 nm).

fibrils contained in the experimentally-induced splenic amyloid were comparable to that found in the patient's spleen as evidenced by electron microscopy. Again mice injected over a comparable period with the non-amyloid-associated κ Bence Jones protein did not develop amyloidosis.

Discussion

The ability to induce amyloidosis AL in an experimental *in vivo* model provides a novel means to study further the pathogenesis of this disease process. When amyloid-associated *human* light chains were injected into another species, namely mice, the recipient animals developed amyloidosis. The deposits had the characteristic tinctorial and ultrastructural features of amyloid and consisted of the human proteins and not mouse proteins. In contrast to the rapid development (within 48 hrs) of Bence Jones protein-containing tubular casts that mimic "myeloma cast nephropathy" (6) and result from the single injection into mice of a relatively small amount of human monoclonal light chains (200-300 mg), we found that under the experimental conditions employed, considerably more protein (~2 gm) given over a much longer period of time (~2 mo) was necessary for amyloid formation. The finding that Bence Jones proteins obtained from patients with amyloidosis AL (as opposed to non-amyloid-associated proteins) were deposited as amyloid in the mouse indicates the inherent "amyloidogenicity" of certain light chains. However, whether amyloid-associated light-chains have common tertiary structural features that permit the formation of the characteristic β-pleated structure (5) remains to be determined. Conceivably, most or all monoclonal light chains are potentially amyloidogenic, as evidenced by the generation of Congophilic, fibrillar V_L fragments (10, 11) and V_L-related peptides (12) through enzymatic digestion of Bence Jones proteins. However, the lack of correlation between the *in vitro* production of "amyloid" and the "amyloidogenicity" of the same protein *in vivo* (11) suggests that additional (host) factors are required for amyloid formation. Our experimental findings indicate that one factor of pathophysiological importance--dehydration--which potentiates myeloma "cast" nephropathy (9), may also promote light-chain amyloid formation. The availability of an *in vivo* model to investigate further the pathogenesis of amyloidosis AL and factors that accelerate, prevent, or reverse its formation is of obvious clinical importance.

Acknowledgments

The assistance of Ms. Teresa Williams, Ms. Bobbie Rush, Ms. Mildred Conley, and Dr. David Gerard in the experimental aspects of this study and Ms. Julie Ottinger in manuscript preparation is gratefully acknowledged. This research was supported in part by NIH Research Grant CA 10056 from the National Cancer Institute and by an Ina M. Barger Memorial Grant for Cancer Research IM-430C from the American Cancer Society.

References

1. Osserman, E.F., Takatsuki, K., and Talal, N. (1964) Multiple myeloma. I. The pathogenesis of "amyloidosis." *Semin. Hematol.* **1**, 3-86.
2. Isobe, T. and Osserman, E.F. (1974) Patterns of amyloidosis and their association with plasma-cell dyscrasias, monoclonal immunoglobulins and Bence-Jones proteins. *N. Engl. J. Med.* **290**, 473-477.
3. Glenner, G.G., Terry, W., Harada, M., et al. (1971) Amyloid fibril proteins: Proof of homology with immunoglobulin light chains by sequence analysis. *Science* **171**, 1150-1151.
4. Zschiesche, W. and Jakob, W. (1989) Pathology of animal amyloidoses. *Pharmac. Ther.* **41**, 49-83.
5. Glenner, G.G. (1980) Amyloid deposits and amyloidosis: The β-fibrilloses. *N. Engl. J. Med.* **302**, 1283-1292.
6. Koss, M.N., Pirani, C.L., and Osserman, E.F. (1976) Experimental Bence Jones cast nephropathy. *Lab. Invest.* **34**, :579-591.
7. Solomon, A. (1985) Light chains of human immunoglobulins. *Meth. Enzymol.* **116**, 101-121.
8. Solomon, A., Frangione, B., and Franklin, E.C. (1982) Bence Jones proteins and light chains of immunoglobuins. Preferential association of the $V_{\lambda VI}$ subgroup of human light chains with amyloidosis AL(λ). *J. Clin. Invest.* **70**, 453-460.
9. Solomon, A. and Weiss, D.T. (1988) A perspective of plasma cell dyscrasias: clinical implications of monoclonal light chains in renal disease. *In* The kidney in plasma cell dyscrasias. Minetti, L., D'Amico, G., and Ponticelli, C., Eds., Kluwer Academic Publishers, Dordrecht, The Netherlands, pp. 3-18.
10. Glenner, G.G., Ein, D., Eaves, E.D., et al. (1971) The creation of "amyloid" fibrils from Bence Jones proteins in vitro. *Science* **174**, 712-714.
11. Linke, R.P., Zucker-Franklin, D., and Franklin, E.C. (1973) Morphologic, chemical, and immunologic studies of amyloid-like fibrils formed from Bence proteins by proteolysis. *Immunol.* **111**, 10-23.
12. Eulitz, M., Breuer, M., and Linke, R.P. (1987) Is the formation of AL-type amyloid promoted by structural peculiarities of immunoglobulin L-chains? Primary structure of an amyloidogenic λ-L-chain (BJP-ZIM). *Biol. Chem. Hoppe-Seyler* **368**, 863-870.

AL AMYLOID, L-CHAIN AND L & H-CHAIN DEPOSITION DISEASES: COMPARISON OF IG SYNTHESIS AND TISSUE DEPOSITION.

BUXBAUM, J., CARON, D. & GALLO, G. DEPARTMENTS OF MEDICINE AND PATHOLOGY NYVA & NYU MEDICAL CENTERS, 423 EAST 23RD ST, NY, NY 10010, USA.

ABSTRACT. Bone marrow cells from 36 patients with AL amyloid and 10 with either light chain or light and heavy chain deposition disease were incubated with radioactive amino acids culture and the Ig-related synthetic products analyzed. All synthesized excess free monoclonal L-chains corresponding to the class found in the tissue deposits. 12 of 32 AL patients had intracellular and/or secreted L-chain fragments. The cells from 5 of 10 deposition disease patients contained L or H fragments or both. H-chain fragments were seen only in the patients with H-chain tissue deposition. There was no evidence for proteolysis of normal sized chains as the mechanism of production of the fragments. Immunofluorescent analysis of tissue P-component demonstrated its presence only in Congo Red positive fibrillar deposits, even in patients whose tissues contained both types of Ig deposition.

Introduction

AL amyloidosis, L-chain deposition disease (LCDD) and L and H-chain deposition disease (LHCDD) are all disorders in which monoclonal immunoglobulins or their fragments are deposited in tissues to a degree sufficient to compromise organ function. While the deposition may be widespread, the most frequently involved organ is the kidney (1). Analyses of the fibrils extracted from the organs of a substantial number of patients with amyloid and a small number with L-chain deposition disease have suggested that in most cases the tissue deposits contain Ig polypeptide fragments rather than intact H or L chains (2-4). While there is much in vitro data supporting a proteolytic origin for the fibrils, our earlier studies showed that bone marrow cells from a significant proportion of AL patients contained Ig fragments, suggesting that the Ig-related molecules found in tissues may have arisen via a synthetic pathway or some combination of aberrant synthesis and proteolysis (5,6).

Materials and Methods

Bone marrow cells were processed and incubated as previously described (6). Analysis of the radioactive Ig related proteins was carried out by electrophoresis of solubilized specific immune precipitates. The nature of the tissue deposits was determined by immunofluorescence, immunohistochemistry and electron microscopy (1). The detection of monoclonal proteins in the serum or concentrated urine samples was performed as in our earlier work (6).

Results

Five of the 36 AL patients and 3 of the 7 LCDD patients had no monoclonal proteins detectable in their serum or urine (Table 1). Monoclonal proteins were found in all of the patients with LHCDD. Free l-chain production, corresponding to the l-chain class found in the tissue deposits, was demonstrated in all patients regardless of the presence of a serum M-protein or urine l-chain. Even in patients whose urine did not contain any detectable free l-chains, but had a detectable M-protein in the serum, free l-chains of the appropriate class were found in the labelling experiments. As in our prior studies, kappa chains tended to exist as monomers intracellularly but as dimers after secretion, while lambda chains were found as both intra and extracellular dimers.

The bone marrow cells of 12 of the 32 AL patients, whose analyses were completed at the time of this meeting, contained radioactive molecules precipitable with anti-l-chain sera which had electrophoretic mobilities consistent with polypeptides smaller than intact l-chains (Table 1). Two of the 7 LCDD patients had similar findings. Both of the LHCDD patients, whose data are complete, had intra and extracellular polypeptides precipitable with anti-h-chain sera, which were smaller than intact chains. One of these was a gamma protein, while the other was an alpha. The cells from all patients containing discrete fragments also contained intact L or H-chains of the same class.

In a few patients we carried out time course experiments, examining the cellular products after short and long periods of radioactive labelling. In each of these the intact chains and the related truncated polypeptides accumulated at about the same rate over the first hour of incubation, indicating that the short Ig polypeptides were not the proteolytic products of intact chains, unless the putative protease acted at a single cleavage site within 5 minutes of synthesis.

Table 1

Immunoglobulins in Monoclonal Ig Deposition Diseases

	Absent M-protein	Labelled Ig Fragments	Kappa/Lambda
AL	5/36	12/32	9/27
LCDD	3/7	2/7	7/0
LHCDD	0/3	2/2	2/1

Discussion

Our data suggest that the synthesis of aberrant Ig peptides may be related to the pathogenesis of the monoclonal Ig deposition diseases. It cannot be the only mechanism since we can demonstrate fragments in approximately 1/3 of such patients, while 90% of deposits yield fragments rather than, or in addition to, intact l-chains. In addition, rapid, discrete, intracellular, post-synthetic proteolysis of intact Ig chains, has not been rigorously eliminated. While "pulse chase" experiments may add to the synthetic argument, the definitive studies require analysis of mRNA isolated from cells producing such fragments. The presence of only a normal sized l-chain mRNA encoding an l-chain of the same class as the deposited molecules would be strong evidence for a post-synthetic origin. However, in all the cases in which we have found fragments, we have also found intact chains. Thus we would expect to find both a full length mRNA and a truncated message of the size appropriate to encode the abbreviated polypeptide.

The demonstration of 2 mRNA species would raise the question of whether the 2 messages represent different transcripts from the same gene in a single cell population, or a biclonal population in which one clone produces a truncated l-chain while the other synthesizes the intact product of the same or another l-chain gene. At the moment we have no evidence for either possibility.

In any case, whether the fragments are synthetic or proteolytic in origin, it is not clear how they relate to the deposited fibril. In vitro studies have shown that treatment with some proteases will generate fragments that will form Congophilic fibrils in the test tube (5,7). The relationship between the propensity of a l-chain to form fibrils in vitro and the presence of AL deposits in vivo is not absolute, hence it is likely that conditions in the test tube do not duplicate those found in vivo. Our prior studies showing similarity of size and antigenicity of a synthetic fragment and the fibril subunit isolated from the same patient, suggest that a newly synthesized amyloidogenic fragment may be deposited with little further processing (8). In contrast, the occurrence of both fibrillar and non-Congophilic deposits, displaying the same l-chain antigenic determinants, in the same patient, suggests that primary protein structure may not be the sole determinant of the tendency to fibril formation (9). These patients may have different forms of the same l-chain, only one of which is fibrillogenic, or different tissues may process the same l-chain differently. The latter may also be true for other forms of amyloid deposition.

Bibliography

1. Buxbaum, J., Chuba, J.V., Hellman, G.C., Solomon, A., Gallo, G. (1990) Monoclonal immunoglobulin deposition disease: light chain and light and heavy chain deposition diseases and their relation to light chain amyloidosis. Ann Intern Med 112, 455-464.
2. Glenner, G. (1980) Amyloid deposits and amyloidosis. N Engl J Med 302, 1283-1293, 1333-1343.
3. Toyoda, M., Kajita, A., Kita, S., Osamura, Y., Shinoda, T. (1988) An autopsy case of diffuse myelomatosis associatd with systemic kappa light chain deposition disease (LCDD). A patho-anatomical, immunohistochemical and immunobiochemical study. Acta Pathol Jpn 38,479-488.
4. Picken, M.M., Frangione, B., Barlogie, B., Luna, M., Gallo, G. (1988) Light chain deposition disease derived from from the kappa I subgroup. Biochemical characterization. Am J Pathol 134, 749-754.
5. Glenner, G.G., Ein, D., Eanes, E.D., Bladen H.A., Terry, W., Page, D.L. (1971) Creation of "amyloid" fibrils from Bence-Jones proteins in vitro. Science 174, 712-714.
6. Buxbaum, J. (1986) Aberrant immunoglobulin synthesis in light chain amyloidosis. J Clin Inv 78, 798-806.
7. Linke, R., Zucker-Franklin, D., Franklin, E.C. (1973) Morphologic, chemical and immunologic studies of amyloid-like fibrils formed from Bence-Jones proteins by proteolysis. J Immunol 111, 10-16.
8. Picken, M.M., Gallo, G., Buxbaum, J., Frangione, B. (1986) Characterization of renal amyloid derived from the variable region of the lambda light chain subgroup II. Am J Pathol 124, 82-87.
9. Gallo, G., Picken, M.M., Frangione, B., Buxbaum, J. (1988) Nonamyloidotic monoclonal immunoglobulin deposits lack amyloid P-component. Mod Pathol 1, 453-456.

GENE REARRANGEMENT STUDIES IN THE DIAGNOSIS OF 'PRIMARY' SYSTEMIC AMYLOIDOSIS AND NODULAR LOCALIZED CUTANEOUS AMYLOIDOSIS

K. GRÜNEWALD,[1] N. SEPP,[2] K.WEYRER,[1] K. LHOTTA,[1] H. FEICHTINGER,[3] G. KONWALINKA,[1] S.M. BREATHNACH,[4] H. HINTNER.[2]

Departments of Medicine,[1] Dermatology,[2] and Pathology,[3] University of Innsbruck, Anichstrasse 35, A-6020 Innsbruck, Austria, and Institute of Dermatology,[4] St. Thomas's Hospital, London SE1, UK.

In approximately 10% of patients with 'primary' systemic amyloidosis neither a B cell neoplasm nor a paraprotein in serum or urine are detectable. Cutaneous lesions of nodular localized cutaneous amyloidosis (NLCA) may be clinically indistinguishable from those seen in systemic amyloidosis L; moreover, in a proportion of patients, progression to systemic amyloidosis L with paraproteinaemia has been reported to occur. Thus there may be difficulty in the classification of patients, with consequent uncertainty as to the appropriate course of management. We have therefore employed gene rearrangement methodology to address this problem.

We investigated patients as follows: patient 1 with 'primary' systemic amyloidosis without evidence of a paraprotein, patient 2 with myeloma-associated amyloidosis, and patient 3 with NLCA. DNA material was prepared from the bone marrow of all three patients and from the excised nodular tumour in patient 3. Bam HI and Hind III digests from this DNA material were hybridized to joining heavy chain (J_H), c lambda chain, c kappa chain, and T cell receptor (TCRcß1) gene probes.

Southern blot analysis demonstrated rearranged bands, in addition to the germline pattern, in bone marrow samples from patients 1 and 2 when hybridized to the J_H probe, indicating monoclonal immunoglobulin gene rearrangement. Rearranged bands with the J_H probe, as well as with the c kappa probe, were also detected in DNA material from the amyloid skin tumour in patient 3. Clonal rearrangement could not be detected in patient 3 when bone marrow cell DNA was hybridized to the J_H probe. The T cell receptor probe failed to document other than germline bands in all instances.

We have been able to demonstrate clonality of bone marrow cells, not only in a patient with overt myeloma-associated amyloidosis and a paraprotein in serum and urine, but also in a patient with 'primary' systemic amyloidosis L in whom neither myeloma nor a paraprotein were detectable by conventional methods. Furthermore, we have demonstrated clonality of the amyloid-producing plasma cells within a skin nodule of a patient with NLCA, in the absence of demonstrable clonal plasma cell proliferation in the bone marrow. This finding not only enabled differentiation from systemic amyloidosis L, but also provides definitive proof that organ-limited nodular cutaneous amyloid deposits arise in relation to cutaneous plasmacytomas. Thus gene rearrangement studies may enable early diagnosis and initiation of treatment in patients with systemic amyloidosis L, as well as differentiating them from patients with organ-limited nodular cutaneous amyloidosis who do not require aggressive therapy.

CLINICOPATHOLOGIC CORRELATIONS IN 109 PATIENTS WITH SYSTEMIC AMYLOIDOSIS STUDIED BY IMMUNOCYTOCHEMISTRY

G. G. Cornwell III[1], B. Thomas[1], R. A. Kyle[2], M. K. Slabinski[1], K. Sletten[3], P. Westermark[4]. Department of Medicine, Dartmouth Medical School, Hanover, NH, 03756[1]; Department of Medicine, Mayo Clinic, Rochester, MN 55905[2]; Department of Biochemistry, University of Oslo, Norway[3]; Department of Pathology, University of Linköping, S-58185-Linköping, Sweden[4].

ABSTRACT

Tissues obtained by biopsy or at autopsy from 266 patients with systemic amyloid were studied with antibodies specific for amyloid fibril proteins. 109 tissues could be characterized as follows: $A\lambda I$ 28%, $A\lambda III$ 7%, $A\lambda VI$ 5%, $A_{\kappa}I$ 28%, $A_{\kappa}III$ 13%, AA 6%, ASc_1 13%. The mean age for A_{λ} and A_{κ} patients was similar (60 yrs), but those with ASc_1 fell into an older group (mean 86 yrs) with heart disease and a younger group (mean 61 yrs) with peripheral neuropathy. The λ/κ ratio of the characterized patients (Group A) was significantly lower than that of the remaining patients with a monoclonal protein (Group B) (1.0 vs 2.4; $p = .003$). There was a significantly higher frequency of nephrotic syndrome ($p = .005$) and lower frequency of myeloma ($p < .0001$) among the λ light chain patients in the total population, when adjustment was made for group membership.

Introduction

The immunologic evaluation of tissues containing AL amyloid has received relatively little attention. This fact is related in part to the difficulties associated with developing antibodies which are specific for the variable regions of immunoglobulin light chain subtypes. Consequently, it has not been clear which AL light chain subtypes are most common and whether individual subtypes are selectively associated with specific clinical syndromes. In an effort to clarify this issue, amyloid-containing tissues from 266 patients with systemic amyloid were evaluated for amyloid fibril proteins AL (5 subtypes), AA and ASc_1. Clinical findings were evaluated for 109 patients in whom specific amyloid proteins could be identified and 114 of the remaining patients with a serum or urine monoclonal heavy or light chain.

Material and Methods

PATIENT POPULATION

Two hundred sixty-six patients in whom a diagnosis of systemic amyloid was made at Mayo Clinic between 1952 and 1987 were studied. The diagnosis was based on positive Congo Red staining of tissues obtained by biopsy or at autopsy. All tissues were fixed in formalin and imbedded in paraffin. A standard set of clinical data was collected for each patient by one investigator (RAK) and stored in computer format.

ANTIBODY STUDIES

Antibodies to amyloid fibril proteins AL (5 subtypes), AA and ASc_1 were raised in New Zealand white rabbits and adsorbed to specificity as previously described [1]. The immunogens consisted of purified amyloid fibril proteins or DAM preparations of fibrils which had previously been characterized by sequencing studies. Immunoperoxidase staining of tissue sections was performed [1] and interpreted independently by 3 or 4 investigators (GGC, BT, PW, MKS).

STATISTICAL METHODS

For comparisons of age, Analysis of Variance (ANOVA) was used. All other variables were categorical; hence chi-square statistics were used to test for associations. In analyses where kappa/lambda and Group A/Group B were both possible variables, the Mantel-Haenszel test was used [2].

Results

IMMUNOLOGIC STUDIES

Amyloid fibril protein subtypes were identified in 109 of the 266 tissues examined (41%). Of the remaining tissues, 91 (34%) contained inadequate amyloid for evaluation, 44 (17%) showed no immunologic reaction and 22 (8%) showed multiple reactions or excessive background reaction.

The 109 tissues were characterized as follows: 30 (28%) $A_\lambda I$, 8 (7%) $A_\lambda III$, 6 (5%) $A_\lambda VI$, 30 (28%) $A_\kappa I$, 14 (13%) $A_\kappa III$, 7 (6%) AA, 14 (13%) ASc_1.

PATIENT GROUPS

The patients were divided into 2 groups: 1) Group A consisted of the 109 patients for whom an amyloid fibril protein was identified; 2) Group B consisted of the remaining 114 patients for whom a monoclonal protein was identified in the serum and/or urine.

AL AMYLOID

There was no significant difference in mean age, sex, frequency of clinical syndromes, mean creatinine, 24-hour urine protein, or incidence of myeloma for individual light chain subtypes in Group A. Consequently, the kappa (κ) and lambda (λ) subtypes were combined for further analysis.

Serum and Urine Monoclonal Proteins in Group A. Serum and urine protein electrophoresis were performed in 76 of the 88 patients identified as having AL amyloid in Group A. 38/40 (95%) of the A_λ group and 30/36 (83%) of the A_κ group (89% overall) had a monoclonal protein in the serum and/or urine.

Lambda/Kappa Ratios. Table 1 shows the λ/κ ratios for Groups A and B. A significantly lower ratio was observed for the A group than for the B group (1.0 vs 2.4; $p = .003$). This difference could be accounted for by the high λ/κ ratio of non reactive tissues in Group B.

TABLE 1. Comparison of λ/κ Ratio for Group A and Group B

Patient Group	λ/κ Ratio	(quotient)	p-value*
Group A	44/44	(1.0)	--
Group B	80/34	(2.4)	p = .003
Inadequate Amyloid	39/21	(1.9)	p = NS
Non Reactive	30/7	(4.3)	p = .001
Other	11/6	(1.8)	p = NS
TOTAL	124/78	(1.6)	--

* χ^2 analysis comparing Group B and Group B subsets with Group A

In light of the relative preponderance of κ light chain amyloid in Group A when compared to the group as a whole, all further analyses were performed on patients from Group A and Group B. Table 2 shows a comparison of the λ/κ ratios of Group A and Group B for various clinical parameters. For comparison of λ and κ chain types, it was necessary to adjust for group membership. In the total group, there was a higher frequency of nephrotic syndrome ($p = .005$) and lower frequency of myeloma ($p < .0001$) among the λ light chain patients. We observed a statistically significant difference in λ/κ for peripheral neuropathy in Group A, but this difference was not observed in Group B or in the total AL population.

The most common cause of death in the AL patients was heart disease (48% in both Group A and Group B). There was no influence of light chain type on the cause of death.

TABLE 2. Comparison of Clinical Parameters for All Patients with AL Amyloid

Clinical Parameter	Group A	Group B	Total		
	λ/κ	λ/κ	λ	κ	p-value
Number of Patients	88	114	124	78	
Creatinine (≥ 2.0 mg%)	1.1	1.8	31.1	35.6	p = NS
Proteinuria (≥ 5.0 g/d)	1.3	1.4	30.0	33.3	p = NS
Syndromes (%)					
Congestive Heart Failure	1.2	1.1	38.7	33.3	p = NS
Nephrotic Syndrome	1.9	2.4	34.6	16.6	p = .005
Carpel Tunnel	.91	.64	20.2	26.9	p = NS
Peripheral Neuropathy	6.0	.85	14.5	9.0	p = NS
Orthostatic Hypotension	2.5	2.0	15.3	6.4	p = NS
Multiple Myeloma (%)	.50	.29	13.7	37.1	p<.0001

AA AMYLOID

Six of the 7 patients with AA amyloid had a chronic underlying illness: osteomyelitis (2), regional enteritis (2) Familial Mediterranean Fever (1) and multiple myeloma (1). The frequency of renal insufficiency (71%) was similar to that observed in patients with AL amyloid.

ASc_1 AMYLOID

Patients with ASc_1 amyloid fell into 2 age groups. Those with predominant heart disease (8 patients) had a mean age of 85.8 yrs whereas those with peripheral neuropathy (4 patients) were younger (60.8 yrs; $p = .002$). The former group is presumed to have senile systemic amyloid, while the latter group may have familial amyloidotic polyneuropathy.

Discussion

The present study extends previous efforts to characterize the immunochemical nature of amyloid deposits on tissue sections [3]. These results provide the first direct correlation between amyloid fibril protein subtype and clinical outcome. Although more extensive studies are required to draw firm conclusions regarding the significance in individual immunoglobulin subtypes, some initial clues are provided.

It appears that $A_{\lambda}I$ and $A_{\kappa}I$ are among the most common immunoglobulin subtypes and that $A_{\lambda}VI$ is not as common as previously reported [4]. Moreover, it appears that $A_{\lambda}II$ and/or $A_{\lambda}IV$ (for which no antibodies were available) may be more common than previously suspected. This conclusion is based on the finding that a) 25% of tissues with adequate or abundant amyloid failed to react with the antibody panel and b) that 30/37 (81%) of this subset of tissues were derived from patients with monoclonal proteins of the λ light chain type.

Since the patients which were successfully characterized by antibodies to light chain proteins (Group A) contained a lower proportion of λ chains than the group as a whole, the remaining patients were also reviewed. It was assumed that those patients with a serum or urine monoclonal protein (Group B) had amyloid of the AL type. When the groups were combined, significant correlations were found between λ chain and nephrotic syndrome and between κ chain and myeloma. The latter result is consistent with data published previously [5].

References

1. Cornwell GG III, Thomas B, Kyle RA, Sletten K, Westermark P. (1988) 'Immunohistochemical typing of tissues from 100 patients with systemic amyloidosis', in Amyloid and Amyloidosis. Tsubura E, Anaki S, Kito S, Uchino F, Isobe T (eds.) Plenum Press, New York, p. 179.

2. Mantel N, Haenszel W. (1959) 'Statistical aspects of the analysis of data from retrospective studies of disease', JNCI 22, 719-748.

3. Cornwell GG III, Husby G, Westermark P, Natvig JB, Michaelson TW, Skogen B. (1977) 'Identification and characterization of different amyloid fibril proteins in tissue sections', Scan J Immunol 6, 1071-1080.

4. Solomon A, Frangione B, Franklin EC. (1982) 'Bence Jones proteins and light chains of immunoglobulins. Preferential association of the $V_{\lambda VI}$ subgroup of human light chains with amyloidosis AL (λ)', J Clin Invest 70,453-460.

5. Kyle RA, Greipp PR. (1983) 'Amyloidosis (AL). Clinical and laboratory features in 229 cases', Mayo Clin Proc 58, 665-683.

Acknowledgments

This work was supported by the Swedish Medical Research Council, the Research Fund of King Gustaf V, the Norwegian Council for Science and the Humanities and the W. P. Cornwell Amyloid Research Fund. The authors are grateful to B. J. Dain for statistical assistance and B. S. Gaull for preparation of the manuscript (Cancer Center Support Grant CA23108).

QUANTIFICATION OF NON-LIGHT CHAIN AMYLOID PRECURSORS AND ACUTE PHASE-RELATED PROTEINS IN AL-AMYLOID SERA.

ALEX W. TONG, DONNA NICODEMUS, AMANDA BURFOOT & MARVIN J. STONE.
Immunology Research Unit, Charles A. Sammons Cancer Center,
Baylor University Medical Center, Dallas, TX 75246 (USA).

Abstract

This study examined the serum concentration of various non-light chain amyloid-related proteins and enzymes in patients (pts) with plasma cell dyscrasia+amyloid (AL, n=13), plasma cell dyscrasia without amyloid (PCD, n=28), pts with non-PCD non-AL disorders (NPCD, n=13), and normal controls (n=30). Compared with normals, AL pts had significantly lower serum levels of prealbumin and plasminogen. β2-microglobulin and protease inhibitors α1-antichymotrypsin, α1-antitrypsin and α2-macroglobulin were significantly elevated. Thirty-eight percent of AL sera (vs. 46% of normal controls) contained ≥0.03 mg/ml of amyloid P-component (SAP). No serum amyloid A (SAA) was detectable in AL pts, despite significant elevation of C-reactive protein (CRP) levels. PCD pts had below normal prealbumin, and elevated values of β2-microglobulin, α1-antichymotrypsin, α2-macroglobulin and CRP. Plasminogen and α1-antitrypsin levels in PCD pts did not differ from normals. NPCD sera contained elevated levels of all three protease inhibitors, whereas the other proteins were within normal limits. Serum levels of interleukin-6 (IL6) were increased in AL and NPCD groups. These observations suggest that AL is accompanied by quantitative changes in serum non-light chain amyloid precursors and acute phase-related proteins; these altered levels may be relevant to amyloid deposition.

Introduction

AL amyloid fibrils comprise intact immunoglobulin (Ig) light chains or fragments from their variable region [1]. The precise amyloidogenic process remains unclear. Not all PCD pts with a fibrillogenic monoclonal light chain subgroup develop AL amyloid [1]. Non-Ig components may be involved in AL amyloid [1,2]. Factors contributing to amyloid deposition include overproduction of amyloid precursor proteins, altered metabolism of precursors, and genetic variants [1]. To explore the possible involvement of non-light chain amyloid precursor proteins in AL amyloidogenesis, this study examined their serum concentration in AL pts. Serum levels of SAP, SAA, β2-microglobulin, and prealbumin were determined and compared with those in PCD, NPCD pts and normal controls. In addition, we measured serum levels of the serine protease precursor plasminogen, protease inhibitors α1-antitrypsin, α1-antichymotrypsin and α2-macroglobulin, CRP and IL6. Based on their concentrations in AL and non-AL sera, this comparative study allowed us to identify other serum proteins that may be potentially involved in AL amyloidosis.

Materials and Methods

Patients. Forty one PCD pts with (13) or without (28) biopsy-proven amyloidosis were studied. Criteria for diagnosis of PCD and AL have been described previously [1,3]. The non-PCD group included non-Hodgkin's lymphoma (7), hypogammaglobulinemia (3), breast carcinoma (1), iron deficiency anemia (1), and asymptomatic familial prealbumin amyloidosis (1). Normal controls were healthy adults. All studies were performed using sera frozen at -20 C for comparable periods.
Serum Protein Quantification. Serum concentrations of plasminogen, α1-antitrypsin, α1-antichymotrypsin, prealbumin, and β2-microglobulin were determined using radial immunodiffusion kits (Binding Site Inc.). Levels of α2-macroglobulin and CRP were measured by nephelometry using an Ouchterlony system with serially-diluted (2-fold) pt serum samples compared with known concentrations of the purified protein (also from Calbiochem). The limit of detection with this technique is 0.03 mg/ml for SAP and 0.15 mg/ml for SAA. Similar evaluations were carried out using the β amyloid protein antiserum Angela (kindly provided by Dr. D. Selkoe) and the β protein precursor antisera C_7 (also from Dr. Selkoe) and anti-XIaI (a gift of Dr. G. Broze). Quantification of serum IL6 was performed by an ELISA assay (R & D Systems).

Results

Serum Concentration of Amyloid Precursor Proteins. The mean serum concentrations of amyloid precursor proteins in each group are listed in Table 1. All AL pts had detectable levels of serum M-protein and/or urine Bence Jones protein. A higher proportion (X^2=11.48; p<0.0007) of AL patients (61.5%) had light chain disease as compared with non-AL PCD pts (7%) [3]. AL sera contained elevated levels of β2-microglobulin (p<0.05) and decreased prealbumin (p<0.001) as compared with normals. Similar fluctuations of these proteins were observed in PCD (but not NPCD) pts. Levels of β2-microglobulin and prealbumin in AL pts did not differ significantly from those of PCD pts. No significant elevations of serum SAA or SAP in AL, PCD, or NPCD pt groups were observed. PreA4 was not detected in normal sera or any of the pt groups. Albumin levels were within the normal range.
Serum Concentration of Acute Phase-related Proteins. Serum enzymes and/or their inhibitors may be involved in amyloid precursor processing and/or degradation [1,4]. AL sera contained elevated levels of the serine protease inhibitors α1-antitrypsin (p<0.01), α1-antichymotrypsin (p<0.001), and α2-macroglobulin (p<0.001) (Table 2). α1-antichymotrypsin was elevated

TABLE 1. Serum Concentration of Amyloid Precursor Proteins.

		AL[a]	PCD	NPCD	NC
M-protein	(g/dL)	0.27±0.65*	1.61±1.52*	ND[a]	ND
β2-microglobulin	(mg/L)	11.7±20.9*	5.2±1.8**	4.0±2.5	2.9±0.7
Prealbumin	(mg/L)	222.8±97.5**	270.6±77.5*	327.6±121.0	327.3±50.4
SAA	(mg/ml)	ND	0.01±0.06	ND	ND
SAP	(mg/ml)	0.04±0.07	0.05±0.08	0.04±0.07	0.02±0.03

[a]Pts are categorized as AL: AL amyloidosis; PCD: plasma cell dyscrasia with no evidence of amyloidosis; NPCD, non-plasma cell dyscrasia; NC: normal controls. Values represent mean ± SD. ND: not detectable.
*Stat. significant from corresponding normal control value ($p<0.05$).
**Stat. significantly from corresponding normal control value ($p<0.001$).

in all 3 pt groups, whereas NPCD sera (but not PCD) had significantly increased α1-antitrypsin. Although α2-macroglobulin levels were elevated in PCD and NPCD sera, this protease inhibitor was present in significantly higher concentration in AL than in other pt groups ($p<0.05$).

AL (but not PCD nor NPCD) sera contained lower than normal ($p<0.02$) levels of plasminogen. This reduced level in AL was unrelated to sample storage duration. Elevated levels of CRP were detected in both AL ($p<0.02$) and PCD ($p<0.05$) (but not NPCD) pt groups (Table 2). Of the PCD pts tested, there was no significant difference in concentration of any of the proteins shown in the Tables between pts with multiple myeloma (MM) versus non-MM PCD. AL sera had elevated levels of IL6 (15.3±16.5 pg/ml; $p<0.05$) compared with normals (3.7±17.2). Similarly, NPCD pts had elevated levels of IL6 (16.0±9.7). Elevated IL6 levels in PCD sera (10.4±11.3) did not differ significantly from normals ($p>0.05$). IL6 levels in MM pts did not differ from non-MM PCD pts.

Discussion

Our study found no significant difference in the concentration of non-Ig amyloid precursors β2-microglobulin, prealbumin, SAA, SAP or preA4 in AL as compared with PCD or NPCD sera. By contrast, there appeared to be distinct fluctuations in serine protease inhibitor and precursor levels in AL sera that were not observed with PCD nor NPCD sera. Whereas α1-antitrypsin and α1-antichymotrypsin were elevated in AL, PCD and NPCD sera, α2-macroglobulin was significantly higher in AL than other pt groups. Acute phase responses may not be the sole contributing factor accounting for these serum protein fluctuations, since the latter did not correlate with CRP levels. α2-macroglobulin is an inhibitor of proteases (plasmin, trypsin, chymotrypsin, kallikrein and elastase) that may be involved in amyloid fibril processing and degradation [1,4]. The significantly increased level of protease inhibitors may reflect abnormal protease activity in AL. Interestingly, AL (but not PCD or NPCD) sera also contained significantly lower levels of plasminogen. Plasmin is effective in degrading SAA or AA fibrils *in vitro* [4]. Pts with AL demonstrated antibodies against casein, a potent AA amyloid inducer in mice [5] and substrate for plasmin. The decreased plasminogen level may reflect altered

TABLE 2. Serum Concentration of Enzymes and Acute Phase-related Proteins.

	AL[a]	PCD	NPCD	NC
Plasminogen(mg/L)	91.9±20.7*	115.3±20.7	133.1±28.2	115.7±27.8
α1-ATRYP (mg/L)	2259.6±559.3*	1986.6±664.1	2238.5±651.0*	1818.8±414.2
α1-ACHYM (mg/L)	804.4±356.4**	677.1±381.9*	741.7±257.5**	472.6±102.7
α2-MACRO (mg/dL)	319.5±44.0**	255.1±95.6*	230.5±95.2*	171.7±30.4
CRP (mg/L)	2.5±3.1*	2.6±4.0*	1.3±1.0	0.4±0.2

[a]same as Table 1; α1-ATRYP: α1-antitrypsin; α1-ACHYM: α1-antichymotrypsin; α2-MACRO: α2-macroglobulin, CRP: C-reactive protein.

homeostasis of plasmin-mediated proteolysis in AL amyloid pts.

The low serum levels of plasminogen and high levels of plasmin inhibitors α1-antitrypsin and α2-macroglobulin raise the possibility of enhanced fibrinolytic activity in AL pts. Hyperfibrinolysis [1,6] with elevated levels of plasmin [6] has been observed in AL pts. The role of hyperfibrinolysis in AL pathogenesis remains to be explored. Our observations suggest that quantitative changes in these enzymes may contribute to (or result from) AL amyloidosis. Further studies to characterize these serine proteases and their inhibitors in AL pts may increase our understanding of amyloidogenesis.

The multiple immunoregulatory activities of IL6 include stimulation of acute phase protein synthesis and autocrine stimulation of human myeloma cell growth [7]. Increased IL6 levels were evident in AL and NPCD sera, with considerable variations in each pt group. Within the PCD group, IL6 levels in MM pts did not differ from non-MM PCD pts. Thus the level of this cytokine may not be a sensitive prognosticator as previously postulated [7]. Among AL pts, IL6 level did not correlate with concentration of any of the amyloid precursors or enzymes. Further investigation is needed in order to define the role of IL6 in AL amyloidosis.

References

1. Stone MJ (1990) 'Amyloidosis: A final common pathway for protein deposition in tissues', *Blood* **75**, 531-545.
2. Tong AW, Lee JC, and Stone MJ (1988) 'Expression of plasma cell-associated non-light chain antigens in patients with plasma cell dyscrasia and amyloidosis', *in*, T Isobe, S Araki, F Uchino, S Kito and E Tsubura (eds.), **Amyloid and Amyloidosis**, Plenum, New York, Pp 185-190.
3. Stone MJ and Frenkel EP (1975) 'The clinical spectrum of light chain myeloma' *Am J Med* **58**, 601-619.
4. Skogen B and Natvig JB (1981) 'Degradation of amyloid proteins by different serine proteases', *Scand J Immunol* **14**, 389-396.
5. Merlini G, Isobe T, Moy PW, et al (1988) 'Anti-casein antibodies in the serum of patients with AL amyloidosis', *in*, T Isobe, S Araki, F Uchino, S Kito and E Tsubura (eds), **Amyloid and Amyloidosis**, Plenum, New York, Pp 17-22.
6. Liebman H, Chinowsky M, Valdin J, et al (1983) 'Increased fibrinolysis and amyloidosis', *Arch Intern Med* **143**, 678-682.
7. Van Snick J (1990) 'Interleukin-6: An overview', *Ann Rev Immunol* 8, 253-278.

INCIDENCE AND EPIDEMIOLOGY OF PRIMARY SYSTEMIC AMYLOIDOSIS (AL) IN OLMSTED COUNTY, MINNESOTA: 1950 THROUGH 1989

Kyle RA*, Linos A**, Beard CM*, Linke R***, Gertz MA*, O'Fallon WM*, Kurland LT*. *Mayo Clinic, Rochester, Minnesota 55905 USA; **University of Athens, Athens, Greece; ***Institüt für Immunologie der Universität, München, West Germany

ABSTRACT. We are unaware of any reported studies of the incidence or prevalence of AL in the US or other countries. The absence of epidemiologic data is probably indicative of the rarity of AL and the diagnostic difficulties in distinguishing AL from secondary amyloidosis (AA), familial amyloidosis (AF), and senile systemic amyloidosis (AS_{C1}). It is difficult to assess the incidence rates over time for AL because of changing criteria of diagnosis, changes in clinical practice, variations in methods of diagnostic indexing of medical records, and differing autopsy rates. Olmsted County, Minnesota provides a rare opportunity to minimize these limitations because medical care for the population of Rochester, Minnesota and the surrounding Olmsted County has been provided primarily by the Mayo Clinic. Virtually all diagnoses made for a significant illness among Olmsted County residents have been compiled in a centralized records-linkage system. The relative stability of the local population, the unusual centralization of high-quality medical care, the high rate of autopsy, and the diagnostic indexing and records-linkage system used for many decades at Mayo Clinic provides an exceptional source for studies of incidence rates and long-term trends in this population.

1. MATERIALS AND METHODS

The records of all Olmsted County residents from January 1, 1950 until December 1, 1989 with a diagnosis of primary, secondary, senile, localized, and familial amyloidosis were obtained from the Mayo Clinic and its affiliated hospitals, the Olmsted Medical and Surgical Group, and the Olmsted Community Hospital. To insure that no cases of amyloidosis were overlooked through the above mentioned system of case ascertainment, we obtained all death certificates or autopsy reports for Olmsted County residents with a diagnosis of amyloidosis and reviewed their medical records. The residency criterion was applied so only those patients who had lived in Olmsted County for at least 1 year before the diagnosis of amyloidosis were considered to be bona fide residents. The diagnosis of AL required the demonstration of amyloid in biopsy or autopsy tissue on the basis of apple-green birefringence when stained with Congo red and viewed under polarized light. The unlabeled immunoperoxidase method was used with antisera against purified amyloid fibril proteins: κ, λ, protein A, prealbumin (transthyretin), β_2-microglobulin, and suitable controls to classify the type of amyloid.

2. RESULTS

Twenty patients fulfilled the criteria for the diagnosis of AL. The median age was 73.5 years with a range of 47 to 92 years. Twelve were male and eight were female. Immunohistochemical stains were performed in 14 cases. Eleven were λ (79%) and three were κ. Tissue was not available for immunohistochemical stains in the remaining six patients. Three of the 6 without tissue for immunostaining had a free monoclonal λ light chain in the urine, while the other 3 had a monoclonal serum protein.

Immunoelectrophoresis/immunofixation revealed a monoclonal (M-) protein in the serum of 15 of 16 patients. Two additional patients (one diagnosed in 1957 and one in 1965) had an M-spike in the serum protein electrophoretic pattern, but immunoelectrophoresis was not done. One had a normal electrophoretic pattern while the remaining patient (diagnosed in 1952) had no electrophoresis. The size of the M-protein was modest with only two >2.0 g/dL at diagnosis. Immunoelectrophoresis/immunofixation of the urine revealed a monoclonal light chain in 9 of 14 cases. Three others had a normal electrophoretic pattern but no urine studies were done in the remaining three patients. An M-protein was identified in the serum or urine in 15 of the 20 patients. All five without an M-protein had immunohistochemical confirmation of AL. Consequently, the diagnosis of AL is firm.

The clinical picture of the 20 Olmsted County patients was very similar to our experience on referral patients with AL. For example, congestive heart failure was present in 30%, nephrotic syndrome in 20%, macroglossia in 15%, and carpal tunnel syndrome in 10%. Rectal biopsy was positive in two-thirds of patients in whom it was performed while the bone marrow biopsy was positive for amyloid in 45%.

Seventeen (85%) of the patients have died. The median survival was 2.3 years (Kaplan-Meier). Cardiac causes (congestive heart failure or arrhythmia) accounted for 12 deaths while two others died of infection.

All but one patient were diagnosed antemortem. Approximately 15 other patients were felt initially to have AL but were proven to have senile systemic amyloidosis when immunohistochemical stains were done. They were excluded from this study.

The overall age and sex adjusted rate was 8.5/million (95% CI, 4.8 to 12.3). The overall sex and age adjusted rate was 6.1/million from 1950 to 1969 (95% CI, 1.2 to 11.1) and 9.9/million from 1970 to 1989 (95% CI, 4.7 to 15.1). The wide confidence interval indicates that the trend noted is consistent with no significant increase over time. We noted an increasing rate of AL in each successive decade of life. This was especially notable in older males.

3. DISCUSSION

Primary systemic amyloidosis (AL) is an uncommon disease that is characterized by the deposition of amyloid fibrils, mainly in the heart, kidney, gastrointestinal tract, peripheral and autonomic nerves, and blood vessels of virtually all organs. The amyloid fibrils consist of the variable portion of an immunoglobulin light chain or fragment thereof. The source of the light chains is a population of monoclonal plasma cells. The designation "AL" reflects the light-chain origin of this type of amyloidosis (Gertz and Kyle, 1989; Kyle and Gertz, 1990).

No other population-based studies on primary systemic amyloidosis (AL) have come to our attention. Primary amyloidosis was found in 6 (0.2%) of 3,414 autopsies conducted from 1937 to 1946 at the Royal Victoria Hospital in Belfast, Ireland and in 43 cases (0.4%) of 11,586 autopsies performed at the same institution from 1961 to 1970 (Thornton, 1983). There was no apparent reason for the increased recognition of primary amyloidosis in the more recent series. Van Rijswijk (personal communication, 1987) estimated the prevalence of primary and secondary amyloidosis at 1/60,000 population. One-third of the patients had primary amyloidosis which amounts to a prevalence of approximately 5/million.

The unique comprehensive medical data source available for the population of Olmsted County, Minnesota has been of great value in determining incidence trends and prevalence rates for a variety of diseases. Previous epidemiologic studies, even for uncommon diseases have produced important and useful epidemiologic data.

The diagnosis of systemic amyloidosis depends upon the demonstration of amyloid in the biopsy specimen of an involved organ. Furthermore, the type of systemic amyloidosis must be determined. The presence of an underlying disease of long duration such as rheumatoid arthritis, tuberculosis, or other inflammatory processes raises the question of AA. However, cases of well-documented AA have been reported in patients without an underlying inflammatory or reactive process (Pras, et al., 1980; Picken, et al., 1987). The diagnosis of AF is apparent when there is a positive family history. We have seen a number of patients in whom no family history or suggestion of hereditary disease was found. Furthermore, some families with AF may have a late onset of their disease. Senile amyloidosis may be confused with AL. We have seen patients with cardiac amyloidosis who were suspected to have AL, but endomyocardial biopsy revealed that the amyloid stained with antisera to transthyretin (Olson, et al., 1987). It is imperative that appropriate histochemical stains be performed on all amyloid tissue in order to confirm the diagnosis of AL. It is especially important to perform appropriate stains of amyloid tissue in patients suspected to have AL but in whom no monoclonal protein is found in the serum or urine.

The increase in rate with increasing age, especially in men as noted here, is indicative of a feature found in many other Olmsted County studies. The very elderly are more likely to be identified as having a specific disease responsible for their illness than in other facilities. Other tertiary centers are more likely to publish their collective experience, but the serious problem of selection or referral bias is unrecognized and therefore ignored. Such selection bias is almost universal in the nonpopulation-based referral centers.

The largest number of patients seen with AL at Mayo Clinic are in the seventh decade of life in contrast to the Olmsted County patients who are a decade older. This may be accounted for by the better surveillance and diagnosis provided for the elderly in Olmsted County and the lower referral practice for the very elderly. This coupled with a large tertiary care center with a major interest in AL may account for the increased incidence in the elderly.

The incidence of AL increased in the last two decades of study (1970 to 1989). However, this increase was not statistically significant. Some of this increase may be due to the more frequent use of immunofixation of serum and urine since 1980. The presence of an M-protein increases the suspicion of AL and is more likely to result in the biopsy of appropriate tissue and the diagnosis of amyloidosis.

In conclusion, this study demonstrates that AL is an uncommon disease with an incidence rate of approximately 8.5/million person years, is rare before age 40, occurs more in men than in women, and shows an increasing incidence rate with advancing age.

4. REFERENCES

Gertz, M.A., Kyle, R.A. (1989) Primary systemic amyloidosis--a diagnostic primer, Mayo Clin Proc, 64:1505.

Kyle, R.A., Gertz, M.A. (1990) Systemic amyloidosis, Crit Rev Oncol/Hematol, 10:49.

Thornton, C. (1983) Amyloid disease: an autopsy review of the decades 1937-46 and 1961-70, Ulster Med J, 52:31.

Pras, M., Zaretzky, J., Frangione, B., Franklin, E.C. (1980) AA protein in a case of "primary" or "idiopathic" amyloidosis, Am J Med, 68:291.

Picken, M.M., Pelton, K., Frangione, B., Gallo, G. (1987) Primary amyloidosis A. Immunohistochemical and biochemical characterization, Am J Pathol, 129:536.

Olson, L.J., Gertz, M.A., Edwards, W.D., et al. (1987) Senile cardiac amyloidosis with myocardial dysfunction. Diagnosis by endomyocardial biopsy and immunohistochemistry, N Engl J Med, 317:738.

LOW INCIDENCE OF AL AMYLOIDOSIS IN JAPAN

T. ISOBE AND T. FUJITA
The Third Division, Department of Medicine,
Kobe University Hospital, Kobe city, Japan

ABSTRACT. Total 179 patients (4.5%) with hematological malignancies were recorded out of 4,017 patients hospitalized in the past. Out of 179, 45 cases (25.1%) were recognized as symptomatic PCD. These 45 cases included 7 cases (15.6%) of AL amyloidosis, 31 (68.8%) of multiple myeloma, and 7 (15.6%) of macroglobulinemia in the present study. Only seven cases of AL amyloidosis were experienced for 16 years of observation. The low incidence of AL amyloidosis in the present study is discussed.

INTRODUCTION

The plasma cell dyscrasias (PCD) represent a group of conditions having as their common feature an abnormal neoplastic prolifeation of plasma cells. The term plasma cell is used to include all cells capable of synthesizing and releasing all classes of immunoglobulins and their subunits. In addition to multiple myeloma which is the most common prototype disease, primary macroglobulinemia, the heavy chain diseases and AL amyloidosis are grouped to be symptomatic (or malignant) PCD. (Osserman (1978)). Since it is known that there has been a low incidence of B cell malignancy including PCD, CLL and hairly cell leukemia in Japan (Blatter (1980)), and the incidence of AL amyloidosis is seldom reported, an attempt to figure out the frequency of AL among PCD in our institution is carried out.

Patients and methods

Myeloma was diagnosed by confirming the presence of plasma cells of more than 10 percent out of nucleated cells in aspirated bone marrow and by identifying a monoclonal immunoglobulin except IgM type in the serum and/or in the urine. The possible association of amyloidosis in myeloma patients was excluded by careful observations during hospitalization and chemotherapy, with daily bed-side examinations along with repeated laboratory tests including ECG, cardiac echograms, bone and bone marrow scintigrams and biopsies either of the stomack or the rectum. Primary macroglobulinemia was on the basis of the presence of a monoclonal IgM in the serum with prolifearions of IgM-producing cells in the marrow or lymphoreticular systems. Diagnosis of amyloidosis was made on the basis of pathohistological identification of Congo-red-stain-positive and green-yellow-birefringent materials at the biopsied specimens from patients (Glenner (1980)). Cases examined in the present study only included patients who were hospitalized at the Third Division, Department of Medicine, Kobe University Hospital from Jan.1, 1974 to Dec.31, 1989.

RESULTS

Total 179 patients (4.5%) associated with hematological malignancies (leukemia-lymphoma-plasma cell dyscrasia) were recorded out of 4,017 patients hospitalized for check-up and treatment. Out of 179 patients 45 cases (25.1%) were recognized as symptomatic PCD. These 45 cases included 7 cases (15.6%) of AL amyloidosis, 31 cases (68.8%) of multiple myeloma with an average of 59.3 (35 to 77 yo) and 7 cases of macroglobulinemia (15.6%) with an average of 67.1 (47 to 77 yo) in the present study (TABLES 1 and 2).

AL amyloidosis included both primary amyloidosis and myeloma-associated amyloidosis. When clinically analyzed, there were 4 cases of primary type AL and 4 cases with myeloma-associated type AL. In fact, one patient of 56 years old male with an monoclonal kappa chains in the urine was found to have an overlapped clinical manifestations, because of his unusual features initially starting as primary type amyloidosis for about 5 years and later developing into osteolytic multiple myeloma. Conversely, as shown in TABLE 3, 2 cases had interesting clinical features starting as straight myeloma and later having signs of systemic amyloidosis. (Details of these 2 cases are also presented in this proceedings, separately. Entitled as CLINICAL INDICATIONS OF SYSTEMIC AMYLOIDOSIS IN MYELOMA PATIENTS).

Myeloma-associated amyloidosis was recorded as 11.4% out of initially diagnosed as straight myeloma. AL amyloidosis was calculated as 15.6% among Symptomatic PCD, as shown in TABLE 4.

DISCUSSION

Myeloma represents a relatively common hematologic malignancy and its incidence rises with age, from approximately 7 per 100,000 at age 50 to over 20 per 100,000 at age. A high incidence of myeloma has been noted in USA, ranging from 514-6.1 males and 4.8-5.3 females per 100,000 residents. However, in Hawaii, Japanese imigrants showed a relatively low incidence 1.1 per 100,000, whereas among Americans living in Hawaii, the incidence was 3.5 per 100,000. Among Japanese living in Japan, the incidence of myeloma is 0.6-0.7 males and 0.4-0.8 females per 100,000 (Blatter (1980)). As to the incidence of residents in Hawaii who in fact included 2 groups, one moved from North-America and the other from Japan. Interestingly, the incidence of myeloma among these 2 groups appeared to reduce among Americans and to rise among Japanese-immigrants, suggestive of the role of circumstantial factors. Thus these low incidence of myeloma among Japanese may possibly be related to circumstantial-dietary differences in the background (Isobe (1987)). As to AL amyloidosis, it is also a disease

TABLE 1. Frequency of AL amyloidosis (1) (1974-1989)

	No. of cases		
AL amyloidosis	7 (0.2%)	(3.9%)	(15.6%)
Symptomatic PCD	45 (1.1%)	(25.1%)	(100%)
Hematological malignancies	179 (4.5%)	(100%)	-
Total hospitalized patients	4,017 (100%)	-	-

TABLE 2. Frequency of Plasma Cell Dyscrasia (1974-1989)

Symptomatic PCD	Out of 45 cases No. of cases	M:F	Average age
Myeloma, plasmacytoma	31	(15:16)	59.3 (35-77)
Myeloma-associated amyloidosis	4*	(1: 3)	58.5 (49-74)
Primary amyloidosis	4*	(4: 0)	58.2 (42-67)
Macroglobulinemia	7	(3: 4)	67.1 (47-77)

*One case overlapped

TABLE 3. AL Amyloidosis 7 cases (1974-1989)

Myeloma-associated Amyloidosis			S-MP BJP
Case 1	Bullous amyloid and GI-tract	74F(Doi)	λ - 0
Case 2	Myeloma into systemic amyloid	55F(Kor)	0 - λ
Case 3	Myeloma into systemic amyloid	50F(Fuk)	Gλ - 0
Primary Amyloidosis			
Case 4	Amyloidosis into myeloma*	56M(Ich)	0 - κ
Case 5	Heart, Skin, GI tract	42M(Ter)	Dλ - λ
Case 6	Heart, Skin, TI tract	67M(Mat)	0 - κ
Case 7	GI tract	64M(Miy)	Aλ - λ

TABLE 4. Frequency of AL amyloidosis (2) (1974-1989)

	Cases	per cent
Myeloma-associated amyloidosis out of straight myeloma	4 out of 35 cases	11.4%
AL amyloidosis out of symptomatic PCD	7 out of 45 cases	15.6%

of middle and advanced age. The mean ages at diagnosis were 55 years and 62 years in two studies (Arapakis and Tribe (1963), Pruzanski and Katz (1976)). It affects men more often than women and whites more often than non-whites.

There have been no published studies of the incidence of AL, except one report. Twenty patients with the diagnosis of AL were collected from records of all Olmsted country residents, Minesota from Jan. 1, 1950 until Dec. 31, 1989. The overall sex and age adjusted rate was 8.5 out of 1,000,000. Comparison of the overall rates between 1950-1969 and 1970-1989 showed no statistical difference, suggesting no significant increase over time (Kyle et al. (1990)).

As to the incidences of AL amyloidosis in different countries have also not been reported in the past. An attempt to define the incidence of

AL amyloidosis has been difficult to investigate, since the diagnosis of amyloidosis as well as the exclusion of possibility of amyloidosis have to be done by organ-biopsies in each patient. It is also required the precise detections of onset (occurance) of AL amyloidosis among patients with plasma cell dyscrasia through repeated clinical and laboratory observations during the period of follow-up study. It is therefore assumed that the study of incidence of AL amyloidosis has to be conducted in one single institution for a long period of time by well-trained physicians.

Compared with the present data in TABLES 1 and 4, high frequency of AL amyloidosis has been reported from Mayo Clinic in USA in which total 229 patients with AL amyloidosis were recorded for 11 years with a range from Jan.1, 1970 to Dec.31, 1980 (Kyle and Greipp (1983)). In Japan, the incidence of AL amyloidosis as well as the incidence of myeloma seemed to be very low compared with those of western countries, probably related to circumstancial-dietary differences. In fact, Japan islands had been politically and geographically isolated for over 2.5 centries (1600-1886). Therefore, customs and diets were very much different from western. After the second world war in 1945, things have been changed markedly along with the changes in increased incidences of lung, rectal, pancreas and mammary cancers in Japan in contrast with lowered incidences of stomach and uterine cancers. These changes also could be ascribed to circumstantial factors.

Although the number of patients in this paper is fairly low compared to these reported in western countries probably due to low incidence of PCD, the results will be helpful to consider the mechanism of pathogenesis of AL amyloidosis.

REFERENCES

1. Osserman EF. (1978) 'Multiple myeloma and related plasma cell dyscrasias', in M. Samter (ed), Immunological Diseases, Little Brown and Co., New York, pp.499-529.
2. Blatter WA. (1980) 'Progress in myeloma', Elsevier, North-Holland, pp.1-65.
3. Glenner GG. (1980) 'Amyloid depostis and amyloidosis. The β-Fibrilloses', N Engl J Med 302, 1283-1292.
4. Isobe T. (1989) 'Chemotherapy for myeloma in Japanese patients', in K. Kimura (ed), Cancer Chemotherpay: Challenges for the Future, Excerpta Medica, Tokyo, pp.243-249.
5. Arapakis G and Tribe CR. (1963) 'Amyloidosis in rheumatoid arthritis investigated by means of rectal biopsy', Ann Rheum Dis 22, 256-262.
6. Pruzanski W. and Katz A. (1976) 'Clinical and laboratory findings in primary generalized and multiple-myeloma related amyloidosis', Can Med Assoc J 114, 906-909.
7. Kyle R., Lines A., Beard CM., Linke R., Gertz MA., and O'Fallon WM. (1990) 'Incidence and epidemiology of primary systemic amyloidosis (AL) in Olmsted country, Minesota: 1950 to 1989', in J.B. Natvig et al (eds.) Amyloidosis (in press).
8. Kyle, RA. and Greipp, PR. (1983) 'Amyloidosis (AL) Clinical and laboratory features in 229 cases', Mayo Clin Proc 58, 665-683.

CLINICAL INDICATIONS OF SYSTEMIC AMYLOIDOSIS IN MYELOMA PATIENTS

T. ISOBE, S. MATOZAKI, T. FUJITA AND T. SHINODA
The Third Division, Department of Medicine
Kobe University Hospital, Kusunoki-cho, Kobe, JAPAN
Tokyo Metropolitan University, Tokyo, JAPAN

ABSTRACT. Among 30 patients of myeloma, 2 cases were recognized to develop manifestations suggestive of amyloidosis during the clinical courses. Both Japanese females, with an age of 50- and 55-year-old, respectively, had been instituted on myeloma chemotherapy of continuous low-dose melphalan-prednisolone administration. Marked changes in the clinical features were noted around 6 to 10 months prior to their deaths. Subjectively, they started to have complaints of lassitude and palpitation. Objective findings included weight loss, decreased both blood pressure and pulse pressure, obvious appearance of macroglossia, cardiac arrythmia and abnormal cardiac echograms.

INTRODUCTION

Myeloma, myeloma-associated amyloidosis, and primary amyloidosis are recognized to be closely related each other on the basis of plasma cell proliferations (Isobe and Osserman (1974)). It is now known that B cell malignancies were seen less frequently in the Orient compared with Western countries (Isobe (1989)). In this regards, it is interesting to know the incidence of systemic amyloidosis which occurs during clinical courses of myeloma in Japanese patients. In the present study, 2 patients were observed in their clinical courses from straight myeloma with a progression to myeloma-associated amyloidosis.

Case presentation

Case 1. K. Kor, 55-year-old Japanese female, visited the orthopedic clinic because of pain in the right hip joint on walking. She was hospitalized with the histological diagnosis of plasmacytoma by an iliac-bone biopsy. Her body weight was 65 Kg. There was no evidence of macroglossia, cardiomegaly or hepatomegaly. Laboratory data included a red blood cell count of $456 x10^4/mm^3$ with hemoglobin 13.6 g/dl, platelet $32.3x10^4/mm^3$, white cell count of $8,800/mm^3$, blood urea nitrogens 13 mg/dl, uric acid 5.9 mg/dl, serum creatinine 0.8 mg/dl, serum calcium 9.3 mg/dl, and an ESR 77 mm/hour. A serum total protein was 6.7 g/dl, including 3.6 g/dl of albumin and γ-globulin 1.1 g/dl with no detectable monoclonal spike. Serum immunoglobulin levels revealed IgG 1,740 mg/dl, IgA 590 mg/dl and IgM 92 mg/dl.

Urinary protein excretion was 1.0 mg a day. An electrophoresis disclosed a monoclonal spike in the urine, which was immunologically identified as BJP of lambda type. X-ray survey showed multiple punched-out lesions in the skull, the right pelvis and the femur, together with a compression fracture of the 1st and 3rd lumbar spines. Bone scintigraphy showed an abnormal accumulation of 99 m Technectium at the lumbar spines, right pelvis and bilateral ribs. With a clinical diagnosis of myeloma, a combination chemotherapy consisting of oral administration of melphalan 2 mg a day and prednisolone 10 mg a day was instituted. There was a response of chemotherapy with decreased amount of daily BJP in the urine. Recovering from her difficulty of walking, the performans status was improved.

In the clinical course with chemotherapy, however, she noted to have complaints of lassitude and palpitation, approximately 6 months prior to her death. Objective findings are shown in Table 1. Her condition deteriorated with cardiac failure. She died about 8 months after the appearance of signs of amyloidosis and about 16 months after the diagnosis of myeloma. Autopsy findings were systemic amyloidosis associated with myeloma. Punched out lesions were found in the sternum and vertebral bodies of Th12 to L3 spines. There were diffuse infiltrations of lambda chain positive plasmacytes. Amyloid deposits were mainly around vessel wall and in the parenchyma in various organs, especially in the tongue and in the heart, where the conductive system was also involved.

Amyloids were also found markedly in kidneys, adrenals and apleen, and moderately in liver, pancreas, lung, thyroid, parathyroid, GI tracts ovaries and several lymph nodes.

Case 2. F.Fuk, 50-year-old Japanese female visited the hospital because of low back pain and difficulty of walk. She was found to have a serum total protein of 10.4 g/dl with an elevated serum γ-globulin of 6.2 g/dl which was immunologically identified as monoclonal IgG (κ). A bone marrow aspiration revealed 67.4% of plasma cells out of nucleated cell counts of $97.5 \times 10^4/mm^3$. There was no evidence of macroglossia, carpal tunnel syndrome, cardiomegaly or hepatomegaly. Clinical diagnosis of multiple myeloma was made. Laboratory data included a red blood cell count of $331 \times 10^4/mm^3$ with a hemoglobin level of 11.9 g/dl, platelet $14.1 \times 10^4/mm^3$, white cell count of 7300 with a normal differential, blood urea nitrogen 13 mg/dl, uric acid 6.9 mg/dl, serum creatinine 1.3 mg/dl, serum calcium 9.5 mg/dl, and an ESR 169 mm/hour. A serum total protein was 11.5 g/dl including 4.9 g/dl of albumin and 6.3 g/dl of γ-globulin fraction, with a monoclonal spike. Serum immunoglobulin measurements revealed IgG 5,210 mg/dl, IgA 31 mg/dl and IgM 24 mg/dl Bence Jones protein in the urine was negative. A X-ray tomography showed lowered density of the bilateral iliac bones. Furthermore, a computed tomography revealed a mass lesion of approximate 10x10x6 cm in size in association with osteolysis with location from the 5th lumbar spine to sacral bone. With a clinical diagnosis of myeloma a combination chemotherapy consisting of oral administration of melphalan 2 mg a day and prednisolone 10 mg a day was instituted. In the clinical course, however, she noted to have complaints of

TABLE 1 Clinical features and their changes

Kor 55F		1981 Sep. Myeloma				1982 Sep. Amyloidosis
Serum						
TP	(g/dl)	6.7		→		4.9
Alb	(g/dl)	3.5		→		2.2
γ-gl	(g/dl)	1.1		→		1.0
Urine						
Protein	(g/day)	0∿0.8				0.5∿1.0
Alb	(%)	39.2				77.8
BJP	(%)	41.2				8.6
Marrow						
NCC		$17.9x10^4$				$21.1x10^4$
Plasma cells (%)		2.4		→		5.6
Bone X-P		Osteolytic		·		Osteolytic
ECG		Normal		→		Junctional rythm
				→		Sick sinus syndrome
Cardiac echogram						
Septal	(mm)	?		→		16
Post. wall	(mm)	?		→		21
BP	(mmHg)	134/96	→	94/78	→	66/52
Tongue		Normal				Macroglossia
Body weight	(Kg)	65		→		48

Fuk 55F		1984 Aug. Myeloma				1987 Dec. Amyloidosis
Serum MP		(+)				(+)
Tp	(g/dl)	13.2	→	9.4	→	7.1
Alb	(g/dl)	4.0	→	3.8	→	3.7
M-P	(g/dl)	8.2	→	4.4	→	2.4
Urine						
Protein		(-)				(-)
BJP		(-)				(-)
Marrow						
NCC		$10.6x10^4$		$12.4x10^4$		$7.1x10^4$
Plasmacells (%)		35.0	→	16.6	→	6.8
Bone X-P		Osteolytic				Osteolytic
ECG		Normal				Low voltage Arrythmia
Cardiac echogram						
Septal	(mm)	?		9	→	15
Post. wall	(mm)	?		9	→	17
BP	(mmHg)	136/84	→	96/70	→	66/52
Tongue		Normal				Macroglossia
Body weight	(Kg)	43	→	55	→	40

lassitude and palpitation, approximately 10 months prior to her death. There was a variety of changes in clinical features similar to those of the 1st case as shown in Table 1. A rectal biopsy revealed amyloid deposits. Her condition deteriorated with cardiac failure. She died about 8 months after the appearance of signs and symptoms of amyloidosis, and about 40 months after the diagnosis of myeloma.

DISCUSSION

AL amyloidosis is a disease of middle and advanced age. It affects men more often than women and whites more often than non-whites. Virtually all patients with AL amyloidosis have evidence of a serum or urinary monoclonal immunoglobulin with a BJP or of a BJP alone, and an excessive numbers of bone marrow plasma cells (Isobe and Osserman (1974), Kyle and Bayrd (1975)). Patients with primary and myeloma-related systemic amyloidosis have a poor prognosis when compared with age-sex-matched controls. Median survival in patients presenting with congestive heart failure was 6 months, and 9 months in those who presented with orthostatic hypotension (Scott (1986)). Poor prognosis are also observed in the present report. Although we speculate on the ability of certain BJPs to make the β-pleated sheet conformation, we cannot predict the amyloidogenicity of a specific BJP. BJP of the first case in the present report were extensively studied. It was grouped into amyloidogenic subsubgroup of $V_\lambda 1$-2 on the basis of amino acid sequence homology. It was also confirmed that this BJP showed in vitro insolubility (Isobe et al (1986)). It is emphasized that early stages of systemic amyloidosis are to be noted by clinicians during the course of myeloma patients, since the early phases of amyloidosis will give us some clues to find out the pathogenesis of systemic amyloidosis (Cohen and Connars (1987)), and hopefully to explore the way of treatment of amyloidosis patients.

REFERENCES

1. Isobe, T. and Osserman, EF. (1974) Patterns of amyloidosis and their association with plasma cell dyscrasia, monoclonal immunoglobulins and Bence Jones proteins. N Engl J Med 290, 473-477.
2. Isobe, T. (1989) AL amyloidosis: A metabolic disease. Haematologica 74, 425-429.
3. Kyle RA, Bayrd ED: Amyloidosis: review of 236 cases. Medicine (Baltimore) 54: 271-299, 1975.
4. Scott PP, Scott WW, Siegelman SS (1986), Amyloidosis: an overview: Seminars in Roentgenol 21, 103-112.
5. Isobe, T, Tonoike H, Kametani F, Shinoda T. (1986) Amyloidogenicity and subgroups of human lambda Bence Jones proteins. In Amyloidosis ed by Glenner GG et al New York, Plenum pp. 477-481.
6. Cohen, A. and Connors, LH. (1987) The pathogenesis and biochemistry of amyloidosis. J Pathol 151, 1-10.

BENCE JONES PROTEINEMIA WITHOUT BENCE JONES PROTEINURIA IN AL AMYLOIDOSIS

T. ISOBE AND G. MERLINI
Department of Medicine, Kobe University Hospital,
Kusunokicho, Kobe, Japan and Department of Medicine,
Pavia University Hospital, Pavia, Italy

ABSTRACT. On the background of systemic amyloidosis with multiple myeloma, unusual manifestations were found in 2 cases, i.e. in a 74 yo female with bullous cutaneous amyloidosis and in a 69 yo female with cutaneous nevus comedonicus and amyloidosis, respectively. In both cases, there were immunochemically unique findings of monoclonal immunoglobulin light chain in the serum, but not in the urine (Bence Jones proteinemia without Bence Jones proteinuria), along with proliferations of plasma cells in the bone marrows of both cases.

INTRODUCTION

Amyloidosis is characterized by a large variety of clinical manifestations, including skin lesions of petechiae, purpura, papules, lichen, nodules, tumors, plaques, scleroderma, poikiloderma, alopecia and xanthomas. Other than these cutaneous changes, unusual types of cutaneous amyloid are reported in 2 cases with myeloma-associated amyloidosis in the present study. A combination of cutaneous amyloid and rare type of plasma cell dyscrasia are discussed.

Case presentation

Case 1. S. Doi. 74 year old Japanese female visited the hospital because of bullous dermal eruptions of milliary to bean size on the chest and abdominal walls, which increased in number for the previous two years. Yellowish eruptions without pain or itching were demonstrated as massive amyloid deposits below dermal papillae and in the dermis by a skin biopsy. A subsequent rectal biopsy realed amyloid in the muscle layer of the rectum, suggesting that the patient had systemic amyloidosis. She was found to have macroglossia. A X-ray survey disclosed the vertebral fractures in the 10th and 12th thoracic spines and osteolytic lesions in the skull, corresponding to abnormal shadows in a bone schintigram. Repeated bone marrow aspirates showed proliferations of plasma cells 21.8% out of an nucleated cell count of $22.3 \times 10^4/mm^3$. A serum total protein was 6.1 g/dl with no prominent spikes in the serum electrophoresis. Immunodiffusion analysis showed low immunoglobulin levels of IgG 410 mg/dl, IgA and IgM 25 mg/dl. Urinary protein was negative by sulfosalicylic acid precipitation method. An immunoelectrophoresis disclosed an abnormal precipitation line in the serum reacted only with antikappa at the alfa2 electrophoretic mobility, whereas there were very faint lines in the 200-times concentrated urine reacted with anti kappa as well as anti lambda at the beta mobility. These findings suggested the presence of monoclonal kappa-chains in the serum, but not in the urine. A peroxidase antibody technique on the paraffinized bone-marrow sections demonstrated positive staining of plasma cells with anti-kappa antiserum, but not with other antisera. A blood urea nitrogen was 21 mg/dl and a serum creatinine level was 1.1 mg/dl. There was no other significant abnormality of laboratory examinations in this patient.

Case 2. R. Ros. 69 year old Cuban woman developed difficulty in keeping her eyes open due to excessive skin around them. She underwent an upper blephoroplasty and excision of milia of the lower eyelids. Pathological specimen revealed amyloidosis. It was noted that the patient had proteinuria, hepatosplenomegaly and pitting edema. The total serum protein was 4.8 g/dl, with decreased albumin and decreased gammaglobulin as shown in Figure 1. In addition, there was Bence

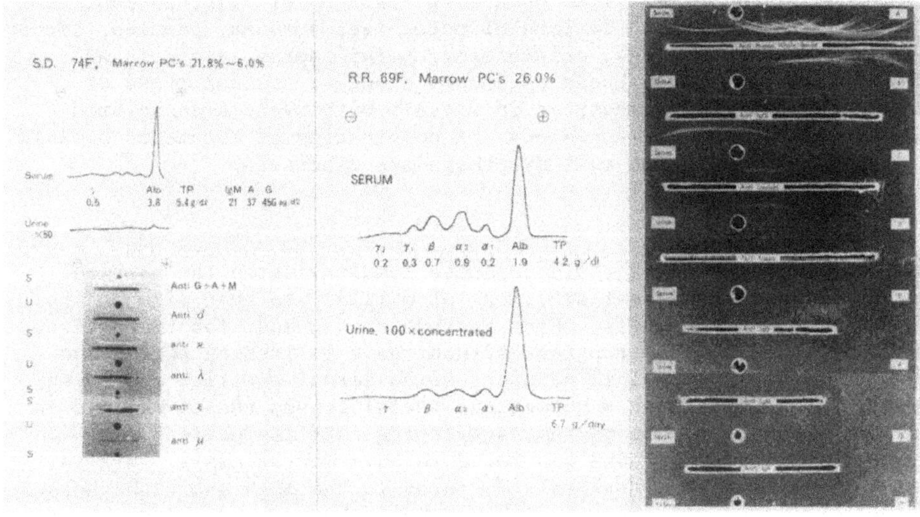

Figure 1. Cellulose acetate electrophoresis of the serum and concentrated urine and agarose immunoelectrophoresis.
Case 1 (left) and Case 2 (center and right)

TABLE 1. BJP emia without BJP uria

	Case 1	Case 2
	S. Doi	R. Ros
Age	74 yo	69 yo
Sex	female	female
Race	Japanese	Cuban
Cutaneous	Bullous eruption	Nevus comedonicus
Amyloid	dermal +	dermal +
	rectal +	rectal +
		perivascular +
	(alive)	(autopsied)
Serum protein g/dl	5.4	4.2
Albumin g/dl	3.8	1.9
γ-globulin g/dl	0.5	0.2
Plasma cells in marrow	21.8%	26.0%
Osteolytic lesion	+	+
Serum	BJPκ	BJPλ
Urine BJP	-	-
Incidence out of		
Amyloid with BJP only	1/55 (1.8%)	1/46 (2.2%)
Amyloid with AL type	1/130(0.8%)	1/88 (1.1%)
Duration of Investigation	1974-1989 (Kobe Univ. Hosp.)	1960-1974 (Columbia Presbyterian Hosp.)

Jones proteinemia without any monoclonal spike in the serum. Repeated urinalysis showed moderate albuminuria without any demonstration of Bence Jones proteins in the urine. Blood urea nitrogen was 19 mg/dl. A bone marrow revealed 26% plasma cells with immature plasmablasts. A chest X-ray revealed enlargement of the heart. A rectal biopsy confirmed the diagnosis of systemic amyloidosis. During the clinical course, she experienced bilateral pleural effusion. She died after approximately 2 years of clinical suffering. At autopsy, widespread systemic amyloid deposition was found predominantly in blood vessel walls. The renal glomeruli were severely affected accounting for the nephrotic syndrome. There was one lytic lesion seen in the lumbar vertebra. A large number of plasma cells were present in the bone marrow. A major pathological diagnosis was systemis amyloidosis associated with multiple myeloma, in a particular association of nevus comedonicus as cutaneous amyloidosis.

In short summary as shown in Table 1, both females, over the age of 65, were found to have osteolytic myeloma with plasma cell proliferations in the bone marrows. In the serum there were low levels of total proteins, decreased albumins, decreased gammaglobulins, and Bence Jones proteins in the serum, but not in the urine in both cases. Unusual manifestations of skin involvement prompted the biopsies to make pathological diagnosis of cutaneous amyloid. Rectal biopsies confirmed systemic amyloidosis. The incidences of BJPemia without BJPuria in two series were recorded as one single case out of 55 AL cases with BJP only (1.8%) and 1 of total 130 AL cases (0.8%) in Kobe series, whereas 1 case out of 46 AL cases with BJP only (2.2%) and 1 of total 88 AL cases (1.1%) in New York series, respectively.

DISCUSSION

The nature of amyloidosis has been extensively explored in the past. (Isobe (1989)). As to skin amyloidosis, it has been reported that involvement of the skin with amyloid deposits can be classified into either an expression of systemic amyloidosis or primary localized skin amyloidosis (Franklin (1976), Isobe et al. (1983)). Primary systemic amyloidosis and myeloma-associated amyloidosis cause clinically detectable cutaneous changes in approximately 10 to 40% of patients (Rubinow and Cohen (1978)). Although purpura, papules, macular and licken are common manifestations among skin amyloidosis, bullae or nevus are rarely found (Beacham et al. (6)) among AL amyloidosis.
It is noted that the incidence of AL cases associated with BJP only (BJPuria without M-proteinemia) was higher than that of straight myeloma-macroglobulinemia group (Isobe and Osserman (1974)). The incidence of BJPemia without BJPuria is very low ranging 0.8 to 1.1% out of AL amyloidosis in 2 series of the present study. It is interesting to note that 2 patients described herein were found to have quite unusual manifestations of cutaneous amyloidosis. In this regards, further clinical study is needed to clarify the relationship between skin deposit of amyloid and "BJPemia without BJPuria".

REFERENCE

1. Isobe, T. (1989) AL amyloidosis: A metabolic disease, Haematologica 74, 425-429.
2. Franklin, EC. (1976) Amyloid and amyloidosis of the skin, J Invest Dermatol 67, 451-456.
3. Isobe, T. Ohashi, M, Masako, K, and Fujita, T. (1983) The significance of urine examination for Bence Jones protein in combination with ultrastructural study in skin amyloidosis, in C.R. Tribe and P.A. Bacon (eds.) Amyloidosis E.A.R.S., John wright & Sons, Bristol, pp.101-103.
4. Robinow, A. and Cohen, A. (1978) Skin involvement in generalized amyloidosis: A study of clinically involved and uninvolved skin in 50 patients with primary and secondary amyloidosis. Ann Intern Med 83, 781-785.
5. Beacham, BE. Greer, KE, Andrews, BS and Cooper, PH (1980) Bullous amyloidosis, An Acad Dermatol 3, 506-510.
6. Isobe, T. and Osserman, EF. (1974) Patterns of Amyloidosis and their assocation with plasma-cell dyscrasia, monoclonal immunoglobulins and Bence-Jones proteins. N Engl J Med 290, 473-477.

SYSTEMIC AMYLOIDOSIS AND MONOCLONAL GAMMOPATHY IN THREE ITALIAN SIBLINGS : A FAMILIAN CASE OF AL-AMYLOIDOSIS?

A.MILIANI[*], F.BERGESIO[a],M.SALVADORI[a],A.M.CICIANI[a],G.P.MERLINI[b], R.DI GUGLIELMO[*],A.MENICUCCI[c],F.TORRICELLI[d],S. DI LOLLO[e],A.AMANTINI[f],M.MANCUCCI[f],A.SODI[g],S.ZUCCARINI[g],T.CAPOBIANCO[d].
Nephrology[a] and Neurophysiopathology[f] Depts,Careggi Hospital and Medical Clinic IV,Ophtalmology[g],Tissue Typing[c],Genetic[d] and Pathology[e] Institutes,University of Florence,Viale Pieraccini 18,50100 Florence; Medical Clinic II[b],University of Pavia,Italy.

ABSTRACT Three italian siblings, two brothers and one sister, two of whom affected from MGUS and one from Waldenström Macroglobulinemia (WM), were found to have sytemic amyloidosis. Two patients showed the same HLA typing and the same light chain (k), but differed in presenting clinical symptoms. Caryotype studies however did not show any peculiar abnormalities shared by the three brothers. Family history and clinical investigations did not account for a typical heredofamilial form, either for reactive or senile amyloidosis. Since evidence of familial occurrance has already been demonstrated for immunoglobulin-related (AL) amyloidosis, we suggest that our three patients may represent a new case of familial AL-Amyloidosis. Routine investigations for amyloidosis in patients with familial MGUS will better define in future the prevalence of such familial form and, eventually, the underlying genetic mechanisms.

Introduction

Familial occurrance of systemic amyloidosis is usually restricted to a heterogeneous group of clinical syndromes also described under the term of heredofamilial amyloidosis (1).

In such a group, apart from familial mediterranean fever (FMF), in which amyloid fibrils are derived from serum amyloid A (SAA), the origin of fibril proteins derives either from genetic variants of plasma prealbumin or it is unknown (1). These syndromes are better known with the name of the organs predominantly affected as "neuropathic", "nephropathic" or "cardiac forms". Until to-date, immunoglobulin-related amyloidosis (AL-A) is still considered as a sporadic disease process.

The only report of familial case of AL-A was published in 1986 and referred to three separate families, each one having two members affected (2).

In this study we discuss the possibility of a new familial case of AL-A occurred in three italian siblings, two of whom affected by MGUS without evidence of multiple myeloma (MM) and one by WM.

Materials and Methods

All three patients underwent the following tests and clinical investigations:

Creatinine clearance, 24 hours urinary protein excretion, serum and urine immunofixation electrophoresis (SIE and UIE), bone marrow aspirate, bone X-ray, abdominal and cardiac ecotomography. A full eye examination (visual acuity, visual field, fundus examination, ocular motility, tonometry, pupillary reflexes, lacrimation tests with corneal staining with fluorescein and evoked potential) was performed together with a detailed electroneurographic study on peripheral motor and sensory nerves (ulnar, posterior tibial and peroneal for motor nerves; ulnar, median and sural for sensory nerves).

In every case the diagnosis of amyloidosis was established histologically on different tissue spicimens on the basis of typical green birefringence after Congo red staining and examination in a polarizing microscope.

Finally, caryotype on peripheral lymphocytes and HLA typing (the latter in 5 members of the family) were carried out.

Reports of cases

Case 1 (T.O.)

A 60 year-old man was first admitted to the hospital because of dyspnea. Physical examination showed bilateral pleural effusion with diffuse adenopathy and hepatosplenomegaly. A MGUS (IgG k) had been diagnosed 3 years before. IgM k monoclonal protein (3.03 g/dl) was detected by SIE, while k light chain (0.4 g/24hours) was found by UIE.

Bone marrow byopsy was typical for WM. Abdominal fat tissue (AFT), pleura and a laterocervical limph node were all found positive for amyloidosis. Altough the patient was asymptomatic, electroneurographic study revealed a bilateral sensorimotor polineuropathy, predominantly axonal, both in the upper and lower limbs. Eye examination was normal and no renal involvement was present.

After 18 months of follow-up a partial remission was obtained by different sequential therapeutic schedules (BACOP, VP 16 + Prednisone

(P), P + Chlorambucil (C)+ P, C + P + DMSO). Serum IgM decreased (1,8 g/dl) and at the time being only a slight organomegaly and right pleural effusion are still present. Bone marrow aspirate is normal and general conditions are relatively good.

Recently,a caryotype examination showed 16% of metaphases with structural rearrangements.

Case 2 (T.A.)

A 74 year -old woman with nephrotic syndrome, sicca syndrome peripheral polineuropathy and orthostatic hypotension was first admitted to the hospital. SIE showed a very slight monoclonal component IgG κ, while UIE revealed 0,3 g/24 hours of BJ excretion. Bone marrow aspirate contained only 2% plasma cells. Neither osteolytic lesions, nor renal failure were present. Amyloid infiltration could be demonstrated in AFT, bone marrow and buccal mucosa. It is noteworthy that a serum IgG k protein had already been observed 10 years before by chance.

Holter registration was normal and so it was cardiac ecotomography. Urinary protein excretion ranged between 4-6 g/24 hours. 4% of metaphases of caryotype showed X deletion.

Treatment with P + Melphalan for 12 months induced disappearance of BJ excretion and reduction of sicca syndrome and neurological symptoms, whereas nephrotic syndrome did not modify much and renal failure occurred.

Case 3 (T.T.)

A 70 year-old man had been showing for 13 years a MGUS IgG λ. Since he was the third in the family history presenting with MGUS and the others were already diagnosed to have systemic amyloidosis, a FTA was performed altough he was apparently asymptomatic.

Diagnosis of amyloidosis was then made. At that time the serum monoclonal component was the same (1,4 g/dl) and BJ excretion was still absent. Routine laboratory tests were within normal range and bone marrow aspirate showed 2% plasma cells. Osteolytic lesions and renal involvement were not evident. Cardiac ecotomography was normal.

Unexpectedly both keratoconjunctivitis sicca and a slight sensorimotor polineuropathy could be shown during clinical investigations. Caryotype was normal while HLA typing showed he was different from the others who shared hydentical HLA typing. The patient has never received any treatment until now.

Discussion

All three brothers shared a common pattern of diffuse polineuropathy, associated in two of them with keratoconjunctivitis sicca and in one also with nephrotic syndrome. Altough renal involvement, sicca syndrome and peripheral neuropathy have all been reported in certain forms of heredofamilial amyloidosis (FAP type I and III), the quite different clinical picture presented by our patients badly account for the same autosomal dominant trait found in these forms (1,3).

Moreover none of the symptoms commonly encountered in heredofamilial amyloidosis were apparent in their kinship. On the other hand none of them suffered from chronic diseases which might account for reactive systemic amyloidosis, or from cardiac involvement which make one think of senile systemic amyloidosis (SSA).

On the contrary,the occurrence of familial cases of AL-A ought not to surprise, since it was well documented in other diseases related to plasma cells dyscrasias (MGUS,MM and WM)(4-). Indeed AL-A was already reported in three family pairs few years ago (2). The hypothesis of a random occurrence of AL-A in all our siblings affected by MGUS seems actually very remote. At present,caryotype and tissue typing did not give a conclusive contribute. In conclusion, altough results of immunohistochemical studies on prealbumin are not yet available, the whole clinical data very likely point to a familial form of AL-A. Besides that, no cases of patients with a heredofamilial form associated with MGUS have yet been reported (5). To evaluate the actual prevalence of familial AL-A, it is desirable that in next future AFT aspirate is carried out routinely in all patients with familial MGUS.

Acknowledgements

We are very gratefull to Dr A.M.Colonna for preparing tissue specimens for examination by light and electron microscopy.

References

1) Pepys M.B. (1988) "Amyloidosis:some recent developments. Quarterly J.Med 252, 283-298.

2) Gertz M.A, Garton J.P and Kyle R.A. " Primary amyloidosis in families" (1986),Am.J.Hematology,22,193-198.

3) Hersch M.I and Mc Leod J.C.(1987) in W.B.Matthews (edt),Handbook of clinical neurology,vol.7(51),Elsevier Science Publ.,pp413-428.

4) Law MIP (1976) "Familial occurrence of multiple myeloma" South Med.J. 69,46-

5) Benson M.D,Brandt K.D,Cohen A.S,Cathcart E.S."Neuropathy,M Components, and Amyloid. (1975) The Lancet,i ,10-12.

PRIMARY SYSTEMIC AMYLOIDOSIS (AL): A RANDOMIZED TRIAL OF COLCHICINE VS. MELPHALAN AND PREDNISONE VS. MELPHALAN, PREDNISONE, AND COLCHICINE.

Kyle RA, Gertz MA, Garton JP, Greipp PR. Mayo Clinic, Rochester, Minnesota 55905 USA

ABSTRACT. Primary amyloidosis is an uncommon disease characterized by deposition of a fibrillar protein often in the heart and kidney resulting in organ dysfunction and death. Treatment for AL is unsatisfactory. The amyloid fibrils consist of the variable portion of monoclonal immunoglobulin light chains and are synthesized by plasma cells. Increased numbers of plasma cells are commonly found in the bone marrow of patients with AL. It is reasonable to attempt treatment with alkylating agents which are known to be effective against plasma cell proliferative processes such as multiple myeloma. We are engaged in a prospective randomized study in which patients have been assigned to melphalan and prednisone or to colchicine or to melphalan, prednisone, and colchicine. This interim analysis suggests the two melphalan-prednisone containing regimens are superior to colchicine.

1. INTRODUCTION

In a placebo-control double-blind study of 55 patients with AL, patients randomized to melphalan-prednisone therapy continued treatment longer and received larger doses than did patients in the placebo group before the code was broken because of progressive disease. Among the 24 patients treated with melphalan-prednisone who had a nephrotic syndrome, proteinuria almost disappeared in two and was reduced by more than 50% in eight others. Renal function remained stable in all 10 responding patients. Among 13 patients who received melphalan-prednisone for more than 12 months, the disease regressed in six, was stable in three, and worsened in four (Kyle and Greipp, 1978).

Colchicine is being used in the treatment of patients with AL. It inhibits casein induction of amyloidosis in mice and has been effective in the control of abdominal pain and the prevention of amyloidosis in patients with familial Mediterranean fever. Colchicine may inhibit amyloidosis by blocking the formation of amyloid-enhancing factor. It also inhibits the secretion of serum amyloid A protein from hepatocytes. Cohen, et al. (1987) reported a median survival of 6 months for 29 patients seen between 1961 and 1983 who were not treated with colchicine and a median survival of 17 months for 53 patients seen between 1976 and 1983 who were treated with colchicine.

In a prospective randomized study of melphalan (0.15 mg/kg/day for 7 days) plus prednisone (0.8 mg/kg/day for the same 7 days) every 6 weeks versus daily colchicine therapy (1 tablet b.i.d. with an increase of 1 tablet each week until side effects occurred), 101 patients were stratified according to their dominant clinical manifestation. If the disease progressed, the other regimen was added. There was no difference in survival when the two groups were compared in total (melphalan-prednisone, 25.2 mos. vs. colchicine, 18 mos.; $P=0.23$). When the survival of patients who received only one regimen was analyzed or when survival was analyzed from the time of entry into the study to the time of death or progression of disease, significant differences ($P<.001$ and $P<.0001$, respectively) favoring melphalan-prednisone therapy were evident. Four patients died of acute nonlymphocytic leukemia and two patients had a myelodysplastic syndrome (Kyle, et al., 1985). Benson (1986) reported that the nephrotic syndrome resolved in 2 of 7 patients with AL who were given melphalan-prednisone and colchicine. Two patients died but three others showed no progression of their disease. Fielder and Durie (1986) reported a survival of 28 months for seven patients with AL and overt multiple myeloma who responded to chemotherapy versus a median survival of 7.5 months for the nine patients without response.

We have developed a prospective a prospective randomized study comparing the effectiveness of melphalan-prednisone versus colchicine versus melphalan-prednisone-colchicine. There is no crossover provision in this study.

2. MATERIALS AND METHODS

Eligibility criteria consisted of tissue diagnosis of primary systemic amyloidosis (AL). Patients with secondary, familial, or localized amyloidosis were excluded. Patients with symptomatic multiple myeloma were excluded as were patients who had diarrhea from autonomic neuropathy or amyloid infiltration of the bowel. Any patient who had prior therapy with melphalan, prednisone, or colchicine was ineligible.

Patients were stratified according to their dominant clinical manifestation--nephrotic syndrome or renal failure, congestive heart failure, peripheral neuropathy, or other. Patients were randomized to regimen I (colchicine, 0.6 mg b.i.d. which was increased gradually to the point of toxicity); regimen II (melphalan, 0.15 mg/kg daily plus prednisone, 0.8 mg/kg daily, both for 7 days every 6 weeks); or regimen III (melphalan, prednisone, and colchicine as in regimens I and II). Leukocyte and platelet values were determined every 3 weeks and the dosage of melphalan adjusted so that leukopenia or thrombocytopenia occurred at mid-cycle. History and physical examinations; blood chemistries; serum and urine electrophoresis, immunoelectrophoresis or immunofixation; bone marrow aspirate and biopsy; prothrombin time; factor X level; serum B12;, carotene; chest x-ray; electrocardiogram; and echocardiogram were performed at appropriate intervals. Patients were continued on therapy for 2 years and treatment was discontinued. The initial therapy was resumed when progression of disease occurred.

3. RESULTS

One hundred sixty-three patients have been entered. Fifty-three were assigned to regimen I, 57 to regimen II, and 53 to regimen III. The median age of patients in regimen I was 64 years (range 35 to 84 yrs), 63 years in regimen II (range 34 to 89 yrs) and 62 years in regimen III (range 33 to 77 yrs). Males were more frequent than females--37 males in regimen I, 40 males in regimen II; and 38 males in regimen III.

The nephrotic syndrome was the most common syndrome (43% in regimen I, 49% in regimen II, and 40% in regimen III) followed by congestive heart failure (15% in regimen I, 14% in regimen II, and 23% in regimen III), and peripheral neuropathy (15% in regimen I, 21% in regimen II, and 19% in regimen III). The frequency of fatigue and presence and amount of weight loss were similar in all three regimens. The incidence of hepatomegaly and macroglossia was not different in the three therapy groups. Values for hemoglobin, leukocytes, platelets, alkaline phosphatase levels, and performance were similar in the three regimens. At the time of entry, the serum creatinine was ≥2 mg/dL in 22% in regimen I, 13% in regimen II, and 13% in regimen III of males and 6% in regimen I, 29% in regimen II, and 7% in regimen III of females. A monoclonal protein was present in the serum and/or urine in 85% of those in regimen I, 81% in regimen II, and 77% in regimen III. The median bone marrow plasma cell level was 4% in regimen I, 5% in regimen II, and 5% in regimen III.

The diagnosis of systemic amyloidosis was made from tissue biopsy from one or more sites. Rectal biopsy was positive in 75% of those in regimen I, 88% in regimen II, and 82% in regimen III, whereas the bone marrow as positive in 60% of those in regimen I, 57% in regimen II, and 54% in regimen III. The subcutaneous fat aspirate was positive in 80% of regimen I, 53% in regimen II, and 75% in regimen III.

Forty-four of the 53 patients in regimen I have died while 40 of the 57 patients in regimen II have expired. Nineteen of the 53 patients in regimen III are alive. The median survival of those receiving colchicine was 9 months; melphalan and prednisone, 16 months; and melphalan, prednisone, and colchicine, 18 months.

4. DISCUSSION

The results of therapy in amyloidosis are difficult to document because the amyloid in a patient cannot be measured accurately. At present, investigators are limited to evaluation of organ function and measurement of the monoclonal protein in the serum and urine. The major measure of therapeutic efficacy is survival.

Colchicine was well tolerated except for the expected gastrointestinal symptoms. Leukopenia and thrombocytopenia did not constitute a serious problem.

Survival was longer in the melphalan-prednisone containing regimens but final evaluation is not possible until the patients are followed longer and the responses analyzed in detail. The incidence of myelodysplasia and acute nonlymphocytic leukemia in the melphalan-containing regimens must be evaluated after all patients have been entered and have beel followed up for a longer period.

5. REFERENCES

Kyle, R.A., Greipp, P.R. (1978) Primary systemic amyloidosis: comparison of melphalan and prednisone versus placebo, Blood, 52:818.
Cohen, A.S., Rubinow, A., Anderson, J.J., et al. (1987) Survival of patients with primary (AL) amyloidosis: colchicine-treated cases from 1976 to 1983 compared with cases seen in previous years (1961 to 1973), Am J Med, 82:1182.
Kyle, R.A., Greipp, P.R., Garton, J.P., Gertz, M.A. (1985) Primary systemic amyloidosis: comparison of melphalan-prednisone versus colchicine, Am J Med, 79:708.
Benson, M.D. (1986) Treatment of AL amyloidosis with melphalan, prednisone, and colchicine, Arthritis Rheum, 29:683.
Fielder, K., Durie, B.G.M. (1986) Primary amyloidosis associated with multiple myeloma: predictors of successful therapy, Am J Med, 80:413.

RESPONSE RATES AND SURVIVAL IN PRIMARY SYSTEMIC AMYLOIDOSIS

M. A. GERTZ, M.D.
R. A. KYLE, M.D.
P. R. GREIPP, M.D.
Dysproteinemia Clinic
Mayo Clinic and Mayo Foundation
200 First Street Southwest
Rochester, Minnesota 55905
United States

ABSTRACT. There were 153 patients with biopsy-proven primary systemic amyloidosis (AL) evaluated for their response to alkylating agent based chemotherapy. There were 27 patients (18 percent) who responded. The serum creatinine had an adverse effect on response rate ($p = 0.05$). In patients with nephrotic syndrome, a normal serum creatinine value, and no echocardiographic evidence of cardiac amyloidosis, the response rate was 39 percent (12 of 31). Of 34 patients with amyloid cardiomyopathy, 5 responded. Two of these five are alive ten years after diagnosis. None of the 18 patients with amyloid peripheral neuropathy showed regression of disease. The median survival of the 27 patients was 89.4 months and 21 of 27 survived five years (78 percent). Eight patients remain alive with a minimum follow-up of 90 months. In the group of 126 patients who showed no response to therapy, the median survival was 14.7 months and 9 (7 percent) survived >5 years. All 126 patients have died. Alkylating agent based chemotherapy for AL is beneficial in a subset of patients.

Introduction

During the past 17 years, there have been two dozen reports describing responses of patients with primary systemic amyloidosis (AL) treated with chemotherapy (1-3). It is unclear which patients with AL derive the greatest benefit from therapy. No series has reported a sufficient number to determine whether responders derive meaningful survival benefit. Response rates remain unknown. This review was undertaken to address these questions.

Materials and Methods

The subjects in this study were 153 patients with AL diagnosed and evaluated at Mayo Clinic. All 153 had biopsy-proven amyloidosis. None of the patients had multiple myeloma. The diagnosis of AL amyloid was verified by the presence of a free monoclonal light chain in the serum or urine in 132 (86 percent) at presentation. In the remaining patients, the diagnosis was made by excluding underlying inflammatory processes that could produce secondary amyloidosis and by excluding a family history of the disease. All patients had been previously untreated. None of the patients have been lost to follow-up. The minimum follow-up is eight years.

Treatment Schema

Patients were treated with melphalan and prednisone. Melphalan therapy was initiated at a dose of 0.15 mg/kg/day in two divided doses. Prednisone therapy was administered at a dosage of 0.8 mg/kg/day in four divided doses. Each cycle of treatment was seven days long. Cycles were repeated every six weeks. The dose of melphalan was adjusted to induce leukopenia. An attempt was made to treat patients for a minimum of 24 months.

Definition of Response

All responding patients were required to have evidence of regression of organ manifestations of amyloidosis. In patients with nephrotic range proteinuria, this required a 50 percent reduction in 24-hour protein loss without an increase in serum creatinine level during follow-up. Patients with hepatic involvement had to have a liver that was no longer palpable and a complete return to normal of the alkaline phosphatase level. Patients with cardiomyopathy had to have total resolution of heart failure. In addition, complete disappearance of an M protein in the serum or urine had to be seen.

Results

A discriminant analysis was performed between the group of responders and non-responders to insure they were homogeneous at the outset of therapy. The analysis was performed using variables known to affect survival: age, presence or absence of hepatomegaly, congestive heart failure, creatinine level, urine light chain, sex, serum β_2 microglobulin, and hemoglobin. None of these factors showed any significant differences between the two groups ($p > 0.1$).

Of the 153 patients treated, 27 (18 percent) responded to melphalan and prednisone therapy. Of the 17 responders with renal amyloid, 11 had complete resolution of the nephrotic syndrome and 6 others had a 50 percent reduction in their urinary protein loss. Of the 17, 2 also had hepatic amyloidosis. In both, hepatomegaly and alkaline phosphatase levels normalized. No patient with a creatinine level >265 micromoles/liter responded to treatment. Renal insufficiency decreases the likelihood of a treatment response ($p = 0.052$). In the 31 patients with amyloid nephrotic syndrome, normal creatinine level, and normal echocardiogram at the time treatment was initiated, the overall response rate was 39 percent. Three additional patients with renal amyloidosis responded to therapy but had insufficient proteinuria at diagnosis to qualify as nephrotic. There were 34 patients with amyloid cardiomyopathy without nephrotic syndrome. Five of these patients responded (15 percent). One patient with isolated hepatic amyloidosis responded. One patient with soft tissue amyloid causing arthropathy, myopathy, and claudication responded. The median time to response was one year. Response rate was independent of the type of monoclonal protein in the serum or urine ($p > 0.1$). The median time from diagnosis to treatment was three weeks, which did not preclude the accrual of patients with poor prognosis destined to have short survival. Although survival in amyloidosis is shorter when multiple organs were involved when compared to those who have a single organ involved, the response rates are not different when involvement is limited to a single organ (response rate 20 percent) versus those with multiple organ involvement (response rate 15 percent, $p > 0.2$). Multivariate analysis was performed on all 153 patients. Age was significant, with older patients having an inferior survival ($p < 0.05$). Of the variables age, sex, creatinine, heart failure, hepatomegaly, neuropathy, and urinary light chain, only neuropathy was significant in predicting lack of response ($p < 0.05$).

Survival

The median survival of the 27 responding patients was 89.4 months and 21 (78 percent) survived five years. The remaining 126 patients had a median survival of 14.7 months with 9 (7 percent) surviving five years. Of the 27 responders, 8 remain alive from 7.5 to 14.4 years after diagnosis. Three have been followed for more than ten years. All 126 non-responders have died. There were nine non-responding patients that survived >5 years. All had a normal creatinine at diagnosis and none had congestive heart failure. Neuropathy was present in five of these nine patients. It has been reported (4) that amyloid neuropathy patients have a better prognosis. We have reported patients with indolent hepatic amyloidosis who survived five years in spite of progressive disease (5).

Discussion

Previous reports have not shown a survival benefit of melphalan and prednisone treated patients compared to either placebo or colchicine. In this report, we demonstrate that a subset of patients will derive benefit from treatment. The percentage of patients who evidence this response is small and is inadequate to shift the median survival. In prospective randomized studies, improved survival for certain subsets may be overlooked. The prolonged survival of the responding group was not due to ancillary factors such as a younger age, absence of congestive heart failure, or a long time between the diagnosis of amyloid and referral for therapy. Although the median survival for patients with congestive heart failure is only 6 months (6) we are currently following two patients with endomyocardial biopy-proven AL alive 10 years after the initiation of therapy. The optimal duration of treatment for patients with amyloidosis is not known. In view of the risk of acute leukemia, one wonders whether a shorter period of melphalan exposure might decrease the risk of damage to the bone marrow. There is no evidence to suggest that if single alkylating agent treatment fails, that patients would derive benefit from more aggressive multi-agent chemotherapy (7). Clear-cut regressions in organ involvement in AL have not been demonstrated with DMSO or colchicine (8,9,10,11).

In conclusion, alkylating agent based chemotherapy for AL can produce regressions of disease in a small percentage of patients. The optimal duration of treatment is unknown. It is not clear that this type of regression has been demonstrated in AL with DMSO or colchicine. Whether combinations of therapy will be of greater benefit remains to be demonstrated with prospective randomized studies.

References

1. Kyle, RA, Greipp, PR. (1978) Blood 52, 818-827.
2. Buxbaum, JN, Hurley, ME, Chuba, J, Spiro, T. (1979) Am J Med 67, 867-870.
3. Kyle, RA, Greipp, PR, Gertz, MA. (1985) Am J Med 79, 708-716.
4. Duston, MA, Skinner, M, Anderson, J, Cohen, AS. (1989) Arch Intern Med 149, 358-360.
5. Gertz, MA, Kyle, RA. (1988) Am J Med 85, 73-80.
6. Kyle, RA, Greipp, PR, O'Fallon, WM. (1986) Blood 68, 220-224.
7. Frustaci, A, Gentiloni, N, Feoli, F. (1981) Minerva Med 72, 957-960.
8. Cohen, AS, Rubinow, A, Anderson, JJ, Skinner, M, Mason, JH, Libbey, C, Kayne, H. (1987) Am J Med 82, 1182-1190.
9. Akoglu, E, Akoglu, T, Erken, E. (1984) Ann Rheum Dis 43, 857.
10. Ravid, M, Shapria, J, Lang, R, Kedar, J. (1982) Ann Rheum Dis 41, 587-592.
11. Wang, WJ, Lin, CS, Wong, CK. (1986) J Am Acad Dermatol 15, 402-405.

URINARY PROTEIN PATTERNS PREDICT SURVIVAL IN PRIMARY SYSTEMIC AMYLOIDOSIS (AL)

M. A. GERTZ, M.D.
R. A. KYLE, M.D.
Dysproteinemia Clinic
Mayo Clinic and Mayo Foundation
200 First Street Southwest
Rochester, Minnesota 55905
United States

ABSTRACT. Serum creatinine level was measured in 153 patients with primary systemic amyloidosis (AL). The median survival of patients with a serum creatinine ≤ 1.3 mg/dL and >1.3 mg/dL was 25.6 and 14.9 months, respectively ($P = 0.007$). Patients with a monoclonal lambda light chain in the urine had an inferior survival compared to those with kappa light chain or no monoclonal protein in the urine. The survivals were 12 months, 30 months, and 35 months, respectively ($P = 0.01$). The total protein excretion had no bearing on survival. Patients with lambda monoclonal protein in the urine excreted 4.56 g of protein per day. Patients with no monoclonal protein and a urinary kappa monoclonal protein excreted 0.52 g/day and 1.09 g/day, respectively. The loss of monoclonal lambda protein in the urine did not result in a higher serum creatinine level. A monoclonal protein was detected in the urine of three-fourths of the patients. The urinary kappa-to-lambda ratio was 1:2.5, but for those patients with nephrotic range proteinuria, the ratio was 1:4.7, suggesting that patients with lambda monoclonal protein in the urine are more likely to have amyloid nephrotic syndrome than patients with no monoclonal protein or kappa monoclonal protein in the urine.

Introduction

In primary systemic amyloidosis (AL), plasma cells produce a monoclonal light chain or fragment thereof which is deposited in the tissues as a nondegradable fibril [3]. Deposition of the fibril interferes with normal organ function and rapidly leads to death. The most common presentation of AL is renal involvement manifested by nephrotic syndrome and is present in one-third of patients at the time of their presentation [6,12]. Histopathologic evidence of AL is found in the kidneys in most patients at the time of postmortem examination [15]. This study was undertaken to determine whether measurements of kidney function and urinary protein parameters were predictive of survival in AL.

Materials and Methods

The study population included 153 patients with biopsy-proven AL. Patients with overt multiple myeloma and other forms of systemic amyloidosis were excluded. All patients were followed to within three months of this analysis or death; none have been lost to follow-up. All patients had immunoelectrophoresis of a concentrated urine specimen to detect the presence of monoclonal light chains. Univariate statistical methods were used to summarize the distribution of each parameter. Survival curves were estimated by the Kaplan-Meier technique [5]. The proportional hazards model of Cox was used to determine the variables that influence survival [4]. All patients gave written informed consent before study entry [7,9].

Results

Of all patients with AL, 45 percent had $\geq$3.0 g/day of protein in the urine and 60 percent excreted in excess of 1 g/day. A urinary protein excretion in the normal range ($<$0.15 g/day) was seen in only 4.6 percent of patients. Immunoelectrophoresis of the urine revealed a monoclonal light chain in 76 percent. The 92 patients who excreted $>$1 g of protein per day had a monoclonal light chain detectable in 86 percent. Patients who had $>$3 g/day proteinuria had a monoclonal light chain detectable in 85 percent.

The overall kappa-to-lambda ratio was 1:2.45. In patients who excreted $>$1 g/day of protein, the kappa-to-lambda ratio was 1:3.38. In patients who excreted $>$3 g/day of protein, the kappa-to-lambda ratio was 1:4.7. This suggests that renal involvement with AL is more common when a lambda monoclonal light chain is produced. The median urinary protein loss in patients excreting a monoclonal urinary kappa protein, monoclonal urinary lambda protein, and no urinary monoclonal protein was 1.09 g/day, 4.56 g/day, and 0.52 g/day, respectively ($P < 0.002$). Lambda light chain loss is clearly associated with nephrotic syndrome. The prevalence of nephrotic syndrome in patients with kappa, lambda, and no monoclonal protein in urine was 30 percent, 58 percent, and 27 percent, respectively. Serum creatinine level was independent of the type of urinary light chain excreted in the urine. The amount of urinary light chain loss was small; the median loss of urinary light chain was 8 percent of the total urinary protein loss.

SURVIVAL ANALYSIS

The 24-hour urinary protein loss had no impact on survival. The median survival of patients with $<$1 g/day and $>$1 g/day urinary protein loss was 2.1 and 1.3 years, respectively ($P > 0.2$). In patients with greater than and less than 3 g of protein in the urine, the median survival was 1.4 and 1.9 years, respectively ($P > 0.05$). The type of monoclonal light chain excreted in the urine had a strong impact on survival. The survival of patients with a urinary kappa, urinary lambda, and no monoclonal light chain in the urine was 2.5, 1.0, and 2.9 years, respectively ($P = 0.01$). The adverse survival impact of a lambda monoclonal protein in the urine was not due to a higher prevalence of heart failure in patients with a monoclonal lambda protein in the urine. The presence of a monoclonal lambda protein in the urine was not associated with a higher prevalence of renal insufficiency. The median creatinine in patients with kappa, lambda, and no monoclonal protein in the urine was 1.2, 1.1, and 1.3 mg/dL, respectively (P = not significant). Serum creatinine had a very important predictive value with regard to survival. The median survival of patients with a serum creatinine $\leq$1.3 mg/dL and >1.3 mg/dL was 25.6 months and 14.9 months, respectively ($P = 0.007$). Multivariate analysis revealed that the prognostic value of serum creatinine was independent of the urinary protein loss and type of urinary monoclonal light chain.

Discussion

Although AL is recognized to be a life-threatening condition, few parameters are recognized that help assess the prognosis of patients with this disorder. Kyle et al. [8] has previously shown that heart failure, hepatomegaly, the presence of urinary light chains, and an elevated creatinine all have adverse effects on survival in AL. Our findings support these conclusions and specifically note that it is the presence of a lambda urinary light chain that accounts for the effect of light chain proteinuria on survival in AL. Shustik et al. [13] previously reported the adverse effect of lambda light chains on survival in myeloma and AL. In addition, the presence of lambda monoclonal protein in the urine is associated with an increase in urinary protein loss without an accompanying increase in serum creatinine. The overall kappa-to-lambda ratio in AL is dependent on the site of organ involvement. Although the kappa-to-lambda ratio in AL is taken to be 1:2, in the presence of nephrotic syndrome, the kappa-to-lambda ratio we found was 1:4.7. In this study, nephrotic syndrome was nearly twice as common in patients with lambda monoclonal protein in the urine compared to those with no monoclonal protein in the urine. This kappa-to-lambda ratio has previously been reported in patients with AL nephrotic syndrome [10]. The measurement of serum creatinine, 24-hour urine protein loss, and immunoelectrophoresis of the urine is essential in the evaluation of patients with AL. Virtually all patients will have proteinuria, and 60 percent will have >1 g of protein per day in the urine. Daniels and Hewlett [2] found proteinuria >1 g/day in two-thirds of their AL patients. Pick et al. [11] detected a urinary monoclonal light chain in the urine in 55 percent of their patient population. This is comparable to the 76 percent positivity found in this study.
Vital Durand et al. [14] found a monoclonal light chain in 63 percent of their patients with AL. Patients with unexplained nephrotic syndrome older than age 30 should have immunofixation/immunoelectrophoresis of the urine since the finding of a monoclonal light chain should increase the suspicion of AL. Measurement of the serum creatinine is mandatory because it correlates directly with survival. Watanabe and Saniter [15]

found a strong correlation between serum creatinine and extensive glomerular amyloid deposits. Browning et al. [1] found renal involvement in 42 percent of their AL patients. In our study, nephrotic syndrome was present in 45 percent of patients. Browning found no relationship between urinary protein loss and amount of glomerular amyloid seen histologically. In that study, the one-year survival was 27 percent with no three-year survivors.

In conclusion, patients with monoclonal lambda light chains in the urine have a higher prevalence of nephrotic syndrome and shorter survival. The serum creatinine has a statistically significant independent effect on survival. Total urinary protein loss does not correlate with survival in AL. All patients with AL should have immunoelectrophoresis and immunofixation of a 24-hour urine specimen and measurement of the serum creatinine level.

References

1. Browning, M, Banks, R, Tribe, C, et al. (1983) Proc Eur Dial Transplant Assoc 20, 595-600.
2. Daniels, JD, Hewlett, JS. (1970) Cleve Clin Q 37, 181-187.
3. Isobe, T, Osserman, EF. (1974) N Engl J Med 290, 473-477.
4. Kalbfleisch, JD, Prentice, RL. (1980) John Wiley and Sons, New York.
5. Kaplan, EL, Meier, P. (1958) J Am Stat Assoc 53, 457-481.
6. Kyle, RA, Greipp, PR. (1983) Mayo Clin Proc 58, 665-683.
7. Kyle, RA, Greipp, PR, Garton, GP, Gertz, MA. (1985) Am J Med 79, 708-716.
8. Kyle, RA, Greipp, PR, O'Fallon, WM. (1986) Blood 68, 220-224.
9. Kyle, RA, Greipp, PR. (1978) Blood 52, 818-827.
10. Pascali, E, Pezzoli, A. (1988) Cancer 62, 2408-2415.
11. Pick, AI, Fröhlichmann, R, Lavie, G, Duczyminer, M, Skvaril, F. (1981) Acta Haematol 66, 154-167.
12. Pruzanski, W, Katz, A. (1976) Can Med Assoc J 114, 906-909. 7
13. Shustik, C, Bergsagel, DE, Pruzanski, W. (1976) Blood 48, 41-51.
14. Vital Durand, D, Touraine, J-L, Levrat, R, et al. (1984) Blut 49, 91-94.
15. Watanabe, T, Saniter, T. (1975) Virchows Arch [A] 366, 125-135.

β_2-MICROGLOBULIN PREDICTS SURVIVAL IN PRIMARY SYSTEMIC AMYLOIDOSIS (AL)

M. A. GERTZ, M.D.
R. A. KYLE, M.D.
P. R. GREIPP, M.D.
J. A. KATZMANN, Ph.D.
Dysproteinemia Clinic
Mayo Clinic and Mayo Foundation
200 First Street Southwest
Rochester, Minnesota 55905
United States

ABSTRACT. Measurement of the serum β_2-microglobulin (β_2-M) is useful in predicting survival in patients with multiple myeloma. Primary systemic amyloidosis (AL) shares many features in common with multiple myeloma. We measured β_2-M levels in 131 patients with newly diagnosed AL. Of those patients, 124 have died, the remaining 7 patients have been followed a minimum of eight years. The median survival of patients with an elevated β_2-M level (>2.7 mcg/ml) was 10.8 months compared to those with a normal β_2-M level of 32.9 months ($p < 0.001$). Multivariate analysis revealed that only the presence of congestive heart failure has a greater impact on survival. Even factoring in congestive heart failure, β_2-M remains a significant predictor of survival. When patients with normal creatinine only are included, the median survival of those with an elevated β_2-M was 9 months versus 39.4 months for those with a normal β_2-M level ($p < 0.001$). Serum β_2-M levels should be measured in all patients with AL since it is a highly significant predictor of survival.

Introduction

β_2-M was first isolated from the urine of patients with proteinuria in 1968 [1,2]. β_2-M is found on the surface of all cells and represents the light chain of the human HLA complex [3]. The serum level of β_2-M is a reliable marker for survival in multiple myeloma [4-10]. The impact of β_2-M on survival in multiple myeloma is significant in a multivariate model [11]. The level of β_2-M will not separate patients with multiple myeloma from those with MGUS [12]. β_2-M is a direct secretory product of the plasma cell [13]. There are, however, exceptions where myeloma cells do not produce β_2-M [14]. Primary systemic amyloidosis (AL). is a plasma cell dyscrasia that shares many features with myeloma. In 229 patients with AL, 21 percent had multiple myeloma [15]. One report indicates that β_2-M predicted response to treatment in patients with myeloma associated amyloid [16]. This study was undertaken to determine whether β_2-M predicts survival or response in patients with AL.

Materials and Methods

The study group consisted of 131 patients with AL. Patients with multiple myeloma were excluded. No patient with ASC_1, AA, AF, or localized amyloidosis was included. No patients were on dialysis at the time of study. All patients had symptomatic disease. The median age of men was 63; the median age of women was 59. The shortest follow-up of surviving patients is eight years. Serum samples stored frozen were used to measure β_2-M level by using the Phadezym β_2-microtest kit (Pharmacia Diagnostics, Uppsala, Sweden). The upper limit of normal for this study is 2.7 mcg/ml.

Results

The median level of β_2-M for all patients was 2.9 mcg/ml. An abnormal serum β_2-M was seen in 54 percent of the patients. The most common amyloid syndrome was nephrotic syndrome in 44 percent of patients. The median urinary protein excretion was 1.9 g/24 hours. The median creatinine was 1.1 mg/dl. A serum creatinine $\geq$2.0 mg/dl was seen in 14 percent of patients. Serum creatinine and 24-hour urine protein are known to have a direct effect on serum β_2-M level [17,18]. These two variables and their effect on the β_2-M were evaluated. Higher levels of urinary protein loss are associated with a higher prevalence of renal failure. All patients with a creatinine $\geq$2.0 mg/dl had an elevated β_2-M level. Of all patients whose β_2-M was elevated, 30 percent had a serum creatinine >2.0 mg/dl. The median urinary protein loss for patients with a normal β_2-M level was 1.1 g/day. In patients with a high β_2-M level, the median urinary protein loss was 4.1 g/day ($p < 0.01$). Even when patients with renal insufficiency were excluded, urinary protein loss was greater in patients with an elevated β_2-M level. Patients with lambda light chain in the urine have a higher incidence of nephrotic syndrome than those with a kappa light chain in the urine or no monoclonal light chain in the urine [19]. Analysis of β_2-M and urinary light chain excretion revealed that there was no relationship between the type of urinary light chain and the serum β_2-M level.

Survival

The median survival of the entire group was 21.1 months. The one-year, three-year, and five-year survivals were 63 percent, 34 percent, and 20 percent, respectively. Patients with an increased β_2-M level had a median survival of 10.8 months and a five-year survival of 14 percent. When the β_2-M level was normal, the median survival was 32.9 months with a five-year survival of 25 percent ($p < 0.001$). Since creatinine is known to have a significant effect on survival in amyloidosis [19], analysis was performed on only those patients with normal serum creatinine. The median survival of 51 patients with a normal β_2-M and normal creatinine was 39.4 months; the five-year survival was 27 percent. There were 32 patients with an elevated β_2-M level and a normal serum creatinine. Their median survival was nine months and their five-year survival was 22 percent ($p < 0.001$). There was no indication that the β_2-M level predicted an improved response to alkylating agent-based chemotherapy ($p = 0.26$).

A multivariate analysis incorporating urinary protein loss, organ involvement, serum creatinine, urine light chain, β_2-M, hemoglobin, sex, and age were analyzed. The most important variable was congestive heart failure. Elevated β_2-M and serum creatinine levels were similarly significant, but not as significant as congestive heart failure. An attempt to identify independent effects was made using a multivariate proportional hazards model. In the best model, congestive heart failure ($p < 0.0001$) and elevated β_2-M ($p < 0.05$) constituted the best model for survival prediction. Adjusting for heart failure, β_2-M remains significant. At this stage, if serum creatinine is assessed it is completely eliminated as a factor ($p = 0.4$). No other variables add significantly to this model.

Discussion

The value of β_2-M in multiple myeloma has been confirmed by many groups. Amyloidosis (AL) like multiple myeloma is a plasma cell dyscrasia. In both diseases there is a clonal population of bone marrow plasma cells. The majority of patients will have a detectable circulating monoclonal protein. Although AL is not a malignancy, the disease can be devastating [20]. The majority of studies report median survivals of two years or less [21]. No system currently exists in which quantitative variables can identify unfavorable subsets of patients with AL. In this study we describe patients with AL and conclude that serum β_2-M is a useful and objectively measurable predictor of survival. In our study, a relationship of elevated urinary protein loss and a high level of β_2-M was recognized. This relationship was not secondary to the higher serum creatinine level in patients with nephrotic syndrome. The increased protein loss associated with elevated β_2-M level does not affect survival. In conclusion, in this study of patients with AL, the three most important factors predicting survival were congestive heart failure ($p < 0.001$), serum creatinine ($p < 0.01$), and β_2-M level ($p < 0.005$). After adjusting for heart failure, β_2-M remains significant ($p < 0.05$) and eliminates serum creatinine level from the model. β_2-M is easily performed, reproducible, and inexpensive. It is commercially available and should be done as part of the evaluation of all patients with AL.

References

1. Berggård, I. and Bearn, AG. (1968) J Biol Chem 243, 4095-4103.
2. Hall, PW. and Vasiljevic, M. (1973) J Lab Clin Med 81, 897-904.
3. Peterson, PA, Cunningham, BA, Berggård, I, Edelman, GM. (1972) Proc Natl Acad Sci USA 60, 1697-1701.
4. Bataille, R, Durie, BGM, Grenier, J. (1983) Br J Haematol 55, 439-447.
5. Fine, J-M, Lambin, P, Desjobert, H. (1988) Acta Med Scand 224, 179-182.
6. Brenning, G, Simonsson, B, Källender, C, Åhre,A. (1986) Br J Haematol 62, 85-93.
7. Scarffe, JH, Anderson, H, Palmer, MK, Crowther, D. (1983) Eur J Cancer Clin Oncol 19, 1361-1364.
8. Cuzick, J, Cooper, EH, MacLennan, ICM. (1985) Br J Cancer 52, 1-6.
9. Alexanian R, Barlogie B, Fritsche H. (1985) Am J Hematol 20, 345-351.
10. Bataille R, Grenier J, Sany J. (1984) Blood 63, 468-476.
11. Greipp PR, Katzmann JA, O'Fallon WM, Kyle RA. (1988) Blood 72, 219-223.
12. Di-Giovanni S, Valentini G, Ravazzolo E, Carducci P, Giallonardo P, Maschio C. (1987) Int J Biol Markers 2, 169-172.
13. Bataille R, Grenier J, Commes T. (1988) Cancer Invest 6, 271-277.
14. Bataille R, Grenier J, Sany J. (1987) Anticancer Res 7, 513-515.
15. Kyle RA, Greipp PR. (1983) Mayo Clin Proc 58, 665-683.
16. Fielder K, Durie BGM. (1986) Am J Med 80, 413-418.
17. Wibell L, Evrin P-E, Berggård I. (1973) Nephron 10, 320-331.
18. Koopman MG, Krediet RT, Zuyderhoudt FMJ, de Moor EAM, Arisz L. (1987) Nephron 45, 140-146.
19. Gertz MA, Kyle RA. (in press) (1990) Am J Clin Pathol.
20. Duston MA, Skinner M, Anderson J, Cohen AS. (1984) Arch Intern Med 149, 358-360.
21. Cohen AS, Rubinow A, Anderson JJ, et al. (1987) Am J Med 82, 1182-1190.

CUTANEOUS AMYLOIDOSIS IN A HORSE. PARTIAL AMINO ACID SEQUENCE ANALYSIS OF AN EQUINE IMMUNOGLOBULIN-LAMBDA LIGHT CHAIN

R.P. Linke, O. Geisel*, D. Mann&

Institute of Immunology, Goethestr. 31 and *Institute of Veterinary Pathology, Veterinärstr. 13, 8000 München, Max-Planck-Institute of Biochemistry, 8033 Martinsried/FRG

Amyloid in animals is mainly of the AA-type with systemic distribution (1). However, another amyloid syndrome with more nodular deposits and organ-limited distribution was described associated sometimes with monoclonal plasmocyte proliferation, indicating the presence of AL-amyloid. We have immunohistochemically identified Aλ-amyloid in two different species, in horse (2) and in a canine extramedullary plasmocytoma (3). Here we report on a cutaneous nodular amyloidosis in a horse associated with a cutaneous plasmocytoma. A 17-year old Haflinger x Islandpony mare was euthanized because of progressive development of multiple nodules covering the entire integument and the joint capsules (4). One cutaneous nodule was frozen for biochemical analysis. Amyloid fibrils were concentrated by the classical water extraction method of Pras. The amyloid fibril proteins were dissolved in 6M guanidine-HCl and separated on Sephadex G-100 in the same solvent. The major retarded protein peak was reduced and alkylated. The N-terminal amino acid was found to be blocked. Digestion with endo-Asp was followed by separation on a RP C18 Vydac HPLC column with a gradient (A: 0.1% TFA; B: 0.1% TFA in 80% acetonitril). The amino acid sequence analysis performed with a gas phase sequenator on one of the peptides is shown below (top sequence). Statistical comparison showed 77% homology to the human VλII immunoglobulin light chain BUR from position 62 to 84 (5).

```
 |                     |
 DRFSASQSGNTATLTISGVQAED
 ::::.:.:::::.:::::.::::
PDRFSGSKSGNTASLTISGLQAEDEADYYCCSYIGSYVFGTGTKVIVLG
 |                     |
```

According to a computer search this sequence is the first published equine immunoglobulin λ-light chain sequence and the first from an equine λ-chain derived amyloid. This data establishes the existence of immunglobulin-light chain-derived amyloid in animals.

1. Zschiesche, W., Jacob, W.: Pharm. Ther. 41, 49-83 (1989)
2. Linke, R.P., Trautwein, G.: Blut 58, 129-132 (1989)
3. Geisel, O., et al.: Vet. Path. (in press)
4. Geisel, O., et al.: Pferdeheikunde 5, 299-234 (1990)
5. Infante, A., Putnam, F.W.: J. Biol. Chem. 254, 9006-9016 (1979)

EXPERIMENTAL AMYLOID CASTS IN MICE INDUCED BY INJECTION OF A HUMAN BENCE JONES PROTEIN

R.P. Linke

Insitute of Immunology, Goethestr. 31, 8000 München/FRG

Amyloidosis can be induced experimentally in mice by injection of a series of different agents such as casein. The ensuing generalized amyloidosis is found to be of the AA-type by chemical and immunochemical analysis. In addition, human serum amyloid-A protein (SAA) has been injected into mice during the induction of experimental amyloidosis and the human precursor has been transformed to amyloid showing the direct precursor-product relationship, by the group of Husby. The question, whether monoclonal immunoglobulin light chains, another amyloid precursor, could induce human AL-amyloidosis in mice is addresse here.

The Bence Jones protein ZIM was purified from the urine of a patient with monoclonal gammopathy and Aλ-amyloidosis, by ammonium sulfate precipitation followed by ion-exchange chromatography. The BJP ZIM was dissolved at 200mg/ml of phosphate buffered saline, centrifuged at 15.000 rpm for 30min and sterile filtered (0.45µm). Mice (C57 BL/6 or C57 BL/6xBalb/c female mice, over 6 months), were injected with an intraperitoneal bolus injection of either 50, 100, 200 or 400 mg ZIM per mouse. After 2 days a second injection of the same amount was given and after three more days the kidneys were examined for the presence of amyloid on formalin-fixed paraffin sections using the classical Puchtler alkaline Congo red staining method. Numerous protein casts were found with approximately 10% of amyloid nature as judged by the affinity for Congo red and by the green birefringence in polarized light, but only in cases when 2 x 100 - 400mg per mouse was given. Immunohistochemical staining using a panel of anti-human amyloid antibodies including antibodies against AA, Aλ, Aκ, AF (TTR), only anti-Aλ was strongly reacting with all casts, including the amyloid casts, demonstrating the deposition of the injected human Bence Jones protein ZIM. When the anti-Aλ antiserum was absorbed with mouse serum, no reduction of the immunohistochemical reaction was seem, proving the presence of the human Bence Jones protein in renal casts. Congo red staining and immunohistochemical reactions were also done on all major organs. There was neither amyloid detectable nor any immunohistochemical staining for λ-light chains, indicating the presence of amyloid restricted to only the renal tubular system, in the absence of generalized amyloidosis, a finding which has also been described in man.

These data demonstrate the possibility of transforming a human λ-light chain into amyloid in mice.

COMMON ELEMENTS IN AMYLOIDOSIS

ROBERT KISILEVSKY
Department of Pathology
Queen's University
Kingston, Ontario, Canada
K7L 3N6

During the past 10-15 years a major focus of amyloid research has been the characterization of the amyloid proteins and their precursors. The amyloid peptides and their precursors have now been correlated with the deposits in the various clinical entities associated with amyloid. At least 12-15 such proteins have now been identified. Clearly of importance, this work nevertheless has emphasized the differences which exist between the amyloids.

The very fact that we have all gathered in Oslo to discuss a subject of common interest resides in the fact that all amyloid deposits have structural similarities. These are characterized by the following features:

1) an amorphous appearance by light microscopy,
2) Congo red positivity,
3) Congo red stained material exhibiting red-green birefringence in polarized light,
4) seven to ten nanometer diameter fibrils by electron microscopy, and
5) fibrils exhibiting large quantities of beta pleated sheeting by infrared and x-ray diffraction spectroscopy.

These features actually define an amyloid deposit. We have only recently begun to realize that not only are there common structural features, but common constituents are now being described with increasing frequency. These common constituents are:

1) amyloid enhancing factor (AEF),
2) the serum amyloid P component (SAP) and,
3) the heparan sulphate proteoglycan (HSPG).

The purpose of my presentation is not to focus on the past but rather place the present in some perspective and bring out directions and unsolved problems in relation to these common elements which are found in amyloids.

Amyloid Enhancing Factor

This element was originally described in the context of AA amyloidosis. One can only define it in a functional sense, as a factor which dramatically shortens the induction time for AA amyloid development. This activity has now been identified in at least four forms of amyloid, these being, the AA, AL, the beta amyloid of Alzheimer's disease, and the transthyretin amyloid in senescence. It is thus, not a specific amyloid protein. To date it has not been possible to identify the cell of origin or the precise nature of this factor. With regard to its origin most work both in the past and that presented at this symposium would suggest that AEF is derived from and exerts its action at the level of the macrophage. We still do not know precisely what AEF is nor how it exerts its dramatic effects. Various groups have been exploring its nature with the idea that it is a specific molecular entity. Its molecular size has been variously reported to range from 5 kd to 30 kd, the smallest being attributed to ubiquitin. Other groups contest this conclusion.

Among additional possibilities is the idea that AEF is not one entity, but one of many, all of which possess the appropriate structure to act as a nidus for the development of amyloid fibrils. A further possibility is that AEF represents a specific macrophage response to several different entities, in much the same way as an inflammatory reaction may be provoked by various noxious agents such as chemicals or bacteria. Approaches and answers to these latter two possibilities have yet to be devised.

Though a lack of resolution of the AEF problem is somewhat discouraging, given the amount of work devoted to this subject, nevertheless, AEF does provide us with a tool to induce amyloid rapidly and some work described at the symposium suggests it may be useful in tissue culture systems to devise ex-vivo models of AA amyloid generation. Such a development would be a major step forward.

Serum Amyloid P Component

SAP has been described in every form of amyloid known. The protein has been well characterized and its gene identified. It is deposited in AA amyloid models as early as the AA peptide, if not earlier. In hamsters there is a striking correlation between the succeptibility to AA amyloid development and the circulating level of SAP. However we have no idea as yet how this molecule plays a role in amyloid induction or development. As described at this meeting several new approaches are being used to examine SAP genetics in hamsters, rats and mice in both amyloid sensitive and resistant strains. This is being done in an attempt to elucidate SAP's role in amyloidogenesis. SAP's normal function is not known either, but SAP does bind free chromatin with the displacemnt of H1 histones which in turn then maintains the solubility of DNA. Thus SAP could function as a means of ensuring that chromatin released at sites of necrosis is maintained in an appropriate state for subsequent removal and disposal.

We have also seen at this meeting presentation of work describing the use of radiolabelled SAP as a diagnostic tool to both delineate the extent of, and follow the turnover of amyloid deposits. Both of these developments should have a significant clinical impact.

Proteoglycans and Glycosaminoglycans

Highly sulphated glycosaminoglycans have been demonstrated in all forms of amyloid examined to date. In the case of AA amyloid these glycosaminoglycans are deposited coincidentally with the AA peptide and have been shown to be of the heparan/heparin sulphate variety and which include the protein core. The heparan sulphate proteoglycan has been described in at least five forms of amyloid which include AA, AL, beta amyloid of Alzheimer's disease, the prion amyloids in experimental scrapie, Creutzfeldt-Jakob disease and Gerstmann Straussler Syndrome as well as the IAPP amyloid of Type II diabetics. The dermatan sulphate proteoglycan has been described in two forms of amyloid, the AA form and the beta protein form seen in Alzheimer's disease. The HSPG observations have been confirmed with isolated amyloid fibrils and as in the case of AA amyloid the heparan sulphate proteoglycan deposition has been shown to be an early event both in Alzheimer's disease and in Down's Syndrome. As reported at this meeting AEF treated macrophages seem to have increasing quantities of glycosaminoglycans on their surface and with it an increase in affinity for the SAA protein. Whether this plays any role in the development of AA amyloidosis in the altered processing of SAA remains to be determined.

It is not yet known if the HSPG is acting alone in terms of its interactions with amyloid peptides or their precursors, and if so how it interacts with such precursors and peptides. It remains to be determined if the presence of the HSPG plays an integral part in fibril generation or simply in fibril stability. The type of HSPG found in the amyloid deposits is that seen in basement membranes. Recent work from at least two groups, as presented at this meeting, have indicated that HSPG is only one element of basement membranes seen in amyloid deposits. The other elements identified have been collagen-type IV, laminin and fibronectin.

Basement Membranes

The presence of the aforementioned basement membrane constituents meshes well with past ultrastructural work describing amyloid deposits in conjunction with basement membranes. In this regard it should also be remembered that SAP has been identified as a normal constituent of basement membranes. This links together, conceptually, many of the structural components as they all relate to basement membranes. This in turn raises several interesting questions about the pathogenesis of amyloids and the potential role of basement membrane function and dysfunction. Little is known about the interactions of the individual basement membrane components with themselves, to give normal basement membranes or for that matter how they interact with various amyloid precursors and peptides. These represent ripe areas for amyloid research.

In summary the common structural features of all amyloids are now being matched by the identification of common structural elements. These are beginning to be explored in much greater depth and hopefully they will elucidate for us how and why amyloid develops and is maintained for such long periods in the affected tissues.

METABOLIC STUDIES OF RADIOIODINATED SERUM AMYLOID P COMPONENT IN NORMAL SUBJECTS AND PATIENTS WITH SYSTEMIC AMYLOIDOSIS

P.N. HAWKINS, R. WOOTTON & M.B. PEPYS
Immunological Medicine Unit, Department of Medicine and Department of Medical Physics, Royal Postgraduate Medical School, Hammersmith Hospital, London W12 0NN U.K.

ABSTRACT. ^{125}I-serum amyloid P component (SAP), injected intravenously into 10 normal subjects, remained predominantly intravascular with mean (SD) T½ in plasma of 24.5 (5.9) hr. The fractional catabolic rate of 68 (19)% of the plasma pool per day was more rapid than other reported human plasma proteins. All radioactivity was excreted in the urine by 14 days. In 16 patients with monoclonal gammopathy or chronic inflammatory diseases, but without amyloidosis, ^{125}I-SAP metabolism was normal. However, among 45 patients with biopsy proven systemic amyloidosis (25, AA type; 20, AL), ^{125}I-SAP was cleared from the plasma more rapidly, accumulated in the amyloid deposits, and persisted there. The T½ in amyloid, measured directly with ^{131}I-SAP, was 24 days. Repeat studies after 6-18 months were notably consistent in normals but changed significantly in amyloid patients, generally correlating with clinical signs of disease progression. Measurements of ^{125}I-SAP turnover may thus be of value for diagnosis and monitoring of amyloidosis. Analysis of SAP metabolism in amyloidosis suggests that plasma SAP is in dynamic equilibrium with a very large amyloid pool, and in two autopsies the total mass of SAP in the amyloid deposits was 2,100 mg and 21,000 mg respectively.

1. INTRODUCTION

Serum amyloid P component (SAP) [1] is a normal plasma glycoprotein of unknown function. It is a calcium-dependent lectin with specificity for the cyclic pyruvate acetal of galactose and related sugars [2], and also binds to sulphated glycosaminoglycans [3]. In addition SAP specifically undergoes calcium-dependent binding to DNA and chromatin *in vitro* [4] and *in vivo* [5] and this may represent a significant part of its normal function. A molecule immunochemically indistinguishable from SAP, so called tissue AP (TAP) [6-8], is a normal constituent of certain extracellular tissue matrices, though it is not known whether TAP is derived from circulating SAP or produced locally. Apart from its normal properties and biological distribution, SAP is important as the circulating precursor of amyloid P component (AP) which is a universal non-fibrillar constituent of all known amyloid deposits [9-11]. This deposition is a consequence of the calcium-dependent binding of SAP to ligands on amyloid fibrils, which has enabled us to use ^{123}I-labelled SAP as a specific agent for radionuclide imaging of amyloid deposits *in vivo* [12-15]. The present studies, which have been reported in full elsewhere [16], detail the distribution, synthesis and catabolism of SAP in normal subjects and patients with systemic amyloidosis using the longer lived isotopes ^{125}I and ^{131}I.

2. METHODS [16]

Pure SAP labelled with ^{125}I or ^{131}I was given by bolus i.v. injection to the following subjects: 1) 10 normal healthy adult volunteers, 5 male and 5 female, aged 22-78 years. 2) 8 patients with chronic inflammatory disorders and 8 with monoclonal gammopathy, diseases associated with systemic amyloidosis but in whom there was no clinical, laboratory or biopsy evidence of amyloid. 3) 25 patients with biopsy proven reactive systemic (AA) amyloidosis complicating chronic inflammatory disease. 4) 20 patients with biopsy proven AL amyloidosis complicating monoclonal gammopathy.

The plasma and whole body clearance of radiolabelled SAP was measured by counting activity in the plasma and urine over 7 days. In 24 amyloid and 18 control subjects plasma activity data was fitted to 1 and 2 compartment models and as a negative power function of time prior to further computed analysis. The *in vivo* persistence of ^{131}I-SAP localised in the amyloidotic liver of an AL patient was measured for 25 days using whole body scintigraphy and the whole body distribution of residual ^{125}I-SAP was determined at autopsy in 2 amyloid patients who died 4 and 12 months after isotope injection. Radioactive SAP was extracted from amyloidotic tissues in these latter patients and characterised *in vitro*.

3. RESULTS

In healthy volunteers plasma activity initially fell relatively rapidly, reflecting distribution and equilibration in the body pool of SAP, leaving at 6 hr, mean (SD) 75 (4)% of the notional starting value in the circulation. Thereafter there was a slower monoexponential decline, throughout the 7 day period of study with T½, mean (SD) 24.5 (5.9) hr; this was paralleled, with a delay of about 24 hr, by urinary excretion of labelled SAP degradation products. At 7 days whole body retention (WBR) of activity was mean (SD) 17 (4)%. The maximum size of the extravascular compartment (EVC), calculated from WBR minus plasma activity, was mean (SD) 29.6 (7.7) and occurred on the first day after injection. Total SAP concentrations were constant in all subjects, enabling various metabolic parameters to be calculated (Table 1).

Table 1. Normal metabolism of SAP (mean ± SD values)

	n	Plasma SAP (mg/l)	Fractional clearance (calculated) (%/24 hr)	Fractional catabolic rate (measured) (%/24 hr)	Synthesis rate (mg/hr)	Distribution vol. (x plasma vol.)
Healthy volunteers	10	29.0±9.6	68±19	74±25	1.93±0.81	1.02±0.04
Patient controls	8	34.8±13.6	72±21	69±10	2.69±1.26	1.05±0.07

In 16 patients with various disorders predisposing to amyloidosis, but in whom the diagnosis had been excluded, all aspects of SAP turnover fell within a reference range of 2 SD in either direction from the mean normal values.

Although patients with amyloidosis had normal plasma SAP levels, in most, the clearance of ^{125}I-SAP was significantly altered. Early plasma clearance of radioactivity was greatly accelerated in the presence of substantial amyloid deposits and in extreme cases over 90% of the injected dose left the circulation within minutes. However, even when clearance was less rapid, urinary excretion of tracer was reduced and WBR at 7 days was increased, as a result of increased accumulation of ^{125}I-SAP in the EVC, i.e. the amyloid deposits. Synthesis rates of SAP were normal or substantially increased. The size of the AP pool within which ^{125}I-SAP accumulated was measured directly at 2100 mg and 21000 mg in 2 patients studied at autopsy. Nevertheless, the fractional catabolic rate (FCR) of SAP was not different from normal indicating that only SAP within the plasma compartment is available for catabolism. Scintigraphic studies using ^{131}I-SAP in one patient with AL hepatomegaly showed the T½ of SAP in the liver amyloid deposits to be around 24 days.

The turnover of ^{125}I-SAP in the amyloid patients as a whole was significantly different from controls, and had considerable diagnostic sensitivity. Sixty-two percent of amyloid patients had significantly increased 6 hr plasma clearance of activity and 89% had increased WBR at 7 days. At least one of these 2 parameters was abnormal in over 90%.

Serial turnover studies in normals gave notably constant results, whereas in amyloid patients the proportion of injected ^{125}I-SAP sequestrated in amyloid deposits frequently increased after a 6-18 month interval suggesting an increased total body load of amyloid.

4. DISCUSSION

We describe here, for the first time, the plasma clearance and metabolism of radioiodinated human SAP. In normals the synthesis rate was 2 mg/hr and the protein was predominantly restricted to the vascular compartment. The FCR of 70% per day was more rapid than has been described for other plasma proteins. Striking alterations of SAP turnover were observed in patients with systemic AA and AL amyloidosis because a substantial proportion of the injected protein, which corresponded with the quantity of amyloid present, specifically localised to a large extravascular pool of SAP in the amyloid deposits and persisted there for long periods. Measurement of SAP turnover has the potential to assist diagnosis and to serially monitor the progress of amyloidosis *in vivo*.

REFERENCES

1. Pepys, M.B. and Baltz, M.L. (1983) Acute phase proteins with special reference to C-reactive protein and related proteins (pentaxins) and serum amyloid A protein. *Adv. Immunol.* **34**: 141-212.
2. Hind, C.R.K., Collins, P.M., Renn, D., Cook, R.B., Caspi, D., Baltz, M.L. and Pepys, M.B. (1984) Binding specificity of serum amyloid P component for the pyruvate acetal of galactose. *J. Exp. Med.* **159**: 1058-1069.

3. Hamazaki, H. (1987) Ca^{2+}-mediated association of human serum amyloid P component with heparan sulfate and dermatan sulfate. *J. Biol. Chem.* **262:** 1456-1460.
4. Pepys, M.B. and Butler, P.J.G. (1987) Serum amyloid P component is the major calcium-dependent specific DNA binding protein of the serum. *Biochem. Biophys. Res. Comm.* **148:** 308-313.
5. Breathnach, S.M., Kofler, H., Sepp, N., Ashworth, J., Woodrow, D., Pepys, M.B. and Hinter, H. (1989) Serum amyloid P component binds to cell nuclei *in vitro* and to *in vivo* deposits of extracellular chromatin in systemic lupus erythematosus. *J. Exp. Med.* **170:** 1433-1438.
6. Dyck, R.F., Lockwood, M., Kershaw, M., McHugh, N., Duance, V., Baltz, M.L. and Pepys, M.B. (1980) Amyloid P component is a constituent of normal human glomerular basement membrane. *J. Exp. Med.* **152:** 1162-1174.
7. Breathnach, S.M., Melrose, S.M., Bhogal, B., de Beer, F.C., Dyck, R.F., Tennent, G., Black, M.M. and Pepys, M.B. (1981) Amyloid P component is located on elastic fibre microfibrils of normal human tissues. *Nature* **293:** 652-654.
8. Breathnach, S.M., Pepys, M.B. and Hinter, H. (1989) Tissue amyloid P component in normal human dermis is non-covalently associated with elastic fiber microfibrils. *J. Invest. Dermatol.* **92:** 53-58.
9. Westermark, P., Shirahama, T., Skinner, M., Noren, P. and Cohen, A.S. (1981) Amyloid P-component (protein AP) in localized amyloidosis as revealed by an immunocytochemical method. *Histochemistry* **71:** 171-175.
10. Pepys, M.B., Baltz, M., de Beer, F.C., Dyck, R.F., Holford, S., Breathnach, S.M., Black, M.M., Tribe, C.R.F., Evans, D.J. and Feinstein, A. (1982) Biology of serum amyloid P component. *Ann. N.Y. Acad. Sci.* **389:** 286-297.
11. Coria, F., Castano, E., Prelli, F., Larrondo-Lillo, M., van Duinen, S., Shelanski, M.L. and Frangione, B. (1988) Isolation and characterization of amyloid P component from Alzheimer's disease and other types of cerebral amyloidosis. *Lab. Invest.* **58:** 454-458.
12. Caspi, D., Zalzman, S., Baratz, M., Teitelbaum, Z., Yaron, M., Pras, M., Baltz, M.L. and Pepys, M.B. (1987) Imaging of experimental amyloidosis with ^{131}I-labeled serum amyloid P component. *Arth. Rheum.* **30:** 1303-1306.
13. Hawkins, P.N., Myers, M.J., Epenetos, A.A., Caspi, D. and Pepys, M.B. (1988) Specific localization and imaging of amyloid deposits *in vivo* using ^{123}I-labeled serum amyloid P component. *J. Exp. Med.* **167:** 903-913.
14. Hawkins, P.N., Myers, M.J., Lavender, J.P. and Pepys, M.B. (1988) Diagnostic radionuclide imaging of amyloid: biological targeting by circulating human serum amyloid P component. *Lancet* **i:** 1413-1418.
15. Hawkins, P.N., Lavender, P.J. and Pepys, M.B. (1990) Evaluation of systemic amyloidosis by scintigraphy with ^{123}I-labeled serum amyloid P component. *New Engl. J. Med.* **323:** 508-513.
16. Hawkins, P.N., Wootton, R. and Pepys, M.B. (1990) Metabolic studies of radioiodinated serum amyloid P component in normal subjects and patients with systemic amyloidosis. *J. Clin. Invest.* (in press).

STRUCTURAL AND FUNCTIONAL STUDIES OF SERUM AMYLOID P COMPONENT

M.B. PEPYS, P.N. HAWKINS, G.A. TENNENT, S.R. NELSON, S. AMATAYAKUL-CHANTLER, R.A. DWEK, T.W. RADEMACHER & P.J.G. BUTLER
Immunological Medicine Unit, Royal Postgraduate Medical School, London, Biochemistry Department, University of Oxford, and Laboratory of Molecular Biology, Cambridge, U.K.

SAP isolated in pure form from pooled normal serum (5000 individual donors), from pooled malignant effusion fluids (500 individual donors) and from single individuals, including one with AA amyloidosis, was characterised with respect to the following properties: 1) its binding activity for the synthetic ligand, phosphoethanolamine-Sepharose and for AL amyloid fibrils; 2) its behaviour on reverse phase chromatography; 3) its isoelectric focussing pattern in urea polyacrylamide gels; 4) its metabolism in normal mice and mice with AA amyloidosis [1]; 5) its complete glycan structure. Remarkably, no heterogeneity or polymorphism was observed. Even the glycan, of which there is a single N-linked biantennary chain per SAP subunit, displays none of the microheterogeneity characteristic of almost all other known glycoproteins. SAP must thus have important function(s) strictly related to its structure. Carbohydrate analysis of AP samples from 3 different individuals predominantly showed a structure identical to SAP but another glycan with terminal N-acetyl glucosamine residues was also present at 3-4% and was not found in normal SAP or SAP from non-amyloid patients.

These studies, which are to be reported in detail elsewhere, add to the list of stable and conserved properties of SAP which include its presence as a very similar serum protein throughout the vertebrate phylum [2,3], the failure so far to detect any individual or species which lacks SAP or any protein polymorphism in SAP, and the stable circulating concentration of SAP seen even in patients with systemic amyloidosis in whom rates of clearance and synthesis may be greatly increased [4,5].

SAP is the single plasma protein which undergoes calcium-dependent binding to DNA *in vitro* [6] and it also binds to extracellular deposits of chromatin *in vivo* [7]. Furthermore, SAP solubilises native long chromatin at physiological ionic strength *in vitro*, selectively and completely displacing H1-type histone [8]. This interaction may contribute to physiological handling of chromatin released from cells *in vivo*, a function potentially of sufficient importance to account for the persistence, stability and homogeneity of SAP.

REFERENCES

1. Hawkins, P.N., Myers, M.J., Epenetos, A.A., Caspi, D. and Pepys, M.B. (1988) Specific localization and imaging of amyloid deposits *in vivo* using ^{123}I-labeled serum amyloid P component. *J. Exp. Med.,* **167:** 903-913.
2. Pepys, M.B., Dash, A.C., Fletcher, T.C., Richardson, N., Munn, E.A. and Feinstein, A. (1978) Analogues in other mammals and in fish of human plasma proteins, C-reactive protein and amyloid P component (protein SAP). *Nature,* **273:** 168-170.
3. Baltz, M.L., de Beer, F.C., Feinstein, A., Munn, E.A., Fletcher, T.C., Taylor, J., Bruton, C., Clamp, J.R., Davies, A.J.S. and Pepys, M.B. (1982) Phylogenetic aspects of C-reactive protein and related proteins. *Ann. N.Y. Acad. Sci.,* **389:** 49-75.
4. Hawkins, P.N., Myers, M.J., Lavender, J.P. and Pepys, M.B. (1988) Diagnostic radionuclide imaging of amyloid: biological targeting by circulating human serum amyloid P component. *Lancet,* **i:** 1413-1418.
5. Hawkins, P.N., Wootton, R. and Pepys, M.B. (1990) Metabolic studies of radioiodinated serum amyloid P component in normal subjects and patients with systemic amyloidosis. *J. Clin. Invest.* (in press).
6. Pepys, M.B. and Butler, P.J.G. (1987) Serum amyloid P component is the major calcium-dependent specific DNA binding protein of the serum. *Biochem. Biophys. Res. Comm.,* **148:** 308-313.
7. Breathnach, S.M., Kofler, H., Sepp, N., Ashworth, J., Woodrow, D., Pepys, M.B. and Hinter, H. (1989) Serum amyloid P component binds to cell nuclei *in vitro* and to *in vivo* deposits of extracellular chromatin in systemic lupus erythematosus. *J. Exp. Med.,* **170:** 1433-1438.
8. Butler, P.J.G., Tennent, G.A. and Pepys, M.B. (1990) Pentraxin-chromatin interactions. Serum amyloid P component specifically displaces H1-type histones and solubilizes native long chromatin. *J. Exp. Med.,* **172:** 13-18.

QUANTIFICATION OF AMYLOID P-COMPONENT IN MULTIPLE TISSUES OF PATIENTS WITH PRIMARY AND FAMILIAL AMYLOIDOIS

Suzanne Curtis Gray
Evangelia C. Mantzouranis *
Alan S. Cohen
Martha Skinner

From the Arthritis Center and Department of Medicine and *Department of Pediatrics, Boston University School of Medicine, Boston, MA 02118 USA

ABSTRACT

Amyloid P component (AP) is a constitutive plasma protein that has been closely linked to deposits of amyloid fibrils. This study examines the amount of AP in three tissues (spleen, liver and heart) of two patients, one with primary (AL) and one with familial (ATtr) amyloidosis. AP was found in all three tissues of both patients. This is the first time it has been quantified in amyloidotic cardiac tissues of any type. The amount of AP in the ATtr heart equaled or exceeded the amounts in the AL heart. The consistently large amount of AP associated with all tissues of all types of amyloidosis may provide a clue to pathogenetic mechanisms involved in light chain and transthyretin (Ttr) fibrillogenesis.

INTRODUCTION

We have previously shown that large amounts of AP can be recovered from the saline and citrate washes of amyloid-rich tissue (Skinner et al, 1983). However, no quantification of AP has been determined in washes from amyloidotic cardiac tissues nor have multiple tissues from one individual been examined.

The availability of autopsy tissues from patients we had evaluated in the Clinical Research Center of the Thorndike Memorial Laboratories at Boston City Hospital allowed us to carry out this study on two patients who both had severe amyloidotic cardiomyopathy.

MATERIALS AND METHODS

Source of AP

Amyloid-rich tissues, heart, liver and spleen, were obtained at autopsy from each of two individuals who died of systemic amyloidosis. One patient had AL amyloidosis with amyloid fibrils composed of lambda light chains. His amyloid disease was diagnosed at age 68 by kidney biopsy and involved his kidneys, heart, gastrointestinal tract and muscles. He survived 16 months and died from congestive heart failure. The second patient had ATtr amyloidosis with the recently identified mutation of alanine for valine at position 30 (Jones, et al 1990). His amyloid disease was diagnosed at age 29 by an abdominal fat aspiration and involved his heart and peripheral and autonomic nervous system. He died 10 years later due to cardiomyopathy.

Isolation of AP

Isolation of AP from the amyloid-rich tissues was performed as previously described (Skinner, et al 1983). Briefly, twenty gram wet weight samples were cut from each of the six tissues which had been fresh frozen at autopsy. Tissues were repeatedly homogenized and centrifuged in 0.14 M saline twice, then in 0.05 M sodium citrate, 0.01 M Tris (hydroxymethyl) aminomethane (Tris) buffered saline (TBS), pH 8.0 twice and then in saline until the optical density of the supernatant solution was less than 0.1 @ 280nm. This usually required 10-15 homogenizations. Supernatants from the first 8 washes were dialyzed and lyophilized for the subsequent isolation and quantification of AP. Amyloid fibrils were isolated from the sediment similar to a procedure previously published by Pras, et al (1968).

Rocket immunoelectrophoresis

Rocket immunoelectrophoresis was performed according to a modified version of the technique of Laurel (1972). Briefly, a gel of 1% agarose in 0.075M veronal buffer, 0.01 M EDTA, pH 8.6 containing 1% goat anti human P component serum was poured between two 11 cm x 20.5 cm glass plates one of which was covered with a sheet of gel bond affixed with glycerol. Ten microliter aliquots of sample material were pipetted into 4 mm wells cut into the agarose gel, arranged in one or two parallel rows. Each sample was tested in triplicate. A standard curve was prepared using serial dilutions of purified human AP.

Electrophoresis was performed for approximately 5 hours at 60 mA using the same veronal buffer. The glass plate which carried the gel bond with agarose was then placed in a glass dish and compressed beneath weighted, veronal buffer soaked paper towels overnight to assure good adherence of the gel to the gel bond. It was then washed three times in 300 ml of 0.14 M saline, twice in 300 ml deionized water, and dried flat with a hand held dryer. The gel was stained with Coomassie blue, destained and dried a final time. A standard curve was prepared using serial dilutions of purified human AP. The height of the rockets was measured and compared to the standard curve to determine the amount of AP in each wash.

RESULTS

Significant amounts of P-component were detected in samples from all tissues tested. From the 20gm wet weight AL tissues we found 16.22 mg AP in the heart, 10.88 mg AP in the spleen, and 2.02 mg in the liver. In the ATtr tissues we found 35.59 mg AP in the heart, 0.69 mg AP in the spleen, and 0.54 mg in the liver. In most tissues the largest amount of AP was found in the citrate washes as might be expected. In addition, the most AP was found in tissues containing the largest amounts of amyloid fibrils (Table 1).

TABLE 1 Quantification of AP in AL and ATtr Amyloid Tissues

Tissue	Fibrils (mg)	AP (mg)	AP/Fibril (%)
AIg lambda			
heart	1492	16.22	1.1
liver	348	2.20	0.6
spleen	409	10.88	2.7
ATtr ala 30			
heart	1898	35.59	1.9
liver	558	0.54	0.1
spleen	478	0.69	0.1

DISCUSSION

This study represents the first time that multiple tissues from one individual have been examined for AP. It is also the first time cardiac tissues have been examined for precise quantification of AP. In addition, detailed data has been obtained on the presence of AP in tissues from a patient with ATtr.

Our results showed that, except in the AL spleen tissue, the greatest amounts of P-component were found in tissues with the largest amounts of amyloid. This confirms the intimate relationship of these two proteins. We also found a large amount of AP in cardiac tissue. It should be noted that both patients we studied had large quantities of amyloid in their heart tissue.

Whether or not AP plays a role in the pathogenesis of amyloidosis is not known. It has been suggested that AP could be the framework on which the amyloid is deposited. Another possibility is that AP simply associates with the amyloid fibrils by a calcium dependent binding much like other charged substances attach to negatively charged amyloid fibrils.

ACKNOWLEDGEMENTS

Supported by grants from the U.S. Public Health Service, NIAMDD (AM 07014), the General Clinical Centers Branch of the Division of Research Resources, National Institutes of Health (RR 533), the Multipurpose Arthritis Center, National Institutes of Health (AM 20613), National Institutes of Health (AR 38551) and the Arthritis Foundation.

REFERENCES

1. Jones LA, Skare J, Harding J, Cohen AS, Skinner M: (1990). A new substitution at position 30 in the transthyretin (TTR) protein associated with familial amyloid polyneuropathy. Arthritis Rheum (in press).
2. Laurell C-B: (1972). Electroimmuno Assay. Scand J Clin Lab Inves. 29, suppl 124, 21-37.
3. Pras M, Schubert M, Zucker-Franklin D, Rimon A, Franklin EC: (1968). The characterization of soluble amyloid prepared in water. The Journal of Clinical Investigation 47:924-933.
4. Skinner M, Shirahama T, Cohen AS, Deal CL: (1983). The Association of Amyloid P-component (AP) with amyloid fibril: An updated method for amyloid fibril protein isolation. Preparative Biochemistry, 12 (5),461-476.

A PRIMED STATE EXISTS *IN VIVO* FOLLOWING REGRESSION OF MURINE AA AMYLOIDOSIS

P.N. HAWKINS & M.B. PEPYS
Immunological Medicine Unit, Department of Medicine
Royal Postgraduate Medical School, Hammersmith Hospital
London W12 0NN
U.K.

ABSTRACT. Using a sensitive, quantitative, and non-invasive *in vivo* method, based on the specific binding of radiolabelled serum amyloid P component to amyloid fibrils, we have directly documented the spontaneous resolution of AA amyloid deposits in mice, and the prolonged existence thereafter of a primed state of enhanced susceptibility to further amyloid deposition. These results may have important implications for understanding and management of amyloidosis in man.

1. INTRODUCTION

Because amyloid has hitherto been demonstrable only by histological examination, the pathogenesis of its deposition is poorly understood, and there is no direct evidence that it can regress. We have lately developed a novel, non-invasive method for *in vivo* detection and quantitative monitoring of amyloidosis using labelled serum amyloid P component (SAP) as a tracer. SAP is the circulating precursor of amyloid P component (AP) [1,2] and undergoes specific non-covalent, calcium-dependent binding to amyloid fibrils *in vitro* [3]; intravenously injected SAP localises rapidly and specifically to amyloid deposits *in vivo* [4-8]. The amount of SAP retained correlates with the overall quantity of amyloid in particular tissues or organs [6-8]. We report here the use of this approach to study the natural history of AA amyloid in the mouse.

2. MATERIALS AND METHODS

2.1. Mice

AA amyloid was induced by i.v. injection of amyloid enhancing factor (AEF) followed by s.c. $AgNO_3$ [9] in 80 female CBA/Ca mice. A similar untreated group served as controls. Amyloid was identified histologically using Congo red [10].

Table 1. Whole body clearance and localisation of ^{125}I-human SAP

	Whole body activity 24 hr after ^{125}I-SAP (% injected dose)	Organ counts at autopsy (% injected dose/gm tissue) Liver	Spleen
6 weeks after AEF/$AgNO_3$			
Treated mice	71.6 (11.2)	21.6 (9.36)	227.2 (66)
Controls	30.4 (3.9)	0.43 (0.14)	0.79 (0.27)
	$P < 0.01$	$P < 0.001$	$P < 0.001$
8 months after AEF/$AgNO_3$			
Treated mice	31.6 (5.8)	0.42 (0.14)	2.47 (0.94)
Controls	29.6 (4.5)	0.39 (0.08)	0.8 (0.24)
	NS	NS	$P < 0.01$
9 months - after limited casein challenge			
Treated mice	73.7 (8.7)	21.1 (4.8)	313.3 (69.2)
Controls	33.1 (5.9)	0.34 (0.13)	1.02 (0.51)
	$P < 0.01$	$P < 0.001$	$P < 0.001$

Values are mean (SD) for each group of 6 mice. Major amyloid was present histologically in the livers and spleens of all treated mice 6 weeks after AEF/$AgNO_3$ treatment, though there was none 8 months later; 3 weeks after limited casein treatment extensive amyloid had re-accumulated. There was no amyloid in any controls.

2.2. SAP clearance studies

Purified human SAP was radiolabelled with ^{125}I and given i.v. to groups of amyloid and control mice [11]. Radioactivity was measured *in vivo* using an ARMAC whole body counter [11] and in the spleen, liver and kidneys following subsequent autopsy [6,11]. The significance of differences in whole body clearance and organ distribution of ^{125}I-SAP was sought using Student's t-test.

3. RESULTS

Six weeks after induction of amyloid, mice injected with ^{125}I-SAP retained over 70% of the injected dose at 24 hr, after which there was a monoexponential decline with a half-time of about 11 days. Approximately 40-45% of the ^{125}I-SAP was localised at 24 hr to the amyloidotic livers and spleens of treated mice, compared to less than 1% in the controls, and there was no uptake elsewhere. The distribution and clearance of ^{125}I-SAP 8 months after AEF/$AgNO_3$ treatment and in further mice from this same cohort 4 weeks later after 5 daily subcutaneous injections of casein is shown in Table 1.

4. DISCUSSION

Heterologous ^{125}I-human SAP provides an excellent marker for monitoring amyloid deposits *in vivo* because the large proportion of SAP which has deposited in mouse amyloid is protected from the rapid breakdown and excretion it undergoes in normal control mice. These studies demonstrated that AEF induced systemic AA amyloid deposits in mice can regress over a 6 month period up to a point where they are no longer demonstrable by light microscopy, using the benchmark Congo red stain. However, despite such apparent resolution, significantly abnormal ^{125}I-SAP localisation remained present and a second limited inflammatory stimulus [12], at a level far below that required in previously untreated animals, was capable of inducing major deposits of new amyloid. This suggests that human AA amyloid might also regress if the provoking stimulus abated or was suppressed, but that, thereafter, careful observation and active anti-inflammatory treatment may be necessary to prevent relapse. Human studies with labelled SAP should objectively document both remission and progression in man.

REFERENCES

1. Pepys, M.B. (1988) Amyloidosis. ***In*** *Immunological Diseases, 4th ed.* (M. Samter, D.W. Talmage, M.M. Frank, K.F. Austen, & H.N. Claman, editors), Little Brown & Co., Boston, pp. 631-674.
2. Coria, F., Castano, E., Prelli, F., Larrondo-Lillo, M., Van Duinen, S., Shelanski, M.L. & Frangione, B. (1988) Isolation and characterization of amyloid P component from Alzheimer's disease and other types of cerebral amyloidosis. *Lab. Invest.* **58**: 454-458.
3. Pepys, M.B., Dyck, R.F., de Beer, F.C., Skinner, M. & Cohen, A.S. (1979) Binding of serum amyloid P component (SAP) by amyloid fibrils. *Clin. Exp. Immunol.* **38**: 284-293.

4. Baltz, M.L., Caspi, D., Evans, D.J., Rowe, I.F., Hind, C.R.K. & Pepys, M.B. (1986) Circulating serum amyloid P component is the precursor of amyloid P component in tissue amyloid deposits. *Clin. Exp. Immunol.* **66**: 691-700.
5. Caspi, D., Zalzman, S., Baratz, M., Teitelbaum, Z., Yaron, M., Pras, M., Baltz, M.L. & Pepys, M.B. (1987) Imaging of experimental amyloidosis with ^{131}I-serum amyloid P component. *Arth. Rheum.* **30**: 1303-1306.
6. Hawkins, P.N., Myers, M.J., Epenetos, A.A., Caspi, D. & Pepys, M.B. (1988) Specific localization and imaging of amyloid deposits *in vivo* using ^{123}I-labeled serum amyloid P component. *J. Exp. Med.* **167**: 903-913.
7. Hawkins, P.N., Myers, M.J., Lavender, J.P. & Pepys, M.B. (1988) Diagnostic radionuclide imaging of amyloid: biological targeting by circulating human serum amyloid P component. *Lancet.* **i**: 1413-1418.
8. Hawkins, P.N., Lavender, P.J. & Pepys, M.B. (1990) Evaluation of systemic AA and AL amyloidosis by scintigraphy with iodine-123-serum amyloid P component. *New Engl. J. Med.* **323**: 508-513.
9. Axelrad, M.A., Kisilevsky, R., Willmer, J., Chen, S.J. & Skinner, M. (1982) Further characterisation of amyloid-enhancing factor. *Lab. Invest.* **47**: 139-146.
10. Puchtler, H., Sweat, F. & Levine, M. (1962) On the binding of Congo red by amyloid. *J. Histochem. Cytochem.* **10**: 355-365.
11. Hawkins, P.N. & Pepys, M.B. (1990) A primed state exists *in vivo* following histological regression of amyloidosis. *Clin. Exp. Immunol.* **81**: 325-328.
12. Janigan, D.T. (1965) Experimental amyloidosis. Studies with a modified casein method, casein hydrolysate and gelatin. *Am. J. Pathol.* **47**: 159-171.

SERUM AMYLOID P-COMPONENT (SAP) REGULATION BY SEX-STEROIDS IN RATS : COMPARED WITH C-REACTIVE PROTEIN (CRP)

Shigeru HASHIMOTO, Yoshihiro TAKAHASHI, Etsuro NISHIDA, and Shunsuke MIGITA *

Department of Obstetrics and Gynecology, Kanazawa University, School of Medicine, 13 - 1, Takara-machi, Kanazawa, 920 JAPAN : * Department of Molecular Immunology, Cancer Research Institute, Kanazawa University, Kanazawa.

ABSTRACT. In order to investigate the effects of sex-steroids on SAP level in rats, SAP was purified from Wistar rats by affinity chromatography of phosphorylcholine. Sample sera were obtained from 180 young and old rats, after which, rats were injected with either estradiol (E2), testosterone (T), or dehydroepiandrosterone (DHA). Sera were serially obtained from the tail vessels until the 8th day after injection. The SAP level was assayed by micro single radial immunodiffusion. As the rats aged, the SAP levels increased from 2.9 mg/dl at 11 weeks to 10.7 mg/dl at 58 weeks. In 37-week-old rats, the SAP levels in females (6.3 ± 1.8mg/dl) were significantly ($p < 0.001$) higher than those in males (3.9 ± 1.0mg/dl), whereas the CRP levels in females (49.8 mg/dl) were lower than those in males (61.5 mg/dl). The SAP levels did not change after T administration, but decreased significantly ($p < 0.001$) to 70% of the prelevel after DHA injection. The SAP levels increased rapidly by E2 administration, especially in young male rats (increased to 189%). Serum E2 levels in young (11wk) male rats were very low before E2 injection, and steeply rose on the 2nd day. From these findings, the different SAP levels in mature female and male rats are attributed to E2.

INTRODUCTION

In opposition to human SAP [1], the SAP in Syrian hamsters is designated as a female protein, being high in females and at almost a zero level in males. These high levels in females decreased through testosterone injection [2]. In rats, SAP and CRP-related pentraxin are both glycoprotein, and which pentraxin is a real SAP is somewhat controversial [3]. We investigated whether the normal levels of SAP in rats differ according to sex, and examined the effects of sex-steroids on SAP concentration comparing with the CRP.

MATERIALS AND METHODS

1. <u>Purification and Antisera.</u> SAP was purified from Wistar rats by affinity chromatography using phosphorylcholine conjugated Sepharose 6B, followed by gel filtration [4]. Contaminating CRP was absorbed using anti-rat CRP antibody. Monoclonal antibody to rat CRP [5] was presented by Dr. W. Nonomura, Tumor Laboratory, Tokyo. Purity of the prepared sample was analysed by SDS PAGE,

revealing a single band of 26,700 dalton corresponding to a SAP monomer. Antisera against purified rat SAP were raised by injections into rabbits.

2. Quantification of Rat SAP. The SAP level was estimated by micro single radial immunodiffusion method using anti-rat SAP serum in 2% agarose gel [6]. A pooled mixture of 15-week-old female rats was used as the standard. The SAP levels measured in 20 lots of the standard were relatively constant at 2.9 to 3.3 mg/dl (95 to 106 %). Groups of 20 normal rats, each of both sexes, were bled by heart puncture at the age of 11, 28, 37, 52, 56, 58, and 73 weeks. Five 11-week-old male rats and five 56-week-old female rats were injected with 0.5ml turpentine oil subcutaneously, and were bled from the tail vein on the 1st, 2nd, 3rd, 5th, and 8th day after the injection. Rat CRP was also quantified as the same schedule.

3. Effects of Sex Steroids. Groups of five 11-week-old male and 56-week-old female rats were given one (0.5mg/0.05ml) subcutaneous injection of estradiol valerate (E2). Each animal was then bled serially until the 8th day after injection. Groups of five 11-week-old and 56-week-old female rats were injected with testosterone oenanthate (T) at amounts of 25mg/0.2ml, or 40mg/0.32ml. A group of five 56-week-old female rats was injected with 3.5mg/0.7ml of dehydroepiandrosterone acetate (DHA). These rats were bled from the tail on the same schedule as those received E2.

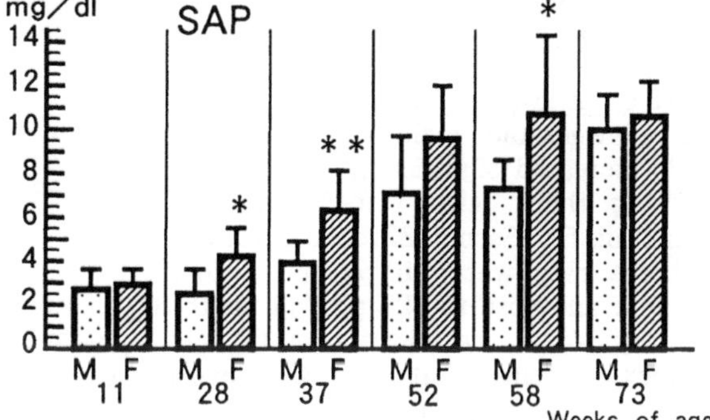

Fig. 1. Serum concentration of SAP in normal rats. Levels of male (M) and female (F) SAP. * P < 0.01, ** < 0.001 compared with male rats. Each value is the mean ± 1SD of 10 normal rats.

RESULTS

1. Serum concentrations of SAP or CRP in Rats. Serum SAP levels in normal rats increased with age (Fig. 1). Significant higher levels in females than in males were observed at 28, 37, and 58 weeks. Whereas, the CRP levels in females were lower than those in males (Fig. 2). In 28-week-old rats, the CRP levels of females (54.6 ± 15.6mg/dl) were significantly ($p < 0.01$) lower than those of males (73.2 ± 13.6mg/dl).

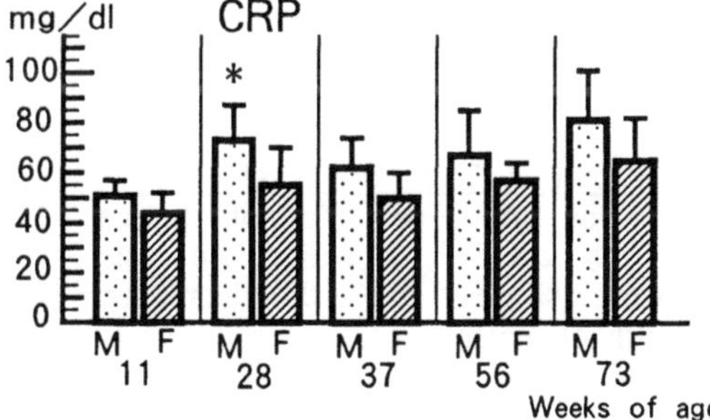

Fig. 2. Serum concentration of CRP in normal rats. Each value is the mean ± 1SD of 10 rats. * P < 0.01 compared with female rats.

2. Effect of a Turpentine injection on the level of SAP or CRP. After a subcutaneous injection of turpentine oil (0.5ml) into 11-week-old male rats, the

SAP levels increased slightly to 123% on the 3rd day, and further increased to 130% compared with the preinjected level of 100% (Fig. 3).

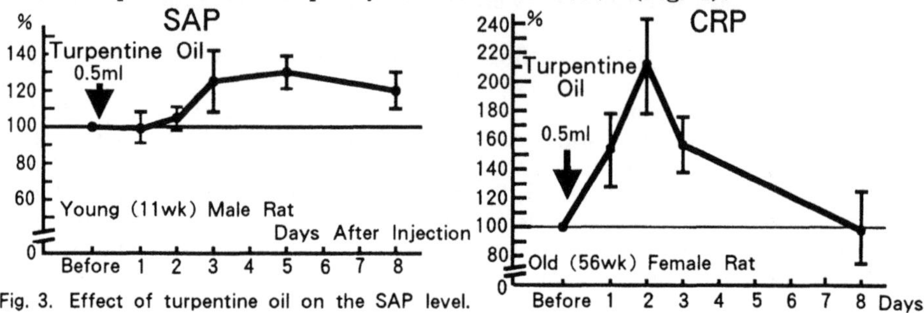

Fig. 3. Effect of turpentine oil on the SAP level. The means and 1SD of 5 rats are shown.

Fig. 4. Effect of a turpentine on the CRP level.

After a injection of 0.5ml turpentine into 56-week-old female rats, the CRP levels steeply increased and reached their peaks on the 2nd day after injection, showing $211 \pm 34\%$ (Fig. 4).

3. Effect of E2 on the level of SAP or CRP. After the injection of 0.5mg E2 into 11-week-old male rats, the SAP levels increased significantly ($p < 0.001$), reaching their peaks (189%) after 5 days (Fig. 5). Serum E2 concentrations of these rats were 10 pg/ml before injection and rose to 227 pg/ml on the 2nd day. After the injection of E2 into 56-week-old female rats, the SAP levels increased reaching their peaks (149%) on the 3rd day. The serum E2 levels were 51 pg/ml before injection and 918 pg/ml on the 3rd day. The estrogen effect to increase the SAP level was greater in young male rats than in old female rats. The CRP levels did not change after E2 administration in 11-week-old male rats.

Fig. 5. Effect of estradiol on the SAP level. The means and 1SD of 5 rats are shown.

4. The Effect of T on the level of SAP or CRP. The SAP levels did not change significantly after T injection, but the levels were slightly ($P < 0.05$) decreased on the 8th day after injection in 11-week-old female rats. The CRP levels did not change after T injection in 56-week-old female rats.

5. The Effects of DHA on the SAP in 56-week-old Female Rats. Serum SAP levels decreased to 78% of the prelevel on the 3rd day, and further decreased significantly ($p < 0.001$) to 70% on the 8th day after DHA injection (Fig. 6).

Fig. 6. Effect of DHA on the SAP level.

DISCUSSION

In humans, older subjects have higher serum SAP levels [1]. In this study, the SAP level in rats showed the same tendency as that of humans. Ponted et al. reported the doubling of rat SAP levels after turpentine injection[3]. Conversely, Beer et al. reported that SAP levels showed no significant increase in rats after croton oil injection [7]. In our study, rat SAP levels increased to 130% of the prelevel on the 5th day after turpentine injection. On the other hand, the CRP levels steeply increased and reached their peaks on the 2nd day after injection. The levels of CRP in 56-week-old rats (57.1mg/dl) are much greater than those of human CRP, and further elevatd to 120.5mg/dl by turpenetine injection. The levels of this greater amount pentraxin (CRP), were higher in males than in females. In Syrian hamsters, the SAP level is higher in females than in females [2]. Although the E2 level in female hamsters fell after ovariectomy, the SAP level did not decrease. In male hamsters, the SAP level increased after orchiectomy, and decreased by T administration. These data indicated that T has a suppressor effect on the SAP level. In hamsters, E2 did not act as a primary stimulus for SAP synthesis. In our study of mature (28wk, 37wk) rats, the SAP levels of females were significantly higher than those of males. The SAP levels increased rapidly by E2 administration, especially in young male rats . However the SAP levels were not changed by T. Serum E2 levels in young (11wk) male rats were very low before E2 injection, and steeply rose on the 2nd day after injection. From these findings, serum level of rat SAP is greatly influenced by E2. The different SAP levels in mature female and male rats are attributed to E2. On the other hand, SAP levels were remarkably decreased by DHA. It is speculated that DHA has other effects besides those of E2 or T. The synthesis of some proteins such as α_1-acid glycoprotein may be controlled by two different routes, namely the acute phase reactant route, which is mediated by interleukin 1, and the sex-steroid hormone route, which is mediated intracellular receptors. It is postulated that the serum concentration of SAP in rats is also regulated by these two routes.

REFERENCES

1. Migita, S., Hashimoto, S., Hisazumi, H., Harada, M., and Okabe, H. (1986) ' Human SAP as an acute phase reactant in the female', in G.G. Glenner, et al.(ed.), Amyloidosis, Plenum Press, New York, pp. 87 – 97.
2. Coe, J.E.(1977) 'A sex-limited serum protein of Syrian hamsters : Definition of female protein and regulation by test.', Proc Natl Acad Sci USA 74, 730 – 733.
3. Pontet, M., D'asnieres, M., Gache, D., Escaig, J., and Engler, R. (1981) 'A new pentraxin (SAP) in the rat : evidence for two quaternary structures and effect of ligands on self-association', Biochim Biophys Acta 671, 202 – 210.
4. Hashimoto, S. , and Migita, S. (1990) 'Serum amyloid P component regulation by sex steroids in rats', Acta Haematol. Jpn 53, 89 – 97.
5. Hirai, H., Nonomura, W., and Hatakeyama, M. (1986) Monoclonal antibodies to human CRP and some characterization of a rat serum protein related to CRP', Protides of the Biological Fluids 34, 283 – 286.
6. Hashimoto, S., and Migita, S. (1979) ' Changes of thirty-nine serum protein components following surgical stress', Acta Haematol Jpn 42, 667 – 677.
7. Beer, F.C.D., Baltz, M.L., Munn, E.A., Feinstein, A., Taylor, J., Bruton, C., Clamp, J.R., and Pepys, M.B. (1982) ' Isolation and characterization of CRP and serum amyloid P component in the rat', Immunology 45, 55 – 70.

ACUTE PHASE PROTEIN RESPONSE TO COLLAGEN INDUCED ARTHRITIS IN MICE

Gonnerman WA[*+], Cathcart ES[‡+], Sipe JD[*], Mortensen RF[&], Hayes KC[#]. Departments of Biochemistry[*] and Medicine[‡], Boston University School of Medicine, Boston MA; Edith Nourse Rogers Memorial VA Hospital[+], Bedford MA; Department of Microbiology[&], Ohio State University, Columbus OH; and Foster Biomedical Laboratories[#], Brandeis University, Waltham MA.

ABSTRACT. Arthritis susceptible B10.RIII mice develop chronic inflammatory arthritis in response to a single immunization with native type II collagen. We have measured plasma levels (by ELISA) of two acute phase proteins in the mouse, amyloid P component (AP) and serum amyloid A protein (SAA), prior to immunization with native bovine type II collagen (100 ug) emulsified in complete Freund's adjuvant and during the development of collagen induced arthritis (CIA). Plasma AP levels were elevated after 1 day, reached a maximum after 2 days and remained elevated at 3, 8, 42 and 63 days after immunization. In contrast SAA levels were elevated at 1 and 2 days, but returned to control levels after 3 and 8 days and increased again at 42 and 63 days. Neither the plasma AP nor SAA levels were related to CIA severity or the presence of arthritis. These differences in responses of AP and SAA suggest that these proteins respond to different control signals and that neither of them are accurate predictors of arthritis severity.

INTRODUCTION

Immunization of genetically susceptible strains of rats [1], mice [2,3], and monkeys [4, 5] with native type II collagen results in development of a chronic polyarthritis. We have measured serum responses of two acute phase proteins, amyloid P component (AP) and serum amyloid A protein (SAA), immediately after immunization with type II collagen (CII), during the early induction phase of CIA and after symptoms of arthritis were apparent.

MATERIALS AND METHODS

Animals: Arthritis-susceptible B10.RIII mice (obtained from Dr. Chella David, Rochester, MN) were maintained under standard conditions. Protocol: Thirty male and thirty female mice were immunized intradermally with 100 ug CII in complete Freund's adjuvant (CFA) (100 ul). Blood samples were taken from the tail vein (4-8 animals/group) immediately prior to immunization, 1, 2, 3, 8, 42 and 63 days after immunization. Beginning 3 weeks after immunization, arthritis severity was assessed twice weekly by a subjective scoring of swelling of each paw on a 0 to 4+ basis. Data are calculated as the mean of the maximum score attained by each animal during the course of the experiment and included all animals.

Measurement of AP and SAA: Plasma AP levels were measured by ELISA [6]. Plasma SAA levels were also measured by ELISA [7].

Statistical Analysis: Statistical significance ($p < 0.05$) of the differences of means between groups was calculated using either Student's t-test or one-way analysis of variance and Duncan's multiple range test.

RESULTS

Plasma AP and SAA Levels: The time course of serum SAA and AP levels is shown in Figure 1. As expected, 1 day after immunization with CII in CFA, circulating SAA and AP levels were markedly elevated ($p < 0.05$). Maximum elevation in AP levels occurred 2 days after immunization but levels remained elevated throughout the course of the experiment. Maximum elevation in SAA levels occurred 1 day after immunization but decreased to control levels by 3 days and were not elevated again until 42 and 63 days.

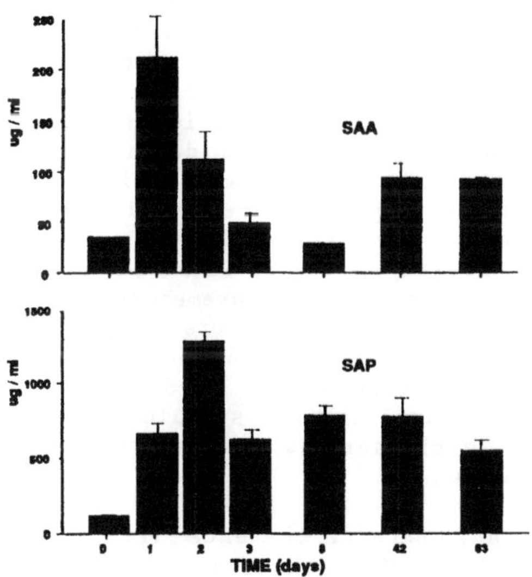

Figure 1. Comparison of time course of increases in AP and SAA following immunization. Values are means ± standard errors.

DISCUSSION

The dichotomy in the time course of response of AP and SAA strongly suggests that the two acute phase proteins are responding to different control signals. In response to an acute inflammatory stimulus, synthesis of both proteins is dramatically increased. If the stimulus were purely inflammatory, one would expect levels of both proteins to return to normal levels as the stimulus diminishes. However, if there is an immunological component to the stimulus as is the case when type II collagen is combined with CFA, then AP levels, but not SAA levels, remain markedly elevated. Precedent for separation of inflammatory and immunological stimuli in the "acute phase response" is established by the demonstration that inflammatory and immunological activities reside in different portions of the Il-1 molecule [8], which, along with IL-6, is one of the primary controlling factors for hepatic synthesis of acute phase proteins [9-11].

The role of acute phase proteins in CIA is somewhat controversial. In studies by Bliven et al [12], AP levels and arthritis severity were poorly correlated. In the MRL/lpr mouse, which develops a spontaneous autoimmune disease resembling human rheumatoid arthritis, the severity of this form of arthritis correlated well with increased AP levels [13]. Inhibitors of eicosanoid synthesis that decrease arthritis severity also decrease SAP levels [14]. In this study we found no correlation between arthritis and AP or SAA levels. At both 42 and 63 days, animals with and without overt symptoms of arthritis were likely to have markedly elevated AP or SAA levels. In general, we do not consider AP to behave in CIA as a classical acute phase protein. The response of acute phase proteins may vary depending upon the activation stimulus, as with expression of mRNA for SAA_3, in which chronic stimuli induce higher levels than do acute stimuli [15].

The key factor in determination of whether the acute phase response to CFA and collagen immunization switches to an systemic polyarthritis may be the level and duration of increased IL-1 production by activated MØs. Administration of IL-1 immediately prior to the expected onset of symptoms increased the incidence of CIA [16].

We have not shown a correlation between increased acute phase protein levels and severity of CIA as we would have expected if MØ IL-1 were a controlling factor for both parameters. However, synthesis of acute phase proteins may depend on factors other than IL-1, e.g., IL-6. Our data also suggest that AP and SAA do not respond to the same signals. Controlling signals may be different in true "acute" situations following an inflammatory stimulus and a "chronic" disease state such as CIA in which there is an antigenic component as well as an inflammatory component.

We gratefully acknowledge the excellent technical support of Louise M. Greene and Greta Knapschaefer. This work was supported by the Veterans Administration and by Public Health Service Grant AG06860.

REFERENCES

1. Trentham, D.E., Townes, A.S., and Kang, A.H. (1977) Autoimmunity to type II collagen: an experimental model of arthritis. J. Exp. Med. 146,857-868.

2. Courtenay, J.S., Dallman, M.J., Dayan, A.D., Martin, A., Mosedale,

(1980) Immunisation against heterologous type II collagen induces arthritis in mice. Nature. 283,666-668.
3. Wooley, P.H., Luthra, H.S, Stuart, J.M, David, C.S. (1981) Type II collagen-induced arthritis in mice. I. Major histocompatibility complex (I region) linkage and antibody correlates. J. Exp. Med. 154,688-700.
4. Cathcart, E.S., Hayes, K.C., Gonnerman, W.A., Lazzari, A.A., Franzblau, C. (1986) Experimental arthritis in a nonhuman primate. I. Induction by bovine type II collagen. Lab. Invest. 54,26-31.
5. Rubin, A.S., Healy, C.T., Martin, L.T., Baskin, G.B., Roberts, E.D. (1987) Experimental arthropathy induced in Rhesus monkeys (Macaca mulatta) by intradermal immunization with native bovine type II collagen. Lab. Invest. 57,524-534.
6. Mortensen, R.F., Shapiro, J., Lin, B.F., Douches, S., Neta, S. (1988) Interaction of recombinant IL-1 and recombinant tumor necrosis factor in the induction of mouse acute phase proteins. J. Immunol. 140,2260-2266.
7. Sipe, J.D., Ignaczak, T.F., Pollock, P.S., Glenner, G.G. (1976) Amyloid fibril protein AA: purification and properties of the antigenically related serum component as determined by solid phase radioimmunoassay. J. Immunol. 116,1151-1156.
8. Boraschi, D., Nencioni, L., Villa, L., et al. (1988) In vivo stimulation and restoration of the immune response by the non-inflammatory fragment 163-171 of human IL-1B. J. Exp. Med. 168,675-686.
9. Sipe, J.D., Vogel, S.N., Sztein, M.B., Skinner, M., Cohen, A.S. (1982) The role of interleukin 1 in acute phase serum amyloid A (SAA) and serum amyloid P (SAP) biosynthesis. Ann. N.Y. Acad.Sci.389,137-150.
10. Ramadori, G., Sipe, J.D., Dinarello, C.A., Mizel, S.B., Colten, H.R. (1985) Pretranslational modulation of acute phase hepatic protein synthesis by murine recombinant interleukin-1 (IL-1) and purified human IL-1. J. Exp. Med. 162,930-942.
11. Gauldie, J., Richards, C., Harnish, D., Lansdorp, P., Baumann, H. (1987) Interferon beta 2 and B-cell stimulation factor-2 shares identity with hepatocyte-stimulating factor and regulates the major acute phase protein response in liver cells. Proc. Natl. Acad. Sci. USA. 84,7251-7256.
12. Bliven, M.L., Wooley, P.H., Pepys, M.B., Otterness, I.G. (1986) Murine type II collagen arthritis. Association of an acute-phase response with clinical course. Arthritis. Rheum. 29,1131-1138.
13. Rordorf-Adam, C., Serban, D., Pataki, A., Gruninger, M. (1985) Serum amyloid P component and autoimmune parameters in the assessment of arthritis activity in MRL/lpr/lpr mice. Clin. Exp.Immunol. 61,509-16.
14. Griswold, D.E., Hillegass, L.M., Meunier, P.C., DiMartino, M.J., Hanna, N. (1988) Effects of inhibitors of eicosanoid metabolism in murine collagen-induced arthritis. Arthritis. Rheum. 31,1406-1412.
15. Rokita, H., Shirahama, T., Cohen, A.S., Meek, R.L., Benditt, E.P., Sipe, J.D. (1987) Differential expression of the amyloid SAA 3 gene in liver and peritoneal macrophages of mice undergoing dissimilar inflammatory episodes. J. Immunol. 139,3849-3853.
16. Hom, J.T., Bendele, A.M., Carlson, D.G. (1988) In vivo administration with IL-1 accelerates the development of collagen-induced arthritis in mice. J. Immunol. 141,834-841.

AN ATTEMPT TO STUDY THE ROLE OF SERUM AMYLOID P COMPONENT IN THE FORMATION OF AMYLOID DEPOSITS IN A TRANSGENIC MOUSE MODEL OF FAMILIAL AMYLOIDOTIC POLYNEUROPATHY

Murakami T[1,2], Nishiguchi S[1,2], Yi S[2,4], Maeda S[1], Araki S[2], Yamamura K[3], Takahashi K[4], and Shimada K[1]
Department of Biochemistry[1], the 1st Department of Internal Medicine[2], Institute for Medical Genetics[3], Department of Pathology[4], Kumamoto University Medical School, Kumamoto 860, Japan

ABSTRACT

To examine the efficacy of the variant transthyretin (TTR) and to elucidate the role of serum amyloid P component (SAP) in the formation of amyloid deposits associated with familial amyloidotic polyneuropathy (FAP), we developed several transgenic mouse lines carrying the human mutant TTR gene. In these mouse lines, human TTR and mouse SAP were deposited as amyloid fibrils. Because SAP is a major acute-phase reactant in the mouse, we asked whether repeated induction of SAP synthesis by injecting *Escherichia coli* lipopolysaccharide (LPS) would stimulate the formation of amyloid deposits in one of these transgenic mouse lines. Contrary to our expectations, there was no significant difference in the onset and extent of amyloid deposition between the LPS-stimulated and unstimulated transgenic mice.

INTRODUCTION

Familial amyloidotic polyneuropathy (FAP) is an autosomal dominantly inherited systemic amyloidosis, characterized by prominent peripheral nerve involvement, and by the extracellular deposition of fibrillar amyloid protein. The amyloid deposit consists mainly of a variant transthyretin (TTR) with a single amino acid substitution and contains a small amount of serum amyloid P component (SAP). We reported that FAP is directly related to a point mutation in the TTR gene [1]. However, the wide span of age at onset suggests the presence of factor(s) other than a mutation in the TTR gene and these would presumably affect amyloid deposition [2]. One such factor may be SAP, because all known types of amyloid deposits so far studied contain SAP [3].

To investigate the molecular pathogenesis of FAP, we developed several transgenic mouse lines carrying the human mutant TTR gene, and found that human TTR and mouse SAP were deposited as amyloid fibrils in these mice [2, 4]. Because SAP is a major acute-phase reactant in the mouse [5], we asked whether the induction of SAP synthesis by acute inflammation would affect the formation of amyloid deposits in one of these transgenic mouse lines.

MATERIALS AND METHODS

Mice and induction of acute inflammation---Acute inflammation was induced in groups of male C57BL/6 mice by intraperitoneal injection of Escherichia coli lipopolysaccharide (LPS). At different times following the injection of 1 μg of LPS/g body weight, blood samples were taken from the ether anesthetized animals.

A transgenic mouse line used in this study was constructed as follows [2, 4]. First, we prepared a 7.8 kb StuI-EcoRI fragment, in which the promoter region of the mouse metallothionein-I gene was ligated to the structural gene of human mutant TTR gene (MT-hTTR30met), for an adequate expression of the human mutant TTR gene in mice. This DNA construct was microinjected into fertilized eggs of C57BL/6 mice and several transgenic mice, expressing the human TTR gene, were obtained. In one of these transgenic mouse lines, amyloid began to deposit in the alimentary tract of even in 6 month-old mice, then increased with aging [2]. In the current study, we used transgenic mice of this line for the following experiments. Groups of the male transgenic mice of the same litter were given injections of LPS every 5 to 6 days, as initiated at age of 2 months.

Specific protein assays---To examine the serum levels of SAP, blood samples were taken from the ether anesthetized mice and the sera were analyzed by the Ouchterlony test or immunoblot analysis, using rabbit anti-mouse SAP antiserum (Calbiochem).

Histochemical analysis---Transgenic mice given repeated injections of LPS, were anesthetized with ether and killed when they were at 5.5 and 13 months of age. Various tissues were examined histochemically. At each time point, two male and one female unstimulated transgenic mice of the same litter were also examined. Tissue sections were stained with Congo red and hematoxylin and examined under polarized light illumination to search for amyloid deposits.

RESULTS AND DISCUSSION

SAP responses to LPS injection in C57BL/6 mice---Levels of SAP were examined in sera taken from male C57BL/6 mice at various times after inducing an acute inflammation, as described under MATERIALS AND METHODS. We confirmed that an injection of LPS markedly elevated the level of circulating SAP. Before injecting LPS, mouse serum SAP was undetectable using the Ouchterlony test. However, after the injection of LPS, a progressive increase in the level of serum SAP occurred and reached a peak at around 44 hr. The elevated level then gradually decreased, but it had not returned to the unstimulated level even 68 hr later (Fig. 1). Immunoblot analysis indicated that the serum level of SAP increased about 20-fold over the unstimulated level within 24 hr (data not shown). Based on the above findings, we decided to repeat injections of LPS every 5 to 6 days.

To determine whether each one of the repeated injections causes a similar change in the serum level of SAP, groups of two male mice were

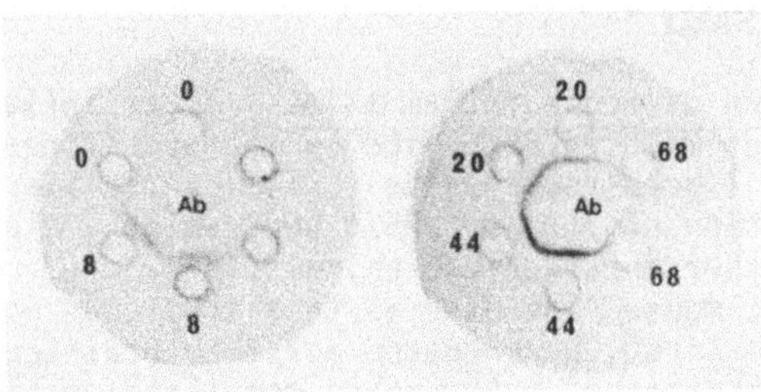

Figure 1. Ouchterlony test
Ten microliters of sera from individual mice were applied at each opening. Numbers indicate time-points examined after the administration of LPS in hours. Ab: rabbit anti-mouse SAP antiserum

given LPS every 5 days, for up to 20 days. Sera samples were taken from two mice of a group at 24 hr after the injection, and the levels of SAP were examined using the Ouchterlony test. We found similar changes in the serum levels of SAP with repeated injections (data not shown).

Induction of SAP synthesis in the transgenic mouse model of FAP---To examine whether the induction of SAP synthesis by acute inflammation would affect the formation of amyloid deposits, we injected LPS every 5 to 6 days into two groups of the male transgenic mice [2, 4]. The injections were initiated when the mice were 2 months of age. After 3.5 months of repeated LPS injections, two mice of one group were killed and examined for the presence of amyloid deposits. We confirmed that the serum level of SAP increased at 24 hr after the last LPS injection and was essentially identical with that observed in the control mice. The serum level of human TTR in the transgenic mice also increased up to about 10-fold within 10 hr after the injection of LPS (data not shown). We expected to find this rapid increase in the serum level of human TTR, because a similar increase in the level of mouse liver metallothionein-I mRNA was observed after the injection of LPS [6]. To compare the degree and extent of amyloid deposition, we also examined histochemically two male and one female unstimulated transgenic mice of the same litter for amyloid deposition. Amyloid deposits were not detected in any of these five 5.5 month-old mice. These data suggest that repeated induction of SAP synthesis by acute inflammation does not cause early deposition of amyloid fibrils.

Eleven months after giving LPS injections, two mice of another group were killed and examined for the presence of amyloid deposits. Amyloid deposits appeared in various tissues, such as small intestine, stomach, heart, thyroid gland, and skin. Similar amyloid deposits were also detected in the same tissues of the two male and one female unstimulated mice of the same litter. In this experiment, the acute-phase response of SAP to the last LPS injection was also essentially identical with that observed in the control mice (data not shown). There was no significant difference in the degree of amyloid deposition in the various tissues between the stimulated and unstimulated transgenic mice (Fig. 2).

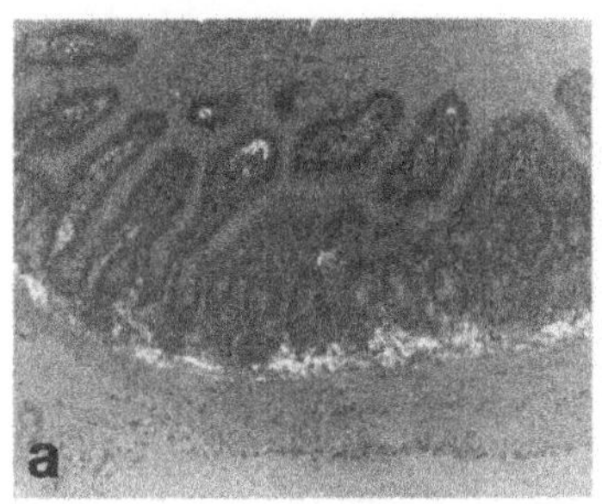

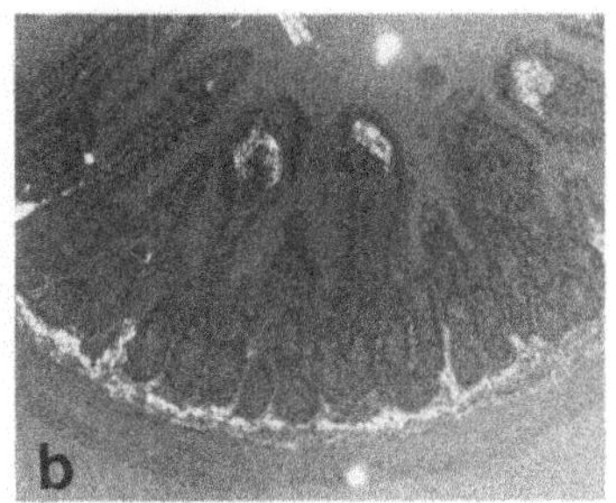

Figure 2. Pathology of the small intestine of 13 month-old transgenic mice carrying the MT-hTTR30met gene. Tissues were stained with Congo red and hematoxylin, then photographed under polarizing light. The amyloid deposits give typical birefringence. Panel (a): LPS-stimulated mouse. Panel (b): unstimulated mouse.

All these observations suggest that the induction of SAP synthesis by acute inflammation does not affect the onset and extent of amyloid deposition. However, these data do not rule out the possibility that SAP has a crucial role in amyloid formation. Normal serum levels of SAP may be sufficient for the formation of amyloid deposits. Site-directed inactivation of the endogenous SAP gene by gene targeting [7] could facilitate elucidation of the role of SAP in amyloid formation.

REFERENCES

1. Shimada, K., Maeda, S. and Araki, S. (1986) 'Genetic basis for familial amyloidotic polyneuropathy', BioEssays 4, 208-212.
2. Shimada, K., Maeda, S., Murakami, T., Nishiguchi, S., Tashiro, F., Yi, S., Wakasugi, S., Takahashi, K. and Yamamura, K. (1989) 'Transgenic mouse model of familial amyloidotic polyneuropathy', Mol. Biol. Med. 6, 333-343.
3. Pepys, M. B. and Baltz, M. L. (1983) 'Acute phase proteins with special reference to C-reactive protein and related proteins (pentaxins) and serum amyloid A protein', in F. J. Dixon and H. G. Kunkel (eds.), Adv. Immunol. 34, Academic Press, pp. 141-211.
4. Wakasugi, S., Inomoto, T., Yi, S., Naito, M., Uehira, M., Iwanaga, T., Maeda, S., Araki, K., Miyazaki, J., Takahashi, K., Shimada, K. and Yamamura, K. (1987) 'A transgenic mouse model of familial amyloidotic polyneuropathy', Proc. Japan Acad. 63(B), 344-347.
5. Pepys, M. B., Baltz, M., Gomer, K., Davies, A. J. S. and Doenhoff, M. (1979) 'Serum amyloid P-component is an acute-phase reactant in the mouse', Nature 278, 259-261.
6. Durnam, D. M., Hoffman, J. S., Quaife, C. J., Benditt, E. P., Chen, H. Y., Brinster, R. L. and Palmiter, R. D. (1984) 'Induction of mouse metallothionein-I mRNA by bacterial endotoxin is independent of metals and glucocorticoid hormones', Proc. Natl. Acad. Sci. USA 81, 1053-1056.
7. Capecchi, M. R. (1989) 'The mouse genetics: altering the genome by gene targeting', Trends Genet. 5, 77-81.

DIFFERENTIAL REGULATION OF SAP GENE EXPRESSION IN SYRIAN AND ARMENIAN HAMSTERS.

S.B.DOWTON
C.N.PETERS
J.MORRISSEY
C.RUDNICK

The Edward Mallinckrodt Department of Pediatrics and the James S McDonnell Department of Genetics, Washington Univ.School of Med., St. Louis, Missouri, U.S.A.

ABSTRACT Studies of the difference in structure and expression of the genes encoding serum amyloid P component in different hamster genera afford unique opportunities to examine the primary structure of SAP monomers and the factors regulating expression of the SAP gene. Accordingly we have isolated and characterized clones for SAP from hepatic cDNA libraries constructed from Syrian and Armenian hamsters.

INTRODUCTION

Serum amyloid P component was originally identified because of cross-reactivity with antisera for amyloid P which is found in all amyloid deposits. SAP is a member of the pentraxin family of proteins. Members of this protein family have been isolated and characterized in several species(1). In all species characterized SAP protein is encoded by a single locus and interspecific variability has been described for the resting serum concentration of this protein as well as with regard to the acute phase responsiveness of the SAP gene. The homologue of SAP in the golden Syrian hamster (*Mesocricetus auratus*)has been termed female protein (FP) since the expression of the gene in that species is modulated by sex-steroids as well as acute inflammatory stimuli(2,3). Serum FP concentration is high in resting female hamsters (1-3 g/L) and, in a manner similar to the change in plasma concentration of human albumin, decreases following administration of an inflammatory stimulus. In male Syrian hamsters a positive acute phase FP response can be elicited(4). Previous studies have shown that the serum levels are reflected in the hepatic levels of FP mRNA accumulation(5).

Armenian hamsters (*Cricetulus migratorius*) are closely related to Syrian hamsters and the expression of the SAP gene has been examined in this species. Although estrogen administration has been reported to cause jaundice and deviation of serum SAP concentrations, no gender divergence of expression SAP levels has been reported.

In order to explore the molecular mechanisms responsible for the difference in regulation of SAP gene expression in these closely related species, we have derived the primary polypeptide structure for Syrian and Armenian hamster SAP from relevant cDNA clones. Availability of SAP probes has also permitted an analysis of hepatic mRNA under conditions of an acute phase response.

METHODS AND MATERIALS

cDNA libraries were constructed in the vector λ ZAP using polyadenylated liver RNA which had been isolated by oligo(Dt) column chromatography as described(6). For each species several clones were isolated and characterized by nucleotide sequence analysis using the dideoxynucleotide chain termination method of Sanger(7). Data derived from clone pFP1 (Syrian hamster SAP) and pArFP1 (Armenian hamster SAP) are depicted in Figure 1 (5,8). Analysis of the sequence data was assisted by the Beckman Microgenie software.

RNA blot studies were performed by standard agarose-formaldehyde gel electrophoresis followed by positive pressure blotting using the Posiblot apparatus(6). Hybridizations were performed using described conditions and radiolabeled pFP1. Probe labeling was by either nick translation or random hexanucleotide primer extension. Autoradiographic signals were analyzed by densitometry using a Beckman DU64 spectrophotometric scanner. Results are displayed as histograms in Figure 2.

RESULTS AND DISCUSSION

The pentraxin proteins have been extraordinarily phylogenetically conserved. Moieties similar to C-reactive protein, the classical pentraxin, or serum amyloid P have been identified in many species including mammals, the dogfish shark, fish and the primitive & ancient marine animal, *Limulus polyphemus*. The regulation of expression of pentraxins has been the subject of intense study, largely because of the profound nature of change of serum CRP levels observed in man during acute inflammation. Several species have offered unusual opportunities to study regulation of pentraxin gene expression as well as the structure of the proteins. In mice the resting level of SAP is genetically determined and in that species a prominent increase in serum concentration is noted after tissue injury or necrosis. In man the serum levels of SAP do not appreciably alter during the course of acute inflammation (9).

Several unique properties of the SAP homologue in the golden Syrian hamster have been described. In this genus SAP was originally identified as female protein (FP) because the expression of FP is gender dependant(2). In the Syrian hamster FP is a prominent serum protein with levels between 1 - 2g/L. In the resting state males have low levels of FP. The divergent sex-limited levels of FP in Syrian hamsters may be manipulated by administration of estrogens and androgens to the animals. Previous studies have shown similar catabolic rates of FP in male and female Syrian hamsters (4) and that the serum levels are reflected in the levels of mRNA specific for FP(5). We have previously analyzed the structure of cDNA clones encoding SAP from Syrian and Armenian hamsters (8). The derived amino acid sequences for these proteins are depicted in Figure 1.

FIGURE 1. SAP AMINO ACID SEQUENCES FOR SYRIAN AND ARMENIAN HAMSTERS

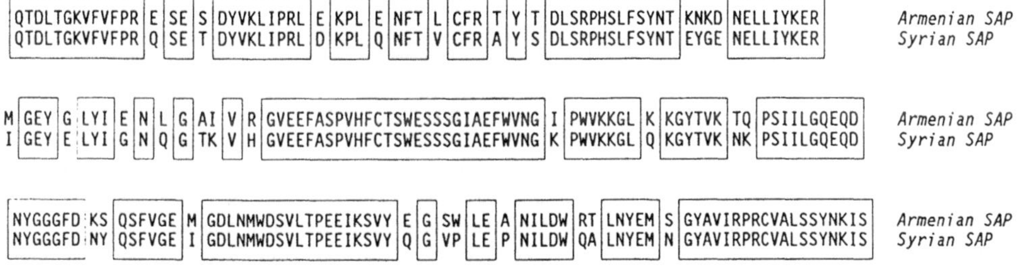

Figure 1. Complete polypeptide sequences for Armenian and Syrian hamster SAP. Top line indicates sequence for Armenian and bottom line in each pair represents Syrian SAP sequence.

These studies reveal that SAP monomers in Syrian and Armenian hamsters share 85% of their residues and are identical in predicted length. In 45% of the remaining differences in predicted primary protein structure a neutral substitution had occurred. Nucleotide sequence identity between SAP clones of these species occurs with 93% frequency. Hamster SAP molecules also share considerable sequence identity with pentraxins of other species and especially with those encoding hamster CRP (S.B.Dowton - unpublished data)

SAP mRNA levels alter during inflammation in both Syrian and Armenian hamsters. After induction of an acute phase response by administration of lipopolysaccharide (25ug/kg) RNA samples were isolated from harvested livers. SAP mRNA levels decrease to approximately 70% of resting levels in female Syrian hamster livers after administration of LPS whereas in male Syrian hamsters the hepatic SAP mRNA levels increase by 20-fold. In Armenian hamsters no gender difference in the direction of the SAP mRNA response was noted and the magnitude of alteration was similar between the sexes.

FIGURE 2. SAP mRNA REPONSES TO LPS ADMINISTRATION

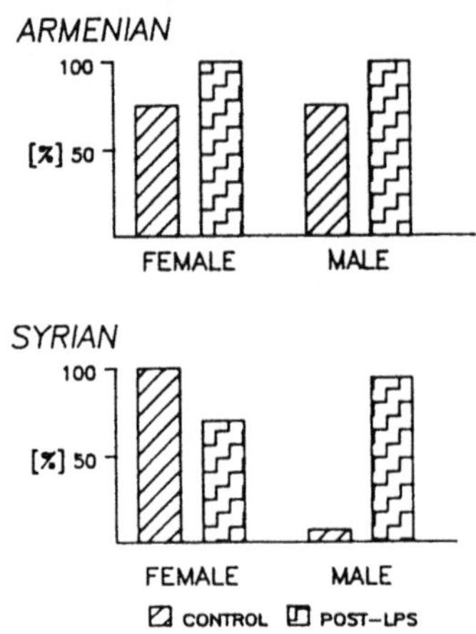

Figure 2. Levels of SAP mRNA was determined densitometrically from RNA blots after hybridization with nick-translated pFP1 probe.

Although the direction of alteration of SAP serum and mRNA levels in male and female Armenian hamsters is the same, an unusual hepatotoxicity of estrogens has been described in this genus as well as in Chinese hamsters (*Cricetulus griseus*). Along with a severe hepatitis, diethylstilbestrol administration to Armenian hamsters causes depression of serum SAP levels - an estrogen receptor dependant phenomenon which is inhibitable by concurrent administration of tamoxifen (10).
Despite differences in the SAP responses to inflammation and estrogen administration, SAP monomers of Syrian and Armenian hamsters are sufficiently similar that hybrid pentamers may be reassembled in the laboratory(11). Future studies will be directed towards elucidation of the molecular details governing regulation of expression of the pentraxins from these species.

Acknowledgement These studies were supported by the National Institutes of Health AI24835 and a Basil O'Connor Starter Scholar Award (5-669) from the March of Dimes Birth Defects Foundation. Drs. J.E.Coe and H.R.Colten provided helpful discussions.

REFERENCES

1. Baltz, M.L., deBeer, F.C, Feinstein, A., Munn, E.A., Milstein, C.P., Fletcher, T.C., March, J.F., Taylor, J., Bruton, C., Clamp, J.R., Davies, A.J.S., and Pepys, M.B. (1982) *Ann NY Acad Sci* **389**, 49-75
2. Coe, J.E. (1977) *Proc Natl Acad Sci USA* **74**, 730-733
3. Coe, J.E., Margossian, S.S., Slayter, H.S., and Sogn, J.A. (1981) *J Exp Med* **153**, 977-991
4. Coe, J.E., and Ross, M.J. (1983) *J Exp Med* **157**, 1421-1433
5. Dowton, S.B., Woods, D.E., Mantzouranis, E.C., and Colten, H.R. (1985) *Science* **228**, 1206-1208
6. Sambrook, J., Fritsch, E.F., and Maniatis, T. (1989) *Molecular Cloning. A Laboratory Manual*, Cold Spring Harbor Laboratory Press, Cold Spring Harbor
7. Sanger, F., Nicklen, S., and Coulsen, A.R. (1977) *Proc Natl Acad Sci USA* **74**, 5463
8. Dowton, S.B., and Waggoner, D.J. (1989) *J Immunol* **143**, 3776-3780
9. Pepys, M.B., Baltz, M.L., DeBeer, F.C., Dyck, R.F., Holford, S., Breathnach, S.M., Black, M.M., Tribe, C.R., Evans, D.J., and Feinstein, A. (1982) *Ann NY Acad Sci* **389**, 286-298
10. Coe, J.E., and Ross, M.J. (1988) *Endocrinology.* **122**, 137-144
11. Coe, J.E., and Ross, M.J. (1987) *Biochemistry* **26**, 704-710

ISOLATION OF cDNA CLONES & EXPRESSION ANALYSES FOR RAT SERUM AMYLOID P (SAP) COMPONENT.

S.BRUCE DOWTON
SCOTT D. McGREW

The Edward Mallinckrodt Department of Pediatrics and the James S McDonnell Department of Genetics, Washington University School of Medicine, St Louis, Missouri, U.S.A.

ABSTRACT SAP is a member of the phylogenetically conserved pentraxin protein family. This study describes isolation of CDNA clones for rat SAP from which the primary structure of this pentraxin has been determined. Rat SAP is 208 residues in length and a sex difference in expression of SAP mRNA in rat liver is documented. The structure and expression of rat SAP is compared with data from other species.

INTRODUCTION

SAP is a member of the pentraxin family of proteins, named for the discoid pentagonal conformation noted when purified serum fractions are viewed by EM. The prototypic member of the pentraxin family of proteins is human C-reactive protein(CRP) (1). In primates and rabbits CRP is a major acute phase reactant since serum concentrations may elevate by 100-1000 fold following administration of an inflammatory stimulus. The alteration in serum concentration of CRP during inflammation occurs as a result of enhanced gene transcription and alteration in efficiency of transport of newly synthesized CRP monomers from the pre-Golgi subcellular compartment (2,3).

Amyloid P (AP) component is a glycoprotein which has been localized in most forms of amyloid deposits. AP contributes approximately 10-15% of the weight of isolated amyloid fibrils and is derived from the circulating form, SAP (1). This protein is also found in glomerular basement membranes and in elastic tissues surrounding blood vessels. Despite the similarities between SAP and CRP, these proteins are distinguished by i.)the fact that assembled SAP is decameric whereas CRP is pentameric, ii.)differences in Ca2+-dependant ligand binding specificities, iii.)the absence of an alteration in human serum SAP concentration during an acute phase reaction iv.)lack of antigenic cross-reactivity and v.)the fact that human SAP is glycosylated and CRP is not. Interspecific differences have been noted in extent of the acute phase response for SAP (Table 1). Plasma concentrations of human SAP do not alter significantly following tissue injury whereas murine SAP is a major acute phase reactant.

Pentraxins have been highly conserved throughout evolution. SAP-like moieties have been identified in mammals, elasmobranchs and fish (4). Availability of molecular probes reflecting the genes and mRNAs encoding SAP from various species have enhanced understanding of the structure and regulation of expression of this pentraxin. Rat SAP has been purified and the approximate M_r of the mature rat SAP monomer is 24,500(5). In order to permit comparison of rat SAP structure with that of other pentraxins this study describes the structure and expression of rat SAP mRNA.

METHODS AND MATERIALS

Several CDNA clones encoding rat SAP were isolated from an acute phase rat hepatic cDNA library, (Dr J.D.Gitlin at Washington University School of Medicine). The λ ZAPII cDNA library was screened as described using a cross-reacting hamster SAP probe, pFP_1 (6,7). The DNA sequence of one clone, $prSAP_1$, containing a 931bp $EcoR_1$ insert, was determined using the dideoxynucleotide chain termination method. Studies of rat SAP specific mRNA were performed by RNA blot analysis as described(7). The expression of rat SAP mRNA in male and female rats and following exposure to LPS (200ug/kg) is shown in Figure 2.

RESULTS AND DISCUSSION

The amino acid sequence of rat SAP derived from $prSAP_1$ is shown in comparison with SAP sequences from other species (Fig.1). Important features of SAP molecules isolated from man, mouse, two genera of hamster (Syrian and Armenian), are listed in Table 1 and contrasted with data regarding rat SAP. SAP moieties have also been described for the dogfish shark, guinea pig, cow and plaice but less detail is available for these species.

TABLE 1. PROPERTIES OF SAP FROM DIFFERENT SPECIES

	Human	Mouse	Hamster(S)	Hamster(A)	Rat
Serum Concentration (mg/L)					
Adult Male	43 ± 14	50*	4 - 20	80 - 320	21 - 40
Adult Female	33 ± 10		1000 - 2000	100 - 300	
Infant	4 + 2		100		
Monomeric Subunit Mr (kD)	28	31	30	32	24.5 - 29
No. of a.a. in mature SAP	204	204	212	212	208
Length of signal peptide	19	20		19	20
Glycosylated	Yes		Yes		Yes
mRNA Size (kb)	1.1	1.1	1.0■	1.0	1.0
Acute Phase Reactant	-	++*	Divergent	+	+/-
Assembled Conformation	Decamer	Decamer	Pentamer	Pentamer	Pentamer Decamer#
Plasma t1/2 (hours)	8.5	7.5-9.5	9.5-14 M 12-16 F		4.8

* strain variability is documented:C57Bl<10mg/ml;C3H,BALB/c,CBA,AJ,SJL 20-80mg/ml;DBA/2 100mg/ml
# C10 symmetric decamers are formed as well as 2 x C5 pentamers
■ Larger size mRNAs are also described; S=Syrian,A=Armenian; M=Male, F=Female

Serum Concentration of SAP

SAP is detectable at low concentrations in the serum of most animals studied. In man serum SAP levels are higher in males (43 ± 14 mg/L) than those observed in females (33 ± 10mg/L). Fetal levels of SAP have not been studied but SAP concentrations in human cord blood samples are 8-10 fold lower than those for adults(4). In the Syrian hamster serum concentrations of SAP[originally termed female protein (FP)], in females are several orders of magnitude higher (1-2 g/L) than those in other species. Serum levels of SAP decrease in female hamsters by 50% during inflammation while in male hamsters serum SAP levels are much lower than females. Serum SAP levels increase in male hamsters following tissue injury. The gender divergence of SAP levels is also able to modulated by sex-steroids and is reflected in hepatic SAP mRNA levels indicating a pre-translational mechanism of regulation of expression(6,8,9).

Murine SAP is a major acute phase reactant in all strains studied. There are, however, genetically determined differences in plasma concentration of SAP between murine inbred strains (Table 1).

The serum concentration of rat SAP increases modestly (1.5 - 2 fold) following tissue injury (10,11). The reported serum concentrations of rat SAP in the resting state have been variable. An initial study reported the serum SAP levels were ~500mg/L(11) whereas further study of several rat strains documented resting serum levels of 21-40mg/L(5).

Structure of SAP

EM studies have demonstrated that pentameric symmetry is assumed during assembly of SAP molecules of all species. Human SAP circulates as a decamer - two identical pentamers apposed face-to-face while hamster SAP travels as single pentamer(1,8). In addition to pentamers rat SAP may exist in single ring C_{10} decameric configuration (11).

Monomeric subunit sizes of SAP have been studied using a variety of techniques including SDS-PAGE, chromatography and high-speed sedimentation gradient ultracentrifugation. The variability of sub-unit M_r noted for some species may reflect different methods of study or glycosylation differences. For man, mouse, hamsters (Armenian and Syrian) and rat, characterization of cDNA clones has permitted prediction of primary structures of SAP monomers. There is considerable conservation of sequence identity (Fig.1) and many amino acid residue differences result from neutral substitutions. The differences in number of amino acids in SAP of each of these species is explicable largely by 3' coding sequence alterations. Typical hydrophobic leader sequences are noted in all available SAP cDNAs.

FIGURE 1. RAT SAP AMINO ACID SEQUENCE COMPARED WITH OTHER SPECIES

```
Rat     MDKLLLWMSVFTSLLSEAFAQ TDL NG KVFVFPR E S ET D Y V K LI PW L E KPL Q NFT L CFR A Y S DLSR SQ SLFSY SVNSRD NELL
H(A)    MDKMLLLLG VSILLSEVFAQ TDL TG KVFVFPR E S ES D Y V K LI PR L E KPL E NFT L CFR T Y T DLSR PH SLFSY NTKNKD NELL
H(S)                          TDL TG KVFVFPR Q S ET D Y V K LI PR L D KPL Q NFT V CFR A Y S DLSR PH SLFSY NTKYGE NELL
Mouse   MDKLLLWMFVFTSLLSEAFCQ TDL KR KVFVFPR E S ET D H V K LI PH L E KPL Q NFT L CFR T Y S DLSR SQ SLFSY SVKGRD NELL
Human   MNKPLLWISVLTSLL*EAFAH TDL SG KVFVFPR E S VT D H V N LI TP L E KPL Q NFT L CFR A Y S DLSR AY SLFSY NTQGRD NELL

Rat     I YK AKLEQ Y S LYI GNSKVTVRGL E EFPS P I H F C TS WESSSGI A EFW V NG KPW VKK G L QKG Y T V KSS P S I V L G QEQD
H(A)    I YK ERMEG Y G LYI ENLGAIVRGV E EFAS P V H F C TS WESSSGI A EFW V NG IPW VKK G L KKG Y T V KTQ P S I I L G QEQD
H(S)    I YK ERIGE Y E LYI GNQGTKVHGV E EFAS P V H F C TS WESSSGI A EFW V NG KPW VKK G L KKG Y T V KNK P S I I L G QEQD
Mouse   I YK EKVGE Y S LYI GQSKVTVRGM E EYLS P V H L C TT WESSSGI V EFW V NG KPW VKK S L QRE Y T V KAP P S I V L R QEQD
Human   V YK ERVGE Y S LYI GRHKVTPKVI E KFPA P V H I C VS WESSSGI A EFW I NG TPL VKK G L RQG Y F V EAQ P K I V L G QEQD

Rat     TY GG G F DKT QSFVGE IA DL Y MWD S VL T P EN I HSVDRGFPPNP NILDW RA LNYE IN GY VV I K P RMWD    NKSS
H(A)    NY GG G F DKS QSFVGE MG DL N MWD S VL T P EE I KSVYEGSWLEA NILDW RT LNYE MS GY AV I R P RCVALSSYNKIS
H(S)    NY GG G F DNY QSFVGE IG DL N MWD S VL T P EE I KSVYQGVPLEP NILDW QA LNYE MN GY AV I R P RCVALSSYNKIS
Mouse   NY GG G F QRS QSFVGE FS DL Y MWD Y VL T P QD I LF*YRDSPVNP NILNW QA LNYE IN GY VV I R P RVWD
Human   SY GG K F DRS QSFVGE IG DL Y MWD S VL P P EN I LSAYQGTPLPA NILDW QA LNYE IR GY VI I K P LVWV
```

Figure 1. Predicted amino acid sequences derived from SAP cDNA clones for rat, Armenian hamster-H(A), Syrian hamster - H(S), mouse (NZ black) & human. Regions of complete homology are enclosed in boxes.

Regulation of SAP Gene Expression

As indicated above there is considerable interspecific variation in resting serum SAP concentration and the degree of alteration of SAP levels during acute inflammation. In mice, strain specific differences in resting expression of SAP are genetically determined whereas in the Syrian hamster the serum levels of SAP may be modulated by estrogens and androgens. Where data are available acute phase differences in serum levels are largely reflected in mRNA suggesting that pre-translational regulation points are important. In addition studies comparing the induction of murine SAP mRNA using azocasein and thioglycollate highlight differences in kinetic responses depending upon the nature of the irritant(12). The catabolism of murine SAP does not alter during acute inflammation (4).

Figure 2 demonstrates that Sprague-Dawley rat hepatic mRNA increases modestly following administration of lipopolysaccharide. In addition, female rats are shown to have a higher level of SAP specific mRNA in the resting state than male animals.

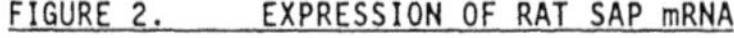
FIGURE 2. EXPRESSION OF RAT SAP mRNA

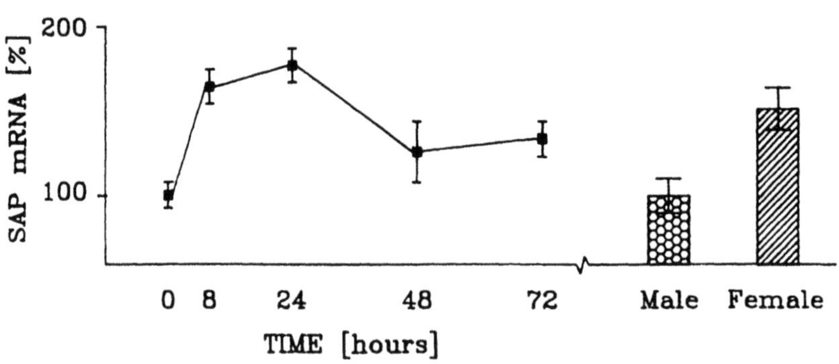

Figure 2. Densitometric analyses of RNA blots of rat hepatic RNA hybridized with radiolabeled prSAP1. Time points reflect number of hours after administration of LPS (200ug/kg).

Genetic Aspects of the SAP Locus

The SAP gene maps to chromosome 1q in man and is linked to the gene for CRP suggesting that these loci may have arisen as a result of gene duplication(13). Physical mapping and genetic studies suggest that a large syntenic segment of human chromosome 1q which encompasses the SAP and CRP loci has been conserved with the distal region of mouse chromosome 1 (14).

Ligands

Ligand binding specificity of pentraxins has been of considerable interest since human CRP was originally identified by its capacity to bind the C-polysaccharide of *S.pneumoniae*. Specific Ca^{2+} dependant interactions of agarose, amyloid fibrils, fibronectin and C4-binding protein with SAP have been defined. Identification that agarose binding by SAP results from interaction with a specific galactopyranoside has defined the stereochemical nature of potentially important *in vivo* ligands (15). An attractive hypothesis, based upon recent demonstrations of high affinity between SAP and DNA at physiologic ionic strength, is that SAP may be an integral component in clearing nucleic acids from sites of inflammation as well as from the circulation (16). Recent studies have focused upon the binding of SAP with glycosaminoglycans which are found in basement membranes and amyloid deposits. Since rats are extraordinarily resistant to amyloidosis studies of interaction of rat SAP with GAGs may provide additional insight into the role of SAP in amyloidogenesis (17).

Acknowledgement

These studies were supported by the National Institutes of Health AI24835 and a Basil O'Connor Starter Scholar Award (No. 5-669) from the March of Dimes Birth defects Foundation. Dr. J.D.Gitlin supplied the rat cDNA library and J.Morrissey provided excellent technical assistance. Dr Harvey Colten provided support and guidance.

References

1. Baltz, M.L., deBeer, F.C, Feinstein, A., Munn, E.A., Milstein, C.P., Fletcher, T.C., March, J.F., Taylor, J., Bruton, C., Clamp, J.R., Davies, A.J.S., and Pepys, M.B. (1982) *Ann NY Acad Sci* **389**, 49-75
2. Goldberger, G., Bing, D.H., Sipe, J.D., Rits, M., and Colten, H.R. (1987) *J Immunol* **138**, 3967-3971
3. MacIntyre, S.S., Kushner, I., and Samols, D. (1985) *J Biol Chem* **260**, 4169-4173
4. Pepys, M.B., Baltz, M.L., DeBeer, F.C., Dyck, R.F., Holford, S., Breathnach, S.M., Black, M.M., Tribe, C.R., Evans, D.J., and Feinstein, A. (1982) *Ann NY Acad Sci* **389**, 286-298
5. DeBeer, F.C., Baltz, M.L., Munn, E.A., Feinstein, A., Taylor, J., Bruton, C., Clamp, J.R., and Pepys, M.B. (1982) *Immunology* **45**, 55-70
6. Dowton, S.B., Woods, D.E., Mantzouranis, E.C., and Colten, H.R. (1985) *Science* **228**, 1206-1208
7. Sambrook, J., Fritsch, E.F., and Maniatis, T. (1989) *Molecular Cloning. A Laboratory Manual*, Cold Spring Harbor Laboratory Press, Cold Spring Harbor
8. Coe, J.E. (1977) *Proc Natl Acad Sci USA* **74**, 730-733
9. Coe, J.E., and Ross, M.J. (1983) *J Exp Med* **157**, 1421-1433
10. Nakada, H., Matsumoto, S., and Tashiro, Y. (1986) *J Biochem* **99**, 877-884
11. Pontet, M., D'Asnieres, M., Gache, D., Escaig, J., and Engler, R. (1981) *Biochim Biophys Acta* **671**, 202-210
12. Zahedi, K., and Whitehead, A.S. (1989) *J Immunol* **143**, 2880-2886
13. Floyd Smith, G., Whitehead, A.S., Colten, H.R., and Francke, U. (1986) *Immunogenetics.* **24**, 171-176
14. Kingsmore, S.F., Watson, M.L., Howard, T.A., and Seldin, M.F. (1989) *Embo J* **7**, 4073-4080
15. Hind, C.R.K., Collins, , P.M., Renn, D., Cook, R.B., Caspi, D., Baltz, M., and Pepys, M.B. (1984) *J Exp Med* **159**, 1058-1069
16. Pepys, M.B., and Butler, P.J.G. (1987) *Biochem Biophys Res Commun* **148**, 308-313
17. Hamazaki, H. (1987) *J Biol Chem* **262**, 1456-1460

ISOLATION OF A 16 KD FRACTION WITH EXTREMELY HIGH AEF ACTIVITY

Tsuranobu Shirahama, Carmela R. Abraham, Shyr-Te Ju,
Katsutoshi Miura and Alan S. Cohen
Arthritis Center, Department of Medicine, Boston University,
Boston, MA 02118, U.S.A.

Robert Kisilevsky
Department of Pathology, Queen's University,
Kingston, Canada K7L 3N6

Erik Gruys
Department of Veterinary Pathology, University of Utrecht,
Utrecht, the Netherlands

ABSTRACT. An AEF extract from amyloidotic mouse livers was fractionated through a very thin tall Sepharose 6B column eluted with 0.01M sodium phosphate buffer (PB) with 0.5M NaCl, pH 8.0. A sharp peak eluted slightly ahead of lysozyme represented the 6th and last protein peak and contained extremely high AEF activity. This fraction revealed 3 bands on SDS-PAGE, all whose N-terminals were found to be blocked in a preliminary amino acid sequencing. Antibodies were raised against this fraction.

INTRODUCTION

Amyloid enhancing factor (AEF) is believed to play a key role in the second phase of amyloidogenesis. In spite of its dramatic biological effects and despite serious efforts by a number of investigators, AEF has so far eluded definitive chemical and immunologic characterization (Abankwa and Ali-Khan, 1988; Axelrad et al, 1982; Baltz et al, 1986; Hardt and Ranlov, 1976; Hol et al, 1985; Kisilevsky, 1983; Shirahama et al, 1990; Varga et al, 1986).

Our collaborated efforts achieved isolation of a small molecular weight fraction into a sharp peak on a gel filtration which contained a very high AEF activity.

MATERIALS AND METHODS

Target: We expected AEF activity to be found spreading in

many fractions whatever the fractionation method is used, and determined, in such a case, to focus our effort to isolate the smallest molecule with a high AEF activity.

Starting Material: In order to carry out a large series of AEF isolation procedures with a starting material of identical quality, more than 100 gm of the lyophilized "glycerol AEF extract" (Axelrad et al, 1982) from amyloidotic mouse livers, of which 50 µg consistently produced amyloidosis in a recipient mouse within 72 hours, was collected and stored at -20°C.

Solvent: After testing many different solvents in order to select a medium that can dissolve AEF well and keep the solubilized AEF from reaggregation (a common problem in AEF isolation procedures) for an extended period of time without adversely affecting its activity, 0.01 M PB with 0.5M NaCl at pH 8.0 was selected for the present study.

AEF Isolation Procedure: The isolation procedure consisted in principle of the following steps.

1. Solubilization of the lyophilized "glycerol AEF extract" into 0.01M PB with 0.5M NaCl at pH 8.0.
2. Precipitation by adding ammonium sulfate to the resultant extract (31.5 gm/100 ml).
3. Re-solubilization of the sediment into the buffer (0.01M PB with 0.5M NaCl, pH 8.0).
4. Fractionation through a 1.2 x 145 cm Sepharose 6B column eluted with the same buffer.

Assay of AEF Activity: AEF activity was assayed by injecting a CBA/J mouse with the test sample intravenously (i.v.) with a simultaneous subcutaneous (s.c.) injection of 1.0 ml of a 1:1 emulsion of 10% aqueous casein and complete Freund's adjuvant (casein-adjuvant emulsion), and by testing splenic amyloid deposition after 72 hours (Shirahama et al, 1990).

RESULTS AND COMMENTS

On gel filtration, an isolated sharp peak (marked in Fig. 1 and designated hereafer as P6) represented the 6th and the last of the recognizable peaks and shoulders and eluted slightly ahead of lysozyme (MW 14,300).

While elevated AEF activity was observed concurrently along many protein peaks, P6 contained the highest per unit AEF activity. Its level was as that an i.v. injection of 10 µg of lyophilized P6 in 0.5 ml of phosphate buffered saline with a concomitant s.c. injection of 1.0 ml of the casein-adjuvant emulsion was consistently capable of inducing amyloidosis in a

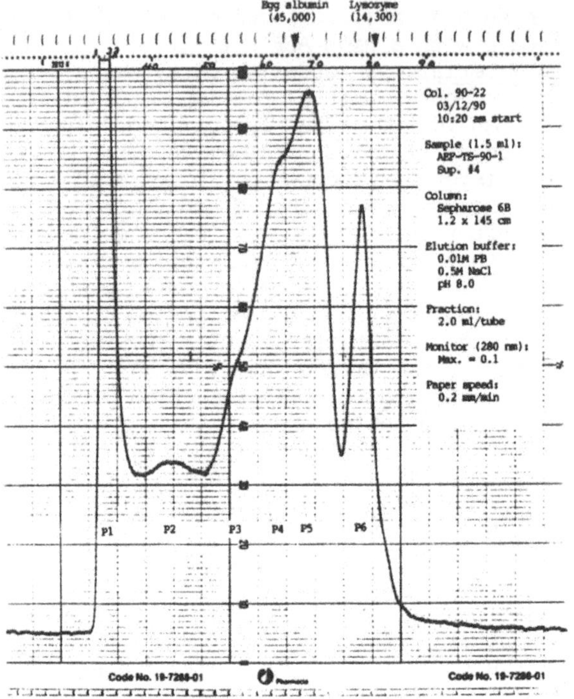

Figure 1. A photograph of an actual recording sheet of a gel filtration profile.

CBA/J mouse within 72 hours, namely a very high AEF activity.

On a sodium dodecyl sulfate polyacrylamide gel electrophoresis (SDS-PAGE), P6 showed 3 bands at molecular weight ranges of 50,000-60,000, 30,000-35,000, and 20,000-25,000.

Amino acid composition of this fraction was:

	% res.		% res.		% res.		% res.		% res.
Asp	6.7	Pro	-	Cys	-	Tyr	2.7	Arg	2.4
Thr	3.9	Gly	12.6	Met	0.9	Phe	3.5		
Ser	16.2	Ala	9.8	Ileu	3.6	His	5.9		
Glu	17.4	Val	4.8	Leu	5.8	Lys	3.6		

In an initial amino acid sequencing, N-terminals of all the

3 bands on SDS-PAGE were found to be blocked.

On a substrate (gelatin) impregnated gel-SDS-PAGE, the bands showed proteolytic activity.

Histocheminical and chemical analyses indicated that this fraction contains a significant amount of non-proteinaceous (namely carbohydrate) component(s).

Antisera generated in rabbits against P6 formed a single precipitin line on Orchterlony plate against the P6 fraction as well as the AEF extract prior to the fractionation on the Sepharose 6B column, and reacted on Western blotting with all the 3 bands formed by P6.

Immunoabsorption with the antisera removed AEF activity from the P6 fraction and significantly reduced the activity of the pre-gel-filtration AEF extract. Further characterization of the antisera is under way.

REFERENCES

Abankwa GV, Ali-Khan Z: Alveolar hydatid cyst induced amyloid enhancing factor (AEF): physicochemical properties and abolition of AEF activity by serine protease inhibitors. Br J Exp Path 69:133-148, 1988

Axelrad MA, Kisilevsky R, Willmer J, Chen SJ, Skinner M: Further characterization of amyloid-enhancing factor. Lab Invest 47:139-146, 1982

Baltz ML, Caspi D, Hind CRK, Feinstein A, Pepys MB: Isolation and characterization of amyloid enhencing factor (AEF). In Amyloidosis, edited by Glenner GG, Osserman EF, Benditt EP, Calkins E, Cohen AS, Zucker-Franklin D. Plemum Press New York, 1986. pp 115-121

Hol PR, van Andel ACJ, van Ederen AM, Draayer J, Gruys E: Amyloid enhancing factor in hamster. Br J Exp Path 66:689-697, 1985

Kisilevsky R: Biology of Disease. Amyloidosis: a familiar problem in the light of current pathogenetic developments. Lab Invest 49:381-390, 1983

Shirahama T, Miura K, Ju S-T, Kisilevsky R, Gruys E, Cohen AS: Amyloid enhancing factor-loaded macrophages in amyloid fibril formation. Lab Invest 62:61-68, 1990

Varga J, Flinn MSM, Shirahama T, Rodgers OG, Cohen AS: The induction of accelerated murine amyloidosis with human spleen extract. Probable role of amyloid enhancing factor. Wirchows Arch B (Cell Pathol) 51:177-185, 1986

AMYLOID ENHANCING FACTOR (AEF) - INDUCED AMYLOIDOSIS LACKS INFLAMMATORY REACTION.

M.M. PICKEN[†], G.R. GALLO[‡] & B. FRANGIONE[‡]

[†]*Loyola University Medical Center*
2160 S. First Avenue
Maywood
IL 60153, U.S.A.

[‡]*New York University Medical Center*
560 First Avenue
New York
NY 10016, U.S.A.

ABSTRACT. Studies were performed on sections of spleens from batches of mice that had been subjected to either of two amyloidogenic protocols: inflammatory stimulus alone or inflammatory stimulus together with AEF. Sections were stained with Congo red to verify amyloid deposition and adjacent sections stained by immunohistochemistry using antibodies against a variety of cellular markers. A striking difference was observed in the degree of inflammatory reaction exhibited by the two groups, being barely noticeable in the AEF-induced group but very strong in the inflammatory stimulus group. This was particularly noticeable using antibodies against lysozyme, α_1-antichymotrypsin, CD 68 and Mac 387 which are markers for myeloid and monocytic/histiocytic cells. We conclude from these findings that AEF-induced amyloidosis lacks an inflammatory component and suggest that AEF may contain factor(s) which are produced by inflammatory cells in "classical" amyloidosis.

Introduction

Amyloid enhancing factor (AEF), isolated from amyloid-laden organs, has been shown to accelerate amyloidogenesis in an experimental setting. Whereas in the classical model of experimental amyloidosis tissue amyloid deposits are detectable within weeks, in AEF-induced amyloidosis the deposits are seen within a few days (1). Although AEF activity has been known for some time, neither its chemical structure nor its mechanism of action is certain. AEF is thus functionally defined as "factor(s) which accelerate deposition of amyloid in experimental models". It has been noted that in the classical model of experimental amyloidosis the process of tissue amyloid deposition is invariably accompanied by an intense inflammatory reaction in the spleen which also is the organ where amyloid deposits are first detectable. For this reason it has been postulated that the inflammatory reaction is involved in the pathogenesis of amyloidosis. No similar histologic comparison, however, was thus far reported on an accelerated model of amyloidosis *i.e.* a model where an inflammatory stimulus is delivered together with AEF (AEF-induced amyloidosis). To this end we have performed comparative studies on tissue sections from AEF-induced amyloidosis and amyloidosis induced by casein alone ("classical" model). We demonstrate that AEF-induced amyloidosis lacks an inflammatory reaction.

Materials and Methods

We performed studies on sections of spleens from two groups of animals. One group was subjected to a protocol for classical amyloidosis and sacrificed after 3-4 weeks (1). The other group received AEF together with an inflammatory stimulus and was sacrificed after 3-4 days (1). The presence of amyloid deposits in the spleens was confirmed by Congo red staining of formalin fixed, paraffin embedded spleen sections; adjacent sections were subsequently studied immunohistochemically. The following antibodies were used for immunohistochemical studies: anti-AA protein (1:1,000)(Calbiochem); anti-murine amyloid P component (1:1,000)(Calbiochem); anti-lysozyme

(1:1,000)(Chemicon); anti-α_1-antitrypsin (AAT)(1:1,000) (DAKO); anti-CD68 (1:100) (DAKO); anti-Mac 387(1:100)(DAKO) and anti-ubiquitin (1:1,000)(DAKO). The immunohistochemical studies were performed as previously described (2). Bound antibody was detected using either the ABC (Vector) or peroxidase-anti-peroxidase system (PAP)(DAKO). Sections incubated with non-immune serum or buffer alone were used as controls. Known positive control sections from mice, as well as sections of spleen from age-matched control mice were stained in parallel. To enhance immunostaining in formalin-fixed, paraffin-embedded tissues, additional sections were pretreated with trypsin followed by washing in buffer.

Results

Both groups developed typical perifollicular deposits of amyloid which were Congo red positive and birefringent under polarized light. The amyloid deposits were reactive with antibodies to amyloid A protein and amyloid P component.

We observed a striking difference in the degree of inflammatory reaction between the two groups; in AEF-induced amyloidosis the inflammatory reaction was barely noticeable while in the "classical" model it was very profound. Although this difference was already appreciable in sections stained with Haematoxylin and Eosin (H&E), it was further enhanced by immunohistochemical stains using antibodies for myeloid and monocytic/histiocytic cells (3). Fig. 1 shows a section of spleen from the "classical" amyloid group with many cells positive for lysozyme. At higher magnification (Fig. 3) many cells are mononuclear and thus presumed to be of monocyte/histiocyte lineage. In contrast, in the AEF group the number of cells positive for lysozyme is much smaller (Figs. 2 and 4), similar to or only slightly higher than, in age-matched control animals (not shown).

Other stains for myeloid and monocytic/histiocytic cells also showed the presence of a distinctive inflammatory reaction in the "classical" group and an apparent lack or paucity of inflammatory reaction in the AEF group (Table 1). The stain for AAT, although less abundant than the stain for lysozyme, demonstrated many strongly positive cells in the "classical" group (Fig. 5 & 6). The AAT positive cells were seen concentrated particularly around the follicles, *i.e.* areas where amyloid is first deposited (Fig. 5). Again in the AEF group, the number of AAT positive cells was smaller than in the "classical" group (Table 1). Similar results were obtained for CD68 and Mac 387, both markers of myeloid and histiocytic cells. The stain for ubiquitin was inconclusive, being essentially negative in the "classical" group and exhibiting weak positivity in the AEF group.

Table 1

Antibody	Classical group	AEF group
Lysozyme	++++	+/-
α_1-antitrypsin	+++	+/-
CD 68	++	+/-
Mac 387	++	+/-
Ubiquitin	-	weak

Discussion

We have demonstrated a striking difference in the degree of inflammatory reaction accompanying amyloid deposition in the spleen between AEF-induced amyloidosis and the "classical" model. Using markers for myeloid and monocytic/histiocytic cells, we showed that in the "classical" model the inflammatory reaction was very pronounced. In contrast, in AEF-induced amyloidosis, the inflammatory reaction was not apparent. We conclude from this that AEF induced amyloidosis lacks an inflammatory reaction.

Based on tissue studies of the "classical" model of experimental amyloidosis, it has been postulated that the inflammatory reaction is involved in the pathogenesis of murine amyloidosis. If this is the case, the fact that AEF-induced amyloidosis lacks an inflammatory reaction suggests that amy-

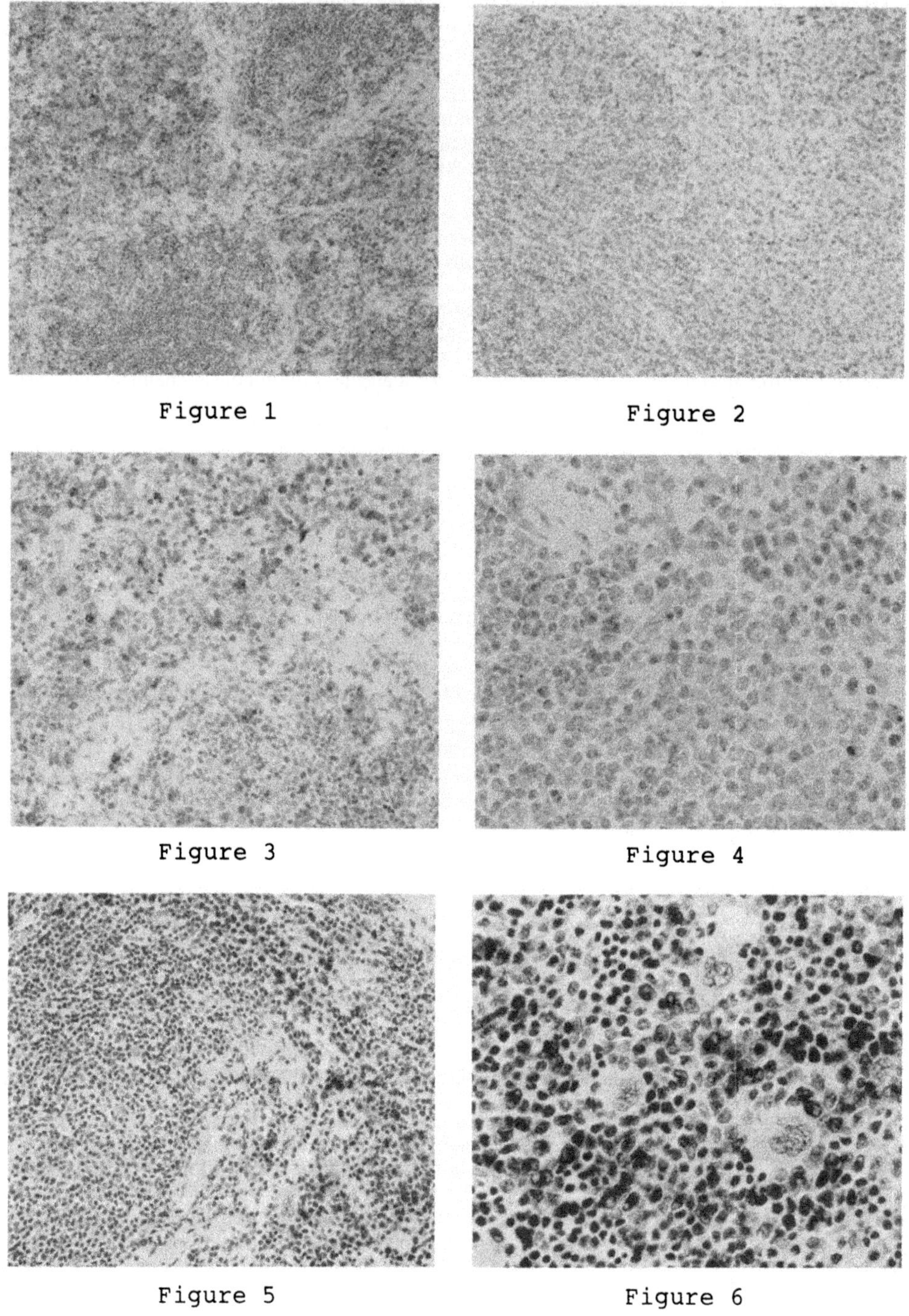

Figure 1

Figure 2

Figure 3

Figure 4

Figure 5

Figure 6

loidogenesis in this model is not associated with inflammatory cells *per se* but rather that AEF may contain factor(s) which are produced by inflammatory cells. Conceivably, AEF itself may be an enzyme(s) and/or inhibitor of inflammatory cell origin.

High AEF activity associated with inflammatory cells has been reported previously. Yokota *et al* (4) reported strong reactivity of antibody raised against partially purified AEF with splenic polymorphonuclear leukocytes. More recently Shirahama *et al* (5), using cell culture experiments, have found high AEF activity in the peritoneal resident cells from amyloidotic mice. In our studies the mononuclear cells, presumed to be of monocytic/histiocytic lineage, comprised a large part of the inflammatory reaction (6, this study). Whether the abundance of stain for two enzymes, *i.e.* lysozyme and AAT, in sections from the "classical" model is related to amyloidogenesis requires further studies. Recently ubiquitin has been reported to have AEF activity (7). Our preliminary tissue studies are inconclusive. The association of enzymes and/or inhibitors with amyloidogenesis has been postulated by previous studies (2, 8).

The effector mechanism(s) of AEF is (are) not known. Whether it induces amyloid fibril formation by direct action on the protein precursor, or indirectly regulates its processing by action at the cellular level, remains to be elucidated. Thus far, the available data suggest that AEF is not simply an accelerating factor, but also plays a crucial role in the deposition of amyloid itself. AEF activity is first detected prior to the deposition of histologically discernible amyloid. It has been shown that A/J mice, which are resistant to the development of "classical" amyloidosis, develop amyloid after prior administration of AEF. Spleen extracts from A/J mice subjected to prolonged injections of casein alone do not have AEF activity. Thus, it appears that the determination of resistance or susceptibility to experimental amyloidosis operates at the level of AEF production (9).

Acknowledgements

Supported in part by Grants from the Kidney Foundation of New York/New Jersey (GRG) & Illinois, the Schweppe Foundation (MMP) and USPHS grants AM-01431 & AM-02594 (BF).

References

1. Axelrod, M.A., Kisilevsky, R., Wilmer, J., Chen, S.J., Skinner, M. (1982). Further characterization of amyloidosis enhancing factor. *Lab. Invest.* **47**, 139-146.

2. Picken, M.M., Larrondo-Lillo, M., Coria, F., Gallo, G.R., Shelanski, M., Frangione, B. (1990). Distribution of the protease inhibitor α_1-antichymotrypsin in cerebral and systemic amyloid. *J. Neuropath. & Exp. Neurol.* **49**, 41-48.

3. Krugliak, L., Meyer, P.R., Taylor, C.R. (1986). The distribution of lysozyme, alpha-1-antitrypsin, and alpha-1-antichymotrypsin in normal hematopoetic cells and in myeloid leukemias: an immunoperoxidase study on cytocentrifuge preparations, smears, and paraffin sections. *Am. J. Hematol.* **21**, 99-109.

4. Yokota, T., Ishihara, T., Kawano, H., Takahashi, M., Yamashita, Y., Gondo, T., Fujinaga, Y., Uchino, F. (1989). Immunocytochemical evidence of amyloid-enhancing factor (AEF) in polymorphonuclear leukocytes. *Acta Pathol. Jpn.* **39**, 349-355.

5. Shirahama, T., Miura, K., Ju, S-T., Kisilevsky, R., Gruys, E., Cohen, A.S. (1990). Amyloid Enhancing Factor-loaded macrophages in amyloid fibril formation. *Lab. Invest.* **62**, 61-76.

6. Picken, M.M., Gallo, G.R., Frangione, B. (1990). Amyloid-Enhancing factor and Inflammatory Reaction. *Lab. Invest.* Letter to the Editor, *in press.*

7. Robitaille, Y., Alizadeh-Khiavi, K., Ali-Khan, Z., Mena, R., Laroche-Cholette, A., Gauvreau, D. (1990). Morphological characterization of a novel antibody against amyloid enhancing factor *(Abstracts of Second International Conference on Alzheimer's Disease Brain Amyloidosis). Neurobiol. of Aging* **11**, 307.

8. Abraham, C.R., Shirahama, T., Potter, H. (1990). α_1-antichymotrypsin is associated solely with amyloid deposits containing the β-protein. Amyloid and cell localization of α_1-antichymotrypsin. *Neurobiol. of aging* **11**, 123-129.

9. Gervais, F., Hebert, L., Skamene, E. (1988). Amyloid-Enhancing Factor: production and response in amyloidosis-susceptible and -resistant mouse strains. *J. Leukocyte Biology* **43**, 311-316.

THE TISSUE ORIGIN OF AMYLOID ENHANCING FACTOR DETERMINES ITS ABILITY TO INDUCE SAA GENE EXPRESSION

I. YOUNG, L. AILLES, S. NARINDRASORASAK, R. KISILEVSKY
Department of Pathology, Queen's University
Kingston, Ontario K7L 3N6 CANADA

INTRODUCTION

Serum amyloid A (SAA) is a family of acute phase proteins whose hepatic synthesis increases 500-1000 fold during inflammation [1]. Murine SAA consists of two markedly homologous apolipoproteins, SAA1 and SAA2, which circulate as components of HDL particles [2-4]. A third less homologous member of the murine SAA gene family, SAA3, is also induced by a variety of inflammatory stimuli [4-6] but a corresponding SAA3 protein has not been identified.

AA amyloidosis is a rare complication of chronic inflammatory disorders in man [7,8] but may be induced readily by persistent inflammation in mice [9]. SAA2 is a known precursor of AA amyloid [10] but the pathogenesis of amyloid formation is not understood. The induction phase of AA amyloidosis can be markedly shortened by the administration of an extract of amyloidotic tissue, termed amyloid enhancing factor (AEF), with a concurrent inflammatory stimulus [9,11]. However, the nature or mechanism of action of AEF has not been defined. This study compares the influence of AEF preparations derived from different tissues on murine hepatic SAA gene expression and plasma SAA protein levels. These effects were correlated with the ability of each AEF preparation to induce AA amyloidosis.

MATERIALS AND METHODS

Animals: Female Swiss white mice were employed in all experiments.
Preparation of AEF: AEF was prepared from amyloidotic murine livers (AEF_L) and spleens (AEF_S), as described previously [9].
Induction Protocols: Subcutaneous inflammation was induced by a single 0.5 ml injection of 2% $AgNO_3$. AEF (100 mg protein) was administered intravenously via the tail. Mice received either AEF_L, AEF_S, $AgNO_3$, AEF_L+$AgNO_3$, AEF_S+$AgNO_3$ or intravenous water (control). At various intervals following treatment, liver tissue was snap frozen for Northern analysis of SAA gene expression. Separate groups of mice received daily injections of AEF_L or AEF_S for 7 days. At various time points splenic amyloid deposition was assessed by Congo red staining of frozen sections.

<u>Plasma SAA Determination</u>: Separate groups of mice were treated with the above protocols and plasma SAA assayed at various intervals by enzyme-linked immunosorbent assay (ELISA) as described elsewhere [12].
<u>Northern Analysis of Hepatic RNA</u>: Total hepatic RNA was isolated as described [13] and Northern blots hybridized with end-labelled oligonucleotide probes specific for SAA1 (5'-ACAAGTGCTCCGAAAGG-3'), SAA2 (5'-AATAACCCCTCCGAAAGG-3') and SAA3 (5'-AGTACTTTCTTCGACCAG-3').

RESULTS

<u>Northern Analysis of Hepatic SAA mRNA</u>

Administration of $AgNO_3$ or AEF_L induced marked accumulation of SAA1 mRNA (Figure 1). Administration of $AgNO_3$+AEF_L resulted in a level of mRNA induction approximately equivalent to the sum of the mRNA inductions produced by each treatment alone (densitometry data not shown). Injection of AEF_S had no effect on SAA1 mRNA levels. Identical results to those seen for SAA1 mRNA were obtained using the SAA2 probe (data not shown). AEF_L induced expression of hepatic SAA3 mRNA in a pattern similar to its induction of SAA1 mRNA. Neither AEF_S nor $AgNO_3$ induced SAA3 mRNA. The molecular weight of each SAA mRNA species decreased progressively following their induction.

<u>SAA Protein Accumulation in Plasma</u>

Injection of $AgNO_3$ or AEF_L alone produced a dramatic increase in plasma SAA (Figure 2). AEF_S alone did not increase plasma SAA nor augment the effect of $AgNO_3$.

<u>Induction of AA Amyloid Deposition</u>

The administration of $AgNO_3$ with either AEF_L or AEF_S resulted in

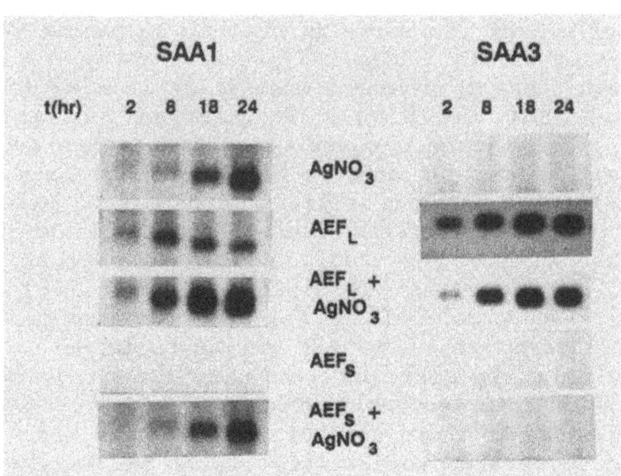

Figure 1: Northern analysis of hepatic SAA mRNA. Northern blots of total hepatic RNA isolated 2,8,18 and 24 hours following treatments were probed for SAA1 and SAA3 mRNA.

an identical pattern of accelerated amyloid deposition (data not shown). Amyloid deposits occurred initially in the perifollicular zones of the spleen within 48 hours of treatment. Daily injection of AEF_L produced amyloid deposition in a similar pattern although amyloid did not appear until the fourth day of treatment. Daily administration of AEF_S alone did not produce amyloid deposition.

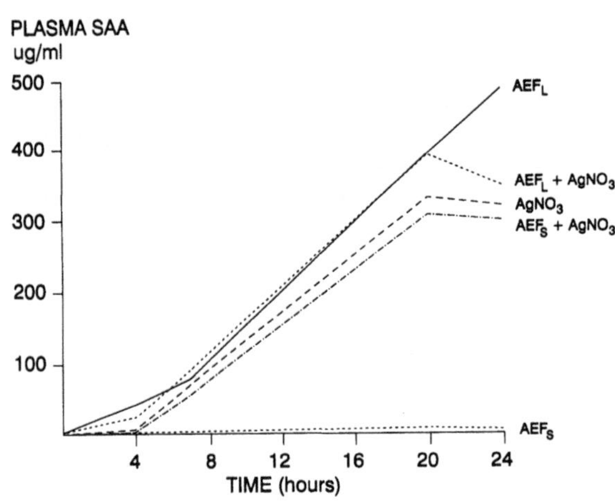

Figure 2: SAA protein accumulation in plasma. Plasma SAA levels were determined by ELISA 4,7,20 and 24 hours following treatments.

DISCUSSION

AEF is defined by its striking ability to markedly accelerate AA amyloid deposition [9,11]. Despite extensive study its nature remains unknown although there is evidence suggesting it may be a glycoprotein [9] or serine protease [14]. This study has shown that AEF preparations differ in their capacity to induce SAA gene expression. AEF_L is a potent inducer of hepatic SAA gene expression. In contrast AEF_S has no effect on SAA gene expression but is as effective as AEF_L in the induction of accelerated amyloid deposition when administered with concomitant $AgNO_3$. These data agree with previous reports which suggested AEF_S has no effect on hepatic SAA mRNA [16] or plasma SAA levels [17,18]. The nature of the SAA gene inducing factor in AEF_L is unclear. Considering that the AEF preparations were extracted from tissues of animals experiencing inflammation it is possible that cytokines such as interleukin-1, which are known to induce SAA gene expression [15], may be components of such preparations.

The capacity of AEF_L to increase plasma SAA levels combined with its ability to precipitate accelerated amyloidosis suggested that administration of AEF_L alone might cause rapid amyloid deposition. This proved to be true as daily AEF_L administration led to amyloid deposition in the spleen within four days. The inability of AEF_S alone to produce amyloidosis is presumably due to its inability to stimulate the synthesis of the SAA precursor of AA amyloid.

There was a transient increase in the molecular weight of each SAA mRNA species following their induction by either AEF_L or $AgNO_3$. We have previously shown that this is due to an alteration in the length of the poly(A) tail of the SAA mRNA [12]. An increase in poly(A) tail length may confer increased stability on mRNA [19,20,21] and so may contribute to the marked accumulation of hepatic SAA mRNA which occurs during inflammation.

ACKNOWLEDGEMENTS

This work was supported by MRC grants MA-11013 (IY) and MT-3153 (RK) and by the Upjohn Company of Canada. We would like to thank Pam Redden for her valuable secretarial assistance.

REFERENCES

1. McAdam KPWJ and Sipe JD. J Exp Med 144:1121, 1976
2. van der Westhuyzen DR, Coetzee GA and de Beer FC (1986) in Amyloidosis (Marrink J, Van Rijswick MH, eds) pp.115, Martinus Nijhoff, The Hague, The Netherlands 3. Husebekk A, Skogen B and Husby G. Scand J Immunol 25:375, 1987
3. Husebekk A, Skogen B and Husby G. Scand J Immunol 25:375, 1987
4. Lowell CA, Potter DA, Stearman RS et al. J Biol Chem 261:8442, 1986
5. Rokita H, Shirahama T, Cohen AS et al. J Immunol 139:3849, 1987
6. Rienhoff HY and Groudine M. Mol Cell Biol 8:3710, 1983
7. Levin M, Franklin EC, Frangione B et al. J Clin Invest 51:2773, 1972
8. Rosenthal CJ, Franklin EC, Frangione B et al. J Immunol 116:1415, 1976
9. Axelrad MA, Kisilevsky R, Willmer J et al. Lab Invest 47:139, 1982
10. Hoffman JS, Ericsson LH, Eriksen N et al. J Exp Med 159:641, 1984
11. Kisilevsky R, Axelrad M, Corbett W et al. Lab Invest 37:544, 1977
12. Brissette L, Young I, Narindrasorasak S et al. J Biol Chem 264:19327, 1989
13. Chomczynski P and Sacchi N. Anal Biochem 162:156, 1987
14. Abankwa GV and Ali-Khan Z. Br J Exp Pathol 69:133, 1988
15. Ramadori G, Sipe JD and Colten HR. J Immunol 135:3645, 1987
16. Sipe JD, Rokita H, Shirahama T et al. Cell Protides Biol Fluids 34:331, 1986
17. Deal CL, Sipe JD, Tatsuta E et al. Ann NY Acad Sci 389:439, 1982
18. Kisilevsky R, Benson MD, Axelrad MA et al. Lab Invest 41:206, 1979
19. Paek I and Axel R. Mol Cell Biol 7:1996, 1987
20. Cochrane AW and Deeley RG. J Mol Biol 203:555, 1988
21. Shiels BR, Northemann W, Grehring MR et al. J Biol Chem 262:12826, 1987

PMSF-SENSITIVE SERINE ESTERASE-ACTIVITY AND FIBRIL-DERIVED AMYLOID ENHANCING FACTOR (FAEF)-ACTIVITY IN HAMSTER ARE NOT RELATED.

Niewold ThA, Kisilevsky R*, Shirahama T#, Gruys E, Dept. of Vet. Pathol., Univ. of Utrecht, The Netherlands. *Dept. of Pathol., Kingston School of Med., Kingston, Canada. #Arthritis Center, Boston School of Med., Boston, USA.

ABSTRACT

The exact nature and the mode of action of the amyloid enhancing factor (AEF) are still not clear. In the present study, the relationship between AEF-activity and serine esterase activity was examined in AEF-preparations of different origin. Hamster FAEF contained a high AEF-activity and a very low serine esterase level. No correlation was found between serine esterase level and AEF-activity in the various AEF-preparations. It was concluded serine esterase activity is not essential for AEF-activity in hamster.

INTRODUCTION

The amyloid enhancing factor (AEF) is an essential factor in experimental AA-amyloidogenesis. AEF-activity was shown to be present in a variety of tissues or extracts of different origin (3,4,6). High levels of AEF are present in amyloidotic tissue and amyloid fibril extracts (3,4,6). Furthermore, AEF-activity is associated with leucocytes (1,2,4) and macrophages (8), the highest activity being found in amyloidotic animals. AEF is described to be a protein (3,4,7), but conflicting data were published on its nature. Initially, the activity was reported to be not inhibited by a variety of protease-inhibitors (amongst which PMSF (phenylmethylsulphonyl fluoride)(3,4), but recently, AEF was described to be a serine esterase (SE), its activity being abolished by PMSF (1,2).

In the present study, the following issues are examined in the experimental hamster model:

A. is fibril AEF (FAEF) activity sensitive to PMSF?
B. is AEF-activity related to serine esterase (SE)-activity?

MATERIALS AND METHODS

Young male Syrian hamsters (Mesocricetus auratus, 100g) received a single intraperitoneal (i.p.) injection of the substance to be tested for AEF-activity on day one, and 7 daily subcutaneous injections of 40 μg LPS in PBS (lipopolysaccharide, E.coli o.127:B8, Difco Labs, Detroit,

Michigan). The hamsters were killed on day 7, and samples of spleen, liver and kidney were fixed in buffered formalin. Paraffin sections (5 µm) were stained with alkaline Congo red and screened for the presence of amyloid. Amyloid involvement was graded as follows: spleen only: 1 point, spleen and liver: 2 points, spleen, liver and kidney: 3 points.

The AEF-preparations used were: fibril AEF (FAEF) prepared as described before (6,7), splenic AEF prepared according to Axelrad et al (3), and lysates of resident or casein-attracted peritoneal cells of amyloidotic and non-amyloidotic animals, prepared according to Abankwa et al (1).

Pretreatment of FAEF with PMSF was performed according to Abankwa et al (1).

Serine esterase activity of injected samples was determined as described before (5) and is given as µM naphthol AS-D liberated/min.

RESULTS

Table 1. Pretreatment of hamster FAEF with PMSF did not abolish its AEF-activity.

treatment (i.p.)	amyloidotic animals/n
FAEF	4/4
FAEF+ 10 mM PMSF	5/5

Figure 1. PMSF-sensitive serine esterase activity and the AEF-activity in preparations of different origin are not related.

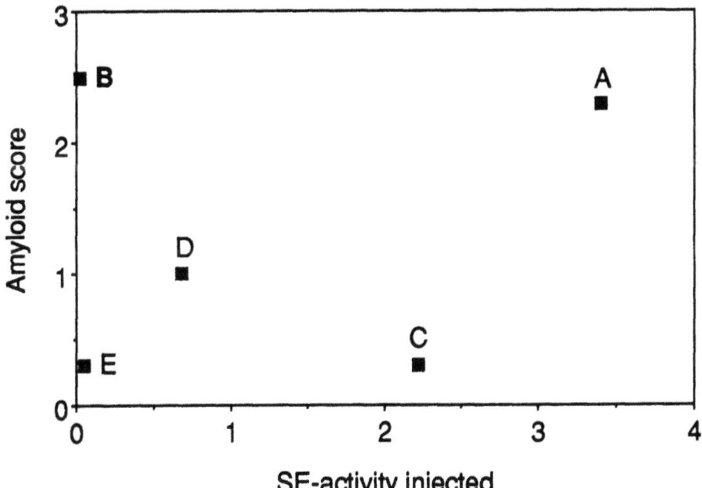

A=splenic AEF, B=fibril AEF, peritoneal cell-lysates from C=amyloidotic, resident ($6x10^6$ cells), D=non-amyloidotic, attracted ($13x10^6$ cells), D=amyloidotic, attracted ($3x10^6$ cells).

FAEF-activity was not sensitive to pretreatment with PMSF (Table 1). No relationship was found between PMSF-sensitive SE-activity and AEF-activity in preparations of different origin. Peritoneal cell-lysates contained a low AEF-activity (Figure 1).

DISCUSSION

AEF was suggested to be a serine esterase (SE), because pretreatment with PMSF abolished its activity (1,2). The putative role of AEF as a protease is not in accord with earlier reports that AEF-activity was not affected by a variety of protease inhibitors (3,4). In the present study, FAEF was not inactivated by pretreatment with PMSF, and no correlation was found between the SE-levels and the AEF-activity in samples of different origin. It is concluded that SE-activity is not essential for AEF-activity, and that SE-activity appears not to be a common characteristic of all AEFs.

REFERENCES

1. Abankwa GV, Ali-Khan ZI: Alveolar hydatid cyst induced amyloid enhancing factor (AEF): physicochemical properties and abolition of AEF activity by serine protease inhibitors. Br.J.Exp.Pathol. 69:133, 1988
2. Alizadeh-Khiavi K, Ali-Khan ZI: Biochemical nature and cellular origin of amyloid enhancing factor (AEF) as determined by anti-AEF antibody. Br.J.Exp.Pathol. 69:133, 1988
3. Axelrad MA, Kisilevsky R: Biochemical characterizations of amyloid enhancing factor. In Amyloid and Amyloidosis, edited by Glenner GG, Costa PP, de Freitas AF, p 527. Amsterdam, Excerpta Medica, 1980
4. Baltz ML, Caspi D, Hind CRK, Feinstein A, Pepys MB: Isolation and characterization of amyloid enhancing factor (AEF). In Amyloidosis, edited by Glenner G, Ossermann EF, Benditt EP, Calkins E, Cohen AS, Zucker-Franklin D, p 115. New York, Plenum Press, 1986
5. Hol PR, van Ederen AM, Snel FWJJ, Langeveld JPM, Veerkamp JH, Gruys E: Activities of lysosomal enzymes and levels of serum amyloid A (SAA) in blood plasma of hamsters during casein induction of AA-amyloidosis. Br.J.Exp.Pathol. 66: 279, 1985
6. Niewold ThA, Hol PR, van Andel ACJ, Lutz ETG, Gruys E: Enhancement of amyloid induction by amyloid fibril fragments in hamster. Lab.Invest. 56:544, 1987
7. Niewold ThA, Tooten PCJ, van Andel ACJ, Gruys E: Induced AA amyloid in hamster: on the amyloid enhancing factor and protein AA-cross reacting components of intermediate molecular weight. In Amyloid and Amyloidosis, edited by Isobe T, Araki S, Uchino F, Kito S, Tsubura E, p 75. New York, Plenum Press, 1988
8. Shirahama T, Miura K, Ju ST, Kisilevsky R, Gruys E, Cohen AS: Amyloid enhancing factor-loaded macrophages in amyloid fibril formation. Lab.Invest. 62:61, 1990

INDUCTION OF AMYLOID DEPOSITION BY SUBFRACTIONS OF THE AMYLOID ENHANCING FACTOR EXTRACTED FROM BRAIN OF PATIENTS WITH ALZHEIMER'S DISEASE.

C. MORISSETTE AND F. GERVAIS
McGill Centre for the Study of Host Resistance and
McGill Centre for Studies in Aging
The Montréal General Hospital Research Institute
1650 Cedar Ave, Montréal, (Québec)
Canada H3G 1A4

ABSTRACT. Crude amyloid enhancing factor (AEF) was extracted from brain samples of patients with Alzheimer's disease (AD) and showed to be capable of inducing amyloidosis. This crude AEF extract was electrophoresed and seven fractions of different molecular weights were isolated by electroelution. Only two out of these seven fractions were found to have AEF activity; one fraction contained high molecular weight proteins (> 90 kDa) and the other was of lower molecular weight (21.5 to 30 kDa). These two fractions could induce accelerated amyloid deposition in experimental animals.

1. Introduction

Cerebral amyloidosis is characterized by localized deposition of amyloid fibril into the brain (Frangione (1989)). The major amyloid component found in Alzheimer's disease (AD), the ß/A4 protein, is a 4.2 kDa polypeptide. cDNA cloning has suggested that the ß/A4 peptide is synthesized as part of a much larger amyloid precursor molecule (APP), an integral membrane protein, coded by a gene located on chromosome 21 (Goldgaber et al. (1987), Kang et al. (1987), Robakis et al. (1987), Tanzi et al. (1987)). ß/A4 protein is derived from parts of the extracellular and membrane-spanning domains of the APP through an unknown mechanism, probably following abnormal proteolytic cleavage and abnormal processing of cell-surface APP (Esch et al. (1990), Glenner (1988), Robakis et al. (1987)). Always found associated with the fibrils are the amyloid P component (AP) and heparan sulfate proteoglycan (HSPG). The reason for their constant association with the amyloid fibrils is however undetermined.

Amyloid enhancing factor (AEF) has also been described in extract of amyloidotic tissues. It has the ability to accelerate the deposition of amyloid fibrils in a model of secondary amyloidosis. AEF is capable of triggering amyloid deposition within 48 hours following its injection concomitantly with an inflammatory stimulus. Amyloid deposition usually takes approximately 15 days before appearing in tissues of animals undergoing sustained inflammation (Kisilevsky et al. (1977), Kisilevsky and Boudreau (1983)). This factor is believed to be produced in the late pre-amyloid phase of the disease to then act on the amyloid phase. It has been found in the spleen, liver and bone marrow of pre-amyloidotic and amyloidotic animals (Axelrad et al. (1982), Kisilevsky and Boudreau (1983)). It has also been reported in amyloidotic tissues of patients with secondary amyloidosis, Familial Mediterranean Fever and Familial Polyneuropathy (Shirahama et al. (1969), Varga et al. (1986)). Its nature and mechanism of action are however still unknown.

We have found that AEF activity is also present in brain extracts of patients with AD. We report here that two out of seven subfractions obtained from the crude AEF extract showed to have the potential to induce accelerated amyloid deposition in experimental animals. One fraction contained high molecular weight proteins (> 90 kDa) while the other fraction contained proteins of 21.5 to 30 kDa.

2. Materials and Methods

2.1. EXTRACTION OF AMYLOID ENHANCING FACTOR

Aliquot of 1.0 to 1.4 gram of thawed coarsely dissected gray matter was homogenized in 8 ml of cold 4 M glycerol-10 mM Tris-HCl, pH 7.5 for 1.5 min. Centrifugation, dialysis and isolation of the AEF extract were conducted as described by Brandwein et al. (1985). The AEF extract was reconstituted in PBS and sonicated. Protein content was determined using the Bio-Rad assay. Biological AEF activity was monitored by injecting C57BL/6N HSD mice with 100 or 500 µg protein i.v. concomitantly with 0.5 ml of 2% $AgNO_3$ solution s.c. Amyloid deposit was determined in the spleen by Congo red staining and by immunofluorescence using anti-amyloid A serum. Presence of AP and ß/A4 protein in the crude extract was determined by Western blot using antibody against human serum AP and against ß/A4 protein, respectively. The anti-ß/A4 protein was an antibody directed against 28 aa synthetic peptide of the ß/A4 protein (generously provided by Dr. Blas Frangione, New York University Medical Centre). HSPG in our crude AEF extract was monitored by assessing the amount of glucosamine by amino acid analysis using Dionex Ion Chromatography system.

2.2. ISOLATION OF THE MAJOR PROTEIN BANDS OF THE AEF EXTRACT

Active AEF extract was electrophoresed (SDS-PAGE). Seven gel fractions comprising the major protein bands were cut from the gel based on their molecular weight. These fractions were then electroeluted from the gel, in dialysis bags in 10 mM CAPS-10% methanol, pH 11 at 50 V for 18 hours. Electroeluted protein solutions were filtered through 0.45 µm membrane and dialyzed against double distilled water (ddH_2O) and lyophilized. Pellets were reconstituted in ddH_2O and precipitated in a 1:4 acetone/methanol solution at -20ºC for 18 hours. Each fraction was centrifuged and dried. After suspension in 0.5 ml PBS and sonication, the fractions were injected i.v. into mice along with a 2% $AgNO_3$ solution s.c. to assess their AEF activity.

3. Results

Three components are always found in association with amyloid deposits: AEF, AP and HSPG. In order to determine if AEF extract contained or could be identified as AP, Western blot assay was done using an antibody directed against serum AP. Furthermore, using the same technique we assessed for the presence of the ß/A4 amyloid peptide in our extract. Both anti-SAP and anti-ß/A4 antibodies did not show any reaction with the AEF extract. Amino acid analysis of the crude AEF did not show to contain more than 2% glucosamine, suggesting that HSPG was not present in our extract preparation. Presence of glucuronic acid was not determined. AEF activity found in our crude extract preparation could thus not be attributed to AP or HSPG.

Seven fractions comprising the major protein bands, designated A through G (Figure 1), were assessed for the AEF activity. Only 2 out of the 7 fractions could induce amyloid A fibril deposition in experimental animals: fraction A comprising high WM proteins (> 90 kDa) and fraction G which contained proteins of 21.5 to 30 kDa (1/2, and 2/2 mice on repeated experiments).

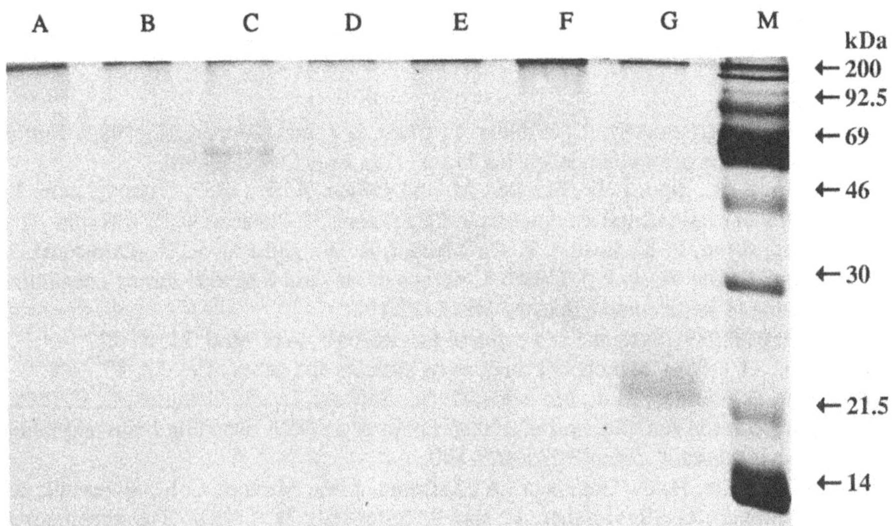

Figure 1. Electrophoresis of the proteins contained in gel segments of the AEF extract.

4. Discussion

AEF was found in brain extracts of patients with AD. Identification of the protein responsible for this activity could shed light on the mechanisms of amyloid deposition and on the pathogenesis of amyloidosis. In order to identify this factor we determined first if the crude extract contained any AP, ß/A4 protein and HSPG. All were absent, suggesting that neither of these components could have the ability to induce accelerated amyloid deposition.

In our attempt to identify within the crude extract which protein is responsible for this AEF activity, seven fractions were obtained following electroelution of the major proteins from the electrophoresed AEF extract. AEF was first observed in the gel segment containing high MW protein only. The following experiments demonstrated that AEF activity resided as well in a fraction containing proteins of 21.5 to 30 kDa. The fact that no activity was present in the G fraction during the first assay probably resulted from the amount of protein contained in this fraction which would have been too low to show any AEF activity. The activity seen with the high molecular weight fraction could originate from aggregation of the lower MW proteins.

Mechanism of action of AEF is still unknown. AEF could affect the cells responsible for degrading the precursor, or it could influence the enzyme system responsible for the complete breakdown of the precursor molecule, or it could act on the precursor itself, or on the fibrils. By purifying the protein responsible for this activity we will be able to understand the mechanism of action of AEF in relation to its ability to trigger amyloid deposition.

5. Acknowledgements

We thank the Brain Tissue Bank, Douglas Hospital Research Centre, Verdun (Québec, Canada) for providing us frozen brain samples from patients with diagnosed AD.
This work was supported by a grant from the Alzheimer Society of Canada (90-05).

6. References

Axelrad, M. A., Kisilevsky, R., Willmer, J., Chen, S. J. and Skinner, M. (1982) 'Further characterization of amyloid-enhancing factor', Lab. Invest. 47, 139-146.

Brandwein, S. R., Sipe, J. D., Skinner, M. and Cohen, A. S. (1985) 'Prostaglandin E_1 inhibition of experimental amyloidosis in CBA/J mice', J. Rheumatol. 12, 418-426.

Esch, F. S., Keim, P. S., Beattie, E. C., Blacher, R. W., Culwell, A. R., Oltersdorf, T., McClure, D. and Ward, P. J. (1990) 'Cleavage of amyloid ß peptide during constitutive processing of its precursor', Science 248, 1122-1124.

Frangione, B. (1989) 'Systemic and cerebral amyloidosis', Ann. Med. 21, 69-72.

Glenner, G. G. (1988) 'Alzheimer's disease: its proteins and genes', Cell 52, 307-308.

Goldgaber, D., Lerman, M. I., Mc Bride, O. W., Saffiotti, U. and Gajdusek, D. C. (1987) 'Characterization and chromosomal localization of a cDNA encoding brain amyloid of Alzheimer's disease', Science 235, 877-880.

Kang, J., Lemaire, H.-G., Unterbeck, A., Salbaum, J. M., Masters, C. L., Grzeschik, K.-H., Multhaup, G., Beyreuther, K. and Müeller-Hill, B. (1987) 'The precursor of Alzheimer's disease amyloid A4 protein resembles a cell-surface receptor', Nature 325, 733-736.

Kisilevsky, R., Axelrad, M., Corbett, W., Brunet, S. and Scott, F. (1977) 'The role of inflammatory cells in the pathogenesis of amyloidosis', Lab. Invest. 37, 544-553.

Kisilevsky, R. and Bourdreau, L. (1983) 'Kinetics of amyloid deposition I. The effects of amyloid-enhancing factor and splenectomy', Lab. Invest. 48, 53-59.

Robakis, N. K., Ramakrishna, N., Wolfe, G. and Wisniewski, H. M. (1987) 'Molecular cloning and characterization of a cDNA encoding the cerebrovascular and the neuritic plaque amyloid peptides', Proc. Natl. Acad. Sci. USA 84, 4190-4194.

Shirahama, T., Lawless, O. J. and Cohen, A. S. (1969) 'Heterologous transfer of amyloid-human to mouse', Proc. Soc. Exp. Biol. Med. 130, 516-519.

Tanzi, R. E., Gusella, J. F., Watkins, P. C., Bruns, G. A. P., St-George-Hyslop, P. H., Van Keuren, M. L., Patterson, D., Pagan, S., Kurnit, D. M. and Neve, R. L. (1987) 'Amyloid beta protein gene: cDNA, mRNA distribution, and genetic linkage near the Alzheimer locus', Science 235, 880-884.

Varga, J., Flinn, M. S. M. , Shirahama, T., Rodgers, O. G. and Cohen, A. S. (1986) 'The induction of accelerated murine amyloid with human splenic extract', Virchows Arch. [B] 51, 177-185.

ISOLATION OF AMYLOID EHANCING FACTOR (AEF)

T.Yokota, T.Ishihara, M.Takahashi, Y.Yamashita, T.Gondo, S.Kawamura, Y. Hoshii, M.Koga, T.Iwata* and F.Uchino
First Department of Pathology, Yamaguchi University School of Medicine, * The School of Allied Health Sciences, Yamaguchi University, Ube, Yamaguchi 755, Japan.

ABSTRACT. After homogenation and centrifugation of the neutrophils and the spleens obtained from mice with an injection of amyloidogen, the supernatants were individually applied to DEAE ion exchange chromatogrophy. AEF activity in each fraction was tested. AEF activity was present in peaks eluted at concentration of 0.17M NaCl. The fractions containing AEF were subjected to gel chromatographic HPLC, and AEF was eluted at about 15KD. Purified-AEF was analyzed by gas chromatography. AEF contained in some saccharides consisting of glucose, mannose, galactosamine and sialic acid, and undefined substance (probably derived from proteins). From the present results, it is suggested that AEF is a glycoprotein in the neutrophilic granules.

INTRODUCTION

Since the initial studies of amyloid enhancing factor (AEF) concerning by Wederin & Ranlov (1966), and Janigan & Druet(1968), a large number of conflicting results have been reported biological and biochemical aspects of this substance. We have reported that strong AEF activity is present in the spleens of aging mice, and AEF has been shown to be a neutrophil-related substance by immunohistochemistry with the use of an anti-AEF antiserum obtained by the immunization of partial purified-AEF from the spleens of the amyloidogen injected-mice(Yokota et al. (1989)).

In this paper, the isolation and the nature of AEF from the neutrophils and the spleens of the amyloidogen injected-mice are described.

MATERIALS AND METHODS

Animals; AKR/J mice were intraperitoneally injected an emulsion of mycobacterium butyricum and Freund's complete adjuvant and were sacrificed under ether anesthesia 11 days after the injection. The blood was drawn into the heparinized-syringe by the heart puncture and the spleens were removed.

AEF activity of the neutrophils; The neutrophils were separated from 50 ml of blood according to the method of Bentwood and Henson (1980). $1x10^8$ cells were obtained, represented morphologically more than 95% neutrophils and were more than 98% viable by trypan blue exclusions.

AEF activity of the neutrophils was examined by injections of

$2x10^3$, $2x10^4$, $2x10^5$, $5x10^5$ and $1x10^6$ cells into tail veins of mice, receiving a series of 3 subcutaneous injections of 10% casein solution beginning on the same day. Control animals were given 3 daily injections of the casein solution.

The release of granule constituents (degranulation) from $2x10^7$ neutrophils activated (15 min, 37 degrees Centigrade) with 1M of the synthetic chemotactic tripeptide (N-formyl-L-methionyl-L-leucyl-L-phenylalanine) and 5 microgram cytocalasin B in a final volume of 1ml physiologic saline was done. After centrifugation at 300 x G, 5min, 0.5ml of the granules-containing supernatant was intraperitoneally injected per a mouse and followed by the injections of casein solution. Control animals were intraperitoneally given the 0.5ml of the solution used for degranulation and followed by the injections of casein solution.

Isolation of AEF from the neutrophils and the spleens; The remainning neutrophils and spleens were homogenized in 10mM phosphate buffered saline (PBS) and dialyzed against 10mM phosphate buffer (PB). After centrifugation, supernatants were respectively applied to an ion-exchange chromatographic column (DEAE-TOYOPEARL, TOSOH, Japan), which was equilibrated with 10mM PB and eluted with a lineal NaCl gradient (0-1M). AEF activity in each fraction (8ml) was tested, and the fractions containning AEF were applied to gel-filtration HPLC using TSKgel G3000SW column (TOSOH, Japan) with the elusion buffer 10mM PB, flow rate 0.5 ml/min, column size 75x300mm.

Gas chromatographic analysis; Purified AEF was analyzed by gas chromatography using a Hitachi 163 apparatus.

RESULT

AEF activity of the neutrophils; Amyloid deposits were observed in the spleens of recipient-mice injected the neutrophils more than $2x10^4$ and the degranulated-solution of the neutrophils. These data are shown in table 1.

TABLE 1. AEF activity of neutrophils and granule-containing solution(GCS)

Number of donor neutrophil and GCS	Splenic amyloid in recipient	
	Degree of amyloid	positive/total recipients
$1x10^6$	III	2/2
$5x10^5$	II	2/2
$2x10^5$	II	2/2
$2x10^4$	I	2/2
$2x10^3$	-	0/2
GCS	I	2/2

The extent of amyloid deposition is graded according to the modified method of Christensen's classification (Hanai et al. 1979).

Isolation of AEF from the neutrophils and spleens; In the ion-exchange chromatography of the neutrophils (Fig. 1), AEF activity was limited in a main peak which eluted at the concentration of 0.17M NaCl. On the other hand, in that of the spleens (Fig. 2), AEF activity was present in the peak A, B, C, and D, and was the strongest in the peak C which was eluted at the concentration of 0.17M NaCl. Subsequently, these peaks were subjected to the gel-chromatographic HPLC, AEF activity was proved in the small peaks (allow) in Fig. 3. These peaks were applied to the same column, again, AEF activity was detected in a single peak eluted at 23 min, and the molecular weights were presumed to be about 15KD from the elusion profile (Fig. 4).

Gas chromatographic analysis; Gas chromatography of the purified-AEF revealed that it contained with some saccharides (glucose, mannose, galactosamine and sialic acid) and undefined substances.

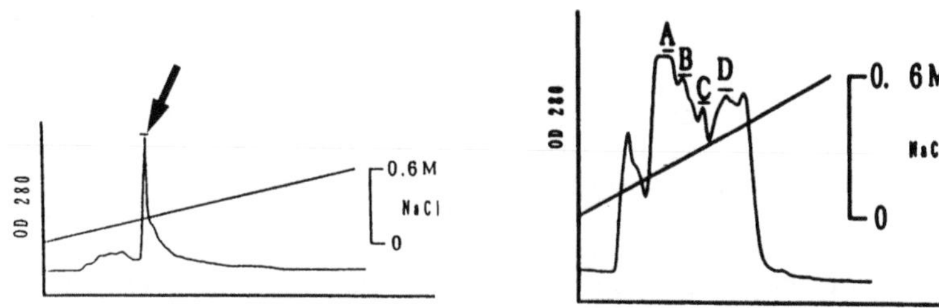

Figure 1 Figure 2.

Figure 1. DEAE-ion exchange chromatography of the preparation from the neutrophils. AEF activity is present in the main peak (allow) eluted at the concentration of 0.17M NaCl.

Figure 2. DEAE-ion exchange chromatography of the preparation from the spleens. AEF activity is detected in the peaks of A, B, C and D, and is the strongest in the peak of C which is eluted at the concentration of 0.17M NaCl.

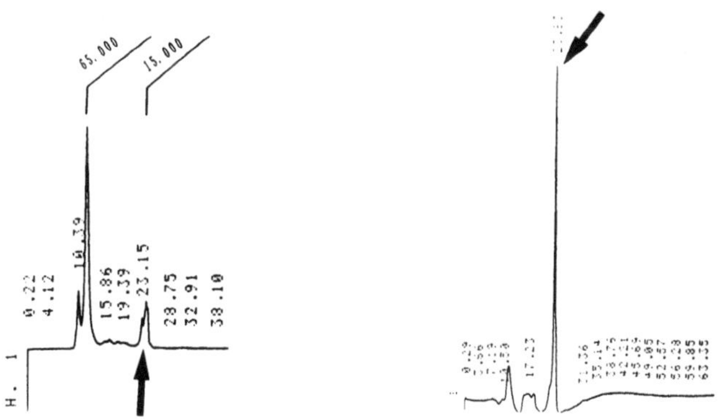

Figure 3. Figure 4.

Figure 3 and Figure 4. Gel chromatographic HPLC. AEF is present in the peak (allow) which is eluted at around 23 min of the retention time and at about 15KD of the molecular weights.

DISCUSSION

In model animals with accelerated amyloid induction, the transfers of various tissues and cells including the spleen, liver, kidney, lung, thymus, bone marrow, lymph node, peritoneal macrophages and peripheral lymphocytes from the amyloidotic donor has been reported. Kedar and Ravid (1980) reported that polymorphonuclear leukocytes from the casein treated-mice were capable of inducing accelerated amyloid formation in the recipient mice. Kisilevsky et al. (1977) reported that there was a striking corelation between the extent of the splenic amyloid deposition and the severity of inflammation at the amyloidogen injected-sites in a model of accelerated experimental amyloidosis. They suggested that AEF was derived from the activating polymorphonuclear leukocytes. Alizadeh-Khiavi and Ali-Khan (1988) reported that the polyclonal AEF antibody reacted positively with the splenic and the peripheral leukocytes from mice injected an amyloidogen. We reported independently that AEF had a close relationship with the neutrophils by the use of immunohistochemistry with anti-AEF antiserum.

In this paper, when varying numbers of the neutrophils from the amyloid laden-mice were injected in the recipient mice with the injections of casein solution, there was a positive correlation between the amount of amyloid in the spleens and numbers of the neutrophils administrated. These findings showed that the amount of amyloid deposition was dependent on the dose of AEF. AEF activity was present in the cell-free and the neutrophilic granules-containing supernatant after the treatment of degranulation. This finding suggests that AEF is present in the neutrophilic granules. On the gel chromatographic HPLC, AEF was eluted at about 15KD, and by gas chromatographic analysis, the several saccharides were detected in the fraction with AEF activity; therefore, AEF is conjectured to be a certain glycoprotein.

ACKNOWLEDGEMENT

This work suported by a Grant-in-Aid for Scientic Research (C02670152) from the Ministry of Education, Science and Culture, and a research grant from the Primary Amyloidosis Research Committe, the Ministry of Health and Welfare.

REFERENCES

Alizadeh-Khiavi K and Ali-Khan Z, (1988) Br J Exp Pathol 69:605-619.
Bentwood BJ and Henson PM, (1980) J Immunol 124:855-862.
Hanai N et al. (1979) Virchows Archiv A Path Anat and Hist 384:45-52
Janigan DT and Druet RL, (1968) Am J Pathol 52:381-390.
Kedar I and Ravid M, (1980) Eur J Clin Invest, 10:63-65.
Kisilevsky R et al. (1977) Lab Invest 37:544-553.
Yokota T et al. (1989) Acta Pathol Jpn 39:349-355.
Yokota T et al. (1989) Virchows Archiv A Path Anat and Hist 414:511-514.
Wedrin O and Ranlov P, (1966) Acta Pathol Microbiol Scandinav 68:1-18.

EFFECTS OF AMYLOID ENHANCING FACTOR ON IN VITRO KUPFFER CELLS

T.IWATA, T.YOKOTA*, M.TAKAHASHI*, J.UEDA, T.ISHIHARA*,
Y.YAMASHITA*, T.GONDO*, S.KAWAMURA* and F.UCHINO*
The School of Allied Health Sciences, Yamaguchi University,
*First Department of Pathology, Yamaguchi University, School of Medicine, Ube, Yamaguchi 755, Japan

ABSTRACT. Kupffer cells (KC) were isolated from amyloid-laden livers of mice (AKC) and non-amyloid livers (NKC). After attachment of AKC to petri dishes, the supernatants containing floating amyloid were centrifuged and the pellet was added to NKC (NKCamy). The deposition of amyloid was observed in many of the AKC and some of NKCamy. After 14 d culture when the deposits of amyloid had almost disappeared, amyloid enhancing factor (AEF) and serum amyloid A (SAA) rich serum were added. The number of amyloid deposits fairly increased in AKC and NKCamy compared with the control cultures. Although no deposit of amyloid was found in the treated NKC, their morphological changes were remarkable. After treatment with AEF, they were swollen and the cell borders became clear. Under the scanning electron microscpy (SEM), stimulated cells displayed prominent petal-like ruffles, ridges and frequent filopodia. After treatent with AEF and SAA-rich liver extract, a fine granular substance was phagocytized, but amyloid fibrils could not be found in the NKC.

Based on these results, we concluded that AEF participates in the second phase of amyloidogenesis, and some other factor in addition to AEF and SAA must be necessary for the synthesis of amyloid fibrils.

INTRODUCTION

Cells of the reticuloendothelial system, particularly KC, have been considered to be responsible for SAA degradation and amyloid protein A (AA) synthesis (1). AEF drastically shortens amyloid induction time in experimental AA-amyloidosis (2, 3). Although this factor is thought to play an important role in the process of amyloid deposition, its functional mechanism is still unclear. In this report, the effect of AEF on KC was investigated using an in vitro system.

MATERIALS AND METHODS

<u>Animals</u>: Animals were AKR or ICR mice weighing over 30g. Mice with amyloidosis had received an intraperitoneal injection of 0.2ml of an emulsion of Mycobacterium butyricum in complete Freund's adjuvant. Mice without amyloidosis were non-treated or had received a subcutaneous injection of the emulsion (stimulated mouse). The spleen and a piece of the liver of each mouse was stained by Congo Red method and the presence

or absence of amyloid was confirmed.

Preparation of SAA rich serum: The serum was collected from the mice that had received an intraperitoneal injection of the emulsion 24 h before.

Preparation of liver extract: The liver was removed from a mouse that had received a subcutaneous injection of the emulsion 24 h before. It was homogenized in 20ml DME and centrifuged at 30,000 rpm for 1 h. The supernatant was used.

Prepatation of AEF: The procedure was performed as described in detail by Yokota in this symposium.

Isolation and culture of KC: KC were isolated with collagenase and pronase. The isolation procedure was modified from procedures described by Iwata(4) and Fuks and Zucker-Franklin(1). The isolated cells were plated on petri dishes on which glass cover slips had been placed. The medium was Dulbecco's modified Eagles's (DME) conaining 10% fetal calf serum, penicillin and streptomycin. After the AKC attached to the petri dishes, the supernatants containing unattached cells, debris and floating amyloid were centrifuged at 5,000 rpm for 40 min. The pellet was added to the NKC isolated from a normal mouse and after incubation at 37C° in 5% CO_2 for 16 h, the supernatants were removed and the medium was replaced with the fresh medium (NKCAmy).

Preparation of specimens for morphology: Glass cover slips layered with cells were fixed in 95% ethanol for light microscpy or with 2% glutaraldehyde, then postfixed with 1% osmium tetroxide solution for SEM and transmission electron microscopy (TEM).

RESULTS

Most of the adherent cells were spread out and many of them were fibroblastic in morphology. Intracellular and extracellular amyloid deposits were easily observed in AKC. In some places, small cell clusters surrounding amyloid nodules were found. In NKCamy dishes, some adherent cells phagocytized small deposits of amyloid. After 14 d culture when the deposition of amyloid had almost disappeared in AKC (4), the medium of AKC, NKCamy and NKC were replaced with DME containing 20% SAA rich serum and 0.3ml AEF. The number of deposits of amyloid became fairly increased in the AKC and NKCamy, as compared with the control cultures. No such deposit was found in NKC.

In order to produce amyloid fibrils experimentally in vitro, NKC were isolated from a stimulated mouse. After 8 d culture, each dish was added 0.2ml AEF and 0.1ml fibronectin, or 0.1ml AEF, 0.2ml liver extract and 0,1ml fibronectin. In several hours the treated cells were swollen and the cell borders became clear and showed a granular appearance under the phase contrast microscopy. Cells maintained in culture in the presence of the above stimuli for 3 d were examined by SEM and TEM. Non-treated NKC had spread out exhibiting a flat appearance with broad transparent veils of cytoplasm with scattered ridges. Some cells had long cord-like extensions which attached onto the underlying transparent cytoplasmic veils (Fig.1). In contrast, AEF stimulated cells showed a great variation in shape and surface feature (Fig.2). The most prominent feature was numerous fine surface ruffles. Many of them looked like the petals of a rose. Ridge-like profiles and more frequent filopodia and intercellular contacts via filopodia were also frequently seen (Fig.3).

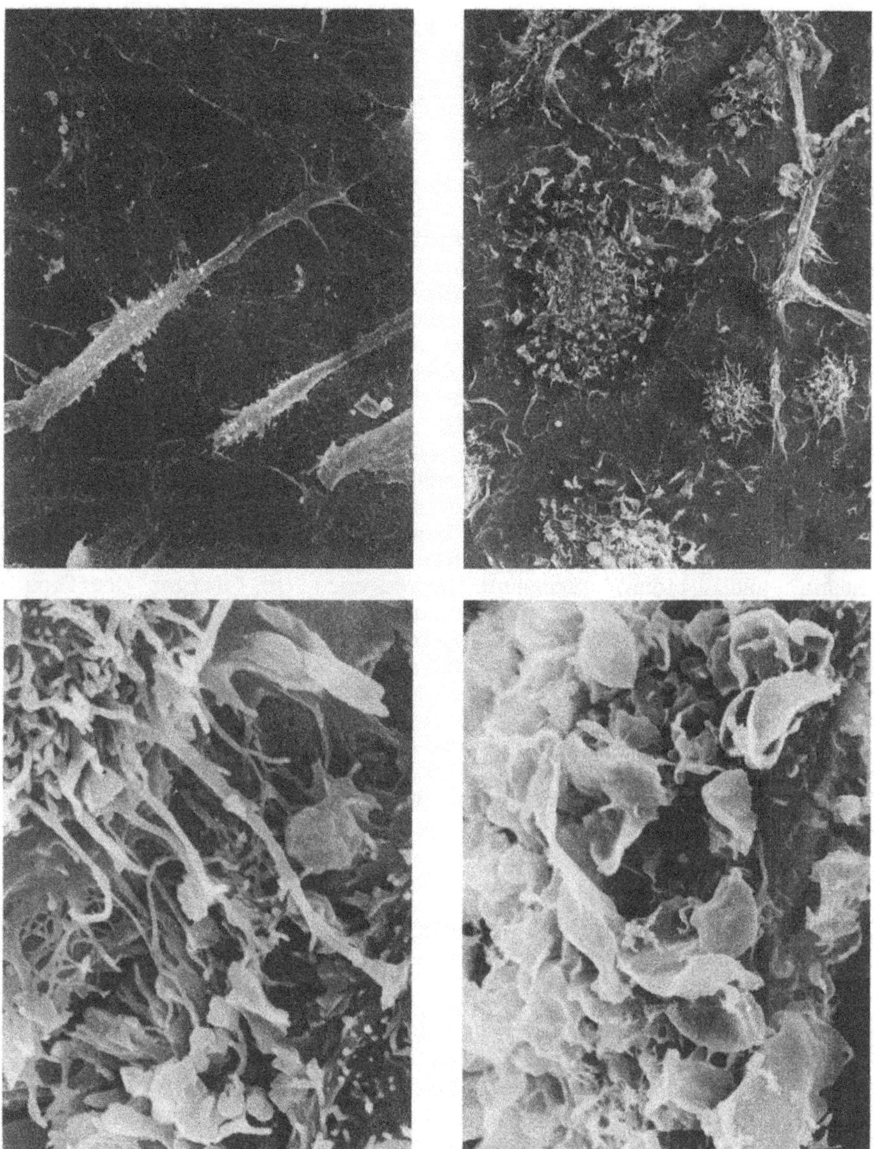

Fig.1 NKC after 12 d in culture, elongated with cord-like extensions attaching onto the underlying transparent cytoplasmic veils. SEM x 720
Fig.2 NKC 3 d after treatment with AEF (12 d in vitro), showing a great variation in shape and surface feature. SEM x 720
Fig.3 NKC 3 d after treatment with AEF (12 d in vitro), showing frequent ruffles and intercellular contacts via filopodia. SEM : x 9,000
Fig.4 NKC, 3 d after treatment with AEF and liver extract (12 d in vitro), having more elaborated surface configuration. SEM x 4,800

TEM revealed numerous lysosomes, some phagosomes, and well-developed endoplasmic reticulum and Golgi apparatus. Treated with AEF and SAA the surface configuration became more elaborate with irregular ridges of different width and shape (Fig.4). Fine granular substances were seen within cytoplasmic invagination, but amyloid fibrils could not be found.

DISCUSSION

By the addition of AEF, in vitro synthesis of amyloid by AKC and NKCamy was activated, but no amyloid fibril could be found in NKC. Amyloidogenesis is believed to be a two phase process and AEF is thought to be involved in the second phase, the process of deposition of amyloid (2). As AKC had been in the second phase in vivo, the reactivation of AKC by AEF seemed to support this hypothesis. The main difference between NKCamy and NKC was a pretreatment by the pellet of AKC supernatant, which contained cell debris of AKC other than amyloid fibrils. Might this pellet contain a factor to accelerate the first stage of amyloidogenesis? If so, NKCamy but not NKC would synthesize amyloid fibrils.

Although amyloid fibrils could not be produced, AEF did stimulated NKC. With regard to the surface morphology of activated macrophages, Polliack and Gordon (5) described the larger surface area with prominent membrane undulations, frequent appearance of larger ruffles and filopodia (6). Petal-like ruffles are said to be characteristic and induced by lipopolysaccharide or macrophage migration inhibitory factor (7). In this study, AEF-stimulated cells showed elaborated ridges and ruffles. Abundant petal-like ruffles were also observed. These findings show morphologic evidence of a high level of membrane activity.

Based on these results, we have concluded that AEF participates the second phase of amyloidogenesis, and some other factor, in addition to AEF and SAA, must be necessary for the synthesis of amyloid fibrils in vitro.

REFERENCES

1. Fuks,A. and Zucker-Franklin,D.(1985) 'Impaired kupffer cell function precedes development of secondary amyloidosis', J.Exp.Med. 161, 1013-1028.
2. Jannigan,D.T. and Druet,R.,L.(1966) 'Experimental amyloidosis: Role of antigenicity and rapid induction', Am. J. Pathol. 48, 1013-1025.
3. Shirahama,T., Miura,K. et al(1990) 'Amyloid enhancing factor-loaded macrophages in amyloid fibril formation', Lab. Invest. 62, 61-68.
4. Iwata,T.(1972) 'Pathological study on amyloidosis: Morphological changes in long-term cultured sinusoidal endothelial cells of normal and amyloid liver of mice', Acta Pathol. Jpn. 22, 231-259.
5. Polliack,A. and Gordon,S.(1975) 'Scanning electron microscopy of murine macrophages', Lab. Invest. 33, 469-477.
6. Parakkal,P., Pinto,J. et al(1974) 'Surface morphology of human mononuclear phagocytes during maturation and phagocytosis', J. Ultrast. Res. 48, 216-226.
7. Homma,Y., Onozaki,K., et al(1982) 'The mechanism of cell surface changes of guinea pig macrophages activated with purified migration inhibitoy factor/macrophage activation factor', Cell.Immunol. 72, 231-238.

MACROMOLECULAR CHARACTERISTICS OF AA TYPE AMYLOID ASSOCIATED POLYSACCHARIDES FROM HUMAN LIVER, KIDNEY AND SPLEEN WITH AA AMYLOID SECONDARY TO RHEUMATIC DISEASE.

MAGNUS J H, STENSTAD T, *KOLSET S O, HUSBY G.

Department of Rheumatology and *Institute of Medical Biology,
University of Tromsø, 9000 Tromsø, Norway.

Abstract

Previous studies have strongly suggested a specific association between glycosaminoglycans (GAGs) and tissue deposits of amyloid. The present study was aimed at investigating this association in purified preparations of amyloid fibrils from liver, kidney and spleen obtained from human protein AA secondary amyloidosis. GAGs were isolated by ion exchange chromatography of amyloid fibril preparations. Significant amount of GAGs were prepared, whereas only trace amounts were detected in the corresponding extract from normal organs. Chemical depolymerization and use of specific enzymes, identified the different GAGs. The composition of GAGs varied within the different organs. We confirm that GAGs are specifically associated with AA amyloid fibrils. The presence of this carbohydrate moiety may play a role in the incorporation of structurally diverse protein precursors into fibrils of identical ultrastructure in the different chemical categories of amyloid deposits.

Introduction

The complete chemical composition of amyloid deposits is unknown, but amyloid fibrils are known to consist largely of specific serum proteins, which systemic appear to determine the clinical category of amyloid disease (1). In addition, studies on the macromolecular components of amyloid have revealed the presence of proteoglycans (PGs) and glycosaminoglycans (GAGs) in the tissue deposits (2). It is not known whether this carbohydrate moiety is an integral part of the of the fibril. Ultrastructural analyses of amyloid fibrils suggest the presence of GAGs on the surface of the amyloid fibrils (3). We have previously reported the presence of GAGs in extracts of AA type hepatic amyloid fibrils associated with juvenile rheumatoid arthritis (4). The present study was aimed at further investigating the GAGs present in amyloid fibril extracts from human organs affected by AA type amyloidosis secondary to rheumatic disease.

Materials and Methods

AMYLOID FIBRIL EXTRACTION

AA type amyloid fibrils were prepared from liver, spleen and kidney from patients with amyloidosis secondary to rheumatic disease using the modified water extraction method of Pras as described (4). The aqueous amyloid fibril supernatant were lyophilised. Corresponding normal organs were subjected to the same extraction procedures.

PROTEOGLYCAN ISOLATION
Lyophilised amyloid fibril and normal extracts were solubilized in 8 M urea 10 mM Tris HCl buffer PH 6.0, with protease inhibitors prior to DEAE-Sephacel ion exchange chromatography (5). The gel was calibrated and eluted with a 6 M urea/10 mM Tris HCl buffer pH 6.0, and a gradient from 0.0 to 1.5 M NaCl. Selected fractions were pooled after determination of hexuronic acid by the carbazole method (6), dialyzed against distilled water, and lyophilised.

BETAELIMINATION
In order to detect possible intact PGs, aliquots of the lyophilised carbazole positive material obtained after ion exchange chromatography was subjected to betaelimination (7) and subsequent Sepharose CL- 6B chromatography using 6 M urea 10 mM Tris HCl pH 6.0 as eluent.

IDENTIFICATION OF GLYCOSAMINOGLYCANS
Enzymatic degradation was performed on lyophilized polysaccharide material after ion exchange chromatography. The galactosaminoglycans chondroitin sulfate (CS) and dermatan sulfate (DS) were degraded by chondroitinase ABC from Seikagaku (8). The chondroitinase ABC resistent material , polysaccharides containing N-sulfated glucosaminoglycans, namely heparin (Hep) and heparan sulfate (HS) were chemically depolymerized by nitrous acid treatment (9).

Results

Amino acid sequencing has previously confirmed the AA nature of the amyloid protein (4,10). The elution profile of carbazole positive material obtained by gradient ion exchange chromatography of urea solubilized amyloid fibrils and the corresponding normal extracts are shown in Fig.1.

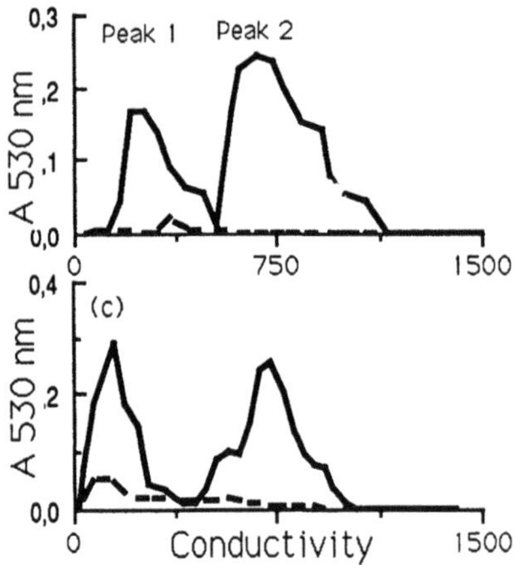

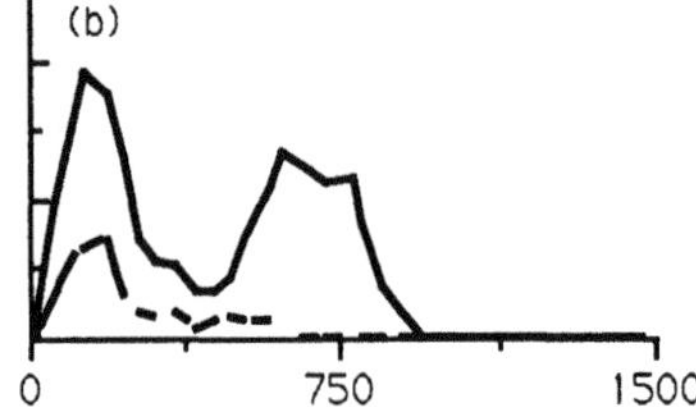

Fig.1 Gradient ion exchange chromatography of amyloid associated GAGs from urea treated AA amyloid fibrils from a) liver, b) spleen and c) kidney (solid line) and corresponding normal extracts (dotted line).

The total amount of GAGs coisolated with these AA fibril preparations estimated by carbazole reactivity is approximately 15 µg per mg lyophilsed fibril material. The amyloid associated GAGs eluted as one major and one minor peak. Peak 1 (salt consentration of 0.15 M NaCl), consisted of material of wich 50% was dialyzable through a membrane with a 6 kD cut off, and the rest, chondroitinase ABC succeptible low molecular weight oligosaccharides.

The material in peak 2 (salt consentration of 0.45M NaCl) thus represent the amyloid associated GAGs, was subjected to different depolymerization procedures prior to gel filtration on Sepharose CL-6B, and the relative amounts of the different types of GAGs in renal, splenic and hepatic AA amyloid fibril extracts are given in Table 1.

TABLE 1 Organ distribution of AA amyloid associated GAGs

	Splenic	Renal	Hepatic
Galactosaminoglycans	70%	100%	60%
N-sulfated glucosamines	30%	0%	40%

Chromatography on Sepharose CL-6B of the high molarity material (Fig.1, peak 2) after betaelimination showed all the material to elute at a Kav of 0.19 identical to that of untreated material (data not shown). The unchanged elution position of this material following betaelimination strongly indicates it to consist of free GAG chains rather than intact PG molecules. According to protein standard a Kav value of 0.19 indicates a molecular weight of approximately 90 kD of these apparently free GAG chains.

Discussion

Previous investigations have provided evidence that GAGs or possibly PGs are associated with amyloid, irrespective of the type of protein making up the fibrils (11). The present study shows by biochemical means that significant amounts of GAGs coisolate with water extracts of amyloid fibrils from human liver, kidney and spleen laden with secondary AA amyloid. In contrast, the corresponding normal control extracts contained only minor amounts of GAGs, thus supporting previous findings (4,12). This also confirms the intimate association of GAGs with the amyloid fibrils in situ, as previously demonstrated using histochemical methods (3).

Few investigations have been performed to answer the question in what form the GAGs are present in amyloid deposits, i.e. whether they are part of intact PGs. The presence of a HSPG core protein in amyloid have been reported emploing immunohistochemistry (13). According to the present biochemical analyses, the amyloid associated GAGs in AA type hepatic, renal and splenic fibril extracts are not present as intact PGs but occure as free GAG chains. However, it cannot be excluded that the amyloid associated GAGs as present in vivo may be part of a larger PG, which eventually disintegrates ex vivo. Although an exact mass determination of GAGs is rather difficult as these linear polysaccharides behave differently under variable conditions (14), the amyloid associatied GAGs chains studied here obviously have relatively high molecular masses.

Discrepant findings have been reported of the distribution of the different GAGs in human amyloid. However, most results derived from crude tissue extracts, whereas our study utilized amyloid fibrils isolated according to the standard water extraction method (15); and this could at least partly explain the difffernces. The kidney and spleen in this study derive from the same individual, and we here demonstrate that the HS : CS/DS ratio in amyloid extracts is differnt when different organs are compared.

Acknowledgments

This work was supported by the Norwegian Council for Science and the Humanities, the Norwegian Cancer Society, the Norwegian Women's Public Health Association and Norsk Revmatikerforbund.

References

1. Husby, G. and Sletten, K. (1986) 'Chemical and clinical classification of amyloidosis', Scand J Immunol 23, 253-256
2. Dalferes, E.R.Jr, Radhakrisnamuerty, B. and Berenson, G.S. (1967) 'Acid mucopolysaccharides of amyloid tissue', Arch Biochem Biophys 118, 284-291
3. Snow, A.,Willmer, J. and Kisilevsky, R. (1987) 'A close ultrastructural relationship between sulphated glycosaminoglycans and AA amyloid fibrils', Lab Invest 57, 687-698
4. Magnus, J.H., Husby, G. and Kolset, S.O. (1989) 'Presence of glycosaminoglycans in purified AA type amyloid fibrils associated with juvenile rheumatoid arthritis', Ann Rheum Dis 48, 215-219
5. Hallen, A. (1972) 'Chromatography of acidic glycosaminoglycans on DEAE-cellulose', J Chromatogr 71, 83-91
6. Bitter, T. and Muir, H. (1962) ' A modified uronic acid carbazole reaction', Anal Biochem 4, 330-331
7. Heinegård, D. and Sommarin, Y. (1987) ' Isolation and characterization of proteoglycans', Methods Enzymol 144, 319-372
8. Kolset, S.O., Kjellen, L. Seljelid, R. and Lindahl, U. (1983) 'Changes in glycosaminoglycan biosynthesis during differentation in vitro of human monocytes', Biochem J 210, 661-667
9. Shively, J. E. and Conrad, H. E. (1976) 'Formation of anhydrosugars in the chemical depolymerization of heparin', Biochemistry 15, 3932-3942
10. Husby, G., Sletten, K., Michalsen, T. and Natvig, J.B. (1972) 'Antigenic and chemical characterization of non-immunoglobulin amyloid proteins', Scand J Immunol 1,393-399
11. Ohishi, H., Skinner, M. Sato-Araki, N., Okuyama, T., Gejyo, F., Kimura, A., Cohen, A.S. and Schmid, K. (1990) 'Glycosaminoglycans of hemodialysis-associated carpal synovial amyloid and of amyloid rich tissues and fibrils of heart, liver, and spleen',Clin Chem 36, 88-92
12. Magnus, J.H., Stenstad, T., Kolset, S.O., Dahl, I.M., Husby, G. and Ranløv, P.J. (1989) 'Presence of polysaccharides in familial cardiac amyloid of Danish origin related to variant transthyretin Met 111'in P.Costa (ed.), Proceedings 1st International Symposium on Familial Amyloidotic Polyneuropathy, Portugal.
13. Norling, B., Westermark, G.T.and Westermark, P. (1988) 'Immunohistochemical identification of heparan sulphate proteoglycan in secondary systemic amyloidosis', Clin Exp Immunol 73, 333-337
14. Wasteson, Å. (1971) 'A method for determination of the molecular weight-distribution of chondroitin sulphate', J Chrom 59, 87-97
15. Pras, M., Schubert, M., Zuker-Franklin, D., Rimon, A. and Franklin, E.C. (1968) 'The characterization of soluble amyloid prepared in water', J Clin Invest 47, 924-933

HEPARAN SULFATE ACCUMULATION IN THE BETA-AMYLOID PROTEIN CONTAINING LESIONS OF DOWN'S SYNDROME OCCURS PRIOR TO THE APPEARANCE OF FIBRILLAR AMYLOID

ALAN D. SNOW,
University of Washington,
Department of Pathology SM-30,
Seattle, WA U.S.A. 98195

ABSTRACT: In the present study, a monoclonal antibody (HK-249) that recognizes a glucosamine sulfate alpha 1⟶4 glucuronic acid-containing determinant in heparan sulfate (HS) chains of a basement membrane derived heparan sulfate proteoglycan was used to identify and localize HS in Downs syndrome (DS) brain, and to determine the sequence of events preceding the formation and accumulation of fibrillar amyloid in DS. Analysis of DS patients at different ages revealed that HS accumulated within neurons of the hippocampus and amygdala, as early as 1 day after birth. Young age-matched controls did not demonstrate similar positive HS immunoreactivity in neurons whereas positive immunostaining for HS was observed in other regions thought to normally contain HS. The earliest deposition of beta-amyloid protein (BAP) was first observed as "amorphous" or "diffuse" cortical deposits in DS brain in patients aged 18 and 24, prior to the accumulation of fibrillar amyloid (observed in DS patients 35 years and older). These cortical deposits also contained positive HS immunoreactivity implying that HS accumulation in conjunction with the BAP is an early event preceding the first appearance of fibrillar amyloid.

INTRODUCTION

Previous studies (1-3) have demonstrated that the amyloid deposits within neuritic plaques (NPs) and congophilic angiopathy contain a specific class of complex carbohydrates known as proteoglycans (PGs). Immunocytochemical studies have recently identified heparan sulfate proteoglycan (HSPG) core protein localized to the amyloid deposits in these lesions (4). However, it was not known whether HSPG accumulation is an early or late event in the accumulation of beta-amyloid protein (BAP). In the present study, a new rat monoclonal antibody recognizing HS glycosaminoglycan chains of the basement membrane derived HSPG was used to determine the sequential appearance of HS, BAP and fibrillar amyloid in the brains of Down's syndrome (DS) patients.

MATERIALS AND METHODS

Brain tissue (including hippocampus and amygdala) was obtained from 12 cases of DS, acquired either from the Dept. of Neuropathology at the Univ. of Washington or from Children's Hospital in Seattle. Eight of these DS cases were under the age of 25 years (and included ages of 1 day, 4 months, 2 yrs., 7 yrs., 15 yrs., 16 yrs., 18 yrs. and 24 yrs) whereas four of these cases were over the age of 35 yrs. Additionally, brain tissue was obtained at autopsy from an 11 yr. old with congenital heart disease, a 13 yr. old with Huntington's disease, a 14 yr. old with cystic fibrosis and a 18 yr. old with cardiopathy. Brain tissue obtained from cases of DS and age-matched controls were fixed in 10% formalin for 24-48 hrs. All tissues were processed routinely and embedded in paraffin.

A monoclonal antibody (known as HK-249), recognizing a specific glucosamine sulfate alpha 1⟶4 glucuronic acid-containing determinant on the GAG chains of the basement membrane derived HSPG (5) was used (at a dilution of 1:5 or 1:10) for immunocytochemical identification and localization of HS in DS and age-matched control brain tissue. Other antibodies used included a polyclonal antibody against the BAP (residues 1-42 of the BAP; used at a dilution of 1:100)(courtesy of Dr. C. Masters). To rule out nonspecific binding and to ensure specificity of the HS antibody, sections were also treated with the HS antibody after pre-incubation (overnight at 4°C) in the presence of excess HSPG antigen.

Both congo red staining (7) and BAP antibodies were used to identify sites of amyloid accumulation. Adjacent serial sections were immunostained with the HS GAG chain antibody.

RESULTS

The brains from all four cases of DS, over the age of 35 years demonstrated the presence of NPs, NFTs and cerebrovascular amyloid deposits, identified by either positive congo red staining (as viewed under polarized light), or by immunostaining with the BAP antibody. Tissue sections immunostained with the HS antibody strongly immunostained amyloid-containing NPs (Fig. 1A) and "primitive" plaques, which on adjacent serial sections were immunostained with the BAP antibody. Additionally, HS immunostaining was observed in DS brain (in patients over 35 years) in the pyramidal neurons of the hippocampus (Fig. 1B) and in the granule cell layer of the dentate gyrus. Additionally, some of the HS positive neurons contained NFTs. Heparan sulfate immunostaining was also observed in DS brains (in patients over 35 years old) in a number of different sites found to contain HS in normal brain (see below).

The brains from DS patients under the age of 30 years (1 day-24yrs) did not contain NPs, NFTs or cerebrovascular amyloid deposits as indicated by negative congo red staining and negative BAP immunostaining for these lesions. However, the 18 and 24 year old DS patients demonstrated "amorphous" or "diffuse" cortical deposits immunostained with the BAP antibody in some areas of the hippocampus and amygdala (Fig. 1C). These regions represented one of the earliest detectable changes observed in the DS brain prior to the appearance of NPs, NFTs and congophilic angiopathy. On adjacent serial sections, these BAP positive cortical deposits were also immunostained with the HK-249 antibody (Fig. 1D).

HS immunostaining in the neurons of the hippocampus, amygdala and cerebellum (ie. Purkinje cells) was observed even in the 1 day and 4 month DS patients. In comparison, immunostaining with the HS in young aged non-DS controls demonstrated weak to no HS immunostaining of pyramidal and granule cell neurons in the hippocampus and amygdala. However, HS immunostaining was demonstrated in non-DS patients in areas normally containing HS such as in the astrocytes in the white matter, the choroid plexus basement membrane, the ependymal lining of the ventricles, and in the walls of meningeal vessels, indicating that the lack of immunostaining of the neurons was not due to preparation artifact. These observations suggest that HS accumulation in neurons of the hippocampus and amygdala is amplified in Down's syndrome brain at an early age (even at 1 day) and not observed to the same extent in non-Down's syndrome patients.

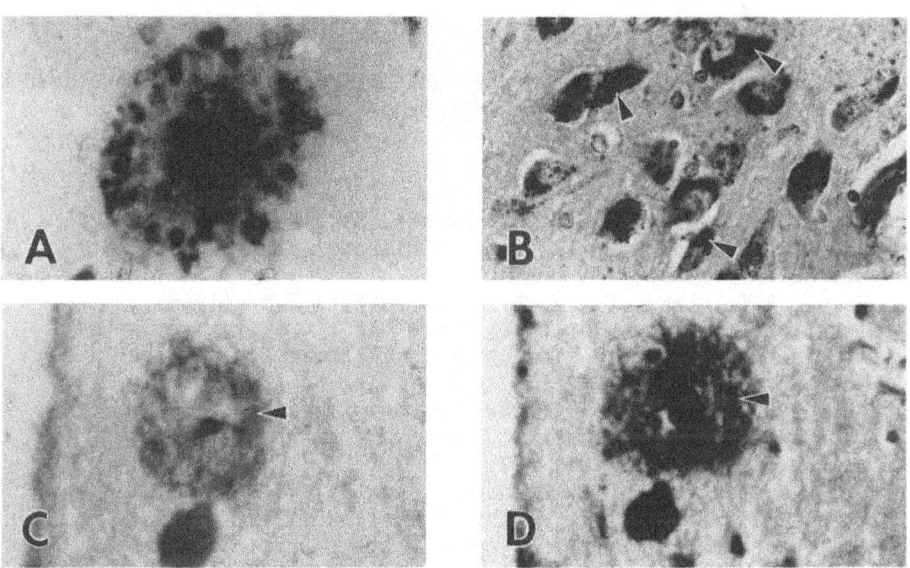

1A: Immunostaining of an amyloid plaque in the hippocampus of a 51 yr. old DS patient using the HS monoclonal antibody. Positive immunostaining is localized to both central amyloid core and periphery. 1B: HS immunostaining (arrowheads) in pyramidal neurons in the hippocampus of a 37 yr. old DS patient. 1C: BAP immunostaining of a diffuse cortical deposit (arrowhead) in the hippocampus of a 24 yr. old DS patient. This represents the earliest appearance of BAP in the DS brain. 1D: Adjacent serial section from Fig. 1C demonstrating the same cortical deposit (arrowhead) immunostained with the monoclonal antibody recognizing HS.

DISCUSSION

In the present study, the DS model was used to determine whether the appearance of HS in conjunction with BAP, preceded or occurred after the initial appearance and accumulation of fibrillar amyloid. The "amorphous" or "diffuse" BAP-positive cortical deposits observed in the brains of DS patients of ages 18 and 24 represented the earliest detectable deposition of BAP, prior to the appearance of fibrillar amyloid (observed in DS patients 35 years and older). These BAP-positive cortical deposits also contained HS suggesting that HS accumulation in conjunction with the BAP occurs prior to the appearance of fibrillar amyloid and is an early event in the pathogenesis of amyloid and/or NP development in Down's brain, and most likely in AD also. The accumulation of HS in both the neurons and BAP cortical deposits in young DS patients may play a pivotal role in predisposing these patients to the early age-related accumulation (ie. observed as early as 35 yrs. of age) of NPs, NFTs and/or congophilic angiopathy.

ACKNOWLEDGEMENTS

This work was supported by the Alzheimer's Disease Research Program of the American Health Assistance Foundation.

REFERENCES

1. Snow, A.D., Willmer, J., Kisilevsky, R. (1987) 'Sulfated glycosaminoglycans in Alzheimer's disease', Lab Invest, 18, 506-510.
2. Snow, A.D., Lara, S., Nochlin, D., Wight, T.N. (1989) 'Cationic dyes reveal proteoglycans structurally integrated within the characteristic lesions of Alzheimer's disease', Acta Neuropath, 78, 113-123.
3. Snow, A.D., Wight, T.N. (1989) 'Proteoglycans in the pathogenesis of Alzheimer's disease and other amyloidoses', Neurobiol Aging, 10, 481-497.
4. Snow, A.D., Mar, H., Nochlin, D., Kimata, K., Kato, M., Suzuki, S., Hassell, J., Wight, T.N. (1988) 'The presence of heparan sulfate proteoglycans in the neuritic plaques and congophilic angiopathy in Alzheimer's disease', Am J Path, 133, 456-463.
5. Kato, Y., Kato, M., Suzuki, S., Kimata, K. (1989) 'A monoclonal antibody against the heparan sulfate of EHS-tumor proteoglycan. IX International Symposium on Glycoconjugates, B8. abstract.
6. Puchtler, H., Sweat, F., Levine, M. (1962) 'On the binding of congo red by amyloid', J Histochem Cytochem, 10, 355-364.

RAPID SYNTHESIS OF cRNA PROBES FOR SAA, SAP AND HEPARAN SULFATE PROTEOGLYCAN mRNAs BY TRANSCRIPTION OF POLYMERASE CHAIN REACTION GENERATED TEMPLATES

I. YOUNG, L. AILLES, K. DEUGAU*, R. KISILEVSKY
Departments of Pathology and Biochemistry*, Queen's University
Kingston, Ontario, K7L 3N6 Canada

INTRODUCTION

The identification of mRNA in tissue sections by in situ hybridization (ISH) has become a standard technique for studying gene expression in individual cells which has been applied to the study of many disorders including amyloidosis [1]. cRNA is the probe of choice for ISH due to its combination of high specificity, specific activity, hybrid stability and detection sensitivity [2,3]. Conventional transcription systems for generating cRNA utilize cloning vectors which contain bacteriophage RNA polymerase promoters [4]. The inherent disadvantage of such systems is the use of cloning techniques to amplify the desired DNA sequence prior to its transcription. We have developed a procedure for synthesizing cRNA probes in vitro which utilizes the polymerase chain reaction (PCR) as the method of DNA amplification rather than DNA cloning. This simple technique allowed the rapid and efficient synthesis of cRNA probes for murine SAA, SAP and basement membrane heparan sulfate proteoglycan (HSPG) mRNAs.

MATERIALS AND METHODS

Strategy

The PCR is a technique in which specific genomic or cloned DNA sequences are enzymatically amplified as directed by two oligonucleotide primers which define the 5'-termini of the amplified sequence [5,6]. Extraneous DNA sequences attached to the 5'-termini of the PCR primers will also be incorporated into the amplified DNA (7-11). In this way, bacteriophage RNA polymerase promoters may be linked to a desired segment of DNA [10,11], thus allowing the subsequent transcription of complementary cRNA from that template by the corresponding RNA polymerase.

Oligonucleotide Primers

The oligonucleotide primers were generated by the Oligonucleotide Synthesis Laboratory at Queen's University, as described previously [12]. The two 20-mer SAA primers define a 140 base pair segment of the 3'-untranslated segment of the SAA1 gene (nucleotides 3179-3318) [13]. The sense and antisense SAA primers were linked at their

5'-termini to the SP6 and T7 bacteriophage RNA polymerase promoters, respectively. The SP6 and T7 sequences were 5'-CGATTTAGGTGACACTATA-3' and 5'-ATTAATACGACTCACTATA-3' respectively. The two 20-mer SAP primers define a 139 base pair segment of the SAP gene (nucleotides 465-603) [14]. The two 20-mer HSPG primers define a 147 base pair segment of the BPG-5 HSPG cDNA clone (nucleotides 301-447) [15]. A separate set of oligonucleotides composed of the SAP and HSPG primers linked to the SP6 promoter were also synthesized. 18-mer oligonucleotides complementary to internal sequences of the antisense strands of the amplified segments of the SAA, SAP and HSPG genes were synthesized.

Polymerase Chain Reaction

PCR was performed for 30 cycles as follows: 94°C, 1 minute; 50°C, 2 minutes; 72°C, 1.5 minutes with 5 second extension during each successive cycle. The composition of the reaction mixture has been described [11]. The genomic DNA extract was prepared by boiling mouse blood in an equal volume of water for ten minutes. Following brief centrifugation, the supernatant was used as the PCR template. BPG-5 (a kind gift from Dr. S. Ledbetter) was used as the template for the HSPG amplification. The amplification products of the PCR were analyzed following PAGE and ethidium bromide staining using standard techniques.

Transcription Reaction

Large quantities of cRNA were synthesized as previously described [11].[α-^{32}P]-rATP was added to some reactions to facilitate transcript analysis. Northern blots of transcripts were probed with [γ-^{32}P]-ATP end-labelled oligonucleotides specific for the antisense cRNAs. High specific activity cRNA probes were transcribed using the following reaction mixture: 1-2 µl PCR product; 1 µl 100 mM DTT; 0.5 µl of 2 mg/ml BSA, 2 µl of 7.5 mM rNTP mixture (2.5 mM each of rATP, rGTP and rCTP); 4 µl of [α-^{35}S]-rUTP (300 µCi at 1320 Ci/mmol); 1 µl of transcription buffer; 0.5 µl RNAsin; 0.5 µl (4-6U) of SP6 or T7 RNA polymerase.

In Situ Hybridization

The SAA antisense cRNA was used to demonstrate hepatic SAA gene expression in mice experiencing inflammation. At intervals following the inflammatory stimulus, sections of liver and spleen were fixed in 4% paraformaldehyde in PBS and embedded in paraffin. After deparaffinization, sections were treated with proteinase K, postfixed in 4% paraformaldehyde and acetylated with acetic anhydride. Sections were prehybridized at 45°C for 2 hours with 50% formamide, 0.3 M NaCl, 20 mM Tris HCl, pH 8.0, 1 mM EDTA, 1 X Denhardt's, 10% dextran sulfate, 100 mM DTT and 0.5 mg/ml yeast tRNA. 2.5-5 X 10^5 dpm ^{35}S-cRNA in prehybridization solution was hybridized to the sections overnight at 45°C. Slides were washed in 4 X SSC, 10mM DTT for 60 minutes at room temperature, dehydrated in ethanol containing 300 mM ammonium acetate, immersed in prehybridization solution for 10 minutes at 65°C, and digested with RNAse A. Slides were then extensively washed in 2 X SSC at room temperature, 0.1 X SSC at 50°C and 0.1 X SSC at room temperature prior to autoradiography.

RESULTS

Amplification of DNA Templates by PCR

Figure 1 demonstrates the amplification products derived from the various PCRs. The 178 base pair sequence resulting from the SAA amplification contains a central 140 base pair SAA sequence which is linked at the 5'-ends of its sense and antisense strands to the SP6 and T7 promoters, respectively. Transcription from this template by the SP6 and T7 RNA polymerases produces 159 base sense and antisense cRNAs which include a 19 base promoter sequence at their 3'-termini. To generate HSPG and SAP antisense cRNA which did not include extraneous 3'-promoter sequences, separate DNA templates were generated which were composed of the SP6 promoter attached to opposite ends of each template. This resulted in two 166 base pair HSPG amplification products (Figure 1), each of which contained the same 147 base pair segment of the HSPG gene. However, the SP6 promoter was attached to the opposite end of the HSPG sequence in each amplification reaction. The same procedure was used to generate the 158 base pair SAP amplification products.

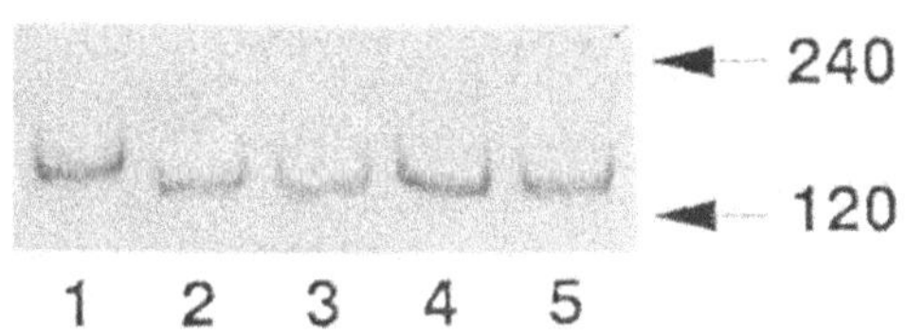

Figure 1. Ethidium bromide stained PAGE of PCR-amplified DNA (negative image). Lane 1, SAA amplification product. Lanes 2 and 4, SAP and HSPG amplification products, respectively, containing SP6 promoter at 5'-end of sense strand. Lanes 3 and 5, SAP and HSPG amplification products, respectively, containing SP6 promoter at 5'-end of antisense strand. Size standards in base pairs are noted.

Synthesis of cRNA Probes

Northern analysis of radiolabelled cRNAs demonstrates that the transcription reactions produced discrete cRNAs (Figure 2A). The SP6 and T7 polymerases transcribed single species of sense and antisense cRNA, respectively, with equivalent lengths of 159 bases. The pairs of sense and antisense HSPG and SAP cRNAs transcribed by SP6 have predicted lengths of 157 and 139 bases, respectively. In contrast to the SAA cRNAs, the HSPG and SAP cRNAs contain no 3'-promoter sequences. Northern blots of the transcripts were probed with end-labelled oligonucleotides complementary to the antisense cRNAs. These oligonucleotides hybridized specifically to the antisense cRNA of each pair of transcripts (Figure 2B).

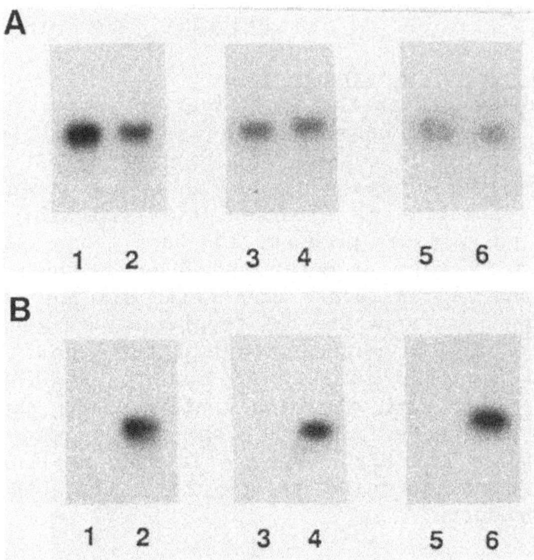

Figure 2. A, Northern analysis of radiolabelled cRNAs transcribed from PCR-amplified DNA. Lane 1, sense SAA cRNA. Lane 2, antisense SAA cRNA. Lane 3, sense SAP cRNA. Lane 4, antisense SAP cRNA. Lane 5, sense HSPG cRNA. Lane 6, antisense HSPG cRNA. B, Northern analysis of unlabelled transcripts hybridized with end-labelled oligonucleotides specific for antisense cRNAs. Lanes contain cRNAs as noted above.

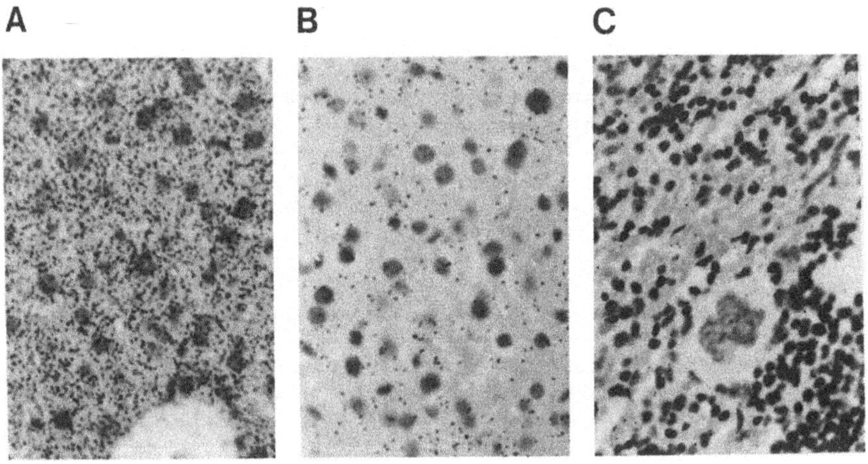

Figure 3. In situ hybridization using ^{35}S-labelled antisense SAA cRNA. A, Murine liver during inflammation. B, Murine liver from an untreated animal. C, Murine spleen during inflammation.

In Situ Hybridization

Antisense SAA cRNA was radiolabelled to high specific activity with ^{35}S-UTP and hybridized to tissue sections following an inflammatory stimulus. Because of the extensive homology between the SAA1 and SAA2 genes, the antisense SAA cRNA synthesized could not discriminate between those two mRNA species. Figure 4 shows the pronounced accumulation of SAA mRNA within the hepatocytes of an inflamed mouse relative to the spleen, where the SAA1 and SAA2 genes are not expressed, and to an untreated control.

DISCUSSION

The requirement of conventional transcription systems for cDNA cloning prior to the transcription of cRNA has restricted the use of cRNA probes to investigators having expertise in, or access to, cloning technology. We have illustrated an alternate technique for synthesizing cRNA probes which replaces the DNA cloning step with PCR. PCR is much simpler than conventional cloning techniques and it is very rapid, an amplification reaction being completed within a few hours. Also, the performance of the amplification and transcription reactions is routine and does not require experience in molecular biology. As a result this methodology will hopefully make mRNA ISH using cRNA probes a generally more accessible research technique.

ACKNOWLEDGEMENTS

This work was supported by MRC grants MA-11013 (IY) and MT-3153 (RK) and by the Upjohn Company of Canada. We would like to thank Pam Redden for her valuable secretarial assistance in the preparation of this manuscript.

REFERENCES

1. Meek RL and Benditt EP. J Exp Med 164:2006, 1986
2. Cox KG, DeLeon DV, Angerer LM et al. Dev Biol 101:485, 1984
3. DeLeon DV, Cox KH, Angerer LM et al. Dev Biol 100:197, 1983
4. Krieg PA and Melton DA. Meth Enzymol 155:397, 1987
5. Mullis KB and Faloona FA. Meth Enzymol 155:335, 1987
6. Saiki RK, Gelfand DH, Stofel S et al. Science 487:985, 1987
7. Higuchi R, Krummel B, Saiki RK. Nucl Acids Res 16:7351, 1988
8. Scharf SJ, Horn GT, Erlich AH. Science 223:1076, 1986
9. Vallette F, Meye E, Reiss A et al. Nucl Acids Res 17:723, 1989
10. Sarkar G and Sommer SS. Science 244:331, 1989
11. Stoflet ES, Koeberl DD, Sarkar G et al. Science 239:491, 1988
12. Archer TK. J Biol Chem 260:1676, 1985
13. Lowell CA, Potter DA, Stearman RS et al. J Biol Chem 261:8442, 1986
14. Nishiguchi S, Maeda S, Araki S et al. Biochem Biophys Res Commun 155:1366, 1988
15. Noonan DM, Horizan EA, Ledbetter SR et al. J Biol Chem 263:16379, 1988

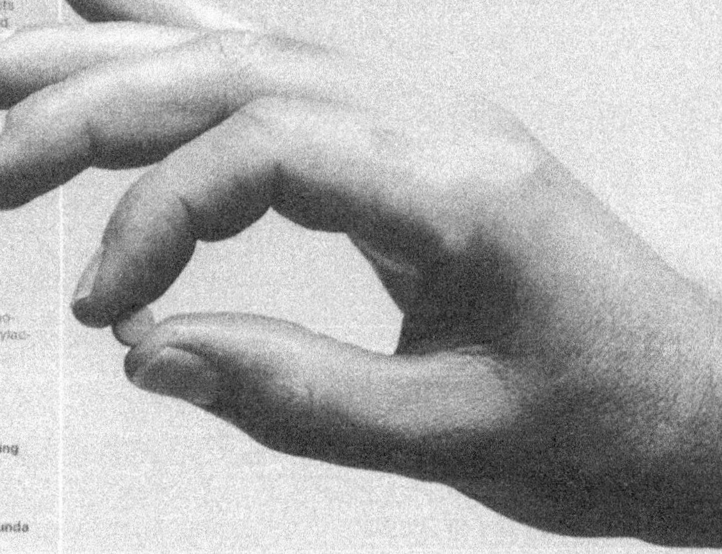

Basement Membrane Components in Addition to HSPG are Present in Murine AA Amyloid Deposits

A. W. Lyon, S. Narindrasorasak, K. J. McCarthy*, J. R. Couchman*, R. Kisilevsky

Departments of Biochemistry and Pathology, Queen's University, Kingston, Ontario, Canada, K7L 3N6; and *Department of Cell Biology and Anatomy, University of Alabama at Birmingham, Birmingham, Alabama 35294

Address all Correspondence:
Dr. R. Kisilevsky
Department of Pathology
Queen's University
Kingston, Ontario, Canada
K7L 3N6

INTRODUCTION

During murine AA amyloidogenesis there is co-deposition of the AA peptide and the basement membrane form of heparan sulfate proteoglycan (HSPG), (1). Recent studies have also demonstrated the HSPG in 5 different types of amyloid. These include AA amyloid in inflammation (1), IAPP amyloid in diabetes (2), beta amyloid in Alzheimer's disease (3), prion amyloid in Gerstmann-Straussler Syndrome (4), and prealbumin amyloid in familial amyloidotic polyneuropathy (5). Although HSPG appears to be a common component of several amyloid deposits, its role in the pathogenesis of amyloids is uncertain and is currently under intense investigation. For example, heparan sulfate as opposed to other glycosaminoglycans influences SAA_2 to adopt a more beta pleated configuration (6), and sulfate ions influence the conformation of AA peptides in AA amyloid fibrils (7).

Basement membranes are composed of a complex organized network of fibronectin, laminin, collagen type IV, HSPG and several minor components including SAP, (8,9). The accumulation of a single basement membrane component such as HSPG, independent of the other components, has not previously been observed. The objective of the present study was therefore to test if the accumulation of basement membrane HSPG in murine AA amyloidosis occurred independent of the other components of basement membranes. To investigate the possibility that the HSPG deposition in AA amyloidogenesis represents a more general disturbance in basement membrane deposition, immunohistochemistry was used to test for the presence of collagen type IV, laminin and fibronectin in early amyloid deposits. The results clearly demonstrate a co-localization of laminin, fibronectin, collagen type IV, HSPG and AA peptide in the perifollicular zone of the spleen during the induction of AA amyloidosis. They indicate that basement membrane components other than the HSPG are also part of AA amyloid deposits. They raise the possibility that an abnormality in basement membrane metabolism may play a role in AA amyloidogeneses.

Materials and Methods

Materials: Vectastain ABC anti-rabbit IgG kit, obtained from Dimension Laboratories Inc., Mississauga, Ontario, CANADA.
Animals and Treatments: Swiss white mice (six to eight weeks old) received either $AgNO_3$, or AEF + $AgNO_3$, for five days. A group of untreated animals served as controls. Animals were killed by cervical dislocation and the spleens were immediately excised and fixed. AEF was prepared as previously described (10), diluted to 1mg protein/ml and 0.5mg administered in a single intravenous injection via the tail vein. Silver nitrate 0.5ml/animal was administered subcutaneously as a 0.2% solution (w/v), (10).
Fixation: The spleens were placed in an acid-alcohol fixitive consisting of 96% ethanol, 1% glacial acetic acid and 3% water, and after 24 hours, the tissues were embedded in paraffin, cut and mounted on poly-L-Lysine coated slides, (11).
Immunohistochemistry: Following the removal of paraffin, slides were treated with 0.5% H_2O_2 in methanol (30 min.) to remove endogenous peroxidase activity and 15,000 U/ml hyaluronidase (30 min.) to enhance the antigenicity of the basement membrane components, (11). Rabbit antisera to the AA peptide and the basement membrane form of HSPG were developed and characterized by this laboratory, (1). Rabbit antisera to Laminin, Fibronectin and Collagen type IV were provided by Dr. J.R. Couchman, University of Alabama at Birmingham (12). The primary antibody-antigen complexes were detected using a biotinylated second antibody and avidinhorseradish peroxidase technique, (Vestastain ABC kit) (13). Control incubations were performed using both normal rabbit serum and saline. All slides were counter-stained with hematoxylin.

Results

Characterization of AA Amyloid: The perifollicular AA amyloid deposit was detected using either the traditional Congo red staining technique or the immunoperoxidase detection of the AA peptide, (Figure1). The interval of five days following the induction protocol was selected to ensure that a large deposit of amyloid was present for this investigation. No amyloid could be detected in either the untreated and inflammation control spleens, (Figure 1a,1b). It has previously been reported that the heparan sulfate proteoglycan could be detected in the amyloid deposit by using the immunoperoxidase staining with anti-heparan sulfate proteoglycan antisera, (1).

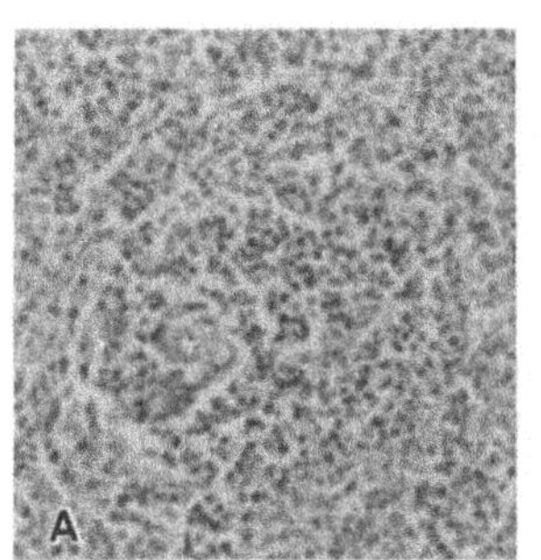

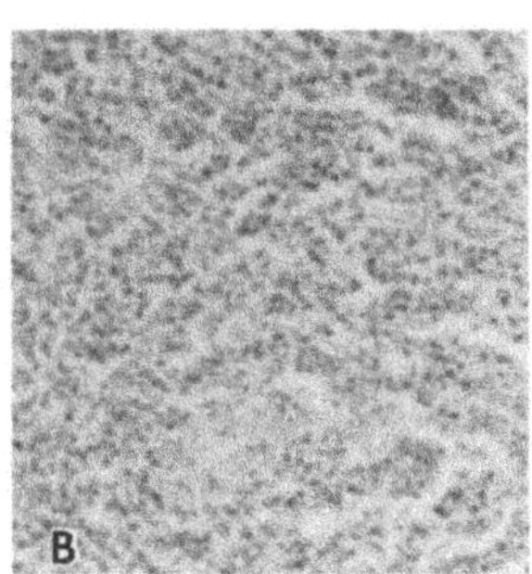

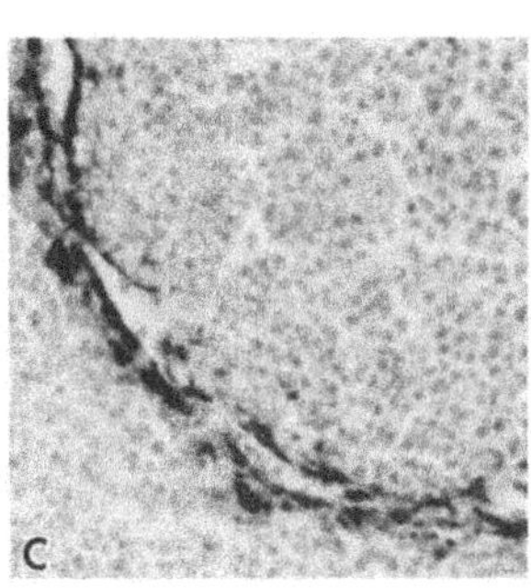

Figure 1: Immunodetection of the AA Peptide. Tissues were stained using the anti-AA peptide antisera with the immunoperoxidase technique and counterstained with hematoxylin. (A) An untreated control splenic perifollicular area. (B) Inflammation control spleen ($AgNO_3$ only). (C) Amyloidotic spleen.

Demonstration of Basement Membrane Components: The use of either anti-fibronectin, anti-laminin or anti-collagen type IV antisera resulted in a strong positive staining of the perifollicular amyloid deposit, (Figure 2). In addition to the amyloid, the antisera to the basement membrane components (including anti-HSPG) also reacted with the basement membranes of blood vessels and demonstrated a weak reaction with megakaryocytes in the tissues from each treatment group. Control incubations with either saline or pre-immune rabbit sera did not demonstrate any positive staining, (Result not shown).

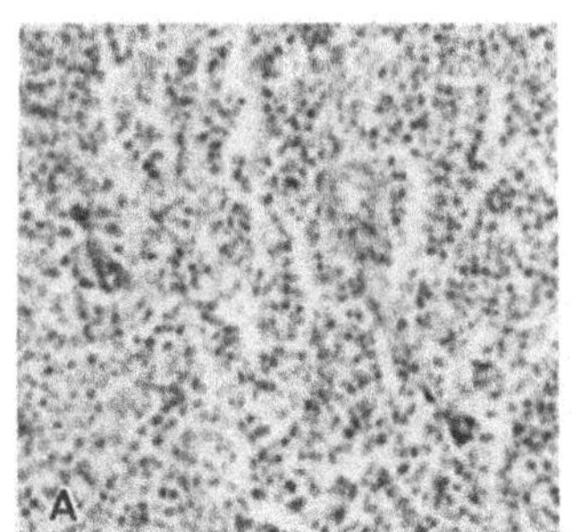

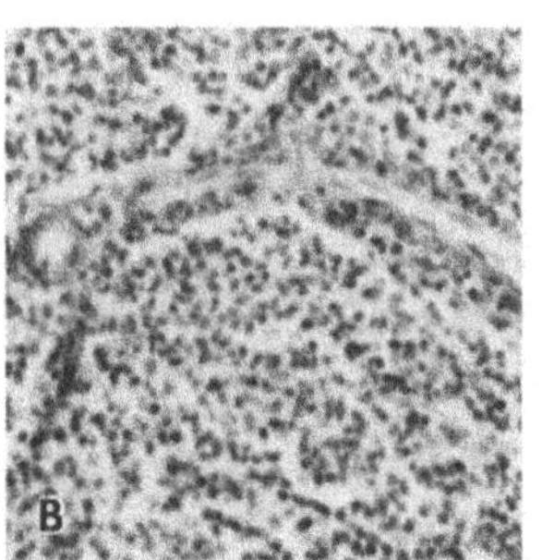

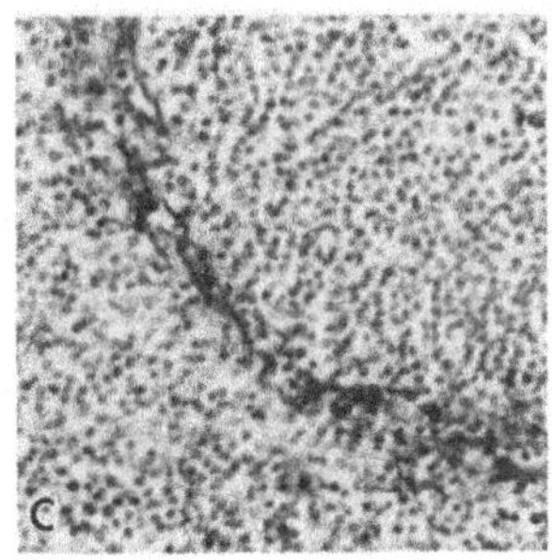

Figure 2: Immunodetection of basement membrane components. Tissues were stained using either anti-fibronectin, anti-laminin or anti-collagen type IV antisera with the immunoperoxiase technique and subsequently counterstained with hematoxylin. (A) An untreated control splenic perifollicular area stained using anti-collagen type IV antisera. (B) Inflammation control stained using anti-collagen type IV antisera. (C) Amyloidotic spleen stained using anti-collagen type IV antisera. The use of anti-fibronectin or anti-laminin as the primary antisera produced an identical positive immunoperoxidase staining pattern to the anti-collagen type IV results presented in this figure.

Discussion

The results of this investigation clearly demonstrate that AA amyloid deposits contain the basement membrane components fibronectin, laminin, collagen type IV and HSPG in addition to the AA-peptide. The precise molecular organization of these basement membrane components and the AA fibers is unknown at this time. However, during the past thirty years, amyloid deposits have been carefully examined by electronmicroscopy and the typical structural elements of basement membranes have not been detected, (14). This suggests that the antigens detected during the present study are not accumulating in an organized basement membrane fashion. They raise the interesting question of why these components are not organizing themselves appropriately.

The inference that the basement membrane may be involved in deposition of amyloid has been suggested by several earlier studies, (1,15,16,17). This is supported by our demonstration of an accumulation of the basement membrane form of HSPG in the perifollicular zone of the spleen during AA amyloidogenesis, (1). Further, fibronectin was recently demonstrated within splenic AA deposits, (17). It is interesting to note that serum amyloid P component, a ubiquitus feature of all amyloids, has been detected in most basement membranes and is also considered to be a basement membrane component, (8,9).

Having demonstrated increased vascular permeability and the lack of an identifiable basement membrane in amyloid ladened capillaries by electronmicroscopy, Schultz and Pitha postulated that AA amyloidosis might be initiated by a lesion to the basement membrane at the site of amyloid deposition, (15,16). This concept amyloid offers a potential explanation for the timing and targeting of AA amyloid and has recently been discussed in relation to the deposition of Alzheimer's amyloid, (18). The current availability of immunohistochemical tools should allow this hypothesis to be tested in amore rigorous manner.

Acknowledgements

This work was supported by grant MT-3153, MA-10477 from the Medical Research Council of Canada and the Upjohn Company. A.W. Lyon was supported by funds from a facilitation award from the Arthritis Society of Canada.

References

1. Snow,A.D., Kisilevsky,R., Wight,T.N. (1989) in Amyloid and Amyloidosis. Edited by I. Isobe, New York, Plenum Press. pp 87-93.
2. Young,I, Ailles,L., Kisilevsky,R. (1990) Human Pathol. submitted
3. Snow,A.D., Mar,H., Nochlin,D., Kimata,K., Kato,M., Suzuki,S., Hassel,J., Wight,T.N. (1988) Am. J. Path. 133 456-563.
4. Snow,A.D., Personal Communication
5. Snow,A.D., Saraiva,M.J., Personal Communication
6. McCubbin,D., Kay,C.M., Narindrasorasak,S., Kililevsky,R. (1988) Biochem. J. 256 775-783.
7. Wong,S., Kisilevsky,R. Scand. J. Immunol. (in press)

8. Timpl,R., Paulsson,M., Dziadek,M., Fujiwara,S. (1987) in Methods in Enzymology vol. 145, Ed. by L.W. Cunningham, Academic Press Inc. New York.
9. Timpl,R., Dziadek,M. (1986) Int. Rev. Exp. Path. 29 1-112.
10. Snow,A.D., Kisilevsky,R., Stephens,C., Anastassiades,T. (1987) Lab. Invest. 56 665-675.
11. Folkvard,J.M., Viders,D., Coleman-Smith,A., Clark,R.A. (1989) J. Histochem. Cytochem. 37 105-113.
12. Couchman,J.R. (1987) J. Cell. Biol. 105 1901-1916.
13. Hsu,S.M., Raine,L., Fanger, H. (1981) J. Histochem. Cytochem. 29 577-580.
14. Snow,A.D., Willmer,J., Kisilevsky,R. (1987) Lab. Invest. 57 687-698.
15. Schultz,R.T., Pitha,J.V. (1985) Am. J. Path. 119 123-137.
16. Schultz,R.T., Pitha,J.V., McDonald,T., Debault,L.E. (1985) Am. J. Path. 119 138-150.
17. Kawahara,E., Shiroo,M., Nakanishi,I., Migita,S. (1989) Am. J. Path. 134 1305-1314.
18. Mooradian,A.D., (1988) Neurobiol. Aging 7 31-39

THE BASEMENT MEMBRANE FORM OF HEPARAN SULFATE PROTEOGLYCAN IS PART OF HUMAN IAPP AMYLOID DEPOSITS IN THE ISLETS OF LANGERHANS

I. YOUNG, L. AILLES, S. AUBIN, R. KISILEVSKY
Department of Pathology, Queen's University,
Kingston, Ontario, K7L 3N6 Canada

INTRODUCTION

Type II diabetes mellitus (DM) is characterized by amyloid deposition within the pancreatic islets of Langerhans [1,2]. The major constituent of islet amyloid is a small protein designated islet amyloid polypeptide (IAPP), or amylin, which is synthesized by beta cells [3,4]. The precise function of IAPP is unknown but it may act as a glucoregulatory hormone [5,6] and may, possibly, play a pathogenetic role in Type II DM. This hypothesis in turn raises the question of the potential role of islet amyloid formation in the pathogenesis of Type II DM.

Little is known about the mechanisms of amyloid fibrillogenesis in general. However, a variety of disparate amyloids examined to date have all been shown to contain highly sulfated proteoglycans [7,9]. In each case where the amyloid-associated proteoglycan has been characterized it has proven to be the basement membrane heparan sulfate proteoglycan (HSPG) [10,12]. The observation that HSPG is a common feature which links disparate forms of amyloid suggests it may play a role in amyloidogenesis. The objective of this study was to determine whether HSPG is a component of islet amyloid in human Type II DM.

MATERIALS AND METHODS

Tissue: Pancreatic tissue was obtained at autopsy from five Type II diabetics and five non-diabetic controls. Tissue blocks were fixed in 10% neutral buffered formalin and embedded in paraffin.
Antisera: A polyclonal antiserum prepared against a synthetic fragment of human IAPP (amino acids 20-29) was a generous gift from Drs. Per Westermark and Ken Johnson. A polyclonal antiserum against the core protein of the basement membrane HSPG produced by the murine EHS tumor was raised in rabbits following standard techniques and affinity purified using a HSPG-sepharose column.
Histochemistry: Sections of pancreas were stained for the presence of islet amyloid using Congo red and sulfated glycosaminoglycans (GAGs) using sodium sulfate Alcian blue (SAB) [13]. Since sulfated GAGs exist covalently bound to proteins as proteoglycans, positive SAB staining

presumptively identifies highly sulfated proteoglycans.
Immunohistochemistry: Immunostaining of tissue sections was performed using the peroxidase-antiperoxidase method. Negative controls included omission of the primary antibody and substitution of normal immune rabbit serum for the primary antibody. Sections of murine spleen containing AA amyloid, which is known to contain abundant HSPG [10], were used as positive controls for the HSPG antiserum.

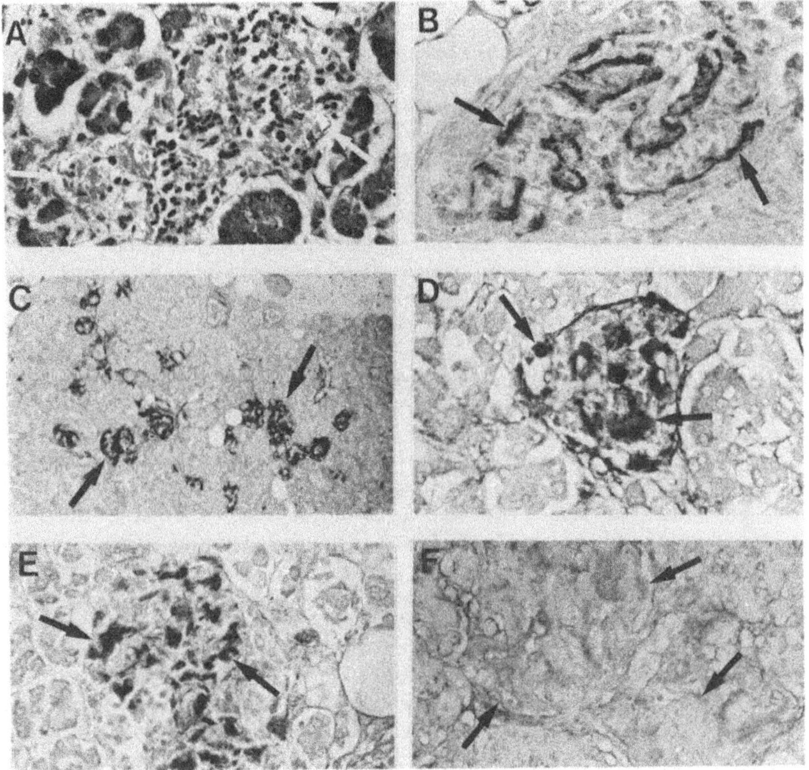

Figure 1: Histochemical and immunohistochemical analysis of human islet amyloid (arrows). Amyloid in a single islet, defined by Congo red (A), shows strong immunoreactivity with antiserum to IAPP (B). Multiple amyloidotic islets stain heavily with SAB (C) and in each islet the SAB staining is localized to the amyloid deposits (D). Positive staining reactions are also evident in islet amyloid treated with antiserum to HSPG (E) but reaction products are not apparent in amyloid in control tissue treated with normal immune serum (F).

RESULTS

In each diabetic pancreas islet amyloid was defined using Congo red (Figure 1A) and in each case the amyloid reacted strongly with the IAPP antiserum (Figure 1B). Whereas no SAB positivity was identified in islets of the control group, islet amyloid stained diffusely and heavily with SAB (Figures 1C and D). The pattern of SAB positivity corresponded to the distribution of the amyloid defined by the Congo red stain. These data suggested that highly sulfated proteoglycans such as heparan sulfate or keratan sulfate were constitutents of the islet amyloid deposit.

Immunohistochemistry using anti-HSPG antiserum was performed to determine whether the presence of the basement membrane HSPG could account for the SAB staining of islet amyloid. Figure 1E shows positive immunostaining of the islet amyloid by the anti-HSPG antiserum, demonstrating the localization of the basement membrane HSPG within the deposit. Immunostaining was not apparent in amyloid deposits in control sections treated with normal immune serum (Figure 1F).

DISCUSSION

In this study we used specific antisera to identify that the basement membrane HSPG is a component of islet amyloid in type II DM. Highly sulfated proteoglycans have been demonstrated within all amyloids examined to date [7,9] and the basement membrane HSPG has been specifically identified in three other forms of amyloid: AA, prion and Alzheimer's beta amyloid [10,12]. The invariable presence of highly sulfated proteoglycans in amyloid deposits suggests they may play an important role in amyloidogenesis in general. This hypothesis is strengthened by ultrastructural investigations which have shown that highly sulfated proteoglycans are intimately related to the amyloid fiber and may be an integral component of it [10-12,14,15]. Furthermore, in a murine model of accelerated AA amyloidosis, HSPG and AA protein are deposited coincidentally at precisely the same location during amyloidogenesis [16].

Although there is a strong association between HSPG and amyloid the nature of a possible role for HSPG in amyloidogenesis remains elusive. The heparan sulfate GAG moiety of HSPG is known to increase the beta-pleated sheet secondary structure of the SAA precursor of AA amyloid [17] suggesting HSPG may exert a conformational effect on amyloidogenic proteins. However, other potential roles such as determining the specific anatomic site of amyloid deposition, stabilization of amyloid fibrils and protection of amyloid against proteolysis have also been postulated (reviewed in [18]).

An internal sequence of the IAPP molecule, encompassing amino acids 20-29, appears to confer amyloidogenicity upon the overall peptide [19]. Species which develop spontaneous Type II DM-like disease show marked homology in this region [20] whereas the rat, which does not develop islet amyloid, shows significant divergence in this region while maintaining marked homology in the amino- and carboxyl termini of the molecule [21]. Investigation of potential molecular interactions between HSPG and the amyloidogenic sequence of IAPP may provide new insights into islet amyloid fibrillogenesis.

ACKNOWLEDGMENTS

This work was supported by MRC grants MA-11013 (IY) and MT-3153 (RK) and by the Upjohn Company of Canada. We would like to thank Pam Redden for her valuable secretarial assistance in the preparation of this manuscript.

REFERENCES

1. Ehrlich JC and Ratner JM. Amer J Pathol 38:49-59, 1961
2. Westermark P and Wilander E. Diabetologia 15:417-421, 1978
3. Westermark P, Wernstedt C, Wilander E et al. Biochem Biophys Res Commun 140:827-831, 1986
4. Westermark P, Wernstedt C, Wilander E et al. Proc Natl Acad Sci USA 84:3881-3885, 1987
5. Cooper GJS, Leighton B, Dimitriadis GD et al. Proc Natl Acad Sci USA 85:7763-7766, 1988
6. Leighton B and Cooper GJS. Nature 335:632-635, 1988
7. Snow AD, Willmer J, Kisilevsky R. Lab Invest 56:120-123, 1987
8. Snow AD, Willmer J, Kisilevsky R. Hum Pathol 18:506-510, 1987
9. Snow AD, Kisilevsky R, Willmer J et al. Acta Neuropathol 77:337-342, 1989
10. Snow Ad, Mar H, Kisilevsky R et al. J Cell Biol 107:160a, 1989 (abstract)
11. Snow AD, Mar H, Nochlin D et al. Amer J Pathol 133:456-463, 1988
12. Snow AD, Nochlin D, DeArmond SJ et al. Alzheimer Dis Assoc Disord 3:40, 1989 (abstract)
13. Lendrum AC, Sidders W, Fraser S. J Clin Pathol 25:373, 1972
14. Snow AD, Willmer J, Kisilevsky R. Lab Invest 57:687-698, 1987
15. Young ID, Willmer J, Kisilevsky R. Acta Neuropathol 78:202-209, 1989
16. Snow AD, Kisilevsky R. Lab Invest 53:37-44, 1985
17. McCubbin WD, Kay CM, Narindrasorasak S et al. Biochem J 256:775-783, 1988
18. Snow AD and Wight TN. Neurobiol Aging 10:481-497, 1989
19. Glenner CC, Eanes ED, Wiley CA. Biochem Biophys Res Commun 155:608-614, 1988
20. Cooper GJS, Day AJ, Willis AC et al. Biochim Biophys Acta 1014:247-258, 1989
21. Leffert JD, Newgard CB, Okamoto H et al. Proc Natl Acad Sci USA 86:3127-3130, 1989

ISOLATION AND CHARACTERISATION OF THE INTEGRAL GLYCOSAMINOGLYCAN CONSTITUENTS OF HUMAN AA AND AL AMYLOID FIBRILS

S.R. NELSON, M. LYON, J.T. GALLAGHER, E.A. JOHNSON & M.B. PEPYS
Immunological Medicine Unit, Royal Postgraduate Medical School, London, Cancer Research Campaign Department of Medical Oncology, Christie Hospital & Holt Radium Institute, Manchester, and National Institute for Biological Standards and Control, Potters Bar, U.K.

ABSTRACT. Amyloid fibrils were isolated by extraction in water from the livers and spleens of 4 patients who had died of monoclonal, AL-type, systemic amyloidosis and 1 with reactive systemic, AA-type amyloidosis. Each fibril preparation contained 1-2% by weight of glycosaminoglycan (GAG) which was tightly associated with the fibrils and not just co-isolated from the tissues with them. After exhaustive digestion of the fibrils with papain and pronase the GAGs were specifically precipitated with cetylpyridinium chloride and were identified by cellulose acetate electrophoresis and selective susceptibility to specific glycosidases. All the preparations contained approximately equal amounts of heparan sulphate and dermatan sulphate together with traces of heparin-like material. There was no evidence for the presence of chondroitin sulphate or other GAGs. Fine structural analysis by oligosaccharide mapping in gradient polyacrylamide gels, following partial digestion with specific glycosidases, showed very similar structures among the heparan sulphates and the dermatan sulphates respectively. GAGs were also extracted by solubilising amyloid fibrils in 4 M guanidinium chloride followed by CsCl density gradient ultracentrifugation. Although a minor proportion of the GAG material obtained in this way was apparently in the form of proteoglycan molecules, most of it was free GAG chains. The presence in amyloid fibrils of different types, in different organs and from different patients of particular GAG classes with similar structures, supports the view that these molecules may be of pathogenetic significance.

1. INTRODUCTION

There has lately been a resurgence of interest in GAGs in amyloid. The demonstration that they are universally present in all forms of amyloid which have been tested [1-7], and that in experimental systems their deposition occurs at the same time as the appearance of amyloid fibrils [8,9], suggest that GAGs may participate in the pathogenesis of amyloid fibril formation and/or persistence. They also suggest that GAGs may be related in some way to the presence of amyloid P component (AP) [10,11], a non-fibrillar serum protein which is also always found in all types of amyloid regardless of the nature of the fibril protein [12].

Hitherto the association of GAGs with amyloid fibrils *per se*, rather than their mere co-deposition in affected tissues, has been surmised from ultrastructural histochemical staining [3,5] and from analysis of fibril preparations [13], in which co-isolation of GAGs was not [14] or could not [15] be excluded.

2. METHODS, RESULTS AND DISCUSSION

The essential features of the present study, which is reported in detail elsewhere [16] were as follows. Both AA and AL fibrils isolated by the water extraction method of Pras [17] contained GAGs even though prior to extraction the tissues had been repeatedly homogenised and washed with physiological saline containing EDTA. These GAGs precipitated completely, together with the fibrils, in the presence of 10 mM NaCl, and only 18% of the GAG could be eluted from the fibrils by exposure to 2 M NaCl. This observation demonstrates that GAGs are tightly associated with amyloid fibrils *per se,* not merely co-isolated with them from amyloidotic tissue nor bound to them by simple polyionic interactions. The GAGs were isolated from amyloid fibrils, both by cetyl pyridinium precipitation [18] after exhaustive proteolysis and by CsCl density gradient ultracentrifugation of guanidine-solubilised fibrils, and were characterised in detail by cellulose acetate electrophoresis [19], digestion by specific glycosidases, refined oligosaccharide mapping [20] and measurement of GluN:GalN ratios [21,22]. All the preparations yielded 1-2% by weight of GAGs and contained approximately equal amounts of heparan sulphate and dermatan sulphate with traces of uncharacterised material with electrophoretic behaviour characteristic of commercial heparin preparations. Furthermore the fine structure of these GAGs was remarkably consistent in different patients with different types of amyloid and in fibrils from different organs from the same patient. Finally, most of the GAG present in amyloid fibrils was in the form of free glycan chains without core protein, and although this may be the result of post-mortem proteolysis it may represent an aberrant pathway of GAG metabolism in amyloidosis.

REFERENCES

1. Snow, A.D., Willmer, J. and Kisilevsky, R. (1987) Sulfated glycosaminoglycans: a common constituent of all amyloids? *Lab. Invest.*, **56**: 120-123.
2. Linker, A. and Carney, H.C. (1987) Presence and role of glycosaminoglycans in amyloidosis. *Lab. Invest.,* **57**: 297-305.
3. Snow, A.D., Willmer, J. and Kisilevsky, R. (1987) A close ultrastructural relationship between sulphated proteoglycans and AA amyloid fibrils. *Lab. Invest.,* **57**: 687-698.
4. Snow, A.D., Kisilevsky, R., Willmer, J., Prusiner, S.B. and DeArmond, S.J. (1989) Sulfated glycosaminoglycans in amyloid plaques of prion diseases. *Acta Neuropathol.,* **77**: 337-342.

5. Young, I.D., Willmer, J.P. and Kisilevsky, R. (1989) The ultrastructural localization of sulfated proteoglycans is identical in the amyloids of Alzheimer's disease and AA, AL, senile cardiac and medullary carcinoma-associated amyloidosis. *Acta Neuropathol.,* **78:** 202-209.
6. Snow, A.D. and Wight, T.N. (1989) Proteoglycans in the pathogenesis of Alzheimer's disease and other amyloidoses. *Neurobiol. Aging,* **10:** 481-497.
7. Perlmutter, L.S., Chui, H.C., Saperia, D. and Athanikar, J. (1990) Microangiopathy and the colocalization of heparin sulphate proteoglycan with amyloid in senile plaques of Alzheimer's disease. *Brain Res.,* **508:** 13-19.
8. Snow, A.D. and Kisilevsky, R. (1985) Temporal relationship between glycosaminoglycan accumulation and amyloid deposition during experimental amyloidosis: a histochemical study. *Lab. Invest.,* **53:** 37-44.
9. Snow, A., Kisilevsky, R., Stephens, C. and Anastassiades, T. (1987) Characterization of serum and splenic glycosaminoglycans during rapid AA amyloid induction. Qualitative and quantitative analysis. *Lab. Invest.,* **56:** 665-675.
10. Pollak, A., Coradello, H., Latzka, U., Lischka, A. and Lubec, G. (1982) Wechelswirkungen Zwischen Amyloid P und Bindegewebsproteinen. *Wiener Klinische Wochenschrift,* **94:** 291-293.
11. Hamazaki, H. (1987) Ca^{2+}-mediated association of human serum amyloid P component with heparan sulfate and dermatan sulfate. *J. Biol. Chem.*, **262:** 1456-1460.
12. Pepys, M.B. (1988) Amyloidosis. In: Immunological Diseases (Samter, M., Talmage, D.W., Frank, M.M., Austen, K.F. and Claman, H.N., eds.), vol. 1, pp. 631-674, Little Brown & Co., Boston.
13. Pennock, C.A. (1968) Association of acid mucopolysaccharides with isolated amyloid fibrils. Nature **217:** 753-754.
14. Magnus, J.H., Husby, G. and Kolset, S.O. (1989) Presence of glycosaminoglycans in purified AA type amyloid fibrils associated with juvenile rheumatoid arthritis. *Ann. Rheum. Dis.,* **48:** 215-219.
15. Ohishi, H., Skinner, M., Sato-Araki, N., Okuyama, T., Gejyo, F., Kimura, A., Cohen, A.S. and Schmid, K. (1990) Glycosaminoglycans of the hemodialysis-associated carpal synovial amyloid and of amyloid-rich tissues and fibrils of heart, liver, and spleen. *Clin. Chem.,* **361:** 88-91.
16. Nelson, S.R., Lyon, M., Gallagher, J.T., Johnson, E.A. and Pepys, M.B. (1990) Isolation and characterisation of the integral glycosaminoglycan constituents of human AA and AL amyloid fibrils. *Biochem. J.* (in press).
17. Pras, M., Schubert, M., Zucker-Franklin, D., Rimon, A. and Franklin, E.C. (1968) The characterisation of soluble amyloid prepared in water. *J. Clin. Invest.,* **47:** 924-933.
18. Scott, J.E. (1960) Aliphatic ammonium salts in the assay of acidic polysaccharides from tissues. *Meth. Biochem. Anal.,* **8:** 145-197.
19. Cappelletti, R., Del Rosso, M. and Chiarugi, V.P. (1979) A new electrophoretic method for the complete separation of all known animal glycosaminoglycans in a monodimensional run. *Anal. Biochem.,* **99:** 311-315.

20. Lyon, M. and Gallagher, J.T. (1990) A general method for the detection and mapping of submicrogram quantities of glycosaminoglycan oligosaccharides on polyacrylamide gels by sequential staining with Azure A and ammoniacal silver. *Anal. Biochem.,* **185:** 63-70.
21. Navratil, J.D., Murgia, E. and Walton, H.F. (1975) Ligand exchange chromatography of amino sugars. *Anal. Chem.,* **47:** 122-125.
22. Johnson, E.A. (1982) Characterization and separation of sulphated glycosaminoglycuronans. *Pharmacol. Res. Commun.,* **14:** 289-320.

BASEMENT MEMBRANE COMPONENTS AND PROTEIN AA IN RENAL AMYLOID DEPOSITS

G.T. Westermark*, B. Norling# and P. Westermark*
Department of Pathology, University of Linköping* and Gustaf Werner Institute, University of Uppsala#, Sweden

Abstract

Frozen thick needle biopsies from patients with systemic secondary (reactive) amyloidosis were used to clarify the ultrastructural colocalization of basement membrane components with protein AA in the amyloid deposits. With the aid of double immunogold labeling, we studied heparan sulphate proteoglycan core protein, laminin, fibronectin, amyloid P component, and collagen IV together with protein AA. All basement membrane components were present in the amyloid deposits except fibronectin and collagen IV.

Introduction

After longterm inflammatory disease with high serum levels of the acute phase serum amyloid protein (apoSAA), some patients develop secondary amyloidosis. It is not yet known why all such patients do not develop this disease. The protein AA that builds up in the extracellularly deposited amyloid are N-terminal fragments of apoSAA. The amino acid sequence of the amyloid protein AA has been established from many different patients. There is no evidence for an amyloidogenic SAA molecule in human, as seen in the murine amyloidosis model. During purification of the amyloid fibrils from the tissue, other components have been found. However, it is not known if they are associated with the fibril itself or result from the purification method. In this ultrastructural study, we have assessed the relationship between basement membrane components (1-3) and the amyloid fibrils.

Patients and methods

TISSUES

Thick needle kidney biopsies were obtained and a portion was stored at -70°C until use. Biopsies from three different patients with secondary (reactive) systemic amyloidosis and protein AA depositions in the renal tissue were used for the study.

Case I: A 65 year old woman with severe rheumatoid arthritis of 45 years duration. Amyloid deposits were seen in the glomeruli and tubular walls.

Case II: A 78 year old man, who was healthy until one year ago. He was found to have AA-amyloidosis with renal involvement, but no underlying disease was diagnosed.

Case III: A 38 year old man with HLA-B27 positive Bechterew's disease since the age of 16. Amyloid deposits involved most of the tissue structures seen in the renal biopsy.

TISSUE PREPARATION FOR IMMUNOELECTRON MICROSCOPY

The renal biopsies were divided into smaller pieces and put into a fixative containing 4% paraformaldehyde and 4% sucrose in 0.1M sodium phosphate buffer, pH 7.4, for 30 minutes at room temperature. Further fixation was performed in the same solution but with a pH of 9.0 overnight at 4°C (4). The tissue was then embedded in Lowicryl (K4M), which was polymerized under ultraviolet irradiation, at -20°C for 24 hours.

IMMUNOGOLD LABELING

For single immunogold staining, the grids were first incubated with a primary polyclonal (rabbit) antibody (Table 1) for four hours and, after washing, treated with 20 nm protein-A gold particles. For double immunogold staining (5), then the grids were rinsed and incubated with a second primary antibody for an additional four hours. In the preceding step, a mouse monoclonal antibody was used, and it was visualized with a biotinylated rabbit anti-mouse antibody and 10 nm streptavidine-gold particles.

Table 1. Primary antibodies used in this study

Antibody to	Dilution	Produced in	Source
Laminin	1:25	rabbit	Authors
Fibronectin	1:100	rabbit	Dako
HSPG	1:40	rabbit	B.Norling (ref. 6)
SAP	1:100	rabbit	Dako
Collagen IV	1:25	mouse	Dako
Protein AA	1:50	rabbit	A.Grubb (ref. 7)
Protein AA	1:100	mouse	Dako

HSPG=Heparan sulphate proteoglycan core protein
SAP=Serum amyloid P component.

Result

Due to the freezing artifacts it was not possible to distinguish between glomerular and tubular basement membrane, but all basement membranes labelled with the antibodies. Specific labeling of the amyloid depositions was found in all cases with both polyclonal and monoclonal antibodies directed against protein AA. Antibodies to laminin, HSPG core protein and amyloid P-component reacted with the basement membranes in material from all three patients. The same antibodies also labelled the amyloid depositions evenly. A reaction with anti-fibronectin antibodies was seen with the basement membrane areas in the material from all three patients. There was no labeling of the amyloid depositions with antibodies to fibronectin in case I or II, while the amyloid deposited in case III reacted strongly. The labeling with antibodies to collagen IV was exclusively seen in basement membranes.

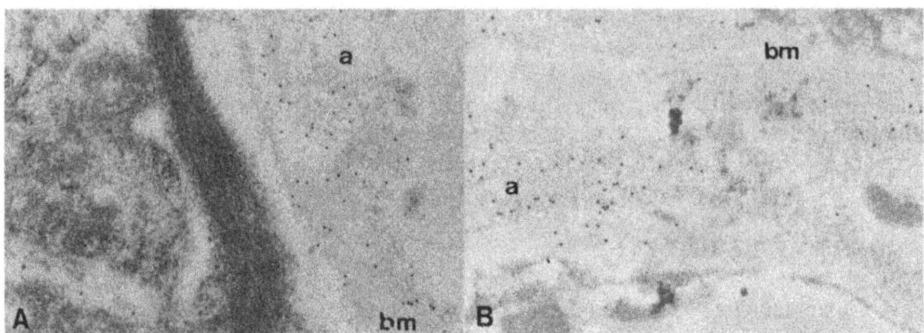

Fig. 1. Basement membrane (bm) and amyloid (a) labelled with anti HSPG (A) and anti laminin (B) visualized with protein-A gold. A = X 25,000 and B = X 28,000.

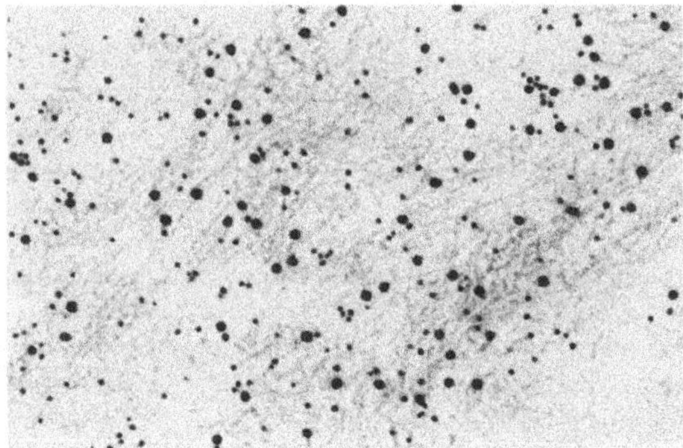

Fig. 2. Double labeling of amyloid of case III with anti protein AA (10 nm gold particle) and anti fibronectin (20 nm gold particle) X 39,000.

Discussion

The pathogenesis of fibrils in reactive amyloidosis is virtually unknown. Protein AA is certainly the main component of the fibrils, but some other protein constituents have been demonstrated in the amyloid deposits. Such constituents are HSPG core protein, amyloid P-component and fibronectin (6,8,9). Whether or not these are integrated in the fibrils or of any importance in the process of deposition is not known.

The present immunogold electron microscopic study, which was undertaken to see if basement membrane components are present in association with the amyloid fibrils, showed that in addition to protein AA, amyloid P-component, HSPG core protein and laminin were present in amyloid deposits of all three patients studied. On the other hand, collagen IV immunoreactivity was never demonstrated in the amyloid. From this study it is impossible to conclude that proteins other than protein AA are present in the fibrils; however, it cannot be excluded that the fibrils have a more complex composition than generally believed. It is also possible that the basement membrane components demonstrated here are of importance for the fibril formation and for the localization of the deposits, even if they are not parts of the fibrils themselves.

Acknowledgements

Supported by the Swedish Medical Research Council, the Research Fund of King Gustaf V and the Östergötland County.

References

1. Courtoy, PJ., Kanwar, YS., Hynes, RO. and Farquhar, MG. (1980) 'Fibronectin localization in the rat glomerulus', J. Cell. Biol. 87, 691-696.
2. Dyck, RF., Lockwood, CM., Kershaw, M., McHugh, N., Duance, VC., Baltz, M. and Pepys, MB. (1980) 'Amyloid P-component is a constituent of normal human glomerular basement membrane', J. Exp. Med. 152, 1162-1174.
3. Scheinman, JI., Foidart, J-M., Gerhron-Robey, P., Fish, AJ. and Michael, AF. (1980) 'The immunohistology of glomerular antigens IV: laminin, a defined noncollagen basement membrane', Clin. Immunol. Immunopathol. 15, 175-189.
4. Kisalus, LL. and Herr, JG. (1988) 'Immunocytochemical localization of heparan sulfate proteoglycan in human decidual cell secretory bodies and placental fibrinoid', Biol. of Reprod. 39, 419-430.
5. Bendayan, M. and Stephen, H. (1984) 'Double labelling cytochemistry applaying the protein A-gold technique' in J. M. Polak and I. M. Varndells (eds.), Immunolabelling for electron microscopy, Elsevier Science Publishers, Amsterdam, pp. 143-154.
6. Norling, B., Westermark, GT. and Westermark, P. (1988) 'Immunohistochemical identification of heparan sulphate proteoglycan in secondary systemic amyloidosis', Clin. Exp. Immunol. 73, 333-337.
7. Grubb, A., Lövberg, H., Thysell, H., Ljunggren, L., Olson, T., Skinner, M., Shirahama, T. and Cohen, AS. (1987) 'Production of an amino acid sequence-specific antiserum against human amyloid A (AA) and serum amyloid A (SAA)', Scand. J. Clin. Lab. Invest. 47, 619-626.
8. Pepys, MB. (1986), 'Amyloid P-component: structure and properties' in J.Marrink and M.H. van Rijswijk (eds.), Amyloidosis, Martinus Nijhoff Publishers, Dordrecht, pp.43-49.
9. Kawahara, E., Shiroo, M., Nakanishi, I. and Migita, S. (1989) 'The role of fibronectin in the development of experimental amyloidosis: Evidence of immunohistochemical codistribution and binding property with serum amyloid protein A', Am. J. Pathol. 134, 1305-1314.

HIGH MOLECULAR WEIGHT POLYSACCHARIDES IN FAMILIAL CARDIAC AMYLOID OF DANISH ORIGIN RELATED TO TRANSTHYRETIN MET 111.

MAGNUS J H, STENSTAD T, KOLSET S O*, DAHL I M, RANLØV P J** AND HUSBY G.

Department of Rheumatology and *Institute of Medical Biology, University of Tromsø, 9000 Tromsø, Norway.
**Department of Medicine B, Central Hospital, Hillerød, Denmark.

Abstract

We have previously demonstrated a strong in vivo association between TTR Met 111 cardiac amyloid fibrils and glycosaminoglycans (1). The present study was aimed at investigating in more detail the macromolecular properties of the polysaccharide moiety of TTR Met 111 cardiac amyloid. Water extracted and lyophilised amyloid fibrils were subjected to treatment with guanidine, and the extracted polysaccharides were isolated by ion exchange chromatography. Significant amount of GAGs were obtained, and further depolymerization by specific biochemic methods and enzymes followed by gelfiltration identified the different GAGs. We conclude that the GAGs in the form of hyaluronic acid, galactosamines and N-sulfated glucosamines as identified in this TTR met 111 cardiac amyloid are specifically associated with the isolated amyloid fibrils, and consist of high molecular weight GAG chains which are not part of intact proteoglycans.

Introduction

Familial amyloid cardiomyopathy of a Danish kindred is the only autosomal dominant inherited form of amyloidosis that have no clinical manifestations but cardiomyopathy (1,2). The transthyretin (TTR) nature of the cardiac amyloid (3) and localization of a methionin for leucine substitution at position 111 (TTR Met 111) have previously been reported (4).

The presence of glycosaminoglycans (GAGs) in tissue deposits of amyloid is confirmed in several reports (5). We have been able to verify, by direct biochemical evidence, the specific association of GAGs with purified TTR Met 111 cardiac amyloid (6). The aims of the present study was to investigate in more detail the macromolecular properties of this polysaccharide moiety.

Materials and Methods

AMYLOID FIBRIL EXTRACTION

Amyloid fibrils were prepared from the myocardium of a 43 year old patient with familial amyloid cardiomyopathy of Danish origin related to variant TTR Met 111 using the water extraction method of Pras et al (7) with a small modification (8). The aqueous amyloid fibril supernatants were lyophilised. Normal myocardium was subjected to the same procedure.

ISOLATION OF GAGS

Lyophilised amyloid fibrils was digested with pronase, and subjected to DEAE-Sephacel ion exchange chromatography (9). The column was calibrated and eluted with a 6 M urea/10 mM Tris HCl buffer pH 6.0, and a gradient from 0 to 1.5 M NaCl. Selected fractions were pooled after determination of hexuronic acid by the carbazole method (10), dialyzed against distilled water, and lyophilised.

PROTEOGLYCAN ISOLATION

Lyophilised amyloid fibril and normal myocardial extracts were solubilized in 8 M urea 10 mM Tris HCl buffer pH 6.0, with protease inhibitors prior to ion exchange chromatography.

BETAELIMINATION

Aliquots of the lyophilised carbazole positive material obtained after ion exchange chromatography was subjected to betaelimination (11) and subsequent Sepharose CL- 6B chromatography with 6 M urea 10 mM Tris HCl pH 6.0 as eluent.

IDENTIFICATION OF GLYCOSAMINOGLYCANS

Enzymatic degradation was performed on lyophilized polysaccharide material after ion exchange chromatography. Galactosaminoglycans, chondroitin sulfate (CS) and dermatan sulfate (DS), were degraded by chondroitinase ABC from Seikagaku. The chondroitinase ABC resistent material , polysaccharides containing N-sulfated glucosaminoglycans, heparin (Hep) and heparan sulfate (HS), were chemically depolymerized by nitrous acid treatment (12). The hyaluronan consentration were determined by a specific radioassay (13).

Results

The TTR Met 111 nature of the amyloid from the patient was confirmed by amino acid sequence analysis of the purified protein (4). The elution profile of carbazole positive material obtained by gradient ion exchange chromatography of pronase digested amyloid fibrils and the corresponding material from normal myocardium is shown in Fig.1.

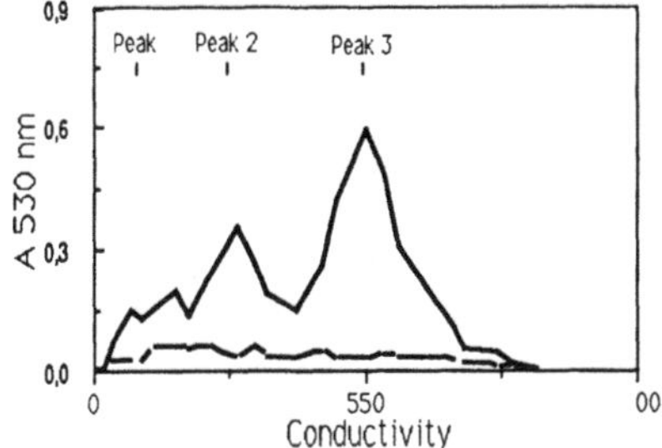

Fig1. DEAE-Sephacel ion exchange chromatography of pronase digested cardiac TTR Met 111 cardiac amyloid fibril and corresponding normal myocardial extracts. Material in peak 1 eluted at 015 M NaCl, that in peak 2 at 0.22 M NaCl and that in peak 3 at 0.45 M NaCl.

The total amount of carbazole positive GAGs coisolated with TTR Met 111 cardiac amyloid was approximately 45 µg per mg of lyophoilised fibril (6).

The amyloid associated GAGs eluted as one major and two minor peaks. Peak 1 (salt consentration of 0.15 M NaCl), consisted of chondroitinase ABC succeptible low molecular weight oligosaccharides. Peak 2 (0.22 M NaCl), consisted of hyaluronan, 3.1 µg per mg lyophilized fibril material. About 57% of the total carbazole positive material eluted at 0.45M NaCl (Peak 3). The depolymerization by chondroitinase ABC and nitrous acid treatment, identified these GAGs as CS/DS and Hep/HS at a 2:1 proportion.

Solubilized amyloid fibrils containing protease inhibitors were similarly subjected to ion exchange chromatography, and GAGs were collected. The elution profile was identical to that ilustrated in Fig.1. Chromatography on Sepharose CL-6B of the high molarity material (Fig.1, peak 3) after betaelimination showed all the material to elute at a Kav of 0.22 identical to that of untreated material, as visualized on Fig.2. The unchanged elution position of this material following betaelimination strongly indicates it to consist of free GAG chains rather than intact PG molecules.

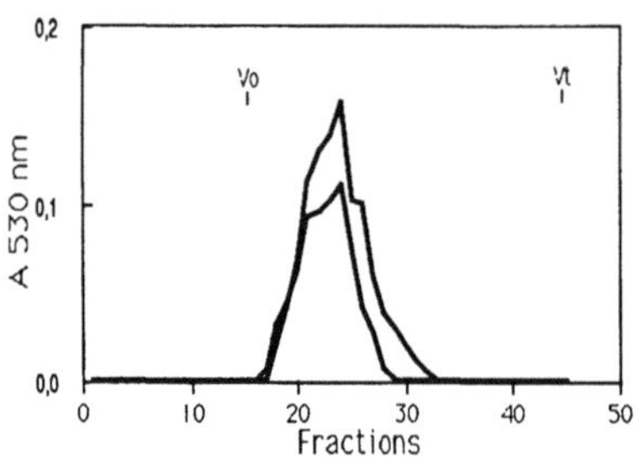

Fig.2 Sepharose CL-6B gel chromato graphy of TTR Met 111 cardiac amyloid associated high molarity GAGs, obtained by ion exchange chromatography (Fig.1, peak 3) before and after betaelimination.

Discussion

The composition of amyloid has been a matter of dispute for more than a century (14). Several investigators have emphasized the presence of GAGs in spontaneous as well as experimental amyloid deposits in addition to the fibril protein (15). Immunohistochemical studies on tissue sections have demonstrated a HS proteoglycan core protein in different types of amyloid, but this PG have not yet been isolated and identified biochemically (15). This study raport the macromolecular properties of the amyloid associated polysaccharides coisoled with TTR Met 111 cardiac amyloid fibril extracts. We conclude that the GAGs in the form of hyaluronan, galactosamines and N-sulfated glucosamines as identified in this TTR met 111 cardiac amyloid are specifically associated with the isolated amyloid fibrils in the form of of high molecular weight GAG chains which are not part of intact proteoglycans (PGs). The high molecular weight GAGs appearing in the amyloid fibril extracts may be part of intact PGs in vivo, which needs further elucidation to better explain the role of GAGs in the fibrillogenesis of amyloid.

Acknowledgments

This work was supported by the Norwegian Council for Science and the Humanities, the Norwegian Cancer Society, the Norwegian Women's Public Health Association and Norsk Revmatikerforbund. The authors wish to thank Ms Kajsa Lilja for skilful technical assistance.

References

1. Varga, J. and Wohlgethan, J. R. (1988) 'The clinical and biochemical spectrum of hereditary amyloidosis', Sem Arthritis Rheum 18, 14-26
2. Benson, M. D. (1988) 'Hereditary amyloidosis - Disease entity and clinical model', Hosp Practice, 165-173
3. Husby, G., Ranløv, P. J., Sletten, K. and Marhaug, G. (1985) 'The amyloid in familial amyloid cardiomyopathy of Danish origin is related to prealbumin', Clin Exp Immunol 60, 207-211
4. Nordlie, M., Sletten, K., Husby, G. and Ranløv, P.J. (1988) 'A new prealbumin variant in familial amyloid cardiomyopathy of Danish origin', Scan J Immunol 27, 119-222
5. Magnus, J.H., Husby, G. and Kolset, S.O. (1989) 'Presence of glycosaminoglycans in purified AA type amyloid fibrils associated with juvenile rheumatoid arthritis', Ann Rheum Dis 48, 215-219
6. Magnus, J.H., Stenstad, T., Kolset, S.O., Dahl, I.M., Husby, G. and Ranløv, P.J. (1989) 'Presence of polysaccharides in familial cardiac amyloid of Danish origin related to variant transthyretin Met 111'in P.Costa (ed.), Proceedings 1st International Symposium on Familial Amyloidotic Polyneuropathy, Portugal.
7. Pras, M., Schubert, M., Zuker-Franklin, D., Rimon, A. and Franklin, E.C. (1968) 'The characterization of soluble amyloid prepared in water', J Clin Invest 47, 924-933
8. Skinner, M., Shirahama, T., Cohen, A. S. and Deal, C.L. (1983) 'The association of amyloid P-component: an update method for amyloid fibril protein isolation', Prep Biochem 12, 461-476
9. Hallen, A. (1972) 'Chromatography of acidic glycosaminoglycans on DEAE-cellulose', J Chromatogr 71, 83-91
10.Bitter, T. and Muir, H. (1962) ' A modified uronic acid carbazole reaction', Anal Biochem 4, 330-331
11.Heinegård, D. and Sommarin, Y. (1987) ' Isolation and characterization of proteoglycans', Methods Enzymol 144, 319-372
12.Shively, J. E. and Conrad, H. E. (1976) 'Formation of anhydrosugars in the chemical depolymerization of heparin', Biochemistry 15, 3932-3942
13.Tengblad, A. (1980) 'Quantitative analysis of hyaluronate in nanogram amounts', Biochem J 185, 101-105
14.Husby, G. (1989) 'Pathogenesis of AA amyloidosis', in M. Pepys (ed.), Argenteuil Symposium 1988: Acute Phase Proteins and the Acute Phase Response, Springer Verlag, pp 169-85.
15.Snow, A.,Willmer, J. and Kisilevsky, R. (1987) 'A close ultrastructural relationship between sulphated glycosaminoglycans and AA amyloid fibrils', Lab Invest 57, 687-698

POINT MUTATION IN AUTOSOMAL DOMINANT FORMS OF AMYLOIDOSIS

Blas Frangione, M.D., Ph.D.
Department of Pathology, New York University Medical Center
550 First Avenue, New York, NY 10016

We have studied three inherited types of amyloidosis: familial amyloidosis, Finnish type (FAF), and the two familial types of cerebral amyloid angiopathy known as hereditary cerebral hemorrhage with amyloidosis: Icelandic (*HCHWA-I*) and Dutch (*HCHWA-D*). *FAF* is an autosomal dominant form of systemic amyloidosis, clinically characterized by lattice corneal dystrophy and progressive cranial neuropathy. The amyloid protein subunit is a degradation fragment of a *variant of gelsolin*, an actin modulating 90 or 93 kDa cytoplasmic and plasma protein. The variant protein is the result of a point mutation in the gelsolin gene.

HCHWA-I and HCHWA-D are also dominant forms of amyloidosis preferentially associated with the small vasculature of the brain and clinically characterized by recurrent strokes leading to premature death. *HCHWA-I* is related to a point mutation in the cystatin C gene, an inhibitor of cysteine proteases, and *HCHWA-D* to a point mutation in the Alzheimer's β precursor amyloid gene. The mutation in the structural gene for these amyloid proteins may be the primary defect, rendering the proteins resistant to normal degradation or alternatively, causing increased susceptibility to abnormal proteolytic breakdown, and acceleration of amyloid deposition.

FAMILIAL AMYLOIDOSIS, FINNISH TYPE (FAF)

The amyloid fibril found in patients with FAF [for more details see Haltia et al., this volume] is a low molecular weight degradation fragment of gelsolin, an actin binding and modulating protein [1-3]. The amyloid protein starts at a position corresponding to residue 173 of the mature plasma gelsolin [1,4] and has an amino acid substitution (asparagine for aspartic acid) at position 187 (position 15 of the amyloid protein). The amino acid replacement is located in a repetitive motif (FXXXDXFIL) of unknown functions that is highly conserved among species [5]. In order to test the possibility that the mutation exists at nucleotide 654 (numbering as for human plasma gelsolin cDNA [4]), genomic DNA was isolated from five unrelated FAF patients. The sequence of the amplified and subcloned fragments demonstrated that all five patients had one allele containing a point mutation, at nucleotide 654, as well as one normal allele (Fig. 1) [Levy et al., submitted). Our preliminary results suggest that the mutation (A instead of G) segregates with the disease, and that slot blot analysis can be used as a diagnostic assay (Fig. 2) for presymptomatic FAF patients and prenatal evaluation. We designate this variant of gelsolin-associated amyloidosis Agel ASN 187.

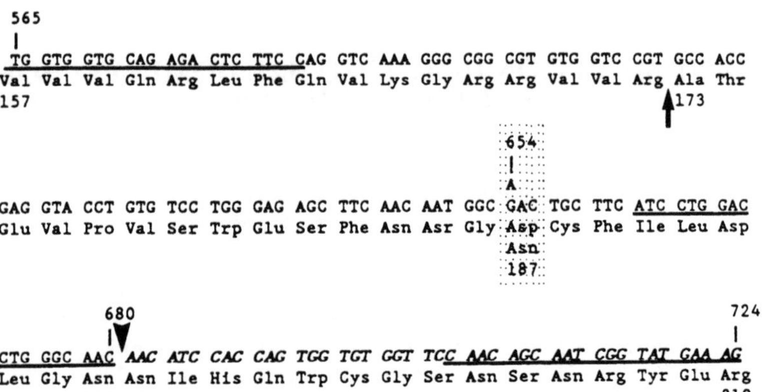

FIGURE 1. The mutation and amino acid substitution found in gelsolin in FAF patients. The nucleotides and predicted amino acids are numbered as reference 4. Underlined sequences: used to synthesize the oligonucleotides; arrows: the amino terminal of the amyloid protein; arrowhead: intron.

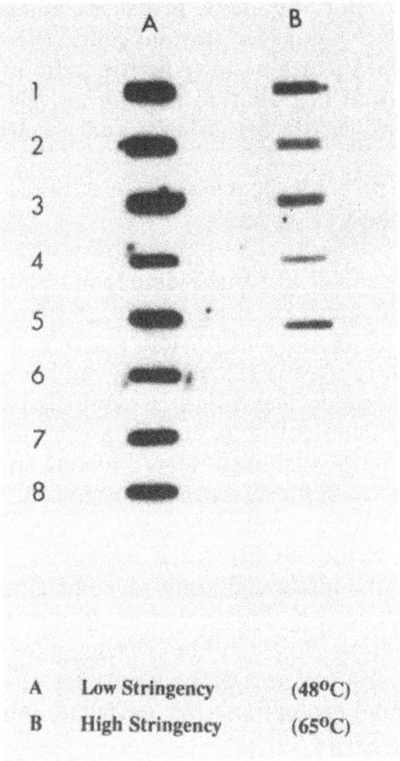

Figure 2. Slot blot analysis demonstrating the existence of a point mutation in DNA isolated from FAF patients (#1-5) and its absence in DNA isolated from two unaffected family members (#6,7) and from normal controls (#8). Genomic DNA sequences 565-680 (Fig. 1) were amplified with the PCR and washed in low stringency (A) and in high stringency (B).

HEREDITARY CEREBRAL HEMORRHAGE WITH AMYLOIDOSIS: ICELANDIC TYPE (HCHWA-I) AND DUTCH TYPE (HCHWA-D)

HCHWA-I is found in patients from Iceland. They have predominantly cerebral amyloid angiopathy, unassociated with neuritic plaques or tangles, that leads to cerebral hemorrhage and thrombotic strokes, causing death before the age of forty [6]. The amyloid protein is homologous to cystatin C (an inhibitor of cysteine protease); it lacks the first ten amino terminal residues and there is an amino acid substitution at position 58 (glutamine for leucine), corresponding to residue 68 of urinary cystatin C [7,8,9]. The cystatin C gene contains three exons and except for a mutation corresponding to nucleotide 281 in the second exon (CAG instead of CTG), the gene cloned from an Icelandic patient is identical to the normal gene [10] (Fig. 3). This mutation abolishes an Alu I restriction site, and loss of this site was detected in HCHWA-I patients; it cosegregates with the disease [11].

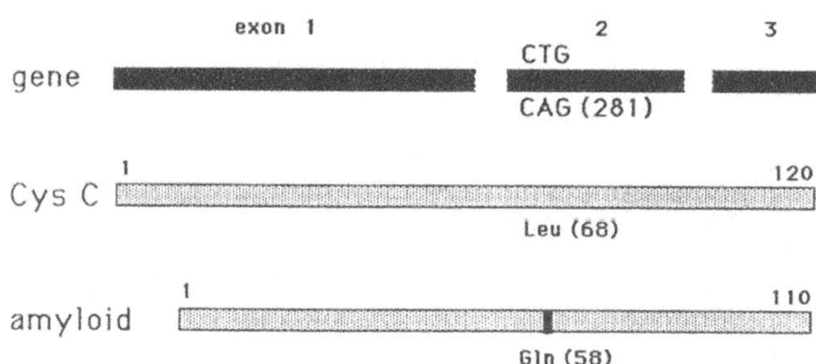

Fig. 3 Schematic representation of the three exons encoding human cystatin C gene. The site of the point mutation found in HCHWA-I and the amino acid substitution present in the amyloid proteins are indicated.

HCHWA-D This form of amyloidosis has been described in four families from two coastal villages in the Netherlands [12,13]. The disease is characterized by amyloid deposition in small leptomeningeal arteries and cortical arterioles, leading to hemorrhage and early death. Apart from the severe amyloid angiopathy, there is an accumulation of parenchymal plaque-like structures resembling preamyloid lesions and the early plaques found in Alzheimer's Disease (AD) [14]. However, very few neuritic plaques and no neurofibrillary tangles have been observed in HCHWA-D patients. Although there are clinico-pathological distinctions between

HCHWA-D and AD, the amyloid fibrils extracted from leptomeningeal vessels are formed by polymerization of a 39-residue peptide similar to the β-protein of AD, Down syndrome, sporadic cerebral amyloid angiopathy and normal aging [15,16]. These observations have led to the suggestion that HCHWA-D may be considered a distinct type of familial AD, with predominantly vascular involvement [14]. Sequence analysis of genomic DNA in HCHWA-D patients demonstrated a point mutation, cytosine for guanine at position 1852 (exon 15), of the precursor β-protein gene, which causes a single amino acid substitution (glutamine for glutamic acid) corresponding to position 22 of the amyloid protein and residue 618 of the precursor protein (Fig. 4). The normal allele was also present in these patients [17]. Both the normal and variant Alzheimer's β-protein alleles are expressed in vascular amyloid in HCHWA-D and may be detected by tryptic peptides mapping [18].

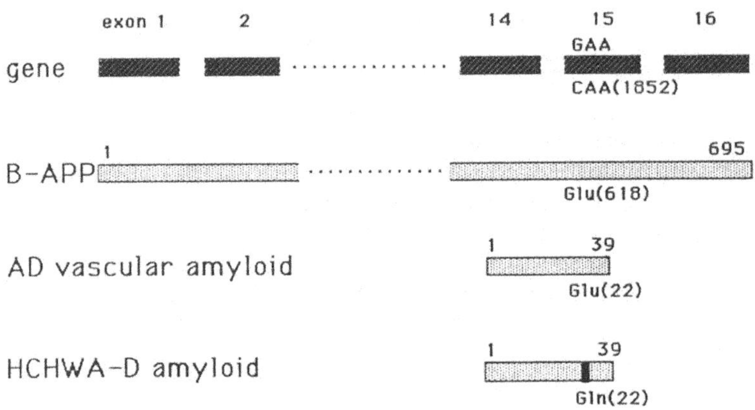

Fig. 4. Schematic representation of the gene encoding (16 exons) the 695 amino acid form of the amyloid β precursor protein [19]. The 39 residue vascular amyloid protein obtained from AD and HCHWA-D patients, the site of a point mutation and the amino acid substitution are indicated [16,20].

The segregation of the HCHWA-D mutation was recently confirmed [Bakker et al., in preparation), and we have developed a diagnostic assay for high risk populations and prenatal evaluation that is based on the existence of the mutation [18].

The mutation in the structural gene for plasma gelsolin, cystatin C and β-protein precursor may be the primary defect in these three autosomal dominant forms of amyloidosis, causing aberrant degradation and polymerization of the resulting β-pleated fragments.

These "disease genes" are important tools for developing animal models in order to study the mechanism(s) and tissue specific factor(s) involved in amyloid fibril formation.

1. Haltia, M., Prelli, F., Ghiso, J., Kiuru, S., Somer, H., Palo, J. and Frangione, B. (1990) Amyloid protein in familial amyloidosis (Finnish type) is homologous to gelsolin, an actin-binding protein. Biochem. Biophys. Res. Commun. 167:927-930.
2. Haltia, M., Ghiso, J., Prelli, F., G., Gloria, Kiuru, S., Somer, H., Palo, J. and Frangione, B. (1990) Amyloid in familial amyloidosis, Finnish type, is antigenically and structurally related to gelsolin. Am J Pathol 136, 1223-1228.
3. Maury, C.P.J., Alli, K., and Baumann, M. (1990) Finnish hereditary amyloidosis. Amino acid sequence homology between the amyloid fibril protein and human plasma gelsoline FEBS Letts 260:85-87.
4. Kwiatkowski, D.J., Stossel, T.P., Orkin, S.H., Mole, J.E., Colten, H.R. and Yin, H.L. (1986) Nature 323:455-458.
5. Way, M. and Weeds, A. (1988) Nucleotide sequence of pig plasma gelsolin: Comparison of protein sequence with human gelsolin and other actin-severing proteins shows strong homologies and evidence for large internal repeats. J. Mol. Biol. 203:1127-1133.
6. Gudmundsson, G., Hallgrimsson, J., Jonasson, T.A. and Bjarnason, O. (1972) Hereditary cerebral haemorrhage with amyloidosis. Brain 95:387-404.
7. Cohen, D.H., Feiner, H., Jensson, O. and Frangione, B. (1983) Amyloid fibril in hereditary cerebral hemorrhage with amyloidosis (HCHWA) is related to the gastroenteropancreatic neuroendocrine protein, gamma trace. J. Exp. Med. 158:623-628.
8. Ghiso, J., Jensson, O. and Frangione, B. (1986) Amyloid fibrils in hereditary cerebral hemorrhage with amyloidosis of Icelandic type is a variant of basic protein (Cystatin C). Proc. Natl. Acad. Sci. (USA) 83:2974-2978.
9. Grubb, A. and Lofberg, H. (1984) Human gamma-trace, a basic microprotein: amino acid sequences and presence in the adenohypophysis. Proc. Natl. Acad. Sci. USA 79:3024-3027.
10. Levy, E., Lopez-Otin, C., Ghiso, J., Geltner, D., and Frangione, B. (1989) Stroke in Icelandic patients with hereditary amyloid angiopathy is related to a mutation in the cystatin C gene, an inhibitor of cysteine proteases. J. Exp. Med., 169:1771-1778.
11. Palsdottir, A., Abrahamson, M., Thorsteinsson, L., Arnason, A., Olafsson, I., Grubb, A. and Jenson, O. (1988) Mutation in cystatin C gene causes hereditary brain haemorrhage. Lancet ii:603-604.
12. Wattendorf, A.R., Bots, G.Th.A.M., Went, L.N., Edtz, L.J. (1982) Familial cerebral amyloid angiopathy presenting as recurrent cerebral haemorrhage. J. Neurol. Sci. 55:121-135.
13. Luyendijk, W., Bots G.Th.A.M., Vegter-vander Vlis M., and Went, L.N. (1986) Familiaire Hersenbloedingen als gevolg van crebrale amyloide angiopathie. Ned Tijdschr Geneekd 130:1935-1940.
14. van Duinen, S.G., Castano, E.M., Prelli, F., Bots, G.Th.A.M., Luyendijk, W. and Frangione, B. (1987) Hereditary cerebral hemorrhage with amyloidosis in patients of Dutch origin is related to Alzheimer disease. Proc. Natl. Acad. Sci. (USA) 84:5991-5994.
15. Glenner, G.G. and Wong, C.W. (1984) Alzheimer's disease and Down's syndrome: sharing of a unique cerebrovascular amyloid fibril protein. Biochem. Biophys. Res. Commun. 122:1131-1135.
16. Prelli, F., Castano, E.M., van Duinen, S.G., Bots, G.Th.A.M., Luyendijk, W. and Frangione, B. (1988) Different processing of Alzheimer's β-protein precursor in the vessel wall of patients with hereditary cerebral hemorrhage with amyloidosis-Dutch type. Biochem. Biophys. Res. Commun. 151:1150-1155.

17. Levy, E., Carman, M.D., Fernandez-Madrid, I., Lieberburg, I., Power, M.D., Van Duinen, S.G., Bots, G.Th.A.M., Luyendijk, W. and Frangione, B. (1990) Mutation of the Alzheimer's disease amyloid gene in hereditary cerebral hemorrhage, Dutch type. Science 248:1124-1126.
18. Prelli, F., Levy, E., van Duinen, S.G., Bots, G.Th.A.M., Luyendijk, W. and Frangione, B. (1990) Expression of a normal and variant Alzheimer's β-protein gene in amyloid of hereditary cerebral hemorrhage, Dutch type: DNA and protein diagnostic assays. Biochem. Biophys. Res. Commun. 170:301-307.
19. Lemaire H.G., Salbaum J.M., Multhaup G., Kang J., Bayney R.M., Unterbak A., Beyreuther K. and Muller-Hill B. (1989) The $PreA4_{695}$ precursor protein of Alzheimer's disease A4 amyloid is encoded by 16 exons. Nucleic Acid Res. 17, 517-522.
20. Prelli, F., Castano, E., Glenner, G.G. and Frangione, B.: (1988) Differences between vascular and plaque core amyloid in Alzheimer's disease. J. Neurochem. 51, 648-651.

Perturbation of processing of cystatin C in monocytes from patients with hereditary cystatin C amyloid angiopathy

L. Thorsteinsson,[1] G. Georgsson,[3] B. Ásgeirsson,[4] M. Bjarnadóttir,[1] Í. Ólafsson,[5] Ó. Jensson,[1] and G. Guðmundsson.[2]

Dept. of Med. Genetics, The Blood Bank [1], Dept. of Neurol.[2] National Univ. Hosp., Inst. for Exp. Pathol., Keldur[3], Science Inst.[4] Univ. of Iceland, Reykjavík Iceland, Dept. of Clin. Chem. Univ. Hosp. Lund Sweden[5].

ABSTRACT. In hereditary cystatin C amyloid angiopathy (HCCAA) a mutation of the cystatin C gene occurs with substitution of a single amino acid in the cystatin C protein, which is deposited as amyloid. The pathogenetic mechanism leading to amyloid deposition is unknown. We have in the pursuit of this question studied the processing of cystatin C in blood monocytes from six carriers of the mutated cystatin C gene (three asymptomatic and three had got repeated strokes). Monocytes from blood donors served as controls. The main finding was that monocytes from asymptomatic and symptomatic individuals accumulated cystatin C intracellularly. Thus the concentration of cystatin C was higher in the cells than in the supernatants whereas the opposite was true for the controls. No difference in the intracellular distribution of cystatin C was found by immunohistochemistry and preliminary results of electron microscopic examination have not revealed any distinct difference in the ultrastructure. As microglia are closely related to monocytes, the observed partial block in the secretion of cystatin C in HCCAA may be of relevance for the pathogenesis of the amyloid deposits in the central nervous system (CNS).

Introduction

Hereditary cystatin C amyloid angiopathy (HCCAA) is a disease inherited in an autosomal dominant way [5]. It is caused by a mutation in the cystatin C gene [9] that leads to formation of cystatin C protein which has glutamin instead of leucine at position 68 of the protein [3], which is deposited as amyloid in the CNS and some other tissues [2,11].

Obviously the substitution of one amino acid changes the physical characteristics of the protein in such a way that it can not be processed in a regular fashion. The fault may either be in the intracellular processing and secretion or in its extracellular breakdown. We decided to look at the former possibility by analysing the kinetics of cystatin C synthesis and secretion from cultured blood monocytes of individuals carrying the mutated cystatin C gene and compare with monocytes from healthy persons. This approach was chosen because cells of monocytic origin (monocytes, macrophages, microgial cells) have been shown to produce cystatin C "in vitro" and may also play a role in the development of some forms of amyloidosis [12].

Material and methods.

Blood samples were taken from six individuals with the mutated cystatin C gene. Three were asymptomatic (age 22-44 years, two studied two times) and three had got repeated strokes (age 19-47 years, one studied two times). Two were studied during the first and second insult respectively but one was studied during the eighth-ninth insult. Ten blood donors served as controls.

Mononuclear cells were isolated from heparinized peripheral blood by the Isopaque/Ficoll gradient centrifugation technique. The adherent cells (monocytes) were incubated in medium RPMI 1640 supplemented with 20% pooled normal human serum for the first 48 hours and then with 10% serum. 24 hours before harvesting the cultures were maintained in serum free RPMI 1640. At harvesting, which was done on day 5, 10 and 15 of culture a serine proteinase inhibitor, bensamidin chloride was added. The supernatant and cells were harvested separately for quantitation of cystatin C by enzyme linked immunosorbent assay [7]. The cells were lysed in 0.05% Triton X-100 and scraped off with a rubber policeman for quantitation of cystatin C.

To establish a measure of the total cell mass the protein content was measured by the Bio-Rad protein assay with an acidic solution of Coomassie-Brilliant Blue G-250.

For the Western blot analysis, lysed monocytes and supernatants were pooled and concentrated by passing through an amicon YM-5 membrane with 50 psi N_2. The lysed cells and supernatants were run separately on a SDS-polyacrylamide gel (PAGE). The gels were blotted onto nitrocellulose membrane [10], incubated with polyclonal rabbit anti-cystatin C antibody, followed by incubation with peroxidase-conjugated goat anti-rabbit IgG antibody [4].

Parallel cultures were fixed in situ either with absolute ethanol for 10 min. at 4°C for immunostaining or 1% glutaraldehyde and 1% paraformaldehyde for electron microscopy. For immunostaining the FITC and the Avidin- Biotin methods were used and the same primary antibody as for the Western blot was applied.

RESULTS

The total amount of cystatin C, i.e. both intra- and extracellular, was comparable in symptomatic individuals and controls, whereas a distinctly lower quantity was detected in cultures from asymptomatic carriers of the mutated gene. This did also hold true when the amount of cystatin C was related to the total cell mass of the cultures as measured by the quantity of proteins, which was 2-3 times lower in the asymptomatic individuals than in the other groups (data not shown).

The relative ratio in the quantity of cystatin C in lysed cells versus supernatant was higher than 1 in carriers of the mutated cystatin C gene independent of whether they were symptomatic or not. This differed markedly from the controls which showed lower values in the cells than in the supernatant (Fig.1). Statistical calculations revealed a significant correlation in both groups although a great individual variation was noted.

In Western blot, cystatin C formed by individuals carrying the mutated cystatin C gene showed the same electrophoretic mobility and similar intensity of immunostaining as found in healthy controls and recombinant cystatin C, which was used as a marker [1] (Fig. 2). The intracellular distribution of cystatin C was according to light microscopy similar in HCCAA and controls. Thus staining was mainly found in the cytoplasm, frequently with perinuclear accentuation but occasionally also in the nucleus. A preliminary electron microscopic survey of the monocyte cultures did not reveal any distinct difference between HCCAA and controls.

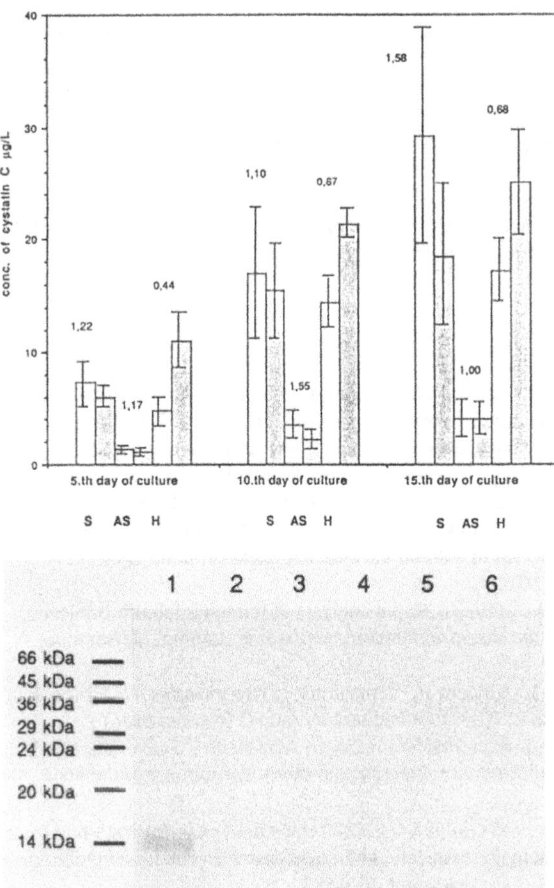

Fig.1 The concentration of cystatin C in lysed monocytes (white column) and supernatant (grey column) isolated from individuals carrying the mutated cystatin C gene (S=symptomatic, AS=asymptomatic), in comparison with healthy individuals (H). The results are presented as mean +/- standard error of the mean.

Fig2. Western blot analysis of monocyte proteins with anti-cystatin C antibody. Detection of bound antibody was performed with peroxidase staining as described in the methods section.
Lane 1 : Cystatin C standard.
Lane 2 : Blank control.
Lane 3 : Supernatant (healthy)
Lane 4 : Lysed monocytes (healthy)
Lane 5 : Lysed monocytes (HCCAA)
Lane 6 : Supernatant (HCCAA)

DISCUSSION

The main finding, i.e. the reversal of the ratio between intra- and extracellular amount of cystatin C in both asymptomatic and symptomatic carriers of the mutated gene as compared with controls, indicates that there is a partial block in the secretion of cystatin C in HCCAA. Apparently the single amino acid substitution of glutamin for leucine at position 68 of the cystatin C protein [3] changes the physical characteristics of the protein in such way that it is secreted to a lesser degree and accumulates intracellularly. Studies of the serine proteinase inhibitor alpha$_1$-antitrypsin have shown that a single amino acid substitution is enough to perturb the cellular processing of that protein in a comparable fashion [6]. We have no indications of a further alteration of the cystatin C protein in our monocyte cultures. Thus the Western blot analysis showed that the cystatin C formed has the same size as the normal protein. This is in accord with recent findings by Olafsson et al. [8] who found cystatin C in the CSF in HCCAA to be of normal size but not truncated as has been reported for the cystatin C in amyloid deposits in CNS [3]

The lower rate of synthesis of cystatin C in asymptomatic carriers of the mutated gene might lead to a slower accumulation of cystatin C and eventually amyloid. This could explain both the difference in the severity of clinical symptoms and the wide variation in the age distribution of the onset of clinical symptoms. The lower cell mass consistently observed in monocyte cultures from the asymptomatic HCCAA individuals may be at least partly due to some defect in their adherance, as it was noted that they showed a greater tendency to detach from the plastic surface, than monocytes from symptomatic individuals and controls, especially during the first two days of culture.

In conclusion the perturbation of the cellular processing observed in the cultured monocytes from HCCAA may be of relevance for the CNS amyloid deposits. In the CNS the microglia, which are closely related to the monocyte/macrophage may play a key role in the amyloidogenesis.

References:

1. Abrahamson M., Dalbøge H., Olafsson I., Carlsen S., Grubb A. (1988) 'Efficient production of native biologically active human cystatin C by Escherichia coli', FEBS Lett, 236, 14-18.
2. Blöndal H., Guðmundsson G., Benedikz E. and Johannesson G. (1989) 'Dementia in hereditary cystatin C amyloidosis', in K. Iqbal, H.M. Wisniewski and B Winblad. (eds.). Alzheimer´s Disease and Related Disorders, Alan R. Liss, New York, pp. 157-164.
3. Ghiso J., Jensson O., Frangione B. (1986) 'Amyloid fibrils in hereditary cerebral hemorrhage with amyloidosis of Icelandic type is a variant of gamma-trace basic protein (cystatin C)', Proc.Natl.Acad.Sci.USA. 8, 2974-2978.
4. Glynn P., Gilbert H. and Newcombe C.M.L. (1982) 'Rapid analysis of immunoglobulin isoelectric focusing patterns with cellulose nitrate sheets and immunoperoxidase staining', J. Immunol. Meth. 51, 251-257.
5. Jensson O., Gudmundsson G., Arnason A., Blöndal H., Petursdottir I.,Thorsteinsson L., Grubb A., Löfberg H., Cohen D. and Frangione B. (1987) 'Hereditary cystatin C (gamma-trace) amyloid angiopathy of the CNS causing cerebral hemorrhage', Acta Neurol. Scand. 76, 102-114.
6. Kalsheker N. (1989) 'Alpha1-Antitrypsin: Structure, function and molecular biology of the gene' Biosci. Rep. 9, 129-138.
7. Olafsson I., Löfberg H., Abrahamsson M., and Grubb A. (1988) 'Production, characterization and use of monoclanal antibodies against the major extracellular human cysteine proteinase inhibitors cystatin C and kininogen', Scand. J. Lab. Invest. 48, 573-582.
8. Olafsson I., Gudmundsson G., Abrahamson M., Jensson O., Grubb A. (1990) 'The amino terminal portion of cerebrospinal fluid cystatin C in hereditary cystatin C amyloid angiopathy is not truncated: direct sequence analysis from agarose gel electropherograms', Scand. J. Clin. Lab. Invest. 50, 85-93.
9. Palsdottir A., Abrahamson M., Thorsteinsson L., Arnason A., Olafsson I., Grubb A. and Jensson O. (1988) 'Mutation in cystatin C gene causes hereditary brain hemorrhage', Lancet ii, 603-604.
10. Taubin H., Staehelin T., and Gordon J. (1979) 'Electrophoretic transfer of proteins from polyacrylamide gels to nitrocellulose sheets: Procedure and some applications', Proc. Natl. Acad. Sci. U.S.A. 76, 4350-4354.
11. Thorsteinsson L., Blöndal H., Jensson O. and Guðmundsson G. (1988) 'Distribution of cystatin C amyloid deposits in the Icelandic patients with hereditary cystatin C amyloid angiopathy' in T. Isobe, S. Araki, F. Uchino, S. Kito and E. Tsubura (eds.), Amyloid and Amyloidosis, Plenum Publishing Corporation, New York, pp. 585-590.
12. Zucker-Franklin D., Warfel A., Grusky G., Frangione B. and Teitel D (1987) 'Novel monocyte like properties of microglial/astroglial cells. Constitutive secretion of lysosome and cystatin C', Lab. Invest.57, 176-185.

MOLECULAR BIOLOGY OF HEREDITARY CYSTATIN C AMYLOID ANGIOPATHY IN ICELAND.

S. JONSDOTTIR[1], A. PALSDOTTIR[1,3], M. ABRAHAMSON[2], A. GRUBB[2] & O. JENSSON[1].

[1]Department of Medical Genetics, The Blood Bank, National University Hospital, P.O. Box 1408, IS-121 Reykjavik, Iceland. [2]Department of Clinical Chemistry, University of Lund, S-221 85 Lund, Sweden. [3]Present address: Institute of Biology, University of Iceland, Grensasvegur 12, IS-108 Reykjavik, Iceland.

ABSTRACT. Hereditary cystatin C amyloid angiopathy, HCCAA, is a fatal dominantly inherited disorder caused by a mutation in the cystatin C gene. The leu-gln mutation at position 68 in exon 2 in the cystatin C gene can be detected as an extra 630 bp Alu I fragment in patients due to a loss of an Alu I restriction site. This mutation has only been found in the 8 HCCAA families originating in the west of Iceland and recently in an additional HCCAA isolate in the south of Iceland. This test has now been carried out on 177 individuals, including a fetus by chorionic villus analysis. 23 patients and 10 asymptomatic at-risk relatives were found to have the mutation. 95 unrelated individuals, 11 spouses and 38 at-risk relatives had normal cystatin C genes. RFLP analysis of three polymorphic restriction sites shows that patients from all the HCCAA families, except one, share an RFLP haplotype which is the most common one in the normal Icelandic population.

1. Introduction

Hereditary cystatin C amyloid angiopathy (HCCAA) is an autosomal dominant disorder characterized by the deposition of cystatin C amyloid fibrils in most investigated tissues. The most serious consequence of the disease is that amyloid deposition in the cerebral arteries leads to a massive brain hemorrhage and death in young adults [1,2]. HCCAA occurring in Icelanders is the first human disorder known to be caused by deposition of cystatin C amyloid fibrils.

The human cystatin C gene has been cloned and sequenced. The gene spans approximately 4.3 kb and contains three exons [3].

HCCAA has been shown to be caused by a point mutation in the codon for leucine at position 68 in exon 2 in the cystatin C gene which results in a leucine-glutamine amino acid substitution in the cystatin C molecule. This mutation can be detected as an extra 630 bp Alu I fragment in patients due to a loss of an Alu I restriction site by using a full length cystatin C cDNA probe and the restriction enzyme Alu I [4]. This 630 bp Alu I marker has been used for the diagnosis of patients, asymptomatic affected individuals and for prenatal diagnosis. The results are reported in this paper.

All the 8 families studied so far, originate from the same geographic area in the west of Iceland [1]. A large family, recently found, originating in the south of Iceland is known to have had many members who died in the prime of life from cerebral hemorrhage. Individuals from this family were analysed for the presence of the 630 bp Alu I marker for HCCAA.

2. Materials and Methods

2.1. PREPARATION OF DNA

DNA of high molecular weight was isolated from 20 ml blood by SDS proteinase K digestion followed by phenol/chloroform extraction [4]. For prenatal diagnosis, DNA was prepared from a chorionic villus biopsy, taken between the 9th and 10th week of gestation. The chorionic villus sample was checked microscopically and any contaminating maternal tissue removed before DNA extraction [6].

2.2 DIAGNOSTIC TEST FOR HCCAA

Genomic DNA (8 μg) was digested with the Alu I restriction enzyme, electrophoresed in 1.3 % agarose and transferred onto a nylon filter (Hybond-N, Amersham). The filter was prehybridized for 2 hrs at 43°C in a hybridization solution (50 % formamide, 1 M NaCl, 10 x Denhard's solution, 10 % dextran sulphate, 50 mM Tris-HCl pH 8.0, 0.5 % SDS, 0.1% sodium pyrophosphate and 0.1 mg/ml heat denatured calf thymus DNA (Sigma)). 25 ng of the cystatin C cDNA probe [5] was labelled with α-^{32}P dCTP to a high specific activity by random oligonucleotide priming using a commercial kit (Amersham). Labelled probe was hybridized to the filters in the same hybridization solution for 16 hrs at 43°C. Filters were washed in 2 x SSC (1 x SSC: 150 mM NaCl, 15 Mm NaCitrate), 0.1 % SDS at 68°C four times for 15 min and finally 10 min in 0.2 x SSC. An X-ray film was then exposed to the filter between two intensifying screens for 2 days.

2.3 RFLP SCREENING

Genomic DNA (8 μg) was digested with restriction enzymes as outlined by the manufactures, electrophoresed in 0.7 % agarose and transferred onto a nylon filter (Hybond-N, Amersham). Hybridization to radiolabelled cystatin C cDNA [5] and C3E2-B genomic probes [3], washing and autoradiography were performed as for the HCCAA diagnostic test.

3. Results

3.1. DIAGNOSIS OF HCCAA

6 members of the family originating in the south of Iceland were analysed for the presence of the 630 bp Alu I marker for HCCAA. In two affected family members, a mother and her daughter who have suffered from severe cerebral hemorrhage, the 630 bp Alu I marker was present. The patients were heterozygous for the mutation in the cystatin C gene and therefore also displayed the 600 bp Alu I fragment which represents the normal cystatin C gene. The healthy parents and two at-risk offspring did not have the 630 bp Alu I marker and therefore have not inherited the disease (Fig. 1a).

The diagnostic test has now been carried out on 177 individuals, including a fetus for prenatal diagnosis. 23 patients and 10 asymptomatic at-risk relatives were found to have the mutation. 38 at-risk relatives, 11 healthy spouses and 95 unrelated individuals had the normal cystatin C genes (Table 1).

Prenatal diagnosis of HCCAA has been performed in one family. The patient, an 18 year old woman, had a two year old asymptomatic daughter with the mutation and requested analysis for her second pregnancy. DNA from chorionic villi, sampled between the 9th and 10th week of gestation, was analysed for the presence of the 630 bp Alu I marker for HCCAA. The fetus did not have the 630 bp Alu I marker and therefore has not inherited the disease (Fig. 1b). This diagnosis was confirmed by analysing DNA from umbilical cord blood after birth (data not shown).

TABLE 1. Individuals analysed for the presence of the 630 bp Alu I marker for HCCAA

	Number of individuals		
	600 bp/600 bp	630 bp/600 bp	Total
HCCAA patients	0	23	23
At-risk relatives	38	10	48
Healthy spouses	11	0	11
Unrelated individuals	95	0	95
Total	144	33	177

600 bp Alu I fragment represents normal gene

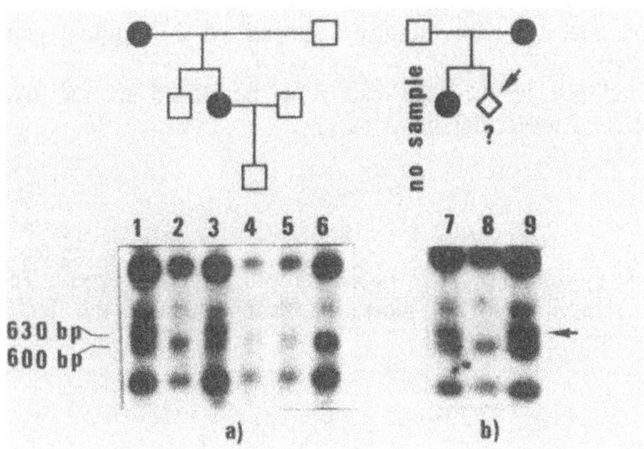

Figure 1. Hybridization of cystatin C cDNA probe to Alu I digested DNA from two HCCAA families. a) Family originating in the south of Iceland.
b) Prenatal diagnosis in a HCCAA family.
Patients are shown as black circles (females).
The 630 bp fragment is the marker for HCCAA (arrow). Unaffected individuals, including a fetus (arrow), have only 600 bp Alu I fragment (lanes 2,4,5,6 and 8) whereas patients also have the 630 bp Alu I fragment (lanes 1,3,7 and 9).

3.2. RFLP ANALYSIS

A study of restriction fragment length polymorphism (RFLP) has been performed with 21 restriction enzymes using the cystatin C cDNA and C3E2-B genomic probes. Three polmorphic restriction sites were found in the 3' region of the cystatin C gene [3,4]: A Pst I RFLP (1.9/2.6 kb), a Sac I RFLP (2.7/8.6 kb) and EcoRI RFLP (18/21 kb).

Haplotype analysis shows that patients from all families available for study share an RFLP haplotype with 1.9 kb Pst I, 2.7 kb Sac I, 21 kb EcoRI fragments, which is also the most common haplotype in the normal Icelandic population. An exception was found in one family originating in the west of Iceland which instead had an RFLP haplotype with 2.6 kb Pst I, 2.7 kb Sac I, 21 kb EcoRI fragments. This suggests that a crossover has occurred between the mutated cystatin C gene and the Pst I restriction site in this family.

4. Discussion

Diagnosis of HCCAA has earlier been based upon immunohistochemical studies of biopsy specimens [2] and measurements of cystatin C in the cerbrospinal fluid (CSF), as HCCAA is characterized by an abnormally low level of cystatin C in the CSF [1].

The 630 kb Alu I marker has been found in all HCCAA patients and co-segregates with the disease in every case. It is also present in some asymptomatic at-risk family members, but is not present in normal spouses and healthy controls (Table 1) [4]. This marker has allowed a simplified and accurate diagnostic procedure for HCCAA. To further simplify the diagnosis of HCCAA, a polymerase chain reaction based procedure has been constructed recently [7].

The presence of the 630 bp Alu I marker in affected members of families in both isolates originating in the west and south of Iceland strongly suggests that the same mutation causes the hereditary cystatin C amyloid angiopathy in both isolates and that all affected are descendants of a common ancestor who initially transmitted this mutant gene to all nine families available for study.

This rare type of hereditary hemorrhage can now be added to the list of diseases diagnosable by the methods of molecular genetics.

5. Acknowledgements

We thank professor Gunnar Gudmundsson for blood sampling and Dr. Reynir Tomas Geirsson for the chorionic villus sampling. This work was supported by the Icelandic Science Foundation and the Heilavernd Society.

6. References

1. Jensson, O., Gudmundsson, G., Arnason, A., Blöndal, H., Petursdottir, I., Thorsteinsson, L., Grubb, A., Löfberg, H., Cohen, D. and Frangione, B. (1987) 'Hereditary cystatin C (γ-trace) amyloid angiopathy of the CNS causing cerebral hemorrhage', Acta Neurol. Scand. 76, 102-114.
2. Thorsteinsson, L., Blöndal, H., Jensson, O. and Gudmundsson, G. (1988) 'Distribution of cystatin C amyloid deposits in the Icelandic patients with hereditary cystatin C amyloid angiopathy', in T. Isobe, S. Araki, F. Uchino, S. Kito and E. Tsubura (eds.), Amyloid and Amyloidosis, Plenum Press, New York, pp. 585-590.
3. Abrahamson, M., Olafsson, I., Palsdottir, A., Ulvsbäck, M., Lundwall, Å., Jensson, O. and Grubb, A. (1990) 'Structure and expression of the human cystatin C gene', Biochem. J. 268, 287-294.
4. Palsdottir, A., Abrahamson, M., Thorsteinsson, L., Arnason, A., Olafsson, I., Grubb, A. and Jensson, O. (1988) 'Mutation in cystatin C gene causes hereditary brain haemorrhage', Lancet ii, 603-604.
5. Abrahamson, M., Grubb, A., Olafsson, I. and Lundwall, Å. (1987) 'Molecular cloning and sequence analysis of cDNA coding for the precursor of the human cysteine proteinase inhibitor cystatin C', FEBS Lett. 216, 229-233.
6. Old, John M. (1986) 'Fetal DNA analysis', in K.E. Davies (ed.), Human Genetic Diseases: a Practical Approach, IRL Press, Oxford, pp. 1-17.
7. Abrahamson, M., Stensmyr, M., Olafsson, I., Jonsdottir, S., Jensson, O. and Grubb, A. (1990) 'Mutation-specific diagnosis of hereditary cystatain C amyloid angiopathy by PCR analysis', VIth International Symposium on Amyloidosis, Aug. 5-8, 1990, Oslo, Norway.

CEREBRAL AMYLOID ANGIOPATHY ASSOCIATED WITH CEREBRAL HEMORRHAGE WITH THE DEPOSITION OF CYSTATIN C : STUDY ON JAPANESE CASES.

S. FUJIHARA, K. SHIMODE, M. NAKAMURA, S. KOBAYASHI
T. TSUNEMATSU, A. PALSDOTTIR* and O. JENSSON*
Third Division of Internal Medicine
Shimane Medical University, Izumo, 693 Japan
*The Blood Bank, P,O. Box 1408, IS-121 Reykjavik, Iceland

ABSTRACT To characterize the cerebral amyloid angiopathy (CAA) in Japan causing cerebral hemorrhage (CH) and consequential vascular dementia (VD), we examined brains of CAA with CH by enzyme immunohistochemistry and gene analysis. We also established enzyme-linked immunosorbent assay (ELISA) to estimate the levels of cystatin C (CC) in cerebrospinal fluid (CSF) from patients with CH comparing with reference cases. Some CAA patients had possible family history of CAA and the others were sporadic. Most of them were aged and normotensive. Amyloid of these Japanese type CAA showed the β-protein (BP) antigenicity coexisting with that of CC. Some of patients with CH showed a low concentration CC in CSF together with clinical manifestations of CAA. Brain tissues from two of them were examined immunohistochemically and amyloid of CAA showed antigenicity of CC and BP. Analysis of CC cDNA of Japanese case did not show the *Alu* I restriction fragment length polymorphism (RFLP) as recognized in the Icelandic HCHWA. The results suggest the presence of not only familial but also sporadic cases of CAA with the deposition of CC associated with CH, causing VD in the normotensive elderly. Abnormal metabolism or malfunction of CC as protease inhibitor may play some roles in CH of CAA. The ELISA method is simple to perform and appears to be useful tool for diagnosing patients with suspected CAA with CH and the deposition of CC.

1. INTRODUCTION

Recently, we have reported Japanese cases of CAA causing CH, of which amyloid shows the antigenicity of CC [1,2]. Some of them had a family history of possible CAA and the others were sporadic[2]. To characterize the Japanese cases of CAA with the deposition of CC and to compare them with hereditary cerebral hemorrhage with amyloidosis (HCHWA) in Iceland [3], we used the immunoperoxidase method, developed ELISA for CC in CSF, and studied the DNA of the CC gene.

2. MATERIALS AND METHODS

We collected brain tissues from 13 Japanese cases of CAA associated with CH, together with clinical and autopsy records. The cases comprised 6 males (average age : 75.6 y.o.) and 7 females (average age :

72.7 y.o.). Control amyloid tissues were those of HCHWA in Iceland [3], and CAA associated with Alzheimer's disease (AD). We applied enzyme immunohistochemistry (avidin: biotinylated enzyme method) for the detection of CC [1,2]. Antisera against CC obtained by courtesy of Dr. Grubb [4] was used, as well as monoclonal antibody raised against synthetic peptide consisting of residues 8 to 17 of amyloid BP of AD, which was donated by Dr. Glenner [5]. We searched for DNA of variant CC by the Southern blot hybridization method. DNA was extracted from frozen brain tissue of case 1 by SDS-proteinase digestion followed by phenol/chloroform extraction. The DNA was digested with *Alu* I and hybridized with the full-length CC cDNA probe after blotting [6]. We established sandwich enzyme immunosorbent assay using monoclonal mouse anti-CC and polyclonal rabbit anti-CC antibodies [7]. CSF specimens were obtained from 29 cases with CH and from 45 reference cases with other neurological diseases (cerebral infarction:27, AD:6, Parkinson's disease:4, amyotrophic lateral sclerosis:5, and epilepsy:3). From the 4 of these CH cases brain tissue sections were available for immunohistochemical examination.

3. RESULTS

Each antisera reacted specifically with the correspondent control amyloid tissues. In 10 of the 13 cases of CAA, amyloid showed a positive reaction with anti-CC. And in all 13 cases amyloid reacted positively with anti-BP, which antibody did not react with the amyloid of HCHWA. Not all the BP-positive areas showed a positive reaction for CC. Although two of the 10 CC-positive cases had a family history of possible CAA, the remaining positive 8 were sporadic cases. 12 of the 13 CAA patients had a history of dementia of cerebrovascular origin. Eight of the CC-positive cases did not have a history of hypertension, whereas the 3 negative cases were hypertensive. DNA extracted from our patient (No.1) showed only the 600-bp *Alu* I fragment, while DNA of the HCHWA patients have two *Alu* I fragments, one 630 bp and one 600 bp (Fig. 1). In 45 reference cases, CSF showed high levels of CC concentration (ranged between 100 and 600 ng/ml). Fifteen patients with CH showed a low concentration CC (< 70 ng/ml) in CSF together with clinical manifestations of CAA (Fig. 2). The histopathological diagnosis of CAA was confirmed in the 2 of these 15 patients. They showed the antigenicity of

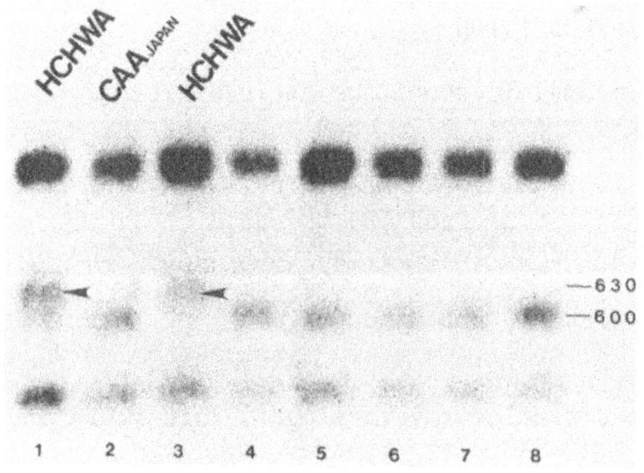

Fig. 1. Southern blot of cystatin C cDNA from Japanese patient (lane 2),patients with HCHWA (lane 1,3), and from normal controls(4-8). Our patient had 600-bp *Alu* I fragment only, while HCHWA patients also had 630-bp fragment (arrowhead), representing a mutation.

CC and BP immunohistochemically (Fig. 3). Remaining 14 patients with CH and high concentration of CC showed clinical manifestations of hypertensive CH. Two of these 14 patients were negative for CAA histopathologically.

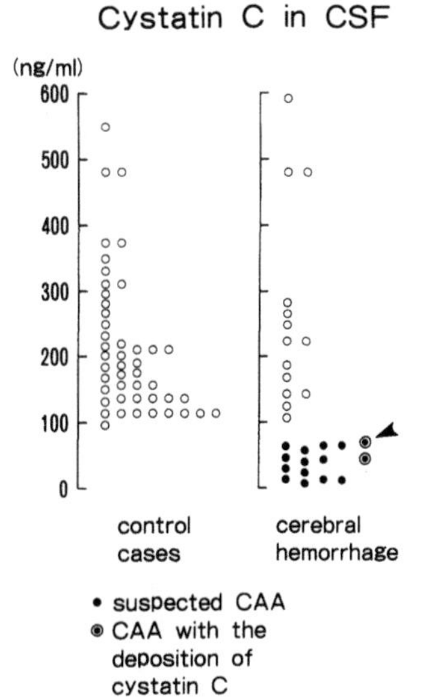

Fig. 2. Concentration of CC in CSF estimated by ELISA.

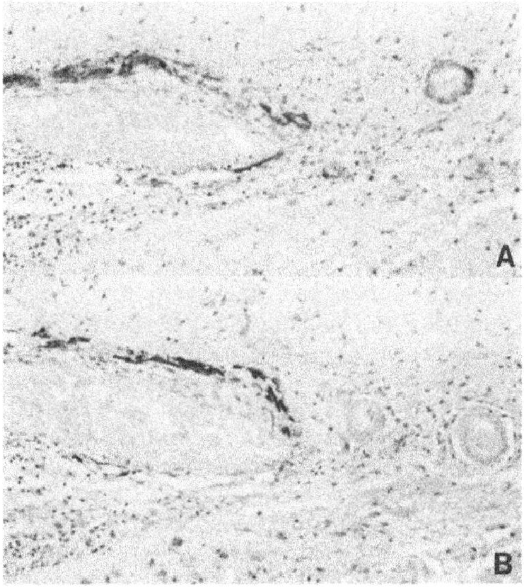

Fig. 3. Immunohistology of the CAA of the case shown in Fig.2 by arrowhead. A; anti-β protein B; anti-cystatin C

4. DISCUSSION

The results suggest the presence of not only familial but also sporadic cases of CAA with the deposition of CC associated with cerebral hemorrhage causing vascular dementia in the normotensive elderly. CAA of the aged without demonstrable Alzheimer-type dementia is related to BP [8]. The average age of our cases was 75 years old. By immunohistochemistry not all parts of the BP-positive amyloid showed the antigenicity of CC, and not all the BP-positive cases were positive for CC [2]. Thus, age-related BP may underlie or precede the deposition of CC which is related to CAA associated with cerebral hemorrhage [2]. Patients with HCHWA in Iceland may develop CAA with BP if they survive till old age. CAA and SP of HCHWA from the Netherlands are related to BP, and CAA of them showed only dubious staining for CC immunohistochemically. In contrast, CAA of our cases showed clear antigenicity of CC as well as of BP [2]. Immunoblotting showed that crude amyloid fibrils from one of our cases contain CC antigens [2]. In addition, we found that patients with CAA with the deposition of CC had low concentration of CC in CSF. We speculate that abnormal metabolism of CC as a cysteine proteinase inhibitor may play some roles in the cause of CH in CAA patients [9]. A cDNA probe was used to identify RFLP which detects a loss of an *Alu* I restriction site because of a mutation in the codon for the position 68 in the CC molecule [6]. This gene analysis did not show the same variant of CC gene of Japanese case as found in the Icelandic HCHWA cases. Further biochemical analysis of the amyloid fibril protein is necessary to clarify if the Japanese cases have the different variation of CC or normal CC. Grubb first suggested that the concentration of CC in CSF would be useful for the diagnosis of HCHWA because of the lower levels of CC in HCHWA patients compared with normal controls [4]. The ELISA method described is simple to perform and appears to be useful tool for diagnosing patients with suspected CAA with CH and the deposition of CC [7].

5. REFERENCES

1. Fujihara, S., Shimode, K., Kobayashi, S., and Tsunematsu, T. (1988) 'Possibly "familial" cerebral amyloid angiopathy in Japan :Immunohisto chemical identification of gamma-trace', in T. Isobe, S. Araki, F. Uchino, S. Kito, E. Tsubura (eds.), Amyloid and Amyloidosis, Plenum Publishing Co., New York, pp. 597-602.
2. Fujihara, S., Shimode, K., Nakamura, M., Kobayashi, S., and Tsunematsu, T. (1989) 'Cerebral amyloid angiopathy with the deposition of gamma-trace (cystatin C) and β-protein', Progress in Clinical and Biological Research 317, 939-944.
3. Jensson, O., Gudmundsson, G., Arnason, A., Blondal, H., Petursdottir, I., Thorsteinsson, L., Grubb, A., Lofberg, H., Cohen, D. and Frangione, B. (1987) 'Hereditary cystatin C (γ-trace) amyloid angiopathy of the CNS causing cerebral hemorrhage', Acta Neurol. Scand. 76,102-114.
4. Grubb, A. and Lofberg, H. (1985) 'Human γ-trace : Structure, function and clinical use of concentration measurements', Scand. J. Clin. Lab. Invest. 45, Suppl 177, 7-13.
5. Allsop, D., Landon, M., Kidd, M., Lowe, J. S., Reynolds, G. P., and Gardner, A. (1986) 'Monoclonal antibodies raised against a subsequence of senile plaque core protein react with plaque cores, plaque periphery and cerebrovascular amyloid in Alzheimer's disease', Neurosci. Letter 68, 252-256.
6. Palsdottir, A., Abrahamson, M., Thorsteinsson, L., Arnason, A., Olafsson, I., and Grubb, A. (1988) 'Mutation in cystatin C gene causes hereditary brain haemorrhage', Lancet ii/8611, 603-604.
7. Shimode, K., Fujihara, S., Nakamura, M., Kobayashi, S., and Tsunematsu, T. (1990) 'Diagnosis of cerebral amyloid angiopathy with cerebral hemorrhage by enzyme linked immunosorbent assay (ELISA) of cystatin C in the cerebrospinal fluid', Clin. Neurol. 30, 288-293.
8. Coria, F., Castano, E. M., and Frangione, B. (1987) 'Brain amyloid in normal aging and cerebral amyloid angiopathy is antigenically related to Alzheimer's disease β-protein', Am. J. Pathol. 129, 422-428.
9. Lofberg, H., Grubb, A. O., Nilsson, E. K., Jensson, O., Gudmundsson, G., Blondal, H., Arnason, A., and Thorsteinsson, L. (1987) 'Immunohistochemical characterization of the amyloid deposits and quantitation of pertinent cerebrospinal fluid proteins in hereditary cerebral hemorrhage with amyloidosis, Stroke 18,431-440.

SEVERAL β_2-MICROGLOBULIN FRAGMENTS IDENTIFIED IN AN AMYLOIDOMA IN A PATIENT WITH LONG-TERM HEMODIALYSIS

R.P. Linke, J. Floege, F. Lottspeich, R. Deutzmann

Institute of Immunology, Goethestr.31, D-8000 Munich
Dep.of Medicine, K.-Gutschowstr. 8, D-3000 Hannover
Max-Planck-Inst. of Biochemistry D-8033 Martinsried
Institute of Biochemistry 31, D-8400 Regensburg

ABSTRACT. Amyloid deposits in patients on long-term hemodialysis are reported to be predominantly of β_2-microglobulin (β_2m) origin. The question, whether amyloidogenesis of this disease represents a mere concentration effect of unmodified β_2m or the deposition of altered β_2m is still controversal. To clarify this issue further, we have analyzed a subcutaneous amyloidoma of a patient on hemodialysis, which was shown to be of β_2m origin. Amyloid fibrils were concentrated, solubilized in 8M guanidine-HCl and separated on Sephadex G-100 in 6M guanidine-HCl according to size. Additional separation by charge yielded several different charge variants of β_2m. N-terminal amino acid sequence analysis showed an uncleaved N-terminus. Cleavage points were found after lysine 6 and 19, and - as novel findings - after glutamine 8, and as minor cleavage sites after residue 9, 10, 11, 14. These results add further weight to the role of proteolytically altered β_2m in the amyloidogenesis in hemodialysis-induced amyloidosis.

1. INTRODUCTION

Various underlaying diseases can promote the deposition of degradation-resistant proteins in amyloid conformation. These diseases cannot only be distinguished on the basis of their clinical features, but also and more precisely by immunohistochemical reactions with appropriate antibodies (1). By contrast to the natural occurring amyloid-diseases, the amyloid deposits in hemodialysis is most probably induced by the consequences of the long-term treatment and may be considered to be iatrogenic (2). The initial chemical (3,4), immunochemical (5), and immunohistochemical (6) analyses have all shown β_2m as the principal amyloidogenic protein. This protein was not found to be the intact β_2m molecule, and the deposition as a function of concentration was put forward to explain amloidogenesis in these patients. The report on amyloid formation in vitro (7) seemed to support this conception. Chemical analysis of amyloid stones of β2m origin in three patients came to a different conclusion, in that β2m-fragments were identified as a major constituent of the amyloid material (8, 10). To determine, whether fragmentation also occurred at extrarenal sites, amyloid obtained from seven additional patients were likewise examined. The result showed β2m fragments, besides molecules with an intact N-terminus (10). However, because of limited amount of tissue available for investigation, only the major polypeptides could be analysed. The preservation of an subcutaneous amyloidoma with masses of amyloid gave us the chance to investigate the fragmentation pattern of β2m more in detail.

2. MATERIAL AND METHODS

2.1 Tissue and amyloid concentration

A subcutaneous tumor of the gluteal region from a 62-year old patient who underwent hemodialysis for 16 years due to chronic glomerulonephritis was obtained on dry ice. The clinical picture and diagnosis have been presented elsewhere (11). The amyloid fibrils were extracted and monitored with the alkaline Congo red staining, reported by Puchtler (9).

2.2 Isolation of polypeptides and characterisation

The lyophilized amyloid fibril concentrate containing almost pure amyloid by Congo red staining, was dissolved in 8M guanidine-HCl and separated in 6M guanidine-HCl on a Sephadex G-100 column. The fractions were dialysed and lyophilized. Immunodiffusion and SDS-polyacrylamide gel-electrophoresis was performed as described (9). Further separation was done by charge following Davis and Ornstein using 12.5% polyacrylamide as described (12). The separated peptides were electrotransferred onto an Immobilon-Membrane (Millipore), and the stained bands excised for sequence analysis. The N-terminal amino acid sequence analysis was determined with a model 470 A gas phase automatic sequenator from Applied Biosystems (Foster City, CA) as described (8).

3. RESULTS

3.1 Separation by size and charge

Most of the amyloid fibril proteins went into solution. The elution profile showed four peaks: a large void volume peak, a smaller one, followed by a 24 kD peak and a large 12 kD peak with a tail. All peaks contained β2m as shown by immunodiffusion and by polyacrylamide gel electrophoresis and Western blotting.
The 12 kD and the trailing fraction were separated by charge into several bands most of which were more acidic than β2m itself, indicating loss of positive charges. When extracted from the gel and separated by SDS-polyacrylamide gel electrophoresis, proteins with slightly different sizes were identified.

3.2 Amino acid sequencing

N-terminal amino acid sequences from some of the charge variants, which were different from intact β2m, showed cleavage in all fractions, besides some intact N-termini. The major truncated molecules commenced at position 7 and 19, both produced by cleavage after lysine and at position 9 after glutamine, another basic amino acid. The minor form commenced at positions 10, 12 and 15.
A summary of these data is given in Fig. 1. A detailed account will be presented elsewhere (manuscript in preparation).

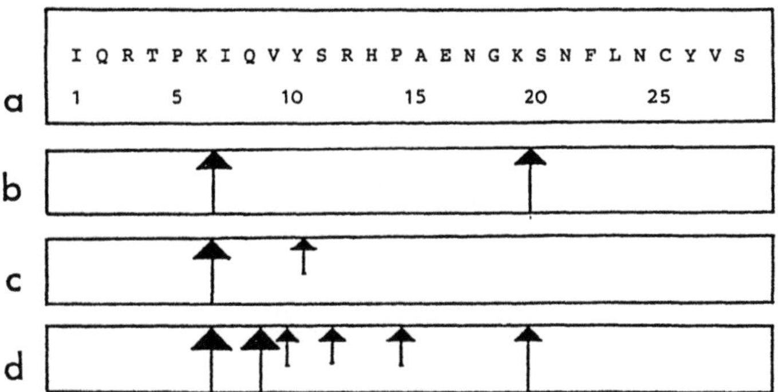

Figure 1: Summary of N-terminal amino acid sequences obtained from amyloid fibril proteins of various patients, inclucding the amyloidoma presented here

a. N-terminal amino acid sequence of β2m
b. Cleavage sites identified in renal amyloid stones (8)
c. Cleavage sites in extrarenal amyloid proteins (9, 10)
d. Cleavage sites in a subcutaneous amyloidoma (this paper)

4. DISCUSSION

Lack of sufficient material leads only to the characterization of the most soluble molecules and the most prominent fragments of β2m. The described results were obtained on an amyloidoma which consisted almost entirely of amyloid. The results show fragmented β2m in amyloid. It was shown earlier that the finding was genuine and not the result of an artifact (10). These results add novel (though minor) fragments to the list of cleaved β2m molecules identified in β2m-derived amyloid. Besides the known cleavage sites published earlier (10), i.e. lysine specific sites, here novel β_2m fragments were identified: the cleavage at position 8/9 (glutamine/valine) follows a basic amino acid, and other cleavage sites 9/10, 11/12 and 14/15 found only as minor fractions with a more unspecific cleavage. These results further strengthen the view and emphasize, that β_2m alteration is important for amyloidogenesis in hemodialysis. In addition, it is shown that, besides the lysine specific proteinases, also other enzymes can be operative in long-term hemodialysis.

5. REFERENCES

1. Linke, R.P.: Nieren- Hochdruckkr. 16, 145-153 (1987)
2. Bardin, T., Zingraff, J, Kuntz, D.,Drüeke: Nephrol. Dial. Transplant. 1, 151-154 (1986)
3. Gejyo, F., Yamada, T., Odani, S., Nakagawa, P., Arakawa, M., Kunimoto, T., Kataoka, H., Suzuki, M., Hirasawa, Y., Shirahama, T., Cohen, A.S., Schmid, K.: BBRC 129, 701-706 (1985)
4. Gorevic, P.D., Casey, T.T., Stone, W.J., DiRaimondo, C.R., Prelli, F.C., Frangione, B.: J. Clin. Invest. 76, 2425-2429 (1985)
5. Linke, R.P.: Appl. Pathol. 3, 18-28 (1985)
6. Shirahama, T., Skinner, M., Cohen, A.S., Gejyo, F., Arakawa, M., Suzuki, M., Hirasawa, Y.: Lab. Invest. 53, 705-709 (1985)
7. Conners, L.H., Shirahama, T., Skinner, M., Fenves, A., Cohnen, A.S.: BBRC 131, 1063-1068 (1985).
8. Linke, R.P.,Bommer, J., Ritz, E., Waldherr, R., Eulitz, M.: BBRC 136, 665-671 (1986)
9. Linke, R.P., Hampl, H., Bartl-Schwarze, S., Eulitz, M.: Biol. Chem. Hoppe Seyler, 368, 137-144 (1987)
10. Linke, R.P., Hampl, H., Lobeck, H., Ritz, E., Bommer, J., Waldherr, R., Eulitz, M.: Kidney Internat. 36, 675-681 (1990)
11. Floege, J., Brandis, A., Nonnast-Daniel, B., Westhoff-Bleck, M., Tiedow, G., Linke, R.P., Koch, K.M.: Nephron 53, 73-75 (1989)
12. Linke, R.P.: Anal. Biochem.141. 55-62 (1984)

6. ACKNOWLEDGMENTS

This study was supported by the Deutsche Forschungsgemeinschaft, SFB 207, project G8. We thank Mss. A. Rail and A. Kerling for technical assistance.

CLINICAL EVALUATION OF OSTEOARTHROPATHY IN 43 PATIENTS ON HAEMODIALYSIS, USING CUPROPHANE MEMBRANES FOR ≥ 5 YEARS

BOUKE P.C.HAZENBERG, WILLEM GEERLINGS*, JORIS GROND&, MARTIN H. VAN RIJSWIJK, GJALT K. VAN DER HEM*
Div. Rheumatology and Nephrology*, Department of Pathology&
State University Hospital, 59 Oostersingel
9713 EZ Groningen, The Netherlands

ABSTRACT. 43 stable patients on chronic haemodialysis (using cuprophane membranes exclusively ≥5 years) were evaluated for symptoms of dialysis associated osteoarthropathy. Median time on dialysis was 120 months (range 60-260). The 16 women and 27 men were included with a median age of 56 years (range 33-76). Shoulderpain was seen in 29 patients (67%) with an actuarial risk of 50% at 134 months. Objective testing showed in 30 patients (70%) some loss of function; of whom 19 (46%) were positive on questioning. Carpal tunnel syndrome (CTS) was present in 16 patients (37%) with a 50% risk at 184 months. Arthritis was seen in 19 patients (44%). Radiological abnormalities were observed in 24 patients (56%). The number of serious symptoms increased with the time on dialysis. Synovial biopsies in 8 out of 11 patients with three serious symptoms established β2M-amyloidosis. Amyloidosis of the β2M-type was found in synovia, small vessels and to a lesser degree in the heart in a post-mortem examination. In conclusion symptoms of osteoarthropathy were frequently present in this group. The number of serious symptoms was related with the time on dialysis. β_2M-amyloidosis was seen in 8 patients. This β_2M-amyloid is one of the types of systemic amyloidosis.

1. INTRODUCTION

Patients undergoing longterm haemodialysis frequently have complaints of carpal tunnel syndrome, arthropathy and spontaneous fractures. Radiologic signs such as cysts, erosions or destructive arthropathy can be detected [1-3]. Amyloid deposition of the β_2-microglobulin (β_2M) type might be causative. Aim of this study was to investigate in 43 selected patients the clinical and radiological signs of this osteoarthropathy.

2. MATERIALS AND METHODS

2.1. Patients

43 stable patients on chronic haemodialysis were evaluated. Patients

with malignancies, arthritis, amyloidosis, diabetes mellitus or on glucocorticoid therapy (>6 months the last 5 years) were excluded. All patients had to be dialysed ≥5 years, using cuprophane membranes exclusively, 2 or 3 times a week (12 hours a week). Median time on dialysis was 120 months (range 60-260). The 16 women and 27 men were included with a median age of 56 years (range 33-76).

Patients were analysed for pain, morning stiffness, loss of function, carpal tunnel syndrome (CTS), arthritis and tendovaginitis with a scoring list.

Standard radiology included the hands, cervical spine, shoulders and hip joints.

A post-mortem examination was performed in a man who had been dialysed for 250 months.

2.2. Definitions

CTS: Clinical signs (typical complaints with Tinell or Phalen sign and a positive EMG) and/or surgery. Arthritis: Chronic (>3 months) or recurrent pain, swelling and loss of function without obvious causes like infection or crystals. Radiologic signs: 1 or more macro-geodes (>1 cm.), 3 or more cysts (>0.5 cm), erosive joint changes or destructive arthropathy. Symptom-score: Numeric summation (ranging 0-3) of CTS, arthritis and radiologic signs; each item 1 point.

2.3. Statistical analysis

The 2 x 2 tables, Mann Whitney U test and Spearman's rank correlation were used where appropriate, with $p<0.05$ as the level of significance.

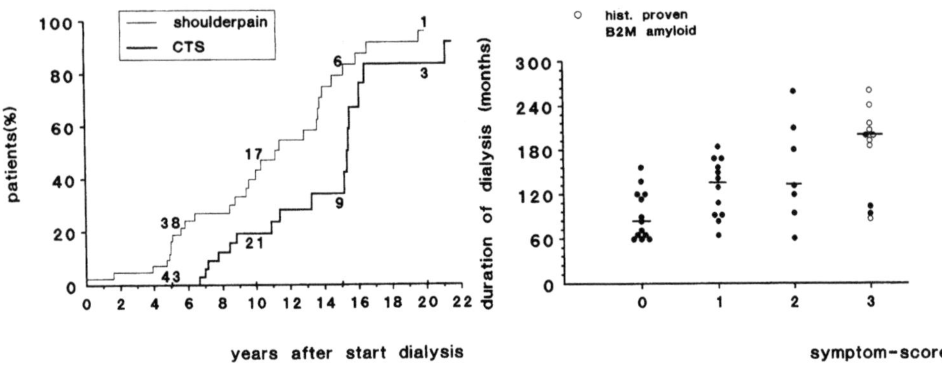

Figure 1. Actuarial risk of CTS and shoulderpain in dialysis patients.

Figure 2. Time on dialysis and symptom-score

3. RESULTS

Men and women did not differ with regard to age (55 resp. 56 years) and time on haemodialysis (135 resp. 133 months). No correlation was apparent as far as age and time on dialysis were concerned. Five patients who had some residual diuresis were dialyzed for less than 65 months.

Chronic or recurrent shoulderpain was observed in 29 patients (67%) and the actuarial risk gradually increased with time on dialysis as shown in figure 1: 50% risk on shoulderpain at 134 months. Morning stiffness was seen in 14 patients (33%) with a median duration of 15 min. (range 5-90). Objective testing showed in 30 patients (70%) some loss of function; of whom 19 (46%) were positive on questioning. CTS was present in 16 patients (37%) and the actuarial risk gradually increased with duration of dialysis as shown also in figure 1: 50% risk on CTS at 184 months. Joint swelling was seen in 22 (51%) and tendovaginitis (crepitans) in 24 patients (56%).

Arthritis was present in 19 patients (44%). Radiological signs were seen in 24 patients (56%): In all 24 patients cystic lesions (macro-geodes in 13 and other cysts in 20), in 9 erosive changes and in 5 a destructive arthropathy. No differences between men and women in the frequency of CTS (33 vs. 44%), arthritis (48 vs. 38%) and radiological signs (67 vs. 38%) could be detected. Three age categories were formed: <50 (N=16), 50-64 (N=12) and ≥ 65 years (N=15). Between the age groups no differences in the frequency of CTS (31, 34 and 47% resp.), arthritis (38, 42 and 53% resp.) and radiologic signs (56, 58 and 53% resp.) were seen.

Figure 2 displays the relation between the symptom-score and the time on dialysis. The median time on dialysis was 83 months for 13 patients with score 0, 138 months for 12 with score 1, 131 months for 7 with score 2 and 198 months for 11 with score 3. The time on dialysis did not differ between the group with score 2 and the other groups; the patients in the groups with score 1 ($p<0.05$) and 3 ($p<0.005$) were dialyzed longer than those with score 0. The patients with score 3 were dialyzed longer than those with score 1 ($p<0.05$). Synovia biopsies were

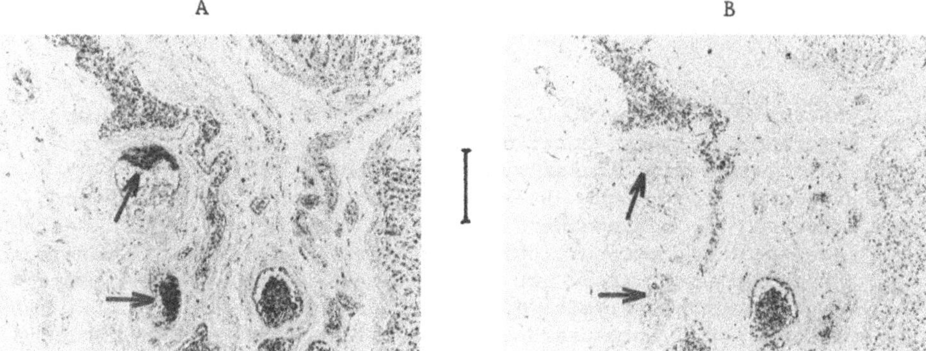

Figure 3. Vascular amyloid depositions in the large bowel (arrows). A) Positive reactivity with anti-β_2M. B) Anti-AA negative. The length of the bar is 0.2 mm.

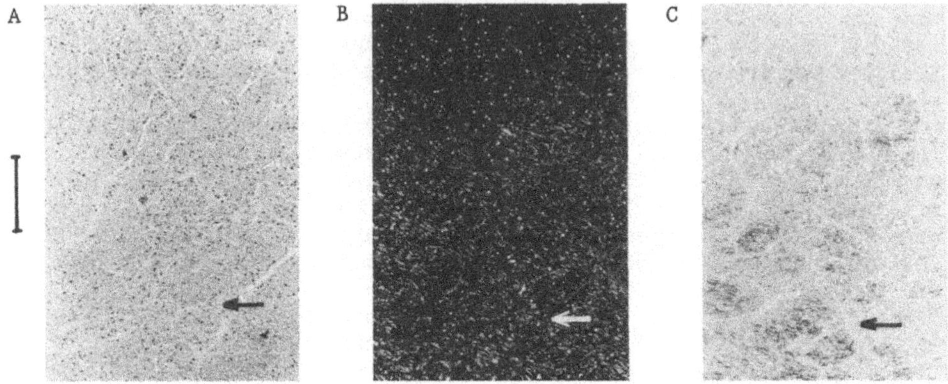

Figure 4. Amyloid deposition in myocardium (arrows). Bar length 0.5 mm. A) Congo red. B) Congo red in polarized light. C) Anti-β_2M.

performed in 8 patients and β2M-amyloidosis could be established. All 8 had a symptom-score of 3 (open dots in figure 2).

Extensive systemic amyloid (anti-β2M positive) deposition was found in the synovia of joints and tendons, in small vessels all over the body (figure 3) and to a lesser degree in the heart (figure 4) in the post-mortem examination of the patient dialyzed for 21 years.

4. DISCUSSION

We were impressed by the high frequency of suffering, disability and radiologic signs of osteoarthropathy in this group of patients. Symptoms were related to the time on dialysis, but not to sex or age. β_2M-amyloidosis was detected in 8 out of the 11 patients with the combination of CTS, arthritis and specific radiological signs. The autopsy emphasized the systemic nature of β_2M-amyloid deposition.

5. REFERENCES

1. Charra, B., Calemard, E. and Laurent, G. (1988) 'Chronic renal failure treatment duration and mode: Their relevance to the late dialysis periarticular syndrome' Blood Purification 6, 117-124.
2. Hardouin, P., Flipo, R.-M., Foissac-Gegoux, P., Thevenon, A., Pouyol, F., Duquesnoy, B. and Delcambre, B. (1987) 'Current aspects of osteoarticular pathology in patients undergoing hemodialysis: study of 80 patients. Part 1. Clinical and radiological analysis' J. Rheumatol. 14, 780-783.
3. Hardouin, P., Lecompte-Houche, M., Flipo, R.-M., et al. (1987) 'Current aspects of osteoarticular pathology in patients undergoing hemodialysis: study of 80 patients. Part 2. Laboratory and pathologic analysis. Discussion of the pathogenetic mechanism' J. Rheumatol. 14, 784-787.

β_2-MICROGLOBULIN-DERIVED AMYLOID AND CALCIUM IN LONG-TERM DIALYSIS PATIENTS

F. Gejyo, S. Maruyama, H. Maruyama, N. Homma,
R. Aoyagi, Y. Suzuki, E. Hoque, M. Arakawa
Department of Internal Medicine(II),
Niigata University School of Medicine,
Niigata 951, Japan

ABSTRACT. β_2-Microglobulin-derived amyloidosis occurs in long-term dialysis patients, causing osteoarthropathic symptoms like carpal tunnel syndrome, trigger finger, bone cyst and destructive spondyloarthropathy. In our patients, we have found that the amyloid co-deposited with ectopic calcification in the heart, urinary and kidney stones was β_2-microglobulin-derived. In order to clarify the distribution of calcium in the amyloid deposits, the mapping analysis of elements contained was performed using an electron probe microanalyzer(Shimazu EPMA-8705). This analysis revealed a co-deposition of calcium and amyloid in the same site, while neither iron nor aluminum was detected to share the same site with amyloid. The serum levels of calcium and phosphate, the product of calcium-phosphate and PTH-C are known to relate to the development of ectopic calcification. However, there was no significant difference in these parameters between the patients with and without amyloid osteoarthropathy in dialysis patients. These results suggest that amyloid deposition of β_2-microglobulin is not related to the serum levels of these factors and that calcium participation in amyloid deposition takes place locally.

1. INTRODUCTION

Amyloidosis is a serious complication in patients with renal failure who are receiving long-term dialysis. The deposition of β_2-microglobulin(β_2-M)-derived amyloid in these patients gives rise to such complications as the carpal tunnel syndrome, bone cysts diagnosed as cystic radiolucencies on bone x-ray, destructive spondyloarthropathy and fractures[1]. However, little is known about how amyloid degeneration of β_2-M is caused or why amyloidosis often affects the bone and joints. In our study of tissue pathology in long-term dialysis patients, we observed several in whom an increase in β_2-M derived amyloid was accompanied by ectopic calcification[2]. We therefore investigated the pathology of tissues from long-term dialysis patients with amyloidosis to understand the role of calcium in the cause of this disorder.

TABLE 1. Analysis of calcifications found in amyloid in 4 long-term hemodialysis patients

Case	Clinical feature	Specimen	Calcium compound (IR spectrum)	Amyloid protein
1	79y. M Nephrosclerosis HD: 2.1y	Kidney stone	Calcium oxalate	β_2-M identified by immunoelectrophoresis
2	53y. M Behcet disease Amyloidosis(AA) HD: 4.2y	Urinary stone	Calcium oxalate	β_2-M identified by N-terminal amino acid sequence
3	36y. M Chronic nephritis HD: 9.5y	Myocardial calcified compounds	Hydroxy apatite	β_2-M identified by immunoelectrophoresis
4	59y. F Chronic nephritis HD: 19.2y	Calcified compounds in synovium	Hydroxy apatite	β_2-M identified by immunoelectrophores

2. MATERIALS AND METHODS

We evaluated specimens obtained at autopsy from the heart and kidney as well as urinary stones from three patients who had received hemodialysis for 2.1, 4.2 and 9.5 years respectively, as well as biopsy specimens of synovial tissue from a patient with carpal tunnel syndrome and a history of dialysis for 19.2 years(Table 1). Calcium compounds were identified by infrared absorbance spectroscopy(Nihon Bunko, Jasco, DS-402G). Soluble proteins were identified by [^{14}C]-HCHO labeling, immunoelectrophoresis and reverse-phase partition chromatography using a C_{18}-bonded vinyl alcohol copolymer gel column(Asahipak ODP-50).

To study the details of the relationship between amyloid and calcium, each sample was analyzed by an electron probe analyzer, Shimazu EPMA 8705. Formalin-fixed tissue specimens were sliced into 4-5 μm sections and placed on a carbon stage for analytical color mapping of calcium(Ca), aluminum(Al), and iron(Fe) at the site of amyloid deposits using the electron probe microanalyzer. In 747 patients undergoing long-term dialysis including 130 cases with carpal tunnel syndrome or cystic radiolucencies, the serum levels of Ca, P, CaxP and PTH-C were measured.

3. RESULTS AND DISCUSSION

Table 1 shows the types of calcium compounds deposited in the amyloid tissues of four different patients. Case 2 had Behçet's disease followed by amyloidosis of the AA type; in this patient β_2-M-derived amyloid was identified in the sandy calcium compounds taken at autopsy from the renal

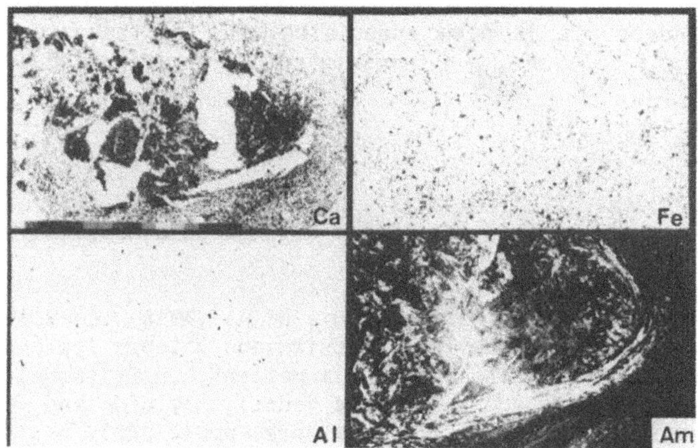

Figure 1. The mapping analysis of elements by an electron probe microanalyzer (Shimazu EPMA-8705). There were significant calcium deposits (Ca) at the sites which were amyloid positive (Am). However, neither iron (Fe) nor aluminum (Al) was detected.

pelvis and urinary bladder. Calcium oxalate was identified by infrared absorbance spectroscopy. The patient should be noted as having the AA and β_2-M types of amyloidosis. The calcium deposits in tissue taken from the heart of a 36-year-old male at autopsy was identified as hydroxyapatite. Details of this case were described previously[2]. In a 59 year-old female with a history of hemodialysis for 19.2 years, synovia were obtained at the fourth operation for carpal tunnel syndrome done because of pain caused by amyloid arthritis. The calcium deposit was identified as hydroxyapatite. This calcium compound was Congophilic and β_2-M-derived amyloid was confirmed immunohistochemically. The chromatographic and electrophoretic characteristics of the extracted protein in these cases were consistent with β_2-M.

In element mapping of the β_2-M-amyloid deposition area, calcium was identified in the sites stained with Congo red, while neither iron nor aluminum was detected as sharing the same site with amyloid (Figure 1). In the patients with urinary and kidney stones, calcium but no iron or aluminum was found in the amyloid layers surrounding a calcium oxalate core. Although no iron or aluminum was detected in the amyloid deposits evaluated in this study, other reports have described cases of amyloidosis complicated by the accumulation on iron or aluminum. The relationship between these metals and amyloidosis remains to be defined.

There were no significant differences in the serum levels of Ca, P, CaxP and PTH-C between the patients with carpal tunnel syndrome or bone cysts and those without such complications. Also, no indicators of ectopic calcification were observed in serum suggesting β_2-M amyloidosis caused.

We confirmed in this study that the deposition of β_2-M amyloid is often accompanied by various calcium compounds and apparently act as nuclei for the formation of amyloid deposits; however, there was no relationship between the deposition of amyloid and the serum parameters of calcium.

This may perhaps be due to the fact that the formation of amyloid occurs within the tissue. It is also speculated that in the presence of high concentration of calcium β_2-M leads to autoaggregation and deposition.

4. REFERENCES

1)Gejyo, F., Odani, T., Yamada, T., et al.(1986) β_2-Microglobulin: A new form of amyloid protein associated with chronic hemodialysis, Kidney Int.30, 385-390.

2)Gejyo, F., Homma, N., Maruyama, H., et al.(1988) Coexistence of β_2-microglobulin-derived amyloid deposits and ectopic calcification in the heart of a chronic hemodialysis patient, in T. Isobe, S. Araki, F. Uchino, S. Kito and E. Tsubura (eds.), Amyloid and amyloidosis, Plenum Publishing Corporation, New York, pp617-622.

IN VIVO METABOLISM OF A MUTANT APOLIPOPROTEIN A-I (ARG-26) ASSOCIATED WITH HEREDITARY AMYLOIDOSIS

Benson, M.D., *Rader, D.J., Schaefer, J.R., Gregg, R.E., Fairwell, T., Zech, L.A., Kindt, M.R., Brewer, Jr., H.B., and Meng, M.S., Indiana University School of Medicine, Department of Medicine, Rheumatology Division, Clinical Building 492, 541 Clinical Drive, Indianapolis, IN 46223; *National Institutes of Health, Bethesda, MD 20892, USA.

ABSTRACT. In the Iowa kindred with amyloidosis (FAP III) the amyloid fibrils contain a variant of apolipoprotein A-I with a Gly to Arg change at position 26. Gene carriers detected by direct DNA testing have hypoalphalipoproteinemia. To investigate a possible role of this finding in amyloid pathogenesis, normal and variant apoA-I metabolism was studied in two gene carriers and two controls.

Kinetic analysis of simultaneously injected ^{125}I-apoA-I$_{Arg-26}$ and ^{131}I-apoA-I$_{Normal}$ revealed markedly faster catabolism of the variant when compared to normal in both of the gene carriers and control subjects. Residence times for the variant apoA-I was 1.7 and 1.8 in the two study subjects compared to 1.6 and 2.1 days in the two control subjects. Residence times for A-I$_{Normal}$ in the study subjects were 3.6 and 3.5 days compared to 4.7 and 4.9 days in the two controls. These data show an increased catabolism of the variant apoA-I in both the heterozygous subjects and the controls and, in addition, show an increased catabolism of A-I$_{Normal}$ in the heterozygous gene carriers when compared to normal subjects. This increase in catabolic rate may explain the hypoalphalipoproteinemia and be a significant factor in the synthesis of amyloid fibrils.

INTRODUCTION

Hereditary amyloidosis is a delayed onset autosomal dominant condition characterized by extracellular accumulation of protein fibrils. Variants of plasma transthyretin are the most common cause of hereditary amyloidosis and to date 10 different mutations in transthyretin associated with systemic amyloidosis have been described [1]. In the clinical syndrome called familial amyloidotic polyneuropathy type III (FAP-III), originally described by Van Allen et al. in an Iowa kindred, the peripheral neuropathy is very similar to the other FAP-I syndromes [2]. However, the Iowa syndrome is associated with amyloid deposits containing an amino terminal fragment of apolipoprotein A-I (apoA-I) [3]. Individuals with this type of amyloidosis are heterozygous for a mutant ApoA-I with an arginine for glycine substitution at position 26 (Arg--26) [4,5]. Initial evaluation of gene carriers in this kindred showed decreased levels of apoA-I compared to normal. This is analogous to the decreased levels of plasma transthyretin in gene carriers for the variant forms of transthyretin associated with amyloidosis. Metabolic turnover studies were done for the variant apoA-I$_{Arg-26}$ and A-I$_{Normal}$ in gene carriers and control subjects to identify the reason for the lowered plasma levels.

MATERIALS AND METHODS

Study Subjects. Two asymtomatic heterozygous gene carriers for apoA-I_{Arg-26} and two healthy young adults were studied. All subjects had normal thyroid, liver and kidney function (Table 1).

Isolation Of Normal And Variant ApoA-I. ApoA-I_{Arg-26} was isolated from the plasma of a heterozygous subject by preparative ultracentrifugation followed by isoelectric focusing on a BioRad 220 dual slab gel unit. The apoA-I was electroeluted and stored lyphilized until used.

Iodination Of ApoA-I. ApoA-I was iodinated by a modification of the iodine monochloride method resulting in approximately 0.5 moles iodine incorporation per mole protein. Labeled proteins were reassociated with autologous lipoproteins prior to use.

Protocol. Patients were maintained on a diet containing 42% carbohydrate, 42% fat, and 16% protein. One day prior to the study subjects were given potassium iodide at a dose of 900 mg per day in divided doses. This was continued for the duration of the study. Subjects were injected intravenously with ^{131}I-apoA-I_{Normal} and ^{125}I-apoA-I_{Arg-26}. Blood samples were obtained at 10 minutes after injection and 1, 3, 6, 9, 12, 16, 24, and 36 hours. Blood samples were then obtained daily through day 6 and on days 8, 10, and 13. Urine was collected throughout the study. Plasma radioactivity decays were analyzed using a multiexponential computer curve-fitting technique. Residence times were obtained from the area under the curve.

RESULTS AND DISCUSSION

Table 1 gives the lipid and apolipoprotein data for all study subjects. Both of the apoA-I_{Arg-26} subjects had HDL cholesterol levels below the 10th percentile for their age and sex. Table 2 gives the kinetic perimeters of apoA-I_{Arg-26} and A-I_{Normal} in all subjects. The residence time for apoA-I_{Arg-26} was significantly shorter than that for A-I_{Normal} in all subjects. The plasma concentration of apoA-I_{Arg-26} was lower than that of A-I_{Normal} consistent with more rapid catabolism. Calculated production rates of both apoA-I proteins are similar indicating that the low concentration of apoA-I_{Arg-26} is not due to decreased production. A-I_{Normal} is also catabolized faster in the apoA-I_{Arg-26} subjects than in normals. This indicates that the decreased total plasma apoA-I concentration in the study subjects is due to increased fractional catabolic rates of both normal and apoA-I_{Arg-26} rather than decreased production. It is obvious then that the hypoalphalipoproteinemia in the subjects with the apoA-I_{Arg-26} mutation is due to increased catabolism of both the normal and Arg-26 apoA-I. While the apoA-I_{Arg-26} is rapidly removed from plasma in both study subjects and normal

Table 1. Characterization of Study Subjects.

SUBJECT	SEX	AGE (yrs)	CHOL	TG	HDL-C	ApoA-I
			(mmol/l)			(mg/l)
$ApoA\text{-}I_{Arg\text{-}26}$ 1	F	31	4.55	1.28	0.70	660
$ApoA\text{-}I_{Arg\text{-}26}$ 2	F	28	4.91	0.69	0.96	940
Control 1	F	20	4.78	1.17	1.22	1190
Control 2	M	20	5.51	0.98	1.47	1130

CHOL - Fasting plasma cholesterol
TG - Fasting plasma triglycerides
HDL-C - Fasting HDL cholesterol

Table 2. Kinetic Parameters of ApoA-I Metabolism.

SUBJECT	PROTEIN	CONC	RT	FCR	PR	
Subject 1	$ApoA\text{-}I_{Normal}$	470	3.6	0.28	5.2	> Total 9.7
	$ApoA\text{-}I_{Arg\text{-}26}$	190	1.7	0.59	4.5	
Subject 2	$ApoA\text{-}I_{Normal}$	670	3.5	0.28	7.6	> Total 13.7
	$ApoA\text{-}I_{Arg\text{-}26}$	270	1.8	0.57	6.1	
Control 1	$ApoA\text{-}I_{Normal}$	1190	4.7	0.21	10.1	
	$ApoA\text{-}I_{Arg\text{-}26}$	-	1.6	0.61	-	
Control 2	$ApoA\text{-}I_{Normal}$	1330	4.9	0.20	10.9	
	$ApoA\text{-}I_{Arg\text{-}26}$	-	2.1	0.47	-	
Historical Controls (n-7)	$ApoA\text{-}I_{Normal}$	1260 $\pm$17	4.9 $\pm$0.4	0.20 $\pm$0.02	10.3 $\pm$1.2	

CONC - Fasting plasma Concentration, mg/l
RT - Residence time, days
FCR - Fractional catabolic rate, pools/day
PR - Production rate, mg/kg - day

subjects, $A\text{-}I_{Normal}$ has a significantly faster catabolic rate in the heterozygous $apoA\text{-}I_{Arg-26}$ subjects than in normals. This suggests that the $apoA\text{-}I_{Arg-26}$ increases the catabolism of intact HDL particles containing both normal and variant apoA-I.

Another interesting finding in this study is that the radioactivity associated with the $apoA\text{-}I_{Arg-26}$, while being rapidly removed from plasma, does not appear in the urine at the rate that is expected. This suggests that the variant $apoA\text{-}I_{Arg-26}$ accumulates in extravascular tissues. This may be associated with biochemical processes which lead to amyloid fibril formation. While the basis for altered metabolism is not known, the Gly to Arg mutation results in a +1 charge difference, and also is predicted to eliminate the reverse turn at residues 24-27 [6]. This change may significantly alter the secondary structure and, therefore, the metabolism of this variant apolipoprotein.

In summary, this study shows altered catabolism of an amyloid precursor apolipoprotein A-I protein with decrease in plasma half life and apparent extracellular sequestration. This altered metabolism may well be an important factor in amyloid fibril formation. Similar mechanisms may be at play in the transthyretin amyloidoses.

ACKNOWLEDGEMENTS

This work was supported by VA Medical Research, the United States Public Health Service (RR-00750, NIDDK-34881, NIAMS-AR20582, AR7448), The Arthritis Foundation, The Grace M. Showalter Trust and The Marion E. Jacobson Fund.

REFERENCES

1. Benson, M.D., Wallace, M.R. (1989) 'Amyloidosis', in A.L. Beaudet, C.R. Scriver, W.S. Sly and D. Valle (eds.), The Metabolic Basis of Inherited Disease, McGraw-Hill, New York, pp. 2439-2460.
2. Van Allen, M., Frohlich, J., and Davis, J. (1969) 'Inherited predisposition to generalized amyloidosis', Neurology 19, 10-25.
3. Nichols, W.C., Dwulet, F.E., Liepnieks, J., and Benson, M.D. (1988) 'Variant apolipoprotein A-I as a major constituent of a human hereditary amyloid', Biochem. Biophys. Res. Comm. 156, 762-768.
4. Nichols, W.C., Gregg, R.E., Brewer Jr., H.B., and Benson, M.D. (1990) 'Characterization of a genetic mutation (apolipoprotein $A\text{-}I_{Iowa}$) associated with familial amyloidotic polyneuropathy type III', Genomics in press.
5. Brewer Jr., H.B., Fairwell, T., Larue, A., Ronan, R., Houser, A., and Bronzert, T. (1978) 'The amino acid sequence of human apoA-I, an apolipoprotein isolated from high density lipoproteins', Biochem. Biophys. Res. Comm. 80, 623-630.
6. Garnier, J., Osguthorpe, D.J., and Robson, B. (1978) 'Analysis of the accuracy and implications of simple methods for predicting the secondary structure of globular proteins', J. Mol. Biol. 120, 97-120.

NEW USA FAMILY HAS APOLIPOPROTEIN AI (ARG26) VARIANT

Lee Anna Jones, M.D.
Jennifer A. Harding, B.S.
Alan S. Cohen, M.D.
Martha Skinner, M.D.

The Arthritis Center, Department of Medicine and the Thorndike Memorial Laboratory, Boston City Hospital, Boston University School of Medicine, Boston, MA, 02118.

ABSTRACT

We have studied a patient from Massachusetts with hereditary systemic amyloidosis significant for renal dysfunction and liver infiltration culminating in hepatic failure and death at the age of 43 years, with no history of peptic ulcer disease or peripheral neuropathy. Amyloid fibrils isolated from this patient were fractionated and the 11 KD product found in the major retarded protein peak was sequenced to reveal a homogeneous apo A-1 variant with arginine for glycine at position 26. This same mutation has been reported in a family from Iowa with a type-III FAP and a 9 KD fragment of a variant apolipoprotein A-1 as the major protein in their amyloid deposits. Peripheral neuropathy and peptic ulcer disease were the prominent symptoms in the Iowan family. The differences between the clinical descriptions of the two kindreds suggest that the apo A-1 mutation of arg26 may have a variety of manifestations.

INTRODUCTION

Familial amyloidotic polyneuropathy (FAP) is a disease which follows a largely autosomal dominant inheritance pattern (Benson and Wallace, 1989). The amyloid deposits are usually composed of an abnormal form of transthyretin (TTR), although there has been one report of an Iowan family of English, Scottish and Irish descent with type-III FAP significant for an 83 amino acid N-terminal fragment of apolipoprotein A-1 (apo A-1) with an arginine for glycine substitution at position 26 deposited in their amyloid fibrils (Nichols et.al., 1988). The clinical aspects of this family included lower limb neuropathy, peptic ulcer disease and renal failure.

We now describe a second kindred of Scandinavian descent living in Massachusetts who had a similiar apo A-1 mutation on N-terminal sequencing of amyloid fibrils.

PATIENT AND FAMILY

The tissues we studied were those of a 43 year old female who has been previously described (Libbey,1987). She had suffered from severe hypertension and chronic renal failure since the age of 25 years. A nephrectomy done prior to her death had established amyloid infiltration as the cause of her renal dysfunction with extensive interstitial deposition of amyloid material about vessels and between tubules but without significant involvement of the glomeruli. Other organs found to be involved at autopsy included her heart, liver, spleen, adrenal medullas, and pituitary gland. Immunofluorescent staining of the tissues revealed no evidence of immunoglobulins. Immunohistochemical studies were inconclusive, with faint staining with the use of monoclonal anti-AA (amyloid protein A) and no staining with with anti-TTR.

The family history was significant for the patient's mother having died of renal amyloidosis at the age of 58 years with an autopsy revealing involvement of the liver, spleen and bone marrow.

METHODS

Amyloid fibrils were isolated and purified from splenic tissue using the technique of Skinner et. al. (1983). To assess their purity, the isolated peaks were run on a 20 cm 15% SDS acrylamide gel at 30 mA for 1 H and 55mA for 1.5 H.

After lyophilization, alkalization and reduction, N-terminal amino acid sequencing was carried out on the major retarded peak of the amyloid fibrils using a 470A gas-phase sequencer equipped with a model 120 PTH analyzer.

RESULTS

Standard isolation of amyloid fibrils followed by purification of components on a Sephacryl S-200 column identified the major retained peak as peak 4 (figure 1). To assess purity prior to sequencing the peaks were run on a SDS gel (figure 2) which showed peak 4 to be a homogeneous band running at a molecular weight of about 11 KD. Direct N-terminal sequencing of this component through position 33 revealed an identical sequence to apo A-1 except for an arginine for glycine at position 26 with no normal sequence present.

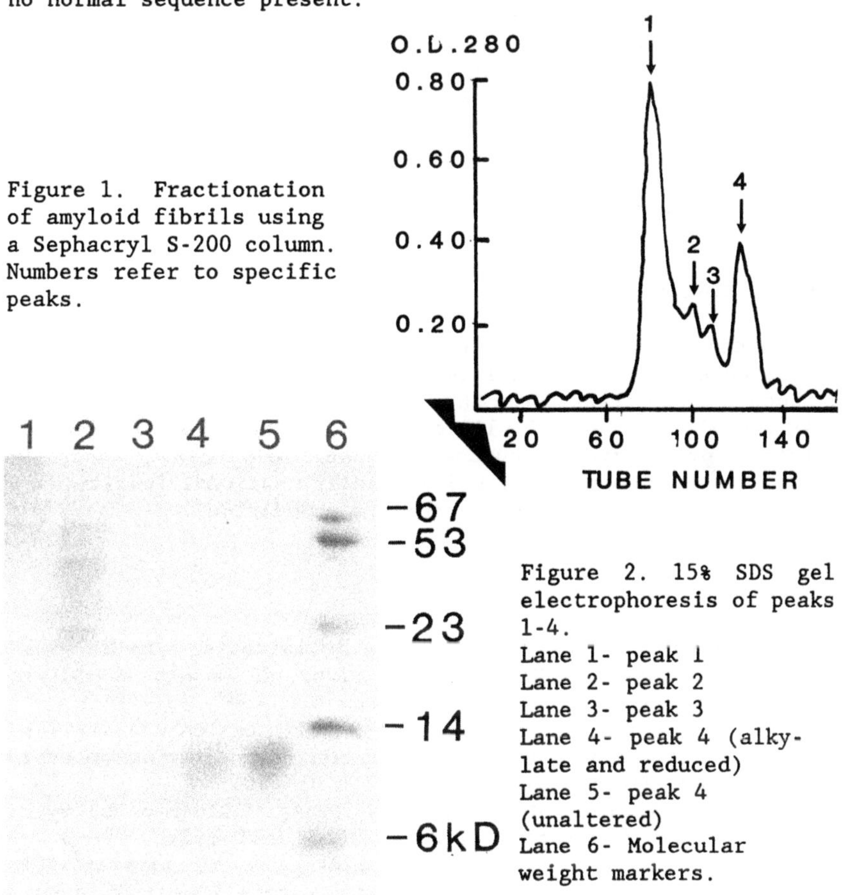

Figure 1. Fractionation of amyloid fibrils using a Sephacryl S-200 column. Numbers refer to specific peaks.

Figure 2. 15% SDS gel electrophoresis of peaks 1-4.
Lane 1- peak 1
Lane 2- peak 2
Lane 3- peak 3
Lane 4- peak 4 (alkylate and reduced)
Lane 5- peak 4 (unaltered)
Lane 6- Molecular weight markers.

DISCUSSION

We report a second kindred to demonstrate a hereditary amyloidosis related to deposition of an abnormal apo A-1. The clinical picture of this family differed from the one previously described, as neither peripheral neuropathy nor peptic ulcers were evident, while renal, hepatic and splenic involvement predominated. The renal disease was unusual for its primary involvement of the tubules while sparing the glomeruli.

Apo A-1 is a 28 KD hepatically synthesized polypeptide of 243 amino acids and is the major component of plasma HDL. It functions as a cofactor for lecithin:cholesterol acyltransferase (Fielding et.al.,1972). There have been 10 apo A-1 variants with base substitutions, 2 of which result in lowered HDL levels while the remainder have no apparent clinical effect (Schonfeld et.al.,1990).

Our finding of a family with an arg26 apo A-1 associated with a non-neuropathic systemic amyloidosis broadens the clinical spectrum of apo A-1 mutations.

ACKNOWLEDGMENTS

The authors would like to thank Dr. Gwendolyn Troxler for her assistance with N-terminal sequencing.

Supported by grants from the U.S. Public Health Service, NIAMDD (AM 07014), the General Clinical Research Centers Branch of the Division of Research Resources, National Institutes of Health (RR 533), the Multipurpose Arthritis Center, National Institutes of Health (AM 20613), and the Arthritis Foundation.

REFERENCES

1. Benson MD and MR Wallace. 1989. Amyloidosis. In Metabolic Basis of Inherited Disease. CR Scriver, AL Beaudet, WS Sly and D Valle, editors. McGraw-Hill, New York, NY, 2439-2460.
4. Fielding C, V Shore and P Fielding. 1972. Lecithin:cholesterol acyltransferase: effects of substrate composition upon enzyme activity. Biochem Biophys Acta 270,513-518.
5. Libbey CA and ML Talbert. 1987. Clinicopathological conference. New Engl Jour Med 317(24),1520-1531.
6. Nichols WC, FE Dwulet, J Liepnieks and MD Benson. 1988. Variant apolipoprotein AI as a major constituent of a human hereditary amyloid. Biochem and Biophys Res Comm 156(2),762-768.
8. Schonfeld G. The genetic dyslipoproteinemias-nosology update 1990. 1990. Athero 81,81-93.
9. Skinner M, T Shirahama AS Cohen and CL Deal. 1986. The association of amyloid P-component (AP) with the amyloid fibril: an updated method for amyloid fibril isolation. Prep Biochem 12,461-476.

Molecular Genetic Study of Mouse Senile Amyloidosis.

K. Higuchi, H. Naiki*, K. Kitagawa, K. Hanada, M. Hosokawa, S. Ishikawa, and T. Takeda.
Department of Senescence Biology, Chest Disease Research Institute. Kyoto University. Sakyo-ku, Kyoto 606, Japan.
*Department of Pathology, Fukui Medical College, Fukui, 910-11, Japan.

ABSTRACT

The apoA-II gene was amplified by polymerase chain reaction (PCR) from chromosomal DNA of nine inbred strains of mice. Sequence analysis of the PCR products indicated the presence of three types of apoA-II genes. Three types of apoA-II proteins (A, B and C) were predicted from the nucleotide sequence of apoA-II cDNA. Substitution of amino acid residues was noted at 4 positions. Each type was identifiable by digestion of PCR amplified apoA-II DNA, using restriction enzyme Cfr13I and MspI. The mouse strains, SAM-P/1, SAM-P/2, SJL/J, A/J had type A apoA-II. These strains generally exhibit amyloid deposition from relatively younger age. Examination of types of apoA-II and amyloid deposition in the F2 hybrid mice showed that apoA-II amyloid deposition was present only in the homozygous mice for type A apoA-II. We postulate that the molecular structure of apoA-II may be an important factor involved in the development of senile amyloidosis in mice.

INTRODUCTION

Senile amyloid protein "AS_{SAM}" was isolated from inbred strains of mice SAM-P/1 (Senescence Accelerated Mouse Prone) established in our laboratory as a murine model of accelerated senescence (1). Biochemical and immunochemical studies indicated that apolipoprotein A-II(apoA-II) in serum high density lipoprotein (HDL) is deposited in tissues in the form of amyloid fibril (AS_{SAM}), without degradation (2). Sequence analysis of apoA-II in the SAM-P/1 strain characterized by a high frequency of severe senile amyloidosis and the SAM-R/1 strain (Senescence Accelerated Mouse Resistant) in which senile amyloidosis occurred with a low incidence revealed amino acid substitution (glutamine in SAM-P/1 and proline in SAM-R/1) at position 5 (3,4). These studies suggested that the molecular type of apoA-II may be linked to the development of murine senile amyloidosis.

In this study, the three molecular types of mouse apoA-II were determined. We developed a procedure making use of PCR for identification of type of apoA-II and a genetic analysis of murine senile amyloidosis was carried out.

MATERIALS AND METHODS

Mice- Strains SAM-P/1, SAM-P/2, SAM-P/6, SAM-P/8, SAM-P/9, SAM-R/1, SAM-R/2, and DDD mice were developed in our laboratory by sister-brother breeding. Strains A/J, AKR/N, BALB/c, B10.BR/Sg, CBA/N, C3H/He, C57BL/6J, NZB/N, were purchased from The Shizuoka Laboratory Animal Center, Shizuoka. SJL/J were purchased from The Gokita Breeding Service, Tokyo. F2 hybrid mice obtained by breeding between SAM-P/9 and C57BL/6J were killed at 12-17 months of age. The liver, kidney, spleen, heart, lung, abdominal skin, stomach, and small intestine were fixed in 10% neutral buffered formaline and embedded in paraffin. DNA was isolated from the liver. These mice had all been raised under conventional conditions at 24$\pm$2°C with a light-controlled regimen (12-hours light/dark cycle) and a commercial chow (CE-2 Nihon CLEA, Tokyo) was provided. Tapped water was given ad libitum.

Isolation of DNA and PCR amplification of apoA-II gene- DNA was isolated from the livers by standard proteinase K digestion. Part of the apoA-II gene was amplified by PCR, using two apoA-II specific primers (SO-AII1; 5'TGAAGCTTCTCGCAATGGTCGCACTGCTGGT 3' and SO-AII2; 5' AGTCATGCTCTGAAAGTACTGTGTG 3')(5) form 1 µg of genomic DNA. The mixture (final volume 100 µl, with conditions as specified in the GeneAmp Kit, Perkin Elmer Cetus, Norwalk) was incubated at 94°C for 6 minutes, followed by 40 cycles of successive denaturation (94°C for 1 minute), annealing (55°C, 2 minutes) and extension (72°C, 2.5 minutes), followed by a final 10 minutes extension at 72°C. The PCR products were digested with restriction enzymes and loaded on 2.5% NuSieve (FMC Bioproducts, Rockland) -1% agarose gel.

Sequence analysis- PCR products of the apoA-II gene were sub-cloned into the pUC19 vector. A cDNA library from livers of C57BL/6J mice in phage λgt11 screened was with a ^{32}P-labeled apoA-II cDNA of SAM-P/1(6). Inserts of positive phages were sub-cloned into pUC19 for sequencing.

Detection of amyloid deposition- Identification of amyloid was made according to evidence of green birefringence in the Congo red stained section under conditions of polarizing microscopy. Immunochemical identification of the deposited amyloid protein was performed using the avidin biotinylated horseradish peroxidase complex (ABC) method with antisera against apoA-II.

RESULTS

Identification of three types of apoA-II- The apoA-II DNA fragment of 424 bp was amplified by PCR from DNA of SAM-P/1, SAM-P/2, SAM-R/1, SAM-R/2, A/J, AKR/N, C57BL/6J, DDD, SJL/J mice and sequenced. The PCR products of SAM-P/1, SAM-P/2, A/J and SJL/J mice had the same sequence(type A). PCR products of SAM-R/1 and DDD (type B) had two nucleotides substitution from type A PCR products. In PCR products of SAM-R/2, AKR/N and C57BL/6J strains (type C), there was a substitution of seven nucleotides from type A PCR product. To determine the structure of the third type apoA-II molecules for which the amino acid sequence had not been determined, we isolated phages which included apoA-II cDNA inserts from the liver cDNA library of the C57BL/6J strain. Substitution of amino acid residues was noted at 4 positions among three types of apoA-II (type A: Gln^{5}, Glu^{20}, Val^{26}, Ala^{38}, B: Pro^{5}, Glu^{20}, Val^{26}, Val^{38}, C: Pro^{5}, Asu^{20}, Met^{26}, Ala^{38}).

Determination of types of apoA-II among inbred mouse strains- For determination of the types of apoA-II among different inbred strains of mice, we used the PCR products of apoA-II gene. Those products were polymorphic to the recognition site of Cfr13I and MspI. PCR products amplified from DNA of 25 different strains of mice were digested with Cfr13I and MspI separately, separated on 3.5% agarose gel electrophoresis. After digestion with Cfr13I, the type A PCR product showed two bands, 272 bp and 152 bp. Type B and C PCR products showed three bands, 272 bp, 106 bp and 46 bp. After digestion with MspI, type A and B PCR products showed two bands, 296 bp and 128 bp and type C PCR products showed three bands, 296 bp, 84 bp and 44 bp. PCR products of the F1 hybrid mice between the strains with different types of apoA-II had all four bands. It became evident that SAM-P/1, SAM-P/2, SAM-P/9, A/J and SJL/J had type A apoA-II, SAM-R/1, SAM-P/6, BALB/C, CBA/N. C3H/He, DDD. NZB/N had type B apoA-II and SAM-R/2, SAM-P/8, C57BL/6J, AKR/N, B10.BR had type C apoA-II.

Senile amyloidosis in F2 hybrid mice- Twenty-two F2 hybrid mice procured by crossing F1 hybrid mice whose parental strain were SAM-P/9 and C57BL/6J were killed at age 12-17 months. The SAM-P/9 strain has the type A apoA-II and the C57BL/6J strain has the type C apoA-II. The genetic type of apoA-II in the individual hybrid mice was determined by PCR amplification. Three mice had type A apoA-II homozygously, six had type C apoA-II homozygously and thirteen had both type A and type C apoA-II heterozygously. Three homozygous mice for type A apoA-II had apoA-II deposition, as senile amyloid fibrils, in the stomach, skin, liver, spleen, kidney, small intestine, lung and heart. A wide variation in the intensity of the amyloid deposition was evident among type A apoA-II homozygous F2 mice.

DISCUSSION

We developed a easy and suitable method to identify three types of apoA-II, using the RFLP of the apoA-II gene amplified by PCR. Since this method is sensitive and only minute amounts of DNA are needed, it should be possible to determine the types of apoA-II using very small masses of tissues such as the tail, blood, sperm and etc. The possibility of the existence of other types of apoA-II in mice should be considered, because the complete cDNA sequence of all inbred strains of mice has not been determined. However RFLP analysis using twenty-two enzymes to all the strains used here indicated no heterogeneity other than three type of apoA-II (Data not shown).

Mouse strains, SAM-P/1, SAM-P/2, SJL/J and A/J which had been reported to exhibit relatively severe senile amyloidosis (7) had type A apoA-II. Genetic analysis using F2 hybrid mice indicated that apoA-II deposition, as senile amyloid fibril, was observed only in mice homozygous for type A apoA-II. Thus the structure of apoA-II may be a major factor which determines the development of senile amyloidosis in mice. Another notion is that type A apoA-II may be prone to construct amyloid fibrils when it presents alone in mouse HDL and the coexistence of type C apoA-II may inhibit fibril formation. With regard to the first point, a comparison of the amino acid sequence of three types of apoA-II may support the idea that the glutamine residue at position 5 is the key residue for the susceptibility to amyloid fibril formation, because three other replacements of amino acid are not specific for type A apoA-II. However the mechanisms of acceleration of amyloid deposition associated with structural difference of apoA-II protein have to be clarified. Age associated phenomena such as senile amyloidosis might be a highly polygenically controlled event and other genetic factors should also control senile amyloid deposition. The possibility that the actual "amyloidogenic gene" located in close proximity to the apoA-II gene might co-segregate with the type of apoA-II in F2 mice was not ruled out. A detailed genetic analysis using larger numbers of hybrid mice, and the construction of congenic strains and transgenic mice are ongoing in our laboratory.

REFERENCES

1. Takeda,T. Hosokawa,M. Takeshita,S. Irino,M. Higuchi,K. Matsushita,T. Tomita,Y. Yasuhira,K. Hamamoto,H. Shimizu,K. Ishii,M, Yamamuro,T. (1981) A new murine model of accelerated senescence. Mech. Ageing Dev. 17, 183-194.
2. Higuchi,K. Yonezu,T. Kogishi,K. Matsumura,A. Takeshita,S. Higuchi,K. Kohno,A. Matsushita,T. Hosokawa,M. Takeda,T. (1986) Purification and characterization of a senile amyloid-related antigenic substance (apoSAS$_{SAM}$) from mouse serum. J. Biol. Chem. 261, 12834-12840.
3. Higuchi,K. Yonezu,T. Tsunasawa,S. Sakiyama,F. Takeda,T. (1986) The single proline-glutamine substitution at position 5 enhances the potency of amyloid fibril formation of murine apoA-II. FEBS Lett. 207, 23-27.
4. Yonezu,T. Tsunasawa,S, Higuchi,K. Kogishi,K. Naiki,H. Hanada,K. Sakiyama,F. Takeda,T. (1987) Molecular-pathologic approach to murine senile amyloidosis, Lab. Invest. 57, 65-70.
5. Yonezu,T. Toda,M. Yamagishi,H. Higuchi,K. Takeda,T. (1989) Structural organization of the gene encoding apolipoprotein A-II in an amyloidotic strain of senescence-accelerated mouse (SAM). Gene 84, 187-191.
6. Kunisada,T. Higuchi,K. Aota,S. Takeda,T. Yamagishi,H. (1986) Molecular cloning and nucleotide sequence of cDNA for Murine senile amyloid protein. Nucleic Acids Res. 14, 5729-5740.
7. Takeda,T. Higuchi,K. Hosokawa,M. (1988) 'AS$_{SAM}$ amyloidosis is present in aging mice of many strains, not only in SAM', in T.Isobe, S.Araki, F.Uchino, S.Kito, E.Tsubura (eds.), Amyloid and Amyloidosis, Plenum Publishing Corporation, New York, pp. 685-690.

FLUOROMETRIC EXAMINATION OF TISSUE AMYLOID FIBRILS IN MURINE SENILE AMYLOIDOSIS: USE OF THE FLUORESCENT INDICATOR, THIOFLAVINE T

HIRONOBU NAIKI[1], KEIICHI HIGUCHI[2], KAORI KITAGAWA[2], ATSUYOSHI SHIMADA[2], WHEN-HSI CHEN[3], MASANORI HOSOKAWA[2], KAZUYA NAKAKUKI[1] and TOSHIO TAKEDA[2]

[1]Department of Pathology, Fukui Medical College, Fukui, Japan and [2]Department of Senescence Biology, Chest Disease Research Institute; [3]Department of Oral and Maxillofacial Surgery, Faculty of Medicine, Kyoto University, Kyoto, Japan

Thioflavine T(ThT), a fluorescent indicator of amyloid fibrils, has been tested in unfractionated tissue homogenates. With 250nM of ThT, liver homogenates from 17-month-old SAM-P/1(senescence accelerated mouse-prone), which contained amyloid fibrils in murine senile amyloidosis(fAS_{SAM}) fluoresced brightly, while normal liver homogenates showed a negligible fluorescence. We determined the concentration of fAS_{SAM} in the tissue, from the fluorescence and using the standard curve for fAS_{SAM} determination. Lower limits of fAS_{SAM} determination were about 1μg/mg tissue. A marked regional heterogeneity of fAS_{SAM} deposition was observed in the liver. We observed a linear correlation between fAS_{SAM} concentration and percentage of amyloid positive area in the liver. Age dependent increases in fAS_{SAM} concentrations and total fAS_{SAM} contents were noted in the liver and spleen of 11 to 15-month-old SAM-P/1.

INTRODUCTION

A novel fluorometric method was developed to examine amyloid fibrils in vitro[1]. This method is based on unique characteristics of thioflavine-T(ThT). In a free form, ThT fluoresces faintly at the excitation and emission maxima of 350 and 438nm, respectively. When ThT binds to specific sites on amyloid fibrils, ThT fluoresces brightly at the excitation and emission maxima of 450 and 482nm, respectively. At a constant ThT concentration, fluorescence change is linear with the increase in amyloid fibril concentration. We thus obtained standard curves for the determination of two murine amyloid fibrils, that is, fAS_{SAM}; amyloid fibrils composed of murine senile amyloid protein(AS_{SAM}) and fAA, amyloid fibrils composed of amyloid protein A(AA). fAS_{SAM} deposits extensively with increasing age in an inbred strain of mice, SAM-P/1(senescence accelerated mouse-prone) [2] and fAA is formed in a secondary amyloidosis. Compared with fAA, fAS_{SAM} showed a much brighter fluorescence with ThT and had a much higher affinity for ThT. Based on these binding characteristics, we attempted to determine the quantity of fAS_{SAM} in unfractionated tissue homogenates, using a low concentration of ThT(250nM). In such cases, ThT binding to fAS_{SAM} was saturated while the ThT binding to fAA and other non-fibrillar compounds was not and the latter showed negligible fluorescence, as low as 1μg fAS_{SAM}/mg tissue could be determined.

We describe herein the method we used to evaluate the extent of fAS_{SAM} deposition, by determining continuous and absolute values with pertinent dimensions(μg fAS_{SAM}/mg tissue). Some quantitative characteristics of fAS_{SAM} deposition in SAM-P/1 were also given attention.

MATERIALS AND METHODS

Determination of Tissue Concentrations of fAS_{SAM}

In the present study, liver and spleen were investigated because these are representative organs of fAS_{SAM} deposition[2] and also are composed of soft tissues which readily sonicate.

Mice were anesthetized with ether and blood samples were taken by cardiac puncture. fAS_{SAM} deposition in the liver was heterogeneous, therefore, after weighing, the whole liever was made into a paste using a ceramic mortar, on ice and no buffer was added. Ten to twenty milligrams of paste were put into an Eppendorf tube(1.5ml) which had been previously weighed, then the tube was weighed using an electrobalance and weight of the paste was calculated from the tube weights, with and without paste. Ice cold distilled water(1.4ml) was added to the tube and samples were sonicated on ice for 30 seconds.

As for spleen, fAS_{SAM} deposition was homogeneous. After weighing, the central portion of the spleen was cut, put into an Eppendorf tube and sonicated.

Ten microliter lots from each sample were added to 1.0ml of the reaction mixture, vortex mixed and applied for the fluorescence spectroscopy as described[1]. Fluorescence intensity per tube(1.4ml) was calculated and divided by the applied paste weight(mg) for standardization. After subtracting the standardized fluorescence of normal tissue, fAS_{SAM} concentration(μg/mg tissue) was calculated, using the standard curve for fAS_{SAM} determination. Total fAS_{SAM} content(mg) was calculated from fAS_{SAM} concentration(μg/mg tissue) and organ weight (mg).

Determination of fAS_{SAM} Distribution in the Liver

Each lobe of the liver was cut along the median line, perpendicular to the tangent line of the edge. Half a lobe was fixed in 10% neutral buffered formalin for immunohistochemistry with anti-apo A-II, the monomer constituent of fAS_{SAM}. The other half, 2mm wide tissue was cut parallel to the cut surface. This slit-like tissue was diced from the edge at 3mm intervals. Each fragment was applied for fAS_{SAM} determination, as described above.

RESULTS AND DISCUSSION

Specific Detection of fAS_{SAM} in Unfractionated Tissue Homogenates

In all determinations we have described, the ThT concentration was fixed at 250nM. fAS_{SAM} deposited liver tissue showed a marked fluorescence, whereas little was seen in normal liver tissue. fAA deposited liver tissue showed almost the same fluorescence as in the normal liver. When the amyloid fibril structure was disrupted by guanidine-HCl treatment, the fluorescence of fAS_{SAM} deposited liver tissue decreased to 1.9% of the non-treated value.

fAS_{SAM} deposited liver tissue from 17-month-old SAM-P/1 was then fractionated according to the method of Pras et al[3]. Eighty seven per cent of the fluorescence was concentrated in fraction 2 with an ionic strength of zero and the amyloid fibrils were suspended in the supernatant, after centrifugation. Thus, the fluorescence in the unfractionated preparations specifically represented fAS_{SAM}.

Distribution of the Heterogeneity of fAS_{SAM} in the Liver

fAS_{SAM} deposited more extensively in median and left lobes and more extensively at the edge than at the central region. Lesser deposits were seen in right and caudate lobes. While we have no clear explanation for this finding, regional differences in blood flow might account for the severity of fAS_{SAM} deposition.

Linear Correlation between fAS_{SAM} Concentration and the Percentage of the Amyloid Positive Area

The higher the fAS_{SAM} concentration the greater the amyloid deposition, as observed morphometrically at the corresponding area. When the fAS_{SAM} concentration was determined to be 1.2μg/mg, the percentage of amyloid positive area was 1.7% and the standardized fluorescence of this sample was about double that of the normal liver. Therefore, the lower limits of the detecting system described in this paper seems to be about 1μg/mg.

There is thus far no documentation concerning the percentage of the weight of amyloid fibrils to the amyloid material, identified as the amyloid positive area on light microscopy. We calculated the value based on the data obtained both from the ThT assay and from the morphometrical analysis. When the fAS_{SAM} concentration was fluorometrically determined to be 50μg/mg tissue, the concentration of the amyloid material was estimated to be 320μg/mg tissue. Therefore, in the liver of animals with murine senile amyloidosis, about 15% weight of the amyloid material seems to be amyloid fibrils and the other 85%, non-fibrilar components; for example, water, lipid, glycosaminoglycans[4] and various proteins, including serum amyloid P component and the precursor of amyloid fibrils.

Age-Related Changes in fAS_{SAM} Concentration and Total fAS_{SAM} Content in the Liver and Spleen

Age dependent marked increases in the severity of fAS_{SAM} deposition in SAM-P/1 have been determined, based only on histological data[2]. We evaluated this change exactly. It was about 11 months old that fAS_{SAM} could initially be detected fluorometrically in the liver and spleen. In 15-month-old SAM-P/1, fAS_{SAM} concentration in the liver and spleen was as high as 50μg/mg tissue.

We have described here a practical method to evaluate the severity of fAS_{SAM} deposition in tissues. This approach should contribute to the development of various in vivo experiments done to elucidate the pathogenesis of age related marked deposition of fAS_{SAM} in SAM-P/1.

REFERENCES

1. Naiki, H., Higuchi, K., Hosokawa, M., and Takeda, T. (1989) 'Fluorometric determination of amyloid fibrils in vitro using the fluorescent dye, thioflavine T', Anal. Biochem. 177, 244-249.

2. Higuchi, K., Matsumura, A., Honma, A., Takeshita, S., Hashimoto, K., Hosokawa, M., Yasuhira, K., and Takeda, T. (1983) 'Systemic senile amyloid in senescence-accelerated mice', Lab. Invest. 48, 231-240.

3. Pras, M., Zucker-Franklin, D., Rimon, A., and Franklin, Edward C. (1969) 'Physical, chemical, and ultrastructural studies of water-soluble human amyloid fibrils', J. Exp. Med. 130, 777-791.

4. Snow, Alan D., Willmer, J., and Kisilevsky, R. (1987) 'Sulfated glycosaminoglycans: A common constituent of all amyloids?', Lab. Invest. 56, 120-123.

THE LOW LEUKOCYTE (LLC) MOUSE, A SECOND MODEL OF "SENESCENCE - ACCELERATED" AMYLOIDOSIS ASSOCIATED WITH APOLIPOPROTEIN AII $PRO^5 \rightarrow GLN$; PREVALENCE OF THIS SUBSTITUTION AMONG INBRED STRAINS OF MICE

C. Warden
L. Bee
A.J. Lusis
Depts. of Medicine & Microbiology
University of California
Los Angeles, California 90024

C. Lerner
C.K. Chai
The Jackson Laboratory
Bar Harbor, Maine 04609

P.D. Gorevic
L.P. Qian
P.C. Munoz
Dept. of Medicine
State University of New York
Stony Brook, New York 11794

ABSTRACT

The LLC/CKC mouse was developed from a hybrid stock derived by cross-breeding C57BL/6J, C57BR/CdJ, A/J, BALB/cJ, LLC/Ckc and SM/Ckc mice screened for low leukocyte counts (4-5000/mm^3) over 22 generations. 100% develop amyloidosis at 10-18 months (spleen>adrenals>kidney>liver). The amyloid subunit protein (A_{LLC}) has a MW of 8.7kD and is distinct from AA protein on 2D Gels and by Western Blot analysis. A_{LLC} has a blocked amino- terminus; following deblocking, the N-terminal sequence of mouse ApoAII was obtained to position 17, with a substitution of Gln for Pro at position 5. The remainder of the sequence of ApoAII was obtained from A_{LLC} following cyanogen bromide cleavage, and by isolation of tryptic peptides by HPLC. A monospecific rabbit antibody to A_{LLC} recognized LLC amyloid in tissue section by immunohistology as well as amorphous forms near reticular cells by immuno EM. Anti-A_{LLC} reacted with a serum protein with alpha globulin mobility that copurified with SAA by formic acid gel filtration. LLC ApoAII was fully sequenced at the DNA level following reverse transcription of polyA+ mRNA isolated from liver and amplification by the Polymerase Chain Reaction (PCR) to further confirm the $Pro^5 \rightarrow$Gln substitution. Anchor PCR amplification and sequencing of ApoAII mRNA from 11 different inbred mouse strains revealed considerable polymorphism of this protein, with common representation of the position 5 Pro$\rightarrow$Gln substitution. SJL, a strain reported to develop non-AA spontaneous amyloidosis (Lab Invest 35:47, 1976) was also found to have this polymorphism. It thus appears that identical variant ApoAII molecules are the major constituents of age-related amyloid developing in SAM/P, LLC/Ckc and possibly SJL mice. Further studies can now be targeted to the physiologic correlates of ApoAII polymorphism, as well as the elucidation of separate but interactive genetic determinants of amyloidogenesis.

INTRODUCTION

An increasing number of experimental models of amyloidosis have been defined biochemically and by molecular techniques, providing systems for the further elucidation of several types of human amyloid (Table I). These models are of interest because they are amenable to studies directed to clarifying the early stages of deposition, as well as manipulations designed to attenuate or reverse this process.

Spontaneous age-related amyloidosis occurs with increased frequency in the SJL/J[(1)], LLC[(2)] and SAM/P[(3)] strains of mice and, in each instance, evidence has accumulated that deposits are non-AA in nature. The LLC mouse was developed as part of a study aimed at elucidating genetic determinants of leukocyte production and was derived by selective breeding from a hybrid population produced by intercrossing six inbred strains through 22 generations by brother-sister matings [(4,5)]; Low leukocyte counts develop progressively after birth, with lymphopenia exceeding neutropenia in severity. There is a 70% incidence of reticular hyperplasia, primarily involving the lymph nodes, which is apparent at 3-6 months, and 100% of these mice develop amyloidosis at 10-18 months[(2)]. Amyloid involves the spleen>adrenals>kidneys>liver, and is not associated with chronic inflammation.

TABLE I:
Animal Models of Amyloidosis

AA/SAA		
"Spontaneous:"	Induced:	
Pekin Duck	Mice (Some Strains)	
Obese-hyperglycemic mice	•Casein	•AgNO3
Abyssinian Cat	•M. Butyricum	•Organ Extracts
(Gray Collie) Dog	Monkey	
Cow	•Chronic Granulomatous Disease	
	Horse	
	•Hyperimmunization	
	Mink	
	•Endotoxin	
	Guinea Pig/Hamster	
	•Casein	
IAPP/Amylin		
Diabetic/Aged Cats		
Diabetic Monkeys		
PrP	ApoAII	
Mice (some strains)	SAM/ P	
Hamster		
Aβ		
Rhesus Monkey	?SJL Mouse	
Polar Bear	?Syrian Hamster	

MATERIALS AND METHODS

A colony of LLC mice has been maintained at SUNY Stony Brook derived from the line developed at Jackson Laboratories in the 1970's. Pathologic features have been described in previous publications[2,6]. Amyloidotic livers, spleens and kidneys from aged (>1 year) LLC mice were processed for extraction, immunohistology or isolation of mRNA following sacrifice. Tissue amyloid was extracted by the water flotation method, and fibrils fractionated under dissociating (5M guanidine) and reducing (0.17M DDT) conditions on Sephadex G-100. Pooled fractions were dialyzed extensively against distilled water and lyophilized[7]. Total RNA was extracted from snap-frozen livers using guanidium thiocyanate and further purified by cesium chloride untracentrifugation; polyA+ RNA was isolated by oligo dT sepharose chromatography.

Rabbits were immunized with denatured amyloid subunit proteins and tested by immunohistology using biotin-avidin conjugates or by Western Blot analysis as previously described[7]. Immunoelectron microscopy was performed on splenic tissue from LLC mice found to have early amyloid deposition; protein A-gold complexes were prepared and electron microscopy carried out as described in a previous publication[8].

Pooled LLC serum was fractionated under physiologic conditions or in 10% formic acid [9]; HDL was isolated by flotation ultracentrifugation, and ApoAII isolated under the same conditions as A_{LLC}. A_{LLC} and ApoAII were deblocked with pyroglutamate aminopeptidase[10], and the N-terminal sequence determined by Edman degradation. Cyanogen bromide cleavage and separation of tryptic peptides followed conditions suggested by Yonezu et al[11]. Individual peptides were characterized by amino acid analysis and direct sequencing, as described[7].

The cDNA (-) strand of ApoAII mRNA was synthesized with moloney murine leukemia virus reverse transcriptase in a mixture containing either oligo (dT) or a specific 3' primer. Primers for amplification of ApoAII were designed based on the sequence of SAM/P ApoAII published by Kunisada et al[12], and cDNA synthesis carried out using the polymerase chain reaction (PCR). Both primers were designed to contain EcoRI sites at their respective 5' ends. The anchored PCR procedure was used to synthesize cDNA corresponding to the 5' end of the ApoAII[13]. Gel purified DNA was directly sequenced as double stranded DNA with the T7 sequencing kit; sequencing primers were nested internal to the PCR primers.

RESULTS

Amyloid fibrils were isolated by water flotation and from the top layer of tissue following homogenization in saline-citrate. These fibrils bound congo red metachromatically and had a typical configuration by electron microscopy. Lyophilized material yielded a retarded peak following fractionation under dissociated and reducing conditions (Figure 1) that was not present in control tissue similarly processed. This peak (A_{LLC}) had a molecular weight of approximately 8kD, and constituted about 30% of the material loaded on the column by dry weight.

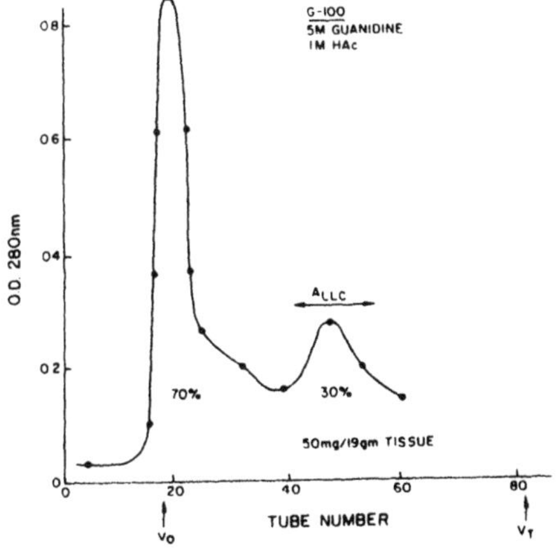

Figure 1: Elution profile of LLC amyloid fibrils fractionated on a Sephadex G-100 Column.

The N-terminal residue of A_{LLC}, found to be blocked, was released with pyroglutamate aminopeptidase, and the sequence of the whole molecule obtained to residue 17. This established that A_{LLC} was ApoAII, with the same $Pro^5 \rightarrow Gln$ substitution as described for the SAM/P mouse[11]. The sequence of the rest of the molecule was derived by placing individual peptides isolated by HPLC following proteolysis. These studies provided the entire sequence of ApoAII, which is compared to published data for the SAM/P, BALB/c, monkey and human proteins in Figure 2.

Figure 2

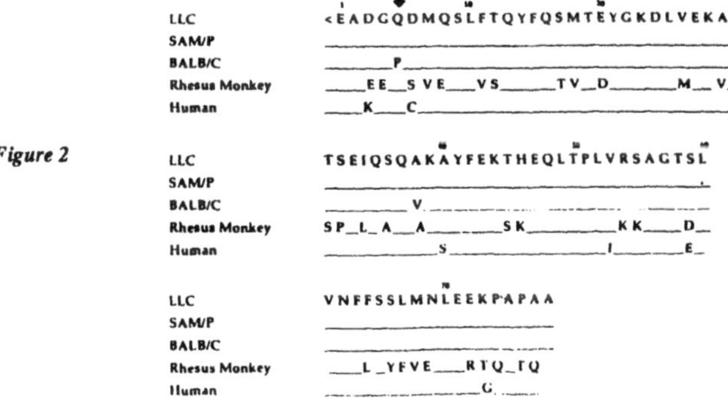

A rabbit polyclonal antibody raised to A_{LLC} recognized LLC amyloid in tissue section, but not AA amyloid deposits induced by casein injection in C57BL/6J mice. Conversely, anti-AA stained the hepatocytes of aged LLC mice injected with endotoxin 24 hours prior to sacrifice, but did not react with the extracellular amyloid. Thus, the two forms of murine amyloid were immunohistologically distinct.

Immunoelectron microscopy using anti-A_{LLC} and protein A-gold complexes demonstrated reactivity with amyloid fibrils, as well as amorphous deposits developing in close association with reticular cells.

Anti-A_{LLC} was found to react by immunoelectrophoresis with a serum protein that had alpha mobility in all mouse strains tested. Immunochemical studies of serum fractionated under physiological conditions, showed that this protein circulated in a high MW fraction, but could be dissociated to a low MW monomer following formic acid treatment of serum[11]. Since it colocalized with Apo SAA (Figure 3), it appeared that the serum form of A_{LLC} was also an apolipoprotein. Apo AII was then isolated from LLC serum by flotation ultracentrifugation and completely sequenced using the approach discribed above for the tissue protein. This established the identity of tissue and serum forms of ApoAII in the LLC mouse which, like SAM/P, is also apparently not modified during fibrillogenesis.

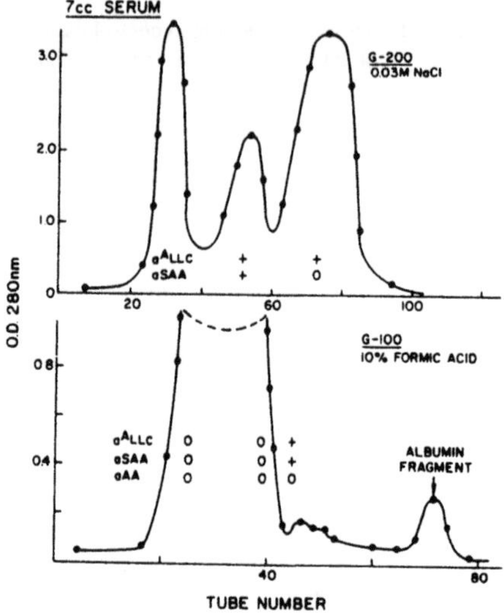

Figure 3: Pooled LLC serum was fractionated under physiologic conditions on Sephadex G-200, and in 10% formic on G-100 (11). Individual fractions were checked for reactivity with antisera to A_{LLC}, murine SAA and AA (C57BL/6) by Western Blot.

Sequencing studies have been confirmed at the DNA level following PCR amplification of reverse transcribed ApoAII mRNA for 20 different strains of mouse. Deduced amino acid sequences for 11 of them are shown in Figure 6. Of note is the presence of glutamine at position 5 of ApoAII in several strains, including A/J, SJL/J and PERA/CAMEi, several of which are known to develop accelerated amyloidosis. These results are in agreement with those reported by Higuchi et al (these proceedings).

```
C57BL/6J 1    MKLLAMVALL VTICSLEGAL VKRQADGPDM QSLFTQYFQS MTDYGKDLME
AKR/J         .......... .......... .......... .......... ..........
DBA/2J        .......... .......... .......... .......... ..........
BALB/cJ       .......... .......... .......... .......... ..E.....V.
C3H/HeJ       .......... .......... ........V  .......... ..E.....V.
SAM-P/1       .......... .......... .......Q.. .......... ..E.....V.
LLC/J         .......... .......... .......Q.. .......... ..E.....V.
A/J           ....T..... .......... .......Q.. .......... ..E.....V.
SJL/J         .......... .......... .......Q.. .......... ..E.....V.
SWR/J         .......... .......... .......Q.. .......... ..E.....V.
PERA/CAMEi    .......... .......... .......Q.. .......... ..E.....V.

C57BL/6J 51   KAKTSEIQSQ AKAYFEKTHE QLTPLVRSAG TSLVNFFSSL MNLEEKPAPA AK
AKR/J         .......... .......... .......... .......... .......... ..
DBA/2J        .......... .......... .......... .......... .......... ..
BALB/cJ       .......... V......... .......... .......... .......... ..
C3H/HeJ       .......... V......... .......... .......... .......... ..
SAM-P/1       .......... .......... .......... .......... .......... ..
LLC/J         .......... .......... .......... .......... .......... ..
A/J           .......... .......... .......... .....
SJL/J         .......... .......... .......... ..S....... ..........
SWR/J         .......... .......... .......... .......... .......... ..
PERA/CAMEi    .......... .......... ......K... .......... .......... ..
```

Figure 4: Amino acid sequences of ApoAII deduced from DNA sequencing of PCR-amplified ApoAII mRNA from 10 different inbred strains of mice. The sequence of SAM-P/1 is from Kunisada et al (12).

TABLE II:

Amyloidogenic Apolipoproteins
(mouse)

	SAA	ApoAII
Concentration (per ml)	<50ug*	0.3-0.5mg
MW (kD)	11.74/11.65	8.7
pI	6.35/6.2	5.0
Chromosome	7	1
Genes	4	1
Polymorphism	yes	yes'
Exons	4	4
Function	Acute-Phase ? immunologic	HDL Structure LCAT Modulation

*May go up to 0.5-1mg/ml during acute-phase response
'Tightly linked to Alp-2 gene (HDL structure)

DISCUSSION

The identification of ApoAII Pro^5→Gln as the major amyloid subunit protein in a second inbred strain of mouse distinct from SAM/P suggests the general importance of this polymorphism in accelerated murine age-related spontaneous amyloidosis. Identification of ApoAII as the major amyloidogenic protein in strains of mice with a low incidence of amyloid, and which do not have this amino acid substitution (e.g. SAM/R)(12,14) suggests that interactive factors other than structural polymorphism are also important in amyloidogenesis.

A number of parallels exist between Apo SAA and ApoAII in regard to amyloidosis (Table II). Both are associated with HDL, and ApoAII has been shown to displace Apo SAA from these particles(15). Both have similar sites of synthesis, and both also appear to deposit as amorphous nonfibrillar forms in tissue. In LLC mice, we found A_{LLC} reactivity in close association with reticular cells in spleen; in SAM/P mice, deposition has been reported in cytoplasm of hepatic cells, in columnar epithelia of the small intestine, and in epithelia of the proximal renal convoluted cells during the preamyloidotic stage of tissue deposition(16. Our observations in the LLC mouse provide the basis for further studies that can now be targeted to defining the intrinsic amyloidogenicity of the Pro^5→Gln substitution, linkage to putative gene or genes responsible for amyloid formation, analysis of the relative effects of aging and genetic milieu on fibril formation and clearance of amyloidogenetic proteins, and elucidation of the full spectrum of ApoAII deposition disease.

REFERENCES

1. Scheinberg MA, Cathcart ES, Eastcott JW, Skinner M, Benson M, Shirahama T, Bennett M: (1976) The SJL/J Mouse: A New Model for Spontaneous Age-Associated Amyloidosis I. Morphologic and Immunochemical Aspects; *Lab. Invest.*, 35:47-54.
2. Chai CK: (1976) Reticular Hyperplasia and Amyloidosis in a Line of Mice with Low Leukocyte Counts; *Amer. J. Pathol.*, 85:49-72.
3. Takeshita S, Hosokawa M, Irino M, Higuchi K, Shimizu K, Yasuhira K, Takeda T: (1982) Spontaneous Age-Associated Amyloidosis in Senescence-Accelerated Mouse (SAM) *Mech Aging and Devel.*, 20:13-23.
4. Chai CK: (1966) Selection for Leukocyte Counts in Mice. *Genetic Res.* 8:125-142.
5. Chai CK, Lerner C: (1985) The Inheritance of Spontaneous Amyloidosis Development in Mice: A Model for Hereditary Threshold Metabolic Disorders; *Amer. J. Med. Gen.*, 22:49-52.
6. Chai CK: (1978) Spontaneous Amyloidosis in LLC Mice: Renal Effect; *Amer. J. Pathol.*, 90:381-398.
7. Gorevic PD, Prelli FC, Wright J, Pras M, Frangione B: (1989) Systemic Senile Amyloidosis. Identification of a New Prealbumin (Transthyretin) Variant in Cardiac Tissue: Immunohistologic and Biochemical Similarity to One Form of Familial Amyloidotic Polyneuropathy. *J. Clin. Invest.* 83:836-843.
8. Chai CK, Lerner C: (1984) Amyloidosis Development in LLC Mice. *Exp. Cell Biol.* 52:301-308.
9. Gorevic PD, Levo Y, Chatpar P, Franklin EC, Frangione B: (1979) Cleavage of Mouse Serum Albumin by an Acid Protease After Administration of Endotoxin. Association with the Generation of Amyloid Serum Component (SAA). *J. Clin. Invest.* 63:254-261.
10. Podell D, Abraham GN: (1978) A technique for the Removal of Pyroglutamic Acid from the Amino Terminus of Proteins Using Calf Liver Pyroglutamate Aminopeptidase; *Biochem. Biophys. Res. Commun.*, 81:176-185.
11. Yonezu T, Higuchi K, Tsunasawa T, Takagi S, Sakiyama F, Takeda T: (1986) High Homology is Present in the Primary Structures Between Murine Senile Amyloid Protein (AS_{SAM}) and Human Apolipoprotein A-II; *FEBS Letters*, 203:149-152.
12. Kunisada T, Higuchi K, Aota S-I, Takeda T, Yamagishi H: (1986) Molecular Cloning and Nucleotide Sequence of cDNA for Murine Senile Amyloid Protein: Nucleotide Substitutions Found in Apolipoprotein A-II cDNA of Senescence Accelerated Mouse (SAM); *Nucl. Acids Res.*, 14:5729-5740.
13. Frohman MA, Dush MK, Martin GR: (1988) Rapid Production of Full Length cDNA's from Rare Transcripts: Amplification Using a Single Gene-Specific Oligonucleotide Primer. *Proc. Natl. Acad. Sci.* 85:8998-9002.
14. Takeda T, Higuchi K, Hosokawa M: (1988) AS_{SAM} Amyloidosis is Present in Aging Mice of Many Strains, Not Only in SAM; In: Isobe T, Araki S, Uchino F, Kito S, Tsubura E (Eds) *Amyloid and Amyloidosis*, Plenum Press, New York, 685-690.
15. Husebekk A, Skogen B, Husby G: (1988) High Density Lipoprotein has Different Binding Capacity for Different Apolipoproteins. The Amyloidogenic Apoproteins are Easier to Displace from High Density Lipoprotein. *Scand J. Immunol.* 28:653-658.
16. Takeshita S, Higuchi K, Hosokawa M, Matsumura A, Higuchi K, Kohno A, Matsuhita M, Yonezu T, Takeda T: (1985) Morphologic Demonstration of Cytoplasmic AS_{SAM}-related Antigenic Substance (SAM_{SAM}) by an Immunoperoxidase Technique; *Amer. J. Pathol.*, 121:455-465.

AGE-RELATED AMYLOID IN THE AORTA

G. Mucchiano*, G.G. Cornwell III$ and P. Westermark*
*Department of Pathology I, University of Linköping, Sweden and
$Department of Internal Medicine, Dartmouth Medical School, Hanover NH

ABSTRACT. Tissue from thoracal and abdominal aorta was taken from 84 autopsy cases. The amyloid deposition in the intima, media and adventitia was studied. Except for one case, medial amyloid was found in all patients above the age of 50. There was an increasing amount of medial amyloid with increasing age. Intimal amyloid was found in 35% of the cases above 50 years of age and seems to be the only variant in the aorta that is related to atherosclerosis. In the adventitia there was amyloid in 2 of the 84 cases. Antiserum against a low molecular weight component labelled medial,but not intimal amyloid, indicating that they may constitute two different entities.

Introduction

The aorta is one of the most common sites for senile amyloid deposition. Three forms of aortic amyloidosis are known: intimal, medial and adventitial [1]. Adventitial amyloid deposits are a manifestation of senile systemic amyloidosis [2]. The purpose of this study was to get a better understanding of the previously basically unknown nature of amyloid in the intima and media.

Material and Methods

Intimal, medial and adventitial amyloid were studied separately by light microscopy (LM), electron microscopy (EM) and immunohistochemistry.

LIGHT MICROSCOPY

Two samples of tissue from the thoracic and two from the abdominal aorta were removed from 84 autopsy cases between 18 and 96 years of age. 54 were male, 30 female.
Sections were stained with Congo Red and examined under polarized light. The quantity of amyloid in the media was evaluated by using a scoring system from 0-3 on each of the four

sections, thus giving a scale from 0-12 in each patient. The sections were scored blindly on two different occasions.

IMMUNOHISTOCHEMISTRY AND ELECTRON MICROSCOPY

Aortic amyloid fibrils were dissolved in 6M guanidine HCl and chromatographed on a Sepharose 6B column. The elution pattern showed a large void volume peak and two smaller retarded peaks.

Proteins corresponding to the lowest molecular weight protein peak (with a molecular weight of 10 kD or less, on SDS- PAGE preparations) was used for raising antibodies in guinea-pig by standard techniques.The antiserum was absorbed with P-component and normal human serum and tested against various tissues containing known and unknown amyloid fibril proteins [3,4] by the peroxidase-antiperoxidase method for light microscopy analysis.

The antibody was also tested by immunogold EM technique on medial amyloid containing aortic tissue. For this study the aortic tissue was fixed in 2.5% glutaraldehyde and embedded in Epon. Sections were incubated for 2 hours with the antiserum, treated with protein A-gold conjugate (15 nm particles) and contrasted with uranyl acetate and lead citrate

Results

LIGHT MICROSCOPY

Intimal amyloid. Amyloid in the intima was found only above the age of 50 and with a frquency of 35% (23 of 63 patients). The lumps of amyloid were irregular and located in close relation to atheromatous lesions.

Medial amyloid.. Medial amyloid was found in 61 out of 63 patients above 50 years old. Among the 21 patients below the age of 50, only one case (a 42 year old male) had amyloid in the media.The amount of medial amyloid increased with increasing age (Fig. 1). No variation was seen between the sexes. There was more amyloid in the thoracic than in the abdominal aorta (total score in thoracic aorta=171 and in the abdominal aorta =127). The amyloid was located to the greatest extent in the inner half of the media and was in the form of nodules and streaks between the smooth muscle cells.

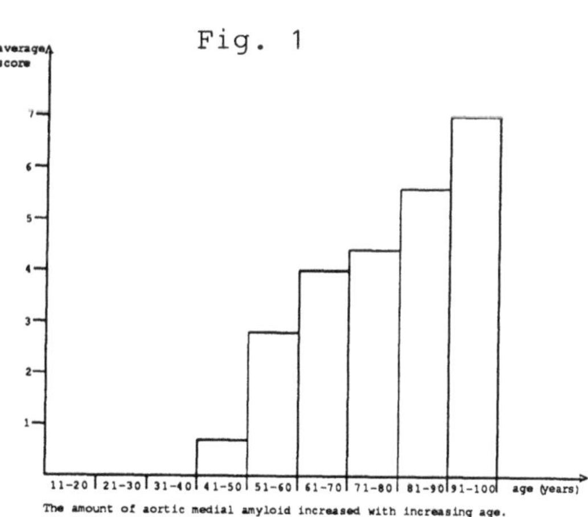

The amount of aortic medial amyloid increased with increasing age.

IMMUNOHISTOCHEMISTRY AND ELECTRON MICROSCOPY

Immunohistochemical studies by light microscopy revealed that the antiserum labelled medial but not intimal amyloid. It also labelled amyloid in a. temporalis and a. carotis communis. It did not label the following kinds of amyloid fibril proteins: AA, AL, ATTR, AANF, Aß, AIAPP, insulin and undetermined amyloid protein deposits in adrenal gland and seminal vesicle.

The amyloid fibrils labelled specifically extracellularly by immunogold electron microscopy studies. The fibrils were about 80 Å in diameter and arranged disorderly in extracellular compact bundles

Discussion

This study confirms the high frequency of aortic amyloid in patients above the age of 50 years [5,6]. There appear to be two separate localized forms of amyloid in the aorta, based on morphological and immunological studies. Of interest is the distinct difference in distribution within the aorta; one is limited to the media, the other to the intima.The intimal form, although clearly less common than the medial, might be of greater clinical importance. It always seems to be in close relation to atherosclerotic plaques. Whether this association reflects cause or effect of atherosclerosis will only be known after further studies.

Acknowledgements

Supported by the Swedish Medical Research Council and the Research Fund of King Gustaf V.

REFERENCES

1. Muckle, T.J.: (1986) 'Peripheral Angiopathy'. Marrink J., Van Rijswijk M.H.,(eds), Amyloidosis, Martinius Nijhoff Publishers, Dordrecht, pp. 271-282.
2. Pitkänen P., Westermark P., Cornwell III G.G. : (1984).'Senile Systemic Amyloidosis'. Am J. Pathol. 117, 391-399.
3. Cornwell III G.G., Husby G., Westermark P., Natvig J.B., Michaelsen T.E., Skogen B.: (1977). 'Identification and characterization of different amyloid fibril proteins in tissue sections'. Scand. J. Immunol. 6:1071-1080.
4. Cornwell III G.G., Natvig J.B., Westermark P., Husby G.: (1978). 'Senile cardiac amyloid : Demonstration of a unique fibril protein in tissue sections'. J. Immunol. 120: 1385-1388.
5. Schwarz P.H., Wolfe K.B., Bath J.S., Ahluwalia H.S., Beuttas J.T.: (1976). 'Amyloidosis in human and pathology: A comparative study'. Wegelius O , Pasternack A., (eds), Amyloidosis. Academic Press, London, pp. 71-102.
6. Battaglia S., Trentini G.P. (1978). 'Aortenamyloidose im Erwachsenalter'. Virchows Arch. A PAth. Anat. and Histol. 378: 153-159.

COMPLETE PRIMARY STRUCTURE OF AMYLOID PROTEIN IN FINNISH HEREDITARY AMYLOIDOSIS. IDENTIFICATION OF A NEW TYPE OF AMYLOID PROTEIN DERIVED FROM VARIANT (ASN-187) GELSOLIN

C. P. J. MAURY, K. ALLI and M. BAUMANN
Fourth Department of Medicine and Department of Medical Chemistry, University of Helsinki, SF-00170 Helsinki, Finland

ABSTRACT. The amyloid protein in Finnish hereditary amyloidosis (familial amyloid polyneuropathy type IV) was isolated and subjected to amino acid sequence analysis as the intact protein and as the alkylated derivative. Peptide fragmentation was carried out by trypsin and endoproteinase (endo-Lys C, endo-Asp, endo-Glu C) digestion. The amyloid protein is a 71-amino acid long fragment of gelsolin corresponding to residues 173-243 of the mature, secreted protein. The amyloid protein contains a single amino acid substitution when compared with the deduced sequence of gelsolin: at position 15 of the amyloid protein an asparagine is found instead of an aspartic acid residue at the corresponding position (187) in the gelsolin molecule. The results show that amyloid subunit protein in Finnish hereditary amyloidosis is a fragment of variant gelsolin that is derived from the actin-binding domain of the precursor molecule.

Introduction

Familial amyloid polyneuropathy (FAP) syndromes are autosomal dominant disorders characterized by extracellular deposits of fibrillar protein with crossed ß-pleated sheet conformation and a clinical syndrome of polyneuropathy. The FAP syndromes differ from each other with respect to distribution and degree of involvement of affected nerves and organs, age of onset, and ethnic origin. The Finnish type of familial amyloidosis (FAP type IV or Meretoja amyloidosis) is a systemic disease characterized by a distinct clinical picture involving progressive cranial neuropathy, corneal lattice dystrophy and distal sensimotor neuropathy (1). Skin, renal and cardiac manifestations may also occur.

The clinically different expression of the Finnish FAP, as compared with the FAP type I, II and III and related syndromes (2) has raised the possibility of a unique amyloid fibril protein in this disease. Indeed, our original studies have shown that the amyloid fibril protein in Finnish FAP is different from all amyloid proteins identified so far, showing amino acid homology with gelsolin, an actin-modulating protein (3). Here we present the complete primary structure of the accumulating renal amyloid protein.

Materials and Methods

Isolation and fractionation of amyloid. Amyloid was isolated from autopsy samples of the kidney of a 71-year-old man with Finnish hereditary amyloidosis. The amyloid was primarily localized to the glomeruli; small amounts were also present in the larger blood vessels and the interstitium. Using the immunofluorescence and peroxidase techniques, the amyloid was specifically stained by antibodies raised against a synthetic docapeptide corresponding to amino acids 231-242 of human plasma gelsolin. The antibodies did not stain amyloid of secondary (amyloid A) or myeloma-associated (AL-kappa) type. For control purposes, Congo-red negative renal and splenic autopsy tissues were subjected to the same extraction procedure as the amyloid tissue. The amyloid was isolated and purified as described previously (3). Gel filtration fractions were studied by gel electrophoresis (15-17% SDS-PAGE) and immunoblot (Western) techniques. The amyloid protein fraction was purified on reverse-phase HPLC (Beckman, System Gold, Programmable Solvent Module 126, SP 8450, UV/VIS detector, Spectra Physics Merck Hitachi D-2500 Chromato-Integration) using a Vydac C_{18} column and a 10-80% acetonitrile gradient in 0.1% trifluoroacetic acid.

Peptide fragmentation and separation on reverse-phase HPLC. The amyloid protein was alkylated and desalted and repurified on HPLC. Tryptic digestion (trypsin-TPCK, Sigma) was carried out in 1% ammonium bicarbonate; incubation with 3% (w/w) of trypsin for 2 h at 37°C was followed by another addition (3%) of the protease and continued incubation overnight at 37°C. The released peptides were separated by reverse-phase HPLC using a Vydac C_{18} column equilibrated with 0.1% trifluoroacetic acid in water, with a linear gradient of acetonitrile (0-60%) in 60 min. Digestion with endoproteinase Lys-C, Asp-N, and Glu-C (Boehringer-Mannheim) was carried out according to the manufacturer.

Amino acid sequence analysis. The sequence analysis was performed by automated Edman degradation using a modified Applied Biosystems 477A/120A on-line pulsed liquid phase/gas sequencer in the gas phase mode. The NBRF Swiss-PROT sequence database was used for computer search of sequence homologies.

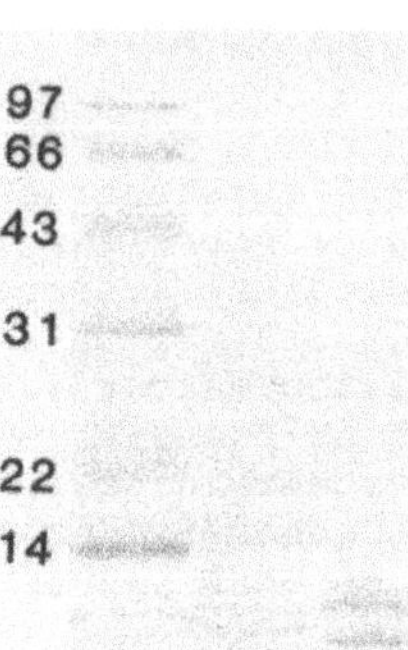

Figure 1. SDS-PAGE (15%) of the renal amyloid protein fraction. Molecular weight markers (Mr x 10^{-3}) are indicated on the left (Bio-Rad).

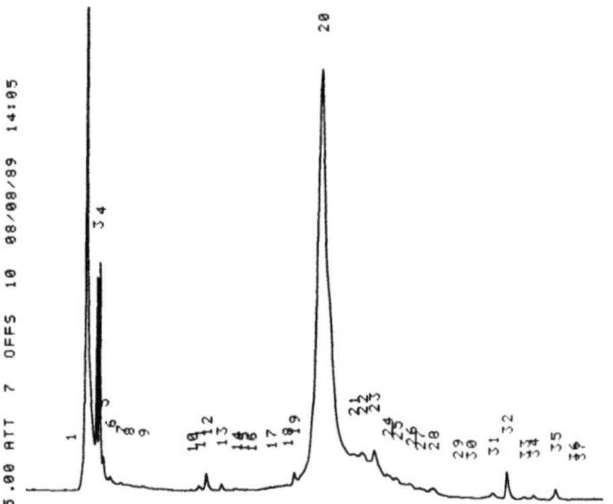

Figure 2. Reverse-phase HPLC of the amyloid protein. Vydac C_{18} and a linear gradient of acetonitrile (0-80%) in 0.1% trifluoroacetic acid.

Results

The extracted amyloid fibril preparations were Congo-red positive and exhibited green dichroism when viewed under polarized light. Electron microscopy of the fibril preparation revealed typical non-branching amyloid fibrils of approximately 8 to 9 nm width. Under dissociating conditions the amyloid subunit protein was eluted in gel filtration as a retarded peak, which was absent in control experiments with material extracted from non-amyloid kidney and splenic specimens. SDS-PAGE of the material eluted in the retarded peak, revealed two bands with Mr of approximately 6000-7000 and 8000-9000, respectively (Fig. 1). Final purification was achieved by reverse phase HPLC (Fig. 2).

Amino acid sequence analyses were carried out on the intact protein and the alkylated derivative. Peptide fragmentation was obtained by trypsin and by endoproteinase Asp-N, Glu-C and Lys-C treatments. By direct automated sequencing 38 amino acids of the N-terminus were identified; the remaining sequence of the molecule was identified by analysing the sequences of the enzymatically derived overlapping peptides. The primary structure of the larger accumulating amyloid protein is as follows:

```
1                 10                 20                 30
A T E V P V S W E S F N N G N C F I L D L G N N I H Q W C G S N S N R Y

     40                 50                 60                 70
E R L K A T Q V S K G I R D N E R S G R A R V H V S E E G T E P E A M
```

Microheterogeneity was present at the N-terminal end of the molecule. In addition to the major form starting with alanine, there were minor forms starting with either threonine (residue 2), glutamic acid (residue 3) or valine (residue 4). In addition to the amyloid protein ending in methionine (residue 71), there were molecules that ended in alanine (residue 70).

The amino acid sequence of the 71-residue amyloid protein is completely homologous to the predicted sequence of human plasma gelsolin (4) in the region of amino acids 173 to 243 of the mature protein (or residues 200 to 270 of the precursor protein) with one exception: at position 15 of the amyloid protein, which corresponds to residue 187 of plasma gelsolin (or 214 of the gelsolin precursor) an asparagine was found instead of an aspartic acid residue.

Discussion

The calculated molecular weight of the larger amyloid protein is 8.1 K, which is consistent with the estimate based on SDS-PAGE. The amyloid protein represents a fragment of the precursor gelsolin molecule and is obviously formed through limited proteolysis of the precursor. The N-terminus showed microheterogeneity, which has also been described in transthyretin-related amyloid proteins and may be a reflection of the amyloid disease process.

The amino acid sequence of the amyloid protein showed identity with the predicted sequence of human gelsolin representing residues 173 to 243 of the mature secreted plasma gelsolin (4) with one exception: at position 15 of the amyloid protein on asparagine was found in contrast to the predicted aspartic acid at the corresponding position (187) in normal secreted gelsolin. The asparagine-for-aspartic acid substitution now demonstrated in the amyloid protein isolated from the kidney is also present in the amyloid protein isolated from the heart (5).

Subsequently to our original report describing the amino acid sequence homology between the amyloid protein and gelsolin in Finnish type hereditary amyloidosis (3), Haltia et al (6) have reported 15 N-terminal amino acids of the amyloid protein confirming the gelsolin-nature of the amyloid. However, in contrast to our finding of the asparagine-for-aspartic acid substitution at position 15 of the amyloid protein (corresponding to residue 187 of gelsolin, this paper and ref. 5), Haltia et al (6) reported a normal aspartic acid residue at position 15 (corresponding to residue 187 of gelsolin).

Gelsolin is an actin-modulating protein found in a variety of mammalian tissues. It binds actin monomers, nucleates actin filament growth, and severs actin filaments (4,7). Plasma gelsolin represents a slightly larger form of gelsolin; both forms are derived by alternative transcriptional initiation sites and message processing from a single gene located on chromosome 9 (7). The function of circulating gelsolin has not been defined, but it may be essential for the clearance of actin filaments released into the circulation during tissue injury and cell senescence.

The sequence of the amyloid protein is part of a functional domain of the gelsolin molecule, and it may be speculated that a disturbed proteolytic degradation of this region of gelsolin and the consequent accumulation of the undegraded fragment into amyloid during fibrillogenesis may lead to disturbance in gelsolin-actin interactions.

References

1. Meretoja, J. (1969) Familial systemic paramyloidosis with lattice dystrophy of the cornea, progressive cranial neuropathy, skin changes and various internal symptoms. A previously unrecognized heritable syndrome, Ann. Clin. Res. 1, 314-324.
2. Araki, S. (1986) Familial amyloidotic polyneuropathies. Portuguese, Japanese, Swedish, British, Jewish, German-Swiss and Finnish forms, in J. Marrink and M. v. Rijswijk (eds.), Amyloidosis, M. Nijhoff Publishers, Dordrecht, pp. 195-218.
3. Maury, C.P.J., Alli, K. and Baumann, M. (1990) Finnish hereditary amyloidosis. Amino acid sequence homology between the amyloid fibril protein and human plasma gelsolin, FEBS Lett. 260, 85-87.
4. Kwiatkowski, D.J., Stossel, T.P., Orkin, S.H., Mole, J.E., Colten, H.R. and Yin, H.L. (1986) Plasma and cytoplasmic gelsolins are encoded by a single gene and contain a duplicated actin-binding domain, Nature (Lond.) 323, 455-458.
5. Maury, C.P.J. Isolation and characterization of cardiac amyloid in familial amyloid polyneuropathy type IV: Relation of the amyloid protein to variant gelsolin (Asn-187), Biochim. Biophys. Acta 1990 (Nov.). In press.
6. Haltia, M., Prelli, F., Ghiso, J., Kiuru, S., Somer, H., Palo, J. and Frangione, B. (1990) Amyloid protein in familial amyloidosis (Finnish type) is homologous to gelsolin, an actin-binding protein, Biochem. Biophys. Res. Commun. 167, 927-932.
7. Kwiatkowski, D.J., Westbrook, C.A., Burns, G.A.P. and Morton, C.C. (1988) Localization of gelsolin proximal to ABL on chromosome 9, Am. J. Hum. Genet. 42, 565-572.

POLYMERIZATION OF GELSOLIN VARIANT FRAGMENT IN TISSUE CAUSES FAMILIAL AMYLOIDOSIS, FINNISH TYPE (FAF)

M. HALTIA, J. GHISO, F. PRELLI, E. LEVY, G. GALLO, S. KIURU, H. SOMER, J. PALO and B. FRANGIONE

From the Department of Pathology and the Kaplan Cancer Center, New York University Medical Center, 560 First Avenue, New York, NY 10016, USA, and the Departments of Pathology and Neurology, University of Helsinki, 00290 Helsinki, Finland.

ABSTRACT. Familial amyloidosis, Finnish type (FAF), is an autosomal dominant form of systemic amyloidosis with progressive cranial neuropathy and lattice corneal dystrophy as principal clinical manifestations. We have shown that the amyloid protein in FAF is a degradation product of gelsolin, an actin-modulating protein. It starts at position 173 of the gelsolin molecule and has an amino acid substitution (Asn for Asp) at position 187. This variant of gelsolin-associated amyloidosis is designated Agel ASN 187. We have established that nucleotide 654 of the gelsolin gene, located in chromosome 9, is mutated (A for G). Antiserum raised against FAF amyloid also reacted with classical and diffuse Lewy bodies in a FAF patient with coexistent diffuse Lewy body disease and Alzheimer type brain lesions.

Introduction

Familial amyloidosis, Finnish type (FAF) [1,2,3], also known as familial amyloid polyneuropathy type IV or the Meretoja type [4], is an autosomal dominant form of systemic amyloidosis showing marked geographic clustering in certain regions of Southern Finland. Cases of FAF also have been reported from the Netherlands, Denmark, and the United States. FAF is clinically characterized by slowly progressive cranial neuropathy and lattice corneal dystrophy. Small deposits of congophilic material with green birefringence in polarized light and fibrillar ultrastructure occur in the blood vessel walls and in association with basement membranes of many tissues throughout the body [1]. Earlier attempts to characterize the FAF amyloid protein have led to inconclusive or conflicting results [5].

Materials, methods and results

Immunoperoxidase studies [3] of autopsy and biopsy specimens from six patients with characteristic clinical, histopathological, and ultrastructural (Fig. 1A) features of FAF did not disclose any immunocytochemical relationship between FAF amyloid and previously identified amyloid proteins or their precursors associated with systemic or cerebral amyloidosis. However, the FAF amyloid deposits were immunolabeled by an antiserum to amyloid P component. Amyloid fibrils were then extracted from the kidney of one patient (VUO) and purified by gel filtration [2]. Rabbit antiserum, raised against a purified low molecular weight subunit of amyloid fibrils, reacted strongly with FAF

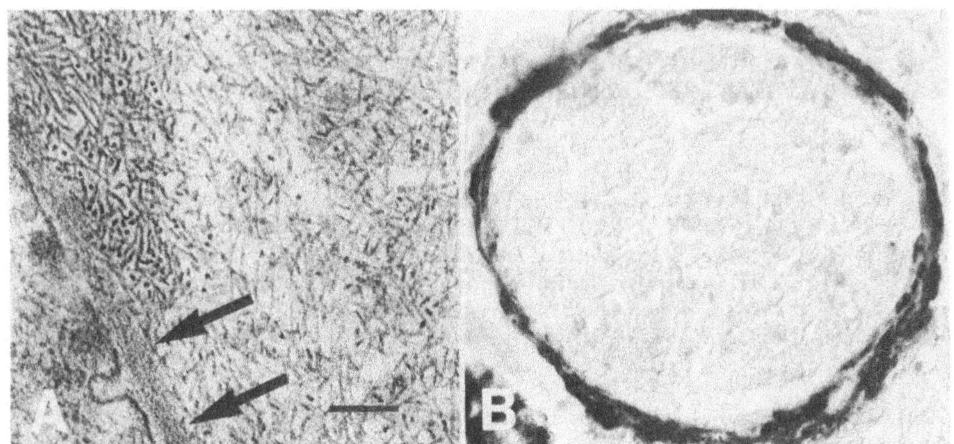

Fig. 1. A. FAF amyloid fibrils associated with the basal lamina (arrows) of a perineurial cell. Sural nerve biopsy of a FAF patient. Electron micrograph, bar 100 nm.
B. Perineurial sheath of a nerve fascicle of a FAF patient shows dark-stained amyloid deposits. Formaldehyde-fixed paraffin section, peroxidase-antiperoxidase method, rabbit antiserum raised against purified low molecular FAF amyloid subunit 1:100.

amyloid deposits in various tissues (Fig. 1B) [3]. This immunoreactivity was completely absorbed by the purified amyloid subunit, and the anti FAF amyloid antiserum did not stain normal glomeruli or amyloid deposits in other types of amyloidosis [3]. The amino terminal sequence of this subunit was homologous to gelsolin [6,7], an actin-modulating protein, starting at position 173 of the gelsolin molecule [2]. Extended amino acid sequence analysis of this original patient [3] showed heterogeneity (Asn and Asp) at position 15, while studies of a second FAF patient (JAA) showed substitution of asparagine for aspartic acid at the same position (Fig. 2), corresponding to amino acid 187 of plasma gelsolin.

The gelsolin variant described here may be due to a guanine to adenine transversion, corresponding to nucleotide 654 of the human plasma gelsolin cDNA [7]. To test this possibility, high molecular weight genomic DNA was isolated from tissues of four autopsy cases of FAF and from fresh lymphocytes of one FAF patient. Fragments containing nucleotide 654 were amplified with the polymerase chain reaction using oligonucleotides that were synthesized based on the cDNA sequences encoding gelsolin. The amplified fragments were subcloned into an M13 bacteriophage vector and sequenced by dideoxy chain termination. The DNA sequences demonstrated that all five patients had one allele containing a point mutation at nucleotide 654, as well as one normal allele. Preliminary results with DNA isolated from affected and unaffected members of the same family suggest that the mutation (G to A) segregates with the disease.

A neuropathological study of our original patient showed that in this patient variant gelsolin coexisted with Alzheimer's β-protein (Fig. 4A) and Alzheimer type brain lesions. The patient also displayed both classical (Fig. 3A) and diffuse (Fig. 4B) Lewy type intraneuronal inclusion bodies, immunoreactive with the anti-FAF amyloid antiserum (Fig. 3B, 4B). Preliminary observations indicate that this antiserum also reacts with Lewy bodies in Parkinson's disease and diffuse Lewy body disease.

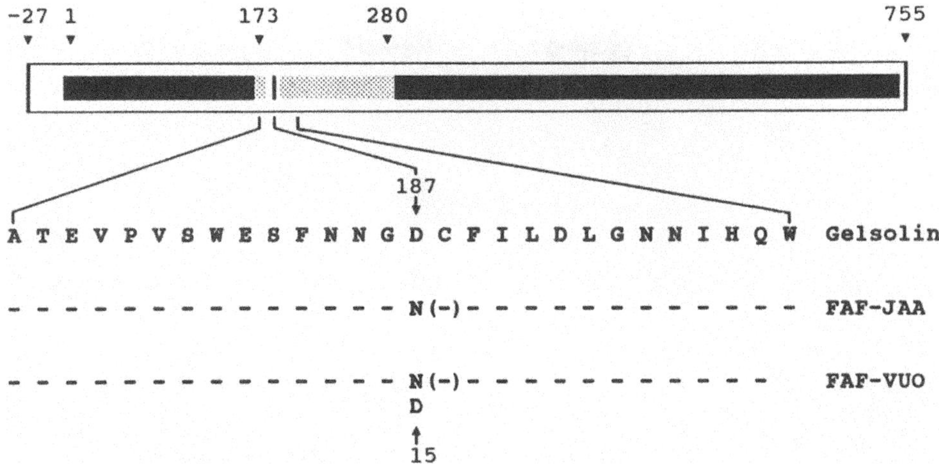

Fig. 2. Schematic representation of human plasma gelsolin, as deduced from cDNA [7], and amino terminal sequences of amyloid proteins derived from the kidneys of FAF patients VUO and JAA in comparison with human plasma gelsolin. Hatched area represents the location of the amyloid protein. Position 187 indicates the site of the amino acid substitution, corresponding to position 15 of the amyloid subunit. Amino acids are expressed in one-letter code. ( ): undetermined. -: homology.

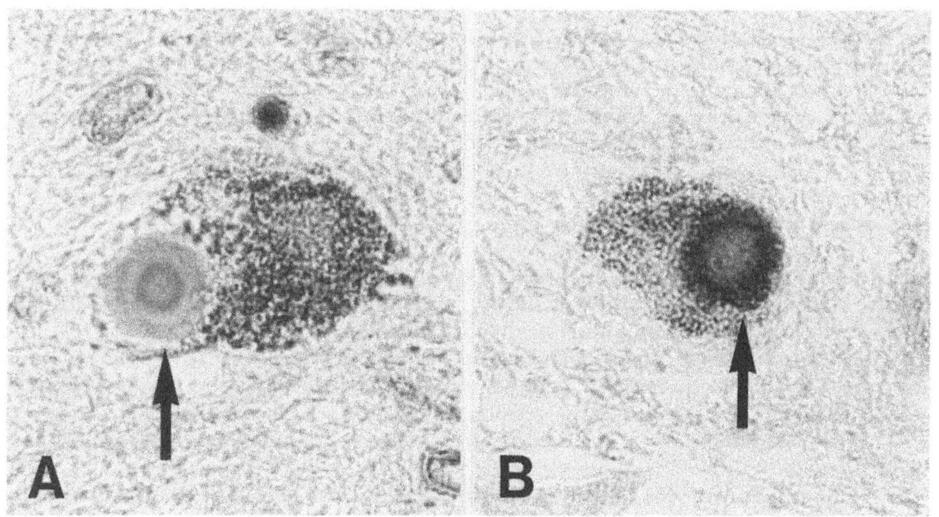

Fig. 3. Classical Lewy bodies (arrows) within nigral neurons of patient VUO. Paraffin sections stained with hematoxylin and eosin **(A)** and rabbit antiserum (1:100) raised against purified FAF amyloid subunit (peroxidase-antiperoxidase method) **(B)**.

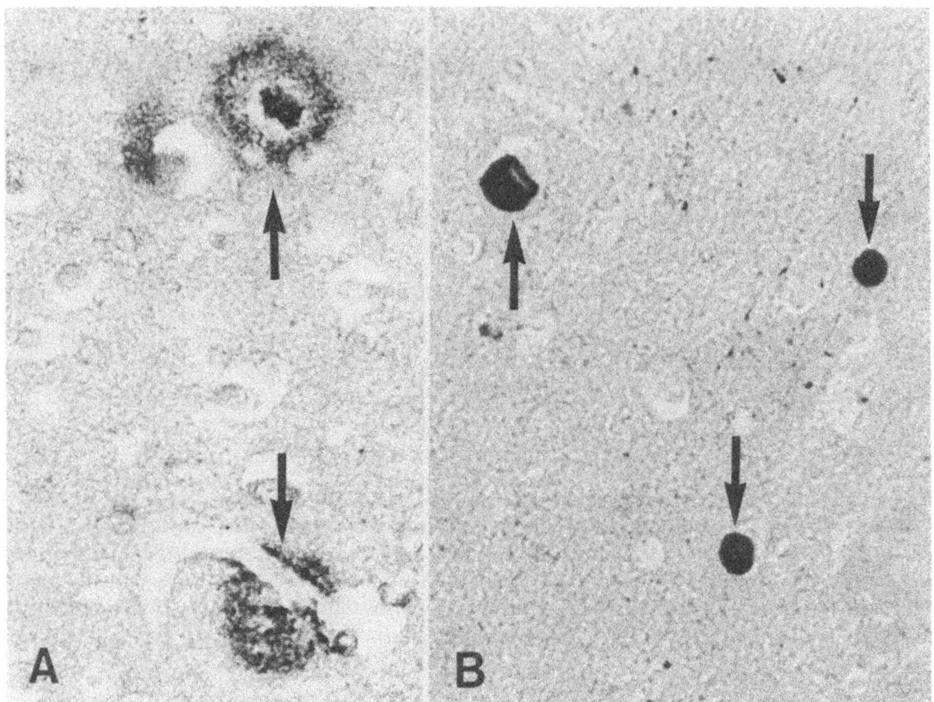

Fig. 4. Temporal neocortex of FAF patient VUO (paraffin sections, peroxidase-antiperoxidase method). **A.** Neuritic plaques (arrows) showing immunoreactivity with an antiserum raised against a synthetic peptide homologous to Alzheimer's β-protein (1:100). **B.** Intraneuronal inclusion bodies (arrows) strongly immunoreactive with an antiserum raised against purified FAF amyloid subunit (1:100).

Discussion and conclusions

Our observations show that the FAF amyloid protein is a degradation fragment of gelsolin, a highly conserved actin-modulating protein [6,7], It starts at position 173 of the gelsolin molecule and has an amino acid substitution (Asn for Asp) at position 187. This variant of gelsolin-associated amyloidosis is designated Agel ASN 187. Other workers have reported homology of tryptic peptides of FAF amyloid to gelsolin (8). We have also established that nucleotide 654 of the gelsolin gene, located in chromosome 9, is mutated (A for G). This mutation seems to segregate with the disease and may provide the basis for a diagnostic test.

Our findings document the deposition of two forms of amyloid-related proteins within the nervous system of the same patient, gelsolin variant and Alzheimer's β protein. Little is known of the simultaneous occurrence of two chemically distinct amyloid proteins in the brain, apart from rare cases with coexistent Creutzfeldt-Jakob and Alzheimer's diseases [9]. The immunoreactivity of both classical and diffuse Lewy bodies with the antiserum raised against FAF amyloid may suggest a role for gelsolin in the pathogenesis of

Parkinson's disease and diffuse Lewy body disease. Acccumulation of gelsolin-related material within neurons is not inconceivable in view of the expression of gelsolin in neurons [10] and its essential function in the modulation of the cytoskeleton [6,11].

References

1. Meretoja, J. (1969) 'Familial systemic paramyloidosis with lattice dystrophy of the cornea, progressive cranial neuropathy, skin changes and various internal symptoms'. Ann. Clin. Res. 1, 314-324.
2. Haltia, M., Prelli, F., Ghiso, J., et al. 'Amyloid protein in familial amyloidosis (Finnish type) is homologous to gelsolin, an actin-binding protein'. (1990). Biochem. Biophys. Res. Commun. 167, 927-932.
3. Haltia, M., Ghiso, J., Prelli, F., et al. (1990) 'Amyloid in familial amyloidosis, Finnish type, is antigenically and structurally related to gelsolin'. Am. J. Pathol. 136, 1223-1228.
4. Cohen, A.S., Rubinow, A. 'Amyloid neuropathy' in, P.J. Dyck, P.K. Thomas, E.H. Lambert and R. Bunge (eds.), Peripheral Neuropathy, vol. II. W.B. Saunders, Co., Philadelphia pp. 1866-1898.
5. Maury, C.P.J., Teppo, A.-M., Kariniemi, A.-L., Koeppen, A.H. (1988) 'Amyloid fibril protein in familial amyloidosis with cranial neuropathy and corneal lattice dystrophy (FAP type IV) is related to transthyretin'. Am. J. Clin. Pathol. 89, 359-364.
6. Stossel, T., Chaponnier, C., Ezzel, R., et al. (1985). 'Non-muscle actin-binding proteins'. Ann. Rev. Cell Biol. 1, 353-402.
7. Kwiatkowski, D.J., Stossel, T.P., Orkin, S.H. et al. (1986) 'Plasma and cytoplasmic gelsolins are encoded by a single gene and contain a duplicated actin-binding domain'. Nature 323, 455-458.
8. Maury, C.P.J., Alli, K., Baumann, M. (1990) 'Finnish hereditary amyloidosis. Amino acid sequence homology between the amyloid fibril protein and human plasma gelsoline'. FEBS Lett. 260, 85-87.
9. Brown, P., Jannotta, F., Gibbs, C.J. et al. (1990) 'Coexistence of Creutzfeldt-Jakob disease and Alzheimer's disease in the same patient'. Neurology 40, 226-228.
10. Petrucci,, T.C., Thomas, C., and Bray, D. (1983) 'Isolation of a Ca^{2+}-dependent actin-fragmenting protein from brain, spinal cord, and cultured neurons'. J. Neurochem. 40, 1507-1516.
11. Forscher, P. (1989). 'Calcium and phosphoinositide control of cytoskeletal dynamics'. Trends in Neuroscience 12, 168-174.

GELSOLIN-RELATED AMYLOIDOSIS. IMMUNOHISTOCHEMICAL STUDIES IN FINNISH HEREDITARY AMYLOIDOSIS WITH ANTIBODIES TO A SYNTHETIC DODECAPEPTIDE OF THE AMYLOIDOGENIC REGION OF GELSOLIN.

C. P. J. MAURY
Fourth Department of Medicine, University of Helsinki,
SF-00170 Helsinki, Finland

ABSTRACT. Our recent studies have shown that the amyloid fibril protein in Finnish hereditary amyloidosis (familial amyloid polyneuropathy type IV) is a new type of amyloid protein that is a fragment of variant gelsolin, a cytoskeletal and plasma protein with actin-modulating properties. Antibodies against a synthetic dodecapeptide of the amyloidogenic region of gelsolin were raised in rabbits and used in immunocytochemistry. The antibodies specifically stained the amyloid deposits in various tissues in patients with Finnish FAP. The staining was completely abolished by absorption of the antiserum with the synthetic dodecapeptide used for immunization. The antibodies did not stain the amyloid of secondary or of the myeloma-associated types. The results provide further evidence for the relation between the amyloid deposited in the systemic tissues of patients with Finnish FAP and gelsolin, and demonstrate the utility of these anti-gelsolin antibodies in diagnostic immunohistochemistry.

Introduction

Gelsolin is a calcium- and polyphosphoinositide-regulated actin-modulating protein that occurs in a cytoplasmic and a secreted form (1-3). Both types of gelsolin are derived by alternative transcriptional initiation sites and message processing from a single gene. Gelsolin binds actin monomers, nucleates actin filament growth and severs actin filaments. Our original studies have shown (4,5) that the inner region of gelsolin is amyloidogenic giving rise to the amyloid subunit protein in familial amyloid polyneuropathy (FAP) type IV (Finnish hereditary amyloidosis). The gelsolin-nature of the amyloid protein has subsequently been confirmed (6). The amyloidogenicity of gelsolin is most probably due to a point mutation in the gelsolin gene resulting in a variant gelsolin molecule characterized by an asparagine-for-aspartic acid substitution at position 187 (5).

By use of a synthetic dodecapeptide corresponding to the amyloidogenic region of gelsolin, anti-gelsolin antibodies were raised in rabbits. It is shown that these antibodies specifically react with the amyloid deposits in various tissues of patients with Finnish FAP. The results provide evidence for the identity of the systemic amyloid tissue deposits in Finnish hereditary amyloidosis with gelsolin, and demonstrate the utility of anti-gelsolin antibodies in diagnostic immunohistochemistry.

Materials and Methods

Cryostat or paraffin sections of tissue samples from 6 patients with Finnish FAP, 2 patients with secondary amyloid A amyloidosis, and 2 patients with amyloid light chain lambda amyloidosis were studied by standard immunofluorescence and immunoperoxidase techniques. The Finnish FAP samples included cryostat sections from the skin (4 cases), rectum (2 cases), kidney (1 case), myocardium (1 case), paraffin sections from the kidney (2 cases), myocardium (2 cases), thyroid gland (2 cases) and salivary gland (1 case). The control amyloid samples included liver and kidney cryostat and paraffin sections (2 cases; amyloid A amyloidosis), and heart and liver cryostat and paraffin sections (2 cases; amyloid light chain lambda). Antibodies to the synthetic docapeptide VHVSEEGTE-PEA-amide, corresponding to residues 231-242 of human plasma gelsolin (Multiple Peptide Systems, San Diego, CA, USA) were raised in rabbits. The peptide was conjugated to keyhole limpet hemocyanin and administered subcutaneously in Freund's complete adjuvant. The antibody titres were studied by enzyme immunoassay. In the absorption experiments 500 µg of uncoupled antigen were added to 200 µl of antiserum and kept at room temperature for 2 h and then at 4°C overnight. Controls in immunohistochemistry included normal rabbit serum, anti-gelsolin antisera absorbed with the peptide used for immunization, anti-transthyretin, anti-immunoglobulin light chain, anti-amyloid-P-component, anti-β_2-microglobulin (all from Dako, Glostrup, Denmark), anti-amyloid A (Calbiochem, La Jolla, CA, USA) and anti-apolipoprotein A-I (Orion Diagnostica, Espoo, Finland).

Results

The anti-(P231-242)gelsolin antibodies strongly reacted with the amyloid deposits in the various tissues of patients with Finnish hereditary amyloidosis (Figs. 1 and 2). The staining was completely abolish-

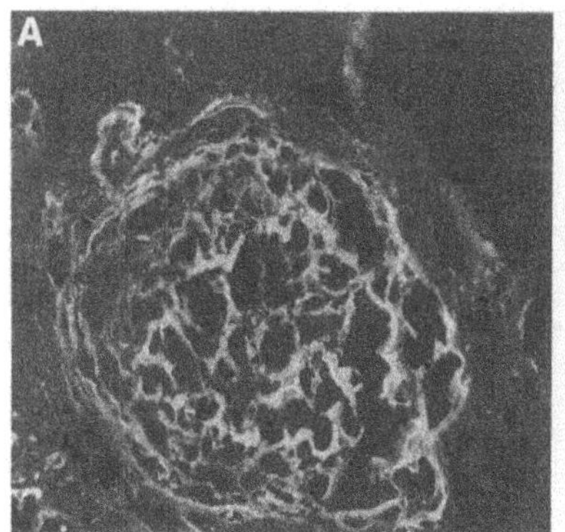

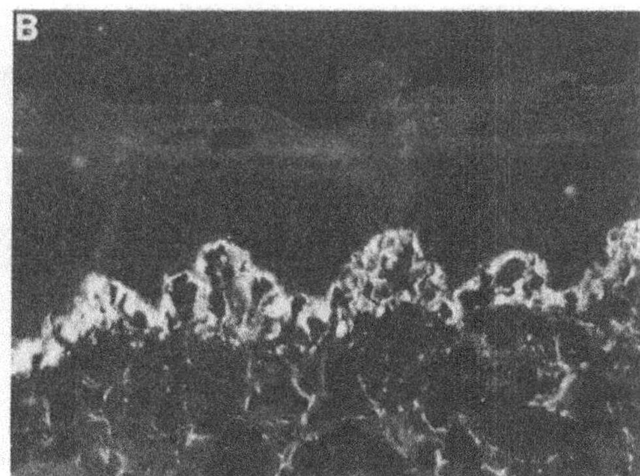

Figure 1. Immunohistochemical examination of tissue amyloid deposits in Finnish FAP with antibodies to the gelsolin docapeptide 231-242. A) Immunofluorescence staining of the amyloid around a sebaceous gland in the skin. B) Immunofluorescence staining of the amyloid in the epidermal-dermal junction in the skin.

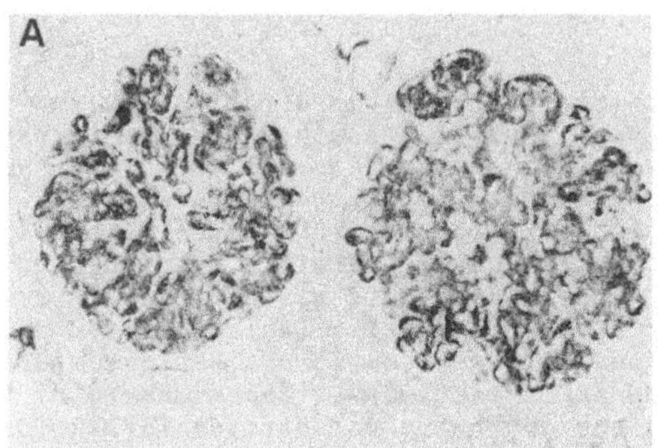

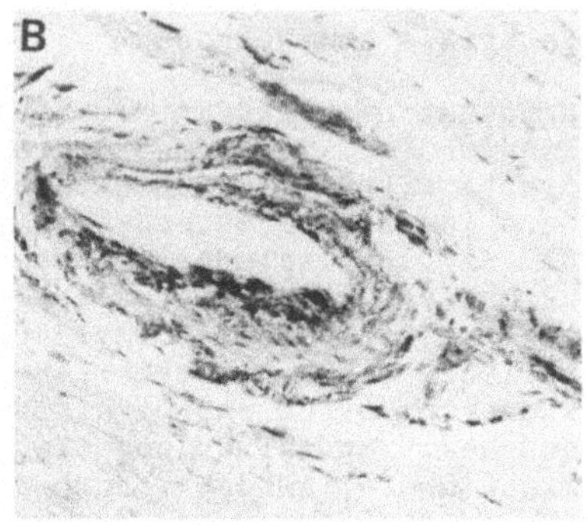

Figure 2. Immunoperoxidase staining of tissue amyloid deposits in Finnish FAP with antibodies to the gelsolin docapeptide 231-242. A) Glomerular amyloid. B) vascular amyloid in the myocardium.

ed by absorption of the antiserum with the synthetic docapeptide P231-242 used for immunization, but not by the peptide P213-221 antigen. The anti-gelsolin antiserum did not stain amyloid of secondary (amyloid A) or of myeloma-associated (amyloid light chain lambda) types.

Discussion

FAP type IV has been described primarily in the Finnish population; by the end of 1970s, more than 300 cases had been recorded (7,8). Cases have also been reported outside Finland, including cases from the United States, The Netherlands and Denmark. The disease is inherited in autosomal dominant mode and, in heterozygous patients, the disease has a late-onset and is slowly progressive. By the age of 20 years, corneal lattice dystrophy is usually manifested, and by the age of 40 years, most patients have developed cranial neuropathy. Renal, cardiac and skin manifestations also occur. Clinically, patients differ from the FAP type I patients who present with polyneuropathy of the lower limbs and severe autonomic dysfunction, and from FAP type II patients who present with cardiomyopathy.

The immunohistochemical studies with the anti-gelsolin antibodies show that the distribution of amyloid is systemic in Finnish FAP; amyloid is found in the intima and media of arteries, in capillary walls, and in the basement membranes of several organs. In the skin amyloid is found around the eccrine sweat glands and the sebaceous glands and at the epidermis-dermis junction.

The anti-gelsolin antibodies used in this study were specific for gelsolin-related amyloid; no staining was seen of amyloid, of amyloid A or amyloid light chain lambda amyloidosis. These antibodies are thus suitable for diagnostic immunohistochemistry and should be included in the panel of antisera used for testing amyloid of unknown type.

A point mutation in the gelsolin gene located on chromosome 9 (1,9) is the probable cause of the disease giving rise to a variant gelsolin molecule containing a single amino acid substitution (5). This substitution presumably leads to a resistance of the inner region of gelsolin to proteolysis resulting in the accumulation and polymerization of the subunit protein to amyloid fibrils.

Finnish FAP is the first human disease shown to be caused by an abnormality in the gelsolin molecule. Since gelsolin is a calcium-regulated actin filament-modulating protein occurring in the cytoskeleton and in the plasma, an abnormality in its degradation and the accumulation of a gelsolin degradation product during fibrillogenesis, may lead to disturbances in actin-gelsolin interactions.

References

1. Kwiatkowski, D.J., Mehl, R. and Yin, H.L. (1988) Genomic organization and biosynthesis of secreted and cytoplasmic forms of gelsolin, J. Cell. Biol. 106, 375-384.
2. Kwiatkowski, D.J., Stossel, T.P., Orkin, S.H., Mole, J.E., Colten, H.R. and Yin, H.L. (1986) Plasma and cytoplasmic gelsolins are encoded by a single gene and contain a duplicated actin-binding domain, Nature (Lond.) 323, 455-458.
3. Yin, H.L., Kwiatkowski, D.J., Mole, J.E. and Cole, F.S. (1984) Structure and biosynthesis of cytoplasmic and secretal variants of gelsolin, J. Biol. Chem. 259, 5271-5276.
4. Maury, C.P.J., Alli, K. and Baumann, M. (1990) Finnish hereditary amyloidosis. Amino acid sequence homology between the amyloid fibril protein and human plasma gelsolin, FEBS Lett. 260, 85-87.
5. Maury, C.P.J. Isolation and characterization of cardiac amyloid in familial amyloid polyneuropathy type IV: Relation of the amyloid protein to variant gelsolin (Asn-187), Biochim. Biophys. Acta 1990 (Nov.). In press.
6. Haltia, M., Prelli, F., Ghiso, J., Kiuru, S., Somer, H., Palo, J. and Frangione, B. (1990) Amyloid protein in familial amyloidosis (Finnish type) is homologous to gelsolin, an actin-binding protein, Biochem. Biophys. Res. Commun. 167, 927-932.
7. Meretoja, J. (1973) Inherited systemic amyloidosis with lattice corneal dystrophy. Dissertation. University of Helsinki, Finland, pp. 1-51.
8. Meretoja, J., Hollmén, T., Meretoja, T. and Penttinen, R. (1978) Partial characterization of amyloid proteins in inherited amyloidosis with lattice corneal dystrophy and in secondary amyloidosis, Med. Biol. 56, 17-22.
9. Kwiatkowski, D.J., Westbrook, C.A., Burns, G.A.P. and Morton, C. (1988) Localization of gelsolin proximal to ABL on chromosome 9, Am. J. Hum. Genet. 42, 565-572.

FAMILIAL AMYLOIDOSIS, FINNISH TYPE

S. KIURU, A-M. SEPPÄLÄINEN, M. HALTIA, H. SOMER, O. VALLE AND J. PALO

Departments of Neurology and Pathology, University of Helsinki, Haartmaninkatu 4, 00290 Helsinki, and Laakso Municipal Hospital, Helsinki, Finland

ABSTRACT. Familial amyloidosis, Finnish type (FAF), previously also known as FAP IV is an autosomal dominant disorder with extracellular deposition of amyloid in several tissues. Neurological examination revealed peripheral facial palsy in 13 of the 14 examined patients. Dysfunction of other cranial nerves and signs of autonomic and peripheral polyneuropathy were also found. Neuropsychological findings were largely normal. Cerebral/cerebellar atrophy was present in some CT scans and a slight, non-specific abnormality was found in brain MRI in two patients. ENMG showed dysfunction of the facial nerve in all, findings of peripheral sensorimotor polyneuropathy, and carpal tunnel syndrome in many patients. Visual, somatosensory, and brainstem auditory evoked potentials and blink reflexes were abnormal in several patients. Ophthalmological examinations showed corneal lattice dystrophy in all patients, some had an abnormal electroretinogram, corneal opacities and erosions. Amyloid was found in skin, muscle and sural nerve in all patients and in several cases in the rectum biopsy. The clinical, neurological and neurophysiological picture of FAF is characteristic and differs from all other amyloidoses.

1. Introduction

Familial amyloidosis of the Finnish type (FAF) is an autosomal dominant form of systemic amyloidosis first described by Meretoja in 1969 [1]. It shows a marked geographic clustering in certain regions of Southeastern Finland [2], and some cases have also been reported from Denmark [3], the Netherlands [4], and the United States[5].

Clinical characteristics of FAF include corneal lattice dystrophy beginning at the age of 20 to 40 years [6], slowly progressive cranial neuropathy starting at about 40 years, and sensorimotor polyneuropathy [1]. Small deposits of congophilic material with a fibrillar ultrastructure are found in most tissues, particularly in association with vessel walls and basement membranes [7].

Recent studies have shown that the amyloid protein in FAF is related to gelsolin [8,9,10] unlike the amyloid proteins in most other types of familial amyloidotic polyneuropathy, which are related to transthyretin variants.

The present study was conducted to clarify the clinical findings, especially the neurological manifestations of FAF.

2. Patients and methods

14 patients (10 women and 4 men) aged between 44 and 74 years were examined at the Department of Neurology, University of Helsinki. All had previously diagnosed corneal lattice dystrophy and genetic background for FAF. Clinical neurological, neuroradiological, neurophysiological and ophthalmological examinations were performed. The presence of amyloid was histologically verified in bioptic material of skin, muscle, rectum and sural nerve.

3. Results

3.1. NEUROLOGICAL FINDINGS

In clinical examination peripheral facial nerve palsy (Fig.1a) with predilection for the upper branch was found in 13 patients. Other signs of cranial neuropathy (Table 1) were loss of the corneal reflex, diplopia with limited ocular motility and defective hearing. The tongue was enlarged, furred, and partly atrophic in some patients. Distal paresthesia, diminished vibration sense and weak tendon reflexes as clinical signs of peripheral neuropathy (Table 2) were found in several patients. Signs of autonomic neuropathy were detected in half of the patients. Neuropsychological tests showed only very slight abnormalities and no signs of dementia.

Table 1. Signs of cranial neuropathy

Trigeminal nerve	4/14
Facial nerve	13/14
Vestibulocochlear nerve	4/14
Hypoglossal nerve	4/14

Table 2. Signs of peripheral neuropathy

Weak reflexes	5/14
Diminished vibration sense	11/14
Distal paresthesia	8/14

3.2. OTHER CLINICAL FINDINGS

Cutaneous changes in the form of thick, soft skin of the scalp were found in 13 of the patients. Many patients had also atrophic skin in the distal parts of the extremities and hypotrichosis. Abnormal echocardiogram and increased serum-creatinine were found in only one patient respectively. Neuroradiological examination showed cerebral or cerebellar atrophy in three of 14 CT scans and a slight, nonspecific abnormality in the two MRI studies performed.

3.3. OPHTHALMOLOGICAL FINDINGS

Ophthalmological examination revealed corneal lattice dystrophy (Fig.1b) in all 14 patients. Corneal opacities were detected in more than half of the patients, and some also had corneal erosions. Only a few patients had an abnormal electroretinogram.

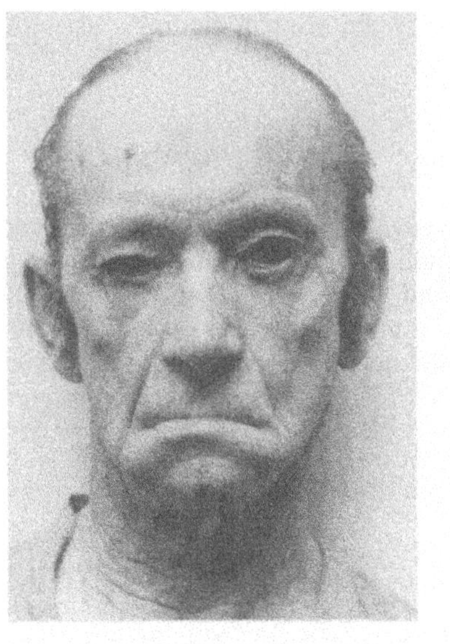

a

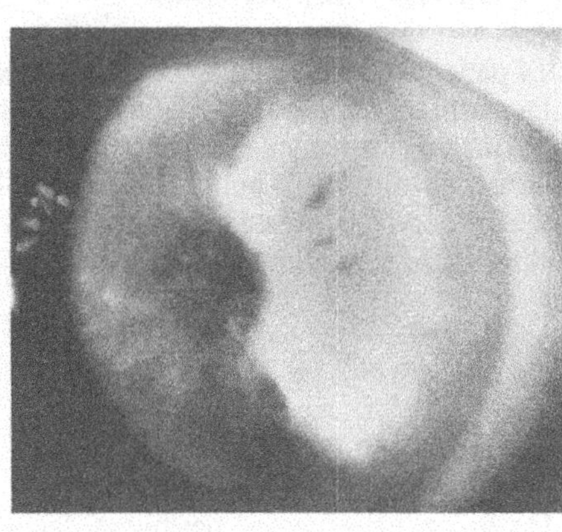

b

Figure 1a. The facial appearance of a 73-year old man. Figure 1b. Corneal lattice dystrophy in the left eye of a 71-year-old woman.

3.4. NEUROPHYSIOLOGICAL FINDINGS

Electroneuromyography revealed dysfunction of the facial nerve in all 14 patients. Six of the patients had findings of distal sensorimotor polyneuropathy, and seven had carpal tunnel syndrome. The central responses were abnormal or delayed in almost half of the examinations of the brainstem auditory evoked potentials. Both visual and somatosensory evoked potentials showed delayed central responses in some patients. Blink reflexes were abnormal in 9 patients.

3.5. HISTOPATHOLOGICAL FINDINGS

All biopsies (Table 3) taken from muscle, skin and sural nerve stained with Congo red and showed green birefringence and red-green dichroism when viewed in polarized light. Rectum biopsies were positive for amyloid only in half of the cases.

Table 3. Amyloid in biopsy samples

Sural nerve		Muscle	
Perineurium	11/11	Vessel walls	14/14
Epineural blood vessels	9/11	Endo-/perimysium	12/14
Skin		**Rectum**	
Epidermal basement membrane	13/13	Vessel walls	6/13
Eccrine sweat glands	13/13		

4. Conclusions

FAF is a progressive systemic disorder with widespread amyloid deposition in the tissues. All examined patients had corneal lattice dystrophy changes and dysfunction of the facial nerve, which are the most characteristic clinical findings and important criteria for the diagnosis. Neurophysiological methods can be used as additional, diagnostic examinations. All biopsies of skin, muscle and sural nerve were diagnostic for amyloid accumulation. Neurological examinations showed that this disorder involves not only the cranial, but also the spinal nerves and the autonomic nervous system. No evidence of dementia was found in the patients studied.

We conclude that Finnish familial amyloidosis differs from the other hereditary amyloidoses by its distinct ophthalmological and neurological manifestations. This is compatible with recent studies which show that the amyloid protein in FAF is homologous to gelsolin with an amino acid sequence clearly different from all other known amyloid proteins.

5. References

1. Meretoja,J.(1969) 'Familial systemic paramyloidosis with lattice corneal dystrophy of the cornea', Ann.Clin.Res.1, 314-324
2. Meretoja,J.(1973) 'Genetic aspects of familial amyloidosis with corneal lattice dystrophy and cranial neuropathy', Clin.Genet.4, 173-185
3. Boysen,G., Galassi,G., Kamieniecka,Z., Schlaeger,J.and Trojaborg,W.(1979) 'Familial amyloidosis with cranial neuropathy and corneal lattice dystrophy', J.Ncurol.Ncurosurg.Psychiatry 42, 1020-1030
4. Winkelman,J.E., Delleman,J.W.,et al (1971) 'Ein hereditäres Syndrom, bestehend aus peripherer Polyneuropathie, Hautveränderungen und gittriger Dystrophie der Hornhaut', Klin.Monatsbl.Augenheilkd. 159, 618-623
5. Darras,B.T., Adelman,L.S., Mora,J.S., Bodziner,R.A., and Munsat,T.L.(1986) 'Familial amyloidosis with cranial neuropathy and corneal lattice dystrophy', Neurology 36, 432-435
6. Meretoja,J.,(1972) 'Comparative histopathological and clinical findings in eyes with lattice corneal dystrophy of two different types', Ophthalmologica 165, 15-37
7. Meretoja,J.and Teppo,L.(1971) 'Histopathological findings of amyloidosis with cranial neuropathy as principal manifestation', APMIS Section A 79,432-440
8. Maury,C.P.K., Alli,K. and Baumann,M.(1990) 'Finnish hereditary amyloidosis, Amino acid sequence homology between the amyloid fibril protein and human plasma gelsoline', FEBS Letters 260, 85-87
9. Haltia,M., Prelli,F., Ghiso,J., Kiuru,S., Somer,H., Palo,J. and Frangione,B.(1990) 'Amyloid protein in familial amyloidosis (Finnish type) is homologous to gelsolin, an actin-binding protein', Biochem.Biophys.Res.Commun.167, 927-932
10. Haltia,M., Ghiso,J.,Prelli,F.,Gallo,G., Kiuru,S.,Somer,H.,Palo,J. and Frangione,B.(1990) 'Amyloid in familial amyloidosis, Finnish type, is antigenically and structurally related to gelsolin', Am.J.Path.136, 1223-1228

SHARED GELSOLIN ANTIGENICITY BETWEEN FAMILIAL AMYLOIDOSIS FINNISH TYPE (FAF) AND ONE FORM OF FAMILIAL LATTICE CORNEAL DYSTROPHY (LCD) WITH POLYNEUROPATHY FROM THE UNITED STATES

P.D. Gorevic
P.C. Munoz
Dept. of Medicine
State University of New York
Stony Brook, New York 11794

M. Rodrigues
Dept. of Ophthalmology
University of Maryland
Baltimore, Maryland 21201

M. Haltia
J. Ghiso
B. Frangione
Department of Pathology
New York Univ. Medical Center
New York, New York 10016

ABSTRACT

Amyloid may involve the cornea in sporadic and familial forms of LCD, as Polymorphic Amyloid Degeneration (PAD), primary gelatinous drop-like dystrophy or, in rare cases, as part of systemic light chain deposition. LCD is prominent in Familial Amyloidosis, Finnish type (FAF), clinical features of which have also been described in rare kindreds from the Netherlands, Denmark and the United States. Previous studies from our laboratories have found AP, but not AA, AL or prealbumin (transthyretin)-reactivity in cases of FAF, hereditary and sporadic LCD from the United States, and PAD examined immunohistologically and by Western Blot analysis of solubilized corneal proteins. Because we have now shown the FAF amyloid to be composed of a 12 kD internal fragment of plasma or cytoplasmic gelsolin, we sought to extend our previous observations using a rabbit antibody developed to the FAF subunit protein, and a commercially-available murine monoclonal antibody to plasma gelsolin. Anti-FAF reacted strongly in tissue section with amyloid deposits from Finnish patients in kidney and cornea, as well as with cornea, conjunctival and skin amyloid deposits from one previously described (Ophthalmology 9:1512, 1983) American case of Meretoja-type familial LCD. No reaction was obtained with cases of sporadic LCD (3), PAD (2) or drop dystrophy (1). The murine antibody, which is specific for a peptide that includes the carboxy terminal actin-binding site of gelsolin, also reacted with amyloid deposits in various tissues of FAF patients (Amer. J. Pathol. 136:1223-1228, 1990). Anti-gelsolin did not react with cases of AL, AA or prealbumin (TTr)-related amyloid in tissue section. It thus appears that sporadic LCD, PAD and drop dystrophy are antigenically distinct from FAF and at least one form of familial LCD; additional studies will be necessary to determine if the former are due to fibril formation involving other gelsolin epitopes, or are due to other amyloidogenic proteins.

INTRODUCTION

Clinical and pathologic studies have delineated several distinct forms of corneal amyloidosis (Table I) [1] Lattice Corneal Dystrophy (LCD) Type II is inherited in an autosomal dominant pattern with most cases presumed to be heterozygous [2]. Although the large majority of patients have been described from Finland [3], additional sibships have been reported from the Netherlands [4], Denmark [5] and in three families in the United States [6-8]. In 1983, Purcell et al described a 79 year-old American male of Irish descent with LCD who had undergone bilateral upper/lower lid blepharoplasties for "flabby eyelids", found to have bilateral peripheral VII nerve palsies; a 23 year-old daughter was found to have asymptomatic early LCD. Immunoperoxidase stains on paraffin sections of corneal tissue, skin and conjunctiva of the propositus were negative using antibodies to AA, transthyretin (prealbumin), as well as immunoglobulin light chain determinants, and it was concluded that amyloid deposition in this disorder likely was due to a unique form of subunit protein [8].

Recent developments have allowed us to reexamine this observation. We [9] and others [10] have now reported the isolation of a novel amyloid fibril subunit protein from cases of familial amyloidosis, Finnish type (FAF), with the amino terminal sequence of gelsolin starting at position 173 of the molecule. This subunit protein appears to be a variant molecule, with a substitution of asparagine for aspartic acid at position 15. Polyclonal antibodies raised to the FAF subunit react with amyloid in tissue (kidney, cornea, skin), whereas anti-TTr/Pa, L-chain and AA do not [11].

Table I

THE CORNEAL AMYLOIDOSES HISTOLOGY

	Age Onset of Symptoms (yrs)	Heredity*	Corneal Lesions	Bowman's Layer-Epithelium	Stroma	Other Ocular Amyloid	Systemic Amyloid
Lattice Dystrophics							
Type I	10-40	D	Central Lattice Dots	++	++ Anterior	No	No
Type II	30-40	D	Peripheral Paracentral Lattice	0	++ Anterior	Conjunctiva Adnexal	Yes
Type III	70-90	R	Thick Lattice	+++	++ Anterior	No	No
Polymorphic Amyloid Degeneration	>50	S	Central/ Peripheral Punctate Filamentous	0	++ Posterior	No	No
Primary Gelatinous Drop-Like Dystrophy	0-20	R	Central	+++	0	No	No

*Autosomal dominant (D) or Recessive (R); Sporadic (S)

MATERIALS AND METHODS

Studies were performed on three cases of LCD Type 1, one case of LCD Type 2 from the United States previously reported [8], and six cases of FAF recently characterized immunohistologically [11]. Corneas were obtained at the time of keratoplasty and other tissue by biopsy or at autopsy. Also studied was fixed tissue from two cases of polymorphic amyloid degeneration (PAD) [12] and one of primary gelatinous drop dystrophy of the cornea [13] (Table I).

Amyloid deposits in formalin-fixed material were studied by congo red staining and by the indirect immunoperoxidase method, using biotin-avidin conjugates. Anti-AA, AP and TTr/Pa were produced in rabbits immunized with denatured subunit proteins (1:100-1:200 division), and anti-FAF as reported.[11,14]. A commercially obtained murine monoclonal antibody to human plasma gelsolin (Sigma) is specific for an epitope located on the 47kD peptide derived from a chymotryptic cleavage of the protein. Controls included normal human cornea, replacements of primary antisera with normal rabbit or normal mouse serum or saline, and concomitant testing of primary antisera at dilutions of 1:50 to 1:1000 on known cases of human secondary (AA), L-chain associated (AL) or senile cardiac (TTr/Pa) amyloidosis.

RESULTS

Rabbit anti-FAF and the murine monoclonal antibody to plasma gelsolin reacted strongly in tissue section with amyloid deposits from Finnish patients in kidney and cornea [11], as well as cornea, conjunctival and skin amyloid deposits from the American case of Meretoja-type familial LCD [18]. Corneal staining showed predominantly stromal deposits, though with some smaller collections of amyloid up to the level of Bowman's layer. Skin and adnexal amyloid prominently involved the subepithelial basement membrane and occurred in a typical distribution surrounding appendages. No reaction was obtained with cases of LCD, Type 1, PAD or drop dystrophy. Furthermore, antigelsolin antibodies did not react with cases of AL, AA or TTr/Pa-related amyloid in tissue section.

DISCUSSION

Our studies indicate that it may be possible to distinguish Type II from other forms of LCD and corneal amyloidosis immunohistologically on the basis of anti-gelsolin reactivity. This may provide a valuable adjunct to clinical distinctions between the three types of LCD on the basis of age of onset, mode of inheritance, location of amyloid deposits within the corneal stroma, configuration and thickness of the lattice lines, incidence of corneal erosions or iritis, and associated facial/peripheral neuropathy and systemic amyloidosis (Table I) (15). Although LCD, Type II appears to be immunohistologically distinct from LCD, Type I, PAD and drop dystrophy, these observations need to be confirmed by biochemical analysis of the subunit proteins of the various forms of corneal amyloid.

ACKNOWLEDGEMENTS

This work was partially supported by a grant from the American Heart Association.

REFERENCES

1. Rodrigues MM, Krachmer JH: (1988) Recent Advances in Corneal Dystrophy and Amyloid Corneal Degeneration; *Amer. J. Ophthamol.*, 98:216-224.
2. Meretoja F: (1973) Genetic Aspects of Familial Amyloidosis with Corneal Lattice Dystrophy and cranial Neuropathy. *Clin. Genetics*, 4:173-185.
3. Meretoja J: (1969) Familial Systemic Paraamyloidosis with Lattice Dystrophy of the Cornea, Progressive Cranial Neuropathy, Skin Changes and Various Internal Symptoms. *Ann. Clin. Res.*, 1:314-324.
4. Winkelman JE, Delleman JW, Ansink BJJ: (1971) Ein Hereditare Syndrom Bestehend Aus Peripherer Polyneuropathie, Haut-Veranderunger Und Gittriger Dystrophie Der Hornhaut; *Klin Monatsbl Augenheilkd*, 159:618-623.
5. Boysen G, Galassi G, Kamieniecka Z, Schlaeger J, Trojaborg W: (1979) Familial Amyloidosis with Cranial Neuropathy and Corneal Lattice Dystrophy; *J. Neurol. Neurosug. Psych.*, 42:1020-1030.
6. Darras BT, Adelman LS, Mora JS, Broziner RA, Munsat TL: (1979) Familial Amyloidosis with Cranial Neuropathy and Corneal Lattice Dystrophy; *Neurology*, 36:432-435.
7. Sack G, Dumars KW, Gummerson KS, Law A, McKosick VA: (1981) Three Forms of Dominant Amyloid Neuropathy; *The Johns Hopkins Med. J.*, 149:239-247.
8. Purcell JJ Jr, Rodgrigues MM, Christi MI, Riner AN, Dooley JM: (1983) Lattice Corneal Dystrophy Associated with Familial Systemic Amyloidosis (Meretoja's Syndrome); *Ophthalmology*, 90:1512-1517.
9. Haltia M, Prelli F, Ghiso J, Kiuru S, Somer H, Palo J, Frangione B: (1990) Amyloid Protein in Familial Amyloidosis (Finnish Type) is Homologous to Gelsolin, An Actin-Binding Protein; *Biochem . Biophys. Res. Commun.*, 167:927-932.
10. Maury CPJ, Alli K, Baumann M: (1990) Finnish Hereditary Amyloidosis, Amino Acid Sequence Homology Between the Amyloid Fibril Protein and Human Plasma Gelsolin; *FEBS Letters*, 260:85-87.
11. Haltia M, Ghiso J, Prelli F, Gallo G, Kiuru S, Somer H, Palo J, Frangione B: (1990) Amyloid in Familial Amyloidosis, Finnish Type, is Antigenically and Structurally Related to Gelsolin; *Amer. J. Pathol.*, 136:1223-1228.
12. Mannis MJ, Krachmer JH, Rodrigues MM, Pardos GJ: (1981), Polymorphic Amyloid Degeneration of the Cornea. A Clinical and Histopathologic Study; *Arch. Ophthalmol*, 99:1217-1223.
13. Weber FL, Babel J: (1980) Gelatinous Drop-Like Dystrophy: A Form of Primary Corneal Amyloidosis; *Arch Ophth.*, 98:144-148.
14. Gorevic PD, Rodrigues MM, Krachmer JH, Green C, Fujihara S, Glenner GG: (1984) Lack of Evidence for Protein AA Reactivity in Amyloid Deposits of Lattice Corneal Dystrophy and Amyloid Corneal Degeneration; *Amer. J. Ophthamol*, 98:216-224.
15. Meretoja J: (1972) Comparative Histopathological and Clinical Findings in Eyes with Lattice Corneal Dystrophy of Two Different Types; *Ophthalmologica*, 165:15-37.

POLYPEPTIDE HORMONES AND AMYLOID

P. WESTERMARK AND K. H. JOHNSON
Department of Pathology, University of Linköping, Sweden
and Department of Veterinary Pathobiology, College of Veterinary Medicine, University of Minnesota, S:t Paul, Minnesota, USA

A stromal hyaline change has been known for a long time to occur in some hormone producing tissues. Most commonly this has been seen in the islets of Langerhans and in medullary carcinoma of the thyroid. The very localized nature of the hyaline change together with some difficulties in staining contributed to the delay in accepting this hyaline change as a form of amyloid. Contemporary analyses and definitions have made it clear, however, that these alterations fullfil the criteria for amyloid. It was not until 1976 that the molecular nature of one of the "endocrine amyloids", that in the medullary carcinoma of the thyroid, was clarified, showing the polypeptide hormone derivation of the fibrils (1). Since then, three other polypeptide hormone-derived amyloid forms have been analyzed by amino acid sequence analysis. This short overview deals with these four amyloid forms (for more detailed reviews, see 2,3). After this brief review of the four forms, I will discuss some possible mechanisms that might be of importance in the pathogenesis of these localized form of endocrine amyloid deposition.

1. Amyloid in medullary carcinoma of the thyroid.

Medullary carcinoma of the thyroid (MCT) is derived from the C-cells and constitutes ≈ 5% of thyroid carcinomas. Amyloid is one of the hallmarks of the tumour but does not occur in all cases. Thus in a recent study of 121 tumours, amyloid was seen in 82% of the tumours (to be published). Amyloid deposits occur typically in the stroma and can constitute a major part of the tumour mass.

The major amyloid fibril protein of MCT is derived from procalcitonin. Partial amino acid sequence analysis of a 6 kDa protein showed identity with calcitonin, but since the protein was larger than calcitonin and had a different amino acid composition, it was concluded to be procalcitonin. As is seen in a recent study (4) on amyloid from another patient, both procalcitonin and mature calcitonin can constitute the amyloid fibrils in MCT. It is possible that mature calcitonin was present also in the first studied material. No fragmentation of the calcitonin was seen. The calcitonin gene is complex and expresses both calcitonin and calcitonin gene-related peptide (CGRP) by alternative splicing (5). Although calcitonin and CGRP are completely different, their precursors contain common N-terminal regions, which is split off at positions of double basic amino acid residues. It is interesting to note that CGRP is related to another amyloid forming protein, IAPP (see below).

There are no data indicating that presence of amyloid has any clinical significance, as for example the prognosis of MCT.

2. Amyloid in islets of Langerhans and in insulinomas.

Islet amyloidosis is one of the most common amyloid forms and is a form of typical "senile amyloidosis" with steadily increasing prevalence with age. In the age group over 60 years some deposits are seen in > 50% of individuals. However, islet amyloidosis is even more common and more extensive in type II diabetes where the majority (> 90%) of the patients have islet amyloid deposits. Islet amyloidosis is not known to occur in type I diabetes, where ß-cells have been destroyed. In type 2 diabetes, the islet amyloid fibrils appear to be a product of the ß-cells. This relationship as well as the common occurrence of amyloid in insulinomas but not in other endocrine pancreatic tumours (e.g. glucagonomas) (6) led to the assumption that islet amyloid fibrils consisted of insulin or proinsulin. Therefore, the finding that the main fibril protein of amyloid of an insulinoma was a previously unknown polypeptide distinct from proinsulin but with partial identity with CGRP was completely unexpected (7). Further studies revealed that the major fibril protein in amyloid of the islets of Langerhans and of insulinomas is a 37 amino acid residue polypeptide, designated islet amyloid polypeptide (IAPP; a commercial term is amylin) (8,9). Human IAPP is expressed as a 89 amino acid residue prepropeptide consisting of a signal sequence and IAPP, which is flanked by two short propeptides linked N- and C-terminally to the mature IAPP by double basic amino acid residues (10-12). Thus, the overall structure of the precursor much resembles that of calcitonin and CGRP. It should also be noted that the processing of proinsulin is similar. Here, a central segment (the C-peptide) is cleaved off in double basic amino acid residues, giving rise to the mature 2-chain insulin molecule (13). It is likely that the conversion of pro-IAPP is performed by the same enzymes as for conversion of proinsulin in the secretory granules.

IAPP is selectively expressed by ß-cells both in humans and in other mammals. It is co-stored with insulin in the secretory granules and is released together with this hormone (14-16) and is also known to be present in the plasma.

Synthetic human IAPP is a strongly amyloidogenic protein in vitro; its amyloidogenic properties most certainly depend on residues in the 20-30 segment of the molecule (11,17). This part of the IAPP molecule is least conserved between species, as is in contrast to the highly conserved N- and C-terminal parts. The interspecies variations at positions 20-29 seem to explain why islet amyloid only occurs in some species like man, cat and monkeys (18,19).

3. Isolated atrial amyloid (IAA).

Amyloid deposits in the heart are very common in aged individuals. The most common form affects only the atria and is designated isolated atrial amyloid (IAA), which is seen in almost 80% of persons over 80 years of age (20,21). The deposits are usually small but can be rather heavy and occur mainly outside and along myocytes. Electron microscopic studies indicate that the fibrils mainly form in close contact with the sarcolemma (22). The atrial myocytes function as endocrine cells which synthesize atrial natriuretic factor (ANF). ANF is the 28 amino acid residue C-terminal part of the 126 amino acid precursor, pro-ANF (23). Pro-ANF is stored in cytoplasmic granules and, within the granules or at the area of release, is cleaved to give rise to ANF. Immunohistochemical and immunocytochemical studies of several cases of IAA have shown that this amyloid binds antibodies to ANF (22,24,25). Amino acid sequence analysis of a major fibril protein of IAA has shown that the protein is ANF (25,26). In one case, the majority of the protein was uncleaved but a small part was N-terminally truncated (25).

IAA is associated with some chronic heart diseases (27,28) but IAA itself is usually of no clinical importance. However, when the deposits are more extensive it cannot be ruled out that they influence the conduction system and and/or the release of ANP.

4. Insulin-derived amyloid forms.

Insulin-derived amyloid was first demonstrated in vivo at the insulin injection site of two patients with diabetes mellitus (29,30). In the single case where the amyloid was purified and analyzed, the fibrils contained whole and uncleaved porcine insulin molecules (30). Formation of such local insulin-derived amyloid masses seems to be a rare event. However, insulin can easily be converted to a fibrillar form in vitro. The fibrils have typical amyloid properties.

Insulin (or proinsulin) was long believed to be the main constituent in human and cat islet amyloid, which later was shown to be IAPP derived. A very recent finding closes the circle; islet amyloid in the degu (a south American rodent) consists of unmodified insulin A and B chains (31).

POSSIBLE FACTORS IN THE PATHOGENESIS OF POLYPEPTIDE HORMONE DERIVED AMYLOID FIBRILS

Why do some polypeptide hormones commonly give rise to amyloid fibrils? There is no definite answer yet, but I will mention a few factors that may be of importance.
1. Size. Amyloid fibril proteins are almost always small molecules which probably are more or less necessary for the fibril formation. Polypeptide hormones have a size that should be suitable for amyloid fibril formation.
2. Local concentration. The local concentrations of the polypeptide hormones are certainly very high in the granules but also extracellularly at the site of release. In vitro studies with synthetic IAPP peptides have shown the importance of concentration in amyloid fibril formation (19). Studies with cat islet amyloid also indicate that overexpression of IAPP is involved in the pathogenesis of islet amyloid (32).
3. Primary structure of the polypeptide. Inherent amyloidogenic amino acid sequences probably exist. This may explain why only some polypeptide hormones in only some species give rise to amyloid fibrils. Using synthetic peptides corresponding to IAPP 20-29 in an in vitro fibril formation system, an amyloidogenic segment (AILS, corresponding to IAPP 25-28 of human and cat) has been identified (19). Proline residues in position 25, 28 and 29 occur in IAPP of species without islet amyloid. Substitutions of Ser 28 with Pro seems to especially protect against fibril formation.
4. Conformation and conformational changes. A high degree of ß-pleated sheet conformation is often present in amyloid precursor proteins - examples being transthyretin and $ß_2$-microglobulin. Interestingly, ANF and insulin have little ß-sheet conformation in solution. However, when insulin is converted into fibrils, a high degree of ß-structure occurs (33). Likewise, ANF, when bound to lipid adopts a substantial amount of ß-structure (34). Therefore, in the latter case, it is possible that fibril formation can occur when ANF binds to lipids, e.g. cell membranes. Similar conformational changes could also be of importance with other polypeptide hormones.
5. Partial degradation of the amyloid precursor. In many forms of amyloidosis, the fibril proteins are partially degraded and often heterogenic. In the polypeptide hormone derived amyloids, degradation of the hormones does not seem to be of importance in fibrillogenesis. Only in one form, IAA, a partial N-terminal truncation was seen in a small portion of the protein. However, this may be a preparation artefact (25).
6. Aberrant processing of the hormone precursor. All studies of polypeptide hormone derived amyloids have indicated that no amino acid substitution is present. However, a defect cleavage of the precursors could theoretically disturb the normal pathways for processing and release. Therefore, the finding that the MCT amyloid consists of a

mixture of procalcitonin and mature calcitonin is of considerable interest. In the sequence analysis of the other polypeptide hormone derived amyloids, no precursors have been found but these may well have been lost in the purification procedure. On the other hand, immune electron microscopical studies have shown the presence of pro-ANF in IAA (unpublished result) and pro-IAPP in islet amyloid (35). The latter finding is especially interesting since proinsulin and pro-IAPP probably are processed by the same enzymes and since one deviation in type 2 diabetes and insulinomas is an increased proportion of proinsulin released from the ß-cells (36). In conclusion, it is possible that a defective processing of the precursors are of importance in the formation of most polypeptide hormone derived amyloids.

7. Interaction with other components. The role of other substances than the hormones themselves in the polypeptide hormone-derived amyloids is not known. However, other components, such as the P-component and proteoglycans, are generally present in the amyloid.

FINAL REMARK

Already in 1938, Gellerstedt (37) pointed out that the "senile" amyloids contain many interesting problems worth while to study. Only lately, the study of polypeptide hormone-derived amyloid forms has proved to be a unique tool for the study of concentrated forms of polypeptide hormones in association with several disease states. For example, IAPP was not known to exist until it was isolated from insulinoma amyloid deposits. Thus, the study of the endocrine amyloids, which for a long time appeared to be mainly of academic interest, has become important in polypeptide hormone research.

References

1. Sletten, K., Westermark, P., Natvig, J.B. (1976) Characterization of amyloid firil proteins from medullary carcinoma of the thyroid. J. Exp. Med. 143:993-998.
2. Westermark, P., and Johnson, K.H. (1988) The polypeptide hormone-derived amyloid forms: Nonspecific alterations or signs of abnormal peptide-processing? APMIS 96:475-483.
3. Johnson, K.H., O'Brien, T.D., Betsholtz, C., and Westermark, P. (1989) Islet amyloid, islet-amyloid polypeptide, and diabetes. N. Engl. J. Med. 321:513-518
4. Sletten, K., Natvig, J.B., and Westermark, P. Chracterization of molecular forms of calcitonin in amyloid fibrils from medullary carcinoma of the thyroid. In J.B. Natvig, Ø. Førre, A. Husebekk, G. Husby, B. Skogen, K. Sletten and P. Westermark (eds.), Amyloid and Amyloidosis, Kluwer Academic Publishers, Dordrect. In press.
5. Amara, S.G., Jonas, V., Rosenfeld, M.G., Ong, E. S., and Evans, R.M. (1982) Alternative RNA processing in calcitonin gene expression generates mRNAs encoding different polypeptide products. Nature 298:240-244.
6. Westermark, P., Grimelius, L., Polak, J.M., Larsson, L.-I., van Noorden, S., Wilander, E., and Pearse, A.G.E. (1977) Amyloid in polypeptide hormone-producing tumors. Lab. Invest. 37:212-215.
7. Westermark, P., Wernstedt, C., Wilander, E., and Sletten, K.A. (1986) A novel peptide in the calcitonin gene related peptide family as an amyloid fibril protein in the endocrine pancreas. Biochem. Biophys. Res. Commun. 140:827-831.

8. Westermark, P., Wernstedt, C., Wilander, E., Hayden, D.W., O'Brien, T.D., and Johnson, K.H. (1987) Amyloid fibrils in human insulinoma and islets of Langerhans of the diabetic cat are derived from a novel neuropeptide-like protein also present in normal islet cells. Proc. Natl. Acad. Sci, USA 84:381-388.
9. Cooper, G.J.S., Willis, A.C., Clark, A., Turner, R.C., Sim., R.B., & Reid, K.B.M. (1987) Purification and characterization of a peptide from amyloid-rich pancreases of type 2 diabetic patients. Proc. Natl. Acad. Sci. USA 84:8628-8632.
10. Sanke, T., Bell, G.I., Sample, C., Rubenstein, A.H., and Steiner, D.F. (1988) An islet amyloid polypeptide is derived from an 89-amino acid precursor by proteolytic processing. J. Biol. Chem. 263:17243-17246.
11. Betsholtz, C., Svensson, V., Rorsman, F., Engström, U., Westermark, G.T., Wilander, E., Johnson, K., and Westermark, P. (1989) Islet amyloid polypeptide (IAPP): cDNA cloning and identification of an amyloidogenic region associated with the species-specific of age-related diabetes mellitus. Exp. Cell. Res. 183:484-493.
12. Mosselman, S., Höppener, J.W.M., Lips, C.J.M., and Jansz, H.S. (1989) The complete islet amyloid polypeptide precursor is encoded by two exons. FEBS Lett. 247:154-158.
13. Nolan, C., Margoliash, E., Peterson, J.D., and Steiner, D.F. (1971) The Structure of Bovine Proinsulin. J. Biol. Chem. 246:2780-2795.
14. Johnson, K.H..,O'Brien, T.D., Hayden, D.W., Jordan, K., Ghobrial, H.K.G., Mahoney, W.C., Westermark, P. (1988) Immunolocalization of islet amyloid polypeptide (IAPP) in pancreatic beta cells by means of peroxidase-antiperoxidase (PAP) and protein A-gold techniques. Am. J. Pathol. 130:1-8.
15. Lukinius, A., Wilander, E., Westermark, G.T., Engström, U., and Westermark, P. (1989) Co-localization of islet amyloid polypeptide and insulin in the B cell secretory granules of the human pancreatic islets. Diabetologia 32:240-244.
16. Clark, A., Edwards, C.A., Ostle, L.R., Sutton, R., Rothbard, J.B., Morris, J.F., and Turner, R.C. (1989) Localisation of islet amyloid peptide in lipofuscin bodies and secretory granules of human B-cells and in isets of type-2 diabetic subjects. Cell Tissue Res. 257:179-185.
17. Glenner, G.G., Eanes, E.D., and Wiley, C.A. (1988) Amyloid fibrils formed from a segment of the pancreatic islet amyloid protein. Biochem. Biophys. Res. Commun. 155:608-614.
18. Betsholtz, C., Christmanson, L., Engström, U., Rorsman, F., Jordan, K., O'Brien, T.D., Murtaugh, M., Johnson, K.H., and Westermark, P. (1990) Structure of cat islet amyloid polypeptide and identification of amino acid residues of pontential significance for islet amyloid formation. Diabetes 39:118-122.
19. Westermark, P., Engström, U., Johnson, K.H., Westermark, G.T., and Betsholtz, C. (1990) Islet amyloid polypeptide: Pinpointing amino acid residues linked to amyloid fibril formation. Proc. Natl. Acad. Sci. 87:5036-5040.
20. Westermark, P., Johansson, B., and Natvig, J.B. (1979) Senile cardiac amyloidosis: Evidence of two different amyloid substances in the ageing heart. Scand. J. Immunol. 10:303-308.
21. Cornwell, G.G.III., Murdoch, W.L., Kyle, R.A., Westermark, P., and Pitkänen, P. (1983) Frequency and distribution of senile cardiovascular amyloid. A clinicopathologic correlation. Am. J. Med. 75:618-623.

22. Johansson, B., and Westermark, P. (1990) The relation of atrial natriuretic factor to isolated atrial amyloid. Exp. Mol. Path. 52:266-278
23. Oikawa, S., Imai, M., Ueno, A., Tanaka, S., Noguchi, T., Nakazato, H., Kangawa, K., Fukuda, A., and Matsuo, H. (1984) Cloning and sequence analysis of cDNA encoding a precursor for human atrial natriuretic polypeptide. Nature 309:724-726.
24. Kaye, G.C., Butler, M.G., D'Ardenne, A.J., Edmondson, S.J., Camm, A.J., and Slavin, G. (1986) Isolated atrial amyloid contains atrial natriuretic peptide: a report of six cases. Br. Heart. J. 56:317-320.
25. Johansson, B., Wernstedt, C., and Westermark, P. (1987) Atrial natriuretic peptide deposited as artrial amyloid fibrils. Biochem. Biophys. Res. Commun. 148:1087-1092.
26. Linke, R.P., Voigt, C., Störkel, F.S., Eulitz, M. (1988) N-terminal amino acid sequence analysis indicates that isolated atrial amyloid is derived from atrial natriuretic peptide. Virchows Arch. B 55:125-127.
27. Johansson, B., and Westermark, P. Isolated atrial amyloidosis. Increased frequency in patients with congestive cardiac failure. In J.B. Natvig, Ø. Førre, A. Husebekk, G. Husby,B Skogen, K. Sletten and P. Westermark (eds.) Amyloid and Amyloidosis, Kluwer Academic Publishers, Dordrecht, in press.
28. Looi, L.M. Raised prevalence of isolated atrial amyloidosis in chronic heart disease. In J.B. Natvig, Ø. Førre, A. Husebekk, G. Husby, B. Skogen, K. Sletten and P. Westermark, Kluwer Academic Publishers, Dordrecht, in press.
29. Störkel, S., Scheider, H.-M., Muntefering, H., and Kashiwagi, S. (1983) Iatrogenic, insulin-dependent, local amyloidosis. Lab. Invest. 48:108-111.
30. Dische, F.E., Wernstedt, C., Westermark, G.T., Westermark P., Pepys, M.B., Rennie, J.A., Gilbey, S.G., and Watkins, P.J. (1988) Insulin as an amyloid-fibril protein at sites of repeated insulin injections in a diabetic patient. Diabetologia 31:158-161, 1988.
31. Hellman, U., Wernstedt, C., Westermark, P., O'Brien, T.D., Rathbun, W.B., and Johnson, K.H. (1990) Amino acid sequence from degu islet amyloid-derived insulin shows unique sequence characteristics. Biochem. Biophys. Res. Commun. 169:571-577.
32. Johnson, K.H., O'Brien, T.D., Jordan, K., Westermark, P. (1989) Impaired glucose tolerance is associated with increased islet amyloid polypeptide (IAPP) immunoreactivity in pancreatic beta cells. Am. J. Pathol. 135:245-250.
33. Burke, M.J., and Rougvie, M.A. (1972) Cross-ß Protein Structures. I. Insulin fibrils. Biochemistry 11:2435-2439.
34. Surewicz, W.K., Mantsch, H.H., Stahl, G.L., and Epand, R.M. (1987) Infrared spectroscopic evidence of conformational transitions of an atrial natriuretic peptide. Proc. Natl. Acad. Sci. USA 84:7028-7030.
35. Westermark, P., Engström, U., Westermark, G.T., Johnson, K.H., Permerth, J., and Betsholtz, C. (1989) Islet amyloid polypeptide (IAPP) and pro-IAPP immunoreactivity in human islets of Langerhans. Diabetes Res. Clin. Pract. 7:219-226.
36. Porte, D., and Kahn, S.E. (1989) Perspectives in Diabetes. Hyperproinsulinemia and amyloid in NIDDM. Clues toetiology of islet ß-cell dysfunction? Diabetes 38:1333-1336.
37. Gellerstedt, N. (1938) Die elektive, insulära (Para=) Amyloidose der Bauchspeicheldrüse. Zugleich ein Beitrag zur Kenntnis der "senilen Amyloidose". Beitr. Path. Anat. 101:1-13.

Islet amyloid polypeptide (IAPP): structure of its cDNA and gene and the identification of species differences of importance for islet amyloid formation.

Christer Betsholtz[1], Lars Christmanson[1], Fredrik Rorsman[1], Viveka Svensson[1], Göran Stenman[2] Kenneth H. Johnson[3] & Per Westermark[4]

[1]*Department of Pathology, University Hospital, S-751 85 Uppsala,* [2]*Department of Oral Pathology, Gothenburg University, Box 33070, S-400 33 Göteborg and* [3]*Department of Veterinary Pathobiology, College of Medicine, University of Minnesota, St. Paul, Minnesota, USA and* [4]*Department of Pathology, University Hospital, S-581 85 Linköping, Sweden.*

The human islet amyloid polypeptide (IAPP) cDNA and gene have been characterized. The cDNA sequence predicts an 89-amino-acid precursor protein from which the 37-amino-acid mature IAPP peptide is formed by N- and C-terminal proteolytic processing. The presence of conserved proteolytic cleavage sites indicate that the IAPP molecule is a normal secretory product of the pancreatic β-cell. Sequence analysis of the normal IAPP gene also indicates that IAPP found in islet amyloid is not mutated. The IAPP gene consists of at least 3 exons of which the first exon is non-coding, the second exon encodes the signal peptide and part of the N-terminal prosequence and the third exon encodes the remainder of that sequence, the IAPP peptide and the C-terminal prosequence. IAPP mRNA was found exclusively in β-cells of the islets of Langerhans. A functional and tissue-specific promoter region was identified in the 5' flanking sequence of the gene. The human IAPP gene mapped to two regions of chomosome 12. Finally, analysis of the IAPP cDNA sequence in several species with or without tendency to develop islet amyloid demonstrated differences in a part of the IAPP molecule which is likely to determine its amyloidogenic properties.

INTRODUCTION

Islet amyloid polypeptide (IAPP) is the main constituent of the amyloid fibrils that occur in the islets of Langerhans of most type 2 diabetics (reviewed in ref 1). Small amounts of islet amyloid also develops in a high percentage of old humans. In other species, islet amyloid is found mainly in primates and cats in conjunction with spontaneous diabetes mellitus In these species, the amyloid fibril also consists of IAPP. Rodents, however, do not develop islet amyloid in association with diabetes mellitus except for the *Octodon degu*. However, in this species, the amyloid consists of insulin and not IAPP (2).

IAPP-derived islet amyloid is deposited in close contact with the β-cells indicating that these cells are the source of the peptide (3). This has been confirmed by immunohistochemistry (4). In addition, IAPP has been localized to the same secretory granules as insulin (5) indicating that the peptide is produced normally and probably cosecreted with insulin. Recently established IAPP radioimmunoassays have demonstrated the release of IAPP from isolated islets of Langerhans and *in vivo* following glucose administration (6-8).

The analyses of cDNA clones corresponding to human IAPP have predicted an 89-amino-acid IAPP precursor including a signal sequence for secretion as well as N- and C-terminal propeptides flanking the mature 37-amino-acid IAPP molecule (9-11). Interestingly, IAPP appears to be a normal and not an abberrant proteolytic cleavage product of the IAPP precursor. This conclusion is supported by the presence of consensus sites for proteolytic cleavage sites similar to those found in proinsulin. In addition, IAPP is homologous to the calcitonin-gene related peptides, CGRP-1 and -2, which are processed at analogous sites. The nature of the C-terminal processing sites in the IAPP and CGRP molecules indicates that the C-termini are amidated, a property which seems essential for the biological activity. Thus, CGRP-NH_2 (and to some extent IAPP-NH_2) induced cAMP production in liver cell membranes whereas CGRP-COOH and IAPP-COOH were inactive (10-12).

The physiological function of IAPP is poorly understood. Inhibitory effects on glycogen synthesis (13) and glucose transport (14) in skeletal muscle cells have been reported as well asthe induction of glucose intolerance in animals injected with IAPP (15-17). However, at present,

```
           signal peptide        N-term. propeptide     C-term. propeptide

IAPP   MGILKLQVFLIVLSVALNHLKA        TPIESHQVEKR      GKRNAVEVLKREPLNYLPL

                              mature peptide

IAPP             KCNTATCATQRLANFLVHSSNNFGAILSSTNVGSNTY -NH2
CGRP-1           A-D----V-H---GL-SR-GGVVKNNFVP-----KAF -NH2
CGRP-2           A------V-H---GL-SR-GGMVKSNFVP-----KAF -NH2
```

Figure 1. The amino acid sequence of the various parts of the IAPP precursor. The mature peptide is shown in comparison with CGRP-1 and -2. Horizontal bars indicate identity.

```
IAPP human        KCNTATCATQRLANFLVHSSNNFGAILSSTNVGSNTY -NH2
     cat          ----------------IR----L-----P-------- -NH2
     rat          -----------------R----L-PV-PP-------- -NH2
     mouse        -----------------R----L-PV-PP-------- -NH2
     hamster      -------------------N--L-PV--P-------- -NH2
     guinea pig   ------------T----R--H-L--A-LP-D------ -NH2
     degu         ------------T----R--H-L--A-PP-K------ -NH2
```

Figure 2. Comparison of the amino acid sequences of IAPP in various mammalian species. Of these, only human and cat develop IAPP-derived amyloid.

it cannot be excluded that these effects are elicited only at pharmacological doses of IAPP and do not reflect a physiological function of the peptide in glucose homeostasis. An interesting possibility is that IAPP participates in the pathogenesis of insulin resistance in type 2 diabetes. Since amyloid appears to be deposited progressively in the course of the disease, an IAPP overexpression situation might be envisioned. However, if IAPP is indeed overexpressed in type 2 diabetes, and to what extent this may influence amyloid formation and the development of insulin resistance, remain to be determined. Some support for an overexpression situation comes from the studies of spontaneous diabetes mellitus in cats, in which IAPP immunoreactivity is increased severalfold in the β-cells of prediabetic animals (18).

The restricted expression of IAPP (in addition to the pancreatic β−cell, which appears to be the principal site of IAPP synthesis, small amounts of IAPP mRNA and immunoreactivity have also been detected in the stomach and gut mucosa, in lung and in dorsal root ganglia (119)) and the potential involvement of the peptide in type 2 diabetes in humans and cats as well as the species-restricted occurence of islet amyloid highlight questions concerning the structure and expression of IAPP which can be addressed using molecular cloning techniques. The present report summarizes data on IAPP cDNA and gene cloning recently published by us and others.

RESULTS AND DISCUSSION

The human IAPP precursor structure as predicted from the cDNA sequence is shown in comparison between with the two members of the CGRP family in Figure 1. Notably, the cysteine residues are conserved indicating a similar tertiary structure. The most dissimilar part of the molecules, residues 20-29, appear to confer the amyloidogenic properties to the IAPP molecule. Thus, a peptide corresponding to this region readily forms amyloid fibrils *in vitro* as does the complete IAPP-peptide (11,20,23). The reason why only certain species develop IAPP-derived amyloid is likely to be explained primarily by differences in IAPP primary structure (Figure 2). Interestingly, the 20-29 regions of the IAPP molecules diverge considerably between the mammalian species investigated to-date, whereas the N- and C-terminal parts of the molecule are essentially conserved. Peptides corresponding to the IAPP 20-29 region in species that do not develop islet amyloid *in vivo*, e.g. hamster, rat and mouse, do not form amyloid fibrils *in vitro* in contrast to the corresponding human and cat peptides, which do (11,20-23). A careful analysis of the *in vitro* amyloidogenic properties of hybrid IAPP 20-29 peptides have indicated that a proline residue at position 28, which is found in e.g. rat and mouse, is strongly protective against amyloid fibril formation. In hamster, which like human and cat carries a serine residue at position 28, the protection against amyloid fibril formation seems to be provided by a combination of proline-valine at positions 25-26 and a proline residue in position 29 (23).

Cloning of the human IAPP gene have revealed that it is composed of three exons of which the first is non-coding, the second exon contains the translation initiation codon and encodes the signal peptide and part of the N-terminal propeptide and the third exon encodes the rest of the IAPP precursor including all of the mature IAPP peptide (10,24-26). Although the structure of the IAPP gene has been unequivocally determined by several groups, the exact positions of the transcription initiation site and promoter/enhancer elements remain controversial. In part, this might be explained by differential promoter usage in the various insulinomas and cell lines analysed. However, a functional and tissue-specific promoter/enhancer activity has been identified within 1500 bp of 5' flanking sequence (26). This sequence does not carry any obvious homology with the insulin promoter/enhancer region indicating that the two genes, although expressed by the same cells, have different transcriptional regulation. This is also supported by observations that insulin and IAPP mRNA levels in the pancreas are affected individually by diabetogenic treatment of rats (27). In addition, studies of primary cultures of pancreatic endocrine cells and established tumor cell lines indicate that IAPP and insulin may not necessarily be expressed by the same cell types (28).

The chromosomal localization of the IAPP gene also remians controversial. Two potential locations have been described on human chromosome 12, 12p12-p13 and 12q13-q14. Whereas Nishi et al (25) and Buckle et al (29) revealed only the former of these two peaks Cockburn and collaborators revealed only the latter (30) and our group revealed both peaks (26). The reason for this discrepancy is unknown. Southern blot analyses indicate the presence of a single IAPP locus in the human genome (24,26). The true position of this locus as well as the potential presence of a related gene on chromosome 12 remain to be determined.

REFERENCES

1. Johnson, K.H., O'Brien, T.D., Betsholtz, C. & Westermark, P. (1989) Islet amyloid, islet amyloid polypeptide and diabetes mellitus. *N.Engl.J.Med.* **321**:513-518.

2. Hellman, U., Wernstedt, C., Westermark, P., O'Brien, T.D., Rathburn, W. & Johnson, K.H. (1990) Amino acid sequence from the degu islet amyloid-derived insulin shows unique sequence characteristics. *Biochem.Biopys.Res.Commun.* **169**:571-577.

3.Westermark, P. (1973) Fine structure of islets of Langerhans in insular amyloidosis. *Virchows Arch (A)* **359**:1-18.

4. Westermark, P., Wernstedt, C., Wilander, E., Hayden, D.W., O'Brien, T.D. & Johnson, K.H. (1987) Amyloid fibrils in human insulinoma and islets of Langerhans of the diabetic are derived from a neuropeptide-like protein also present in normal islet cells. *Proc.Natl.Acad.Sci USA* **84**:3881-3885.

5. Lukinius, A., Wilander, E., Westermark, G.T., Engström, U. & Westermark, P. (1989) Co-localization of islet amyloid polypeptide and insulin in the β-cell secretory granules of human pancreatic islets. *Diabetologia* **32**:240-244.

6. Kanatsuka, A., Makino, H., Ohsawa, H., Tokuyama, Y., Yamaguchi, T., Yoshida, S. & Adachi, M. (1989) Secretion of islet amyloid polypeptide in response to glucose. *FEBS Lett.* **259**:199-201

7. Kahn, S.E., D'Alessio, D.A., Schwartz, M.W., Fujimoto, W.Y., Ensinck, J.W., Taborsky, G.J. & Porte Jr, D. (1990) Evidence of cosecretion of islet amyloid polypeptide and insulin by β-cells. *Diabetes* **39**:634-638.

8. Mitsukawa, T., Takemura, J., Asai, J., Nakazato, M., Kangawa, K., Matsuo, H. & Matsukura, S (1990) Islet amyloid polypeptide response to glucose, insulin and somatostatin analogue administration. *Diabetes* **39**:639-642.

9. Sanke, T., Bell, G.I., Sample, C., Rubenstein, A.H. & Steiner, D.F. (1988) An islet amyloid peptide is derived from an 89-amino-acid precursor by proteolytic processing. *J. Biol. Chem.* **263**:17243-17246.

10. Mosselman, S., Höppener, J.W.M., Lips, C.J.M. & Jansz, H.S. (1989) The complete islet amyloid polypeptide precursor is encoded by two exons. *FEBS Lett.* **247**:154-158.

11. Betsholtz, C., Svensson, V., Rorsman, F., Westermark, G.T., Wilander, E., Johnson, K.H. & Westermark, P. (1989) Islet amyloid polypeptide: cDNA cloning and identification of an amyloidogenic region associated with the species-specific occurence of age-related diabetes mellitus. *Exp.Cell Res.* **183**:484-493.

12. Morishita, T., Yamaguchi, A., Fujita, T. & Chiba, T. (1990) Activation of adenylate cyclase by islet amyloid polypeptide with carboxyterminal amid via calcitonin gene-related peptide receptors on rat liver plasma mambranes. *Diabetes* **39**:875-877.

13. Leighton, B. & Cooper, G.J.S. (1988) Pancreatic amylin and calcitonin gene-related peptide cause resistance to insulin in skeletal muscle in vitro. *Nature* **335**:632-635.

14. Zierath, J.R., Andréasson, K., Galuska, D., Engström, U., Johnson, K.H., Betsholtz, C., Westermark, P. & Wallberg-Henriksson, H. (1990) Rat islet amyloid polypeptide inhibits insulin-stimulated glucose transport in rat skeletal muscle without affecting glycogen content. *Submitted.*

15. Johnson, K.H., O'Brien, T.D., Jordan K., Betsholtz, C. & Westermark, P. (1990) The putative hormone islet amyloid polypeptide (IAPP) induces impaired glucose tolerance in cats. *Biochem.Biophys.Res.Commun.* **167**:507-513.

16. Molina, J.M., Cooper, G.J.S., Leighton, B. & Olefsky, J.M. (1990) Induction of insulin resistance *in vivo* by amylin and calcitonin gene-related peptide *Diabetes* **39**:260-265.

17. Sowa, S., Sanke, T., Hirayama, J., Furuta, H., Nishimura, S. & Nanjo, K. (1990) Islet amyloid polypeptide amide causes peripheral insulin resistance *in vivo* in dogs. *Diabetologia* **33**:118-120.

18. Johnson, K.H., O'Brien, T.D., Jordan, K., & Westermark, P. (1989) Impaired glucose tolerance is associated with increased islet amyloid polypeptide (IAPP) immunoreactivity in pancreatic beta cells. *Am.J.Pathol.* **135**:245-250.

19. Ferrier, G.J.M., Pierson, A.M., Jones, P.M., Bloom, S.R. Girgis, S.I. & Legon, S. (1989) Expression of the rat amylin (IAPP/DAP) gene. *J.Mol.Endocrinol.* **3**:R1-R4.

20.Glenner, G.G., Eanes, E.D. & Wiley, C.A. (1988) Amyloid fibrils formed from a segment of the pancreatic islet amyloid protein. *Biochem.Biophys. Res.Commun.* **155**:608-614.

21. Betsholtz, C., Christmanson, L., Engström, U., Rorsman, F., Svensson, V., Johnson, K.H. & Westermark, P. (1989) Sequence divergence in a specific region of islet amyloid polypeptide (IAPP) explains differences in islet amyloid formation between species. *FEBS Lett.* **251**:261-264.

22. Betsholtz, C., Chistmanson, L., Engström, U., Rorsman, F., Jordan, K., O'Brien, T.D., Murtaugh, M., Johnson, K.H. & Westermark, P. (1990) Structure of cat islet amyloid polypeptide and identification of amino acid residues of potential significance for islet amyloid formation. *Diabetes* **39**:118-122.

23. Westermark, P., Engström, U., Johnson, K.H., Westermark, G.T. & Betsholtz, C. (1990) Islet amyloid polypeptide: Pinpointing amino acid residues linked to amyloid fibril formation. *Proc.Natl.Acad.Sci.USA* **87**:5036-5040.

24. Mosselman, S., Höppener, J.W.M. Zandberg, A.D.M., VanMansfeld, A.H.M., Geurts van Kessel, C.J.M. & Jansz, H.S. (1988) Islet amyloid polypeptide: Identification and chromosomal localization of the human gene. *FEBS Lett.* **239**:227-232.

25. Nishi, M., Sanke, T., Seino, S., Eddy, R.L., Fan, Y.-S., Byers, M.G., Shows, T.B., Bell, G.I. & Steiner, D.F. (1989) Human islet amyloid polypeptide gene: complete nucleotide sequence, chromosomal localization and evolutionary history. *Mol.Endo.* **3**:1775-1781.

26. Christmanson, L., Rorsman, F., Stenman, G., Westermark, P. & Betsholtz, C. (1990) The human islet amyloid polypeptide (IAPP) gene: Organization, chromosomal localization and functional identification of a promoter region. *FEBS Lett.* **267**:160-166.

27. Bretherton-Watt, D., Ghatei, M.A., Bloom, S.R., Jamal, H., Ferrier, G.J.M., Girgis, S.I. & Legon, S. (1989) Altered islet amyloid polypeptide (amylin) gene expression in rat models of diabetes. *Diabetologia* **32**:881-883.

28. Madsen, O.D., Nielsen, J.H., Michelsen, B., Westermark, P., Betsholtz, C., Nishi, M. & Steiner, D.F. (1990) slet amyloid polypeptide (IAPP/amylin) and insulin expression are controlled differently in primary and transformed islet cells. *Mol. Endo.* in press.

29. Buckle, V.J., Marsland, A.M., Mosselman, S. & Höppener, J.W.M. (1989) Localization of the human islet amyloid polypeptide (IAPP) gene to 12p11.2-p12.3. *Cytogenet.Cell.Genet.* **51**:972.

30. Cockburn, D., Holt, S.M., Roberts, A.N., Cooper, G.J.S., Reid, K.B.M. & Boyd, Y. (1989) Localization of the amylin locus to chromosome 12. *Cytogenet.Cell.Genet.* **51**:977.

HUMAN ISLET AMYLOID POLYPEPTIDE (IAPP): IDENTIFICATION IN HUMAN PANCREAS, ESTABLISHMENT OF RADIOIMMUNOASSAY, AND ITS RESPONSE TO PHYSIOLOGICAL STIMULATION

M. NAKAZATO, J. ASAI, M. MIYAZATO, T. MITSUKAWA, H. TOSHIMORI, J. TAKEMURA, K. KANGAWA*, H. MATSUO#, and S. MATSUKURA
Third Department of Internal Medicine and Department of Biochemistry*, Miyazaki Medical College, Kiyotake, Miyazaki 889-16, and National Cardiovascular Center Research Institute#, Suita, Osaka 565, Japan.

ABSTRACT. Islet amyloid polypeptide (IAPP) was isolated from a soluble peptide fraction of pancreata of non-diabetic patients and from normal human plasma using immunoaffinity chromatography, gel filtration and reverse-phase high performance liquid chromatography (RP-HPLC) coupled with radioimmunoassay (RIA). IAPP[1-37], IAPP[17-37], and other two IAPP-related peptides which were putative pro-IAPPs or different processing products of IAPP, were identified. Complete amino acid sequence of IAPP[1-37] was identical to that of IAPP identified in islet amyloid in the pancreas of patients with non-insulin-dependent diabetes mellitus (NIDDM) and in insulinoma amyloid. IAPP[1-37] is a major molecular form of IAPP in the pancreas, but it accounted for as little as 20-31% of immunoreactive IAPP in the plasma. IAPP was also found in the lower portion of the mucosa of the gastrointestinal tract, suggesting its endocrine or paracrine role in the gut. Plasma concentration of IAPP in normal individuals increased in response to glucose load. IAPP is a novel pancreatic hormone secreted from B cells under glucose stimulation. Amyloid deposition in the islets might be responsible for development of NIDDM.

Introduction

Amyloid deposits in the islets of Langerhans are observed in over 90% of NIDDM patients and are also quite common in insulinoma. Recently, a polypeptide constituting islet amyloid has been isolated from pancreata of patients with NIDDM and insulinoma. This peptide, designated islet amyloid polypeptide (IAPP) (1) or amylin (2), is 37-amino acid long and has 46% amino acid sequence homology with human calcitonin gene-related peptide (CGRP). The purpose of this study is to elucidate the physiological function of IAPP and amyloidogenesis in NIDDM.

Materials and Methods

RIA FOR HUMAN IAPP: An antiserum was raised against a synthetic C-terminal tetradecapeptide corresponding to subsequence of human IAPP[24-37]. RIA procedure was described elsewhere (3). IC_{50} of standard curve was 22 fmol/tube, and minimum detection level was 2.5 fmol/tube. The antiserum did not exhibit any cross-reactivities with human CGRPs, insulin, glucagon, somatostatin, or pancreatic polypeptide.

ISOLATION OF IAPP FROM AMYLOID DEPOSIT- FREE HUMAN PANCREAS: Pancreas in which amyloid was not observed was extracted as described elsewhere (4). The extract was applied to an octadesylsilica column, washed with 0.5M acetic acid and then 0.1% trifluoroacetic acid (TFA) solution. The adsorbed materials were eluted with a 60% acetonitrile (CH3CN) solution containing 0.1% TFA. The eluate was evaporated and loaded on an SP- Sephadex C- 25 column, pre- equilibrated with 1M acetic acid. The column was washed with 1M acetic acid, then eluted successively with 2M pyridine and 2M pyridine- acetate (pH 5.0). After lyophilization, the pyridine- acetate fraction was subjected to gel filtration on a Sephadex G- 50 fine column. All fractions were monitored by RIA for human IAPP. Fractions containing immunoreactive (ir)- IAPP were pooled and subjected to immunoaffinity chromatography on an anti- IAPP IgG- Affi- Gel 10 column (4). Peptides adsorbed on the column were separated by RP- HPLC on a diphenyl column. Human IAPP was finally purified by RP- HPLC on a Chemcosorb 3ODS- H column.

CHROMATOGRAPHIC CHARACTERIZATION OF IAPP IN HUMAN PANCREAS: An extract of normal human pancreas was chromatographed by RP- HPLC on a TSK ODS SIL 120A column. All fractions were monitored by RIA.

CHROMATOGRAPHIC CHARACTERIZATION OF IAPP IN HUMAN PLASMA: Plasma was applied to Sep- Pak C- 18 cartridges, then the column eluate was subjected to IAPP immunoaffinity column. The column eluate was subjected to RP- HPLC system under the same condition used in analysis on pancreatic extract.

IAPP RESPONSE TO GLUCOSE: Eight subjects were given 75 glucose orally, seven subjects were given 10 g glucose intravenously, and eight subjects were given an intravenous bolus injection of insulin (0.1 U/kg). Six subjects were given 10 g of glucose intravenously with pretreatment of subcutaneous injection of 50 μg somatostatin analogue (SMS 201 - 995) 30 min before glucose injection. All experiments were performed after an overnight fast. Plasma IAPP was measured by RIA after extraction with a Sep- Pak C- 18 cartridge.

MEASUREMENT OF IAPP IN TISSUE AND PLASMA: Tissues were resected 6 non- diabetic patients and homogenized. The extract, except for the pancreas, was applied to a Sep- Pak C- 18 cartridge and human IAPP IgG immunoaffinity column, then submitted to RIA. Pancreatic extract was directly subjected to RIA. Plasma was obtained after an overnight fast. Plasma IAPP was extracted using a Sep- Pak C- 18 cartridge and then submitted to RIA.

Results

IDENTIFICATION OF IAPP IN NORMAL HUMAN PANCREAS: Human IAPP was isolated by cation exchange chromatography on an SP - Sephadex C - 25 column, Sephadex G - 50 gel filtration, IAPP IgG affinity chromatography, and finally RP - HPLC. At positions corresponding to 4- 5K and 2K daltons, 95% and 5% of ir- IAPP eluted (4). Their amino acid sequences were determined by amino acid analyses and sequence analyses using a gas- phase sequencer linked with RP- HPLC for identification of released PTH amino acids. Amino acid sequences of IAPPs thus determined are shown in Fig. 1. C- terminal amidation of IAPP was confirmed by the finding that the peptide emerged at an elution position on HPLC identical to that of synthetic IAPP with C- terminal amide. IAPP of 4K daltons was 37- amino acids long, with a sequence identical to that of IAPP deposited as islet amyloid in NIDDM and insulinoma. IAPP of 2K daltons was found to correspond to subsequence [17- 37] of human IAPP.

	5 10 15 20 25 30 35
Human IAPP [1-37]	**KCNTATCATQRLANFLVHSSNNFGAILSSTNVGSNTY-NH_2**
Human IAPP [17-37]	**VHSSNNFGAILSSTNVGSNTY-NH_2**

Figure 1. Amino acid sequences of human IAPP[1 − 37] and IAPP[17 − 37] isolated from normal human pancreas.

CHARACTERIZATION OF IAPP IN PANCREAS: Ir- IAPPs in human pancreas were identified by RP- HPLC. IAPP[1- 37] and IAPP[17- 37] accounted for 65% and 4% of ir - IAPP in the pancreas, respectively (5). At positions 5.5 and 3.5 min earlier than that of IAPP[1- 37] on the chromatogram of HPLC, 24% and 5% of immunoreactivity was detected, respectively. These four ir- IAPPs were also observed in human plasma as described below, indicating that the IAPPs were secreted into the circulation from the pancreas.

CHARACTERIZATION OF IAPP IN PLASMA: IAPPs in human plasma were isolated by a preparative C- 18 column, immunoaffinity column, and finally RP- HPLC. Approximately 31% of ir- IAPP emerged at an elution position identical to that of human IAPP[1- 37] and 50% and 18% of immunoreactivity emerged at positions 5.5 and 3.5 min earlier than that of human IAPP[1- 37] (5). IAPP[17- 37] accounted for 4% of ir - IAPP in the plasma.

TISSUE CONTENT AND PLASMA CONCENTRATION OF HUMAN IAPP: IAPP content in the pancreas of 6 non- diabetic patients was 865.2 ± 305.4 (SD) pg/mg wet weight and a small amount of ir- IAPP was detected in the stomach, duodenum, and jejunum (3). Immunohistochemical studies revealed that IAPP was co- localized with insulin in B cells of the pancreas and was observed in the lower portion of the mucosa of the gastrointestinal tract. No IAPP - immunoreactivity was present in any systemic organs including central nervous system. Mean plasma concentration of IAPP in 10 normal individuals was 18.5 ± 4.8 (SD) pg/ml.

PLASMA IAPP RESPONSE TO GLUCOSE: Plasma IAPP level progressively increased after oral glucose load, reaching a peak value of 54.3 ± 4.2 pg/ml 60 min after glucose load, then declining (6). Plasma IAPP level at 180 min remained elevated, being significantly higher ($p<0.01$) than basal level. A significant positive correlation was observed between plasma levels of IAPP and insulin ($r=0.50$, $P<0.01$) and between IAPP and glucose ($r=0.55$, $P<0.01$). After 10 g glucose bolus injection, plasma IAPP level reached a peak value of 46.4 ± 3.6 pg/ml 5 min after injection. Somatostatin analogue completely abolished plasma IAPP response to intravenous glucose injection. Aftrer insulin injection, plasma IAPP levels gradually decreased, reaching a nadir of 11.6 ± 1.6 pg/ml 60 min after injection. Significant correlation was observed between plasma IAPP and C- peptide levels.

Discussion

IAPP is a normal constituent of human pancreas, although the peptide was originally isolated from islet amyloid deposits in patients with insulinoma and NIDDM. The present sequence determination indicates that amyloid deposition in the islets of NIDDM and insulinoma does not result from a variant molecular form of IAPP. Islet amyloid is mostly situated at the capillary wall of the islets and is adjacent to the capillary endothelial cells. We also found that IAPP is secreted at a higher rate in impaired glucose tolerance and in the early stage of NIDDM, which may result in amyloid deposition in the islets (unpublished observations). Impaired catabolism or aberrant processing of IAPP in degenerated B cells might be also related to amyloid fibril formation since islet amyloid was often observed in non-diabetic aged individuals as well. Amyloidogenesis in insulinoma is probably associated with overproduction of IAPP by tumor cells, as is the case with calcitonin-producing tumor. In the pancreas of IDDM patients, IAPP-immunoreactivity in B cell secretory granules and islet amyloid were not observed (unpublished observations). IAPP[1-37], IAPP[17-37] and other two molecular forms of IAPPs were isolated in the plasma and soluble peptide fraction of human pancreas. Further study is needed to clarify which molecular form of IAPP moiety participates in amyloid fibril formation in the islets.

Identification of IAPP promises to help elucidate the regulatory system for carbohydrate metabolism and to clarify amyloidogenesis in NIDDM and insulinoma.

References

1. Westermark, P., Wernstedt, C., Wilander, E., and Sletten, K. (1986) 'A novel peptide in the calcitonin gene related peptide family as an amyloid fibril protein in the endocrine pancreas', Biochem. Biophys. Res. Commun. 140, 827-831.
2. Cooper, G.J.S., Willis, A.C., Clark, A., Turner, R.C., Sim, R.B., and Reid, K.B.M. (1987) 'Purification and characterization of a peptide from amyloid-rich pancreases of type 2 diabetic patients', Proc. Natl. Acad. Sci. USA. 84, 8628-8632.
3. Nakazato, M., Asai, J., Kangawa, K., Matsukura, S., and Matsuo, H. (1989) 'Establishment of radioimmunoassay for human islet amyloid polypeptide and its tissue content and plasma concentration', Biochem. Biophys. Res. Commun. 164, 394-399.
4. Nakazato, M., Asai, J., Miyazato, M., Matsukura, S., Kangawa, K., and Matsuo, H. 'Isolation and identification of islet amyloid polypeptide in normal human pancreas', Regul. Pept. in press.
5. Nakazato, M., Miyazato, M., Asai, J., Mitsukawa, M., Kangawa, K., Matsuo, H., and Matsukura, S. (1990) 'Islet amyloid polypeptide, a novel pancreatic peptide, is a circulating hormone secreted under glucose stimulation', Biochem. Biophys. Res. Commun. 169, 713-718.
6. Mitsukawa, T., Takemura, J., Asai, J., Nakazato, M., Kangawa, K., Matsuo, H., and Matsukura, S. (1990) 'Islet amyloid polypeptide response to glucose, insulin, and somatostatin analogue administration', Diabetes 39, 639-642.

RAT ISLET AMYLOID POLYPEPTIDE (IAPP): ISOLATION AND SEQUENCE DETERMINATION, IMMUNOHISTOCHEMICAL STUDY, AND ITS SECRETION FROM PANCREAS

J. ASAI, M. NAKAZATO, M. MIYAZATO, T. MITSUKAWA, H. TOSHIMORI, J. TAKEMURA, K. KANGAWA*, H. MATSUO#, and S. MATSUKURA
Departments of Internal Medicine and Biochemistry*, Miyazaki Medical College, Kiyotake, Miyazaki 889- 16, and National Cardiovascular Center Research Institute#, Suita, Osaka 565, Japan

ABSTRACT: We isolated and identified IAPP[1- 37] and IAPP[19- 37] in normal rat pancreas by sequence analyses. Regional distribution and molecular forms of rat IAPP were studied by a highly sensitive and specific radioimmunoassay (RIA) for the peptide. IAPP[19- 37], accounting for 57% of IAPP- immunoreactivity in rat pancreas, is a major molecular form of rat IAPP moiety. A large amount of IAPP (328.5 $\pm$ 25.0 pmol/g wet weight) was found in rat pancreas and the peptide was also detected in pyloric antrum of stomach, duodenum, jejunum, ileum, and colon at 0.1- 0.8% of the level of pancreas. IAPP was immunohistochemically observed in B cells in the islets and the lower portion of the mucosa of gastrointestinal tract of the rat. IAPP was secreted from perfused rat pancreas in response to glucose. The distribution and secretion of IAPP suggest a possible endocrine or paracrine function in pancreas and gastrointestinal tract.

Introduction

Islet amyloid polypeptide (IAPP) (1), also designated amylin (2), is a 37- amino acid polypeptide which constitutes insulinoma amyloid and islet amyloid in the pancreas of patients with non- insulin- dependent diabetes mellitus. We isolated rat IAPP from normal rat pancreas by utilizing the cross- reactivity of an antiserum raised against human IAPP with rat IAPP, and have determined its amino acid sequence (3). Both rat and human IAPPs are 37 amino acids long and their sequences are 84% identical. We established a sensitive and specific RIA system for rat IAPP based on its sequence. To delineate the physiological function of IAPP, we studied regional distribution, molecular forms and secretion of rat IAPP. Furthermore, localization of IAPP was demonstrated immunohistochemically.

Materials and Methods

RIA FOR RAT IAPP: An antiserum was raised against a pentadecapeptide, which corresponds to subsequence [24- 37] of rat IAPP with an additional arginine at the N-terminus. Rat IAPP[1- 37] was used as a standard peptide for RIA. Half- maximum inhibition by rat IAPP[1- 37] was observed at 16 fmol/tube, and the peptide was detectable at a low level of 2 fmol/tube. Rat IAPP[19- 37] showed 100% cross-reactivity with the antiserum.

ISOLATION OF RAT IAPP IN PANCREAS: IAPPs were isolated by gel filtration on a Sephadex G- 50 fine column, immunoaffinity chromatography on an anti- rat IAPP IgG - Affi - Gel 10 column, and finally by reverse - phase high performance liquid chromatography (RP - HPLC) on a diphenyl column (4). All fractions of above chromatographies were monitored by RIA. Rat IAPPs thus purified were subjected to sequence analyses using as a gas - phase sequencer linked with RP - HPLC for identifying PTH amino acids.

DETERMINATION OF TISSUE CONTENT OF IAPP: Tissues were obtained after decapitation from 3 male Sprague Dawley rats weighing 230- 250 g that had been fed a diet of standard rat chow ad libitum. Pancreas was also extracted from 3 rats fasted 4 days. Tissues were extracted and IAPP was measured by RIA.

IMMUNOHISTOCHEMISTRY: Immunohistochemical staining was performed by the avidin biotin peroxidase complex (ABC) method (5). The antiserum for rat IAPP was used at a final dilution of 1/2,000- 4,000.

IAPP RESPONSE TO GLUCOSE IN PERFUSED RAT PANCREAS: Four pancreata from Sprague Dawley rats were perfused for 30 min with 80 mg/dl glucose, 40 min with 320 mg/dl glucose, and then 10 min with 80 mg/dl glucose. The flow rate was 2 ml/min. Perfusate was applied to a Sep- Pak C- 18 cartridge and then submitted to RIA.

Results

IDENTIFICATION OF IAPP IN RAT PANCREAS: Two immunoreactive (ir) IAPPs were observed at positions corresponding to molecular weight (Mr) of 4,000 and 2,000 on Sephadex G- 50 gel filtration. The IAPPs were purified as a single peak by RP- HPLC. Rat IAPP of Mr 4,000 emerged at an elution position exactly identical to that of authentic rat IAPP[1- 37] whose amino acid sequencing analysis has been reported (3). Rat IAPP of Mr 2,000 was found to correspond to the subsequence [19- 37] of rat IAPP by amino acid analysis and sequence analysis.

TISSUE CONTENT OF IAPP: IAPP content in rat pancreas was 328.5 ± 25.0 pmol/g wet weight. IAPP content in the pancreas fell to 54% of control after fasting for 4 days. Molecular forms of IAPP in the pancreas of fed and fasted rats were compared by RP- HPLC coupled with RIA. The mean ratio of IAPP[19- 37] to IAPP[1- 37] was 1.3 in 3 fed rats, and increased to 2.4 in 3 fasted rats. IAPP was detected in pyloric antrum of stomach at 0.8% of the level of pancreas and was found in duodenum, jejunum, ileum, and colon at approximately 0.1% of the level of pancreas. No IAPP- immunoreactivity was found in any of the other tissues examined including central nervous system.

HISTOCHEMICAL LOCALIZATION OF RAT IAPP: A large number of cells in the islets were immunoreactive for both IAPP and insulin. In the stomach, IAPP- cells were chiefly located in the pyloric antrum. Processes of the cytoplasma extended from the bipolar peripheral region of the cell like a neuronal process. Some long processes reached the surface of the lumen, and others appeared to make contact with other IAPP- cells. Fragments of immunoreactive processes were also often seen next to non- IAPP cells at the base of the glands. IAPP- cells were scarce in the body of the stomach and intestine.

SECRETION OF IAPP FROM PANCREAS: IAPP concentration in perfusate rose in typical biphasic fashion in response to glucose as shown in Fig. 1. During 320 mg/dl glucose perfusion IAPP rose to a maximum level of 155.2 ± 49.7 pg/ml. IAPP concentration rapidly returned to the basal level by 80 mg/dl glucose perfusion.

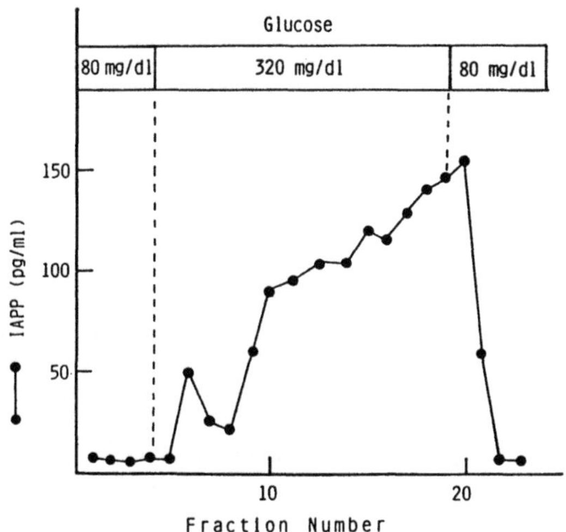

Figure 1. IAPP response to glucose in perfused rat pancreas.

Discussion

We identified IAPP[1- 37] and IAPP[19- 37] in normal rat pancreas with the latter being the major molecular form. From human pancreas, IAPP[17- 37] in addition to IAPP[1- 37] was isolated; however, IAPP[17- 37] constituted as little as 2- 6% of IAPP - immunoreactivity in human pancreas (6). These results suggest that processing of IAPP in pancreas differs between human and rat. An enzyme that specifically cleaves an Arg18- Ser19 bond in rat IAPP must act on processing of IAPP[19- 37] from IAPP[1- 37]. Subsequence [25- 29] of IAPP molecule is a critical site for forming amyloid fibrils (7). Rat IAPP has 84% amino acid sequence homology with human IAPP, whereas, subsequence [25- 29] of rat IAPP, except for Leu 28, differs from that of human IAPP. The structure of rat IAPP is not hydrophobic, which may explain the lack of amyloid fibril formation in rat pancreas.

IAPP[1- 37] inhibited both basal and insulin- stimulated rates of glycogen synthesis in stripped rat soleus muscle. IAPP[1- 37] also inhibited insulin release from isolated rat pancreatic islet. Further study is needed to clarify the physiological significance of rat IAPP[19- 37] since IAPP[19- 37] comprises the major component of IAPP moiety.

IAPP is a possible product of the ancestral gene of calcitonin gene- related peptide (CGRP) which is a neuromodulator ubiquitously existing in nerve fibers. IAPP is mainly localized in the pancreas, is present in the gastrointestinal tract at very low level, but is not found in nerve tissues. The distribution of IAPP, which is markedly different from that of CGRP, suggests that IAPP serves as a hormone.

IAPP was found in pyloric antrum of stomach, which was also demonstrated by immunohistochemical studies. A large number of IAPP- containing cells were seen in the lower portion of the antropyloric mucosa. Extention of IAPP - immunoreactive processes to the surface of the lumen and contact of IAPP- cells with other non- IAPP cells indicate that IAPP may play an endocrinal or paracrine role in the gastrointestinal tract.

The distribution and secretion of IAPP in response to glucose suggest a possible role for the control of carbohydrate metabolism. Abnormal synthesis, secretion and/or impaired catabolism of IAPP could be responsible for amyloid deposition in the islets of NIDDM.

References

1. Westermark, P., Wernstedt, C., Wilander, E., and Sletten, K. (1986) 'A novel peptide in the calcitonin gene related peptide family as an amyloid fibril protein in the endocrine pancreas', Biochem. Biophys. Res. Commun. 140, 827- 831.
2. Cooper, G.J.S., Willis, A.C., Clark, A., Turner, R.C., Sim, R.B., and Reid, K.B.M. (1987) 'Purification and characterization of a peptide from amyloid- rich pancreases of type 2 diabetic patients', Proc. Natl. Acad. Sci. USA. 84, 8628- 8632.
3. Asai, J., Nakazato, M., Kangawa, K., Matsukura, S., and Matsuo, H. (1989) 'Isolation and sequence determination of rat islet amyloid polypeptide', Biochem. Biophys. Res. Commun., 164, 400- 405.
4. Asai, J., Nakazato, M., Miyazato, M., Kangawa, K., Matsuo, H., and Matsukura, S. (1990) 'Regional distribution and molecular forms of rat islet amyloid polypeptide', Biochem. Biophys. Res. Commun., 169, 788- 795.
5. Toshimori, H., Mashita, R., Nakazato, M., Asai, J., Mitsukawa, T., Kangawa, K., Matsuo H., and Matsukura S. 'Islet amyloid polypeptide (IAPP)in the gastrointestinal tract and pancreas in man and rat', Cell Tissue Res., in press.
6. Nakazato, M., Miyazato, M., Asai, J., Mitsukawa, M., Kangawa, K., Matsuo, H., and Matsukura, S. (1990) 'Islet amyloid polypeptide, a novel pancreatic peptide, is a circulating hormone secreted under glucose stimulation', Biochem. Biophys. Res. Commun. 169, 713- 718.
7. Westermark, P., Engström, U., Johnson, K., Westermark, G.T., and Betsholtz, C. (1990) 'Islet amyloid polypeptide: Pinpointing amino acid residues linked to amyloid fibril formation', Proc. Natl. Acad. Sci. USA., 87, 5036- 5040.

FACTORS AFFECTING DIABETOGENESIS AND AMYLOIDOGENESIS ARE PROVIDED BY STUDIES OF IAPP IN THE DOG AND CAT

K.H. JOHNSON*, K. JORDAN*, T.D. O'BRIEN, M.P. MURTAUGH*, C.WERNSTEDT**, C. BETSHOLTZ*** AND P. WESTERMARK****
Department of Veterinary Pathobiology*, College of Veterinary Medicine, University of Minnesota, St. Paul, MN 55108 USA; Ludwig Institute for Cancer Research**, Uppsala Branch, Uppsala, Sweden; Department of Pathology***, University of Uppsala , Uppsala, Sweden; and Department of Pathology****, University Hospital, Linköping, Sweden

ABSTRACT. We show that dog IAPP, like human and cat IAPP incorporates the putative amyloidogenic **AILS** sequence at positions 25-28. However, dogs do NOT develop IAPP-derived islet amyloid but DO form IAPP-derived amyloid deposits in insulinomas. These studies in dogs, together with our semiquantitative immunohistochemical studies in cats, suggest that beta cell aberrations, leading to increased production and localized concentration of IAPP, provides a second prerequisite for the aggregation of IAPP to form amyloid.

Introduction

Islet amyloid polypeptide (IAPP) [1] or amylin [2], is a 37 amino acid C-terminally amidated polypeptide that is the major protein constituent of amyloid deposits in insulinomas and islet amyloid deposits in pancreatic islets of Type 2 diabetic humans and adult diabetic cats. IAPP has been shown by immunohistochemical and immunoelectron microscopic studies to be stored with insulin in beta cell secretory vesicles [3] and is cosecreted with insulin in response to glucose or arginine. IAPP immunoreactivity and/or IAPP mRNA expression has been demonstrated in the pancreatic islets of many species but it is both interesting and curious that IAPP-derived islet amyloidosis develops in association with age-related diabetes mellitus in only a certain few species (e.g., humans, non-human primates and cats [4].

Several avenues of <u>in vitro</u> and <u>in vivo</u> investigations have provided important clues to the interrelationships between IAPP, IAPP-derived islet amyloid, and diabetes mellitus in these certain species. For example, normal inherent differences in the primary structure within the 20-29 region of IAPP between different species appear to be importantly linked to the ability of IAPP to aggregate and form amyloid fibrils. Synthetic peptides corresponding to the human and cat sequence in this region have been shown to aggregate and form Congophilic amyloid-like fibrils <u>in vitro</u> whereas synthetic IAPP 20-29 of the hamster, rat and mouse lacked the ability to form fibrils [5]. The 25-28 region of human and cat IAPP is identical in structure (i.e., AILS) and appear to be the most important amyloidogenic sequence common to human and cat IAPP [6]. IAPPs from species which do not form islet amyloid diverge substantially from the human and cat in this 25-28 region.

With respect to the relationship of IAPP to development of diabetes mellitus, recent <u>in vitro</u> and <u>in vivo</u> studies have suggested that IAPP may inhibit insulin secretion and induce an insulin resistance state [2]. However, further studies are needed to clarify the physiological role(s) of IAPP and its possible relationships to Type 2 diabetes.

Additional and potentially important clues regarding the relationships of IAPP to amyloidogenesis and diabetogenesis have been obtained from our recent studies in cats [9] and dogs [7,8]. We show that a specific IAPP structural motif alone is obviously not adequate for the conversion of IAPP to amyloid fibrils in vivo but that beta cell aberrations, leading to increased production and localized concentration of IAPP, provides a second prerequisite for the aggregation of IAPP to form amyloid.

Materials and Methods

IMMUNOHISTOCHEMISTRY: IAPP immunoreactivity in cat pancreatic islets was evaluated [9] using the peroxidase antiperoxidase (PAP) method. Rabbit antisynthetic undecapeptide corresponding to positions 7-17 of human IAPP was used as the primary antiserum.

IAPP immunoreactivity in seven normal cats and six cats with impaired glucose tolerance was evaluated using the following dilutions of rabbit antisynthetic IAPP 7-17: 1:2000, 1:10,000, 1:15,000, 1:20,000, and 1:25,000.

Three canine pancreatic endocrine tumors [8], confirmed by Congo red staining to have potassium permanganate-resistant amyloid deposits, were also evaluated for IAPP immunoreactivity using the PAP technique and anti-synthetic human IAPP 7-17.

MOLECULAR BIOLOGY: Total cellular RNA was prepared from dog pancreas [7] using the acid guanidiniun/phenol method. Poly(A)$^+$, selected on oligo (dT)-cellulose, was used to generate single-stranded cDNA using AMV Reverse Transcriptase and oligo (dT_{12-18}) primers. The cDNA was used as template for PCR using the following two mixtures of oligonucleotide primers:

5'-AAGTG(C/T)AACACNGC(C/T)ACNTG(C/T)GC-3'
and 5'-TANGTGTT(A/G)(C/G)(A/T)(C/G/T)CC(CG)ACGTT-3'

Amplifications were carried out for 30 cycles consisting of 1.5 minute denaturation at 94 C, 1.5 minute annealing at 37 C, and 1.5 minute extension at 72 C. The amplification products were identified on a polyacrylamide gel, eluted and sequenced directly by the dideoxynucelotide chain termination procedure with ^{32}P end-labeled PCR primers used as sequencing primers.

Results

IMMUNOHISTOCHEMISTRY OF CAT PANCREATIC ISLETS. Using the PAP method and a series of incrementally increasing dilutions of anti-synthetic IAPP 7-17 under constant and uniform conditions, beta cells from cats with impaired glucose tolerance had stronger IAPP immunoreactivity than beta cells from normal cats [9]. As shown in Table 1, six of six cats with impaired glucose tolerance and only one of seven normal cats elicited IAPP immunoreactivity at the 1:15,000 dilution.

cDNA-PREDICTED AMINO ACID SEQUENCE OF DOG IAPP. PCR amplification and DNA sequence analysis provided unambiguous cDNA and predicted amino acid sequence seen for positions 10-35 of dog IAPP [7] (Table 2). It can be seen that dog IAPP, like human and cat IAPP, incorporates the putative amyloidogenic AILS sequence at positions 25-28.

IMMUNOHISTOCHEMISTRY OF DOG PANCREATIC ENDOCRINE TUMORS. Interstitial amyloid deposits present in the three tumors [8] showed strong immunoreactivity with anti-synthetic IAPP 7-17.

TABLE 1: IAPP IMMUNOREACTIVITY IN PANCREATIC ISLETS OF NORMAL AND IMPAIRED GLUCOSE TOLERANT CATS USING INCREASING DILUTIONS OF ANTI-IAPP 7-17 AND THE PAP METHOD

	ANTI-IAPP 7-17 DILUTIONS				
	1:2,000	1:10,000	1:15,000	1:20,000	1:25,000
NORMAL CATS					
FIA 202	+	+	-	-	-
FIA 205	+	+	-	-	-
FIA 206	+	+	-	-	-
FIA 208	+	+	-	-	-
FIA 212	+	+	-	-	-
FIA 216	+	+	-	-	-
FIA 218	+	+	+	-	-
IMPAIRED GLUCOSE TOLERANT CATS					
FIA 203	+	+	+	-	-
FIA 213	+	+	+	-	-
FIA 225	+	+	+	-	-
FIA 230	+	+	+	-	-
FIA 235	+	+	+	-	-
FIA 236	+	+	+	-	-

TABLE 2: PREDICTED DOG IAPP AMINO ACID SEQUENCE (POSITIONS 10-35) AND COMPARISON WITH IAPP FROM HUMANS AND OTHER ANIMALS

	10 15 20 25 30 35
DOG	Q R L A N F L V R T S N N L G **A I L S** P T N V G T N
HUMAN	Q R L A N F L V H S S N N F G **A I L S** S T A V G S A
CAT	Q R L A N F L I R S S N N L G **A I L S** P T A V G S A
HAMSTER	Q R L A N F L V H S N N N L G P V L S P T A V G S A
RAT/MOUSE	Q R L A N F L V R S S N N L G P V L P P T A V G S A
G. PIG	Q R L T N F L V R S S H N L G A A L L P T D V G S A

Discussion

The results of these immunohistochemical studies of cat pancreatic islets indicate an apparent increase in IAPP content in cats with impaired glucose tolerance as compared to normal cats. The increase in IAPP content in beta cells from cats with impaired glucose tolerance may be due to increased production or decreased secretion of IAPP. Increased production and release of IAPP by beta cells could thus play a significant role in the progressive deposition of islet amyloid that is strongly associated with the development of impaired glucose tolerance or overt diabetes in cats.

This study also indicates that dog IAPP, like human and cat IAPP, contains the putative amyloidogenic AILS sequence at positions 25-28 [7]. However, to the best of our knowledge and experience, dogs do not develop IAPP-derived islet amyloid. The lack of occurrence of islet amyloid in dogs is supported by a review of our pathology files at the

University of Minnesota, College of Veterinary Medicine, over a 25 year period (1964-1989). Amyloid restricted to the pancreatic islets was not observed in any of the 6,828 non-diabetic or diabetic dogs which were autopsied and evaluated histologically.
It is interesting that although dogs do not develop IAPP-derived islet amyloid, IAPP-derived amyloid deposits in dog pancreatic endocrine tumors [8] were confirmed immunohistochemically in this study. This is consistent with our molecular biology study indicating that dog IAPP does incorporate the putative amyloidogenic sequence at positions 25-28.

These studies in dogs and cats indicate that a specific IAPP structural motif alone is obviously not adequate for the conversion of IAPP to amyloid fibrils in vivo but that beta cell aberrations leading to increased production and localized concentration of IAPP provides a second prerequisite for the conversion of IAPP to amyloid.

References

1. Westermark, P., Wernstedt, C., Wilander, E., Hayden, D.W., O'Brien, T.D., and Johnson, K.H. (1987) Amyloid fibrils in human insulinoma and islets of Langerhans of the diabetic cat are derived from a neuropeptide-like protein also present in normal islet cells. Proc. Natl. Acad. Sci. USA 84, 3881 - 3885.
2. Cooper, G.J., Leighton, B., Dimitridadis, G.D., Parry-Billings, M., Kowalchuk, J.M., Howland, K., Rothbard, J.B., Willis, A.C., and Reid, K.B.M. (1988) Amylin found in amyloid deposits in human type 2 diabetes mellitus may be a hormone that regulates glycogen metabolism in skeletal muscle. Proc. Natl. Acad. Sci. USA 85, 7763 - 7766.
3. Johnson, K.H., O'Brien, T.D., Hayden, D.W., Jordan, K., Ghobrial, H.K.G., Mahoney, W.C., and Westermark, P. (1988) Immunolocalization of islet amyloid polypeptide (IAPP) in pancreatic beta cells by means of peroxidase-antiperoxidase (PAP) and protein A-gold techniques. Am. J. Pathol. 130, 1 - 8.
4. Johnson, K.H., O'Brien, T.D., Betsholtz, C., and Westermark, P. (1989) Islet amyloid, islet-amyloid polypeptide, and diabetes mellitus. N. Engl. J. Med. 321, 513 - 518.
5. Westermark, P., Engström, U., Johnson, K.H., Westermark, G.T., and Betsholtz, C. (1990) Islet amyloid polypeptide: pinpointing amino acid residues linked to amyloid fibril formation. Proc. Natl. Acad. Sci. USA. In presS.
6. Betsholtz, C., Christmanson, L., Engström. U., Rorsman, F., Jordan, K., O'Brien, T.D., Murtaugh, M., Johnson, K.H., and Westermark, P. (1990) Structure of cat islet amyloid polypeptide and identification of amino acid residues of potential significance for islet amyloid formation. Diabetes 39, 118 - 122.
7. Jordan, K., Murtaugh, M.P., O'Brien, T.D., Westermark, P., Betsholtz, C., and Johnson, K.H. (1990) Canine IAPP cDNA provides clues regarding diabetogenesis and amyloidogenesis in type 2 diabetes. Biochem. Biophys. Res. Commun. 169, 502 - 508.
8. O'Brien, T.D., Westermark, P., and Johnson, K.H. (1990) Islet amyloid polypeptide and calcitonin gene-related peptide immunoreactivity in amyloid and tumor cells of canine pancreatic endocrine tumors. Vet. Pathol. 27, 194 - 198.
9. Johnson, K.H., O'Brien, T.D., Jordan, K., and Westermark, P. (1988) Impaired glucose tolerance is associated with increased islet amyloid polypeptide (IAPP) immunoreactivity in pancreatic beta cells. Am. J. Pathol. 135, 245 - 250.

ISLET AMYLOID POLYPEPTIDE: SYNTHETIC PEPTIDES FOR STUDY OF THE PATHOGENESIS OF ISLET AMYLOID

Per Westermark, Kenneth H. Johnson, Ulla Engström, Gunilla T. Westermark, Hel.lena Dominguez, Lars Christmansson and Christer Betsholtz

Department of Pathology, Universities of Linköping and Uppsala, Ludwig Institute for Cancer Research, Uppsala Branch, Uppsala, Sweden and Department of Veterinary Pathobiology, College of Veterinary Medicine, University of Minnesota St. Paul, Minnesota

ABSTRACT

Studies have indicated that the 20-29 segment of islet amyloid polypeptide (IAPP) determines the fibril formation. Variations between species in this region explain why only some species develop islet amyloid. This assumption is strongly supported by our study where we have used synthetic peptides in an fibril formation test system. The sequence AILS ($IAPP_{25-28}$) is the most important amyloidogenic part of the IAPP molecule.

INTRODUCTION

Islet amyloid polypeptide (IAPP) is the main constituent of islet amyloid (IA) (1-3). Only a few species including man and cats develop this form of amyloid. The 20-29 segment of the human IAPP molecule has capacity to form amyloid fibrils *in vitro* and may be responsible for the formation of IA (4-7). Amino acid sequence variations in this evolutionary least conserved part of the IAPP molecule correlates with the occurrence of amyloid in different species. In order to test the hypothesis that the $IAPP_{20-29}$ segment determines the fibril formation capacity of the IAPP molecule, we have studied the ability of different synthetic $IAPP_{20-29}$ peptides to form fibrils in vitro.

MATERIAL AND METHODS

Peptides corresponding to $IAPP_{20-29}$ of different animals, decapeptides with amino acid substitutions (see Table 1), human IAPP1-37 and the peptide GAILSS were synthesized by automatic solid phase synthesis. Rat 1-37 IAPP was purchased from Multiple Peptide Systems (San Diego, CA).

In vitro fibril formation

Synthetic peptides, dissolved in 10 % acetic acid, were kept at +20°C over night and studied for fibril formation. Tubes with little fibril formation were neutralized with NH_4OH. Smears of all solutions were stained with Congo red and studied in polarized light. Samples were also negatively stained and studied electron microscopically.

RESULTS

The results are given in Table 1. Full length human IAPP (positions 1-37) dissolved in acetic aced spontaneously formed fibrils with amyloid properties in vitro. These fibrils were straight and resembled native amyloid fibrils. On the other hand, rat $IAPP_{1-37}$ did not give rise to any fibrils even after neutralization and concentration. The studies with the $IAPP_{20-29}$ peptides of five different species showed that only human and cat peptides had amyloidogenic properties and gave rise to gels with Congophilia and green birefringence. Human $IAPP_{20-29}$ had a exceptionally strong tendency to form fibrils. These resembled ultrastructurally those formed from full length IAPP. Rat, hamster and degu $IAPP_{20-29}$ did not give rise to fibrils in any of the conditions tested. Human $IAPP_{24-29}$ also gave rise to rigid fibrils with amyloid staining properties.

TABLE 1. Amino acid sequences and amyloidogenic properties of synthetic peptides used in the present study

Peptide	Sequence	Fibril
Human IAPP 24-29	G A I L S S	++
Cat IAPP 20-29	S N N L G A I L S P	++
Rat IAPP 20-29	S N N L G P V L P P	-
Hamster IAPP 20-29	N N N L G P V L S P	-
Degu IAPP 20-29	S H N L G A A L P P	-
Human IAPP 20-29	S N N F G A I L S S	+++
Human IAPP 20-29, L23	S N N L G A I L S S	+++
Human IAPP 20-29, P25	S N N F G P I L S S	++
Human IAPP 20-29, V26	S N N F G A V L S S	++
Human IAPP 20-29, P28	S N N F G A I L P S	-
Human IAPP 20-29, P29	S N N F G A I L S P	++
Human IAPP 20-29, L23, P25	S N N L G P I L S S	++
Human IAPP 20-29, P25, V26	S N N F G P V L S S	+++
Human IAPP 20-29 P28, P29	S N N F G A I L P P	-
Hamster IAPP 20-29, A25, I26	N N N L G A I L S P	++
Rat IAPP 20-29, A25, I26	S N N L G A I L P P	–

Human $IAPP_{20-29}$ with amino acid substitutions

Human $IAPP_{20-29}$ peptides with one or two positions exchanged for rodent residues and rat and hamster $IAPP_{20-29}$ with human residues at position 25 and 26 were also tested for fibril formation. All the substitutions reduced the amyloidogenic properties of the human $IAPP_{20-29}$ peptide but there was considerable differences with the different substitutions. Thus, replacement of serine with proline at position 28 ($IAPP_{20-29}$ P28) almost completely abolished fibril formation while the same substitution in position 29 had minor effects. In contrast, substitution of proline for alanine at position 25 or substitution of proline for serine at position 29 had only minor effects.

Fibrils formed with full length human IAPP and human $IAPP_{20-29}$ resembled each other and native amyloid fibrils. Also fibrils from human $IAPP_{20-29}$ L23, human $IAPP_{20-29}$ V26 and human $IAPP_{20-29}$ P25 V26 had this morphology. Fibrils from human $IAPP_{20-29}$ P25, human $IAPP_{20-29}$ P29 and human $IAPP_{20-29}$ P28 P29 were long, slender and curvy. The few fibrils formed from human $IAPP_{20-29}$ P28, did not resemble native amyloid fibrils.

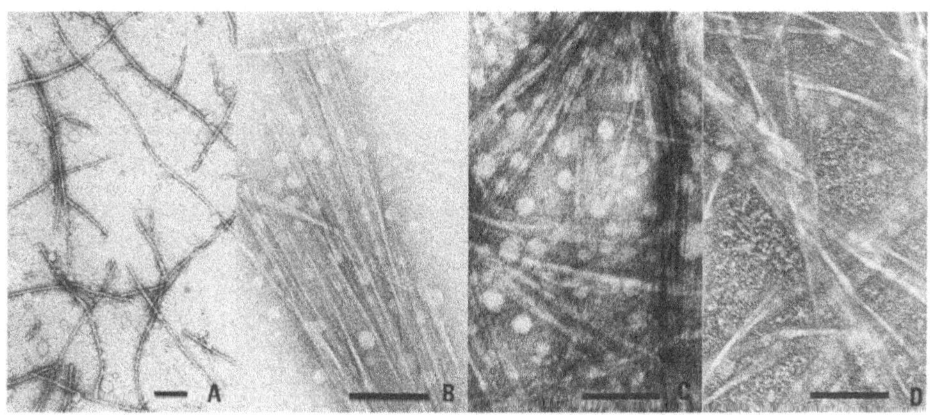

Fig. 1. Fibrils formed from human IAPP1-37 (A), human $IAPP_{20-29}$ (B), human $IAPP_{20-29}$, V26 (C) and human $IAPP_{24-29}$ (D). Bar = 100 nm.

DISCUSSION

This study shows that human and cat but not rat IAPP has intrinsic amyloidogenic properties. The study also strongly indicates that the 20-29 segment contains the important amyloidogenic sequence since human and cat $IAPP_{20-29}$, but not rat and hamster $IAPP_{20-29}$ give rise to amyloid-like fibrils. The experiments with hybrid peptides show that the amyloidogenic value of the different residues in the 20-29 segment is varying. Thus, an exchange of proline for serine in position 28 has much stronger influence than substitutions with proline for alanine in position 25 or proline for serine in position 29. The study therefore strongly supports the theory that amino acid sequence variations in positions 20-29 of IAPP of different species determines whether or not IAPP-derived IA can form (5, 6). The primary structure of IAPP is not the only factor of importance for amyloid formation since dogs never get IA and the AILS sequence is present in canine IAPP.

Most work was performed with the 20-29 segment. However, in this study we also found that the very short peptide GAILSS, corresponding to human $IAPP_{24-29}$ had amyloidogenic properties supporting our other findings.

The finding that the Chilenian rodent degu, which often acquires IA does not have an amyloidogenic IAPP can seem contradictory to the other results. However, degu IA consists of insulin rather than IAPP.

Supported by the Swedish Medical Research Council, the Nordic Insulin Fund, Louis-Hansen's Memorial Fund, and the National Institute of Diabetes and Digestive and Kidney Diseases.

REFERENCES

1. Westermark, P., Wernstedt, C., Wilander, E. and Sletten, K. (1986) A novel peptide in the calcitonin gene related peptide as an amyloid fibril protein in the endocrine pancreas. Biochem. Biophys. Res. Commun. 140, 827-831.
2. Westermark, P., Wernstedt, C., Wilander , E., Hayden, D.W., O'Brien, T.D. and Johnson, K.H. (1987) Amyloid fibrils in human insulinoma and islets of Langerhans of the diabetic cat are derived from a neuropeptide-like protein also present in normal islet cells. Proc. Natl. Acad. Sci U.S.A. 84, 3881-3885.
3. Cooper, G.J., Willis,A.C., Clark, A., Turner, R.C., Sim, R.B. and Reid, K.B. (1987) Purification and characterization of a peptide from amyloid-rich pancreases of type 2 diabetic patients. Proc. Natl. Acad. Sc. U.S.A. 84,8628-8632.
4. Johnson, K.H., O'Brien, T.D., Betsholtz, C. and Westermark, P. (1989) Islet amyloid, islet-amyloid polypeptide, and diabetes mellitus. New Engl. J. Med. 321, 513-518.
5. Glenner, G.G., Eanes, E.D. and Wiley, C.A. (1988) Amyloid fibrils formed from a segment of the pancreatic islet protein. Biochem. Biophys. Res. Commun. 155, 608-614.
6. Betsholtz, C., Svensson, V., Rorsman, F., Engström, U., Westermark, G.T., Wilander, E., Johnson, K.H. and Westermark, P. (1989) Islet amyloid polypeptide (IAPP): cDNA cloning and identification of an amyloidogenic region associated with the species-specific occurrence of age-related diabetes mellitus. Exp. Cell. Res. 183, 484-493.
7. Westermark, P., Engström, U., Johnson, K.H., Westermark, G.T. and Betsholtz, C. (1990) Islet amyloid polypeptide: Pinpointing amino acid residues linked to amyloid fibril formation. Proc. Natl. Acad. Sci. U.S.A. 87, 5036-5040.

INTRACELLULAR FORMATION OF AMYLOID FIBRILS IN B-CELLS OF HUMAN INSULINOMA AND PRE-DIABETIC MONKEY ISLETS.

A. CLARK[1], J.F. MORRIS[1], L.A. SCOTT[1], A McLAY[2],
A.K. FOULIS[2], N.L. BODKIN[3], B.C. HANSEN[3]
[1]Department of Human Anatomy, Oxford, UK,
[2]Pathology Department, Glasgow Royal Infirmary, UK,
[3]Department of Physiology, University of Maryland, Baltimore, USA.

ABSTRACT. Amyloid formed from islet amyloid polypeptide (IAPP) is present in pancreatic islets of spontaneously diabetic humans, monkeys and cats and in some insulinomas. The factors which cause amyloid deposition are unknown but may be related to abnormal processing or catabolism of the peptide. To determine the sites at which fibrils are formed, immunoreactivity for IAPP (IAPP-IR) was examined electron microscopically in 16 specimens of insulinoma and in pancreatic autopsy specimens from two pre-diabetic monkeys. In 9/16 insulinomas, IAPP-IR was detected on extracellular amyloid and in 6 of these, IAPP-IR was located on intracellular fibrils some of which were membrane bound. IAPP-IR was found on the radially arranged islet amyloid of pre-diabetic monkey islets. IAPP-IR on fibrils at intracellular sites suggests that amyloidosis may commence inside the cell. Subsequently, the fibrils would be extruded from the cell or become extracellular as a result of cell death.

1.0. Introduction

Amyloid deposits are a characteristic feature of the islets of type 2 diabetic man [1,2] and of spontaneous diabetes in cats [3] and monkeys [4]. The amyloid fibrils are formed from a 37 amino acid peptide known as islet amyloid polypeptide (IAPP) [5] or `amylin'[6]. This peptide is a natural constituent of the islets and is located in the insulin granules and lysosomes of B-cells in both diabetic and non-diabetic individuals [7,8]. Amyloid formed from IAPP is also a feature of some insulinomas [9]. Conversion of the peptide from the native form to the insoluble beta-pleated conformation is critically dependent upon the amino acid sequence [10] but the mechanisms which cause amyloid to be deposited are as yet unknown. Islet amyloid may either be a primary feature of aberrant B-cell function, as present in insulinomas, or be related to the abnormal secretory activity of B-cells which accompanies insulin resistance in diabetes. To determine possible mechanisms responsible for amyloid production, tissue from human insulinomas and pancreatic islets from *Macaca mulatta* monkeys exhibiting physiological characteristics of pre-diabetes have been examined by means of immunoelectron microscopy.

2.0 Materials and Methods

Human insulinoma tissue was obtained by surgical resection from 16 patients. Pancreatic tissue was obtained at necropsy from 2 *Macaca mulatta* which had symptoms of prediabetes (glucose intolerance and obesity [11]). Small blocks of the tissue were fixed in

0.5% glutaraldehyde + 2.5% paraformaldehyde or in 2.5% glutaraldehyde and some specimens were post–fixed in 1% osmium tetroxide. Tissue was dehydrated and embedded in Spurr's resin or LR gold (London Resin Company, UK). Ultrathin sections of tissue mounted on nickel grids were immunogold labelled for IAPP by use of a polyclonal antiserum to IAPP $_{7-37}$, and for insulin by use of a polyclonal antiserum to bovine insulin. Antibody binding sites were localised with protein–A gold.

3.0 Results

3.1. INSULINOMAS

Extracellular amyloid deposits were clearly visible in 9 of the 16 cases of insulinoma, occupying 2–10% of the tumour material. Immunogold labelling for IAPP identified amyloid fibrils which were arranged in random masses between the insulinoma cells. Invaginations in the plasma membrane at the margins of the B–cells were filled with fibrils arranged in a parallel orientation.

3.1.1 *Figure 1.* Electron micrographs of amyloid fibrils in an insulinoma and monkey islet (a). Parallel intracellular fibrils in insulinoma B–cell IAPP–IR, labelled with 10nm gold particles, arrows; I, insulin granule; M, mitochondrion; scale bar, 0.5 μm (b) 'starburst pattern of intracellular amyloid fibrils in insulinoma B–cell; I, insulin granules; scale bar, 1.0 μm (c) radial orientated of extracellular amyloid fibrils in monkey pancreatic islet; scale bar, 1.0 μm.

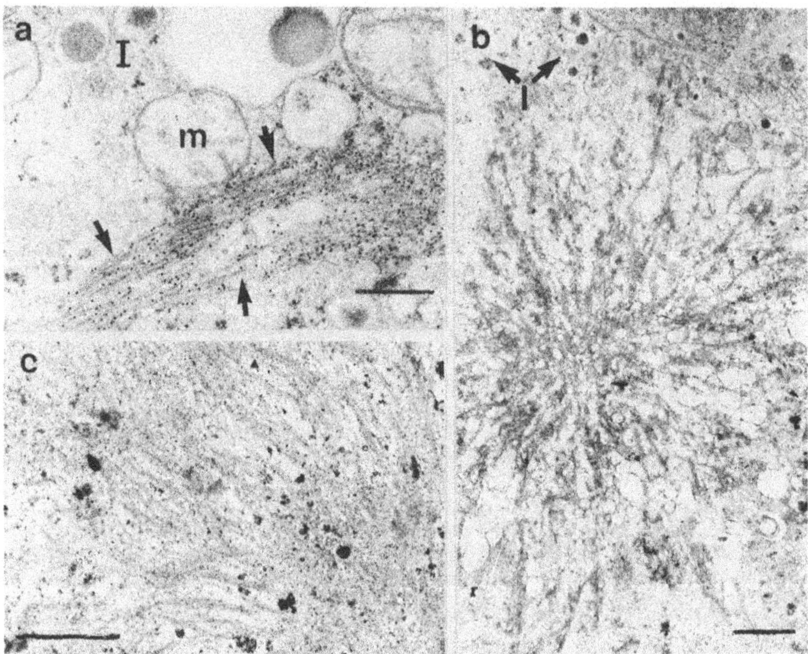

IAPP–IR was present within the profiles of B–cells in 6 specimens of insulinoma. This intracellular IR was located on fibrillar material which was either arranged randomly or in parallel arrays within the cytoplasm (Figure 1a). The fibrils were usually enclosed within membranes which were poorly defined, but which did not have the appearance of rough endoplasmic reticulum. In one specimen a 'starburst' pattern of radially arranged membrane bound IAPP–IR fibrils extended across the cell (Figure 1b); insulin granules and cytoplasmic vesicles were associated with these radially arranged fibrillar structures.

Insulin granules in insulinoma tissue were often atypical: many were non–crystalline and not always surrounded by the characteristic clear halo. Many granules showed poor imunoreactivity for insulin compared to that found in granules of pancreatic islet B–cells. IAPP–IR was found in some insulin granules

3.2. MONKEY PANCREAS

Extracellular IAPP–IR amyloid was present in islets from both of the monkeys. The deposits were often circular, 15–30 μm in diameter and situated adjacent to islet capillaries and the endocrine cells. The amyloid occupied less than 30% of the islet mass. Invaginations of the B–cell plasma membrane were filled with bundles of parallel fibrils as in the insulinomas. The extracellular fibrils were arranged either in irregular masses or, more commonly, in a symmetrical pattern, radiating from a central point (Figure 1c). Smaller masses of immunoreactive material were present adjacent to, or within, insulin–containing B–cells. The lack of clearly defined membranes (an unwanted effect of the fixative regime required to preserve IAPP–IR), prevented identification of the exact location of the amyloid. No intracellular IAPP–IR was found on insulin granules or lysosomes in monkey pancreas.

4.0 Discussion

Formation of amyloid from IAPP requires conversion of a naturally occurring soluble peptide into an insoluble beta–pleated form which polymerises to form amyloid fibrils. Processing of IAPP involves proteolytic cleavage of the peptide from the larger propeptide [12] which would probably occur within the B–cell. Immunoreactivity for the N–terminal flanking peptide of IAPP has been found within the amyloid; this could suggest that abnormal processing of the peptide is involved amyloidosis [13]. Formation of fibrils inside the cell would further support this hypothesis.

Identification of the membranes enclosing the intracellular fibrillar bodies was difficult. When close to the margin of the cell profile, they were not distinguishable from cross–sections of the invaginations at the cell surface. However, many fibrillar bodies were obviously not related to the cell surface and were considered to be truly intracellular.

The mechanisms responsible for fibril formation may be related to the physiological characteristics of B–cells in insulinoma and in diabetic islets; in both, B–cell products are hypersecreted [14] and abnormal processing of insulin results in secretion of proinsulin [15]. Since IAPP is co–located [7] and co–secreted with insulin [16], processing of pro–IAPP and proinsulin could be similar. Thus, intracellular amyloidogenesis might be due to (a) aberrant processing of IAPP or (b) IAPP accumulation within intracellular compartments resulting from aberrant insulin processing. The finding of radial arrays of extracellular amyloid in the monkey islets and a similar pattern of intracellular fibrils in an insulinoma suggests a common mechanism of amyloid deposition: accumulation of fibrils within the cell may develop from a nidus (perhaps a lysosome) and polymerise progressively , eventually resulting in cell death. Compression of the radially arranged extracellular amyloid in the islets would convert the symmetrical array to the irregularly arranged fibrils characteristic of most deposits. Deposition of more amyloid might then occur on pre–existing extracellular fibrils.

ACKNOWLEDGEMENTS: We are grateful to Mr. B.J Britton, Consultant Surgeon, (Oxford) for helpful collaboration in the collection of insulinoma tissue and to T. Alexander and S. Fluck, (Baltimore) for assistance with the experimental animals and to I. Samuel for her help with manuscript preparation. We thank the British Diabetic Association for support (AC and JFM), the National Institutes of Health, USA for a grant (BCH No:DK37717) and the Royal Society, London for a travel grant for AC to attend the Amyloidosis Symposium.

5.0 References

1. Clark, A., Wells, C.A., Buley, I.D., et al. (1988) 'Islet amyloid, increased A–cells, reduced B–cells & exocrine fibrosis: quantitative changes in the pancreas in type 2 diabetes', Diabetes Res. 9, 151–159.
2. Bell, E.T. (1952) 'Hyalinization in the islets of Langerhans in diabetes mellitus', Diabetes 1, 341–344
3. Yano, B.L., Hayden, D.W., and Johnson, K.H. (1981) 'Feline insular amyloid association with diabetes mellitus', Vet Pathol. 18, 621–627.
4. Howard, C.F. (1986) 'Longitudinal studies on the development of diabetes in individual Macaca nigra', Diabetologia 29, 301–306.
5. Westermark, P., Wernstedt, C., Wilander, E., et al. (1987) 'Amyloid fibrils in human insulinoma & islets of Langerhans of the diabetic cat are derived from a neuropeptide–like protein also present in normal cells', Proc. Natl. Acad. Sci USA 84, 3881–3885.
6. Cooper, G.J.S., Willis, A.C., Clark, A., et al. (1987) 'Purification & characterization of a peptide from amyloid–rich pancreas of type 2 diabetic patients', Proc Natl Acad Sci USA 84, 8628–8632.
7. Clark, A., Edwards, C.A., Ostle, L.R., et al. (1989) 'Localisation of islet amyloid peptide in lipofuscin bodies and secretory granules of human B–cells and in islets of Type II diabetic subjects', Cell Tiss Res. 257, 179–185.
8. Lukinius, A., Wilander, E., Westermark, G.T., et al. (1989) 'Co–localisation of islet amyloid polypeptide and insulin in the B–cell secretory granules of human pancreatic islets', Diabetologia 32, 240–244.
9. Westermark, P., Grimelius, L., Polak, J.M., et al. (1977) 'Amyloid in polypeptide hormone producing tumours', Lab Invest. 37, 212–215.
10. Betsholtz, C., Christmanson, L., Engstrom, U., et al. (1990) 'Structure of cat islet amyloid polypeptide & identification of amino acid residues of potential significance for islet amyloid formation', Diabetes 39,118–122.
11. Hansen, B.C. and Bodkin, N.L. (1986) 'Heterogeneity of insulin responses: phases leading to type 2 (non–insulin–dependent) diabetes mellitus in the rhesus monkey', Diabetologia 29, 713–719.
12. Sanke, T., Bell, G.I., Semple, C., et al. (1990) 'An islet amyloid peptide is derived from an 89–amino–acid precursor by proteolytic processing', J Biol. Chem. 263, 17243–17246.
13. Westermark, P., Engstrom, U., Westermark, G.T., et al. (1989) 'Islet amyloid polypeptide (IAPP) & pro–IAPP immunoreactivity in human islets of Langerhans', Diabetes Res. Clin Prac. 7, 219–226.
14. Ward, W.K., LaCava, E.C., Paquette, T.L.,et al. (1987) 'Disproportionate elevation of immunoreactive proinsulin in Type 2 (non–insulin dependent) diabetes mellitus & in experimental insulin resistance', Diabetologia 30, 698–702.
15 Turner, R.C. and Heding, L.G. (1977) 'Plasma proinsulin, C–peptide & insulin in diagnostic suppression tests for insulinomas', Diabetologia 13, 571–577.
16. Kanatsuka, A., Makino, H., Ohsawa, H., et al. (1989) 'Secretion of islet amyloid polypeptide in response to glucose', FEBS Lett 259, 199–201.

A COMPARATIVE STUDY BETWEEN HUMAN B-CELL INSULIN AND ISLET AMYLOID POLYPEPTIDE (IAPP) STORAGE AND AMYLOID DEPOSITION IN TYPE 2 DIABETES MELLITUS AND IN NON-DIABETICS

Berends, M.J.H.*, Nieuwenhuis, M.G.#, Lips, C.J.M.#, Blok, A.P.R.*, Ooms, E.C.M.*, Veldhuizen, R.W.*
* Department of Pathology, Westeinde Hospital, PB 432, 2501 CK The Hague
# Department of Internal Medicine, University Hospital, PB 85500, 3508 GA Utrecht, The Netherlands

INTRODUCTION

Islet amyloid polypeptide is a recently discovered pancreatic polypeptide hormone which is produced by the B-cells of the islets of Langerhans and is co-secreted with insulin. IAPP is the formative protein in islet amyloid depositions in type-2 diabetes patients and in some non-diabetics.

We performed a retrospective immunohistochemical investigation on surgical and autopsy pancreatic tissue specimens in order to get answers to questions concerning:

1. the distribution pattern of IAPP-immunoreactivity (IR) in normal islets and in islets of type-2 diabetic patients.
2. the influence of autolytic processes on the IR of IAPP and insulin.
3. the relationship between the cytoplasmatic IAPP-IR and the pattern and/or the amount of amyloid deposited in the islets.

MATERIAL AND METHODS

From 160 autopsied patients and 10 surgical patients one specimen of pancreatic tissue per patient was screened for the presence of amyloid with the Sulfated Alcian Blue (SAB) staining method. All the positive specimens (confirmed by Congo red staining) and a selection of the negatives were stained with the indirect ABC immunoperoxidase method, using rabbit anti-synthetic human amylin (Peninsula) and anti-human insulin (Dako). All samples were routinely fixed in 4% formaldehyde, dehydrated in acetone and embedded in paraffin (Paraclean). The specimens were then divided into groups according to their state of autolytic damage.
For tissues obtained surgically: fixation within one hour after removal, with or without frozen section procedure for other pathology during operation.
For autopsy material: fixation within 1 hour after autopsy and autopsy within 12 hours after death: day 0, resp. after one day, after two days and after three days.
In addition, some samples were immunostained with rabbit antisera to a synthetic rat Calcitonin Gene Related Peptide (CGRP) fragment (23-37,Amersham), to human glucagon and with a monoclonal antibody to AA-amyloid (Dako).

RESULTS

The SAB-screening results of 160 autopsies and 10 surgical pancreatic tissue sections to detect amyloid are shown in table 1.

Sulfated Alcian Blue staining

10 surgical	
1 positive	9 negative
1 DM-2	9 non-DM*

160 autopsies				
54 positive		106 negative		
21 non-DM-2*	33 DM-2	2 DM-2	3 DM-1	101 non-DM*

Table 1a

* not known as overt diabetic (DM)

Of 35 DM-2 and 21 non-DM-2 patients the number of amyloid positive islets and the total number of islets per cm^2 of examined tissue are given in table 1b.(**fat**:number of amyloid-positive islets:thin:total number of islets per cm^2.

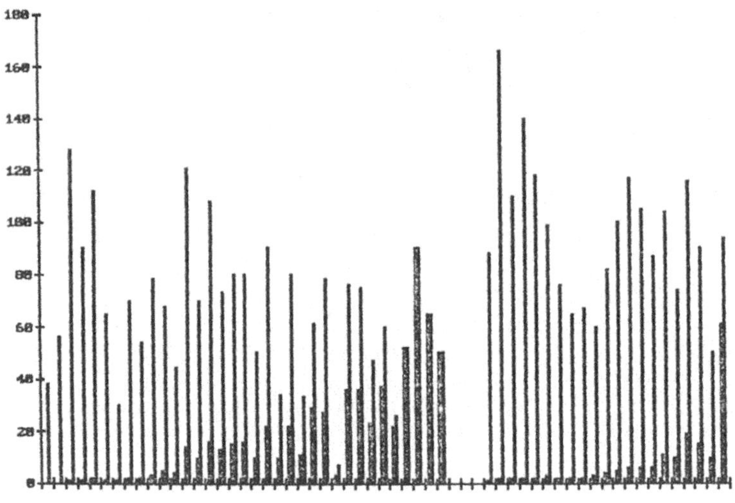

Table 1b

In 32 of 86 cases from all patient groups, the tissue appeared to be well preserved. The results of the influence of the preservation state concerning IR are given in table 2.

INFLUENCE of AUTOLYTIC PROCESSES on IR to:					
INSULIN	CGRP	AMYLIN		GLUCAGON	
B-cells	amyloid	amyloid		B-cells	A-cells
insensitive to lytic processes				sensitive to lytic processes	

Table 2

ISLET STAINING PATTERN IN AMYLOID NEGATIVE PANCREAS
Normal cell counts (5 micron section): about 200 cells in an islet of average diameter.
Immunoreactive B-cells (IAPP and insulin): 70-90% of the islet cells.
IR-insulin:
- strong and diffuse staining
- high storage capacity
- **resistant** to autolytic damage

IR-IAPP:
- variable staining intensity; often stronger staining in the cytoplasm facing the capillary wall
- compared to insulin less storage capacity
- very sensitive to autolytic processes and freeze-thawing

ISLET STAINING PATTERN IN AMYLOID POSITIVE PANCREAS
Cell counts in general normal; cell reduction - to 10-20% - occurs only in case of massive amyloid deposition.
Immunoreactive B-cells: 70-90% of the islet cells.
IR-insulin:
- staining pattern normal
- in spite of cell reduction there are always immunoreactive B-cells left

IR-IAPP in amyloid:
- strong reaction in amyloid depositions
- amyloid always appears to be deposited extracellularly between the B-cell and the capillary wall, surrounding these walls and never between B-cells
- amyloid positive islets can be seen evenly distributed throughout the section, but occur more often in clusters.

IR-IAPP CYTOPLASMATIC STAINING PATTERN (in well preserved tissue)

- in amyloid negative islets : staining as in normal amyloid negative pancreatic specimens
- in amyloid positive islets : smaller number of positive staining cells (fig.1)
- INVERSE RELATIONSHIP between amyloid deposits and percentage

INFLUENCE of AUTOLYTIC PROCESSES on IR to:				
INSULIN	CGRP	AMYLIN		GLUCAGON
B-cells	amyloid	amyloid	B-cells	A-cells
insensitive to lytic processes			sensitive to lytic processes	

Table 2

ISLET STAINING PATTERN IN AMYLOID NEGATIVE PANCREAS

Normal cell counts (5 micron section): about 200 cells in an islet of average diameter.

Immunoreactive B-cells (IAPP and insulin): 70-90% of the islet cells.

IR-insulin:
- strong and diffuse staining
- high storage capacity
- **resistant** to autolytic damage

IR-IAPP:
- variable staining intensity; often stronger staining in the cytoplasm facing the capillary wall
- compared to insulin less storage capacity
- very sensitive to autolytic processes and freeze-thawing

ISLET STAINING PATTERN IN AMYLOID POSITIVE PANCREAS

Cell counts in general normal; cell reduction - to 10-20% - occurs only in case of massive amyloid deposition.

Immunoreactive B-cells: 70-90% of the islet cells.

IR-insulin:
- staining pattern normal
- in spite of cell reduction there are always immunoreactive B-cells left

IR-IAPP in amyloid:
- strong reaction in amyloid depositions
- amyloid always appears to be deposited extracellularly between the B-cell and the capillary wall, surrounding these walls and never between B-cells
- amyloid positive islets can be seen evenly distributed throughout the section, but occur more often in clusters

IR-IAPP CYTOPLASMATIC STAINING PATTERN (in well preserved tissue)

- in amyloid negative islets : staining as in normal amyloid negative pancreatic specimens
- in amyloid positive islets : smaller number of positive staining cells (fig.1)
- INVERSE RELATIONSHIP between amyloid deposits and percentage

of cytoplasmatic IAPP-IR staining cells
- the amount of cytoplasmatic IAPP-IR is inversely related to the surface of the capillary walls covered with amyloid.

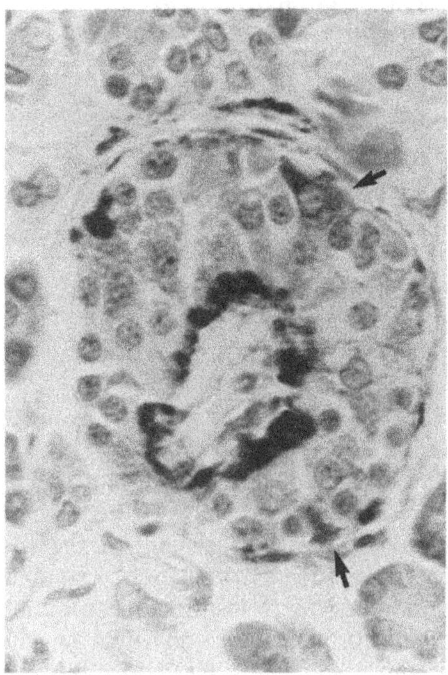

Figure 1. IR-IAPP amyloid deposits surrounding a central capillary wall; two cells (arrow) show strong cytoplasmatic IR-IAPP.

CONCLUSIONS:
1. There is no difference in IR-patterns - concerning IAPP and insulin - between non-diabetic and type-2 diabetic amyloid negative pancreatic islets.
2. IR to insulin and to IAPP in amyloid is not affected by autolytic damage, in contrast to cytoplasmatic IAPP-IR, which is lost very easily.
3. In both, non-diabetic and type-2 diabetic IAPP-amyloid-positive islets, cytoplasmatic IAPP-IR is inversely related to the amount of surface of capillary walls covered with amyloid.

HYPOTHESES:
- Adequate stimulation of B-cells to secrete IAPP and insulin may be hampered by a layer of amyloid deposits surrounding the lamina basalis of the capillary walls. IAPP is not stored and the release of small amounts is directly apposited to the amyloid layer. The process of IAPP amyloid deposition is slowly progressive, at least in type-2 diabetes patients, eventually resulting in insulin deficiency.
- The finding of the presence of amyloid positive islets often clustered together among normal islets may render support to a new hypothesis of a genetic B-cell defect: two recessive mutations in homologous alleles are required to express the abnormality in B-cells: in most cases the first mutation is inherited.

Pancreatic Islet Amyloid in the Degu Is Derived from Insulin

Timothy D. O'Brien*, Ulf Hellman+, Per Westermark¶, Christer Wernstedt+, William B. Rathbun§, and Kenneth H. Johnson*

Department of Veterinary Pathobiology, University of Minnesota, St. Paul, MN 55108*; Department of Pathology, Linköping University, Linköping, Sweden¶; Ludwig Institute for Cancer Research, Uppsala Branch, Uppsala, Sweden+; and Department of Ophthalmology, University of Minnesota, Minneapolis, MN§.

Abstract

Pancreatic islet amyloid was isolated from pooled degu (Octodon degus) pancreases and purified by gel chromatography and reversed phase HPLC. Amino acid sequence analysis revealed that the major protein component of the islet amyloid was insulin. In tissue sections, the degu islet amyloid lost congophilia following oxidation with $KMnO_4$; had immunoreactivity to insulin antiserum; and lacked immunoreactivity to IAPP and other hormones. Degu islet amyloid, therefore, represents a distinct form of islet amyloid which is derived from insulin rather than islet amyloid polypeptide (IAPP).

Introduction

The occurrence of islet amyloid in the degu is curious and unique in that it is the only rodent species known to develop islet amyloid [1]. A rodent model would be a very useful tool in the study of the pathogenesis of islet amyloidosis. Therefore, the current study was conducted to characterize the islet amyloid deposits that occur in the degu, and to determine whether the islet amyloid in this species is related to islet amyloid polypeptide (IAPP)(as are human and feline islet amyloids)[2] or other islet hormones. Another goal was to determine whether IAPP is present in pancreatic islet cells of the degu, as has been demonstrated in several other species previously studied [3].

Materials and Methods

Pancreases from 8 female and 4 male degus (age 2.5 to 3.5 years) were fixed in

10% neutral buffered formalin, processed by standard techniques, and stained with hematoxylin and eosin, Congo red, and Congo red following oxidation with $KMnO_4$. Immunoperoxidase staining on pancreatic sections (with and without formic acid pretreatment) for insulin, IAPP, glucagon, somatostatin, pancreatic polypeptide and calcitonin gene-related peptide was done as previously described [3,4]. Positive and negative controls were then performed with antisera and techniques as previously described [3].

Pancreases pooled from 8 aged degus were used to isolate islet amyloid as previously described [2]. Lyophilized islet amyloid protein was purified on a Sephadex G50 Fine column [5]. The fractions containing the small single retarded peak protein were pooled and an aliquot dialyzed exhaustively against distilled water and lyophilized. Sodium dodecyl sulphate polyacrylamide gel electrophoresis (10-20% gradient) was performed on this gel purified protein. An aliquot of the partially (gel chromatography) purified islet amyloid protein was then sequenced for 18 steps on an automatic sequence analyzer. Since initial amino acid sequencing indicated that the islet amyloid protein was insulin, additional aliquots of the gel purified islet amyloid protein were reduced, pyridylethylated, and separated by reversed phase HPLC [5], which resulted in separation of the insulin A- and B-chains. The purified insulin chains were then subjected to complete amino acid analysis [5].

Results

Amyloid was identified by typical Congo red staining in 10 of 12 degu pancreases. Congo red staining of the islet amyloid was partially to completely eliminated following oxidation by $KMnO_4$. Immunohistochemical staining showed that degu islet amyloid had moderate immunoreactivity with anti-porcine-insulin serum, whereas, little or no immunoreactivity was detected with antisera directed against other hormones. Formic acid treatment markedly increased islet amyloid immunoreactivity with antiserum to insulin, but had no effect on immunoreactivity with the other antisera. IAPP immunoreactivity was noted in islet cells of 11 of 12 degus. The distribution of IAPP immunoreactivity compared to insulin indicated that it was present in the beta cells as reported in other species [3]. CGRP immunoreactivity was not detected in islet cells.

Amyloid in the initial pellet readily dissolved in 6M guanidine HCl in 0.1 M Tris-HCl buffer solution. SDS-PAGE of material from the single small protein peak obtained by gel chromatography revealed only one retarded protein band with apparent molecular weight less than 6 kDa. Reduction, pyridylethylation and reversed phase HPLC separation of the gel purified material resulted in complete purification of the insulin A- and B-chains. Amino acid analysis of the two major HPCL peaks showed that these fractions corresponded to the A- and B-chains of degu insulin respectively (Fig. 1).

```
Insulin A-Chain

1     5       10      15      20
G-I-V-D-Q-C-C-N-N-I-C-T-F-N-Q-L-Q-N-Y-C-N-V-P      Degu

G-I-V-D-Q-C-C-T-N-I-C-S-R-N-Q-L-M-S-Y-C-N-D        Coypu

G-I-V-D-Q-C-C-T-N-I-C-S-R-N-Q-L-L-T-Y-C-N          Casiragua

G-I-V-E-Q-C-C-T-S-I-C-S-L-Y-Q-L-E-N-Y-C-N          Human


Insulin B-Chain

1     5       10      15      20      25      30
Y-S-S-Q-H-L-C-G-S-N-L-V-E-A-L-Y-M-T-C-G-R-S-G-F-X-Y-R-P-H-D  Degu

Y-V-S-Q-R-L-C-G-S-Q-L-V-D-T-L-Y-S-V-C-R-H-R-G-F-X-Y-R-P-N-D  Coypu

Y-V-G-Q-R-L-C-G-S-Q-L-V-D-T-L-Y-S-V-C-K-H-R-G-F-X-Y-R-P-S-E  Casiragua

F-V-N-Q-H-L-C-G-S-H-L-V-E-A-L-Y-L-V-C-G-E-R-G-F-F-Y-T-P-L-T  Human
```

Figure 1. The complete amino acid sequence of the A- and B-chains of degu insulin, purified from islet amyloid. Amino acid sequence comparisons are made with human, coypu, and casiragua insulins (homologous residues shown in bold type).

Discussion

In this study we have shown immunohistochemically and by amino acid sequence analysis that insulin and not IAPP is the precursor protein for islet amyloid in the degu. This is in contrast to human and cats, where islet amyloid has been shown to be derived from IAPP [2]. Several other findings are consistent with a non-IAPP origin of degu islet amyloid including: insulin and not IAPP immunoreactivity, partial to complete loss of congophilia following $KMnO_4$ oxidation, and solubility in 6 M guanidine HCl solution [2]. The findings of this study are also consistent with recent findings indicating that the cDNA predicted degu IAPP amino acid sequence (Nishi M, Steiner DF, personal communication) lacks the putative amyloidogenic sequence which is present in the 20-29 region of human and cat IAPP [6], and would therefore not be expected to form amyloid fibrils.

The primary amino acid sequence of the degu insulin A-chain is unique, in that it is comprised of 23 amino acids (Fig. 1), whereas, in most species except the Coypu (Myocastor coypus, another hystrichomorph) it is 21 amino acids in length [7]. The degu insulin B-chain is comprised of 29 amino acid residues whereas, in most species it is comprised of 30 amino acids [7]. The deletion occurs most likely at position 25, as in the coypu and casiragua [7]. The degu insulin B-chain has 63% and 57% homology to the coypu and casiragua respectively and has 60% homology to the human B-chain. Whether the distinctive amino acid sequence of degu insulin causes it to have an increased tendency to form amyloid fibrils is unknown at this time.

References

1. Murphy JC, Crowell TP, Hewes KM, Fox JG, Shalev M: Spontaneous lesions in the degu. In Symposium of Comparative Pathology of Zoo Animals. Smithsonian Institute Press, 1979, p. 437-44

2. Westermark P, Wernstedt C, Wilander E, Hayden DW, O'Brien TD, Johnson KH: Amyloid fibrils in human insulinoma and islets of Langerhans of the diabetic cat are derived from a novel neuropeptide-like protein also present in normal islet cells. Proc Natl Acad Sci USA 84:3881-85, 1987

3. Johnson KH, O'Brien TD, Hayden DW, Jordan K, Ghobrial HKG, Mahoney WC, Westermark P: Immunolocalization of islet amyloid polypeptide (IAPP) in pancreatic beta cells using peroxidase antiperoxidase (PAP) and protein A-gold techniques. Am J Pathol 130:1-8, 1988

4. Kitamoto T, Ogomori K, Tateishi J, Prusiner SB: Formic acid pretreatment enhances immunostaining of cerebral and systemic amyloids. Lab Invest 57:230-36, 1987

5. Hellman U, Wernstedt C, Westermark P, O'Brien TD, Rathbun WB, Johnson KH: Amino acid sequence from degu islet amyloid-derived insulin shows unique sequence characteristics. Biochem Biophys Res Comm 169:571-577, 1990

6. Westermark P, Engström U, Johnson KH, Westermark GT, Betsholtz C: Islet amyloid polypeptide: Pinpointing amino acid residues linked to amyloid fibril formation. Proc Natl Acad Sci USA 87:5036-5040, 1990.

7. Halldén G, Gafvelin G, Mutt V, Jörnvall H: Characterization of cat insulin. Comp Biochem Biophys 247:20-27, 1986

ISOLATED ATRIAL AMYLOID DEPOSITS. IMMUNOCHEMICAL EVIDENCE FOR THE PRESENCE OF POLYPEPTIDES WITH MOLECULAR WEIGHTS HIGHER AND LOWER THAN ATRIAL NATRIURETIC PEPTIDE ANP

R.P. Linke, H.O. Klein, S. Modrow, M. Marin-Grez

Institute of Immunology, Goethestr. 31, 8000-Munich
Department of Physiology, Pettenkoferstr. 12, 8000-Munich
Pettenkofer-Institute of Microbiology, Pettenkoferstr. 9

ABSTRACT. Isolated atrial amyloid deposits were shown by immunohistochemistry and by N-terminal amino acid sequencing to be derived from the atrial natriuretic peptide (ANP). To find out whether only the ANP monomer (3.5 kDa) was present, an atrial amyloid fibril concentrate was solubilized and separated by size. All fractions were examined for the presence of ANP-antigenic material by radioimmunoassay. The result shows that besides monomeric ANP also molecules of approximately 7 kDa and those smaller than ANP could be detected. The larger fractions could represent ANP-dimers or a precursor of ANP, and the molecules smaller than ANP could represent degradation products.

1. INTRODUCTION

The frequency of isolated atrial amyloid deposits increases steeply with advancing age. Most of the individuals over 85 years are affected. The clinical significance, however, has not definitively been evaluated (1). Amyloid deposits of this disorder were shown to be derived from ANP, by immunohistochemistry (2), and by N-terminal amino acid sequence analysis (3, 4). ANP is known to be synthesized in atrial myocytes and secreted into the plasma by atrial filling presure, in order to regulate the blood volume by diuresis and sodium uresis (5). It is the purpose of this report to find out whether only monomeric ANP or molecular species of different molecular weight are present in the ANP-derived amyloid. To this end, amyloid fibril proteins were separated by size and the individual fractions were radioimmunoassayed for the presence of ANP.

2. MATERIAL AND METHODS

2.1 Separation by size

The amyloid fibrils of amyloid-containing atrial tissue of a 67-year-old woman were extracted and concentrated as previously described (4). The major proportion of amyloid was not found in the water extracts, but in the final sediment. After reduction with dithiothreitol in 8M guanidine-HCl, the sample was acidified with formic acid and the solubilized proteins were applied to an Ultropac TSK G2000SW column (7.5 x 300 mm, LKB, Freiburg/FRG) and separated in 60% formic acid and 10% isopropanol.

2.2 Radioimmunoassay

Aliquots of the fractions obtained by HPLC were radioimmunoassayed using polyclonal antibodies against alpha human ANP (αhANP) and radiolabelled ^{125}J-αhANP (both from Amersham Buchler, Braunschweig/FRG). Standard was $\alpha hANP_{1-28}$ (Bissendorf Biochemicls GmbH, Hannover/FRG). Bound tracer was separated from free tracer by double antibody technique. Samples were measured at the straight part of the standard curve (4-50ng/ml).

2.3 Polyclonal anti-ANP antibodies

To identify ANP-derived amyloid in tissue sections, we induced anti-ANP antibodies in four rabbits (Deutsche Riesenschecken) using two automatically synthesized ANP-analogues (Applied Biosystems, 430A): ANP, **desCys 121: 105-123** CFGGRMDRIGAQSGLG-NS, and **ANP 111-123**: DRIGAQSGLGCNS. The peptides were coupled to bovine thyreoglobulin (Sigma, Taufkirchen/FRG) and tetanustoxoid (Behring-Werke, Marburg/FRG) (5mg + 2.5mg + 0.1mg, respectively) using 1-ethyl-3-(3-dimethyl-aminopropyl) carbodiimide-HCl (6). The dialysed and lyophilized conjugate was dissolved in 0.9% NaCl and emulsified with an equal volume of complete Freund's adjuvant (Behring-Werke) and injected at 200µg per rabbit intradermally at multiple sites. Booster injections were given one month later and monthly thereafter for approximately 6 months. The antibody response was examined on fixed paraffin sections for the reaction with atrial myocytes. The antibody titer of the best bleedings was determined by the binding of ^{125}JαANP to serial dilution of antibodies. The dilution with 50% maximal binding was taken as the value for the titre.

3. RESULTS AND DISCUSSION

3.1 Chromatography of amyloid fibril proteins

The elution profile of the size separation of atrial amyloid fibrils is shown in Fig. 1. The protein elution curve displayed three peaks, one void volume protein and one at the position of salt. At position of 3.5 kDa, around fraction 25, the small protein peak was found to represent ANP by partial sequence analysis (4). Monitoring each of the fractions for the presence of ANP-antigenic material, fractions around 25 gave the strongest signal coinciding with the position of ANP, which was also identified with a synthetic ANP and monitored at 280nm. By contrast to synthetic ANP, polypeptides from the atrial amyloid showed larger and smaller ANP-antigenic molecular species. These additional molecules could either represent ANP-aggregates, possibly dimers, and the small ones degradation products of ANP. The additional molecules are either adsorbed to the amyloid fibril or they are indeed incorporated into the amyloid fibril.

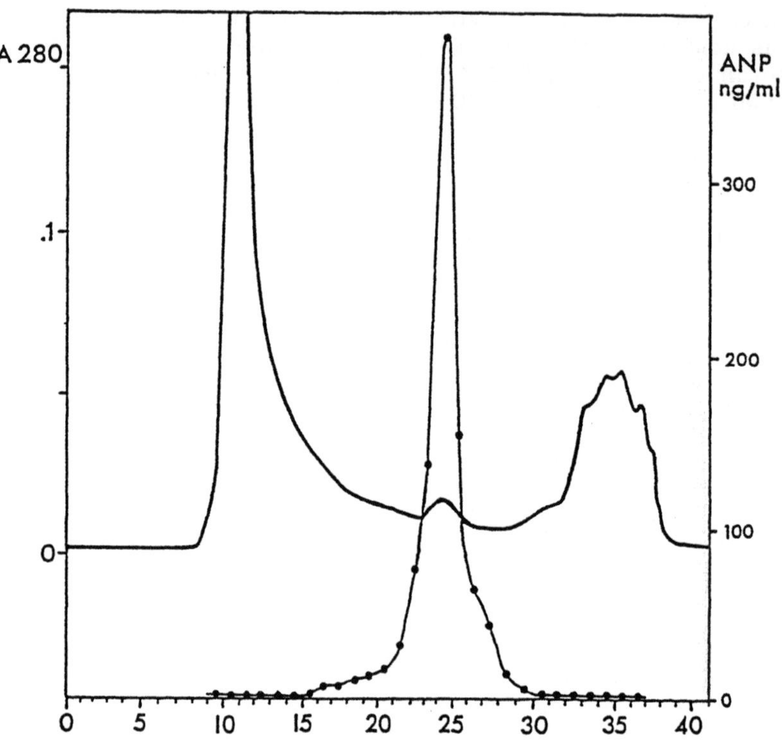

Fig. 1: Size separation by HPLC of isolated atrial amyloid fibril proteins and analysis for ANP-antigenic material by radio-immunoassay.

Fraction number is seen at the abszissa and continuous protein determination at the ordinate left, and ANP concentration at the ordinate right. The small peak at approximately 3.5 kDa comprises most of the immunoreactivity.

Fig.: 2: Results on anti-ANP performance

Rabbit Bleeding	991 7.7.88	992 21.5.88	992 7.7.88	993 7.7.88	
ANP on myocytes	++	+++	++	+	
Amyloid in tissue sect.	0	(+)	++	0	
RIA-Titer (50% max.) n:	4000	10000	4000	<200	1/n

Antibody response to ANP and the amyloid in tissue sections was very different in the four rabbits. Only one rabbit, injected with the first ANP synthetic peptide reacted very strong on atrial myocytes in tissue sections and with ANP by radioimmunoassay. This rabbit also reacted with atrial myocates of other vertebrates (dog, goat, mouse, frog, chicken). Only serum obtained from one of the two rabbits injected with the second peptide moderately stained amyloid. A summary of the performance of the peptid antibodies against ANP is given in Fig. 2. The four rabbits show a heterogeneous response to ANP. The divergence between reactivity towards ANP and atrial amyloid is intriguing. Different from other amyloid types with a more uniform staining, some amyloid deposits are less stained than others. These data may indicate, that the ANP in amyloid has a different conformation as compared to the native molecule. Alternatively, the atrial amyloid is not antigenically identical in all patients and all deposits of one patient.

4. REFERENCES

1. Westermark, P., Johannson, B., Natvig, J.B.: Senile cardiac amyloidosis; evidence of two different amyloid substances in the aging heart.
Scand. J. Immunol. 10, 303-308 (1980)
2. Kaye, G.C., Butler, M.G., D'Ardenne, A.J., Edmonson, S.J., Camm, A.J., Slavin, G.: Isolated atrial amyloid contains atrial natriuretic peptide: a report of six cases.
Brit. Heart J., 56, 317-320 (1986)
3. Johannsson, B., Wernstedt, C., Westermark, P.: Atrial natriure9tic peptide deposited as atrial amyloid fibrils.
Biochem. Biophys. Res. Comm. 148, 1087-1092 (1987)
4. Linke, R.P., Voigt, C., Störkel, F.S., Eulitz, M.: N-terminal amino acid sequence analysis indicates that isolated atrial amyloid is derived from atrial natriuretic peptide.
Virchows Archiv 55, 125-127 (1988)
5. Flynn, G., Davis, P.L.: The biochemistry and molecular biology of atrial natriuretic factor. Review article.
Biochem. J. 232, 313-321 (1985)
6. Goodfriend, T.L., Levine, L., Fasman, G.D.: Antibody to bradykinin and angiotensine: a use of carbodiimid in immunology.
Science 144, 1344-1346 (1964)

4. ACKNOWLEGMENT

This work was supported by the Deutsche Forschungsgemeinschaft, Sonderforschungsbereich 207, G8, DFG Li 247/7-2, and Ma 948/1-2. We thank Mss. U. Kunert and A. Kerling for technical assistance.

RAISED PREVALENCE OF ISOLATED ATRIAL AMYLOIDOSIS IN CHRONIC HEART DISEASE

L.M. LOOI
Department of Pathology
Faculty of Medicine
University of Malaya
59100 Kuala Lumpur, Malaysia

ABSTRACT

Congo red screening of 211 consecutive cardiac biopsies obtained during cardiac surgery from 167 patients revealed 26 (16%) instances of isolated atrial amyloidosis (IAA). IAA-positive patients ranged from 25 to 52 years in age with a mean of 39 years. Controls consisted of 247 healthy adults autopsied for traumatic deaths, with an age range of 18 to 89 years and a mean of 38 years. Only 7 (3%) control subjects were IAA-positive, all above 40 years of age. 23 (88%) IAA-positive biopsies were from patients with chronic rheumatic heart disease (CRHD) and 3 (11%) atrial septal defect (ASD). The prevalence of IAA in CRHD was 23%, appreciably higher than that in ASD (15%) and other patients with atrial biopsies. The prevalence in both CRHD and ASD was significantly higher ($P<0.001$) than in the controls. IAA deposits were permanganate-resistant and immunohistochemically negative for AA protein. They were observed in intramyocardial vessel walls, along the myocardial sarcolemma and the subendocardium. There was associated myocyte hypertrophy but no atrophy. Electron microscopy demonstrated typical non-branching amyloid fibrils. It is postulated that mechanical and physiological stress to the atria results in a raised prevalence of IAA. The association of atrial natriuretic peptides with IAA would support this view.

INTRODUCTION

It is recognised that senile cardiac amyloidosis is not a single entity and that histomorphologically and chemically different forms occur. Conventional senile cardiac amyloidosis (SCA) can be associated with amyloid deposits in other organs, such as the lungs, forming a feature of senile systemic amyloidosis [1]. Another form of senile cardiac amyloidosis, named isolated atrial amyloidosis (IAA), is localized to the atria and has been shown to contain atrial natriuretic peptide (ANP) [2,3]. A third form of age-related cardiovascular amyloid, senile aortic amyloid, is usually localized to the aorta [4]. An increased prevalence of IAA has been observed in Malaysian patients who underwent cardiac surgery for a variety of heart ailments. The study is reported below.

MATERIALS AND METHODS

During a 5.5-year-period, 27,052 surgical biopsies received by the Department of Pathology, University of Malaya were screened histologically, using alkaline Congo red, for amyloid to determine the pattern of amyloidosis among Malaysians. Among these were 211 consecutive cardiac biopsies obtained during cardiac surgery from 167 patients. Controls consisted of tissues from both atrial appendages, the interventricular septum and the roots of the aorta and pulmonary artery removed at autopsy from 247 healthy adults (above 17 years old) with sudden traumatic deaths and no evidence of heart disease.

Sections from formalin-fixed, paraffin-embedded tissues were stained with H&E and alkaline Congo red with and without prior treatment with $KMnO_4$. Further sections from amyloid positive cases were stained for human AA protein, human AP protein and human immunoglobulin lambda and kappa light chains using immunoperoxidase methods. Paraffin-embedded material from 19 positive cases were reprocessed for electron microscopy.

RESULTS

Prevalence: Of 167 patients screened, 80 were Chinese, 58 Malay, 28 Indian and 1 other. There was no significant difference in the prevalence of IAA among the various ethnic groups. The distribution of biopsies by location were: 80 right atrium, 71 left atrium, 27 mitral valve, 17 infundibular wall, 3 interatrial septum, 5 aortic valve and 8 other. IAA was detected in 26 biopsies, all atrial tissues. Since atrial biopsies were obtained from 154 of the 167 patients screened, the overall prevalence of IAA in atrial biopsies was 16.9% (26/154). 2 mitral valves and 1 aortic valve exhibited the typical irregular plaques of dystrophic amyloidosis and were hence excluded from further analysis.

Prevalence in atrial appendages: 80 patients had left atrial appendage biopsies (Table 1). 78 (98%) underwent closed mitral valvotomy for chronic rheumatic mitral valve disease. 1 had a left atrial myxoma and the other, a ventricular septal defect (VSD). There were 19 IAA-positive cases, giving an overall prevalence of 24% and a range of 13% in the 3rd decade of life to 67% in the 6th decade. Their ages ranged from 25 to 52 years with a mean of 36 years. All IAA-positive left atrial biopsies were from patients with chronic rheumatic heart disease (CRHD).

71 patients had right atrial appendage biopsies. 21 had CRHD, 17 atrial septal defect (ASD), 9 VSD, 8 pulmonary stenosis, 8 Fallot's tetralogy and the remaining a variety of other cardiac problems. 6 had IAA, suggesting a prevalence in right atrial appendages of 8% (6/71). Of these, 4 had CRHD and 2 had ASD. The age distribution of IAA-positive cases in relation to these ailments is shown in Table 1. All IAA-positive cases were females. Their ages ranged from 39 to 52 years with a mean of 46 years. All 3 biopsies from the interatrial septum were from

patients with ASD; the sole biopsy positive for IAA was from a 52-year-old Chinese female.

<u>Prevalence in relation to disease conditions</u>: All 26 IAA-positive biopsies were from patients with either CRHD or ASD. The prevalence of IAA in CRHD was about 23% (23/90), appreciably higher than that of 15% (3/20) in ASD. In both CRHD and ASD, the prevalence was significantly higher ($p<0.001$) than the prevalence of 3% observed in healthy controls.

<u>Controls</u>: The ages of controls ranged from 18 to 88 years with a mean of 38 years. IAA was detected in 3% (7/247), ranging from 3% in the 5th decade to 33% in the 9th decade. There was no ethnic or sex predilection in IAA-positivity. IAA was only detected in individuals older than 40 years and involved 5 right atrial appendages and 4 left atrial appendages. The interventricular septum and aorticopulmonary vessels were spared.

TABLE 1. Age distribution of IAA-positivity in test subjects and controls

Age (yr)	Left atria		Right atria*		Controls	
	Positive	Screened	Positive	Screened	Positive	Screened
0-9	0	0	0	4	0	0
10-19	0	6	0	4	0	11
20-29	5 (13%)	39	0	13	0	100
30-39	8 (38%)	21	1	9	0	41
40-49	4 (36%)	11	4	5	3 (9.4%)	32
50-59	2 (67%)	3	1	3	1 (3.4%)	29
60-69	0	0	0	0	1 (6.3%)	16
70-79	0	0	0	0	1 (6.7%)	15
80-89	0	0	0	0	+1 (33.3%)	3
>90	0	0	0	0	0	0
Total	19 (24%)	80	6	38	7 (2.8%)	247

* Only patients with CRHD or ASD
+ Also had senile aortic amyloid

<u>Staining characteristics, morphology and clinical features</u>: IAA was not discernible on the routine H&E stain but showed definite rose-pink Congophilic deposits with characteristic apple-green birefringence. They were either permanganate-resistant or partially resistant. AA protein and immunoglobulin light chains were not detectable. AP protein was usually present.

IAA deposits occurred in the subintima and media of small intramyocardial arteries and arterioles and along myocardial sarcolemma. Irregular small nodular or streaky deposits were often present in the subendocardial tissues. There was associated myocardial hypertrophy but no myocyte atrophy. Electron microscopy demonstrated non-branching amyloid fibrils in all 19 cases for which ultrastructural examination was performed.

IAA-positive subjects had decreased effort tolerance of a

mean duration of 5 years by the time of surgery. This was attributable to their respective cardiac disease. There were no features suggestive of systemic amyloidosis. One patient died postoperatively; no deposits were found outside the heart. Similar limitation of deposits to atria was noted in controls.

DISCUSSION

Though IAA is known to begin at a slightly younger age than conventional SCA, this study shows its occurrence at an even younger age-group than expected. The obvious difference between this Malaysian study and others is that here, one is investigating a group of patients with cardiac ailments serious enough to warrant cardiac surgery. Thus, it is reasonable to infer that chronic heart disease contibutes significantly to a higher prevalence of IAA. The duration of heart disease, besides age, may well have a role to play in the rising prevalence observed with age.

That chronic heart disease, in particular CRHD and ASD, can result in an earlier and more frequent occurrence of IAA is an important observation. It implies that factors other than age are active in the pathogenesis of IAA. It is conceivable that recurrent and chronic inflammation in rheumatic heart disease, as well as physiological stress on the atria due to abnormal haemodynamics, such as in mitral valve disease or ASD, can contribute to an increase in IAA formation. Alternatively, the damaged atria may have a reduced capacity to degrade and remove amyloid deposits. The recent finding that IAA contains atrial natriuretic peptide [2,3] would support a direct role of the atrial myocyte in IAA formation. Although IAA appears relatively "silent" clinically, it is premature to regard it as harmless. Whether IAA in patients with heart disease will progress and lead to acclerated cardiac damage or contribute to the development of troublesome arrhythmias, digoxin sensitivity or cardiac failure, need to be clarified. These aspects will have obvious clinical relevance in the care of these patients.

REFERENCES

1. Pitkanen P, Westermark P and Cornwell III GG. (1984) Senile systemic amyloidosis. Am J Pathol, 117: 391-399.

2. Kayle GC, Butler MG, D'Ardenne AJ, Edmondson SJ, Camm AJ and Slavin G. (1986) Identification of immunoreactive atrial natriuretic peptide in atrial amyloid. J Clin Pathol, 39: 581-582.

3. Johansson B, Wernstedt C and Westermark P. (1987) Atrial natriuretic peptide deposited as atrial amyloid fibrils. Biochem Biophys Res Commun, 148: 1087-1092.

4. Cornwell III GG, Murdoch WL, Kyle RA, Westermark P and Pitkanen P. (1983) Frequency and distribution of senile cardiovascular amyloid. A clinicopathologic correlation. Am J Med, 75: 618-623.

ISOLATED ATRIAL AMYLOIDOSIS. INCREASED FREQUENCY IN PATIENTS WITH CONGESTIVE CARDIAC FAILURE.

B Johansson and P Westermark
Department of Rehabilitation Medicine, University of Uppsala and Department of Pathology, University of Linköping, Sweden

The major subunit protein in isolated atrial amyloid (IAA) is ANF. Patients with congestive cardiac failure have high levels of ANF. The main objective was to study if there was a correlation between cardiac failure and IAA. Eighty autopsied patients were investigated; 48 with congestive cardiac failure were compared with 32 without cardiac failure. Congo red stained sections from both atria and left ventricle were studied under polarized light. Statistical analysis revealed an age-adjusted 4.3-fold increase in the risk of having amyloidosis of IAA type if cardiac failure was present. IAA could be a consequence of cardiac failure. However, since a few patients without cardiac failure had rather heavy amyloid infiltration, there must be other factors of importance in the pathogenesis of IAA.

Introduction

Isolated atrial amyloid (IAA) is an amyloid restricted to the atria of the heart, seen in a majority of older patients [1-3]. The major subunit protein is atrial natriuretic factor (ANF) [4, 5]. The concentration of ANF in serum and atrium is increased in patients with congestive cardiac failure [6, 7]. Consequently, one could expect an increased frequency of IAA in patients with cardiac failure.

Material and Methods

Consecutive patients autopsied during 1989-90 were investigated. Inclusion criteria were a history of heart failure noticed in the patient record at least 6 month before death and signs of chronic congestion at autopsy. As a control group, patients without clinical history of heart failure and with no signs of chronic congestion or heart disease other than mild cardiosclerosis at autopsy were choosen from the same period. Eighty patients remained for the study, 48 with heart failure and 32 controls. As the frequency of IAA increases with age [3] the patients were divided into three groups <70, 70-80 and >80 years old (Tables I and II).

Pieces from left ventricle and both atria were sectioned, stained with alkaline Congo red and studied in polarized light. A typical appearance of amyloid distributed in a linear pattern along the muscle fibres of the atria only [1] was taken as evidence that the amyloid was of IAA origin. The amount of amyloid was considered as minor if only small local deposits were noticed; otherwise the amount was considered as major (Table I and II). In the statistical analysis, patients with isolated atrial amyloid were compared with patients with no amyloid deposits (Table III).

Results

The frequency and amount of IAA increased with age as expected. Statistical analysis [Mantel-Haenszel statistics] revealed an increased risk of having amyloidosis in patients with cardiac failure, compared to the control group, by 4.3 in the entire material. This increase in risk was most obvious in the eldest group (Table III). However, there were a few patients without cardiac failure who had rather heavy atrial amyloid infiltration.

TABLE I. Frequency and amount of amyloid of IAA type in the atria of 48 patients with congestive heart failure

Age (Mean)	No amyloid deposit (No.)	Minor amyloid deposits (No.)	Major amyloid deposits (No.)
<70 (60.4)	5	0	3
70-79 (75.2)	6	3	8
≥80 (86.3)	3	9	11

TABLE II. Frequency and amount of IAA in the atria of 32 patients without heart failure

Age (Mean)	No amyloid deposit (No.)	Minor amyloid deposits (No.)	Major amyloid deposits (No.)
<70 (64.9)	9	1	1
70-79 (73.9)	5	2	1
≥80 (84.9)	7	3	3

TABLE III. Occurrence of IAA in 32 patients without and 48 patients with congestive heart failure and calculated increase in risk of amyloidosis when cardiac failure occurs

Age	Amyloid	Cardiac failure (No.)	No cardiac failure (No.)	Relative risk*
<70	Yes	3	2	2.7
	No	5	9	
70-79	Yes	11	3	3.1
	No	6	5	
≥80	Yes	20	6	7.8
	No	3	7	

*Relative risk= increase in risk of having amyloidosis in the presence of cardiac failure when compared to the absence of cardiac failure. In the entire patient population the age-adjusted relative risk (95% confidence limits) = 4.3 (1.5-12.4). χ^2 (Mantel -Haenszel); 6.83; $p<0.01$.

Discussion

The fibrilogenesis in amyloidosis is not fully understood, but a high concentration of the subunit protein is considered to be an important factor [8]. We now show that congestive cardiac failure, a condition with high ANF levels, is correlated to a high incidence of IAA, thus supporting the presumption above. This suggests a probable high incidence of IAA in other heart affections associated with high ANF levels. Consistently, preliminary results from a study of patients with hypertension show increased frequency of IAA. Moreover, another paper in this book reports a raised prevalence of IAA in chronic heart disease [9]. The clinical significance of IAA, if any, is not known, but it might reflect an impaired ANF release or processing which could weaken the compensation mechanisms in cardiac failure. Large amounts of IAA might also have a deleterious impact on atrial function resulting in e.g. atrial fibrillation.

Acknowledgements

We thank Anna-Helena Forsberg and Marie-Louise Eskilsson for valuable technical assistance and Hemming Johansson for expert help with the statistical analysis. Supported by the Swedish Medical Research Council (project No. 5941), the Research Fund of King Gustaf V and the Swedish Society of Medicine.

References

1. Westermark, P., Johansson, B., and Natvig, J.B. (1979). Senile cardiac amyloidosis: evidence of two different amyloid substances in the ageing heart. Scand. J. Immunol. 10, 303-308.
2. Cornwell, G.G. III., Murdoch, W.L., Kyle, R.A., Westermark, P., and Pitkänen, P. (1983). Frequency and distribution of senile cardiovascular amyloid. A clinicopathologic correlation. Am. J. Med. 75, 618-623.
3. Steiner, I. (1987). The prevalence of isolated atrial amyloid. J. Pathol. 153, 395-398.
4. Johansson, B., Wernstedt, C., and Westermark, P. (1987). Atrial natriuretic peptide deposited as atrial amyloid fibrils. Biochem. Biophys. Res. Commun. 148, 1087-1092.
5. Linke, R.P., Voigt, C., Störkel, F.S., Eulitz, M. (1988). N-terminal amino acid sequence analysis indicates that isolated atrial amyloid is derived from atrial natriuretic peptide. Virchows Arch. B 55, 125-127.
6. Akimoto, K., Miyata, A., Kangawa, K., Koga, Y., Hayakawa, K., and Matsuo, H. (1988). Molecular forms of atrial natriuretic peptide in the atrium of patients with cardiovascular disease. J. Clin. Endocrin. Metabol. 67, 93-97.
7. Fyhrquist, F and Tikkanen, I. (1988). Atrial natriuretic peptide in congestive heart failure. Amer. J. Cardiol. 62, 20A-24A.
8. Johansson B. Senile Cardiac Amyloidosis [Dissertation]. Acta Universitatis Upsaliensis, 1990. 28 pp. Uppsala, Sweden, ISBN 91-554-2571-2.
9. Looi, M.L. Raised prevalence of isolated atrial amyloidosis in chronic heart disease. Sixth International Symposium on Amyloidosis, Oslo, Norway, 1990.

CHARACTERIZATION OF MOLECULAR FORMS OF CALCITONIN IN AMYLOID FIBRILS FROM MEDULLARY CARCINOMA OF THE THYROID

K. SLETTEN, J.B. NATVIG and P. WESTERMARK
Department of Biochemistry, University of Oslo, Norway, Institute of Immunology and Rheumatology, Oslo, Norway and Department of Pathology, University of Linkøping, Sweden

INTRODUCTION

The thyroid medullary carcinoma (MCT) are C-cell neoplasms which express calcitonin. In a study of 122 cases of MCT, 82% were found to have amyloid deposit. The amyloid exhibits the same histochemical feature as other amyloid material. In an earlier report (1) of amyloid in MCT we showed that the main fibril protein was derived from procalcitonin, but were unable to determine the exact size of the molecule. Our intention is to elucidate why these tumor producing cells express procalcitonin molecules prone for amyloid fibrils.

MATERIALS AND METHODS

Preparation of amyloid fibrils and protein purification

About 5 gm of amyloid-rich tumor tissue from a patient (MCT-Vås*) with sporadic type of MCT was sent to the laboratory. The material was homogenized repeatedly in 0.15 M NaCl containing 0.01 M sodium citrate and 0.02% sodium azide. After washing in distilled water and centrifugation, the pellet, containing most of the amyloid, was lyophilized. 50 mg of this material was dissolved in 6 M guanidine HCl containing 0.1 M dithiothreitol and applied to a 1.6 x 65 cm Sepharose CL-6B column from which material was eluted with 5M guanidine in distilled water. Registration was performed at 280 nm. Suitable fractions were pooled, dialysed against deionized water and lyophilized. Further purification was obtained by gel filtration through a 1.6 x 90 cm Sephacryl S-300 column.
*) Thanks is due to Dr. Hans Nordgren, Vasterås, Sweden.

Immunochemistry

A previously characterized antiserum (anti ACal) against the subunit fibril protein of MCT-amyloid of patient Fr (1) with the peroxidase-anti-peroxidase method was used on paraffin-embedded material of MCT-Vås.

SDS-Polyacrylamide gel electrophoresis (SDS-PAGE)

SDS-PAGE was performed as described (2).

Structural studies
Polypeptide samples were hydrolysed and analysed on an automatic amino acid analyser (Biotronic LC 5000). N-terminal analyses were performed using an automatic protein sequence analyser (Model 477A and 120A, Applied Biosystems).

RESULTS AND DISCUSSION

Immunohistochemical staining of sections of MCT-Vås with anti ACal showed reaction with amyloid and with the cytoplasm of the tumor cells (Fig.1). This antiserum has previously been shown not to react with amyloid of other types, including insulinomas (unpublished observation). SDS-PAGE of the extracted amyloid fibrils revealed two faint bands in the low molecular weight region (Fig.2).

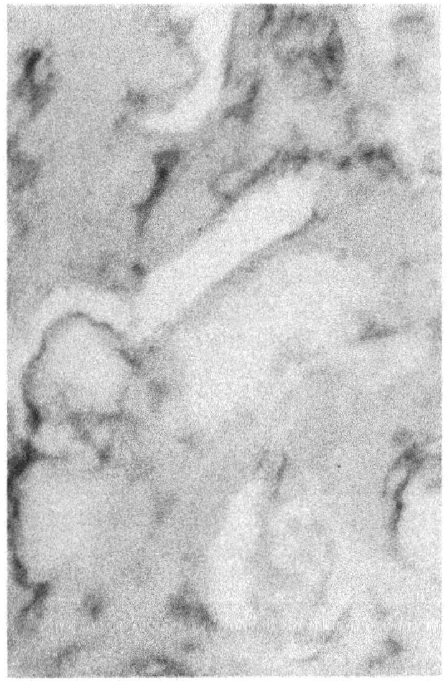

Fig. 1. Medullary carcinoma amyloid labelled with anti protein ACal antiserum.

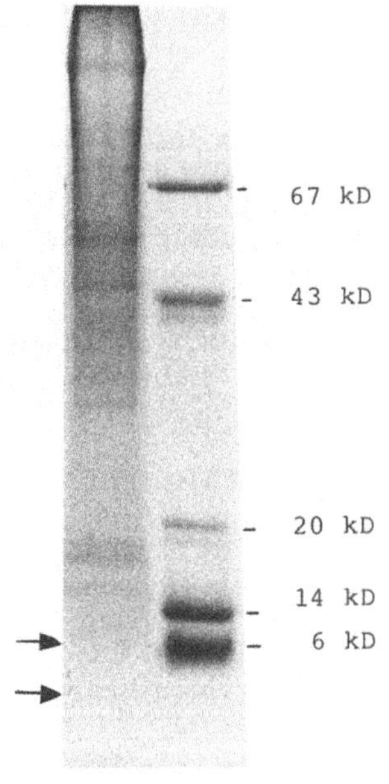

Fig. 2 SDS-PAGE of amyloid fibrils.
Lane 1: Amyloid fibrils
Lane 2: Protein calibration standard.
The arrows indicate where the faint bands appear.

Their molecular weights were estimated to be about 3 and 6 kD. Gel filtration of amyloid degraded material revealed a major Vo peak and a retarded broad two shouldered peak. Selected fractions from the retarded peak were rerun on a column of Sephacryl S-300.

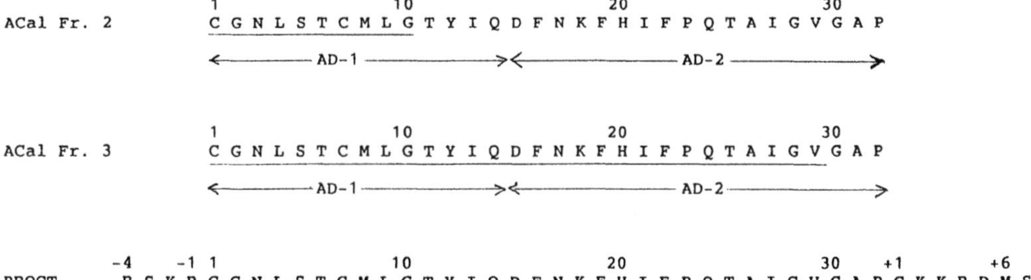

Fig. 3. The amino acid sequence of polypeptides purified from human medullary carcinoma amyloid fibrils and of proforms of human calcitonin.
PROCT: human procalcitonin forms (4).
The lines indicate Edman degradation on polypeptides. Peptides marked AD are peptides obtained from digestion with endoproteinase Asp-N.

Table 1

AMINO ACID COMPOSITION ON CALCITONIN-DERIVED POLYPEPTIDES OBTAINED FROM AMYLOID FIBRILS OF A PATIENT WITH MEDULLARY CARCINOMA OF THYROID

Residues/Molecules

	Fr.2	Fr.3	Calcitonin Res. 1-32
Asp	3.36	3.09	3
Thr	3.59	4.89	5
Ser	2.28	1.5	1
Glu	3.75	2.53	2
Pro	2.0	2.0	2
Gly	4.12	4.03	4
Ala	2.41	2.09	2
Cys	0.5	1.2	2
Val	1.47	1.00	1
Met	0.85	0.96	1
Ile	1.05	0.91	1
Leu	2.62	2.02	2
Tyr	1.07	0.93	1
Phe	2.34	2.86	3
His	1.00	0.96	1
Lys	1.46	0.96	1
Arg	1.04	-	0

N-terminal analyses of the two main fractions 2 and 3 revealed that the major protein in both fractions started in position 1 of calcitonin (Fig.3). Fraction 3 was analysed for 29 cycles and the amino acid sequence of 27 residues of the calcitonin molecule was confirmed. The two cysteine residues in positions 1 and 7 could not completely be established. Fraction 2 was run for 10 cycles which established the same results as for fraction 3 (Fig.3). As the gel filtration indicated a higher molecular weight of the material in fraction 2, the result suggested an extension of the polypeptide in the C-terminal region. However, digestion of fractions 2 and 3 with endoproteinase Asp-N, followed by N-terminal analyses, resulted in the amino acid sequence of positions 1 - 32 of calcitonin in both fractions. As the N-terminal analyses of Asp-N digested fractions, gave a higher yield of the C-terminal peptides, the results indicated a partially blocked or ragged N-terminus. The amino acid composition of the material in fractions 2 and 3 was determined and the results are shown in Table 1 together with that reported for calcitonin (3). The results of fraction 3 confirm the composition of calcitonin, positions 1-32, while fraction 2 seems to contain a proform of calcitonin extended to 2 to 3 residues in the N-terminal region.
The results confirm our earlier studies (1) that the amyloid fibrils of medullary carcinoma contains prohormone forms as well as the hormone itself.

ACKNOWLEDGEMENTS

The work was supported by the Norwegian Council for Science and the Humanities, by the Swedish Medical Research Council and the Research Fund of King Gustav V.

REFERENCES

1. Sletten, K., Westermark, P. and Natvig, J.B. (1976) Characterization of amyloid fibril proteins from medullary carcinoma of the thyroid. J. Exp. Med. 143, 993-998.
2. Blobel, G. and Dobberstein, B. (1975) Transfer of proteins across membranes. I. Presence of proteolytically processed and non processed nascent immunoglobulin light chains on membrane-bound ribosomes of murine myeloma. J. Cell Biol. 67, 835-851.
3. Neher, R., Riniker, B., Rittel, W. and Zuber, H. (1968) Menschliches Calcitonin. III. Struktur von Calcitonin M und D. Helv. Chim. Acta. 51, 1900-1905.
4. Le Moullec, J.M., Jullienne, A., Chenais, J., Lasmoles, F., Guliana, J.M., Milhaud, G. and Moukhtar, M.S. (1984) The complete sequence of human preprocalcitonin. FEBS Lett. 167, 93-97.

PATHOFIBRILLOGENESIS AND AMYLOID PROTEINS

Benson, M.D.
Indiana University School of Medicine
Department of Medicine
Rheumatology Division, Clinical Building 492
541 Clinical Drive
Indianapolis, IN 46223, USA.

"The terms amyloid and amyloidosis are generic ones embodying a spectrum of related proteins and their corresponding disorders..."

(Heller et al., 1966) [1]

The amyloidoses are a group of diseases or conditions which by definition share the common property of the amyloid beta fibril. This classification on the basis of a physical property brings together diseases of very diverse etiologies, a fact we have come to appreciate with our increasing knowledge of amyloid protein chemistry and molecular biology. Genetic, neoplastic, metabolic, and perhaps normal physiologic mechanisms can all lead to forms of amyloidosis. The question then is whether an understanding of the pathogenesis of any one of these conditions can be obtained by looking at factors which are common to them all. In addition, are pathogenic factors which are obvious in one form of amyloidosis worthy of consideration in other forms as well? For this unitarian approach to pathofibrillogenesis we must start with the common properties.

All forms of amyloid and amyloidosis have two things in common. First, the amyloid deposits are composed of fibrils which have a beta structure. These fibrils are usually 80 to 100A in diameter and are of indeterminate length. The ordered nature of the fibril is responsible for the birefringence of amyloid deposits and the Congo red binding. The second factor common to all forms of amyloidosis is the fact that, in each, the beta fibrils have a homogeneous subunit protein. This subunit protein may be as small as 4,000 daltons or as large as an intact immunoglobulin light chain (23,000 daltons). Most AA proteins are 8,000 to 9,000. The majority of immunoglobulin light chain amyloid proteins are 15,000 to 20,000 and the transthyretin subunit proteins are usually the intact monomer which is approximately 14,000 daltons. The Alzheimer subunit protein, on the other hand, is usually only 42 amino acid residues with a molecular mass between 4,000 and 5,000. In all cases it would appear that the subunit protein specific for each disease aggregates or polymerizes to form the backbone of the beta fibril.

Since the beta fibril defines the disease, we need to look to the second factor, the subunit proteins of the fibrils, in our consideration of common pathofibrillogenic mechanisms. Characteristics of these proteins which need to be considered include structure, metabolism, function, and inducers of synthesis. Also we need to consider in our analysis of pathofibrillogenesis other fibril constituents and, finally, factors which make the fibril resistant to degradation.

The structure of the subunit protein is obviously of paramount importance and has been the subject of most of the recent work on pathofibrillogenesis. The major amyloid subunit proteins include the variants of transthyretin, immunoglobulin light chains, protein AA. Other amyloid subunit proteins include apolipoprotein A1, A2, cystatin C, Alzheimer beta protein, and gelsolin. Some of these proteins have been the subject of extensive structural analysis at the primary, secondary, tertiary, and quaternary levels while other structures are relatively unknown. The most thoroughly studied amyloid subunit protein is transthyretin [2]. At the primary structural level we now recognize 10 separate amino acid substitutions which are associated with hereditary systemic amyloidosis (Figure 1). These include the methionine-30, isoleucine-33, histidine-58, alanine-60, tyrosine-77, serine-84, asparagine-90, methionine-111, cysteine-114, and isoleucine-122 transthyretins. While all of these substitutions can be hypothesized to alter the secondary and tertiary structure of the transthyretin monomer in such ways as to promote fibril formation, crystallographic data so far have only been reported for the methionine-30 variant where a significant increase in cell size has been found. These data were generated with the use of variant transthyretin isolated from the plasma of patients homozygous for the methionine-30 mutation. The other mutations which are usually present in the heterozygous state give a mixture of normal and variant transthyretin and, therefore, have not been studied by X-ray diffraction. Now that recombinant variant transthyretins are being produced, we will be able to analyze in more depth the effects of each substitution on secondary and tertiary structure. Certainly the studies of Blake et al. show that prealbumin has extensive beta pleated sheet structure and should, therefore, be conducive to beta fibril formation [3].

Immunoglobulin light chains are another amyloid subunit protein with extensive antiparallel beta pleated sheet structure. There are certain other observations which suggest that structure is of prime importance in immunoglobulin light chain amyloidosis. First, there are more lambda than kappa amyloid proteins. In addition, the lambda VI subtype is particularly prone to amyloid fibril formation. If we consider immunoglobulin amyloid in a manner similar to transthyretin, we could hypothesize that the amyloid fibril subunit protein is the Bence-Jones protein or light chain dimer, which, when produced in excess, is the prevailing form in the plasma of patients with monoclonal plasma cell dyscrasias. Two factors then become important in Ig amyloid fibril synthesis. First, it is important that the two immunoglobulin light chains forming the dimer have a high enough affinity so that the dimer structure is not easily disrupted. Studies on light chain dimers, indeed, show that lambda light chains have a higher association constant in general than do kappa light chains. This then could be a factor in the predominance of lambda light chain amyloid. Looking at the crystallographic data for kappa I light chain proteins gives us a model to consider in which residues spanning the regions of residues 36 to 49 and residues 94 through 98 may participate in interactions to stabilize the dimer (Figure 2) [4]. Key substitutions in these areas could increase the association of the kappa I dimer. A second factor in light chain amyloid fibril formation could be external residues on the beta pleated sheet strands which, if they undergo hydrophobic for hydrophilic substitutions would give areas of association and allow polymerization of the dimeric structures. In this model key changes may be in the outer strands at residues 4 and 5, 20, 72 and 76 [5]. A third structural factor which may be of importance in 2 of 10 kappa I amyloid proteins that we have studied is the presence of asparagine linked carbohydrate at position 61. Usually this position has an arginine. Position 61 is on the outside of the molecule facing toward the constant domain giving space for the carbohydrate so as not to disrupt aggregation. Indeed, the carbohydrate may be a factor in dimer association.

Less is known of the structure of AA molecules in reactive amyloidosis. While diffraction patterns of lyophilized fibrils show a cross beta pattern, no crystallographic analysis of the SAA or AA proteins has been accomplished. Structure, however, may be an important determinant in fibril formation. In the mouse only one form (SAA2) is found in the amyloid fibrils, although SAA1 and SAA2 would appear to be synthesized in equal amounts. In the human the amyloid fibrils usually show a predominance of SAA1 with 10% or less of SAA2. Phylogenetic analysis of the SAA proteins has shown high degrees of conservation, a fact consistent with the importance of structure in amyloid fibril formation [6].

Apolipoprotein AI is projected to have considerable alpha structure, but a significant portion (residues 1 through 55) of the 83 residue amino terminal fragment that forms amyloid fibrils is predicted to have beta structure. X-ray diffraction studies on synthetic peptides homologous to the Alzheimer beta protein have shown beta structure as well.

Metabolism of the subunit protein may well be important in amyloid fibril formation and includes synthesis, degradation and deposition of the subunit protein. Significant factors in synthesis include the fact that 1) in immunoglobulin amyloidosis a plasma cell dyscrasia must be present where monoclonal protein is synthesized. No evidence has ever been presented of amyloid being made from polyclonal immunoglobulin. In reactive amyloidosis elevated plasma levels of SAA are presumed to be important in generation of the amyloid fibrils. In the transthyretin amyloidoses increased production has not been shown for transthyretin in general, but, obviously, the genetic mutants are produced and are the cause of the disease. Cleavage or modification of transthyretin would not appear to be of great importance in amyloid fibril formation but, in both immunoglobulin and reactive amyloidosis, partial degradation of the precursor protein is the rule. The majority of immunoglobulin light chain amyloid subunit proteins include the entire variable region (V_L) plus a small portion of the constant domain. While no specific enzyme sites have been demonstrated, it could be hypothesized that this is the subunit size that fits nicely into the amyloid fibril structure. SAA is usually cleaved between residue 76 and 77, although much smaller and larger AA subunit proteins have been identified. Again no definite enzyme cleavage has been defined although elastase type enzymes have been hypothesized to be important in fibril synthesis.

Finally, local factors affecting deposition may be important in the generation of amyloid deposits. Possible factors in this process include blood circulation and the accumulation of subunit proteins in the extravascular space. Some hint of the importance of catabolism in amyloid fibril synthesis can be seen in our recent studies on the hereditary amyloidosis associated with a mutant of apolipoprotein AI [7]. In this condition we have been able to show that the plasma residence time of the mutant protein is approximately half of the normal protein in both gene carriers and in normal controls. This increased catabolism of the variant protein explains the low level of HDL cholesterol seen in these patients. Of greater interest in these studies is that the radiolabel associated with variant apoA-I was lower in the urine than the radiolabel associated with normal apolipoprotein AI. This is strong evidence for extravascular accumulation of the variant apolipoprotein AI. This may be an important factor in amyloid fibril formation. While purely conjecture, similar mechanisms may be at play in the transthryetin amyloidoses where plasma levels of the variant are usually lower than the normal.

It is not clear whether the **function** of amyloid subunit proteins plays a major factor in fibril synthesis. There is no evidence that immunoglobulin has an immune function in Ig amyloidosis. The function of SAA is not known, although a role in tissue response to injury and, therefore, presence in the extravascular space, has been proposed. Transthyretin has transport properties for thyroxine and vitamin A, but whether these roles are important in the localization of amyloid fibrils within nerve, vitreous, and other organs is not known.

Induction of amyloid subunit protein synthesis is of major importance in several types of amyloidosis. There is not definite evidence that antigenic stimulation is a factor in the generation of monoclonal immunoglobulin synthesis in immunoglobulin amyloidosis. In patients with multiple myeloma, whatever factors are involved in the neoplasia obviously play a role. SAA is synthesized in response to cytokines such as IL1 and IL6 and the increased synthesis is a factor in amyloid fibril formation. The transthyretin amyloidoses have a genetic origin and, obviously, without the point mutations present in each disease these specific subunit proteins, namely the transthyretin mutants, would not be synthesized. In dialysis amyloidosis beta-2 microglobulin synthesis would appear to be related in the actual process of hemodialysis and this may be mediated by factors associated with the dialysis membranes. Certainly in these patients, very high levels of beta-2 microglobulin are seen.

Other constitutents of amyloid fibrils include P component which is present in all types of amyloid deposits and many investigators feel is important in amyloid fibril synthesis. Although the possibility of its affect on proteolytic enzymes may be important, no definite structural role in the amyloid fibril has been shown for this globular

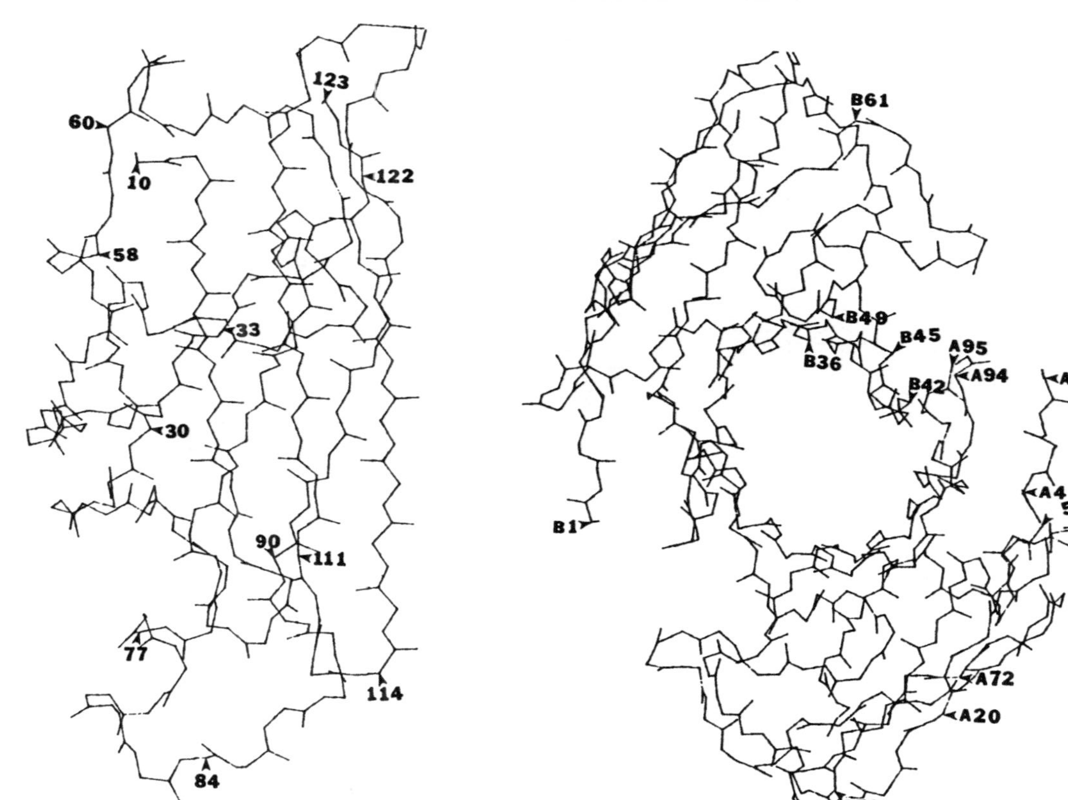

Figure 1. Computer generated model of transthyretin monomer showing positions of amyloid associated residues. Data extends from residues 10 to 123. [3]

Figure 2. Computer generated model of Kappa I dimer showing residues that may be important in dimer stability and fibrillogenesis. [4]

protein. A number of studies have shown sulfated proteoglycan association with amyloid fibrils and, indeed, these contribute much to the staining properties of amyloid deposits. It is very likely that these are important to the integrity of the fibril. Amyloid enhancing factor has been shown to be important in the animal model of reactive amyloidosis. What this entity is and how it functions to promote amyloid deposit formation is still a subject of investigation.

Finally, a characteristic of the fibrils is their **resistance to degradation**. Once they are formed it is uncommon for amyloid deposits to resolve. A number of factors may be at play including the fact that the fibrils are essentially inert. They are not foreign and the body does not recognize them as something to reject. The fibrils are extracellular and protected from proteolytic enzymes that are associated with cells. The possibility of protease inhibitors protecting the fibrils has been raised. In addition, many proteins such as SAP are associated with the fibrils in a calcium dependent fashion. This binding of calcium may be important in the resistence of amyloid fibrils to degradation.

CONCLUSIONS

In conclusion it is obvious that no single unifying factor is involved in amyloid fibril synthesis. Instead there appear to be a number of factors which may be at play in the different diseases. These factors may interact and have varying degrees of importance in generating the structural parameters, the synthesis, the degradation, and the preservation of the entity we call the amyloid fibril.

REFERENCES

1. Heller, H. Gafni, J., Sohar, E. (1966) 'The Inherited Systemic Amyloidoses', in J.B. Stanbury, J.B. Wyngaarden, D.S. Fredrickson (eds.), The Metabolic Basis of Inherited Disease/Second Edition, McGraw-Hill Book Company Publishers, New York, NY, pp. 995-1014.
2. Benson, M.D. and Wallace, M.R. (1988) 'Amyloidosis', in C.R. Scriver, A.L. Beaudet, W.S. Sly, and D.Valle (eds.), The Metabolic Basis of Inherited Disease/Sixth Edition, McGraw-Hill Information Services Company, New York, NY, pp. 2439-2460.
3. Blake, C.C.F., Geisow, M.J., Oatley, S.J., Rerat, B., and Rerat, C. (1978) 'Structure of prealbumin: Secondary, tertiary and quaternary interactions determined by fourier refinement at 1·8 A', J. Mol. Biol. 121, 339-356.
4. Epp, O., Lattman, E.E., Schiffer, M., Huber, R., and Palm, W. (1975) 'The molecular structure of a dimer composed of the variable portions of the Bence-Jones protein REI refined at 2·0-A resolution', Biochemistry 14, 4943-4952.
5. Liepnieks, J.J. (1990), VIth International Symposium on Amyloidosis, Oslo, Norway.
6. Harats, N. (1990), VIth International Symposium on Amyloidosis, Oslo, Norway.
7. Benson, M.D. (1990), VIth International Symposium on Amyloidosis, Oslo, Norway.

THE SULPHATE AND CHLORIDE IONS HAVE DIFFERENT EFFECTS ON THE STRUCTURE OF AA AMYLOID FIBRILS

S. Wong and R. Kisilevsky
Departments of Pathology and Biochemistry
Queen's University
Kingston, Ontario, Canada
K7L 3N6

INTRODUCTION

During the past 4 to 5 years we have realized that glycosaminoglycans as part of proteoglycans may be playing more than a passive role in amyloid deposition. In inflammation associated amyloid (AA amyloid) there is coincidental deposition of the AA peptide and the GAG (1). This coincidental deposition has been observed regardless of the nature of the inflammatory stimulus, the length of time between the onset of inflammation and the subsequent deposition of the amyloid, or which tissue has been depositing amyloid. Evidence has accumulated to indicate that the proteoglycan is the basement membrane form of heparan sulphate proteoglycan (HSPG) (2,3). This same molecule has been demonstrated in several other forms of amyloid which include the beta amyloid in Alzheimer's disease (4), the IAPP amyloid in Diabetes (5), the prealbumin form of amyloid in familial amyloidotic polyneuropathy (6), and the prion amyloid in Gerstmann-Straussler Syndrome (7). In addition, highly sulphated glycosaminoglycans have been demonstrated in all forms of amyloid examined to date (8). In at least two forms of amyloid, AA, and that associated with the beta protein in Alzheimer's disease the GAGs appear to be intimately related to the structure of the amyloid fibril (9,10).

The above observations suggest that sulphated glycosaminoglycans or HSPG may play a role both in the pathogenesis and the structure of the amyloid fibrils. One way in which this might occur is through an ionic interaction between the amyloid peptides or its precursor and the sulphate moieties on the glycosaminoglycans. Theoretical binding sites have been identified both on SAA and the beta amyloid precursor (11).

We have examined the accessibility of human AA peptides in isolated human AA fibrils to labelling in media containing NaCl at varying ionic strengths, and compared this with the accessibility of these peptides to such labelling in the presence of Na_2SO_4. If sulphate on GAGs plays a role in maintaining fibril structure, exogenous sulphate should compete with the sulphate which is part of the GAG, potentially displacing such molecules and altering fibril structure. Thus the labelling accessibility of the AA peptides in the presence of sulphate should be different from that seen in NaCl.

The results indicate that sulphate is effective in opening amyloid fibril structure at concentrations as low as 70 mM while chloride concentrations as high as 0.5 M are ineffective. Concentrations of chloride in the range of 1 M appear to reduce labelling accessibility of the AA peptides in such fibrils. These results infer that sulphate probably as part of the GAG moieties plays a significant role in maintaining the structure of the AA amyloid fibril.

MATERIALS AND METHODS

Preparation of Human AA Amyloid Fibrils

Human spleen from a patient with longstanding rheumatoid arthritis and which contained AA amyloid was used. The amyloid fibrils were isolated according to the procedure of Pras as modified by Skinner et al (12,13). The isolated amyloid fibrils were stored in 20% glycerol at $-20^{o}C$ until ready for use.

Incubations of AA Amyloid Fibrils in Different Salt Solutions

An aliquot of the glycerol stored amyloid fibrils sufficiently large to be used under all salt conditions was dialysed against 50 mM borate pH 8.5 for 48 hours at $4^{o}C$ with 5-6 changes of buffer. The protein concentration was approximately 1 mg/ml. The dialysed preparation was aliquoted into test tubes containing the appropriate amount and type of salt in 50 mM borate. The conditions used were 50 mM borate alone, or containing various concentrations of sodium chloride up to 1 M, or 70 mM sodium sulphate. The pH of each preparation was maintained at 8.5. Each sample remained at 4° C for 24 hours with periodic vortexing, after which the samples were radio labelled. The above procedure was repeated with 4-5 replicates so that statistical comparisons could be made between the groups.

Reductive Methylation and Double Isotope Labelling

Reductive methylation with both ^{14}C and ^{3}H was performed by the technique of Means and Feeney as described by Kisilevsky et al (14). The ^{14}C labelling was done with the fibrils intact following which the fibrils were denatured and relabelled with ^{3}H. Thus, each peptide was doubly labelled.

Two Dimensional Gel Electrophoresis

Following reductive methylation, dialysis, and lyophilization the samples were taken up in 1 ml of 6 M urea, 20% glycerol, pH 9.3 with Bromphenol blue as a marker. Approximately 50 ug of protein were used in the first dimension. Electrophoresis in the first dimension occurred on the basis of charge, using the techniques of Ornstein and Davis (16,17). Separation of the samples in the second dimension occurred in a 12.5% separating gel measuring 0.3 x 14 x 15 cm using the technique of Laemmli (18).

Two dimensional gel electrophoretograms of reductively methylated and unaltered AA peptides were compared. No shift in positioning of the peptides could be determined.

After electrophoresis the gels were stained in Coomassie Blue, destained in 20% methanol, 10% acetic acid and the AA peptides cut from the gel to determine the extent of ^{3}H and ^{14}C labelling in each of the peptides.

Western Blotting

Some unlabelled samples were used for Western blotting using the procedure of Burnette (19). The presence of human AA proteins was detected by the use of a rabbit anti human AA antibody, a generous gift of Dr. M. Skinner, Thorndike Memorial Laboratories, Boston University School of Medicine.

Data Analysis

The two dimensional electrophoretograms indicated that there were seven peptides consistently present, five of which were positive on Western blotting with the anti AA antisera. The tritium $^3H/^{14}C$ ratio of the individual AA peptides was determined and normalized to each of the other AA peptides on that gel. This was done for each of the quadruplicate or quintuplicate gels for a given salt condition. Thus the isotope ratio and its statistical variance could be determined for each normalization and for each peptide. The reasons for such normalizations has been adequately described in previous publications (14,20). A high tritium $^3H/^{14}C$ ratio indicated poor accessibility of the peptide to ^{14}C labelling in its native state, while a low $^3H/^{14}C$ ratio indicated the converse. A comparison could then be made between the labelling accessibility of the fibrils in the various salt solutions and the standard condition of 50 mM borate. This allowed us to examine which peptides underwent significant conformational change in the various salt solutions. The direction of ratio shift, increasing or decreasing would also indicate whether the peptides were becoming more or less exposed.

RESULTS

Two Dimensional Electrophoresis of Peptides from AA Fibrils

Figure 1 demonstrates the peptides observed after two dimensional gel separation of the AA fibril constituents. Seven peptides are present. All were adequately labelled. The ones designated P1 - P5 reacted with anti AA antisera for which reason for we considered and analysed only the data relating to peptides 1-5.

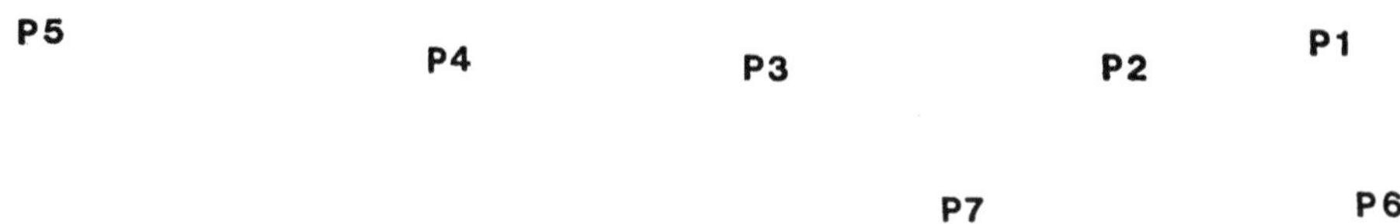

Figure 1 Two dimensional gel separation of human splenic AA peptides. Peptides P1-P5 react with rabbit anti-human AA antisera. The peptides were separated first horizontally, from left to right, by charge, and then vertically on a slab gel according to molecular weight. The molecular weight of the peptides, determined on other gels, were 55-8500.

Table 1
Comparison of normalized $^{3}H/^{14}C$ Values in 50 mM Borate vs 70 mM Na_2SO_4 which generated a $p \leq 0.05$ and Direction of Ratio Shift*

	NORMALIZER				
	P1	P2	P3	P4	P5
AA Peptides					
P1	-				I
P2	D	-	D	D	I
P3		I	-		I
P4		I		-	I
P5	D	D	D	D	-

* "D" represents a significant ($p \leq 0.05$) decrease in ratio and therefore a significant increase in labelling accessibility of the peptides when they are in undenatured AA fibrils. "I" represents the converse.

Table 2
Comparison of normalized $^{3}H/^{14}C$ Values in 50 mM Borate vs 1 M NaCl which generated a $p \leq 0.05$ and the Direction of Ratio Shift*

	NORMALIZER				
	P1	P2	P3	P4	P5
AA Peptides					
P1		I	I	I	I
P2	D			D	
P3	D				
P4	D				I
P5	D				

* "D" and "I" are defined in the legend to Table 5.

Tables of the relative accessibility to reductive methylation of the AA peptides in the various salt solutions have been constructed and are in press (21). Summary tables representing these data are shown in Tables 1 and 2. In Table 1 we have compared the labelling accessibility of the peptides in 50 mM borate vs that seen in 50 mM borate plus 70 mM Na_2SO_4. In Table 2 a similar comparison has been made against 1 M NaCl. The direction of shift of the normalized ratios is indicated. "D" represents a significant ($p \leq 0.05$) decrease in ratio and therefore an increase in the labelling accessibility while "I" represents the converse. Note that in Table 1 there is a repeating pattern of behaviour of peptides 2 and 5. The amino groups of each of these two peptides are more accessible to labelling in Na_2SO_4 than in 50 mM borate alone. A similar comparison of the data in Table 2 shows that only peptide 1 is undergoing a decrease in accessibility. Comparisons of all other salt solutions (0.15, 0.25 and 0.5 M NaCl) fail to reveal any repeatable symmetrically significantly differences.

DISCUSSION

We have shown previously that using double label reductive methylation, it is possible to simultaneously examine more than 50 proteins in a macro molecular complex. In this way one can to determine whether conformational differences are taking place in the individual constituents making up the complex as the state of the macro molecular complex is changing (14,20,22). Using reductive methylation, large changes in labelling ratio can occur if but a single accessible amino group is exposed or concealed in different physical states (14). In contrast to ribosomes which is the organelle which we have previously examined, AA amyloid fibrils are composed of polymeric associations of individual AA peptides. It is difficult to know precisely how many peptides make up a fibril, whereas in a ribosome each each protein is present in one copy. We cannot therefore determine the number of free amino groups available for reductive methylation in such amyloid fibrils. Be that as it may, each AA deposit has a particular family of AA peptides which seems to characterize a deposit in that tissue (23). This is thought to be due to the characteristic proteolytic enzymes present in each tissue which cleave the AA precursor, SAA, at particular locations.

In the present study 5 specific AA peptides were examined in human AA amyloid fibrils. We have been able to demonstrate that in the presence of 70 mM sulphate two of these peptides undergo significant increases in their accessibility to labelling. In contrast equivalent concentrations of chloride had no effect. In fact, chloride had little effect until concentrations greater than 0.5 M were encountered. Further, the effect that 1 M sodium chloride had was in a direction opposite that seen 70 mM sulphate. These results are in keeping with our postulate that GAGs interact with the AA peptides through their sulphate moieties, but they do not preclude additional interactions which occur between the protein core of the proteoglycan and the AA peptides themselves.

It is unfortunate that the proteoglycan component of the AA fibril could not be resolved in the two dimensional gel procedure. HSPG of the basement membrane variety has a molecular weight of greater than 600,000 (24), and it likely remained that the origin during electrophoresis. No data are therefore available on the exposure or behaviour of the proteoglycan in the various salt solutions.

ACKNOWLEDGEMENTS

This work was supported by grant MT-3153 for the MRC of Canada. Sharon Wong was an Ontario Graduate Scholar during the performance of this work. The authors thank Mrs. A. Northcott for her able administrative assistance and Mrs. B. Latimer and Ms. K. Wowk for their able secretarial assistance.

REFERENCES

1. Snow AD, Kisilevsky R. Lab Invest 1985; 53:37
2. Snow AD, Kisilevsky R, Wight TN. In Amyloid and Amyloidosis: (eds. Isobe T, Araki S, Uchino F, Kito S, Tsubura E). Plenum Press, New York (1988) pp 87-93
3. Norling B, Westermark GT, Westermark P. Clin Exp Immunol 1988; 73:333
4. Snow AD, Mar H, Nochlin D, Kimata K, Kato M, Suzuki S, Hassell J, Wight TN. Amer J Pathol 1988; 133:456
5. Young I, Ailles L, Narindrasorasak S, Kisilevsky R. Human Pathol (submitted for publication)
6. Snow AD, Saraiva M. (personal communication)
7. Snow AD. (personal communication)
8. Snow AD, Willmer J, Kisilevsky R. Lab Invest 1987; 56:120
9. Snow AD, Lara S, Nochlin D, Wight TN. Acta Neuropathol 1989; 78:113
10. Young I, Willmer JP, Kisilevsky R. Acta Neuropathol 1989; 78:202
11. Kisilevsky R. Neurobiol Aging 1989; 10:499
12. Pras M, Schubert M, Zucker-Franklin D, Rimon A, Franklin EC. J Clin Invest 1968; 47:924
13. Skinner M, Shirahama T, Cohen AS, Deal CL. Prep Biochem 1983; 12:461
14. Kisilevsky R, Weiler L, Treloar MA. J Biol Chem 1978; 253:7101
15. Means GE, Feeney RE. Biochemistry 1968; 7:2192
16. Ornstein L. Ann N Y Acad Sci 1965; 121:321
17. Davis BJ. Ann N Y Acad Sci 1964; 121:404
18. Laemmli UK. Nature 1970; 227:680
19. Burnette WN. Anal Biochem 1981; 112:195
20. Kisilevsky R, Treloar MA, Weiler L. J Biol Chem 1984; 259:1351
21. Wong S, Kisilevsky. Scand J Immunol (in press)
22. Kisilevsky R, Gore J. Biochim Biophys Acta 1987; 910:282
23. Westermark GT, Sletten K, Westermark P. In Amyloid and Amyloidosis: (eds. Isobe T, Araki S, Uchino F, Kito S, Tsubura E). Plenum Press, New York (1988) pp 199-203
24. Ledbetter SR, Tyree B, Hassell JR, Horigan E. J Biol Chem 1985; 260:8106

KINETIC PROPERTIES OF AMYLOID FIBRIL POLYMERIZATION IN VITRO

Hironobu Naiki[1], Keiichi Higuchi[2],
Kazuya Nakakuki[1] and Toshio Takeda[2]

[1]Department of Pathology, Fukui Medical College,
Fukui 910-11, Japan and [2]Department of Senescence
Biology, Chest Disease Research Institute, Kyoto
University, Kyoto 606, Japan

We investigated the polymerization kinetics of murine senile amyloid fibrils(fAS_{SAM}) in vitro. When sonicated fAS_{SAM} was incubated with its constituent monomer protein(AS_{SAM}), the extension of amyloid fibrils was observed in an electron microscopic analysis. Quantitative fluorometric analysis with thioflavine T revealed that 1) extension of amyloid fibrils occurred by a pseudo-first-order exponential increase in the fluorescence of thioflavine T; 2) rate of extension was maximal around pH7.5 and inhibited with the increase in KCl or NaCl concentration in the reaction mixture; 3) rate of polymerization was proportional to the product of the fAS_{SAM} number concentration and the AS_{SAM} concentration; 4) net rate of extension was the sum of the rates of polymerization and depolymerization. These results show that extension of amyloid fibrils proceeds by consecutive association of precursor proteins onto the ends of existing fibrils.

INTRODUCTION

Various precursors of amyloid fibril proteins have been isolated [1,2]. To better comprehend the pathogenesis of amyloidosis, it is essential to study of vitro, the kinetics and processes by which these precursor proteins form amyloid fibrils.

We developed a novel fluoremetric method to examine amyloid fibrils in vitro[3,4], as based on the unique characteristics of thioflavine T(ThT). The availability of this method prompted us to analyze the polymerization kinetics of murine senile amyloid fibrils (fAS_{SAM}), in vitro. Age dependent severe fAS_{SAM} deposition is one of the chief characteristics in the senescence accelerated mouse-prone (SAM-P/1) strain[4].

We now report a system in which AS_{SAM} and sonicated fAS_{SAM} are incubated at 37°C, in the presence of 300mM urea. Extension of amyloid fibrils, which results from the consecutive association of AS_{SAM} onto the ends of fAS_{SAM}, is monitored by electron microscopy and fluorometric analysis with ThT.

MTERIALS AND METHODS

Purification of fAS_{SAM} and AS_{SAM} - fAS_{SAM} was purified from the livers of 14- to 15-month-old SAM-P/1 mice, as described elsewhere[3].

AS_{SAM} was purified from a pellet of ultracentrifugation of crude fAS_{SAM} derived at a second step of the above mentioned purification procedure. The following procedures were all performed at 4°C. Six molar urea polyacrylamide gel electrophoresis was performed on a 16.2 × 13 × 0.4-cm slab gel with 7.5% acrylamide. The lyophilized sample(about 2.5mg of protein) was dissolved in 2.0ml of sample buffer containing 6M urea and incubated for 8h, which allowed for the depolymerization of fAS_{SAM} into AS_{SAM}. It was then applied onto a gel and electrophoresed overnight at 12.5mA. AS_{SAM}-containing bands located by stained reference gels were excised, diced into small pieces and suspended in 10mM NH_4HCO_3. AS_{SAM} was eluted for 24h with stirring. The elution buffer was dialyzed against the same elution buffer for 24h and lyophilized.

Polymerization Assay and Fluorescence Spectroscopy - In all experiments, size of the reaction mixture was 40μl. Preparation of the reaction mixture was performed on ice. First, distilled water was put into a tube to make the final concentration of the reaction mixture 40μl. Second, 250mM phosphate or Tris-HCl buffer was added to yield the final buffer concentration of 25mM. Third, 400mM AS_{SAM} solution dissolved in 600mM urea(3.48mg protein/ml) was added to yield the final AS_{SAM} concentration of 0 to 200mM. Six hundred millimolars of urea was then added to yield the final urea concentration of 300mM. fAS_{SAM} solution was finally added to yield the final fAS_{SAM} concentration of 0 to 50ng protein/μl.

The reaction was started by placing these mixtures in an incubator set at 37°C, it was carried out for 10 to 210min, then was stopped by moving them back onto the ice. From each mixture, 5μl lots were derived in triplicate, just before and after the polymerization reaction. The preparation was then used for fluorescence spectroscopy as described[3].

We confirmed that the fluorescence was proportional to the mass concentration of fAS_{SAM}(i.e. the concentration of AS_{SAM} in polymeric form) and independent of the number concentration of fAS_{SAM}.

RESULTS

Extension Kinetics of fAS_{SAM}

When AS_{SAM} was incubated with fAS_{SAM} at 37°C, the extension of amyloid fibrils was observed in an electron microscopic analysis. In this reaction, the fluorescence of ThT increased with no lag and proceeded to equilibrium. Fluorescence increase was linear over 40min. Therefore, in the following experiments, fluorescence increase at 30min after the initiation of the reaction was regarded as the initial rate of extension.

When AS_{SAM} was incubated with fAS_{SAM} on ice, or when AS_{SAM} was incubated without fAS_{SAM} at 37°C, no increase of the fluorescence was observed over 3h of the reaction.

Effect of pH and Salt Concentration on the Initial Rate of Extension

The initial rate of fAS_{SAM} extension was maximal around pH7.5 and decreased with increase in the NaCl or KCl concentrations. KCl exhibited a more potent inhibitory effect for the extension than did NaCl.

Effect of AS_{SAM} and fAS_{SAM} Concentrations of the Initial Rate of Extension

The initial rate of extension was linear to the seed fibril concentration. Moreover, the initial rate increased twice when the sonicated fAS_{SAM} was incubated with AS_{SAM} instead of the equal protein concentration of purified fAS_{SAM}. With sonication, the average length of fAS_{SAM} decreased by about 50%, thus the number concentration of fAS_{SAM} increased about double. Therefore, we concluded that at a constant AS_{SAM} concentration, the initial rate of extension was proportional to the number concentration of fAS_{SAM}.

At a constant fAS_{SAM} concentration, a perfect linearity was observed between the AS_{SAM} concentration and the initial rate of fAS_{SAM} extension($r = -0.999$). Below the AS_{SAM} concentration of 20nM the fluorescence decreased during the reaction and the initial rates were graphed as negative values. This indicated that the seed fAS_{SAM} depolymerized during the reaction. When the AS_{SAM} concentration is zero, the net rate of extension was governed by the rate of depolymerization. Therefore, 1) the initial rate of polymerization is proportional to the AS_{SAM} concentration 2) at each AS_{SAM} concentration, the net rate of fAS_{SAM} extension is the sum of the rates of polymerization and depolymerization.

DISCUSSION

We now assume that the kinetic properties of amyloid fibril polymerization can be described as:

$$[\,P\,] + [\,M\,] \underset{k_{-1}}{\overset{k_2}{\rightleftharpoons}} [\,P\,] \qquad (1)$$

where [P] is the number concentration of seed fibrils, [M] is the concentration of AS_{SAM}, k_2 and k_{-1} are the apparent rate constants for polymerization and depolymerization, respectively.

If t is the time, f(t) is the concentration of newly polymerized AS_{SAM}, $[\,M\,]_0$ is the initial AS_{SAM} concentration, then Eq. 1 is described as

$$f'(\,t\,) = k_2[\,P\,][\,M\,] - k_{-1}[\,P\,] \qquad (2)$$

$$[M] = [M]_0 - f(t) \quad (3)$$

The following results are consistent with Eq. 2. First, at a constant AS_{SAM} concentration, the initial rate of extension was proportional to the number concentration of fAS_{SAM}. Second, at a constant fAS_{SAM} concentration, the initial rate of polymerization was proportional to the AS_{SAM} concentration and finally, at each AS_{SAM} concentration, the net rate of fAS_{SAM} extension was the sum of the rates of polymerization and depolymerization.

It is well established that the formation of protein polymers such as bacterial flagella, actin filaments and microtubles involves at least two steps: nucleation and elongation[5]. We now focus on the elongation process. As shown for bacterial flagella, actin filaments and microtubles, the elongation process is described by the condensation polymerization model shown as Eq. 1. It is interesting that this model originally introduced to explain elongation of the physiological polymers can also explain elongation of the essentially pathological polymers, i.e. amyloid fibrils. Therefore, this model may have generality to explain the noncovalent protein polymerization in both physiological and pathological states.

REFERENCES

1. Castaño, Eduardo M., and Frangione, B. (1988) 'Biology of disease; Human amyloidosis, Alzheimer disease and related disorders', Lab. Invest. 58, 122-132.

2. Higuchi, K., Yonezu, T., Kogishi, K., Matsumura, A., Takeshita, S., Higuchi, K., Kohno, A., Matsushita, M., Hosokawa, M., and Takeda, T. (1986) "Purification and characterization of a senile amyloid-related antigenic substance ($apoSAS_{SAM}$) from mouse serum', J. Biol. Chem. 261, 12834-12840.

3. Naiki, H., Higuchi, K., Hosokawa, M., and Takeda, T. (1989) 'Fluorometric determination of amyloid fibrils in vitro using the fluorescent dye, thioflavine T', Anal. Biochem. 177, 244-249.

4. Naiki, H., Higuchi, K., Matsushima, K., Shimada, A., Chen, W-H., Hosokawa, M., and Takeda, T. (1990) 'Fluorometric examination of tissue amyloid fibrils in murine senile amyloidosis: Use of the fluorescent indicator, thioflavine T', Lab. Invest. 62, 768-773.

5. Oosawa, F. and Asakura, S. (1975) Thermodynamics of the polymerization of protein, Academic Press, Inc., London.

IN VITRO ASSEMBLY OF MURINE AMYLOID A PROTEIN, TWO MURINE SERUM AMYLOID A PROTEINS, AND NORMAL HUMAN TRANSTHYRETIN TO FORM AMYLOID-LIKE FIBRILS

SATOSHI BABA, KATSUTOSHI MIURA, and HARUYUKI SHIRASAWA
2nd Department of Pathology
Hamamatsu University School of Medicine
3600 Handa-cho, Hamamatsu 431-31, Japan

ABSTRACT. Murine amyloid A protein (AA), two isotypes of murine serum amyloid A protein (SAA_1 and SAA_2), and normal human transthyretin (TTR) were examined whether they polymerize into amyloid-like fibrils in vitro. The proteins were dissolved in solution containing 6 M-guanidine hydrochloride and the solutions were diluted into the solvents of various pH values. All the four proteins were assembled into amyloid-like fibrils in acidic conditions without proteolytic enzymes or any other co-existents such as amyloid P component or glycosaminoglycans. The fibrils bound Congo red and were curvilinear, twisted, and 5-10 nm wide by electron microscopy. The results suggest that proteolytic processing of amyloid precursors is not necessary for fibril assembly and a microenvironment of low pH is possibly related to amyloid formation.

INTRODUCTION

Serum amyloid A protein (SAA) is the precursor of amyloid A protein (AA) in the reactive amyloidosis. In mice, both SAA_1 and SAA_2 are found in acute-phase HDL, but only SAA_2 is deposited as AA-amyloid fibrils [1]. In familial amyloidotic polyneuropathy (FAP), only variant transthyretin (TTR) constitutes amyloid fibrils [e.g., 2], although both normal and variant TTR are found in the circulation [3]. Senile cardiac amyloidosis (SCA)/senile systemic amyloidosis (SSA) have been considered to be related to normal TTR [4].

Many successful attempts have been reported of in vitro formation of amyloid fibrils. As to AA, however, one failed in re-constituting amyloid fibrils [5], whereas the others succeeded [6,7]. No such attempt has been reported about either normal or variant TTR. We hence tried to determine whether amyloid-like fibrils are formed in vitro from murine AA, SAA_1, SAA_2, and normal human TTR, and here we report success in forming amyloid-like fibrils from all the four proteins in acidic conditions.

MATERIALS AND METHODS

Murine AA-amyloid fibrils were extracted with distilled water and SAA-rich HDL was prepared from the serum of LPS-treated mice by sequential ultracentrifugation. The AA-fibrils and SAA-rich HDL were dissociated with 6 M guanidine-HCl/0.1 M Tris (pH 8.0)/0.1 mM EDTA, and fractionated on a column of Sephacryl S-200. AA- and SAA-fractions were further purified by reversed-phase HPLC (Senshu pak ODS-H-1251 column; SSC, Tokyo, Japan) with an acetonitrile gradient (30-50%) in 0.1% trifluoroacetic acid. Normal human TTR was commercially obtained (Sigma).

The purified proteins were verified by 8 M urea/SDS-PAGE followed by N-terminal amino acid sequencing for SAAs and AA, or fast atom bombardment mass spectrometry

(FAB/MS) for TTR. N-terminal amino acid sequences of AA, SAA_1 and SAA_2 were analyzed by automatic Edman degradation by a Beckman 890M sequencer. FAB/MS of TTR was carried out [8] on a JMA-AX505H mass spectrometer (JEOL). Triptic digest of TTR was directly loaded onto the mass spectrometer.

The four proteins were solubilized (2.5 mg/100 μl) in 6 M guanidine-HCl, 10 mM Tris-HCl (pH 7.4), 1 mM EDTA, and 5 mM dithioerythritol. In addition, undissociated solution of TTR (2.5 mg/100 μl) in 10 mM Tris-HCl (pH 7.4) was prepared. After incubation for 4 h at room temperature, the solution was diluted 50-fold with following buffers: 5 mM glycin-HCl (pH 2.2 and 3.0), 5 mM sodium acetate buffer (pH 3.6, 4.4, 5.2, and 5.6), 5 mM Tris-HCl(pH 7.2 and 8.0), and 5 mM glycin-NaOH (pH 9.0 and 10.0). By regulating the concentration of KCl, the ionic strength of the each buffer was adjusteted to 0.16. After incubation (6-12 h) at room temperature, the preparations were negatively stained with 1% uranyl acetate and examined by electron microscopy.

RESULTS

On the reversed phase HPLC of SAA fraction, two large peaks were observed, and they were found to be SAA_1 and SAA_2 from the mobilities on urea/SDS-PAGE. N-terminal amino acid sequences purified SAA_1, SAA_2, and AA were as follows:

SAA_1: Gly-Phe-Phe-Ser-Phe-Val-His-Glu-Ala-Phe-
SAA_2: Gly-Phe-Phe-Ser-Phe-Ile-Gly-Glu-Ala-Phe-
AA: Gly-Phe-Phe-Ser-Phe-Ile-Gly-Glu-Ala-Phe-

They were all identical to the data reported by Hoffman et al. [1]. On FAB/MS of TTR, tryptic peptides were detected as protonated ion at m/z 672 (T3: The peptide number is based on the previous report [8].), m/z 690 (T2), m/z 704 (T8), m/z 832 (T1), m/z 1267 (T8+T9), m/z 1366 (T4), and m/z 1394 (T6). These spectora all coinside with expected peptides from the sequence of normal TTR [8] and no abnormal peptides such as T4 [Met^{30}] [2] were observed.

The purified SAA_1, SAA_2, AA, and TTR formed amyloid-like fibrils in the acidic conditions (Table 1 and Fig. 1). Fibrils observed at pH -3.6 were 5 to 10 nm wide and of variable length. They frequently have periodic twists or narrowings and appeared more curvilinear than native amyloid fibrils. At pH 4.4-5.6, similar fibrils were observed, but they were less yielded and tended to aggregate nonspecifically. At pH 7.2-, non-fibrillar aggregates were observed in the preparations of AA and SAAs, and few aggregates in those of TTR. As to TTR, the same results occured even when it was initially dissolved in 10 mM Tris-HCl (pH 7.4). Fibrillar structure was still observed at least 24 h after neutralization of pH by addition of NaOH into the acidic solutions. Congo red staining of the fibrillar preparations showed green birefringence under polarized light, although the intensity of the green color was less than that observed in tissue sections presumably due to irregular orientation of the fibrils formed in vitro.

DISCUSSION

We observed that murine AA, SAA_1, SAA_2, and normal human TTR are all capable of forming amyloid-like fibrils without proteolytic processing or any other co-existents. As to TTR, the data provided supporting evidence that amyloid fibrils of SCA/SSA consist of normal TTR.

The significance of limited proteolysis of precursor molecules has been emphasized in the pathogenesis of amyloidosis. It is now controversial, however, because intact precursors are also deposited in diverse amyloidoses such as FAP [4]. In addition, deposition of SAA possibly precedes its conversion to AA [9]. Our success in fibril formation from both

TABLE 1. Assembly of amyloid-like fibrils from murine AA, SAA_1, SAA_2, and normal human TTR observed by electron microscopy after dilution with the solvents of various pH values.

Solvent conditions		AA	SAA_1	SAA_2	TTR
50 mM Gly-HCl	(pH 2.2)	++	++	++	++
50 mM Gly-HCl	(pH 3.0)	++	++	++	++
50 mM NaOAc-AcOH	(pH 3.6)	++	++	++	++
50 mM NaOAc-AcOH	(pH 4.4)	+	+	+	+
50 mM NaOAc-AcOH	(pH 5.6)	+*	+*	+*	-
50 mM Tris-HCl	(pH 7.2)	-	-	-	-
50 mM Tris-HCl	(pH 8.0)	-	-	-	-
50 mM Gly-NaOH	(pH 9.0)	-	-	-	-
50 mM Gly-NaOH	(pH 10.0)	-	-	-	-

* A few fibrils were observed, but it was not reproducible.

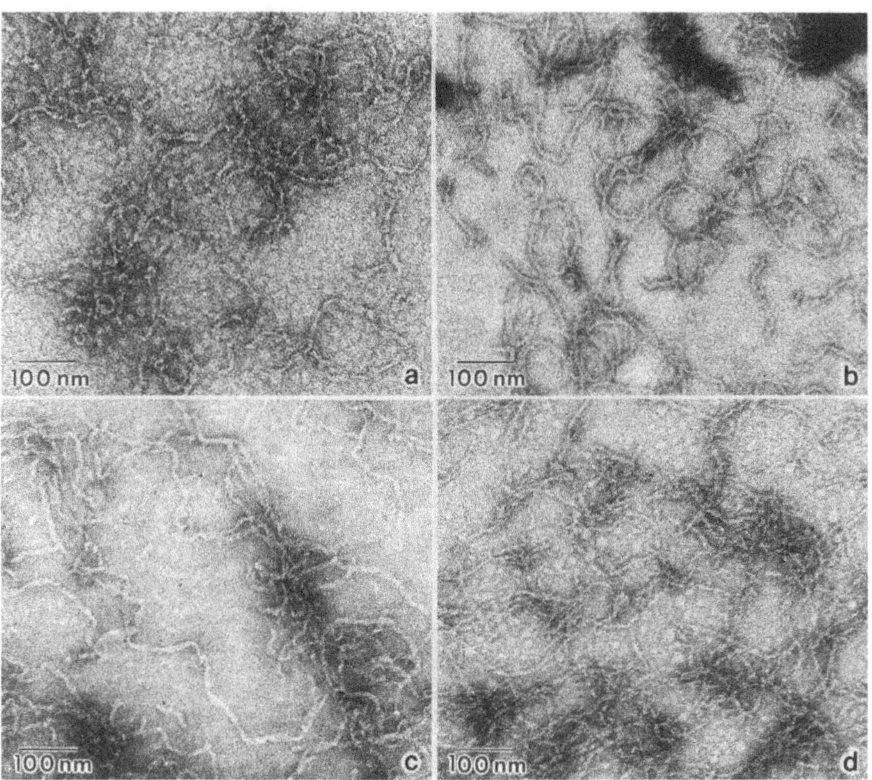

Figure 1. Electron micrographs of negatively stained amyloid-like fibrils: (a) AA, (b) SAA_1, and (c) SAA_2 in acetate buffer (pH4.4); and (d) TTR in acetate buffer (pH 3.6).

intact SAAs and TTR supports the suggestion that cleavage of precursor proteins is not always essential to amyloid fibril formation. Moreover, it is indicated that other materials such as amyloid P component or glycosaminoglycans which coexist in amyloid deposits are not essential for fibrillogenesis at least under acidic conditions.

Of interest in this study is the acidic conditions under which fibrils were formed, and because fibrils were still observed after neutralization of the acidic solutions, fibril assembly seems nearly irreversible. Under an acidic condition, proteins may undergo denaturation. Because these protiens have intrinsic β-structure (especially, TTR is rich in β-structure), it is likely that denaturation is accompanied by fibril assembly resulting from stacking of β-sheets. We can not yet answer whether an acidic condition is actually related to the development of amyloid in vivo. However, concerning of the fact that amyloid fibrils frequently appear in membrane-bound channels closely associated with the lysosomes of reticuloendothelial cells, we suppose that low pH in the microenvironment such as in endosomes or lysosomes triggers the formation of minute fibrils which play a role of nuclei for additional fibril formation.

It is also of primary significance in the pathogenesis of amyloidosis why SAA_2 and TTR variants are readily deposited as amyloid in vivo. Against the expectation that SAA_1 were less fibrillogenic than SAA_2 and AA, our data indicated that SAA_1 and normal TTR can also form amyloid-like fibrils. Although further comparative studies are necessary about the properties for fibril polymerization of SAAs and TTRs, it is possible that minor structural differences between amyloid protein and their non-amyloidgenic relatives are related to some factors other than property of fibril polymerization itself.

REFERENCES

[1] Hoffman, J.S., Ericsson, L.H., Erikson, N., Walsh, K.A., and Benditt, E.P. (1984) 'Murine tissue amyloid protein AA—NH_2-terminal sequence identity with only one of two serum amyloid protein (ApoSAA) gene products', J. Exp. Med. 159, 641-646.

[2] Tawara, S., Nakazato, M., Kangawa, K., Matsuo, H., and Araki, S. (1983) 'Identification of amyloid prealbumin variant in familial amyloidotic polyneuropathy (Japanese type)' Biochem. Biophys. Res. Commun. 116, 880-888.

[3] Nakazato, M., Kangawa, K., Minamino, N., Tawara, S., Matsuo, H., and Araki, S. (1984) 'Identification of a prealbumin variant in the serum of a Japanese patient with familial amyloidotic poluneuropathy' Biochem. Biophys. Res. Commun. 122, 712-718.

[4] Cornwell III, G.G., Sletten, K., Olofsson, B.O., Johansson, B., and Westermark, P. (1987) 'Prealbumin: its association with amyloid' J. Clin. Pathol. 40, 226-231.

[5] Hol, P.R., Langeveld, J.P.M., van Beuningen-Jansen, E.W., Veerkamp, J.H., and Gruy, E. (1984) 'A second component in bovine AA amyloid fibrils not identical with protein AA is essential for AA amyloid fibrillogenesis', Scand. J. Immunol. 20, 53-60.

[6] Zuckerberg, A., Gazith, J., Rimon, A., Reshef, T., and Gafni, J. (1972) 'The structural subunit of amyloid—Isolation & characterization of a polypeptide capable of fibril-formation', Eur. J. Biochem. 28, 161-165.

[7] Prelli, F., Pras, M., and Frangione, B. (1987) 'Degradation and deposition of amyloid AA fibrils are tissue specific', Biochemistry 26, 8251-8256.

[8] Wada, Y., Matsuo, T., Takakuse, I., Suzuki, T., Azuma, T., Tsujino, S., Kishimoto, S., Matsuda, H., and Hayashi, A. (1986) 'Mass spectrometric detection of the plasma prealbumin (transthyretin) variant associated with familial amyloidotic polyneuropathy' Biochim. Biophys. Acta 873, 316-319.

[9] Shiroo, M., Kawahara, E., Nakanishi, I., and Migita, S. (1987) 'Specific deposition of serum amyloid A protein 2 in the mouse' Scand. J. Immunol. 26, 709-716.

SECONDARY STRUCTURE CHANGES IN MUTANT TRANSTHYRETINS AFTER PROTEOLYSIS BY NEUTROPHILIC SERINE PROTEASES

Martha Skinner
Mary T. Walsh * +
Phillip J. Stone +
Lawreen Heller Connors
Alan S. Cohen

From the Arthritis Center, Department of Medicine, * Department of Biophysics + Department of Biochemistry, Boston University School of Medicine Boston MA 02118.

ABSTRACT

The secondary structure of plasma transthyretin (TTR) from patients with familial amyloidotic polyneuropathy was studied with respect to alteration in the amount of beta conformation after exposure to proteolytic enzymes of the neutrophilic serine protease family. We examined TTR from four affected individuals, each with a different mutation or at a different stage of disease. After exposure to human neutrophilic elastase (HNE) or cathepsin G, circular dichroic (CD) spectra for each was compared to normal.

The mutant TTR's exhibit marked alterations in beta conformation after digestion. The degree of CD alteration of mutant TTR digested with HNE correlates with the severity of disease in each kinship.

INTRODUCTION

In this study, we have examined the secondary structure and, in particular, the alteration in the amount of beta conformation of TTR after exposure to proteolytic enzymes of the neutrophilic serine protease family. Major disruption in the structure of TTR isolated from patients with FAP was found by CD analysis.

MATERIALS AND METHODS

Source of TTR

TTR was isolated from the plasma of 4 patients with familial amyloidotic polyneuropathy (TTR_{FAP}) who were seen and evaluated in the Clinical Research Center. Two of these patients have the TTR_{FAP} with methionine for valine at position 30 as previously reported (Whitehead, et al 1984 and Saraiva, et al 1986). The first, of Swedish origin, developed neuropathy at age 39 and lived with FAP until age 52. The second, of Greek origin, has the mutant gene but is not yet symptomatic at age 37. The third patient, of German origin, developed autonomic neuropathy at age 29, had a rapidly progressive course of disease and died at age 39. This patient's TTR_{FAP} had a new mutation of ala for val at position 30 (Jones, et al 1990). The fourth is of German/English ancestry and has the TTR_{FAP} of tyrosine for serine at position 77 (Skinner, et al 1989). This patient developed neuropathy and cardiomyopathy at age 63 and has been symptomatic for ten years.

Enzyme digestions and circular dichroism analysis

TTR was isolated by ion-exchange and molecular sieve chromatography as previously described (Skinner, et al 1988). HNE and Cat G were purified from purulent sputum.

Each TTR (TTR_{FAPs} and TTR_{N}) was solubilized in 0.15 M NaCl, 0.02 M Tris, pH 7.4 at a concentration of 1 mg/ml and was divided into 2 or 3 aliquots. One aliquot was untreated. HNE was added to a second aliquot in an enzyme to substrate (w/w) ratio of 1:50. To the third aliquot, Cat G was added in an enzyme to substrate ratio of 1:25. All samples were incubated at 37^{0}C for 18 hrs. Digestion was stopped by freezing. CD spectra of TTR_N and TTR_{FAP} with and without enzyme treatment were recorded at ambient temperature on a Cary 61 CD Spectropolarimeter (Varian; Palo Alto, CA) calibrated from 500 to 190nm with d-10-camphorsulfonic acid (1 mg/ml in ethanol). The spectrum reported for each sample represents the average of three individual spectra for each preparation and has been corrected for baseline contribution due to buffer (0.15M NaCl, 0.02mM Tris-HCl, pH 7.4) or buffer plus enzyme.

Molar ellipticity values, [θ], were calculated according to the following equation: $[\theta]$ (deg cm^2/decimol) = θ x MRW/10 x 1 x c, where 0 represents the displacement from the baseline value x full range in degrees, MRW equals the mean residue weight of an amino acid, 1 is the pathlength of the cell in cm, and c equals the concentration of protein in g/ml (Greenfield and Fasman 1969). The [θ] values reported are ±1% for each sample after averaging over multiple preparations and scans.

RESULTS AND DISCUSSION

Highly purified plasma TTR_{FAP} in a 30% yield was obtained following ion exchange and gel chromatography. On SDS-PAGE the TTR_{FAP} resolved primarily as a 14kda monomeric unit, indicating comigration of the mutant and normal TTR components.

Normal untreated TTR exhibited a negative minimum at 214nm ($[\theta]$=-7248). The spectrum after treatment with HNE was similar, however with a broadened trough from 208 to 220nm and slightly increased ellipticity from 215 to 200nm with respect to the untreated. The negative minimum was at 211nm ($[\theta]$=-7582). Cat G treatment altered the spectrum to a greater extent. The minimum remains at 212nm ($[\theta]$=-(6400), however, the ellipticity was diminished over the entire spectrum. Although the spectra and secondary structures of all untreated TTR_{FAPs} appeared to be similar to the TTR_N, HNE or CatG treatment of all mutant TTRs, with the exception of the one from the Tyr 77 patient altered the spectrum significantly and more extensively, than for normal TTR.

The degree of CD alteration correlates with the clinical information in patients with the mutations we studied. In the Swedish patient with the met 30 mutation a marked disruption was found. In the Greek patient who has the same met 30 mutation but is asymptomatic and does not have amyloid deposition on abdominal fat aspiration, the CD analysis showed less disruption of the beta conformation. This patient at age 37, is at the approximate age when symptomatology was evident in members of her kinship with FAP.

In the third patient with a newly defined alanine for valine mutation at the same position 30, a markedly unusual CD spectrum is observed even before digestion with HNE. This pattern is even more pronounced after digestion. This patient is from a kinship which has had very early development of symptoms and very aggressive disease. All FAP family members in this kinship, except for the patient, have died before age 35. In the fourth patient with a tyrosine for serine mutation at position 77 the alteration in the beta conformation of the TTR_{FAP} was very minimal. In this patient's family, amyloid develops at an older age, usually the seventh decade.

It must be noted that the TTR from FAP patients used in this study was isolated from persons heterozygous for the mutant TTR. Therefore, a portion of the molecules were normal and a portion were mutant. Thus the changes in CD pattern with respect to the mutant TTR are even more pronounced.

ACKNOWLEDGEMENTS

Supported by grants from the U.S. Public Health Service, NIAMDD (AM 07014), the General Clinical Centers Branch of the Division of Research Resources, National Institues of Health (RR 533), the Multipurpose Arthritis Center, National Institutes of Health (AM 20613), National Institutes of Health (HL 26335) (HL 19717) and the Arthritis Foundation.

REFERENCES

1. Benson, M.D., and Wallace, M.R. (1989) The metabolic Basis of Inherited Disease. Ed by CR Scruver, AL Beaudet, WS Sly, D Valle. (ed) McGraw-Hill, pp 2439-2460.
2. Greenfield, N., and Fasman, G.D. (1969) Computed circular dichroism spectra for the evaluation of protein conformation. Biochemistry 10,4108-4116.
3. Jones LA, Skare J, Harding J, Cohen AS,and Skinner M (1990) A new substitution at position 30 in the transthyretin (TTR) protein associated with familial amyloid polyneuropathy. Arthritis Rheum (in press).
4. Saraiva, M.J.M., Sherman, W., and Goodman, D.S. (1986) Presence of a plasma transthyretin (prealbumin) variant in familial amyloidotic polyneuropathy in a kindred of Greek origin. J Lab Clin Med 108,17-226.
5. Skinner M., Connors L.H., Kagan H.M., Stone P., and Cohen A.S. (1988) Degradation studies on plasma prealbumin In Amyloid and Amyloidosis. ed by T. Isobe, S. Araki, F. Uchino, S. Kito, E.T. Subura. Plenum Press New York pp 125-130.
6. Skinner, M., Libbey, C.A., Skare, J.C., Benson, M.D., Milunsky, A., and Cohen, A.S. (1989) Tyrosine for serine 77 is the variant transthyretin in a United States family of German/English ancestry with familial amyloidotic polyneuropathy. Arquivos de Medicina. 3,189.
7. Whitehead, A.S., Skinner, M., Bruns, G.A.P., Costello, W., Edge, M.D., Cohen, A.S., and Sipe, J.D. (1984) Cloning of the human prealbumin cDNA: localization of the gene to chromosome 18 and detection of a variant prealbumin allele in a family with familial amyloid polyneuropathy. Mol Biol Med 2,411-423.

PRODUCTION OF AMYLOIDOGENIC PEPTIDES FROM HUMAN IMMUNOGLOBULIN LIGHT (L)-CHAINS

MANFRED EULITZ*, MICHAEL BREUER*, ABY EBLEN§, DEBORAH T.WEISS§ AND ALAN SOLOMON§

* GSF Institut für Klinische Molekularbiologie und Tumorgenetik, Marchioninstr.25, 8000 München 70, Germany, § University of Tennessee Medical Center at Knoxville, 1924 Alcoa Highway, Knoxville/Tn. 37920/USA

Abstract: Structural studies were performed on three human immunoglobulin L-chains isolated from the urine of patients with generalized amyloidosis. The complete amino acid sequence of the V-regions was established for all three proteins. According to their amino acid sequence all proteins belong to Subgroup I of human κ-L-chains. Heavy precipitates were formed during the tryptic digestion of the reduced and carboxymethylated chains. These precipitates resemble amyloid in many ways as they stained positive with Congo red, showed the typical green birefringence in polarized light, were insoluble in most solvents and indigestible by the usual proteolytic enzymes. Amyloidlike fibrillar structures were demonstrable by electron microscopy in the precipitates of all three proteins. These amyloid forming peptides, which aggregate in the precipitate derive in all three chains from the same regions within the variable and constant parts in the three L-chains. Generally there is some evidence that the capability for amyloid formation resides in certain hydrophobic regions within the human immunoglobulin L-chains.

Introduction:

It was first shown by Glenner et al.(1) that monoclonal immunoglobulin L-chains are the main constituents of AL-type amyloids. Subsequent studies showed that either intact κ- and λ-L-chains or, more often, fragments thereof are detectable in AL-amyloid(2-4), although the number of completely sequenced AL-type amyloid proteins is still scarce. It has been shown in some studies that only 6-15% of patients with plasma cell dyscrasias develop amyloidosis.(2,5) This observation, and the fact that L-chains of the lambda-type, especially of the subgroup λ-VI (6), predominate in amyloid deposits might point to structural pecularities in amyloidogenic L-chains. In an attempt to further characterize these pecularities we undertook structural studies on Bence Jones proteins from patients suffering from generalized amyloidosis. In the course of this studies we observed the formation of heavy precipitates during tryptic digestion. These precipitates show many characteristics commonly found in amyloid.

MATERIAL AND METHODS

Isolation, purification, reduction and carboxymethylation of the Bence Jones proteins were done as described(7). Tryptic digestion was performed in 0.1 mol methylmorpholine/acetate buffer ph 8.0 with TosPheCH_2-treated trypsin. Precipitates formed during digestion were separated by centrifugation at 12 000 rpm. Peptides from the supernatant or the precipitate were isolated by HPLC on a C_{18}-reversed phase column(Vydac). Electron microscopy of precipitated peptides was done after negative staining with 2% phosphotungstic acid, pH 5.0. Amino acid analysis of the tryptic peptides was done after 24^h hydrolysis in constant boiling HCl at 105°C using an automatic amino acid analyzer (Model 5000,Biotronik Franfurt/M.). The amino acid sequence of the undigested proteins or their tryptic peptides was established with a model 470A gas phase sequenator connected on line to a model 120A PTH-amino acid analyzer(Applied Biosystems, Foster City,Cal.).

RESULTS

Amino acid sequence of the V-regions of the proteins GRI, CRO and KING: The amino acid sequence of the three V-regions of this proteins was established by automatic degradation of the undigested carboxymethylated proteins and of tryptic peptides deriving from these proteins (see fig.1).It was possible to align all tryptic peptides unequivocally within the chain. By comparison with already published V-region sequences in the compilation of Kabat et al.(8),all three L-chains show the closest similarity to the proteins of subgroup I of human κ-L-chains. Amino acid exchanges among the three chains concentrate in the complementary determining regions(CDR). With exchange rates between 14.8% (proteins GRI/ROY) and 27,8% (proteins GRI/KING and ROY/KING) the degree of variability does not exceed the limits of about 25% which can be seen between individual members of one subgroup. There were some rare amino acid substitutions in the three proteins, but in general neither the position nor the type of exchange allows the distinction between amyloidogenic and non-amyloidogenic immunoglobulin L-chains.

Amyloid generating peptides rising by tryptic digestion of carboxymethylated human κ-immunoglobulin L-chains: Heavy precipitates were formed during the tryptic digestion of all three reduced and carboxymethylated L-chains. These highly insoluble precipitates consist of peptide material, which stained strongly positive with congo red and showed the green birefringence in polarized light typically found in amyloid deposits.

Examination of the precipitates by electron microscopy after negative staining exhibited fibrillar structures indistiguishable from typical amyloid fibrils (see also fig.2). The

PRIMARY STRUCTURE OF THE AMYLOIDOGENIC BENCE JONES PROTEINS GRI, CRO AND KING

```
                       10                  20                  30
ROY   D I Q M T Q S P S S L S A S V G D R V T I T C Q A S Q D I S
GRI   - - - - - - - - - - - - - - - - - - - - - - - - - - - - - -
CRO   - - - - - - - - - - - - - - - - - - - - - - - R - - - S F N
KING  - - - - - - - - - T - - - - - - - - - S - - - R - - - N - N

                       40                  50                  60
ROY   I F L N W Y Q Q K P G K A P K L L I Y D A S K L E A G V P S
GRI   S Y - - - - - - - - - - - - E - - - - A G - T - - T - - - -
CRO   N - - - - - - - - - - - - - - - - - - - - - T - - S - - - -
KING  - W - A - - - - - - - T - - - - - M - K - - V - - N - - - -

                       70                  80                  90
ROY   R F S G T G S G T D F T F T I S G L Q P E D I A T Y Y C Q Q
GRI   - - - - S - - - - - - - - - - - S - - - - - V - - - - - - -
CRO   - - - - S - - - - - - - L - - - S - - - - - F - - - - - - -
KING  - - - - S - - - - E - A L - - A S - - - D - F - - - - - - -

                      100             108
ROY   F D N L P L T F G G G T K V D F K R
GRI   Y L - - I F - - - P - - - - - I - -
CRO   T Y T G - I - - - Q - - - L E I - -
KING  Y T S Y - Y - - - Q - - T L E I - -
```

Fig.1: Amino acid sequence of the V-regions of the Bence Jones proteins GRI, CRO and KING. The amino acid sequence of protein ROY was taken from the compilation of Kabat et al.(7). The amino acids are given in the one letter code. Concordant amino acids in corresponding positions are lined, substitutions marked by letters.

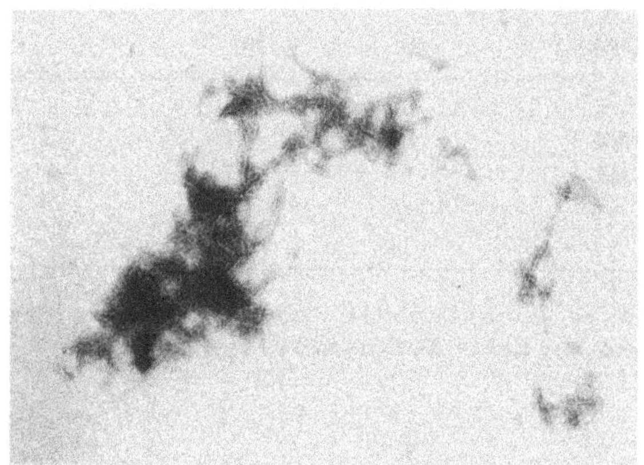

fig.2
Fibrillar structures in the precipitate from protein GRI demonstrated by electron microscopy after negative staining

picture shown resulted from the precipitate of protein GRI, but the precipitates of the proteins CRO and KING showed the same pattern.

Attempts to separate the peptides in the precipitates by high performance liquid chromatography failed completely, because the aggregates were insoluble in the solvents used for this purpose. They were also indegestible by proteases other than trypsin, such as chymotrypsin, pepsin, subtilisin, thermolysin and the protease of the V_8-strain of Staphylococcus aureus. The precipitates were dissolved finally only by the use of a mixture of formic acid/isopropanole/water (50:10:40 v/v). Thereafter the peptides of this solution were separated completely by gradient elution on a reversed phase column. Their amino acid composition was estimated after hydrolysis and their amino acid sequence established by extended runs on the sequenator. Surprisingly peptides derived from the same positions in all three proteins could be identified as main constituents of the precipitates. Two peptides in particular,derived from the positions 62-104 of the V-region and positions 127-142 of the constant part, represented more than 60% of the material of the precipitates as calculated from the amino acid content in the separated peptide peaks (see also table 1). Two additional peptides from the variable part (e.g. position 1-18 and position 25-42) were found to be admixed to the aggregates,formed during the digestion of proteins GRI and CRO, but to a much lesser extent. No other peptides from the C-region were found in the precipitates.

Table 1

Position of the peptide in the L-chain	Content of the peptides in the Precipitate (Percent)*		
	GRI	CRO	KING
1-18	9%	7.8%	absent
25-42	10%	22.6%	12.5%
62-104	37.6%	38.4%	43.5%
127-142	43.2%	31.2%	44.0%

* calculated from the amino acid content of the peptides in the precipitate after separation by HPLC and hydrolysis in HCl

Discussion:

The results of this study indicate, that certain tryptic peptides from human immunoglobulin κ-L-chains are capable of forming aggregates which resemble amyloid in many aspects. Morphologically they appeared in the electron microscop as fibrillar structures indistinguishable from true amyloid fibrils. Furthermore the aggregates stained positive with congo red, showed the green birefringence in polarized light, were insoluble in most solvents and indegestibel by common proteolytic enzymes. Thus they share many properties which were generally accepted as characteristic of amyloid (2-4).

Surprisingly, we found that the amyloid-like precipitates in all three proteins studied consisted uniformly of the same peptides, which derive from certain regions of immunoglobulin-L-chains. These peptides comprise the amino acid residues spanning the positions 62-104 of the variable region and positions 127-142 of the constant part. Peptides comprising the positions 1-18 and 25-42 were found in a lesser amount in the precipitates of proteins GRI and CRO, but not in protein KING. Therefore this peptides were not regarded as essential for the formation of the fibrillar aggregates.

X-ray crystallographic studies of Bence Jones proteins(9) revealed that these proteins were folded in antiparalell ß-pleated sheets in a sandwich type structure, with hydrophobic amino acid side chains filling the internal space netween both layers. According to the model provided by Lesk and Chothia (10), the amyloid generating peptides enumerated above form the ß-strands E, F and G and the CDR3 of the V-domain and the ß-strnd B of the C-domain. This native conformation could no longer be existent in the amyloid generating eptides, because the carboxymethylation abolishes the fixation of the antiparalell ß-strands by disulfide bridges. Nevertheless the peptides forming the precipitate must regain ß-structures to a certain extent, since this conformation is a prerequisite for the formation of amyloid fibrils. In a previous paper (11) we described the formation of amyloid generating peptides for an amyloidogenic human immunoglobulin L-chain of the subgroup λ-I. Thus both classes of human immunoglobulin L-chains seem to be capable to release amyloid generating peptides during digestion with trypsin.

It was shown by other authors (12-14) that in vitro digestion of Bence Jones proteins leads to the precipitation of fibrillar material. But these experiments were conducted with native L-chains rather than reduced and alkylated proteins as in our experiments. Furthermore the fragments are included in this in vitro amyloids seem to comprise much larger parts of the V-region. It has to be cleared by further experiments if the potential to form amyloid like precipitates is a property of all human immunoglobulin-L-chains or whether it is restricted to certain subclasses and amyloidogenic L-chains.

Acknowledgement: We wish to express our appreciation to Dr.R.P.Linke for performing the congo red staining of the precipitates and for helpful discussions. We thank Miss M.Darsow and Miss M.Knonsalla for expert technical assistance. This work was supported in part by the Sonderforschungsbereich 207 of the Deutsche Forschungsgemeinschaft.

References:

1. Glenner,G.G., Harbaugh,G., Ohm, J.J., Harada,M. and Cuatrecasas, P.(1970) Biochem.Biophys.Res.Commun.41, 1287-1289
2. Glenner, G.G. (1980) N.Engl.J.Med. 302,1283-1292;1333-1343
3. Pepys,M.B. (1988) Quart.J.Med., 252, 283-298
4. Stone,M.J. (1990) Blood, 75, 531-545
5. Kyle, R.A. and Greipp,P.R., (1983) Mayo Clin.Proc.,58, 665-683
6. Solomon,A., Frangione,B. and Franklin,E.C.(1982), J.Clin. Invest. 70, 453-460
7. Eulitz,M. (1974), Eur.J.Biochem. 50, 49-69
8. Kabat,E.A., Wu,T.T., Reid-Miller, M., Perry,H.M. and Gottesmann,H.M., eds.,(1987) Sequences of Proteins of Immunological Interest (National Institutes of Health, Bethesda, MD),4th Ed.
9. Epp,O., Lattmann,E.E., Schiffer,M., Huber,R. and Palm,W.(1975) Biochem. 14, 4943-4952
10. Lesk, A.M. and Chothia, C. (1982) J.Mol.Biol., 160, 325-342
11. Eulitz,M. and Linke,R.P. (1987) Biol.Chem.Hoppe Seyler, 368, 863-870
12. Glenner,G.G., Ein,D., Eanes,E.D., Bladen,H.A., Terry, W. and Page,D.L. (1971) Science 174, 712-713
13. Linke,R.P., Tischendorf,F.W., Zucker-Franklin,D. and Franklin, E.C. (1973) J.Immunol. 111,24-26
14. Epstein,W.V., Tan,M. and Wood,I.S.(1974) J.Lab.Clin.Med. 84, 107-112

PREDOMINANCE OF ONE SAA ISOTYPE (SAAI) IN HUMAN REACTIVE AMYLOID

Liepnieks, J.J., Leagre, C., Kluve-Beckerman, B., and Benson, M.D.
Veterans Affairs Medical Center (583/111RH), 1481 West 10th Street, Room #A772, Indianapolis, IN 46202; Indiana University School of Medicine, Department of Medicine, Rheumatology Division, Clinical Building 492, 541 Clinical Drive, Indianapolis, IN 46223, USA

ABSTRACT. Three forms of SAA each consisting of 104 amino acids have been identified in human plasma. To elucidate whether one of these forms predominates in the formation of AA amyloid deposits, the amino acid sequence of the subunit protein in amyloid in five cases of reactive amyloidosis was investigated. The subunit protein was obtained from isolated fibrils by chromatography on Sepharose CL6B in 4M guanidine hydrochloride, digested with trypsin, and fractionated by reverse phase HPLC. SAAI contains Val, Ala, and Asp at residues 52, 57 and 60 respectively, while SAAIIα and SAAIIβ contain Ala, Val, and Asn. These residues are contained in the tryptic peptides from residues 47-62 and 48-62. The relative amounts of these peptides present in the tryptic digest of amyloid subunit protein as determined by sequence analysis of the peptides suggested that SAAI was the predominant form in AA amyloid deposits. SAAII peptides represented only trace to 10% of the total in four cases and approximately 30% in the fifth case.

INTRODUCTION

Serum amyloid A protein (SAA) is the plasma precursor for amyloid A protein (AA), the major subunit protein in amyloid deposits of secondary or reactive amyloidosis [1]. Human SAA isolated from plasma is polymorphic, and three forms of SAA each consisting of 104 amino acids have been identified [2-7]. SAAI differs from SAAIIα and SAAIIβ in 7 and 8 residues respectively [2,3]. SAAI contains Val, Ala, Asp, Phe, Phe, Glu, and Lys at positions 52, 57, 60, 68, 69, 84 and 90 respectively, while SAAIIα and SAAIIβ contain Ala, Val, Asn, Leu, Thr, Lys, and Arg [2,3]. In addition, SAAI and SAAIIα have His at position 71 while SAAIIβ has Arg [2,3]. Two forms of SAA have been identified in mouse plasma, but only one was present in amyloid deposits [8]. To elucidate whether one of the three human SAA forms predominates in the formation of AA amyloid deposits, the amino acid sequence of the subunit protein in five cases of reactive amyloidosis was investigated. Sequence analysis of the tryptic peptides arising from residues 47 to 62 where SAAI and SAAII differ at three positions was used to identify the peptide as arising from SAAI or SAAII, and to determine the relative amounts of the peptides. The results suggest that SAAI is the predominant form in human AA amyloid deposits.

MATERIALS AND METHODS

Isolation Of Amyloid Fibrils And Subunit Protein. Amyloid fibrils were isolated from tissues by the procedure of Pras et al. [9] as previously described [10]. Fibrils were isolated from the spleens of CIC, GIB, JAC, and HEA, and from formaldehyde fixed lymph nodes of WAR. Fibrils were reduced, alkylated, and fractionated on a Sepharose CL6B column as previously described [10].

Trypsin Digestion And Peptide Separation. The subunit protein was digested with TPCK-treated trypsin at pH 8.0, and peptides were fractionated on an Altex Ultrasphere C-18 column eluted with 0.1% TFA and an acetonitrile gradient as previously described [10].

Sequence Analysis. Peptides were sequentially degraded on a Beckman 890C sequenator and PTH-amino acids were identified by HPLC as previously described [2,3].

RESULTS AND DISCUSSION

SAAI differs in amino acid sequence from SAAIIα and SAAIIβ at 7 and 8 residues respectively [2,3]. Three of these differences occur in tryptic peptides T9 and T8-9 as indicated by the boxed residues below:

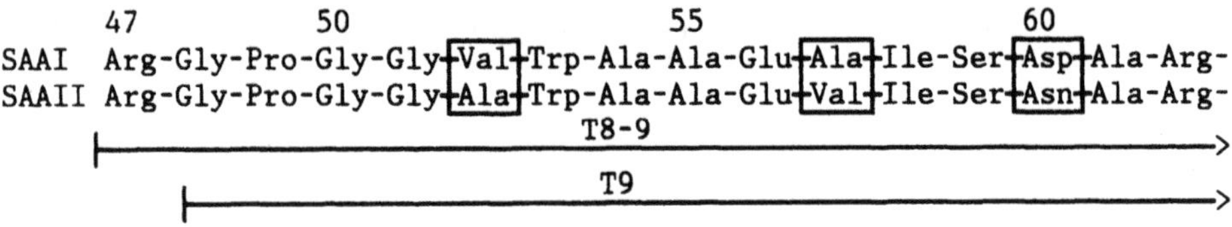

In addition, SAAI has Phe, Phe, Glu, and Lys at positions 68, 69, 84, and 90 respectively while SAAIIα and SAAIIβ have Leu, Thr, Lys, and Arg. SAAI and SAAIIα have His at position 71 while SAAIIβ has Arg. Human AA protein isolated from amyloid usually consists of the N-terminal 76 residues of SAA, but shorter N-terminal fragments have been reported [1]. Thus, residues 68, 69, 71, 84, and 90 where SAAI and SAAII differ, may or may not be present in all amyloid deposits. Therefore, we have used the presence of tryptic peptides T8-9 and T9 for determining and quantitating the relative amounts of SAAI and SAAII in amyloid deposits.

Digestion with trypsin of the subunit proteins isolated from the amyloid of the five patients and separation of the resulting peptides by reverse phase HPLC gave a pattern similar to that obtained with human SAA except the carboxyl terminus peptides of SAA were absent [2,3]. In addition, several minor peaks eluted before and after the major T8-9 peptide peak in varying amounts for the five amyloid samples. Sequence analysis of these peptides from CIC revealed that they arose from peptides T9 and T8-9 from both SAAI and SAAII, and from partial peptides T9 and T8-9 comprising residues 48-59 and 47-59 from both SAAI and SAAII. Similar results were obtained with GIB and WAR subunit protein. HEA was also similar except the partial T9 and T8-9 peptides may have ended at residue 58. One sample, JAC, contained only SAAI peptides. A very small peak eluted at the SAAII peptide T9 and T8-9 position, but it was not sequenced. Thus, JAC may contain traces of SAAII in amyloid. Table I summarizes the results of the relative amounts of SAAI and SAAII present in the amyloid of the five patients. SAAI comprised almost all the AA in amyloid in JAC, approximately 90% in GIB, WAR, and HEA, and about two-thirds in CIC. Thus, SAAI is the predominant form in human AA amyloid deposits. Whether the SAAII present in these deposits is the α or β form is being investigated.

TABLE 1. Percentage of SAAI and SAAII complete or partial peptides T9 and T8-9 present in tryptic digests of amyloid subunit protein

Patient	% SAAI	% SAAII
JAC	~100	trace
GIB	92	8
WAR	89	11
HEA	89	11
CIC	67	33

ACKNOWLEDGEMENTS

This work was supported by VA Medical Research, The United States Public Health Service (RR-00750, NIDDK-34881, NIAMS-AR20582, AR7448), The Arthritis Foundation, The Grace M. Showalter Trust and The Marion E. Jacobson Fund.

REFERENCES

1. Glenner, G.G. (1980) 'Amyloid deposits and amyloidosis: the beta-fibrilloses,' N. Engl. J. Med. 302, 1283-1292 and 1333-1343.
2. Dwulet, F.E., Wallace, D.K., and Benson, M.D. (1988) 'Amino Acid structures of multiple forms of amyloid-related serum protein SAA from a single individual,' Biochemistry 27, 1677-1682.
3. Kluve-Beckerman, B., Dwulet, F.E., and Benson, M.D. (1988) 'Human serum amyloid A, three hepatic mRNAs and the corresponding proteins in one person,' J. Clin. Invest. 82, 1670-1675.
4. Eriksen, N., and Benditt, E.P. (1980) 'Isolation and characterization of the amyloid-related apoprotein (SAA) from human high density lipoprotein,' Proc. Natl. Acad. Sci. U.S.A. 77, 6860-6864.
5. Bausserman, L.L., Herbert, P.N., and McAdam, K.P.W.J. (1980) 'Heterogeneity of human serum amyloid A proteins,' J. Exp. Med. 152, 641-656.
6. Parmalee, D.C., Titani, K., Ericsson, L.H., Eriksen, N., Benditt, E.P., an Walsh, K.A. (1982) 'Amino acid sequence of amyloid-related apoprotein (apoSAA) from human high-density lipoprotein,' Biochemistry 21, 3298-3303.
7. Sletten, K., Marhaug, G., and Husby, G. (1983) 'The covalent structure of amyloid-related serum protein SAA from two patients with inflammatory disease. Hoppe-Seyler's Z. Physiol. Chem. 364, 1039-1046.
8. Hoffman, J.S., Ericsson, L.H., Eriksen, N. Walsh, K.A., and Benditt, E.P. (1984) 'Murine tissue amyloid protein AA. NH_2-terminal sequence identity with only one of two serum amyloid protein (apoSAA) gene products,' J. Exp. Med. 159, 641-646.
9. Pras, M., Schubert, M., Zucker-Franklin, D., Rimon, A., and Franklin, E.C. (1968) 'The characterization of soluble amyloid prepared in water,' J. Clin. Invest. 47, 924-933.
10. Kluve-Beckerman, B., Dwulet, F.E., DiBartola, S.P., and Benson, M.D. (1989) 'Primary structures of dog and cat amyloid A proteins: Comparison to human AA,' Comp. Biochem. Physiol. 94B, 175-183.

A HISTOCHEMICAL MODEL OF THE AMYLOID FIBRIL

John H. Cooper, Department of Pathology,
Dalhousie University, Halifax,N.S., Canada.

Abstract. A previous histochemical construct of the dye-binding amyloid fibril has been revised by use of computer graphics to include the usual twisted form of beta-sheet molecules. The resulting model is a bilaminar, twisted-ribbon filament, whose edges form macrohelical, regularly-stepped, 10A-wide, hydrophobic binding strips, to which the long, narrow, planar, rotatable Congo red molecule, and other amyloidophilic dyes or drugs of similar shape, hydrophobicity and rotational capacity, are bound by close-range forces. The modelling also affords preliminary insight into an analogous close-range bonding arrangement of amyloidogenic monomers to yield stable, directionally straight, twisted filaments.

Introduction. The definitive histological property of amyloid is its red staining, and associated green birefringence, with Congo red(CR). Histochemical analysis of this reaction shows that it involves binding of the dye molecules in the fibrils' axis, and is dependent on their conformational integrity [1,2], but is unaffected by blockades of potential chemical binding groups[2,3]. Instead, CR has been shown to resemble other amyloid dyes of similar elongated planar shape, width, and hydrophobicity (Thioflavine S and T, Sirius red F3B) in having close-range, van der Waals[5], binding affinity for similarly dimensioned, hydrophobic sites, which, in amyloid, should extend along the fibril axis[4].

This histochemical prescription has been correlated with physicochemical data on amyloid proteins[6], and on the presence in known examples, such as Ig light chain[7], serum prealbumin[8] and β-2 microglobulin[9], as in many other beta sheet proteins[7], of a core structure of two sheets forming a sandwich, in which the middle layer, 9.5A thick, of interfacing hydrophobic residues, is exposed only at the edges. The correlation produced a construct of the amyloid filament as a linear, hydrogen-bonded assembly of beta-sheet-sandwich monomers, in which the dye molecules are bound to hydrophobic grooves between the lateral edges of the apposed sheets of each bilaminar monomeric unit[4]. However, this model must be refined to recognize the presence in most beta-sandwich molecules[7], including those of the amyloid proteins noted above [7,8,9], of a marked twisting of the strands in each sheet, with consequent twisting (averaging 20° per strand) of the sheets themselves, and with an anticlockwise rotation of their sandwich alignment[10].

Material and Methods. The new model was fashioned by programs individually designed to produce graphic three-dimensional computer images of the protein and dye molecules involved, using standard data on molecular structure and dimensions. While various beta-sheet sandwich forms were simulated, the the archetypical model filament was fashioned from sandwich pairs of identical sheets rotated anticlockwise by 30° [7], with each sheet consisting of four similar strands of seven residues, having a left-handed interstrand twist-angle of 20° except at monomer interfaces (as in prealbumin dimer[8].

Results. It was found that twisting gives the model polymeric filament the form of a bilaminar twisted ribbon, with the the postulated lateral binding strip forming a kind of spiral staircase, whose floor regularly changes its slope to match the twist angle of its parent strand(Fig.1). Such stepwise angulation of the binding site requires complementary segmental twisting (at around 5A intervals) of CR or other dye molecules that are to be bound to it by close-range forces. Since the CR molecule can effect segmental twisting by rotation at the C-N and C-C single bonds between its rigid aromatic rings[10], and since the other amyloid dyes noted above, despite their variable length, have a similar spacing of rotatable bonds, it was possible to accommodate the dyes in the binding site (Fig.1). Two drugs, Nifedipine and Digoxin, reported to be taken up by amyloid fibrils, were also found to have molecules compatible with the dye-binding site, with the smaller, rotatable, Nifedipine molecule having greater binding potential, in agreement with the quantitative data reported[11,12].

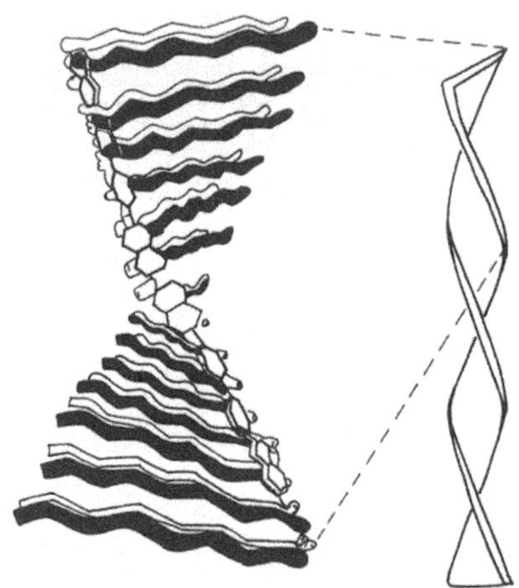

Fig.1 The enlargement of the twisted-ribbon filament on the left shows two CR molecules in the helical binding site.

Discussion. The postulated binding of CR and analogous dyes as spiral arrays of segmentally twisted molecules on a macrohelical hydrophobic site, forming the edge of a bilaminar twisted-ribbon filament, is consistent with, or even explains various previous findings. Firstly the reported resemblance of the optical rotatory dispersion of CR-amyloid fibril complexes with that of CR-alpha-helical poly-L-lysine(PLL), but not that of the CR -beta-PLL complex[13] is explained by the helicity of the filament's hydrophobic binding site, in contrast to the absence of such a site in either of the hydrophilic polylysine complexes, which may simply bind the dye ionically or by H-bonding in the pattern of their respective conformations. Secondly, a rotationally-twisted molecular deformation of bound CR, similar to that of the model, has been demonstrated previously in spectroscopic studies of CR bound to certain enzymes, which have a beta-sheet domain in their coenzyme binding sites[14]. Thirdly, the fluorescence of CR bound to amyloid, which indicates interruption of molecular conjugation[15], can be explained by involvement of the dye's azo double bonds as well as its single bonds in the molecular rotation.

Finally, concerning fibrillogenesis, it should be noted that, while the initial assembly of amyloidogenic monomers presumably involves the action of some template, such as proteoglycan [16]; and while the monomers may ultimately be linked by H-bonding between vicinal edge chains[4]; the computerized study indicated the need for a more precise alignment-bonding mechanism to produce stable, directionally straight, twisted-ribbon filaments from such markedly assymmetrical, twisted sandwich units, as β-2-microglobulin, or Ig light chain. Therefore the possiblity of an analogy between adsorptive (dye-binding) and crystal (fibrillogenic) forces was explored, with formulation of a mechanism, analogous to the dye-binding, involving close-range binding to hydrophobic sites of the amyloidogenic monomers themselves in a stable, directionally straight filamentous array[17].

While details of this construct await subsequent publication the arrangement entails alignment of monomers in filamentous array, with their beta-strands normal to the array axis, and with successive units rotated in the strand axis so as to have alternately obverse and reverse postures. In this way corresponding, rotationally exposed, hydrophobic corners of the inner sheet faces of neighboring monomers are brought into register, and may be overlapped as structurally complementary, close-range-binding surfaces to produce stable and straight alignment. The histochemical construct, be it noted, is of a single **filament** in an amyloid fibril complex, which appears usually to comprise at least two such filaments, possibly bound together by other components, such as proteoglycans[16].

REFERENCES.

1.Glenner GG, Eanes ED, Page DL. The relation of the properties of Congo red-stained amyloid fibrils to the beta conformation. J Histochem Cytochem 1972;20:821-826.
2.Cooper JH. Selective amyloid staining as a function of amyloid composition and structure. Lab Invest 1974;31:232-238.
3.Puchtler H, Sweat F, Levine M. On the binding of Congo red by amyloid. J Histochem Cytochem 1962; 10:355-364.
4.Cooper JH. A histochemical construct of the amyloid fibril. In Tribe CR, Bacon PA, eds. Amyloidosis E.A.R.S. Bristol: John Wright & Sons Ltd. 1983:31-34.
5.Horobin RW, Bennion PJ. The interrelation of the size and substantivity of dyes; the role of van der Waals attractions and hydrophobic bonding in biological staining. Histochemie 1973; 33:191-204.
6.Glenner GG, Eanes ED, Bladen HA, Linke RP, Termine JD. b-pleated sheet fibrils; a comparison of native amyloid with synthetic protein fibrils. J Histochem Cytochem 1974; 22:1141-1158.
7.Cohen FE, Sternberg MJE, Taylor WR. Analysis of the tertiary structure of protein beta-sheet sandwiches. J Mol Biol 1981; 148:253-272.
8.Blake CCF, Geisow MJ, Oatley SJ. Structure of prealbumin: secondary, tertiary, and quaternary interactions determined by Fourier refinement at 1.8A. J Mol Biol 1978;121:339-356.
9.Becker JW, Reeke GN Jr. Three-dimensional structure of β2-microglobulin. Proc Nat Acad Sci USA 1985; 82:4225-4229.
10.Griffiths J. Colour and Constitution of Organic Molecules. London: Academic Press. 1976:105.
11.Gertz MA, Skinner M, Connors LH, Falk RH, Cohen AS, Kyle RA. Selective binding of Nifedipine to amyloid fibrils. Amer J Cardiol 1985; 55:1646.
12.Rubinow A, Skinner M, Cohen AS. Digoxin sensitivity in amyloid cardiomyopathy. Circulation 1981; 63:1285-1288.
13.Benditt EP, Eriksen N, Berglund C. Congo red dichroism with dispersed amyloid fibrils, an extrinsic Cotton effect. Proc Nat Acad Sci 1970; 66:1044-1051.
14.Edwards RA, Woody RW. Spectroscopic studies of Cibacron blue and Congo red bound to dehydrogenases and kinases. Biochemistry 1979; 18: 5197-5204.
15.Puchtler H, Sweat F, Gropp S. An investigation into the relation between structure and fluorescence of azo dyes. J Microsc Soc 1967; 87: 309-328.
16.Snow AD, Willmer J, Kisilevsky R. Sulfated glycosaminoglycans: a common constituent of all amyloids? Lab Invest 1987;56:120-123.
17.Cooper JH. A histochemical model of the amyloid fibril. Computer presentation. VIth International Symposium on Amyloidosis. Oslo 1990.

HIGH MOLECULAR WEIGHT PROTEINS, SENSITIVE TO COLLAGENASE DIGESTION ARE INTIMATE CONSTITUENTS OF AMYLOID DEPOSITS.

V. BELLOTTI °, A. PUCCI *, E. ARBUSTINI *, G. MERLINI °,
M. STOPPINI^, G. FERRI ^, E.F. OSSERMAN §.
*° Institute of Clinical Medicine II, * Dept. Pathologic Anatomy, IRCCS Policlinico S. Matteo, Pavia ^ Department of Biochemistry University of Pavia, Italy; § Inst. Cancer Res., Columbia University, 10032 New York, USA.*

ABSTRACT. Proteins with molecular weight (MW) higher than 100 kD are present in the fibrils extracted from amyloid deposits of patient And (λ VI AL amyloidosis). These proteins (MW 135-140 kD) have a high content of glycine (21%) and can be proteolyzed by bacterial collagenase. Electron microscopy study demonstrates that collagenase induces a significant modification of the supramolecular organization of the AL amyloid fibrils.

Introduction

Amyloid deposition in extracellular compartments is a biological phenomenon probably regulated by different and interdependent mechanisms. The role of the true amyloidogenic proteins [1] like light chains, SAA, β-2-microglobulin, prealbumin etc., can be probably differentiated from the role of other proteins detectable in minimal but significant amount in every amyloid deposit, like P-component [2], interalpha trypsin inhibitor [3], and proteoglycans [4]. Furthermore it has been reported that proteins with MW higher than 100 kD are always present in aqueous extracts of amyloid fibrils [5-8] .

We think that the characterization of the structure and function of these proteins may be important for a better comprehension of the amyloid biology.

Materials and Methods

Amyloid fibrils extraction was performed according to Pras et al [9] from tissues stored at - 80°C.

Carboxymethylation and aminoacid analysis was performed as previously reported [10].

Collagenase digestion: Clostridium histolyticum enzyme (type VII, SIGMA) was used at a ratio 1:100 protein, pH 7.1 (Tris HCl-$CaCl_2$, 10 mM) 37°C, overnight.

Electron microscopy analysis: Samples were fixed in Karnowsky's solution, post fixed in 1.5% osmium tetroxide and embedded in Epon. A frame of 100 points was used for morphometric analysis according to Gundersen et al.[11].

Results and Discussion

The amyloid fibrils extracted from the spleen of patient AND (λ VI AL amyloidosis) were constituted by multiple proteins preliminarly purified by gel filtration (Figure 1).The characterization of the proteins eluted under peak II of Fig. 1 was the aim of the present work. Further purification of this peak II by SDS-PAGE and blotting on immobilon, shows the presence of two bands corresponding to a MW of 135 and 140 kD respectively (inset of Fig.1). Immunological analysis carried out on both the whole protein mixture and the electrophoretically purified proteins, gives the results reported in Table 1.

Table 1. Immunoreactivity of high molecular weight proteins to different antisera.

Antiserum	reacts with 135 and 140 kD bands	present in peak II
γ–α–μ	no	no
complement	no	no
fibrinogen	no	no
fibronectin	no	no
interalpha trypsin inhib.	no	yes (traces)
P-component	no	yes (traces)
lipoproteins	no	no
whole plasma proteins	yes	yes
λ light chains	no	yes
k light chains	no	yes

Since the failure in immunological characterization of this proteins, we tried to identify their chemical properties. The amino acid content of the material eluted under peak II was determined and the isolated 135 and 140 kD proteins were submitted to N-terminal sequence determination (Table 2).

Table 2. Amino acid content and amino terminal sequence of the high molecular weight proteins

Amino acid	residues %	Amino acid	residues %
Cys	1.25	Val	4.66
Asp	8.23	Met	1.14
Thr	4.63	Ile	2.56
Ser	7.00	Leu	6.60
Glu	10.88	Tyr	0.90
Pro	7.76	Phe	2.42
Gly	21.8	His	1.71
Ala	9.92	Lys	4.45
Arg	4.40		

NH_2 sequence: X-F-M-L-I-E -V

The aminoacid analysis shows an unusually high concentration of glycine consistent with a fibrous protein probably related to proteins of connective tissue matrix.
The aminoterminal sequence did not match with any known protein sequence, however the amount available for sequencing was very low and we cannot exclude that the obtained sequence belongs to a contaminant associated to a NH_2 blocked protein.
The susceptibility of these proteins to proteolysis from different enzymes was tested. These experiments showed that collagenase from Clostridium histolyticum was able to selectively digest the two proteins of 135-140 kD leaving intact the remaining ones (Fig.2). This finding suggests that these molecules have repetitive X-Gly sequences in area exposed to hydrophilic solvents; furthermore the specificity of collagenase led us to investigate if the protease caused any effect on the supramolecular structure of fibrils.

Figure 1. Gel filtration and SDS-PAGE of AND amyloid fibrils.

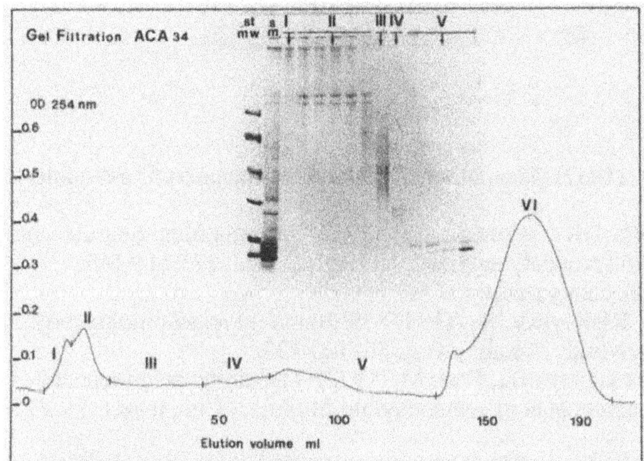

Figure 2. SDS PAGE amyloid fibrils a= control b=collagenase treated.

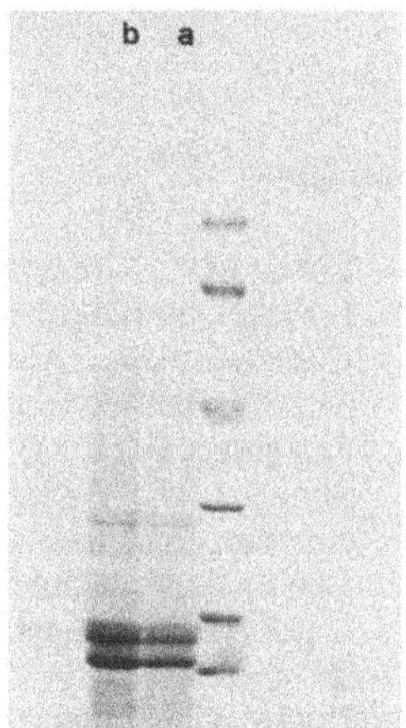

Electron microscopy analysis of fibrils incubated with collagenase was performed in this case and on fibrils of four additional AL amyloid patients. In all of them the electron microscopy analysis showed that fibrils were constituted by both a single and double filament; both configurations were present before and after collagenase treatment.

Untreated fibrils showed a continuous network pattern whereas treated samples did not (Fig.3). By morphometry, points overlying fibrils in untreated samples were significantly higher than those of treated fibrils ($p< 0.02$). It is likely that collagenase acts as a lytic agent on the double filaments interrupting bridges among fibrils.
The structural characterization of this protein, sensitive to collagenase digestion, will explain its function on the supramolecular organization of amyloid fibrils.

Acknowledgements

Study supported by the C.N.R. Target Project on Biotechnology and Bioinstrumentation.

Figure 3. Electron microscopic study: fibrils network before (**a**) and after (**b**) collagenase digestion.

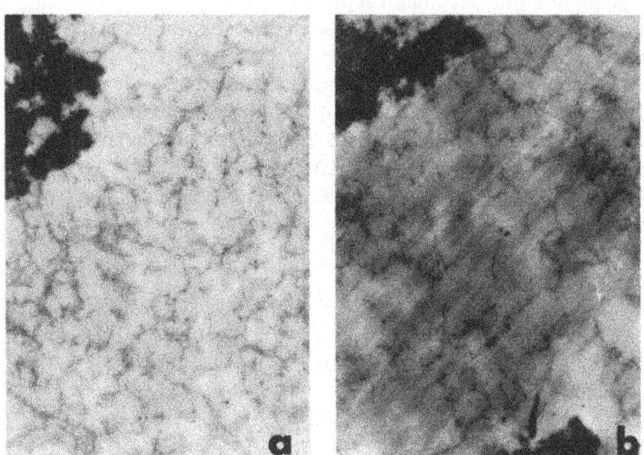

References

1. Cohen, A.S., Connors, L.H. (1987) 'The pathogenesis and biochemistryof amyloidosis', J. Pathol. 151, 1-10 .
2. Cathcart, E.S., Comerford, F.R., Cohen, A.S. (1965) 'Immunologic studies on a protein extracted from human secondary amyloid', N. Engl. J. Med. 273,143-146.
3. Frangione, B. (1988) Personal communication.
4. Snow, A.D., Willmer, J., Kisilevsky, R. (1987) 'Sulfated glycosaminoglycans : a common constituent of all amyloids ?', Lab. Invest. 56, 120-123.
5. Levin, M., Franklin, E.C., Frangione, B.,, Pras, M. (1972) 'The amino acid sequence of a major non immunoglobulin component of some amyloid fibrils', J. Clin. Invest. 51, 2773-2776.
6. Husby, G., Sletten, K., Michaelsen, T.E., Natvig, J.B. (1972) 'Antigenic and chemical characterization of non-immunoglobulin amyloid proteins', Scand. J. Immunol. 1, 393-400.
7. Husby, G., Sletten, K. (1977) 'Structural similarities between a protein extracted from normal human tissues and a component of amyloid fibrils', Acta Path. Microbiol. Scand. 85,153-160.
8. Scott ,D.L., Marhaug, G., Husby, G. (1983) 'Comparative studies of the high molecular weight amyloid fibril proteins and similar components from normal tissues', Clin. Exp. Immunol. 52, 693-701.
9. Pras, M., Schubert, M., Zucker-Franklin, D., Rimon, A., Franklin, E.C. (1968) 'The characterization of soluble amyloid prepared in water', J. Clin. Invest. 47,924-933.
10. Ferri, G., Stoppini, M., Iadarola, P., Bellotti, V., Merlini, G. (1989) 'Structural characterization of k II Inc, a new amyloid immunoglobulin', Biochim. Biophis. Acta 995,103-108.
11. Gundersen, H.J.G., Bendtsen, T.F., Korbo L., et al. (1988) ' Some new, simple and efficient stereological methods and their use in pathological research and diagnosis', A.M.P.I.S. 96,379-394.

INTRAPERITONEAL AMYLOID FORMATION BY AMYLOID ENHANCING FACTOR RICH MACROPHAGES IN ASCITIC FLUID

KATSUTOSHI MIURA*, SATOSHI BABA*, HARUYUKI SHIRASAWA*,
SHYR-TE JU**, ALAN S. COHEN**, AND TSURANOBU SHIRAHAMA**
*The Department of Pathology, Hamamatsu University School of Medicine, Hamamatsu, Japan and **the Department of Medicine and the Arthritis Center, Boston University School of Medicine, and the Department of Medicine and Thorndike Memorial Laboratory, Boston City Hospital, Boston, Massachusetts, USA.

ABSTRACT. Amyloidotic peritoneal resident cells were packed in a microchamber and cultured in ascites with additional inflammatory stimuli which increased SAA concentration to 10% of the serum highest level. On the 7th day, Congo red positive structures which showed green birefringence under polarized light were found inside and occasionally outside the chamber. By anti-AA or -SAA immunostaining, cell surface of macrophages as well as amyloid deposits were positively stained. Immunologic depletion of T and B lymphocytes from amyloidotic peritoneal cells did not adversely effect the amyloid formation in microchambers. These results suggest that either ascitic fluid containing sufficient amount of SAA or peritoneal macrophages with high AEF activity are indispensable agents for AA amyloid fibrillogenesis in the peritoneum.

INTRODUCTION

We recently reported that peritoneal macrophages from amyloidotic mice (amyloidotic peritoneal macrophages) contained very high AEF activity and were capable of processing SAA to amyloid fibrils (4). However, why no amyloid is deposited in the peritoneum? Is the supply of SAA to the peritoneal cavity insufficient or does the peritoneal cavity contain inhibitory factor(s) for amyloidogenesis? If enough SAA is supplied, will peritoneal cells produce amyloid in situ? To address these questions, we induced ascites in mice and cultured the amyloidotic peritoneal cells in it. To keep the donor peritoneal cells from migration and from mingling with the recipient's cells, we confined them in a microchamber. We present here our successful results which support that the amyloidotic peritoneal macrophages can produce amyloid in ascitic fluid.

MATERIALS AND METHODS

ASCITIC INDUCTION AND AEF ACTIVITY

Ascites was induced in mice by weekly intraperitoneal injections of 0.2 ml of a 9:1 emulsion of CFA and PBS. AEF activity was assayed by the method previously described (4) by i.v. injecting 0.5 ml of ascitic fluid and $1x10^5$ cells to a mouse respectively.

EFFECTS OF ASCITES ON AEF ACTIVITY

AEF extract from amyloidotic liver (1) was dissolved in 0.5 ml of ascitic fluid and incubated for 30 min at room temperature. The mixture was i.v. injected to a mouse. As a control PBS was used in place of ascitic fluid.

SODIUM DODECYL SULFATE-POLYACRYLAMIDE GEL ELECTROPHORESIS (SDS-PAGE), WESTERN BLOTTING, AND DOT BLOT ASSAY FOR SAA

For comparing the contents of proteins of ascites and serum, we used SDS-PAGE and western blotting. Ascites collected from mice more than a week after the last i.p. injection of emulsion of CFA and PBS (stable ascites), ascites collected from mice at 22 h after s.c. injection of 50 ug of LPS (stimulated ascites), normal mouse serum and serum from mice at 22 h after receiving LPS (inflammatory serum) were electrophoresed through a 15 % SDS-PAGE and immunoblotted with anti-SAA antiserum (2).

For titration of SAA, dot blot enzyme immunoassay was used by the method of Ogata (3). Serially diluted samples were blotted on a nitrocellulose disc and reacted with anti-SAA antiserum. Samples tested were stable and stimulated ascites, and normal and inflammatory mouse serum.

CONFINING CELLS IN MICROCHAMBERS AND TRANSPLANTATION

Plastic microchambers with one side hole (Millipore, Bedford, MA) were shielded with 0.45 um filter membrane using MF cement made of ethylene dichloride and methyl ethyl ketone mixture (Millipore). Cells were injected from the side hole using 25 G needle with 1 ml syringe and plugged with sealing clay (Cristoseal, Fisher Scientific, Springfield, NJ). About $5x10^5$ cells were confined in a microchamber.

Mice were anesthetized by i.v. injection of 2,2,2-tribromoethanol (Avertin)(Aldrich, Milwaukee, MI). A chamber was inserted through the abdominal opening which was then sutured with 3.0 silk thread.

HISTOLOGICAL PREPARATION OF THE CELLS IN THE MICROCHAMBERS AND AMAYLID DETECTION

Seven days after operation mice were sacrificed by cervical dislocation and microchambers and ascites were collected from the peritoneal cavity. The filter membranes of the microchamber were cut, enucleated with surgical blade and the internal surfaces were gently touched on glass slides. The ascites was centrifuged at 3000 rpm for 10 min and the sediment was smeared on glass slides.

The slides were quickly air dried and stained with Hematoxylin-Congo red and anti-SAA or anti-AA(2).

DEPLETION OF B AND T LYMPHOCYTES

Amyloidotic peritoneal cells were incubated with anti Thy 1.2 (HO-13-4, no.TIB 99, American Type Culture Collection (ATCC), Rockville, MD) and anti B cell (J11d.2, no.TIB 183, ATCC) monoclonal antibodies for 45 min at 37°C, centrifuged down and reacted with rabbit complement (25% rabbit serum in culture medium) for 30 min at 37°C. Treated cells were washed 3 times before use.

OTHER CONTROL EXPERIMENTS

As a control, similar microchamber experiments were carried out by using peritoneal cells from normal mice in place of amyloidotic peritoneal cells. To evaluate the effects of additional inflammatory stimuli, control mice received neither LPS nor emulsion of casein and CFA after the operation.

RESULTS

ASCITIC INDUCTION AND AEF ACTIVITY

Most mice developed ascites after four injections of the CFA and PBS emulsion. The volume of stable ascites collected from a mouse was 5 to 18 ml (average 12.27 ml). The ascitic fluid contained numerous macrophages, lymphocytes and polymorphonuclear (PMN) leukocytes in varying percentages among individual mice. Ascitic fluid and cells had weak AEF activity. No amyloid was detected in the ascitic fluid of any of these mice.

NO INHIBITORY FACTORS FOR AEF IN ASCITES

AEF activity was unchanged or slightly increased by the additional ascitic fluid.

SAA AND PROTEIN CONTENTS IN ASCITES

Ascites and serum contained almost same proteins (Fig. 1). However, concentration of SAA of ascites was very low compared with that of the acute inflammatory serum. Additional inflammatory stimulation increased SAA concentration to a 10 % of the level of acute inflammatory serum (Fig. 2).

AMYLOID FORMATION IN TRANSPLANTED CHAMBERS

The touch smears of the inside surface of the filter membrane of the chamber containing the amyloidotic peritoneal cells displayed small fibrillar structures which showed apple-green birefringence on Congo red staining (Fig. 3, Table 1). Macrophages with large mononuclear nuclei and rather plump cytoplasm were often present close by the Congo red positive structures. By immunohistochemistry, anti-AA and anti-SAA antibodies stained the Congophilic materials (Fig. 4).

Depletion of B and T lymphocytes from amyloidotic peritoneal cells did not adversely effect the amyloid formation. Amyloid deposits were occasionally observed in the chambers containing the amyloidotic peritoneal cells even when additional inflammatory stimuli to the recipient mice were omitted. Amyloid was not detected in a chamber in which peritoneal cells from normal mice were replaced (Table 1).

DISCUSSION

The development of amyloid deposits in the peritoneal chamber under the conditions of the present study indicates that either ascitic fluid containing sufficient amount of SAA or peritoneal macrophages with high AEF activity are indispensable agents for AA amyloid fibrillogenesis in the peritoneum. Yet, ascites after inflammatory stimuli contained only 10% concentration of SAA in acute inflammatory serum, which suggests that this concentration of SAA may be sufficient enough for AA fibrillogenesis by the amyloidotic peritoneal macrophages. In the present results cell surface of the amyloidotic peritoneal macrophages close to the amyloid deposits was positively stained with anti-SAA. SAA might be retained on the cell surface and processed to AA protein.

It is possible that ascites may contain unknown factors that affect amyloidogenesis. We attempted to culture the AEF-rich macrophages in SAA-rich medium and succeeded in making amyloid although the amount of the products was minute and temporary. Comparative studies of the in vitro and the peritoneal microchamber systems will contribute for studying the precise mechanism of amyloidogenesis.

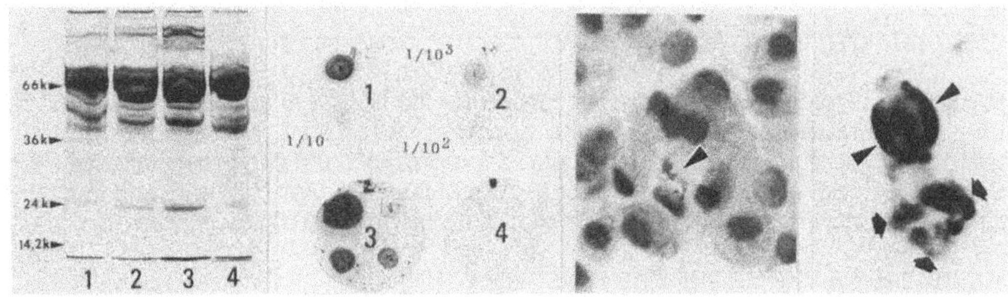

Fig. 1 Fig. 2 Fig. 3 Fig. 4

Fig. 1. SDS-PAGE of ascites and serum. Samples tested were stimulated ascites (lane 1), stable ascites (lane 2), inflammatory mouse serum (lane 3) and normal serum (lane 4).
Fig. 2. Dot blot assay for SAA. Serially diluted samples were blotted on a nitrocellulose disc and reacted with anti-SAA antiserum. Samples were same as those in Fig. 1.
Fig. 3. An amyloid deposit in a microchamber. A fibrillar structure in the vicinity of the macrophage is Congo red positive with green birefringence (arrowheads).
Fig. 4. An anti-SAA antibody stains cell surface of macrophages (arrowheads) and a Congophilic deposit (arrows) in a microchamber.

TABLE 1. INTRAPERITONEAL CHAMBER EXPERIMENTS

Donar cells or condition	Amyloid in a chamber
Amyloidotic peritoneal cells (APC)	+
Normal peritoneal cells	-
T and B cell depleted APC	+
APC without additional inflammation#	+/-

+,detected; -,not detected; +/-,rarely detected.
#without post-operational injections of LPS and the casein-CFA emulsion.

REFERENCES

1. Axelrad, MA., Kisilevsky, R., Willmer, J., Chen, SJ., and Skinner, M. (1982) 'Further characterization of amyloid enhancing factor', Lab Invest 47,139-146.
2. Miura, K., Ju, S-T., Cohen, AS., and Shirahama, T. (1990) 'Generation and use of site specific antibodies to SAA for probing AA amyloid development', J. Immunol 144,610-613.
3. Ogata, F. (1989) 'Quantitative dot-blot enzyme immunoassay for serum amyloid A protein', J. Immunol Methods 116,131-135.
4. Shirahama, T., Miura, K., Ju, S-T., Kisilevsky, R., Gruys, E., and Cohen, AS. (1990) 'Amyloid enhancing factor-loaded macrophages in amyloid fibril formation', Lab Invest 62,61-68.

HISTOCHEMICALLY RECOGNIZABLE CHANGES OF AMYLOID FIBRILLOGENIC MACROPHAGES

Tsuranobu Shirahama, Katsutoshi Miura, Shyr-Te Ju
and Alan S. Cohen
Arthritis Center, Department of Medicine, Boston University,
Boston, MA 02118, U.S.A.

Erik Gruys
Department of Veterinary Pathology, University of Utrecht,
Utrecht, the Netherlands

Robert Kisilevsky
Department of Pathology, Queen´s University,
Kingston, Canada K7L 3N6

ABSTRACT: We examined whether any recognizable changes occur in the characteristics of macrophages when they become "amyloid fibrillogenic", by comparing the normal and the amyloid fibrillogenic macrophages by means of histochemical and immunohistochemical staining. Two changes appeared particularly interesting. 1. The amyloid fibrillogenic macrophages tended to carry thicker glycosaminoglycan (GAG) coatings more frequently than the normal. 2. The amyloid fibrillogenic macrophages displayed a stronger tendency to attract SAA to their surface.

INTRODUCTION

We recently reported that peritoneal resident macrophages from amyloidotic mice were loaded with amyloid enhancing factor and were ready to process SAA into amyloid fibrils (amyloid fibrillogenic macrophages), but bore no amyloid with them (Shirahama et al, 1990). This system has provided us with an excellent model with which the nature of the amyloid fibrillogenic macrophages can be studied.

In the present study, we have sought to delineate the changes that occur in the characteristics of macrophages when they become amyloid fibrillogenic, through comparative studies of the normal and the amyloid fibrillogenic peritoneal resident macrophages, in special reference to the histochemical and immunohistochemical changes in the cellular surface coatings by SAA and GAG both of which are receiving increasing attention in regard to their roles in amyloidogenesis (Kisilevsky, 1989; Shirahama, 1989; Snow and Wight, 1989).

MATERIALS AND METHODS

Induction of Amyloidosis: Amyloidosis was induced in CBA/J mice, by weekly subcutaneous (s.c.) injections of 0.5 ml of a 1:1 emulsion of 10% aqueous casein and complete Freund's adjuvant (casein-adjuvant emulsion)(Shirahama et al, 1990).

Peritoneal Resident Cells: From amyloidotic and normal mice, peritoneal resident cells were collected by gentle washing of the peritoneal cavity with phosphate bufferred physiological saline (PBS). A drop of the cell suspension was applied to a gelatinized microscope slide and air dried. The slides were fixed in bufferred 10% formalin for 10 min.

Exposure to SAA Rich Serum: An aliquot of the cells on the slides were covered with SAA rich or normal mouse serum and incubated at 37°C for 30 min in a wet chamber. SAA rich serum was collected from mice 18 hours after they received a s.c. injection of 0.5 ml of the casein-adjuvant emulsion. The slides were then washed in PBS and fixed in bufferred 10% formalin.

Histochemical and Immunohistochemical Preparations: An aliquot of the slides were reacted with periodic acid Schiff (PAS) reagent. Another aliquot of the cells were stained with 0.1% Alcian blue in 0.05M acetate buffer at pH 5.7 containing graded concentrations of magnesium chloride; 0.0 M, 0.1 M, 0.2 M, 0.3 M, 0.4 M, 0.5 M and 0.6 M (Mowry and Scott, 1967). The third set of the slides were reacted with anti-SAA antibodies (Miura et al, 1990) which were subsequently localized immunohistochemically.

RESULTS

GAG Surface Coating of Macrophages:

Thin surface coatings that stained positively with PAS and Alcian blue were observed on most of the normal macrophage-monocyte population. This GAG coating was remarkably denser and thicker on the peritoneal macrophages from amyloidotic mice when compared to the normal. With the differential staining of Alcian blue, the coating stained more intensely with the higher magnesium chloride concentrations, suggesting the involvement of highly sulfated GAGs.

SAA Surface Coating of Macrophages:

Thin coating by SAA, as demonstrated immunohistochemically using anti-SAA antibodies, was observed on some macrophages. Differences of the coatings in quality and quantity were not discernible between the normal and the amyloid fibrillogenic macrophages.

<u>SAA Surface Coating of Macrophages Incubated with SAA Rich Serum:</u>

SAA coating of the amyloid fibrillogenic macrophages significantly increased by incubating them with SAA rich serum (Fig. 1), while such increase was not remarkable on the normal macrophages.

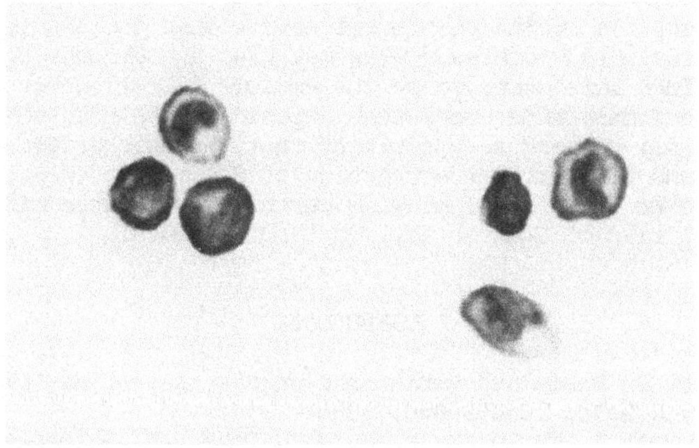

Fig. 1. Peritoneal resident cells incubated with SAA rich serum and then immunohistochemically reacted with anti-SAA.

DISCUSSION

The present results have revealed two interesting aspects of amyloidotic peritoneal resident macrophages. 1. They carry thicker GAG coatings than the normal. 2. They display a stronger tendency to attract SAA to their surface.

Potential role of proteoglycans (PGs) and GAGs in amyloidogenesis has recently been receiving increasing attention (Kisilevsky, 1989; Shirahama, 1989; Snow and Wight, 1989). The thicker GAG surface coatings on the amyloid fibrillogenic macrophages which did not bear amyloid suggest that this change may occur prior to amyloid deposition. Further, if GAGs are indeed involved in amyloid fibril formation, they likely play a causative role in amyloid fibril formation rather than occurring as the results of amyloid deposition.

The present findings regarding the SAA coatings of the macrophages are of interest in relation to our recent observation (Shirahama et al, 1990). We were puzzled when we found no amyloid deposits in the peritoneal cavity of amyloidotic mice, the original residence of the amyloid fibrillogenic macrophages. We attributed this lack of amyloid to a possible lack of supply of SAA. This assumption has found a support from our more recent study (Miura et al, 1990) which revealed that ascites contained very low levels of SAA and that the amyloid fibrillogenic macrophages were indeed capable of forming amyloid in the peritoneal cavity when the SAA levels of the ascites were elevated. This may also explain why thicker SAA coatings were observed on the amyloid fibrillogenic macrophages only after they were exposed to SAA rich serum.

One may suspect a possibility that the thicker GAG surface coating and the stronger attraction of SAA may be related. If it is proven to be true, it will certainly strengthen the potential role of GAGs in amyloid fibrillogenesis.

REFERENCES

Kisilevsky R: Theme and variations on a string of amyloid. Neurobiol Aging 10:499-500, 1989

Miura K, Baba S, Shirasawa H, Ju S-T, Cohen AS, Shirahama T: Intraperitoneal amyloid formation by amyloid enhancing factor rich macrophages in ascitic fluid. Submitted for publication, 1990

Miura K, Ju S-T, Cohen AS, Shirahama T: Generation and use of site-specific antibodies to serum amyloid A for probing amyloid A development. J Immunol 144:610-613, 1990

Mowry RW, Scott JE: Observations on the basophilia of amyloids. Histochemie 10:8-32, 1967

Shirahama T: Proteoglycans in amyloidogenesis. Neurobiol Aging 10:508-510, 1989

Shirahama T, Miura K, Ju S-T, Kisilevsky R, Gruys E, Cohen AS: Amyloid enhancing factor-loaded macrophages in amyloid fibril formation. Lab Invest 62:61-68, 1990

Snow AD, Wight TN: Proteoglycans in the pathogenesis of Alzheimer´s disease and other amyloidoses. Neurobiol Aging 10:481-497, 1989

ULTRASTRUCTURAL ASPECTS OF CELL MEMBRANE IN AA-AMYLOIDOGENESIS.

Niewold ThA, Ultee A, Gruys E.
Department of Veterinary Pathology, University of Utrecht,
Postbox 80158, 3508 TD, The Netherlands.

ABSTRACT

In systemic AA-amyloidosis amyloid deposition takes place in different organs. Cells of the mononuclear phagocytic system (MPS) are generally thought to be the common factor between organs in amyloid formation. However, in some reports amyloidogenesis was suggested to be related to membrane alterations in various cell-types. Here, ultrastructural evidence is presented, supporting the latter hypothesis.

INTRODUCTION

In the pathogenesis of AA-amyloidosis, MPS-cells were suggested to play a crucial role, based on their close ultrastructural relationship with amyloid deposits. MPS-cells were possibly the common factor between the different organs in which amyloid is deposited (8). Furthermore, MPS-cells are a likely source of proteolytic enzymes that could converse SAA to AA, a step thought to be essential in AA-amyloid fibrillogenesis. The MPS-concept of AA-amyloidogenesis received wide acceptance, in spite of ultrastructural observations of amyloid deposits lacking a clear relationship with MPS-cells (4,6). In one report, amyloid formation was suggested to be a membrane associated process that could occur at a variety of cell-types (4).

In this study, we re-examined the ultrastructure of early amyloidogenesis in experimental hamster amyloidosis, with special attention to the kidney.

MATERIAL AND METHODS

Young male Syrian hamsters (Mesocricetus auratus, 100g) received a single intravenous injection of fibril AEF (FAEF) (5) on day one, and daily subcutaneous injections of 40 μg LPS in PBS (lipopolysaccharide, E. coli o.127:B8, Difco Labs, Detroit, Michigan). One group of hamsters received daily LPS-injections only. The hamsters were killed on day 7, and samples of spleen,liver and kidney were taken for routine histology and electron microscopy.

Paraffin sections (5 μm) of buffered formalin fixed tissues were stained with alkaline Congo red for the presence of amyloid.

Electron microscopical samples were fixed in 2.5% glutaraldehyde, post-fixed with 2% osmium tetroxide and embedded in Durcupan. Ultrathin sections were stained with uranyl acetate and lead citrate.

Immuno-electron microscopical examination of kidney was performed on buffered formalin fixed tissue samples (0.5 mm^3), incubated overnight at $4^{o}C$ either with undiluted normal rabbit serum or undiluted rabbit anti-hamster AA antiserum. Samples were then washed with PBS, followed by 2 h incubation at room temperature with 1:5 diluted peroxidase labeled goat anti-rabbit antibodies (GAR/PO, ICN Biochemicals, Cleveland, Ohio). Samples were washed in PBS and reacted with a 0.1% diaminobenzidine (DAB) solution without hydrogen peroxide for 30 min, followed by 50 min in DAB-solution with hydrogen peroxide. PBS-washed tissue samples were post-fixed with 2% osmium tetroxide, embedded in Durcupan, and ultrathin sections were viewed not contrasted.

RESULTS

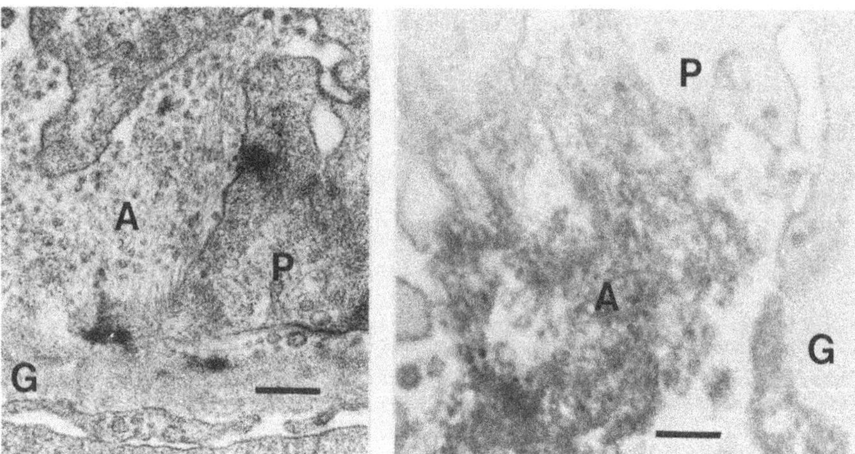

Figure 1 (left). Electron micrograph of amyloidotic glomerulus. Amyloid deposition (A) at the podocyte (P) aspect of the glomerular basement membrane (G). Note the presence of spherical microparticles (SMP) found intermingled with amyloid fibrils. (Uranyl acetate and lead citrate). Bar= 0.2 µm.

Figure 2 (right). Anti-AA immunoelectron micrograph of the same specimen as in Figure 1. The amyloid mass (A) is heavily stained. The SMPs and parts of the cellular membrane of the podocytes show a positive reaction at the rim. The reaction product is also found in membrane bound vesicles in the podocyte cytoplasm. Bar= 0.2 µm.

In the organs of the hamsters that received 7 daily injections of LPS only, no amyloid was found. In the animals that also received FAEF, amyloid deposits were found in spleen, liver and kidney.

Splenic amyloid was found in close association to sinus macrophages. In the liver, amyloid deposits were found perivascularly and along the sinusoids. In the latter location, subendothelial amyloid deposits were found in close association with hepatocytes. Deep invaginations into the cellular membrane of the hepatocytes were often observed, containing bundles of well-oriented amyloid fibrils (not shown).

In the kidney, glomerular amyloid deposits were found in the mesangium. Furthermore, amyloid deposits were present at the podocyte side of the glomerular basement membrane (GBM) (Fig.1).

In all three organs, in the amyloid deposits small vesicle-like particles (35-100 nm) were found in close association with amyloid fibrils. This was most prominent in the renal amyloid deposits located at the podocyte side of the GBM. Immuno-electron microscopy of amyloidotic kidney showed that in these locations, DAB-staining was found on the amyloid fibrils, the vesicle-like particles, and the podocyte cellular membrane neighboring the amyloid deposits (Fig.2). Furthermore, membrane-bound vesicles in the podocyte cytoplasm showed a positive reaction. No significant staining was found in the normal serum treated control.

DISCUSSION

MPS-cells were thought to be primarily involved in the formation of AA-amyloid fibrils, based on their intimate spatial relationship with amyloid deposits. MPS-cells showed typical amyloid-related membrane changes, described as indentations and invaginations, often containing well-oriented tufts or bundles of amyloid fibrils. These locations were considered to represent the actual site of amyloid formation and were thought to occur with MPS-cells only (8). However, similar cell membrane changes in close relationship with amyloid deposits, were also observed with cells of non-MPS nature. In several species, this was found to occur with hepatocytes, endothelial cells, renal epithelium and various other cell-types (4,6). Based on these observations, it was concluded that there are no specific cells, but many cells in various organs and tissues that may produce amyloid. The synthesis of amyloid was surmised to occur at the cellular membrane showing the characteristical membrane changes that are possibly one of the important conditions for amyloid deposition (4).

Another constant companion of amyloid deposition are the small vesicle-like particles. These structures were often described as lipid droplets, globules or vesicles, but are in size and appearance very similar to the so-called spherical microparticles (SMP) described to occur in a variety of diseases. SMPs were associated with a form of cell atrophy and remodelling of the cell surface (1). Few authors discussed SMPs, and they were thought to be a change secondary to amyloid deposition, but the co-occurrence and co-localization with amyloid fibrils could indicate a more direct relationship.

Immunostaining with anti-AA antibodies revealed that in the kidney not only the amyloid fibrils were positive, but also the cellular membrane of the neighboring podocyte, and the membrane surrounding SMPs. Similar observations were made in the murine model (2). Hepatocytes and renal epithelium showed a similar staining of the cell surface that was thought to be caused by accumulation of SAA in the cellular membrane (2,3,7).

Macrophages in amyloidosis seemed to accumulate SAA at the cell surface as a possible first step to fibrillogenesis (3). The accumulation of AA-cross reactive material in the cellular membrane as found here to occur in renal podocytes, indicates that this phenomenon is likely not exclusive to MPS-cells.

In conclusion, amyloid formation appears to take place with a variety of cell-types. These cells show typical membrane changes in close association with the amyloid fibrils and fibrillogenesis occurs in close relationship to the cellular membrane. In the cellular membrane in these locations, AA-cross reactive material (likely SAA) accumulates and may thereby provide locally the high SAA concentration that is thought to be an important factor in amyloid fibrillogenesis. The subsequent formation of amyloid fibrils apparently influences the structure of the cellular membrane causing destabilization of latter, leading to the characteristic membrane changes and the generation of membrane fragments (SMPs) in the extracellular space.

REFERENCES

1. Ferrans VJ, Thiedemann KU, Maron BJ, Jones M, Roberts WC: Spherical microparticles in human myocardium. An ultrastructural study. Lab.Invest. 35:349, 1976
2. Miura K, Takahashi Y, Shirasawa H: Immunohistochemical detection of serum amyloid A protein in the liver and the kidney after casein injection. Lab.Invest. 53:453, 1985
3. Miura K, Ju ST, Cohen AS, Shirahama T: Generation and use of site-specific antibodies to serum amyloid A for probing amyloid A development. J.Immunol. 144:610, 1990
4. Nakagawa S: Ultrastructural investigation of amyloidosis. Pathogenesis of systemic amyloidosis. Appl.Pathol. 2:328, 1984
5. Niewold ThA, Hol PR, van Andel ACJ, Lutz ETG, Gruys E: Enhancement of amyloid induction by amyloid fibril fragments. Lab.Invest. 56:544, 1987
6. Shirahama T, Cohen AS: Ultrastructural studies on renal peritubular amyloid experimentally induced in guinea pigs. I. General aspects. Lab.Invest. 19:122, 1968
7. Shirahama T, Cohen AS: Immunocytochemical study of hepatocyte synthesis of amyloid AA. Am.J.Pathol.118:108, 1985
8. Sorenson GD, Bari WA: Murine amyloid deposits and cellular relationships. In amyloidosis, edited by Mandema E, Ruinen L, Scholten JH, Cohen AS, p58. Amsterdam, Excerpta Medica, 1968

AMYLOID FIBRIL FORMATION IN THE ROUGH ENDOPLASMIC RETICULUM OF PLASMA CELLS FROM A PATIENT WITH LOCALIZED Aλ AMYLOIDOSIS.

Tokuhiro Ishihara, Mutsuo Takahashi, Mayumi Koga, Tadaaki Yokota, Yoshimi Yamashita, Fumiya Uchino and *Takako Iwata

First Department of Pathology, Yamaguchi University School of Medicine, Ube 755, Japan. *Yamaguchi University The School of Allied Health Sciences, Ube 755, Japan.

ABSTRACT. Evidence for amyloid fibril formation in rough endoplasmic reticulum (rER) of plasma cells from a patient with localized Aλ amyloidosis is described. The inclusions in rER of plasma cells were composed of tightly packed, regular arrays of fibrils cut in both longitudinal and cross section. The fibrils, measuring 10 nm in width, were always oriented parallel to the long axis of the inclusions. By immunoelectron microscopy with anti-human Aλ antiserum, gold particles labeled the amyloid fibrils located both in the rER of plasma cells and in the extracellular space. In addition electron-dense material in the dilated rER was occasionally labeled. These findings suggest that at least some amyloid fibrils are unequivocally created in the rER of plasma cells.

INTRODUCTION

Although the precise sites of amyloid fibril formation are still controversial, several cells, including Kupffer cells, macrophages, fibroblasts and so on, are thought to be involved in the fibrillogenesis (1-4). To our knowledge, there is no reports showing amyloid fibrils in the rER. Using immunoelectron microscopy, we describe immunolabeled amyloid fibrils in the rER of plasma cells with Aλ amyloidosis.

MATERIALS AND METHODS

The patient, a 62-year-old man, was diagnosed as having Aλ amyloidosis 13 years ago. The tissue fragments from the duodenum were fixed in 10% formalin solution for light microscopy and in buffered 2.1% glutaraldehyde for electron microscopy. The paraffin sections were stained with hematoxylin and eosin and with Congo red. Congo-red-positive material showing green birefringence under polarized light was identified as amyloid. The paraffin-embedded tissue sections were stained for amyloid deposits using the avidin-biotin-peroxidase complex (ABC) technique. The protein A-gold immunocytochemical study was performed using ordinary processed blocks for electron microscopy according to the method of Bendayan and Zollinger(5).

RESULTS

Amyloid deposits were demonstrated in the interstitium of the mucosa and in the muscularis mucosae of the duodenum and stomach. The deposits reacted only with anti-human Aλ antiserum. A moderate number of plasma cells were noted in the interstitium of the mucosa. Some plasma cells were located close to amyloid deposits. These plasma cells reacted with either anti-immunoglobulin λ or κ light chain antisera. No amyloid deposits were seen in the rectum, skin, bone marrow, or urinary bladder examined. Electron microscopically, fusiform to irregular-shaped inclusions, 0.5-1.0 μm wide and 1-5 μm long, were noted in the cytoplasm of a plasma cell (Fig. 1). These inclusions were always surrounded by a unit membrane bearing ribosomes on its outer surface, indicating that it was rER. They were composed of tightly packed, regular arrays of fine fibrils cut in both longitudinal and cross section. The fibrils were always oriented parallel to the long axis of the inclusions, and measured 10 nm in width. On cross section, the distance between the centers of adjacent fibrils was 20 nm. Serial sections of the plasma cell with fibrils in the rER showed no fibrils in other organelles, including the Golgi apparatus and lysosomes. The reaction product (gold particles) to anti-human Aλ antiserum was always associated specifically with the extracellular amyloid deposits. Numerous gold particles also labeled the fibrils in the rER of plasma cells (Figs. 2,3). In addition, gold particles occasionally labeled electron dense nonfibrillar material in the dilated oval-shaped rER of plasma cells (Fig. 4).

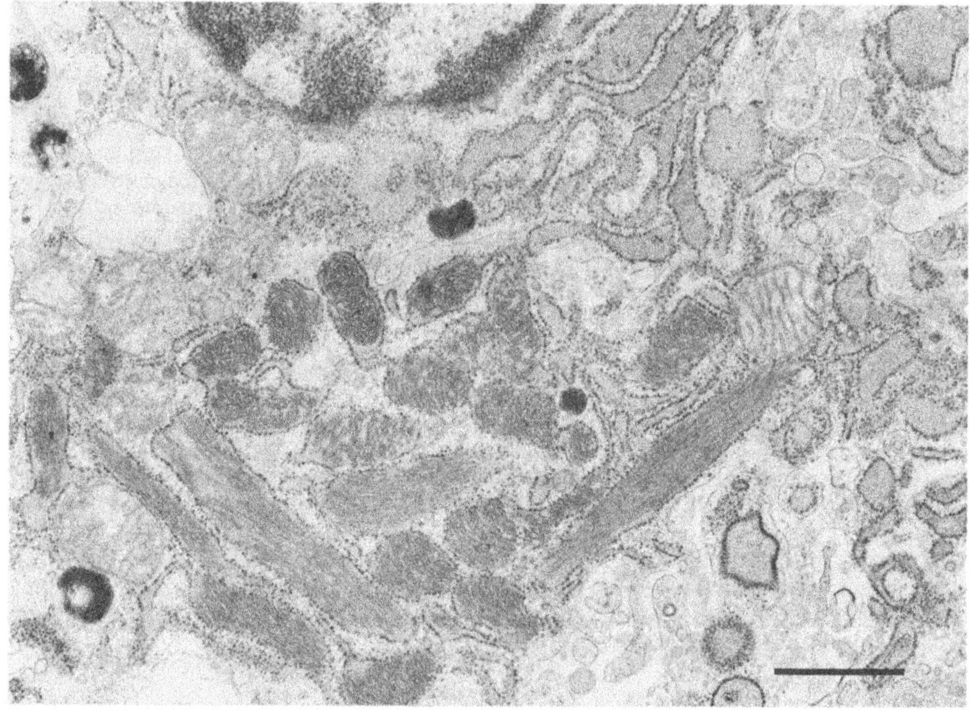

Fig.1 A plasma cell with well-developed rough endoplasmic reticulum has many fusiform to irregular-shaped inclusions containing regular arrays of fibrils. The inclusions are surrounded by a unit membrane bearing ribosomes on its outer surface.

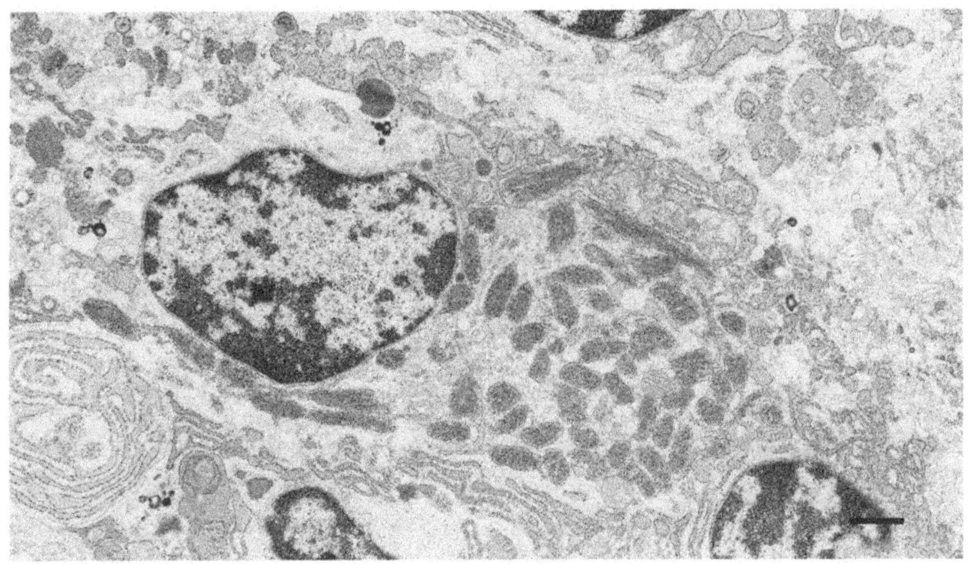

Fig.2 A plasma cell has a large number of inclusions. In the inclusions, there are many fibrils labeled gold particles to anti-human Aλ antiserum.

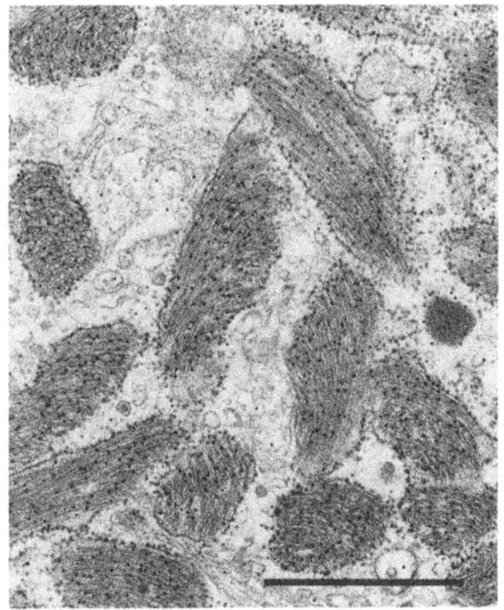

Fig.3 Numerous gold particles labeled the fibrils in the rough endoplasmic reticulum of a plasma cell.

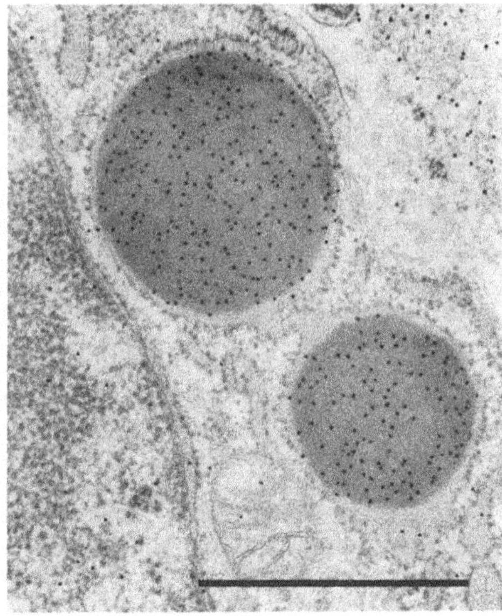

Fig.4 Gold particles labeled electron-dense nonfibrillar materials in the dilated rough endoplasmic reticulum of a plasma cell.

DISCUSSION

We clearly demonstrated fibrils in the rER of plasma cells. Both the fibrils in the rER of plasma cells and extracellular amyloid fibrils reacted to anti-human Aλ antiserum, and are identified as Aλ fibrils. The electron-dense nonfibrillar material in oval-shaped rER also reacted to anti-human Aλ antiserum, and is considered to be the precursor protein of Aλ fibrils. The amyloid fibrils protein in Aλ amyloidosis is derived primarily from immunoglobulin light chains(6). Amino acid sequence analysis has demonstrated areas of homology between some amyloid fibril proteins and the variable region of the immunoglobulin light chain. Zucker-Franklin and Franklin, using electron microscopy and immunofluorescence microscopy, demonstrated the presence of amyloid fibrils within plasma cells and histiocytes(7). They postulated that amyloid or its precursor protein is elaborated through the rER and that polymerization of the fibrils takes place in the Golgi apparatus. Kjeldsberg et al. reported that most of the inclusions in myeloma cells and macrophages in a case of multiple myeloma had a distinct fibrillar appearance, and that the cisternae of the rER were not dilated and did not contain any fibrillar structures(8). They suggested that amyloid fibrils may form in the Golgi apparatus or in lysosomes.

From these findings in the present and past papers we suggested that the Aλ fibrils are created in the rER of plasma cells due to polymerization or degradation of the precursor protein, and are deposited in the extracellular space by the mechanism of holocrine of the plasma cell.

REFERENCES

1. Uchino, F.(1967) Pathological study on amyloidosis. Role of reticuloendothelial cell in inducing amyloidosis. Acta Pathol. Jpn. 17,49-82.
2. Ishihara, T. and Uchino, F. (1975) Pathological study on amyloidosis. Amyloid formation and resorption in Kupffer cell. Recent Adv. RES Res. 15,145-171.
3. Shirahama, T. and Cohen, A.S. (1975) Intralysosomal formation of amyloid fibrils. Am. J. Pathol. 81,101-116.
4. Takahashi, M., Yokota, T., Kawano, H., Gondo, T., Ishihara, T., and Uchino, F. (1989) Ultrastructural evidence for intracellular formation of amyloid fibrils in macrophages. Virchows Arch. A 415,411-419.
5. Bendayan, M. and Zollinger, M. (1983) Ultrastructural localization of antigenic sites on osmium-fixed tissues applying the protein A-gold technique. J. Histochem. Cytochem. 31,101-109.
6. Glenner, G.G., Ein, T., and Terry, W.D. (1972) The immunoglobulin origin of amyloid. Am. J. Med. 52,141-147.
7. Zucker-Franklin, D. and Franklin, E.C. (1970) Intracellular localization of human amyloid by fluorescence and electron microscopy. Am J. Pathol. 59,23-41.
8. Kjeldsberg, C.R., Eyre, H.J., and Totzke, H. (1977) Evidence for intracellular amyloid formation in myeloma. Blood 50,493-507.

A COMPARATIVE STUDY OF AMYLOID FORMATION AND RESORPTION USING IMMUNOELECTRON MICROSCOPY

Mutsuo Takahashi, Tadaaki Yokota*, Tokuhiro Ishihara*, Hiroo Kawano*, Toshikazu Gondo*, Yoshimi Yamashita*, Fumiya Uchino*, and Takako Iwata**

Department of Clinical Laboratories and *Pathology, Yamaguchi University School of Medicine, Ube, Yamaguchi 755, Japan. **The School of Allied Health Sciences, Yamaguchi University.

ABSTRACT. Amyloid formation and resorption in the murine liver were examined by the technique of protein A-gold immunoelectron microscopy using anti-mouse AA antiserum. The liver biopsy was done 4 days after the injections of amyloid enhancing factor (AEF) and casein solution, and the mice were sacrificed 1 and 2 weeks after the biopsy. In the biopsied liver, gold particles labeled several inclusions within the cytoplasm of the Kupffer cells. These inclusions, being round to fusiform in shape, were constantly membrane-bounded. Some of them contained fibrillar structures, corresponding to amyloid fibrils, while most were composed of a homogeneous, granular matrix. In the stage of amyloid resorption, gold particles labeled irregularly-shaped phagosomes in the Kupffer cells. These phagosomes also contained flocculent and phagocytized membranous structures. The present results provide an additional support for the concept that some amyloid fibrils are formed within lysosome-derived organelles of the Kupffer cells.

INTRODUCTION

It is well known that in experimental amyloidosis Kupffer cells play an important role in the formation of amyloid fibrils in the liver. This concept is based partly on the observations of amyloid fibrils in the cytoplasm of Kupffer cells by electron microscopy [1,2]. However, there has been still controversy whether amyloid fibrils are actually polymerized within the cytoplasm of Kupffer cells or an intracellular location of amyloid fibrils merely represents a phagocytized phenomenon.

Our purpose is to elucidate the role of the Kupffer cells in the formation and resorption of amyloid fibrils by comparing the features of both stages in experimental amyloidosis using immunoelectron microscopy.

MATERIALS AND METHODS

Amyloid enhancing factor (AEF) was extracted according to the method of Axelrad and Kisilevsky [3] from the spleens of amyloid-laden mice. ICR mice were given a single intraperitoneal injection of 0.5 ml of AEF and daily subcutaneous injections of 0.5 ml of a 10% casein solution in 0.3 M $NaHCO_3$. Wedge biopsy of the liver was performed 4 days after the amyloidogenic stimuli and the mice were sacrificed 1 or 2 weeks after the biopsy. The liver was removed under ether anesthesia, and the tissue fragments were fixed in a 5% buffered formalin solution for light microscopy. Small pieces of the liver were fixed in a 2.1% glutaraldehyde solution for electron microscopy.

Antiserum to murine protein AA was prepared in white rabbits as previously described [4]. Protein A-colloidal gold particles (15 nm in diameter) were purchased from EY Laboratories (San Mateo, USA).

Paraffin-embedded sections of the liver were stained for amyloid deposits by the avidin-biotin-peroxidase complex method. The protein A-gold immunocytochemical study was performed using ordinary processed blocks for electron microscopy as previously described [5].

RESULTS

Light Microscopic Immunohistochemistry

Four days after the administrations of AEF and casein solution, the biopsied liver showed small amounts of amyloid deposits around the vessels and Disse's space, which positively reacted with anti-mouse AA antiserum. The amyloid deposits in the liver obtained from autopsy were considerably decreased in amount but trace amounts of the deposits were still discernible in some of the mice.

Immunoelectron Microscopy

In the biopsied liver, gold particles labeled amyloid fibrils located extracellularly in the Disse's space or cytoplasmic invaginations of the Kupffer cells and hepatocytes. Gold particles also labeled round to fusiform dense bodies in the cytoplasm of the Kupffer cells. These dense bodies were uniform in shape, constantly membrane-bounded, and measured 0.5-1.0 μm in width and 1.0-3.0 μm in length. Some of the dense bodies contained fibrillar structures corresponding to amyloid fibrils. The others were composed of a homogeneous, granular matrix and did not contain any recognizable fibrils (Fig. 1).

In the autopsied liver, small amounts of amyloid deposits were observed extracellularly and often showed felt-like appearance. In the cytoplasm of the Kupffer cells, gold particles labeled variable-shaped organelles. Some of them were similar to the dense bodies as seen in the biopsied liver but they were more irregular in shape. The others were membrane-bounded vacuoles which contained flocculent and fibrillar structures often intermingled with phagocytized membranous materials (Fig. 2).

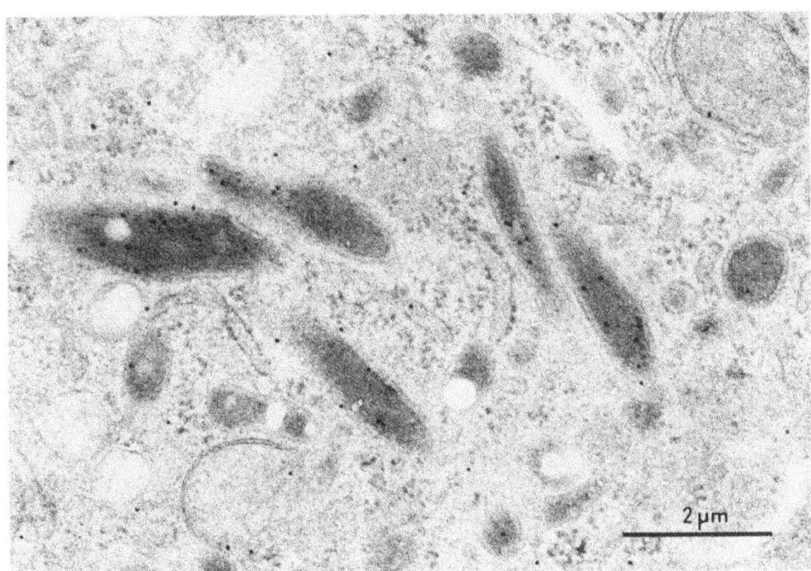

Fig. 1 Four days after the administration of AEF and casein solution, gold particles label regularly-shaped, oval to fusiform dense bodies composed of a homogeneous, granular matrix in the cytoplasm of a Kupffer cell. Immunoelectron microscopy

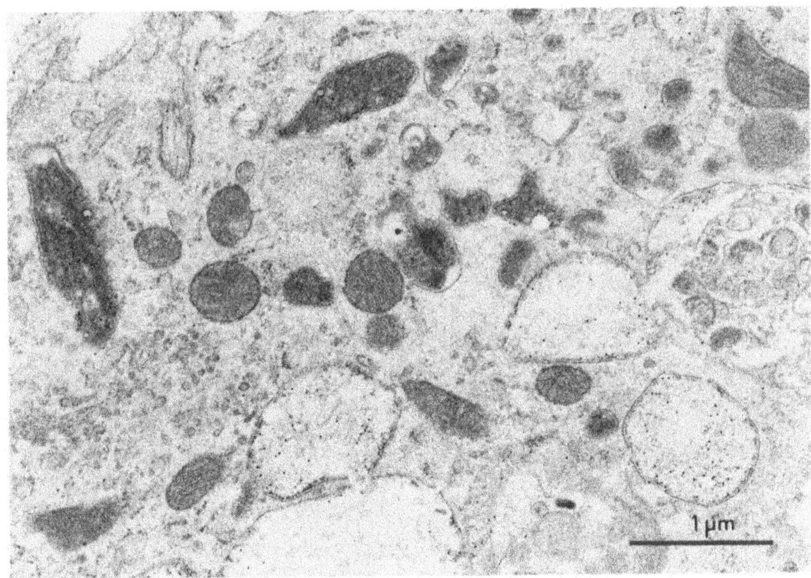

Fig. 2 One week after the biopsy, at the resorption stage of amyloid deposits, immunolabeled inclusions are variable in shape. Some of them contain flocculent and fibrillar structures intermingled with phagocytized membranous structures. Immunoelectron microscopy

DISCUSSION

In the present study, small amounts of amyloid deposits were detected in the biopsied liver 4 days after AEF and casein injections. This model of rapid amyloid induction could afford us an opportunity to observe the amyloid fibril formation prior to its resorption by phagocytosis. By immunoelectron microscopy, it was clearly demonstrated that some Kupffer cells in the biopsied liver contained a homogeneous, granular matrix as well as fibrillar structures labeled with gold particles within the dense bodies. These inclusions are consistent with those reported by us [5] in histiocytes in the spleen at the stage of amyloid induction. Thus, the inclusions are thought to be lysosome-derived organelles resulting from previously pinocytized serum amyloid A protein by the Kupffer cells. On the other hand, the Kupffer cells in the autopsied liver contained not only immunolabeled dense bodies but also flocculent and fibrillar inclusions often intermingled with phagocytized membranous structures. These inclusions in the autopsied liver are interpreted as heterophagosomes in which phagocytized amyloid fibrils were processed in various stages of digestion.

The present results provide an additional support for the concept that some amyloid fibrils are formed within lysosome-derived organelles of the Kupffer cells.

This work was supported by a Grant-in-Aid for Scientific Research of the Ministry of Education [C01570195] and by The Ichiro Kanehara Foundation [K88172].

REFERENCES

1. Shirahama, T. and Cohen, A.S. (1975) 'Intralysosomal formation of amyloid fibrils', Am. J. Pathol. 81, 101-116.
2. Uchino, F., Takahashi, M., Yokota, T., and Ishihara, T. (1985) 'Experimental amyloidosis: Role of the hepatocytes and Kupffer cells in amyloid formation', Appl. Pathol. 3, 78-87.
3. Axelrad, M.A. and Kisilevsky, R. (1980) 'Biological characterization of amyloid enhancing factor', in G.G. Glenner, P.P. Costa, and A.F. de Freitas (eds.), Amyloid and Amyloidosis, Excerpta Medica, Amsterdam, pp. 527-533.
4. Imada, N. (1981) 'Pathological study on amyloidosis: Isolation and purification of amyloid fibril protein and biochemical and immunological analysis' Yamaguchi Med. J. 30, 149-161 (in Japanese).
5. Takahashi, M., Yokota, T., Kawano, H., Gondo, T., Ishihara, T., and Uchino, F. (1989) 'Ultrastructural evidence for intracellular formation of amyloid fibrils in macrophages' Virchows Arch. A 415, 411-419.

A HISTOCHEMICAL, IMMUNOHISTOCHEMICAL, ULTRASTRUCTURAL AND IMMUNOELECTRON MICROSCOPICAL CHARACTERIZATION OF CEREBROVASCULAR AMYLOID AND DIFFUSE PLAQUES IN AUTOPSIED AGED DOGS.

Tokuhiro Ishihara, Toshikazu Gondo, Mutsuo Takahashi, Tadaaki Yokota, Yoshimi Yamashita, Fumiya Uchino, Matsuo Kajiyama, *Shu-ichi Ikeda, **David Allsop, and ***Kohzoh Imai.

First Department of Patholgy, Yamaguchi University School of Medicine, Ube 755, Japan. *Department of Medicine (Neurology), Shinshu University School of Medicine, Matsumoto, Japan. **Division of Biochemistry, School of Biology and Biochemistry, The Green's University of Belfast, Northern Ireland, U.K.. ***Department of Internal Medicine (Section 1), Sapporo Medical College, Sapporo, Japan.

ABSTRACT. Amyloid deposits were seen in the arteries and capillaries in the leptomeninges and superficial brain cortices in 19 (67.9%) of 28 aged dogs. Immunohistochemically, cerebrovascular amyloid was reactive to anti-ß protein (ß/A4) antibody. Additionally, a variable number of diffuse plaques reacted with anti-ß/A4 antibody were also noted throughout the cerebral cortex in 24/28 dogs (85.7%). These diffuse plaques were not detected by Congo red or silver impregnation. Electron microscopically, amyloid fibrils, measuring 10 nm in width were located in the tunica media of the arteries. A few aggregations of amyloid fibrils were noted in the diffuse plaques. Immunoelectron microscopically, gold particles labeled the amyloid fibrils in the blood vessels and brain cortex. These findings demonstrated that aged dogs provide a useful animal model for many aspects of ß/A4 amyloidosis.

INTRODUCTION

The mechanism of amyloid fibril formation in cerebral blood vessels and senile plaques is still unclear, and establishment of an animal model is necessary for the clarification. We examined the cerebrum and cerebellum as well as visceral organs from 28 aged dogs using an immunohisto- che mical method with antibody to ß/A4. Ultrastructural and immunoelectron mic roscopic (immunogold method) studies were also carried out.

MATERIALS AND METHODS

Specimens were taken from the frontal, parietal, temporal, and occipital lobes, and visceral organs of 28 aged dogs (10 to 22 years of age). Sections were stained with hematoxylin-eosin, Hirano's silver method, and Congo red. Congo red-positive material showing green birefringence under polarized light was identified as amyloid. Immunohistochemical studies were performed on paraffin-embedded sections using the avidin-biotin-peroxidase complex (ABC) technique. The sections were stained with anti-ß/A4 antibody(1,2). For the demonstration of ß/A4, sections were pretreated with 90% formic acid for 30 min to enhance amyloid staining. For immunoelectron microscopy, semithin and ultrathin sections were cut serially. After removal of epon, semithin sections were pretreated with 0.5% periodic acid solution for 15 min, with 99% formic acid for 5 min, and with 10% normal goat serum for 1hr. Sections were then immunostained for ß/A4 using TB2 antiserum(2).

RESULTS

Cerebrovascular amyloid deposits were seen in 19 (67.9%) of 28 aged dogs. They were seen in the walls of the arteries and capillaries in the leptomeninges and the superficial brain cortices. In the arteries of the leptomeninges, amyloid deposits were located in the media. Cerebrovascular amyloid was found most frequently in the frontal and parietal lobes. We did not find any senile plaques at all with the Congo-red stain. The cerebrovascular amyloid reacted only with anti-ß/A4 antibody (Fig.1); occasionally, Congo red-negative vessels also reacted. Formic acid pretreatment often enhanced the immunostaining in the cerebral vessels and cortices. The intensivity of the immunoreaction for ß/A4 tended to be increased in the adventitia of arteries in the leptomeninges. A large number of nodular, immunoreactive diffuse plaque lesions were also noted throughout the cerebral cortex in 24 (85.7%) out of the 28 aged dogs(Fig.2). These diffuse plaques, ranged in size from 50 to 250 μm were not detected by Congo red stain or by silver impregnation. In serial sections stained with Congo red and ß/A4 immunohistochemistry, a similar distribution of amyloid deposits in the cerebral vessels was found, although the positive area detected by the former method was less than the latter.

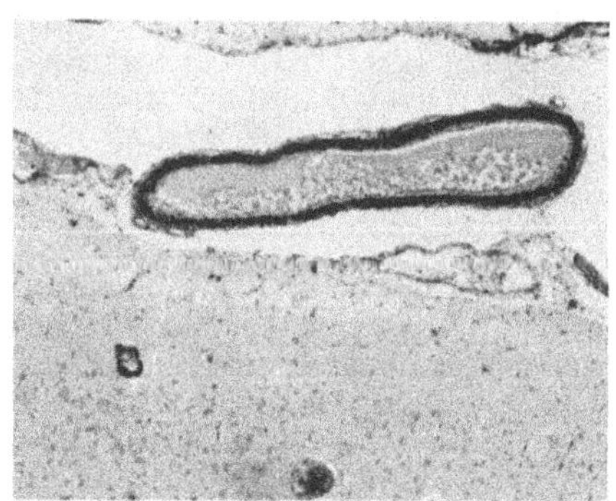

Fig.1 Cerebrovascular amyloid reacts with anti-ß/A4 antibody.

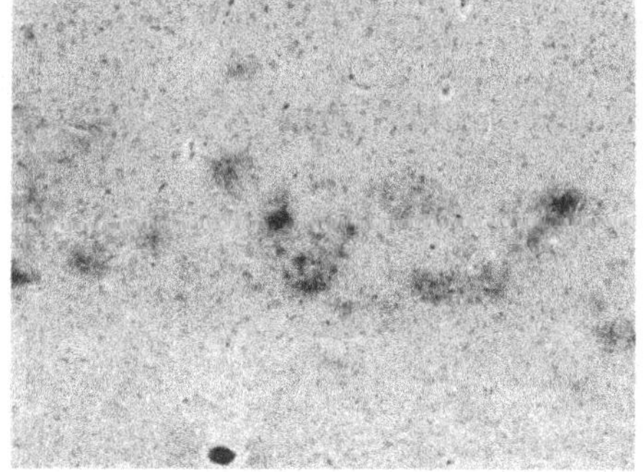

Fig.2 Diffuse plaques react with anti-ß/A4 antibody.

Electron microscopically, amyloid fibrils, measuring 10 nm in width were observed in the media of the arteries. In less involved vessels, small amounts of amyloid fibrils were found among the smooth muscle cells in the media and the collagen fibers in the adventitia, while severely involved arteries showed a replacement of the media and adventitia by the fibrils. A few bundles of amyloid fibrils were noted among the neurites in all diffuse plaques examined. In semithin sections, small vessels and a few diffuse plaques were also reactive to anti-ß/A4 antibody. Immunoelectron microscopically, gold particles labeled amyloid fibrils in the tunica media of leptomeningeal (Fig. 3) and cortical arteries. These sparse amyloid fibrils labeled by the gold particles were often intermingled with damaged cell organella in the diffuse plaques (Fig. 4).

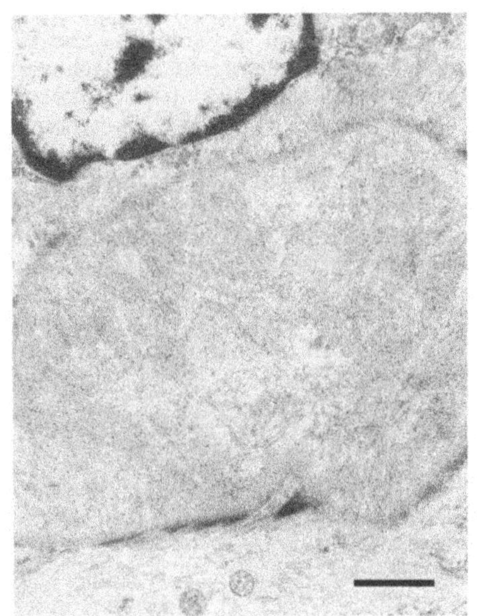

Fig.3 Gold particles label amyloid fibrils in the media of an artery.

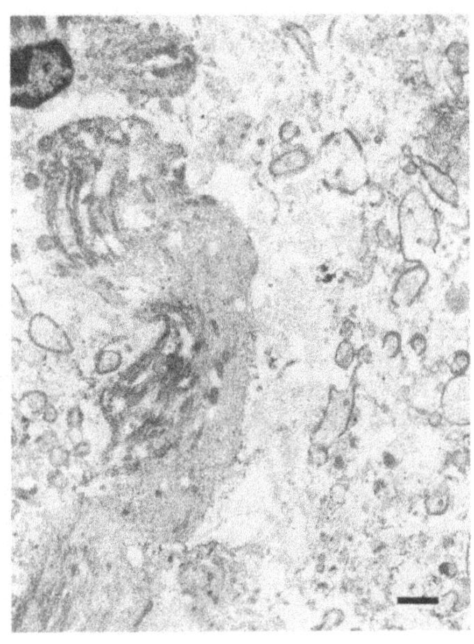

Fig.4 Sparse amyloid fibrils labeled with gold particles are seen in the cortex.

DISCUSSION

Cerebrovascular amyloid found in 19 (67.9%) of 28 brains of aged dogs. The cerebrovascular amyloid was consistently reactive for anti-ß/A4 antibody. Some of Congo red-negative vessels were ß/A4 immunoreactive. We have previously observed the same phenomenon in human brains. This might be due to the presence of small amounts of amyloid fibrils not detectable by Congo red, or to the accumulation in the vessel walls of non-fibrous forms of ß/A4 or its precursor. In addition to the cerebrovascular amyloid deposits, large numbers of ß/A4-immunoreactive plaque lesions were often found in the cerebral cortex after formic acid pretreatment. They resemble diffuse plaques, lacking any obvious amyloid deposits or abnormal neurites, that recently have been emphasized in the literature by many authors(3,4,5). Immunoelectron microscopy revealed gold particles located only on amyloid fibrils. In diffuse plaque areas we found small scattered bundles of a few amyloid fibrils specifically labeled with the gold particles. Such a sparse accumulation of fibrils is presumably below the threshold level that can be detected by Congo red at the light microscope level. These findings are similar to those reported by Ogomori et al.(4) in human with Alzheimer's disease. Tagliavini et al.(5) have suggested that ß/A4-immunoreactive materials not detected by Congo red may contain ß/A4 or its precursor in a non-fibrous pre-amyloid form. In these aged dog brains we could not find any non-fibrous materials labeled by gold particles and so could not provide evidence in support of this proposal. Molecular biological studies of the precursor of ß/A4 (APP) indicate that mRNAs encoding APP are expressed not only in brain but also in many other tissues throughout the body. This finding, together with analogies with systemic amyloidoses, has been interpreted to suggest a serum origin for ß/A4 amyloid in Alzheimer's disease. However, in other systemic amyloids of circulating origin (e.g. AA nd AL forms) amyloid deposits in the brain occur only in areas where there is an inherent increase in the permeability of the blood brain barrier (e.g. choroid plexus, area postema) and they do not accumulate in the brain parenchyma and vessels(6). Recent observations of early diffuse plaques in the brain of patients with Down's syndrome support the concept of a neuronal origin for senile plaque amyloid rather than a serum origin, although an origin of cerebrovascular amyloid from a circulating serum precursor cannot as yet, be ruled out(7). Regardless of the exact pathological processes involved, it is clear from our observations that aged dogs can serve as a useful animal model for some aspects of ß/A4 brain amyloidosis. Although there are no neurofibrillary tangles in the dogs, these animals often develop cerebrovascular amyloid deposits and diffuse plaques that are remarkably similar to those observed in the human brain.

REFERENCES

1. Allsop, D., Landon, M., Kidd, M., et al. (1986) Monoclonal antibodies raised against a subsequence of senile plaque core protein react with plaque cores, plaque periphery and cerebrovascular amyloid in Alzheimer's disease. Neurosci. Lett. 68:252-256.
2. Yachi, A., Imai, K., Saito, N. and Yamashita, T. (1989) Preparation and application of monoclonal antibody to ß-protein. Annual Report of the Primary Amyloidosis Research Committee, The Ministry of Health of Welfare of Japan, pp 64-66. (in Japanese)
3. Ikeda, S., Allsop, D. and Glenner, G.G. (1989) Morphology and distribution of plaque and related deposits in the brains of Alzheimer's disease and control cases: an immunohistochemical study using ß-protein antibody. Lab Invest 60:113-122.
4. Ogomori, K., Kitamoto, T., Takahashi, J., et al. (1989) ß-protein amyloid widely distribution in the central nervous system of patients with Alzheimer's disease. Am. J. Pathol. 134:243-251.
5. Tagliavini, F., Giaccone, G., Frangione, B. and Bugiani, O. (1988) Preamyloid deposits in the cerebral cortex of patients with Alzheimer's disease and nondemented individuals. Neurosci. Lett. 93:191-196.
6. Ishihara, T., Nagasawa, T., Yokota, T., et al. (1989) Amyloid protein of vessels in leptomeninges, cortices, choroid plexuses, and pituitary glands from patients with systemic amyloidosis. Hum. Pathol. 20:891-895.
7. Allsop, D., Haga, S., Haga, C., et al. (1989) Early senile plaques in Down's syndrome brains show a close relationship with cell bodies of neurons. Neuropathol. Appl. Neurobiol. 15:531-542.

INCREASED BINDING OF ACUTE PHASE LIPOPROTEINS BY PERITONEAL MACROPHAGES (MØs) IN MICE

Gonnerman, W.A., Cathcart, E.S., Sipe, J.D., Hayes, K.C.
Departments of Medicine and Biochemistry, Boston University School of Medicine, Boston MA; EN Rogers Memorial VA Hospital, Bedford MA; Foster Biomedical Laboratory, Brandeis University, Waltham MA.

ABSTRACT. Serum amyloid A protein (SAA), synthesized in response to an acute inflammatory stimulus, is transported in serum in association high density lipoprotein. We have compared peritoneal macrophage binding of lipoprotein fractions isolated from normal mice with those isolated from mice 18 hrs after intraperitoneal injection of 100 ug purified endotoxin. Lipoproteins were isolated by ultracentrifugation at d > 1.21 g/ml and the apolipoproteins labelled with ^{125}I by the iodine monochloride method. Labelled lipoproteins were incubated with adherence purified peritoneal macrophages and cell associated radioactivity measured. Cellular uptake of acute phase lipoproteins was six to seven-fold greater that uptake of lipoproteins from normal animals. Treatment of the cells with glutaraldehyde prior to exposure to the lipoproteins abolished the difference in uptake.

Introduction.

Partial degradation of serum amyloid A (SAA) protein to an 8500 kd fragment is necessary for deposition of amyloid fibrils into tissue [1,2]. The proteolytic step responsible for this selective degradation has been isolated to an elastase-like enzyme on the surface of Kupffer cells [3] and mononuclear phagocytic cells [4,5]. We have hypothesized that tissue macrophages (MØs) may also control degradation at specific sites within affected tissues and that repeated injections of casein or azocasein may induce amyloid deposition by overwhelming the degradative system of the MØ. Amyloid P component (AP) may also play a pivotal role in this process since it acts an an acute phase reactant in the mouse and has been proposed to be an elastase inhibitor [6]. We have initiated studies to investigate the control of the MØ degradative system for SAA using peritoneal MØs and ^{125}I labelled SAA.

Materials and Methods

<u>Isolation of plasma lipoprotein fractions</u>: Blood was collected by cardiac puncture 18-20 hrs following i.p. injection of 100 ug purified

endotoxin (RIBI). After centrifugation, plasma was removed by aspiration and pooled. The density of the plasma was adjusted to 1.21 g/ml by addition of KBr. Aliquots of the plasma were then overlayed with KBr (density 1.21 g/ml) in centrifuge tubes and centrifuged for 35 hrs at 40,000 rpm in a SW41 swinging bucket rotor. Pooled plasma from normal mice was treated identically. ApoSAA was isolated from the HDL complex by electrolution of SAA after SDS PAGE.

Radiolabelling of Lipoprotein: Aliquots of the lipoprotein fraction from acute phase and normal plasma and the electroeluted apoSAA containing 25 ug total protein were labelled with ^{125}I by the iodine monochloride method. Free iodine was removed by column chromatography on Sephadex G25.

Isolation of peritoneal macrophages (MØs): Either resident or thioglycolate elicited peritoneal MØs were harvested and purified by adherence as previously described [7]. Adherent cells were cultured for 24 hrs in either 12, 24 or 96 well tissue culture plastic plates. Equivalent amounts of radiolabelled lipoproteins were added to the cultures at the end of the adherence period. After 24 hrs, the media were removed from the cell layers, the cells were washed three times with phosphate buffered saline (PBS) which was then pooled with the culture media. The cell layer was harvested into 0.1 N NaOH. Radioactivity was measured in both the combined media and wash aliquots and the cell layers.

Results

Cell Binding of Labelled Lipoprotein: Thioglycolate elicited macrophages from female CBA/J mice were incubated for either 20 or 44 hrs with either the lipoprotein fraction from normal or from acute phase mice or with normal lipoprotein plus electroeluted SAA (5 x 10^5 cpm of each). Matching sets of cells were treated with glutaraldehyde prior to addition of the radiolabelled material. The total radioactivity measured in the cell lysate is shown in table 1. There was approximately a seven-fold increase in radioactivity in cells incubated with the acute phase lipoproteins compared with either normal total lipoprotein or with purified apoSAA. When 50% of the counts were added as normal lipoproteins and 50% as apoSAA there was only a slight increase over cells incubated with either of these fractions alone. Glutaraldehyde fixation abolished the increase in cell-associated radioactivity seen with acute phase sera.

Table 1. Cell-associated Radioactivity (CPM x 10^{-3})

Fraction	Normal cells		Glutaraldehyde cells	
	20 hr	44 hr	20 hr	44 hr
normal Lipoprotein	3.6	3.4	2.3	3.4
apoSAA	4.0	4.2	2.7	3.9
AP Lipoprotein	36.7	27.4	3.1	3.3
nLipo (0.5) + apoSAA	4.5	5.7	3.5	4.5

<u>Effect of Different Eliciting Agents (Activators) on Binding</u>. In order to determine if activation of peritoneal MØs would alter binding of lipoproteins, male CBA/J mice were given i.p. injections of either casein (1 ml of a 10% w/v solution), casein + 100 ug bacterial endotoxin (LPS), or thioglycollate. Non elicited (resident) MØs were used as controls. Cell associated radioactivity was measured as above and expressed as cpm/10^6 cells. The cell associated radioactivity is shown in table 2.

Table 2. Cell-associated Radioactivity (CPM x 10^{-3})

Fraction	Resident	Casein	Casein +LPS	Thioglycolate
Normal Lipo	3.6	4.6	6.5	6.4
Acute Lipo	24.4	24.6	26.1	35.4
apoSAA	6.8	5.7	6.5	7.8

Casein by itself did not increase the yield of MØs although there was a marked increase when LPS was added to the casein. Thioglycolate caused a significant increase in the number of recovered cells. None of these eliciting protocols significantly altered the amount of cell-associated lipoprotein.

Discussion

Since SAA is transported in the plasma as a complex with high density lipoprotein (HDL) we have isolated the lipoprotein fraction from normal and acute phase sera and have iodinated the apoproteins while complexed to the HDL particle. This should provide a more physiological substrate for the MØ since this is probably the form in which the SAA would be presented to the cell. When we have incubated this material with MØs in culture we have seen marked differences in cell association of the lipoprotein fraction from normal compared to acute phase sera.

Similar differences have been noted for the HDL_3 fraction of human serum when incubated with normal human neutrophils [8]. In this study the chemical composition of the HDL_3 fraction was similar between normal and acute phase sera but SAA was the major apolipoprotein in acute phase sera. Acute phase HDL was degraded 5-10 times more rapidly than normal sera when incubated with normal human neutrophils. SAA was the major cell associated apolipoprotein when cells were incubated with acute phase sera while apo-AI was the predominant lipoprotein when cells were incubated with normal sera.

Other studies have suggested that in the mouse the composition of the lipoprotein fraction is altered following endotoxin administration. Very low density lipoprotein (VLDL) increased markedly 8-24 hr after LPS while the HDL fraction decreased in a dose related fashion following LPS (Sakaguchi, 1982).

These results suggest that acute phase lipoproteins containing high levels of SAA may have increased affinity for MØs which could lead to increased SAA degradation at specific tissue sites.

We gratefully acknowledge the excellent technical support of Louise M Greene. This work was supported by Public Health Service Grant AG06860.

References

1. Husebekk, A., Skogen, B., Husby, G., and Marhaug, G. (1985) Transformation of amyloid precursor SAA to protein AA and incorporation in amyloid fibrils in vivo. Scand. J. Immunol 21,283-287.
2. Meek, R.L., and Benditt, E.P. (1986) Amyloidogenesis. One serum amyloid A isotype is selectively removed from the circulation. J. Exp. Med. 163,499-510.
3. Fuks, A., Zucker-Franklin, D. (1985) Impaired Kupffer cell function precedes development of secondary amyloidosis. J. Ex. Med. 161,1013-1028.
4. Lavie, G., Zucker-Franklin, D., Franklin, E.C. (1978) Degradation of serum amyloid A protein by surface-associated enzymes of human blood monocytes. J. Exp. Med. 148,1020-1031.
5. Skogen, B., Thorsteinsson, L., and Natvig, J.B. (1980) Degradation of protein SAA to an AA-like fragment by enzymes of monocytic origin. In G. G. Glenner, P. P. Costa, and F. deFreitas (eds.), Amyloid and Amyloidosis, Oxford-Princeton, Amsterdam, pp 165-170.
6. Vachino, G., Heck, L.W., Gelfand, J.A., Kaplan, M.M., Burke, J.F., Berninger, R.W., and McAdam, K.P.W.J. (1988) Inhibition of human neutrophil and Pseudomonas elastases by the amyloid P-component: A constituent of elastic fibers and amyloid deposits. J. Leukocyte Biol. 44,529-534.
7. Leslie, C.A., Gonnerman, W.A., Ullman, M.D., Hayes, K.C., Franzblau, C., and Cathcart, E.S. (1985) Dietary fish oil modulates macrophage fatty acids and decreases arthritis susceptibility in mice. J. Exp. Med. 162,1336-1349.
8. Shephard, E.G., de Beer, F.C., de Beer, M.C., Jeenah, M.S., Coetzee, G.A., and van der Westhuyzen, D.R. (1987) Neutrophil association and degradation of normal and acute-phase high-density lipoprotein 3. Biochem. J. 248,919-926.
9. Sakaguchi, S. (1982) Metabolic disorders of serum lipoproteins in endotoxin-poisoned mice: the role of high density lipoprotein (HDL) and triglyceride-rich lipoproteins. Microbiol. Immunol. 26,1017-1034.

CHARACTERIZATION OF NON-AA PROTEINS IN AMYLOID FIBRILS OBTAINED FROM A COW WITH CHRONIC INFECTION

Veiby O.P.*, Sletten K.¤, Husby G#. & Nordstoga K.
*Hafslund Nycomed Bioreg A/S, ¤Dep. of Biochemistry University of Oslo, #Dep. of Rheumatology University of Tromsø and National Veterinary Institute, Oslo, Norway.

1. Abstract

The elution pattern obtained when amyloid fibrils from amyloid-laden bovine kidneys were subjected to gelfiltration under dissociating conditions, revealed a larger amount of non-AA material than usually seen from other species. SDS-PAGE of this non-AA fraction yielded several Coomassie blue stained bands. The most distinctive ones gave estimated molecular weights of 15 kDa, 18 kDa, 33 kDa and 43 kDa. These molecular species were further characterised by electroblotting, cyanogen bromide cleavage and N-terminal analysis. The results revealed that the non-AA fraction consisted of histones H2B, H3 and H4 in addition to protein AA.

2. Introduction

Most of the work on the amyloid fibrils have so far been concerned with the low molecular weight proteins (1). In this study on an AA type of amyloidosis, we have analysed the fractions immediately following the void volume material.

3. Materials and Methods

Amyloid fibrils were obtained from the kidney of a cow with amyloidosis associated with recurrent bacterial infections. The renal amyloid fibrils were isolated according to Pras et al.(2) and Skinner et al. (3), and dissolved in a buffer with 6M guanidine-HCl, pH 8.3 containing reducing agents. The dissociated fibrils were gel filtered on a column of Sephadex G-100 in 5 M guanidine-HCl/ 0.1 M acetic acid. Fractions were dialysed against distilled water and lyophilized. Selected fractions were subjected to a second gel filtration on a column of Sepharose 4B-CL under the same conditions as above. Sodium dodecylsulphate-polyacrylamide slab gel electrophoresis (SDS-PAGE) was performed according to Laemmli (4). Protein bands were electroblotted to polyvinylidene difluoride membranes (PVDF). Electroblotted and stained polypeptides on PVDF membranes were used for N-terminal analyses, cyanogen bromide cleavages, acid hydrolyses followed by amino acid analyses and eluted material for reverse phase high performance liquid chromatography (HPLC) as described (5). The amino acid sequences were compared with proteins in the UWGCG Protein Data Base for identification.

4. Results

4.1. GELFILTRATION

The elution profile obtained when crude bovine amyloid fibril extract was gel filtered on Sephadex G-100 followed a normal pattern. Most of the material was eluted in the void volume and in the immediately following fractions, which could indicate that the material contained higher concentrations of factors involved in fibrillogenesis. The fractions corresponding to peaks III and IV, making up distinct shoulders on the declining part of the void volume peak, were rechromatographed on a column of Sepharose 4B CL. The elution profile revealed two well separated protein peaks, one at the void volume of the column (V_0) and the other slightly retarded, here referred to as the non-AA fraction.

4.2. CHARACTERISATION

SDS PAGE of the non-AA fraction resulted in several bands (Fig. 1). Estimated molecular masses for the most distinct protein bands were 43 kDa, 33 kDa, 18 kDa and 15 kDa. The material in these bands were electroblotted onto PVDF membrane for further characterisation.
The amino acid composition of the 43 and 33 kDa proteins showed a relative high content of glutamic acid/glutamine, while the 18 and 15 kDa proteins showed a high level of lysine and arginine. The four proteins were all found to contain methionine. Cysteine could only be traced in the 18 kDa protein. N-terminal analyses of the electroblotted bands showed blocked N-terminii for all of them. Cyanogen bromide cleavage followed by HPLC and N-terminal analyses of selected fractions revealed the results shown in Table 1. A search in the Protein Data Base (7) showed that the

amino acid sequence data obtained from the 43 kDa protein band could not be recognized. No amino acid sequence data could be elucidated from the 33 kDa protein band. The 18 kDa protein band was found to contain both histone H2B and H3 (Table 1) and the 15 kDa protein band contained histone H4 and a small amount of protein AA (Table 1).

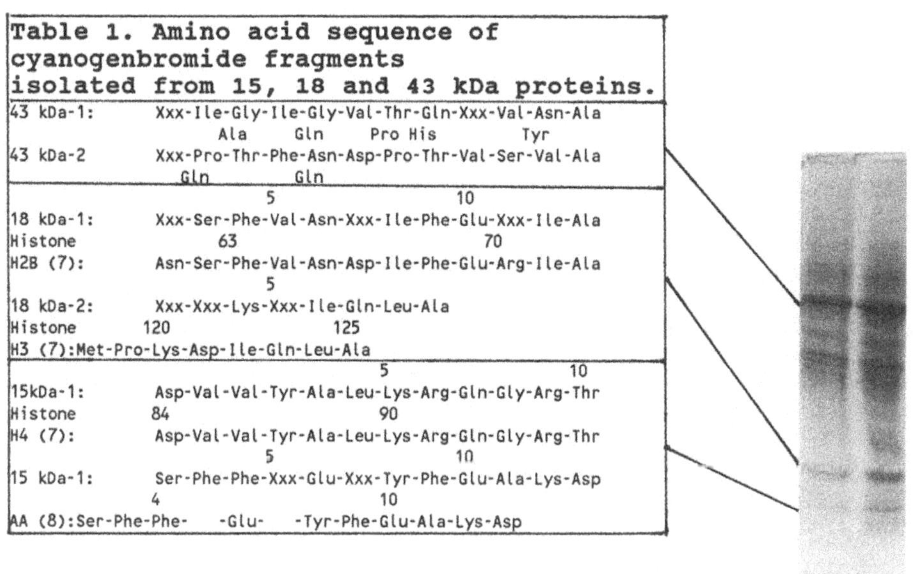

Table 1. Amino acid sequence of cyanogenbromide fragments isolated from 15, 18 and 43 kDa proteins.

43 kDa-1:	Xxx-Ile-Gly-Ile-Gly-Val-Thr-Gln-Xxx-Val-Asn-Ala
	Ala Gln Pro His Tyr
43 kDa-2	Xxx-Pro-Thr-Phe-Asn-Asp-Pro-Thr-Val-Ser-Val-Ala
	Gln Gln
	5 10
18 kDa-1:	Xxx-Ser-Phe-Val-Asn-Xxx-Ile-Phe-Glu-Xxx-Ile-Ala
Histone	63 70
H2B (7):	Asn-Ser-Phe-Val-Asn-Asp-Ile-Phe-Glu-Arg-Ile-Ala
	5
18 kDa-2:	Xxx-Xxx-Lys-Xxx-Ile-Gln-Leu-Ala
Histone	120 125
H3 (7):	Met-Pro-Lys-Asp-Ile-Gln-Leu-Ala
	5 10
15kDa-1:	Asp-Val-Val-Tyr-Ala-Leu-Lys-Arg-Gln-Gly-Arg-Thr
Histone	84 90
H4 (7):	Asp-Val-Val-Tyr-Ala-Leu-Lys-Arg-Gln-Gly-Arg-Thr
	5 10
15 kDa-1:	Ser-Phe-Phe-Xxx-Glu-Xxx-Tyr-Phe-Glu-Ala-Lys-Asp
	4 10
AA (8):	Ser-Phe-Phe- -Glu- -Tyr-Phe-Glu-Ala-Lys-Asp

Fig.1. SDS-PAGE of non-AA. NonAA was dissolved in 0.125 M Tris-HCl pH 6.8, 2% SDS, 5% 2-mercaptoethanol. 15% polyacrylamide gels were run. Both lanes contained non-AA.

5. DISCUSSION

In our study to characterise the proteins in the high molecular weight fractions (nonAA), no amyloid P component could be detected. This was, however, expected since the use of sodium citrate in the initial saline washes would eliminate any proteins, including the P component, that were bound to the amyloid extract in a calcium dependent

fashion (3). We were, however, surprised to find the histone proteins H2B, H3 and H4 eluting immediately after the non-AA. SDS-PAGE of the Vo fractions revealed these protein bands only after treatment with reducing agents, which would suggest that the proteins were packed within disulphide bridges. To our knowledge, it has never been shown any association between chromatin proteins and amyloid fibrils. However, Pepys and Butler (6) have shown that there exists a specific interaction between serum amyloid P component and chromatin.
They also suggest that SAP may play a role in the handling of chromatin released from damaged and dying cells in vivo. In our case, as mentioned above, the calcium was removed and still we find the chromatin protein associated.

6. REFERENCES:

1) Kisilevski R. (1987) 'From arthritis to Alzheimers disease: current concepts on the pathogenesis of amyloidosis.' Can.J.Physiol.Pharmacol.,65,1805-1815
2) Pras M., Schubert M., Zucker-Franklin D., Rimon A. and Franklin E.C.(1968)'The characterization of soluble amyloid prepared in water.' J.Clin.Invest.,47, 924.
3) Skinner M. Cohen A.S., Shirahama T. and Cathcart (1974) 'P-component (pentagonal unit) of amyloid:isolation, characterization and sequenceanalysis.' J.Lab.Clin.Med.,84,604
4) Laemmli U.K.(1970) 'Cleavage of structural proteins during the assembly of the head of bacteriophage T4.' Nature,227,680
5) Veiby O.P., Sletten K., Husby G. & Nordstoga K.(1990) 'Amino acid sequence analysis of non-AA protein material in AA-type amyloid fibril extracts from bovine kidney.' In preparation.
6) Pepys M.B. & Butler P.J.I (1987) 'Serum amyloid P component is the major calcium dependent specific DNA binding protein of the serum.' Biochem.Biophys.Res.Commun. 148,308-13
7) UWGCG Protein Data Base Nucleic Acids Research (1984) 12 (1),387
8) Rossevatn K., Andresen P.K., Sletten K., Husebekk A., Huseby G., Nordstoga K., Johnsen K.H., Westermark I. and Westermark P. In preparation.

COMPOSITIONAL ANALYSES OF AMYLOID FIBRILS

ALMENDINGEN, M.*, SYVERSEN, P .V.*, SLETTEN, K.* and HUSBY, G.**

* *Department of Biochemistry, University of Oslo, Norway*
** *Department of Rheumatology, University of Tromsø, Norway*

ABSTRACT

Amyloid fibrils extracted from patients with primary AL and secondary AA amyloidosis, as well as AA fibrils from a cow, were completely solubilised and analysed for macromolecular components. The proteins were separated by SDS-polyacrylamide slab-gel electrophoresis and by SDS high performance electrophoresis. The main protein components were quantitated from amino acid analyses of hydrolysates. Data for the content of proteins, nucleic acids and glucosamino-glucans, as well as the content of high and low molecular mass proteins, are presented.

1. Introduction

During the last two decades extensive studies have been made to clarify the construction of the amyloid fibrils. From different amyloid cases, completely unrelated proteins have been found to be constituents of the amyloid fibrils. However, the mechanism of the fibrillogenesis itself is still obscure.

2. Materials and methods

The following materials obtained from patients with primary and secondary amyloidosis were used :

Type	Patient	Organ	Age	Sex
	AR	Speen	57	M
AL	AL-612	Spleen	82	F
	EPS	Liver	62	M
	JL	Liver	25	M
AA	RHan	Liver	10	M
	Cow	Kidney		

The amyliod fibrils were extracted from the above mentioned organs with distilled water according to Pras (1968). The amyloid fibrils were completely solubilised in 3% sodium-dodecylsulphate (SDS) containing 3 % dithiothreitol (DTT). SDS-polyacrylamide slab gel electrophoresis (PAGE) was performed as described by Laemmlie (1970). The fibrils were also separated and characterised on SDS high performance electrophoresis coloumn (HPEC) using a 230A HPEC system from Applied Biosystem. Protein quantitation was detemined on acid hydrolysed materials using a Biotronic LC 500 amino acid analyzer. DNA was analysed as described by Burton (1956) and RNA analysis as described by Mejbaum (1939). Glycosaminoglycan analysis was carried out according to Dische (1947).

3. Results and discussion

The amyloid fibrils from all cases were found to dissolve very nicely in a solution of 3 % SDS containing 3 % DTT, and aliqoutes were taken out for determination of the contents of proteins, nucleic acids and glucosaminoglycans. The results are shown in Table 1.

TABLE 1. Macromolecular composition of amyloid fibrils.

	AL-fibrils				AA-fibrils		
Sample	AR	AL-612	EPS		JL	RHan	Cow
%-Protein	65	68	67		56	56	55
%-DNA	1	1	1		2	0,5	
%-RNA	2	2	5		3	2	
%-GAGs	11	15	16		10	13	12
Total	79%	86%	89%		71%	72%	67%

The analyses revealed that the macromolecules accounted for 79 to 89 % in the AL-fibrils, while the corresponding data for the AA-fibrils were about 70 %. The major difference observed is due to a higher protein content in the AL-fibrils. The significance of this difference of fibrils obtained from AL and AA amyloidosis is not clear. The contents of RNA, DNA and glucosamino-glycans are of the same magnitude in all cases. The SDS slab PAGE of the different fibrils revealed quite distinct protein bands (Fig. 1) and the estimated molecular weight ranged from 14 to 42 kDa (Table 2). In addition to the low molecular AA-protein bands and the AL-protein bands, a protein with molecular mass of about 30 kDA is seen in five of the six cases. Although this protein band is faint it is seen in both AA- and AL-type amyloid fibrils obtained from the spleen, the liver and the kidney. The SDS slab PAGE showed also that the AA- and AL-proteins are the major components of the fibrils.

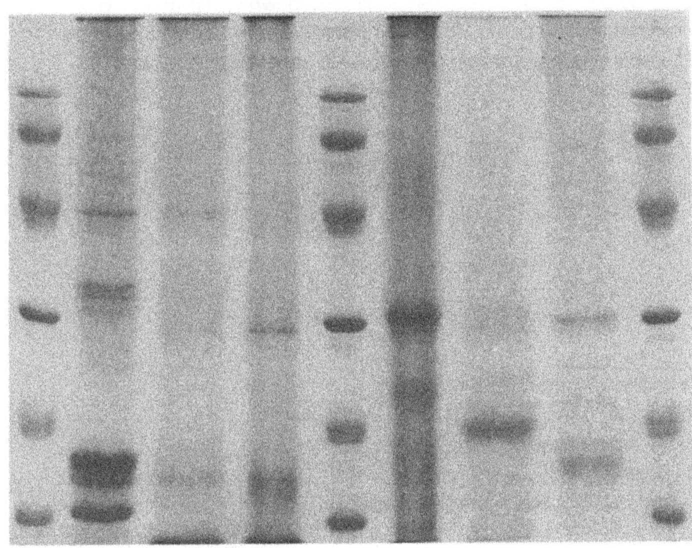

Fig. 1. SDS PAGE of amyloid fibrils.
Lane 1, 5 and 9 are marker proteins as marked in kDa (from left to right)
Lane 2 : amyloid fibrils from Cow
Lane 3 : " RHan
Lane 4 : " JL
Lane 6 : " AR
Lane 7 : " EPS
Lane 8 : " AL-612
100 ug of each amylod fibrils were applied

TABLE 2. Molecular weight estimation of the proteins from the different amyloid fibrils (kDa).

AA-fibrils			AL-fibrils		
Cow	RHan	JL	AR	EPS	AL-612
42,1	42,1				
32,7					
31,3					
30,5	29,8		29,8	29,8	29,1
	27,9	27,9		27,8	
					24,3
22,4			21,9	20,1	21,9
16,2	16,6	16,2			18,6
14,8	>14	>14			

Preparative SDS polyacrylamide gel HPEC of amyloid fibrils, as shown for RHan in Fig. 2, revealed one major low molecular weight peak. Fractions from this peak, as marked, were collected and quantitated by amino acid analyses. The results are shown in Table 3.

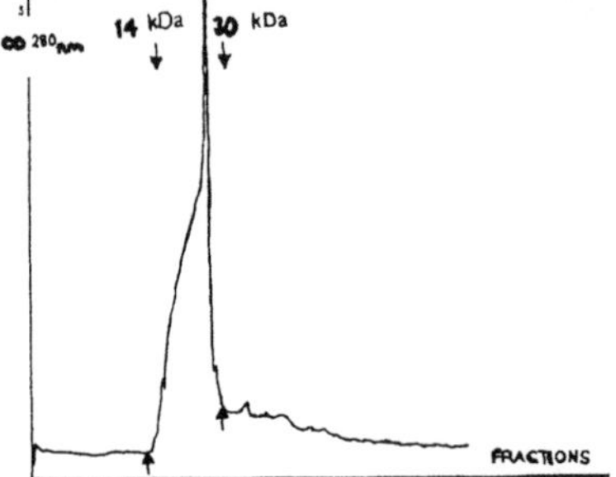

Fig.2 Electropherogram of amyloid fibrils (RHan) separated on HPEC.
Coloumn type : 3,5 x 50 mm
Gel type : 5% acrylamide, 3% SDS
Sample : RHan
Amount applied: 100 ug solubilised amyloid fibrils

TABLE 3. The yield of the different low molecular weight protein obtained from HPEC.

	AL-fibrils				AA-fibrils		
Sample	AR	AL-612	EPS		JL	RHan	Cow
%-low mol. protein	54	62	58		80	64	69

The results obtained shows that the low molecular weight material accounts for about 55% or more of the total amyloid fibril protein. It remains to be shown whether the other material present in the amyloid extract are integrated in the fibrils themselves, are non-fibrillar amyloid components or merely represent contaminants co-extracted with the fibrils.

5. References

Burton, K., (1956) `A study of the conditions and mechanism of the diphenylamine reaction for the colorimetric estimation of deoxyribonucleic acid` Biochem.J. 62,315.

Dische, Z. (1947) `A new specific colour reaction of hexuronic acids` J.Biochem.147,189.

Laemmlie, U.K.,(1970)`Cleavage of structural proteins during the assembly of the head of bacteriophage T-4` Nature.227, 680-685.

Mejbaum, W. (1939)´Über die bestimmung kleiner pentosenmengen, inbesondere in derivaten der adenylsaúre` Z.Physiol.Chem.117-120.

Pras, M.,(1968)`The characterisation of soluble amyloid prepared in water`J.Clin.Invest. 47,924.

INTRATUMOUR AMYLOIDOSIS IN PRIMARY AND METASTATIC NASOPHARYNGEAL CARCINOMA: AN IMMUNOHISTOCHEMICAL AND ULTRASTRUCTURAL STUDY.

L.M. LOOI
Department of Pathology
Faculty of Medicine
University of Malaya
59100 Kuala Lumpur, Malaysia

ABSTRACT

Congo red screening of consecutive diagnostic biopsies from 497 primary nasopharyngeal carcinoma (NPC) and 113 metastatic NPC revealed amyloid deposits in 65 (13%) primary and 14 (12%) metastatic tumours. There was no age, sex or ethnic difference between amyloid-positive and amyloid-negative patients. Amyloid was present in all three histological subtypes of the tumour, the prevalence being higher in non-keratinising (20%) than squamous (12%) and undifferentiated (10%) carcinoma. There was good concurrence in amyloid status between primary tumours and their respective metastasis: 88% of amyloid-positive metastatic tumours had amyloid-positive primaries and 95% of amyloid-negative metastatic tumours had no detectable amyloid in the primary biopsies.

Histologically, the amyloid deposits were similar in both primary and metastatic tumours. Amyloid was observed both within tumour cells, often distending the cytoplasm and pushing the nucleus aside, and as extracellular globules among tumour cells and in the stroma. It often assumed a peculiar spicular appearance. The deposits were Congophilic, exhibited green birefringence, permanganate-resistant and non-immunoreactive for AA protein and immunoglobulin light chains. Faint positivity for AP protein was observed. Electron microscopy revealed the non-branching fibrils of amyloid. In one instance, collections of fibrils were observed within the tumour cell cytoplasm.

The histomorphological and ultrastructural characteristics of the deposits support the hypothesis that this type of amyloid is of neoplastic origin.

INTRODUCTION

The association of amyloidosis with nasopharyngeal carcinoma (NPC) is not well-known and has been mainly reported from the East [1]. Congo red screening of routine biopsies received by the Department of Pathology, University of Malaya over a 5.5 year period revealed that localised NPC-related amyloidosis accounted for 27% of all types of amyloidosis encountered [2]. In view of the frequent occurrence of NPC in South-East Asia and in the Chinese throughout the world [3], it may well prove to be an important form of tumour amyloidosis. The following is an investigation into the morphological and immunohistochemical characteristics of this form of amyloidosis.

MATERIALS AND METHODS

Biopsies from the primary tumour of 497 consecutive subjects with NPC received by the Department of Pathology, University of Malaya, during the 16-year period between 1967 and 1982 were reviewed. Inadequate biopsies and those showing lesions other than NPC, such as adenocarcinoma or lymphoma, were excluded from this study. Where a patient had multiple biopsies, only the first diagnostic biopsy was included in the analysis. In addition, 113 consecutive lymph node biopsies with metastatic NPC were also reviewed.

Tissues were fixed in 10% buffered formalin, blocked in paraffin and sections stained with H&E and alkaline Congo red with and without prior treatment with $KMnO_4$. Further sections from amyloid positive cases were stained for human AA protein, human AP protein and human immunoglobulin lambda and kappa light chains using immunoperoxidase methods. Paraffin-embedded material from 2 positive cases were reprocessed for electron microscopy.

Tumours were categorised histologically according to the WHO classification. Any inflammatory host response present was noted.

RESULTS

<u>Prevalence in primary tumours</u>: Amyloid deposits were detected in 65 (13%) primary tumours. The ages of the patients ranged from 8 to 88 years with a mean of 45 years. NPC was more common in males and among the Chinese rather than the Indians and Caucasians. However, there was no significant age, sex and ethnic predilection in amyloid-positivity.

<u>Pathological features</u>: The deposits were inconspicuous because of their patchy distribution. Amyloid was detected within tumour cells and extracellularly (Fig. 1). Within tumour cells, the eosinophilic amyloid spherules would distend the cytoplasm, flattening and pushing the nuclei aside as the deposits became more abundant. Some deposits assumed a stellate, radially orientated fibrillar appearance. Extracellular deposits of similar appearance were observed in the stroma, often in close contact with neoplastic cells and associated with plasma cells, lymphocytes and macrophages.

Amyloid was present in all three histological subtypes of NPC i.e. undifferentiated (UC), non-keratinising (NKC) and differentiated squamous cell carcinoma (SCC). The prevalence was highest (20% or 25/123) in NKC while it was observed in 12% (18/149) of SCC and 10% (22/225) of UC. A lymphoplasmacytic stroma infiltrate was common in NPC but it bore no association with the presence of amyloid ($0.90>P>0.80$).

Staining and electron microscopic characteristics: The amyloid stained rose-pink with Congo red and showed green birefringence. The intensity of Congophilia, however, varied among deposits and was sometimes weak. 14 cases investigated for KMnO4 sensitivity were resistant. AA protein was not detected in 11 cases for which it was tested. In 3 of 9 instances, a weak immunoreactivity for AP protein was noted. Similarly, weak positivity for both lambda and kappa light chains were observed in 3 of 11 cases. Ultrastructurally, collections of randomly arrayed, non-branching fibrils were observed between tumour cells. In 1 case, clumps of such fibrils were present within the cytoplasm of tumour cells.

Amyloid deposits in metastatic NPC: 14 (12%) of 113 metastatic NPC in lymph nodes contained amyloid. This positivity rate concurred with that of primary NPC. As in the primary tumour, NKC was the subtype with the highest frequency (17.4%) of amyloid. Furthermore, amyloid was observed both within and amidst the tumour cells. In 30 patients, biopsies of both the primary and metastatic tumours were performed at the same time or a few weeks apart (Table 1). There was excellent concurrence in amyloid-positivity (and negativity) between primary tumours and their respective metastasis (McNemar's test; P=0.5).

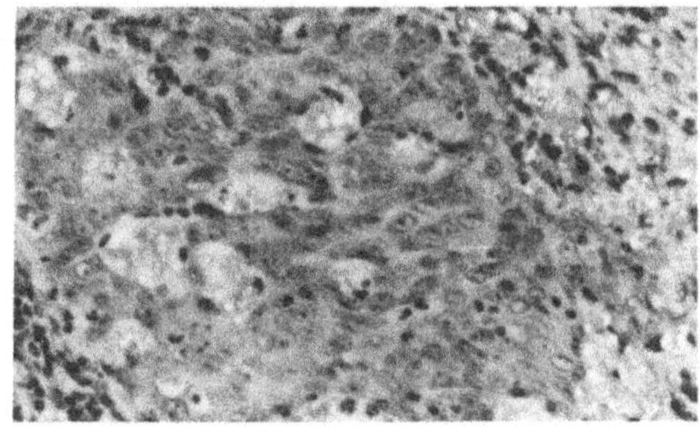

Figure 1. Birefringent amyloid deposits within NPC cells and in the stroma. Congo red - cross polarised light.

TABLE 1. Correlation of amyloid in primary and metastatic NPC

Primary NPC	Metastatic NPC Amyloid present No. (%)	 Amyloid absent No. (%)	Total
Amyloid present	7 (87.5)	1 (12.5)	8
Amyloid absent	1 (4.5)	21 (95.5)	22
Total	8 (26.7)	22 (73.3)	30

DISCUSSION

This investigation draws attention to the occurrence of amyloid in close assocaition with NPC cells. This phenomenon has probably gone unnoticed because the deposits were small and patchy in location and easily missed on routine examination. In this centre, biopsies performed as early as 1967 contained amyloid but were missed until the present study was carried out. The true prevalence of amyloid in NPC is likely to be higher than the 13% shown here, as many of the biopsies were small and amyloid, being patchy in distribution, may not have been sampled in many instances.

One can infer from its resistance to KMnO4 and the lack of reactivity for AA protein that NPC amyloid is not "reactive" or "secondary" in nature. Inconsistent and weak staining for AP protein and light chains suggest that these are not major components of this form of amyloid. In the case of AP protein, this is surprising AP protein is known to be a ubiquitious protein in most forms of amyloid [4].

The histological and ultrastructural features, and the finding of similar deposits in metastatic tumours, suggest that the amyloid is a product of the neoplastic cells. It was noted that some tumour cells contained only a small amount of amyloid. In others, almost the entire cytoplasm was occupied by the substance, suggesting a gradual increase in the amount of intracellular amyloid with eventual release of amyloid into the extracellular space. A similar mechanism has been postulated for amyloid in medullary carcinoma of the thyroid [5].

In both primary localized cutaneous amyloidosis and basal cell carcinoma, there are indications that amyloid originates in the keratogenous epithelial cells [6,7]. This is not surprising since keratin and amyloid share a beta-pleated configuration on X-ray diffraction [8]. The appearance of NPC amyloid is somewhat similar to amyloid in basal cell carcinoma and it is feasible that they share similar pathogenetic mechanisms. In view of these observations, NPC can be viewed as a amyloidogenic tumour.

REFERENCES

1. Prathap K, Looi LM, Prasad U (1984). Localized amyloidosis in nasopharyngeal carcinoma. Histopathology, 8: 27-34.

2. Looi L.M. (1986). Amyloidosis in Malaysians: a histopathological and immunohistochemical study of the various tyles of amyloidosis in a Malaysian patient population. MD thesis, University of Malaya.

3. Shanmugaratnam K. (1982) Nasopharynx. In: Schottenfeld D, Fraumeni JR Jr., eds. Cancer epidemiology and prevention. Philadelphia: WB Saunders, pp 536-553.

4. Pepys M (1988) Amyloidosis: some recent developments. Q J Med,252: 283-298.

5. Ljungberg O (1972). On medullary carcinoma of the thyroid. Acta Pathol Microbiol Scand, Sect A, Pathol, 231 (suppl): 1-57.

6. Yoneda K, Watanabe H, Yanagihara M, Mori S (1989). Immunohistochemical staining properties of amyloids with anti-keratin antibodies using formalin-fixed, paraffin-embedded sections. J Cutan Pathol, 16: 133-136.

7. Looi LM (1983). Localised amyloidosis in basal cell carcinoma: a pathologic study. Cancer, 52: 1833-1836.

8. Gueft B (1972). The analogy of amyloid and keratin as suggested by X-ray, amino acid, and ultrastructural analysis. Mt Sinai J Med, 39: 91-102.

INTRATUMOUR AMYLOIDOSIS IN CARCINOMA OF THE CERVIX

L.M. LOOI
Department of Pathology
Faculty of Medicine
University of Malaya
59100 Kuala Lumpur, Malaysia

ABSTRACT

Congo red screening of 161 invasive squamous cell carcinomas of the uterine cervix revealed 2 (1.2%) instances of intratumour amyloidosis. The amyloid deposits occurred as Congophilic, green-birefringent globules among carcinoma cells and in the connective tissue stroma between invasive tongues of tumour. Some deposits exhibited a distinctive spicular appearance. The deposits were permanganate-resistant and failed to exhibit immunoreactivity with AA protein, AP protein and immunoglobulin light chains. The histochemical and morphological characteristics of these deposits were similar to amyloid deposits found in nasopharyngeal carcinoma (NPC) in an earlier study. As with NPC, it is possible that the amyloid fibrils are composed of products of the tumour cells, such as keratin or keratin-related intermediate filaments. However, although carcinoma of the cervix is morphologically similar to NPC, the occurrence of amyloid in carcinoma of the cervix is a relatively rare phenomenon unlike its occurrence in about 13% of NPC.

INTRODUCTION

The occurrence of amyloid within tumours has been known for a long time. In a recent study based on Congo red screening of 27,052 routine surgical biopsies received by the Department of Pathology, over a 5.5 year period, localized intratumour amyloidosis constituted the largest category (58%) of amyloidosis encountered [1,2]. The presence of amyloid in calcifying epithelial odontogenic tumours and apudomas is generally known but its occurrence within epithelial tumours such as carcinomas of the nasopharynx, lung, gastrointestinal tract and cervix has not received much attention. This study describes the occurrence of amyloid deposits within carcinoma of the cervix and provides some insight into its pathogenesis.

MATERIALS AND METHODS

Biopsies from 161 primary invasive squamous carcinomas of the cervix received by the Department of Pathology, University of Malaya were reviewed. Inadequate biopsies and those showing other histological types of neoplasia, such as adenocarcinoma and sarcomas, were excluded from this study. Where a patient had multiple biopsies, only the first diagnostic biopsy was included in the analysis.

Tissues were fixed in 10% buffered formalin, blocked in paraffin and sections stained with H&E and alkaline Congo red with and without prior treatment with $KMnO_4$. Further sections from amyloid positive cases were stained for human AA protein, human AP protein and human immunoglobulin lambda and kappa light chains using immunoperoxidase methods.

Tumours were categorised histologically into large cell non-keratinising (LNK), keratinising (KSCC), small cell (SSCC) and adenosquamous (ASCC) types.

RESULTS

Prevalence and clinical features:

Of the 161 carcinoma of the cervix screened, 70% were LNK, 17% KSCC, 7% SSCC and 6% ASCC. Amyloid deposits were detected in 2 tumours, indicating a prevalence of 1.2% One patient was a 72-year-old Iban woman with a large-cell non-keratinising carcinoma and the other, a 62-year-old Chinese woman with a keratinising squamous carcinoma. Both did not have evidence of systemic amyloidosis.

Pathological features:

The amyloid deposits were patchy in distribution and generally inconspicuous. They appeared as globules and spherules among and in close contact with tumour cells, as well as in the connective tissue stroma between tongues of tumour (Fig. 1). No intracellular deposits were noted. The deposits often exhibited a stellate, radially orientated fibrillar appearance.

Tinctorial and immunohistochemical characteristics:

The amyloid stained rose-pink with Congo red and exhibited typical apple-green birefringence under cross-polarized light. The intensity of Congophilia, however, was generally weak. The deposits were metachromatic with crystal violet. They were permanganate-resistant and failed to exhibit immunoreactivity for AA protein, AP protein and both lambda and kappa immunoglobulin light chains.

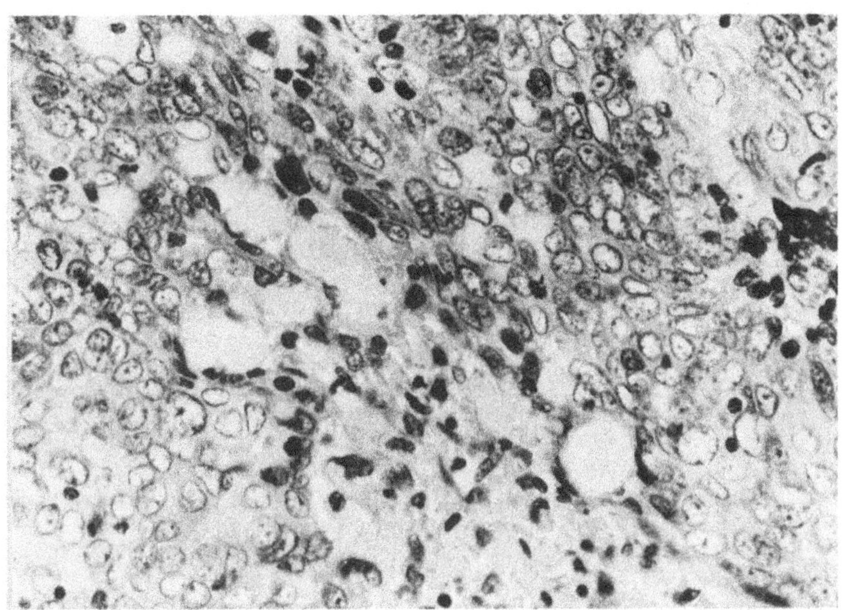

Figure 1. Globules of amorphous, eosinophilic amyloid deposits among tumour cells of an invasive large-cell non-keratinising squamous cell carcinoma of the uterine cervix. H&E X 300.

DISCUSSION

The immunohistochemical and morphological characteristics of the amyloid encountered here are remarkably similar to that described in nasopharyngeal carcinomas (NPC) [3] and precludes the possibility of AA amyloid. It is noteworthy that both types of neoplasia are of squamous mucosal surfaces and are histologically very similar. It is likely that the formation of amyloid within both types of neoplasia have similarities in their pathogenesis. As with NPC and other epithelial tumours such as basal cell carcinoma [3,4], it is likely that the amyloid fibrils are composed of products of the tumour cells such as keratin or keratin-related intermediate filaments.

It is of interest that AP protein was not detected in these amyloid deposits, an observation that is also similar to NPC amyloid. It may be that AP protein has a minor role, or perhaps no role, to play in the formation of these tumour amyloids. This is important to our understanding of amyloidogenesis as, so far, AP protein has been a constant constituent of most amyloids [5].

Another point of note is that although carcinoma of the cervix is an extremely common malignancy, the occurrence of amyloid within it is an uncommon phenomenon. This is in contrast to NPC, which though morphologically similar, has a high prevalence (13%) of intratumour amyloid [4]. The reason for this is not clear but would indicate some differences in their pathogenetic pathways.

REFERENCES

1. Looi LM (1986). Intratumour amyloidosis in Malaysians: an immunohistochemical study. Ann Acad Med Singapore, 15: 52-56.

2. Looi L.M. (1986). Amyloidosis in Malaysians: a histopathological and immunohistochemical study of the various tyles of amyloidosis in a Malaysian patient population. MD thesis, University of Malaya.

3. Prathap K, Looi LM, Prasad U (1984). Localized amyloidosis in nasopharyngeal carcinoma. Histopathology, 8: 27-34.

4. Looi LM (1983). Localised amyloidosis in basal cell carcinoma: a pathologic study. Cancer, 52: 1833-1836.

5. Pepys M (1988) Amyloidosis: some recent developments. Q J Med,252: 283-298.

MOLECULAR BIOLOGY OF AMYLOIDOGENESIS IN THE TRANSTHYRETIN RELATED AMYLOIDOSES

M.J.M. Saraiva[1,2], P.P. Costa[2]
[1]Instituto de Ciências Biomédicas
Universidade do Porto
[2]Centro de Estudos de Paramiloidose
Hospital de Santo António
4000 Porto, Portugal

ABSTRACT. In the past few years molecular biology has contributed to the ongoing research on the transthyretin (TTR) related amyloidoses. Several non exclusive intervening factors in amyloidogenesis are investigated by these techniques; they include the amyloidogenic potential of TTR, due to either modifications on the conformation of the protein and/or proteolysis at specific and constant sites, and finally interaction with tissue or circulating factors. Newer tools like PCR technology, genetic engineering in bacteria and transgenic animals are now used to approach the pathogenic mechanisms underlying these diseases.

INTRODUCTION

During the last decade, molecular biology has played a fundamental role in medicine, with contributions towards the establishment of pathogenic mechanisms underlying diseases. This is certainly true in the case of the TTR related amyloidoses. Sophisticated molecular biology technology is being applied in the lines of ongoing research in the several labs in the world which are trying to answer the crucial question of why TTR is an amyloidogenic protein with clinically heterogeneous pathogenic consequences.

This report gives a summary account of the recent advances on this topic.

Genetic and clinical heterogeneity in the TTR related amyloidoses

That there exists a genetic and clinical heterogeneity in the TTR associated amyloidoses is very evident by the impressive list of TTR variants that have been found associated with this group of diseases. Substitutions at positions 30, 33, 42, 45, 49, 50, 58, 60, 64, 77, 84, 90, 111, 114 and 122 have been characterized both by protein structural data and DNA analyses. A variety of clinical syndromes have been associated with these several TTR mutations. Most of them have neuropathy as a major clinical manifestation. The other clinical manifestation vary, reflecting differences in organ distribution and involvement with amyloid deposits . Within the neuropathies, some affect predominantly the lower limbs, others the upper limbs, autonomic neuropathy is a feature in some of them and vitreous involvement is important in some forms (Benson and Wallace, 1989). Three TTR mutations have been associated predominantly with cardiac amyloidosis, characterized by prominent cardiomyopathy and the absence of neuropathy; these are TTR mutations with Thr 45, with Met 111 and Ile 122 substitutions. In the so called senile systemic amyloidoses (SSA), normal TTR has been implicated (Westermark et al., 1990); SSA is a common disease that affects about 25% of individuals over the age of 80 and the heart is a major organ of massive TTR amyloid infiltration (Pitkanen et al.,1984).

The clinical heterogeneity also extends to the onset of the disease. For instance, in the Met 30 amyloidoses, the onset is very variable among patients, ranging from the 3rd decade to the 7th decade or even later; gene dosage does not influence the onset, as homozygous individuals can be asymptomatic late in life (Holmgreen et al., 1988); homozygous and heterozygous individuals have also been found for the Ile 122 related amyloid cardiomyopathy affecting the black population and again, gene dosage has no effect on the clinical expression (Jacobson et al., 1990, Saraiva et al., 1990).

The intervening factors in amyloidogenesis

In the TTR amyloidoses it is clear that amyloid formation preceedes the onset of clinical symptoms, being difficult to assess the timing relationship between the two events. At this point, the intervening factors in amyloidogenesis are largely unknown, but it is commom sense among researchers that we are in the presence of a multifactorial process where possible hypotheses are not exclusive; they could be summarized as follows:

First, we have the TTR amyloidogenic potential which can be related hypothetically to either or both the conformation of TTR or to proteolysis of the protein. In addition to the amyloidogenic potential, binding to tissue might influence the deposition and the presence of GAGs for instance in this type of amyloid has been documented and could explain why some tissues are prone to amyloid deposition, whereas others are not. Finally, one should not exclude also the possibility of interference in the process of circulating factors (which could be hypothetically related to aging).

The amyloidogenic potential of TTR

Conformational hypothesis

A conformational hypothesis implies a conformational modification introduced by an aminoacid substitution or post-translationally. This would lead to the formation of a new critical structural domain in the protein, that assumes an "amyloidogenic" conformation. In this hypothesis, some mutations in TTR would not produce an "amyloidogenic" conformation. Due to the late onset nature of this group of diseases, it will take sometime to definetely prove that some mutant TTRs are not in fact amyloidogenic, but screening studies of the general population by IEF have revealed mutant TTRs without apparent pathogenic consequences (Altland et al.,1987).These include a basic variant with an Arg for Pro substitution at position 102, and an acidic variant, with an Asn for His substitution at position 90 (Saraiva et al., 1989); this last acidic variant appeared in 4 out of 1,200 healthy subjects, one of them homozygous for the substitution. A neutral variant of TTR with a Ser for Gly substitution at position 6 was also described, detected due to its abnormal binding properties for T4, without being amyloidogenic to date (Fitch et al.,1989).

The proven amyloidogenic substitutions are located in disparate positions of the molecule, as represented in figure 1, making it difficult to predict a common amyloidogenic domain . Without X-ray analyses of crystals of these mutants it will be premature to define exactly the structural modifications introduced by the mutations and see whether this modification is common among them. Crystals of mutant TTR Met 30 have been obtained from TTR isolated from plasma of an homozygous individual (Hamilton et al., 1989) and will certainly give insights into this issue.

In heterozygous individuals,tetrameric mutant hybrid species with distinct conformations possibly circulate. A great variation in the ratio of mutant to

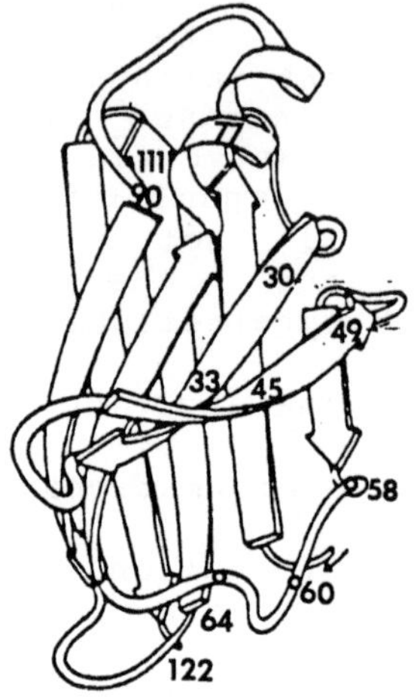

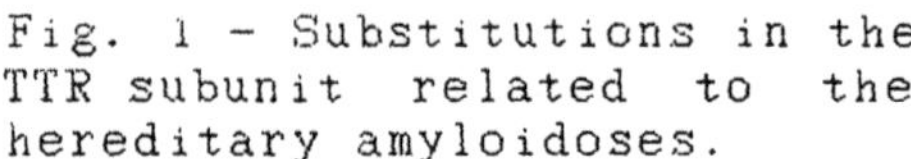
Fig. 1 - Substitutions in the TTR subunit related to the hereditary amyloidoses.

normal monomer in amyloid has been found by several labs, and variation of this ratio in tissues from the same patient is also observed, meaning that hybrid species can have amyloidogenic potential. The amyloidogeneicity may vary among the hybrids and might be affected by the presence of additional modifications. For instance, an asymptomatic Met 30 carrier has been found who possesses a second mutation, of Asn for His at position 90, lacking the normal monomer (Saraiva et al., 1989); it will be interesting to follow up this case and observe the effect of the second mutation in the amyloidogenic potential. In this context, another situation that is now being investigated in depth concerns the finding of the same genetic defect giving rise to different phenotypic expressions; in one case, the protein is amyloidogenic (Skare et al.,1990) in the other apparently not; the same asparagine for histidine substitution at position 90 appears to be involved, but the IEF pattern obtained is different; the possibility exists that post-translational events operate that affect the amyloidogeneicity of the protein.

One of the consequences that have been raised for the TTR amyloidogenic potential concerns changes in TTR subunit self assembly properties. It has been hypothesized that amyloidogenic TTR circulates as a tetrameric protein, but the interaction between the subunits is slightly weaker. Polymerization could occur by special bonding forces such as disulfide bonds, via the cysteine residue located in each monomer (Migita et al., 1989). If, in fact the self assembly of amyloidogenic TTR is altered, what is stil hard to envisage is the pathway of polymerization, that can occur via mono, di, tetra or even polymeric species.

Proteolytic hypothesis

Fragmentation of TTR has been also implicated to explain its amyloidogenic potential. This concept is based on the finding of TTR fragments in amyloid fibrils where the positions of cleavage are constant . They include mainly residues 46, 49 and 52 of TTR and fragments of TTR starting at these points have been demonstrated in fibrils from patients with substitutions 30, 33,111, 122 and in SSA patients . If, in fact, proteolysis of TTR triggers fibril formation, this is an unifying mechanism between the hereditary amyloidoses and the common SSA . Aging could possibly influence the proteolysis of both mutant and normal TTR in the vulnerable region encompassing residues 46 to 56 of TTR. The proteolytic process could then originate fragments that aggregate. At this point, we do not know if proteolysis preceedes amyloid fibril formation, or whether is a secondary event. The same is true for the role of tissue components that have been identified in fibrils, such as GAGs, fibronectin , etc.

Molecular biology tools to investigate the amyloidogenic potential of TTR

As referred to previously, the possible intervening factors in fibril formation are complex and unknown and molecular biology again provides us with newer tools to confirm or exclude hypotheses. Thus, the amyloidogenic potential due to conformational changes will be further expanded through screening and characterization of TTR variants; screening of variants by IEF in immobilized gradients (Altland et al.,1987) will add to the list of amyloidogenic and non- amyloidogenic TTR variants. The recent PCR technology will permit easily to identify newer mutations through DNA sequencing of amplified TTR exons (Nichols et al., 1989). Furthermore, PCR technology is and will be applied for diagnosis at the pre-natal, pre-symptomatic and symptomatic levels through RFLP, ASO analyses or other variations of the method.

The other important tool to investigate amyloidogenesis is synthetic TTR produced by recombinant DNA (Furuya et al., 1989). This permits the availability of mutants in large quantities for studies of conformation and polymerization. For instance, crystals have been obtained from TTR Met 30 isolated from secretion media of E.coli that will allow 3D studies and comparisons with other mutants obtained by the same procedure. The involvement of thiols in polymerization will be possible with synthetic mutants lacking cys 10 and TTR Ser 10 has been constructed for this purpose (Furuya et al., this series).

Finally, "in vivo" studies, through transgenic animals is crucial for the investigation of the intervening factors, specially of tissue and circulating nature. These animals are available for Met 30, produce amyloid in several organs and tissues (except choroid plexus and nerve)(Shimada et al.,1989) and will be instrumental also to test agents that interfere with amyloid deposition.

REFERENCES

Altland, K.,Becher, P., Banzhoff, A (1987), Electrophoresis 8, 293-297.

Benson, M.D., Wallace, P. (1989), in Scriver, C.R., Beaudeat, A., Sly, W., Valle, D (eds), The metabolic basis of inherited disease, 6th edition, McGrow Hill, New York, pp. 2439-2460.

Fitch, N .J .S., Akbari, M.T., Sheppard, M.C., Ramsden, D.B. (1989), Arq. Med. 3, 189-A9.

Furuya, H., Nakazato, M., Saraiva, M.J.M., Costa,PP Sasaki, H., Matsuo, H., Goto, I.,Sakaki, Y.(1989) Biochem. Biophys. Res. Commun. 163, 851-859.

Hamilton, J. A., Steinrauf, L.K., Holmgren, G., Benson, M.D. (1989), Arq. Med. 3, 194 - A32.

Holmgren, G., Haettner, E., Nordenson, I., Sandgren, O. , Steen, L. , Lundgren, E. (1988), Clin. Genet. 34, 333-338.

Jacobson, D.R., Gorevic, P.D., Buxbaum, J.N. (1990), Am. J. Hum. Genet. 47, 127-136.

Migita, S., Takegami, M., Ikegawa, S. (1989), Arq. Med. 3, 195 - A35.

Nichols, W. C., Liepnieks, J. J., McKusick, V.A., Benson, M.D. (1989), Genomics 5: 535-540.

Pitkanen, P., Westermark, P., Cornwell, G.G. III, (1984), Am. J. Pathol. 117, 391-396.

Saraiva M.J.M.,Almeida,M.R.,Costa,P.P., Altland,K., Gawinowicz, M.A. (1989), Arq. Med. 3, 188 - A8.

Saraiva, M.J.M. Sherman, W., Marboe, C., Figueira, A. Costa, P.P., Freitas, A.F., Gawinowicz, MA.,(1990) Scand. J. Immunol. In press.

Shimada,K., maeda, S., Murakami, T., Nishiguchi, S., Tashiro, F., Yi, S., Wakasugi, S., Takahashi, K., Yamamura, K.. (1989) Biol. Med. 6, 333-343.

Skare,J.,Milunsky,J.,Milunsky,A.,Skare,I.B. Cohen, A.S., Skinner, M. (1990), Clin. Genet.In press

STUDIES ON THE MOLECULAR ARRANGEMENT IN TRANSTHYRETIN-RELATED FAMILIAL AMYLOIDOTIC POLYNEUROPATHY FIBRILS

C.J.Terry & C.C.F.Blake, Laboratory of Molecular Biophysics, Rex Richards Building, South Parks Road, Oxford. OX1 3QU. UK

1. Abstract

The involvement of transthyretin (TTR) in Familial Amyloidotic Polyneuropathy (FAP) has been widely documented. Extensive biochemical studies on the TTR from Portuguese FAP-diagnosed patients and the TTR from control patients have revealed them to be indistinguishable with respect to many physical parameters (Mascarenhas,M.J. (1983)). However, further sequence analysis studies exposed a Val 30 → Met substitution. Since then, 7 further FAP-related TTR mutations have been discovered all of which result in the same fatal amyloid deposition. In an effort to understand how a single substitution can result in extensive fibril formation we have carried out a computer graphics analysis of each mutation by subsituting it into the high resolution structure of native TTR and studying the molecule for any subsequent changes imposed on it. This resulted in the discovery of a region in the TTR molecule in which all the mutations lie that overlaps the interacting surface in the crystallographic unit cell. This suggested a similar arrangement of molecules within the fibrils and crystals. To obtain experimental evidence for the orientation of molecules within the fibrils we have implemented x-ray fibre diffraction techniques using Met 30 fibrils extracted from human kidney tissue. Preliminary results support the proposed orientation of molecules within the fibrils indicating that the thyroxine-binding channel lies parallel to the fibre axis.

2. Materials and Methods

2.1 FIBRILS

Met 30 FAP fibrils extracted from human kidney tissue were kindly provided by Dr.A.M.Damas from the University of Porto, Portugal.

2.2 COMPUTER GRAPHICS ANALYSIS

The coordinates for native human transthyretin were accessed from the Daresbury Databank and each of the 14 known mutations were in turn substituted into the structure. The molecule was viewed on an Evans & Sutherland PS300 Graphics system using the program package FRODO (Jones,T.A. et al (1985).

2.3 X-RAY FIBRE DIFFRACTION

Met 30 FAP fibrils, as above, were mounted by evaporation from a water droplet such that maximum fibril alignment was achieved in the beam. High angle patterns were recorded at the Daresbury Synchrotron Source station 7.2 on x-ray film during exposure times of 35 minutes at a relative humidity of 66%. The specimen to film distance was 483.00mm, determined by recording the diffraction from the known standard silica. The optical densities of the films were determined on a SCANDIG densitometer using a 50-μ raster. The programme GUCK2 (Ladner,J.E. (1979) mod.Clifton,I. (1984)) was used to obtain radial scans through the films.

3. Results

3.1 COMPUTER GRAPHICS ANALYSIS

The molecule was analysed for any obvious changes imposed on the structure by the substitutions eg. steric clashes on internal substitutions; the substitution of a surface hydrophobic residue for a hydrophilic sidechain producing a 'sticky' patch on the surface of the protein (as is the case for haemoglobin in sickle cell anaemia). In only one case was it likely that any gross change in the structure would result from the substitutions and that was for the Portuguese Met 30 variant. There is clearly insufficient space to accommodate this significantly larger sidechain.

Treating the FAP fibril-forming mutations as a group within the molecule resulted in the discovery of a region within the protein in which all the FAP mutations lie. This region is 3-dimensional in so far as the substituted residues can be buried aswell as lie on the surface.

It is interesting to note that when compared with the transthyretin crystallographic unit cell the region overlaps the region in the molecule which forms one of the interacting surfaces in the crystal (Fig.1). It appears that the mutations are each capable of making an area of the protein which is 'sticky' at the high crystallising concentrations 'sticky' at the lower physiological concentrations. This points to a similar arrangement of transthyretin tetramers within the fibrils as within the crystal.

3.2 X-RAY FIBRE DIFFRACTION

Preliminary results point to the stacking of the tetramers such that the thyroxine-binding channel is parallel to the fibre axis. The high angle diffraction pattern shows several discrete reflections and some more diffuse. The 4.7Å and 12Å reflections are easy to assign and contribute towards the characteristic cross-β pattern displayed by amyloid fibrils (Fig.2). This is in good agreement with the proposed orientation of transthyretin tetramers since this would result in the β strands lying perpendicular to the fibre axis and the β sheets lying parallel to it.

We are about to collect further medium and low angle data to establish the longer

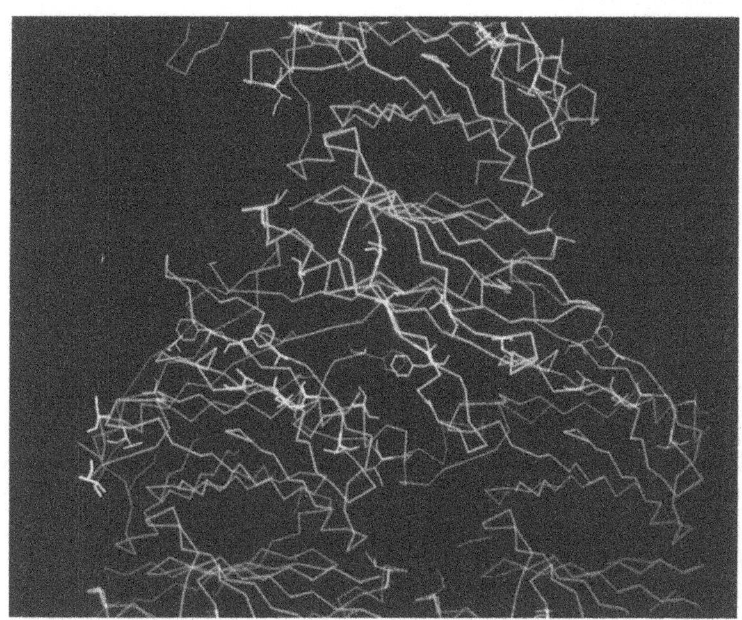

Fig.1 Interface region of the TTR crystallographic unit cell overlaps the region containing the FAP-associated mutations. (Mutation sites are highlighted by the native sidechains).

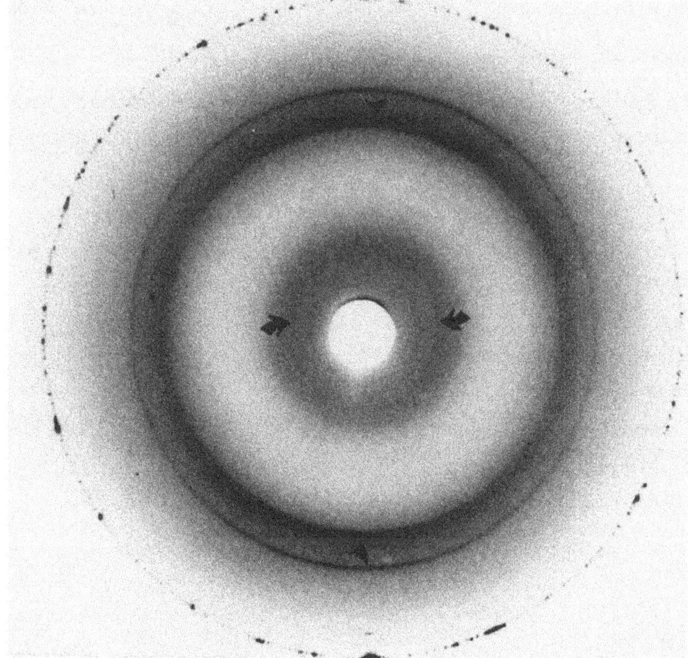

Fig2. High angle diffraction pattern of Met 30 FAP fibrils. Arrowheads and arrows indicate the 4.7Å and 12Å reflections respectively.

repeat distances within the fibrils.

4. Discussion

The reflections on the high angle x-ray diffraction pattern agree well with the proposed orientation of transthyretin tetramers within the fibrils and, together with the computer graphics analysis, provide good evidence for the stacking of TTR molecules such that the thyroxine-binding channel is parallel to the fibre axis. They are also remarkably similar to the diffraction patterns from other forms of amyloid fibrils (Kirschner et al (1986)) showing the high resolution structure to be consistent with general amyloid characteristics.
The fibrils also stained red with congo-red and exhibited green birifringence under crossed polars. This indicates that the congo-red molecules bind parallel to the fibre axis (Wolman & Bubis (1965)). If the binding site of congo-red on the transthyretin molecule were determined conclusive evidence for the molecular orientation would be provided. To this end we are to start crystallographic experiments, binding congo-red to crystals of native transthyretin. A difference map between the complex and native structure should identify the binding site.
The ability of such a diverse range of substitutions to produce the same physical result leads one to ponder on the nature of the molecule surface in the region of the mutations. One possible reason for a single mutation having such a profound effect on the aggregating properties of transthyretin is that the hydrophobic character of this region is held in a very fine balance.

Acknowledgements

The authors wish to thank Dr Trevor Forsythe and Paul Langan of Keele University for their help and advice during x-ray data collection and analysis.

References

Jones,T.A. et al., "Methods in Enzymology", (*eds. H.W.Wycoff, C.H.W. Hirs & S.N.Timasheff*) Acad. Press, London, 115, 157-171 (1985).
Kirschner,D.A., Abraham,C. & Selkoe,D.J., P.N.A.S., 83, 503-507 (1986).
Ladner,J.E., Heidelburg (1979), version 5 modified by Clifton,I. Daresbury (Sept 1984)
Mascarenhas,M.J., Costa,P.P. & Goodman,D.S., J. Lab. Clin. Med., 102(4), 590-603 (1983).
Wolman,M & Bubis,J.J., Histochemie, 4, 351-356 (1965).

X-RAY CRYSTAL STRUCTURE OF THE MET-30 VARIANT OF HUMAN PREALBUMIN (TRANSTHYRETIN)

JEAN A. HAMILTON, L.K. STEINRAUF, J. LIEPNIEKS AND M. BENSON
Departments of Biochemistry, Medicine, and Medical Genetics
Indiana University School of Medicine
Indianapolis
USA

and

G. HOLMGREN, O. SANDGREN AND L. STEEN
Departments of Clinical Genetics, Ophthalmology and Clinical Medicine
University of Umea
Sweden

ABSTRACT. The molecular structure of the Met-30 variant of human serum prealbumin (transthyretin) has been determined by x-ray crystallography to 2.3 A resolution. Refinement using XPLOR and the Konnert-Hendrickson constrained least-squares programs has now reached the crystallographic residual R = 23%. All 127 residues of both independent protein molecules are present, including low density for residues 1-9 and 124-127, which were not found by Blake, et al. in the structure of normal human prealbumin. At the present stage of refinement the two protein molecules in the crystallographic asymmetric unit are still constrained to obey a local 2-fold rotation axis. The mutated residue (30) is securely positioned in the interior of the molecule. In the vicinity of residue 30, the beta sheets have been shifted from 0.5 to 1.0 Angstroms in comparison to the structure of normal prealbumin and the size of the thyroxine binding site has been increased by about 0.8 A.

Introduction

Prealbumin (transthyretin) is a natural component of blood plasma, and the Met-30 variant has been shown to be involved in Type I familial amyloidotic polyneuropathy. Dwulet and Benson [1] have identified this variant in both plasma and in amyloid deposits of Type I individuals; for a review of this disease see Benson and Wallace, 1988 [2].

The crystal structure of normal plasma prealbumin was completed by Blake et al. [3]. The structure was found to have two protein molecules in the asymmetric unit, closely bonding together through extensive contacts of beta sheets, and being related by a non-crystallographic two-fold axis closely parallel to the crystallographic b axis. The tetramer is formed from the dimer by the true crystallographic two-fold axis with much less extensive contacts and with a cavity through the center. Each monomer consists of eight beta strands, connected by turns of 3-10 residues, and with two turns of alpha-helix between the E strand and the E-F turn, as may be seen in the diagram in Fig. 1. The site of thyroxine binding was found by Blake, et al. [4] to be between dimers in the central cavity, while it is presumed that the retinol-binding protein is associated with the exterior of the tetramer.

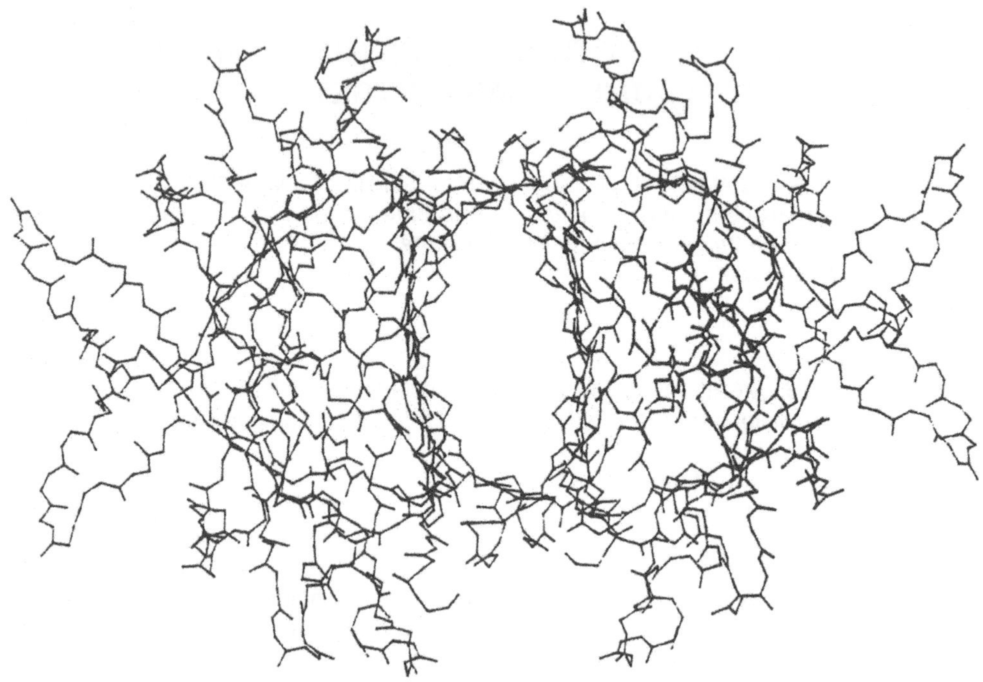

Fig. 1 A backbone plot of the tetramer of the Met-30 variant showing the hollow core which corresponds to the thyroxine-binding site in normal prealbumin.

Materials and Methods

Prealbumin (transthyretin) was isolated from the plasma of an individual homozygous for the methionine-30 variant associated with amyloidosis. Crystallization conditions were investigated by the hanging drop, vapor diffusion method. Optimal conditions were found to be 38-45% ammonium sulfate, 100 mmolar citrate buffer, pH 4.8 to 6.0. Two crystal forms, diamonds and needles, were observed. Diamonds suitable for x-ray diffraction analysis were grown from 43% ammonium sulfate at pH 5.3.

The space group was $P2_1 2_1 2$, with dimensions $\underline{a}$ = 44.07 $\underline{b}$ = 86.92 $\underline{c}$ = 65.90 A (normal prealbumin as given by Blake: $\underline{a}$ = 43.2 $\underline{b}$ = 85.3 $\underline{c}$ = 65.3 A), and the crystals diffracted to spacings beyond 2.0 A. Data to 2.3 A resolution were collected on the area detector at the Department of Biophysics, Johns Hopkins University, Baltimore to give 10,500 independent reflections.

The crystal structure of the Met-30 variant was found to be isomorphous to that of natural prealbumin as described by Blake, although there has been an obvious increase in volume of the unit cell by 4.9%. Structure factor calculation, based on the coordinates from Blake, gave an initial R value of 44% for the shell between 8.0 A and 4.0 A. A preliminary account has been previously published (5). Missing atoms and residues in Blake's structure were built using QUANTA (6) and refined using the XPLOR system of programs (7) to R = 26% for all data. Electron density maps were calculated and residues 1-10, 30, 38-40, 60-66, 98-104, and 123-127 were rebuilt using TOM (8) on the Silicon Graphics computer to give better agreement with the observed density. Refinement has been continued using the Konnert-Hendrickson constrained least-squares program (9), and the R value now stands at 23% for the 6.0 - 2.3 A data. All residues in both molecules of the asymmetric unit are now well behaved, except for the glycyl residues in the 1-8 segment and for residue 124.

Results

The differences between the structures of normal prealbumin and the Met-30 variant are not large but are very extensive. The changes may be described as global rather than local. Residue 30 is situated in the interior of the molecule, at the beginning of the B strand. The B strand is in antiparallel alignment with strands C and E, and there is extensive hydrogen bonding between the backbone carbonyl oxygen and amino hydrogen atoms. The side group of residue 30 makes contacts of 3.5 A or less with residues Val-14 of the A strand, Ser-46 of the C strand, Leu-55 of the D strand, and Ile-73 of the E strand.

Both protein molecules in the asymmetric unit have been shifted by 0.3 to 0.5 A in the negative x and negative y direction with respect to Blake's coordinates. These shifts cause the cavity of the tetramer to increase by about 1 A, resulting in what could be a less specific site for the binding of thyroxine. Recent studies have shown that the Met-30 variant is unable to bind thyroxine (Benson, Personal Communication).

The expansion of the tetramer has caused a decrease in the number of interactions for the dimer-dimer association, but not for the monomer-monomer association. The number of dimer-dimer contacts found from the coordinates of normal prealbumin is much more than those found in the Met-30 variant. However, the number for normal prealbumin is severely inflated because of many impossibly close contacts between neighboring protein molecules. A critical comparison will not be possible until the structure of normal prealbumin has been refined to the same extent as that of the Met-30 variant.

Each prealbumin molecule can be divided into four parts: interior, monomer-monomer interface, internal cavity surface, and exterior. Interior and interface residues have high electron density and have refined to low temperature factors. Interior surface residues have higher temperature factors but still very recognizable electron density, while exterior residues have still higher temperature factors and low electron density for the side chains. Residues 1-10 (pre-A strand), 39-40 (BC turn), 60-66 (DE turn), 98-104 (FG turn), and 123-127 (post-H strand) were either not found by Blake, et al., or have refined to positions 1-4 A away from the positions reported thereby.

We have found that residues 1-11 are not a continuous extension of the A strand and that residues 145-127 are not the continuous extension of the H strand. Residues Pro-11 and Pro-125 contribute to these breaks in continuity. Residues 1-11 are partly stabilized by an interaction of Lys-9 with Glu-61 and the peptide atoms of residue Val-123 is involved in hydrogen bonds in the continuation of the interaction of strand G with strand H. The sulfhydryl group of Cys-10 is probably making a weak hydrogen bond with His-31.

Acknowledgements

This research has been supported by an equipment grant from the Indianapolis Research Support Committee and a research grant from the Biomedical Research Committee of Indiana University School of Medicine. The authors wish to thank medical student Mark Albrechts for assistance with computer graphics.

References

1 Dwulet, F. E. and Benson, M. D. (1984) 'Primary Structure of an Amyloid Prealbumin and its Plasma Precursor in a Heredofamalial Polyneuropathy of Swedish Origin', Proc. Natl. Acad. Sci. USA, 81, 694-698.

2 Benson, M. D. and Wallace, M. R. (1988) in C. R. Scriver, A.L. Beaudet, W.S. Sly, W. and D. Valle (eds.) The Metabolic Basis of Inherited Disease, McGray-Hill Publishers, pp 3647-3681.

3 Blake, C. C. F., Geisow, M. J., Oatley, S. J, Rerat, E., and Rerat, C. (1978) 'Structure of Prealbumin, Secondary, Tertiary, and Quaternary Intreractions Determined by Fourier Refinement at 1.8 A', J. Mol. Biol., 121, 339-356.

4 Blake, C. C. F. and Oatley, S. J. (1977) 'Protein-DNA and Protein Hormone Interactions in Prealbumin: a Model of the Thyroid Hormone Nuclear Receptor' Nature (London), 268, 115-120.

5 Hamilton, J. A., Steinrauf, L. K., Liepnieks, J. J., Benson, M. D., Holmgren, G., Sandgren, O., and Steen, L. (1989) 'Crystallization and Preliminary X-Ray Structural Investigation of Variant Met-30 Prealbumin' Proceedings 1st Internat. Symp. on Familial Amyloidotic Polyneuropathy.

6 QUANTA: A Protein Modeling Software Package, Polygen Corporation, 200 Fifth Avenue, Waltham, Mass., 02154, USA.

7 XPLOR: Brunger, A. T., in N. W. Isaacs and M. R. Taylor (eds), Crystallographic Computing, 4, Techniques and New Technologies, Oxford University Press Publishers.

8 TOM: A Version of the Jones Electron Density Display Package, Christian Cambillau, L. C. C. M. B., Faculte Nord, Boulevard Pierre, Dramard, 13326 Marseille, France. Silicon Graphics Computer Systems, 200 North Shoreline Boulevard, Mountain View, Cal., 94043, USA.

9 Konnert, J. H. and Hendrickson, W. (1980) 'A Restrained-parameter Thermal-factor Fourier Refinement Procedure', Acta Cryst., A36, 344-350.

DISULFIDE BOND FORMATION OF TRANSTHYRETIN (TTR) AS POSSIBLE INITIAL STEP OF FAMILIAL AMYLOID POLYNEUROPATHY (FAP)

Shunsuke MIGITA, Miyako TAKEGAMI and Merrill D. BENSON*
Department of Molecular Immunology, Cancer Research Institute, Kanazawa University, Takara-machi, Kanazawa, 920, JAPAN: *Department of Medicine and Medical Genetics, Indiana Univ. School of Medicine, Indianapolis, Indiana, 46223, USA

ABSTRACT: FAP is a molecular disease due to a point mutation within the TTR gene. However, several amino acid substitutions of TTR have been reported as amyloidogenic. We examined seven different types of FAP sera by SDS- PAGE. The 77Tyr TTR tetramer is cleaved to a monomer form by pretreatment with 0.1 % of SDS, 30Met, 60Ala and 84Ser require 0.3 % SDS, 58His and 122Ile types require 0.4% SDS, while normal TTR is cleaved with 0.5 % SDS. The 122Ile homozygote type is more sensitive to SDS than the heterozygote type. This indicates that the tetramer binding forces are weaker in amyloidogenic TTR than the normal TTR. Newly formed disulfide bonds among TTR molecule was confirmed as a possible result of the weaker tetramer binding forces. This could be an initial step for amyloidogenesis in FAP.

INTRODUCTION

Amyloid is a regularly polymerized beta structural protein. Since we expected the TTR in FAP patient sera to polymerize more easily than normal, we used SDS-PAGE for the detection of these polymer. Previously we found a clear difference between normal and 30Met TTR with a selected condition of sample pretreatment(1). Then this method was expanded to other types of TTR to check whether the same differences can be observed or not.

MATERIALS AND METHODS

1. Materials: Seven different types of FAP TTR, heterozygote sera of 30Met, 58His, 60Ala, 77Tyr, 84Ser and homo- and heterozygote sera of 122Ile were obtained.
2. SDS-PAGE: Electrophoresis in gels containing SDS was performed as described by Laemmli(2). However, the protocol of sample pretreatment was modified. In the original method, the samples were diluted with pH 6.8 Tris HCl buffer containing 0.8 % SDS and 5 % 2-mercaptoethanol (2ME) and were heated for 3 min. at 100°C. We modified this protocol as

follows: 1) absence of 2ME and use of 0.1 % to 0.5 % SDS in the same buffer. 2) 5 min. heating at 90°C.

3. Western blotting: Fractions transferred electrophoretically on a nitrocellulose sheet were visualized with rabbit anti-human TTR(Behring Werke) and swine anti-rabbit IgG conjugated with peroxidase (Dako) as described previously(1). For the detection of retinol binding protein (RBP) or fibronectin(FBN), rabbit antisera to these proteins were used.

4. Diagonal SDS-PAGE: In order to confirm the presence of disulfide bond form of the protein, diagonal SDS-PAGE was performed(1).

RESULTS

1. Differences Between Normal and 7 Abnormal TTRs

Seven different FAP sera were tested under serial concentration of SDS in the pretreatment step. As shown in Fig.1, 77Tyr TTR was cleaved to a monomer form using concentration of SDS as low as 0.1%. 60Ala and 84Ser TTR were cleaved with 0.3 % of SDS like 30Met FAP. 58His and 122Ile are cleaved with 0.4 % SDS, while normal TTR is cleaved with 0.5 % SDS. 122Ile type homozygote serum was slightly more sensitive to SDS cleavage into the monomer form than was the 122Ile type heterozygote serum.

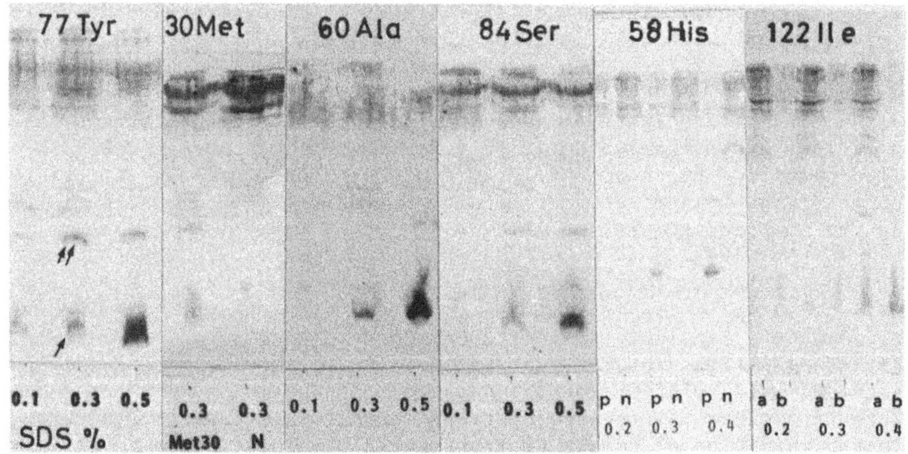

Fig. 1. Cleavage of TTR tetramer with 0.1 to 0.5 % of SDS shown by SDS PAGE. N or n:normal , p:58His, a:122Ile hetero, b:homozygote, arrow:monomer, 2 arrows:trimer, Note that amyloidogenic TTR are more easily cleaved at low SDS concentration than normal TTR.

2. Formation of Disulfide Bonds

When 30Met type of TTR was cleaved with 0.3 % SDS, we noticed the appearance of intermediate polymers of TTR, like dimer, trimer, tetramer and so on. Presence of disulfide bonds was analysed by diagonal SDS-PAGE. Almost all polymers changed to monomer after treatment with 2ME, indicating the presence of disulfide bonds between the monomer as shown in Fig. 2. In addition of this, faint spots remained on the diagonal line, revealing that a part of the polymer formation does not involve disufide bonds. After 0.3 % SDS treatment, sera were left at 4°C for 4 days, to allow the intermediate polymers to change in the more higher molecular weight polymer form. Most of these polymers were cleaved by 2ME, but not 10 % SDS treatment. This phenomenon occured in abnormal as well as normal TTR (Fig.3). Whether inhibition of disulfide bond formation inhibits TTR polymerization was examined with the disulfide bond inhibitors, iodoactic acid(IA) or L-penicillamine(LP). IA or LP were mixed with sample serum and treated with 0.3 % SDS and heat. TTR polymerization was inhibited proportionally with the concentration of IA or LP (Fig.4). These results indicate that the disulfide bonds are involved for the formation of higher molecular weight polymers of TTR.

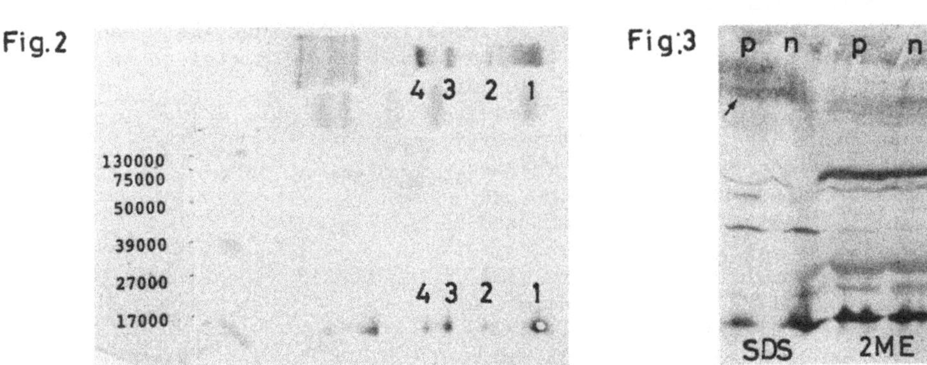

Fig. 2. Intermediate polymers (2, 3 and 4mer) produced from 30Met TTR by 0.3 % SDS are shown on the top row. Changing pattern of these to monomer by diagonal PAGE is shown.
Fig. 3. Higher molecular weight TTR polymers(arrow) produced in vitro (n:normal, p:30Met) are cleaved by 2ME, but not 10 % SDS, indicating that the polymers are formed by SS-bond.

3. Role of FBN or RBP for the Polymerization of TTR

In the process of TTR polymerization, other proteins like FBN or RBP may participate as constituent of amyloid fiber. Whether these proteins are involved in the formation of TTR polymer in vitro was examined by Western blotting using antisera against these proteins. The locations of these proteins within the gel depended upon their molecular weight and no association was observed between these proteins and TTR (Fig.5).

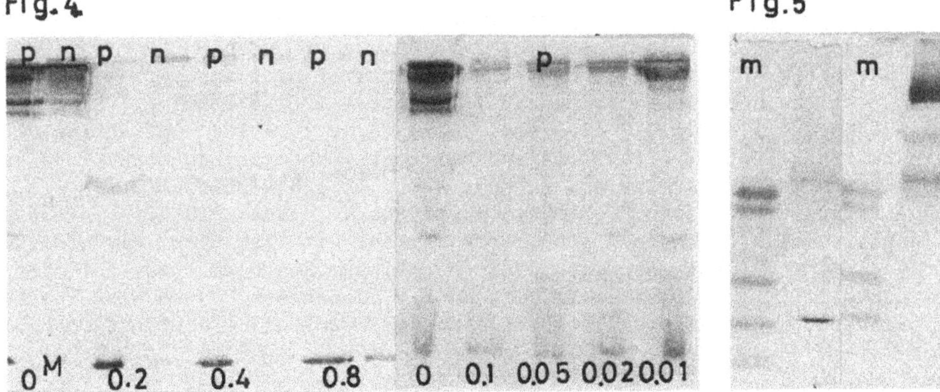

Fig. 4. L-penicillamine(left) and iodoacetic acid(right) inhibit polymer formation of TTR in proportion with the molar concentration indicated.
Fig. 5. Western blotting of anti-RBP(left) and anti-FBN(right) on SDS induced TTR polymer forming process. m:molecular weight marker. No association of TTR and RBP or FBN was find.

DISCUSSION

Why many types of amino acid substitution of TTR cause the same disease? SDS concentration required for tetramer cleavage was different according to the position of the amino acid substitution. However, all FAP TTR were cleaved at lower SDS concentration than the normal TTR. Since the tetramer formation is an essential character of TTR, many amino acids will more or less participate to the tetramer formation. One amino acid substitution may reduce the binding force of tetramer. TTR monomer has one free cystein in No.10 from the N terminal. However, strong noncovalent forces, such as 9 hydrogen bonds between 2 monomers, may inhibite the disulfide bridge formation. Distances between two sulphur atoms of Cys in the TTR tetramer could be calculated to AB 44.8, AC 5.3 and AD 44.7 Å, if each sulphur of tetramer is A, B, C and D(3). The distance should be within 2Å for disulfide bond and AC has a steric hindrance. Possible bindinding could occur at contact of another monomer arranged on the same axis (Fig.6). Whether amyloid fibril is a polymer of abnormal TTR alone or a mixed polymer of normal and abnormal TTR is controversial(4). We show here that even normal TTR can make higher molecular polymerform, suggesting that a normal TTR may change to cardiac or senile amyloid (5) by the same mechanism and as later onset.

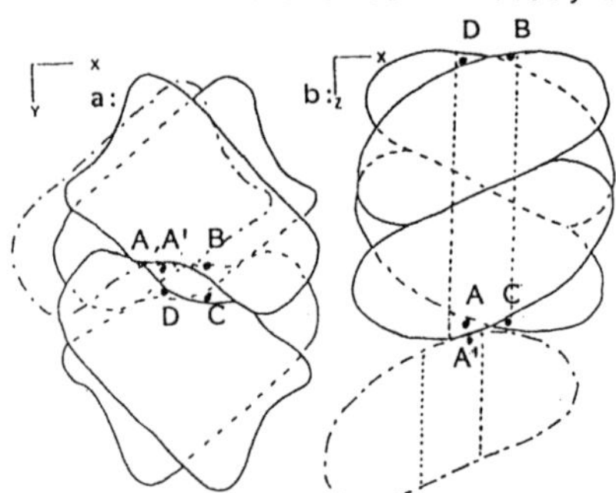

Fig.6. TTR pentamer by disulfide bond. a;from Z,b;from Y axis, A--D;S of Cys. (modified from Blake(3))

This in vitro experiments may differ from in vivo mechanism of amyloidogenesis. Since SDS is not present in vivo, however, the weaker binding forces of the tetramer may help to induce higher molecular movement and will induce disulfide bond between TTR monomer as a consequence.

REFERENCES

1) Migita,S.,Takegami,M.,Ikegawa,S.,Araki,S.,Nakashima,A.and Hamaguchi, K. (1989) 'A new simple screening method of the sera containing abnormal transthyretin by SDS-PAGE', 1st International FAP Symposium in Portugal in press

2) Laemmli,U.K. (1970) 'Cleavage of structural proteins during the assembly of the head of bactriophage T4', Nature 227, 680-685.

3) Blake,C.C., Geisow,M.J. and Oatley,S.J. (1978) 'Structrue of prealbumin: Secondary, tertiary and quaternary interaction determined by Fourier refinement at 1.8 A', J. Mol. Biol. 121, 330-356.

4) Tawara,S.,Nakazato,M.,Kangawa,K.,Matsuo,H. and Araki,S. (1983) 'Identification of amyloid prealbumin variant in familiar amyloidotic polyneuropathy (Japanese type)', Biochem.Biophy.Res.Comm. 116, 880-888

5) Conwell III,G.G.,Sletten,K.,Olfsson,B.O.,Johansson,B. and Westermark, P. (1987) 'Prealbumin; its association with amyloid'. J.Clin.Path. 40, 226-231

STRUCTURE OF TRANSTHYRETIN MOLECULES IN AMYLOID FIBRILLS FROM THE VITREOUS BODY IN INDIVIDUALS WITH THE MET30 MUTATION.

J. WAHLQUIST, C. THYLÉN, E. HÆTTNER, O. SANDGREN, G. HOLMGREN and LUNDGREN, E.
Inst. Cell Mol. Biol., Dept. Ophthalmology and Dept. Clin. Genetics, Univ. Umeå. S-901 85 Umeå, Sweden.

ABSTRACT. Amyloid fibrils were isolated from the vitreous body from a heterozygous and and a homozygous individual diagnosed as FAP I (transthyretin met-30) by RFLP. On SDS-PAGE the intact TTR monomer (17 kDa) as well as a dimer was seen. The dimer form was more prominent under nonreducing conditions. Two other bands were also found. The larger 14 kDa band was identified by protein sequencing to correspond to amino acids 49-127, possibly cleaved at a putative serine protease site between amino acids 48 and 49 (lys-thr). A smaller fragment containing a cystein group probably represents the 1-48 fragment or parts of it.

1. INTRODUCTION

Several point mutations of transthyretin (TTR) have been described, causing deposits of amyloid. (Review by Benson and Wallace, 1989). The substitution of methionine for valine in position 30 is typical of type 1 familial amyloidotic polyneuropathy (FAP) occurring in Japanese (Tawara et al., 83), Portuguese (Saraiva et al. 1984) and Swedish patients (Holmgren et al., 1988a).

The mechanism for fibril formation as a result of this amino acid substitution is not known. Some of the patients develop manifestations as vitreous opacities. Most of the patients are heterozygous as expected for an autosomal dominant trait, although among the Swedish patients several homozygous individuals have been found (Holmgren et al, 1988a, Sandgren et al, 1990). Saraiva et al. (1984) showed that the fibrils selectively accumulated the mutated protein. In this study, we have studied fibrils from the vitreous body from a homozygous and a heterozygous individual. TTR proteins dominated and a significant part of the material was truncated with a fragment starting at amino acid position 49. There was moreover an illegitimate intersubunit SS-bridge formed engaging the cystein at position 10.

2. MATERIALS AND METHODS

2.1. Clinical data

The patients examined had vitreous opacities of amyloid-like appearance and were treated surgically with pars plana vitrectomy. The TTR-met30 mutation was identified by RFLP analysis as previously described (Holmgren et al 1988 b).

2.2 Methods

The vitreous material was collected in 0.9 % NaCl following

vitrectomy and was stored frozen in 1 ml portions at -20 0 C. Upon thawing the fibrils were centrifuged (15.000 rpm, 25 min, 4 0 C) and dissolved in buffer (3M urea, 2.5 % SDS, 0.05 M Tris pH 6.8) and run on 20 % SDS polyacrylamide gels (SDS-PAGE) under reducing (0.1 M dithiotreitol) and non-reducing conditions. The samples were run in duplicate; one gel was used for silverstaining of the proteins (See and Jackowski, 1989) and one gel for immunoblotting . The primary antibody was rabbit antihuman TTR (DAKO, Denmark), and the secondary antibody was goat anti rabbit IgG horseradish peroxidase (Bio-rad, USA), developed with 4-chloro-1-naphol (Bio-Rad, USA).

For protein sequence analysis, the amyloid material was run on a 15% SDS-PAGE under reducing conditions, the proteins were transferred to a Immobilon PVDF membrane (Millipore, Bedford, Massachusetts, USA) and subjected to sequence analysis.

3. RESULTS

Figure 1A and B shows the results from SDS-PAGE and immunoblotting under reducing and non reducing conditions of the material from the two individuals, one heterozygous and the other homozygous. TTR from plasma was used as controls.

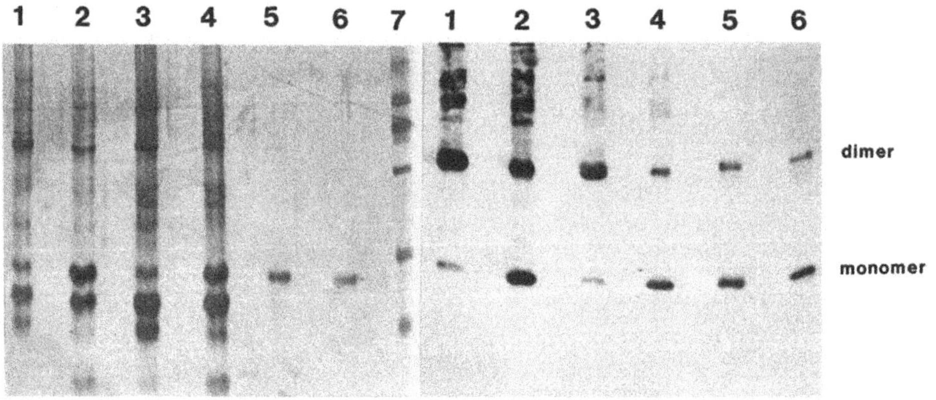

Figure 1A 20 % SDS-PAGE ,1B immunoblotting.
Lanes 1-4 Vitreous samples from individuals carrying the TTR met-30 mutation (1=heterozygous, non-reducing conditions, 2=heterozygous, reducing conditions, 3=homozygous, non-reducing conditions, 4=homozygous, reducing conditions, lane 5= molecular weight standards, proteins between 14.400 and 97.300 kDa (omitted in the gel for the immunoblotting), lane 6-7 =TTR from plasma (6=non-reducing conditions, 7= reducing conditions.

Under reducing conditions the TTR monomer identified by immunoblotting migrated as a 17 kDa protein. A second prominent band migrated as a 14 kDa protein, and it has only been showed to stain with the antihuman-TTR antibody in material purified by HPLC (data not shown).

For further identification protein sequence analysis was performed. The 14 kD band was found to be a fragment of TTR as the NH2-terminal amino acid corresponded to thr^{49} followed by 9 other amino acids in the published sequence (Kanda et al., 1974)). We also tried to sequence the 17 kDa protein which however failed due to end terminal blocking.

Under non reducing conditions we found the same bands as above of 14 and 17 kDa, however, with a decrease in the intensity of the 17 kDa band in the homozygous individual as compared to the heterozygous individual. The intensity of a band corresponding to the TTR dimer in size increased, which also was detected by the antibody.

Also a smaller fragment was seen, which shifted to a larger size mobility under non-reducing conditions. This fragment was more prominent from the homozygous material. As this peptide obviously contained a cystein it was interpreted to represent at least part of the 1-48 kDa fragment.

Identical results were obtained from studies on another homozygous and heterozygous individual (data not shown).

4. DISCUSSION

In this study we could take advantage of the presence of amyloid fibrils from the protein poor environment of the vitreous from an individual, which was homozygous with respect to the amino acid substitution at position 30 in TTR (type 1 FAP). We therefore had the unique opportunity to study pure mutated amyloid fibrils from homozygous individuals to which the normal, non-mutated protein did not contribute. Comparison was made with material from heterozygous individuals, carrying both mutated and non-mutated TTR.

We made two main findings; first, one disulphide-bond was detected as shown by differences in migration behaviour in SDS-PAGE under reducing and non-reducing conditions. The intact 17 kD monomer detectable under reducing conditions, showed less staining intensity under non-reducing conditions, and a band with the size of the TTR dimer was seen. The 14 KDa band (49-127 fragment) and the 1-48 fragment were most conspicuous in the homozygous individual, however, the same principal pattern was found in the heterozygous individual. As there is only one cystein (at position 10) per monomer, it must therefore be an illegitimate covalent bond between two subunits.

The second observation is a cleavage between the amino acids at positions 48 and 49, i.e. the peptide bond lys-thr, fitting with a serine protease cleavage site. The same finding has been described previously (Gorevic et al., 1987) in a patient without family history of amyloidosis, and the genotype of this individual is not known. Cornwell et al. (1988) and Westermark et al.(1990) also demonstrated other size fragments; in the TTR associated form of senile amyloidosis, peptides starting at postions 46 and 52 were detected. The presence of both the normal monomer, the 49-127 and the putative 1-48 peptide in a homozygous individual, is proof that the assumed proteolytic cleavage is not complete and suggests that the full size subunit in fibrills from heterozygous individuals is not just the presence of the non-mutated protein. The fact that the proteolytic cleavage also may occur in non-mutated TTR (Cornwall op.cit.) shows that the met-30 mutation is not a prerequisite for the proteolytic cleavage.

The finding of a covalent bond via a cysteinyl residue between subunits was described already by Felding et al. (1985). Our study shows that this really occurs between mutated proteins, and also exist in the smaller putative 1-48 fragment. This was seen by the mobility shift of the 1-48 fragment under non-reducing conditions and more strongly in the homozygous individual, where the protein with the size of the normal dimer was weakly staining, and there was a shift in mobility of the assumed 1-48 fragment.

The interesting possibility that the fibrill formation is facilitated by iuxtaposition of two cysteins as a result of change in structure due to the amino acid substitution can be experimentally tested. The protease cleavage can obviously affect both normal and mutated protein, and might be a secondary phenomenon. However, as it has been repeatedly seen in amyloid fibrills, its role in fibrill formation requires further studies.

5. ACKNOWLEDGEMENTS

This study was supported by grants from the Swedish Medical Society, the patient organization FAMY and FAP Medical Research AB.

6. REFERENCES

Benson, M. and Wallace, M. R. 1989. In The Metabolic Basis of inherited Disease, pp 2439-2460. Mc Graw Hill Book Co, New York, USA.

Costa P. P., A. S. Figura, F. R., Proc Natl Acad Sci USA 75, 4499-4503.

Holmgren G., E. Haettner, I. Nordensson, O. Sandgren, L. Steen, E. Lundgren (1988a), Clin Genet 34, 333-338.

Holmgren G., Holmberg, E., Lindström, A, Lindström, E, Nordenson I., Sandgren, O, Svenson, B., Lundgren, E. and von Gabain, A. (1988b). Clin. Gen. 32, 289-294.

Gorevic P. D., M. M. Rodrigues, W. H. Spencer, P. C.Munoz, A. W. Allen, A. Z. Verne (1987), Ophthalmol. 94, 792-798.

Cornwell III G. G., K. Sletten, B. Johansson, P. Westermark (1988), Bioch Biophys Res Commun. 154, 648-653.

Felding P., G. Fex, P. Westermark, B. O. Olofsson, P. Pitkänen, L. Benson (1985), Scand J Immunol. 21, 133-140.

Kanda, Y., de Witt, G, Canfield, R. E. and Morgan, F. J.(1974), J Biol Chem, 249, 6796-6805.

Saraiva M. J. M., S. Birken, P. P. Costa, D. S. Goodman (1984), J Clin Invest. 74, 104-119.

Sandgren,O., Holgren, G. and Lundgren, E. (1990), Arch. Opthalmol. In press.

See, Y. P. and Jackowski, G (1989), In Protein Structure,Ed. By T E Creighton , IRL Press London.

Tawara , S. Nakazato, M., Kangawa, K., Matsuo and Araki, S. (1983),Bioch. Biophys. Res. Com. 116, 880-883.

Westermark, P., Sletten, K., Johansson, B. and Cornwell III, (1990), Proc. Natl. Acad. Sci., USA 87, 2843-2845.

FORMATION OF FIBRILS BY NORMAL TRANSTHYRETIN AND SYNTHETIC TRANSTHYRETIN FRAGMENTS *IN VITRO*.

Å. Gustavsson, U. Engström, and P. Westermark
Department of Pathology I, University of Linköping, S-581 85 Linköping and Ludwig Institute of Cancer Research , Uppsala Branch, Uppsala, Sweden

Abstract

In both senile systemic amyloidosis and familial amyloidotic polyneuropathy the amyloid fibrils are made up by full-length transthyretin (TTR) as well as fragments of the molecule. It has been demonstrated that other amyloid fibril proteins, e.g. atrial natriuretic factor and islet amyloid polypeptide can form amyloid-like fibrils *in vitro*. In the present study we have used both normal TTR, purified from plasma, and synthetic polypeptides, corresponding to segments of TTR. We show that normal TTR and two of the studied synthetic TTR segments easily form amyloid-like fibrils *in vitro*.

Introduction

Senile systemic amyloidosis (SSA) and familial amyloidotic polyneuropathy (FAP) are two forms of amyloidosis in which the amyloid fibrils consist of transthyretin (TTR) (Sletten *et al.*, 1980, Costa *et al.*, 1978, Tawara *et al.*, 1983). The fibrils are built up by a mixture of full-length TTR and fragments of TTR (Felding *et al.*, 1985, Westermark *et al.*, 1987).

In FAP there is often an amino acid substitution in the TTR molecule, e.g. methionine for valine at position 30, as in the Swedish form (Dwulet and Benson, 1984), whereas in SSA there has only been found normal TTR in the amyloid fibrils (Cornwell *et al.*, 1988, Westermark *et al.*, 1990). An intermolecular ß-sheet conformation seems to be of importance in the formation of amyloid fibrils (Glenner, 1980), but nothing is known at present about the exact mechanism of fibrillogenesis.

It has previously been demonstrated that some amyloid fibril proteins e.g. islet amyloid polypeptide and atrial natriuretic factor form amyloid-like fibrils *in vitro* (Johansson and Westermark, 1990). The aim of the present study was to investigate if normal transthyretin and synthetic polypeptides, corresponding to different parts of the TTR molecule, form amyloid-like fibrils *in vitro*.

Materials and methods

In the present study we used normal transthyretin, purified from human plasma using an affinity column containing retinol binding protein.

Polypeptides were synthesized by automatic solid phase synthesis on an Applied Biosystems model 430 A peptide synthesizer (Applied Biosystems, Foster City, CA). Each peptide represented an 11 residues long segment of the transthyretin molecule. The sequences of the peptides are shown in Fig 1. In the tertiary structure of transthyretin ß-sheet strands A and G are homologous with peptide 175 and 177, respectively. Peptide 176 contains the very short ß-strand D flanked by two and five residues.

TTR 10 - - - - - - - - - - 20
Peptide 175 Cys-Pro-Leu-Met-Val-Lys-Val-Leu-Asp-Ala-Val-NH_2

TTR 50 - - - - - - - - - - 60
Peptide 176 Ser-Glu-Ser-Gly-Glu-Leu-His-Gly-Leu-Thr-Thr-NH_2

TTR 105 - - - - - - - - - - 115
Peptide 177 Tyr-Thr-Ile-Ala-Ala-Leu-Leu-Ser-Pro-Tyr-Ser-NH_2

Figure 1. Amino acid sequences of the three synthetic polypeptides 175, 176 and 177. The corresponding segment of the transthyretin amino acid sequence is indicated above.

Transthyretin and synthetic peptides were dissolved in 10% acetic acid in a concentration of 10 mg/ml. After one night at room temperature the samples were neutralized with ammonia to pH 7. Both before and after neutralization aliquots were removed, placed on formvar coated coppergrids and negatively stained with 2% uranyl acetate. The amount of fibril formation was determined by electron microscopy in a JEOL 100 S-X TEM microscope.

Samples were also stained with Congo red and examined in a Zeiss polarization light microscope.

Results

When normal TTR was dissolved in acetic acid, fine nonbranching fibrils occurred spontaneously (Fig. 2). These fibrils, although curvy, resembled native amyloid fibrils. In the same way, peptide 175 gave massive fibril formation (Fig. 3). When peptide 177 was studied, massive

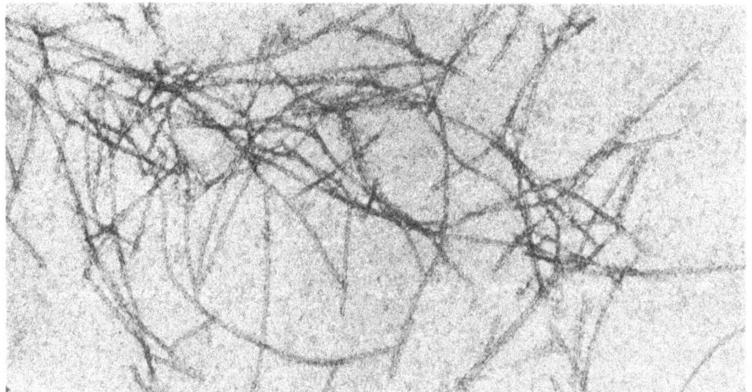

Figure 2. Electronmicrograph of fibrils formed by normal TTR.

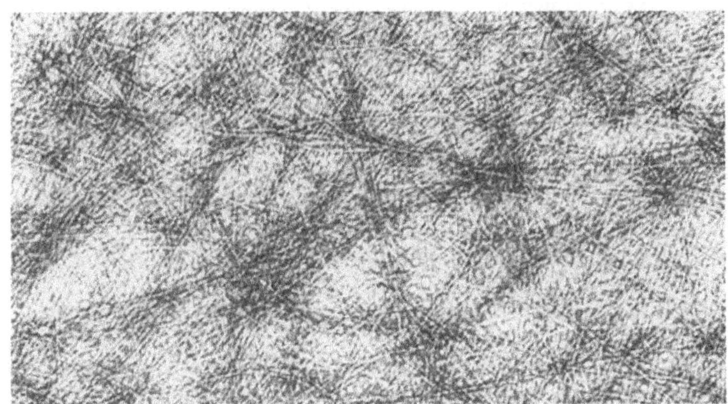

Figure 3. Electronmicrograph of fibrils formed by peptide 175, corresponding to amino residues 10-20 in the TTR amino acid sequence.

fibril formation occurred only after neutralization. In contrast, peptide 176 was not fibrillogenic in the system used here.

Fibrils formed from both 175 and 177 had affinity for Congo red and exhibited green birefringence in polarized light.

Discussion

There is increasing evidence that almost any amino acid substitution occurring in the TTR molecule can give rise to amyloid fibril formation *in vivo* (Dwulet and Benson, 1986, Pras *et al.*, 1983, Saraiva *et al.*, 1984, Wallace *et al.*, 1986). It is therefore of interest, as shown here, that TTR, purified from normal human plasma, can easily be converted to amyloid-like fibrils *in vitro*. However, it has also been shown that TTR without any substitution is involved in the amyloid formation in SSA, which is the most common TTR-derived amyloid form (Westermark *et al.*, 1990). How this fibril formation occurs is unknown but the finding that the peptides corresponding to the two ß-strands A and G were fibrillogenic *in vitro* supports the view that one or several of the ß-strands in TTR are involved in amyloid fibril formation.

Acknowledgements

This work was supported by the Swedish Medical Research Council and the Research Fund of King Gustaf V.

References

Cornwell III, G. G., Sletten, K., Johansson, B. and Westermark, P. (1988) 'Evidence that the amyloid fibril protein in senile systemic amyloidosis is derived from normal prealbumin', Biochem. Biophys. Res. Commun. 154, 648-653.

Costa, P. P., Figueiras, A. S. and Bravo, F. R. (1978) 'Amyloid fibril protein related to prealbumin in familial amyloidotic polyneuropathy', Proc. Natl. Acad. Sci. USA 75, 4499-4503.

Dwulet, F. E. and Benson, M. D. (1984) 'Primary structure of an amyloid prealbumin and its plasma precursor in a heredofamilial polyneuropathy of Swedish origin', Proc. Natl. Acad. Sci. USA 81, 694-698.

Dwulet, F. E. and Benson, M. D. (1986) 'Characterization of a transthyretin (prealbumin) variant associated with familial amyloidotic polyneuropathy type II (Indiana/Swiss)', J. Clin. Invest. 78, 880-886.

Felding, P., Fex, G., Westermark, P., Olofsson, B.-O., Pitkänen, P. and Benson, L. (1985) 'Prealbumin in Swedish patients with senile systemic amyloidosis and familial amyloidotic polyneuropathy', Scand. J. Immunol. 21, 133-140.

Glenner, G. G. (1980) 'Amyloid deposits and amyloidosis. The ß-fibrilloses', N. Engl. J. Med. 302, 1283-1292.

Johansson, B and Westermark, P. (1990) 'The relation of atrial natriuretic factor to isolated atrial amyloid', Exp. Mol. Path. 52, 266-278.

Pras, M., Prelli, F., Franklin, E. C. and Frangione, B. (1983) 'Primary structure of an amyloid prealbumin variant in familial polyneuropathy of Jewish origin' Proc. Natl. Acad. Sci. USA 80, 539-542.

Saraiva, M. J. M., Birken, S., Costa, P. P. and Goodman, D. S. (1984) 'Amyloid fibril protein in familial amyloidotic polyneuropathy, Portuguese type' J. Clin. Invest. 74, 104-119.

Sletten, K., Westermark, P. and Natvig, J. B. (1980) 'Senile cardiac amyloid is related to prealbumin' Scand. J. Immunol. 12, 503-506.

Tawara, M., Nakazoto, M. K., Kangawa, K., Matsuo, H. and Araki, S. (1983) 'Identification of amyloid prealbumin variant in familial amyloidotic polyneuropathy (Japanese type)' Biochem. Biophys. Res. Comun. 116, 880-888.

Wallace, M. R., Dwulet, F. E., Conneally, P. M. and Benson, M. D. (1986) 'Biochemical and molecular genetic characterization of a new variant prealbumin associated with hereditary amyloidosis' J. Clin. Invest. 78, 6-12.

Westermark, P., Sletten, K. and Olofsson, B.-O. (1987) 'Prealbumin variants in the amyloid fibrils of Swedish familial amyloidotic polyneuropathy', Clin. exp. Immunol. 69, 695-701.

Westermark, P., Sletten, K., Johansson, B. and Cornwell III, G. G. (1990) 'Fibril in senile systemic amyloidosis is derived from normal transthyretin', Proc. Natl. Acad.Sci. USA 87, 2843-2845.

FIRST TURKISH FAMILY WITH FAP HAS HOMOZYGOUS MET 30 TTR

Eren Erken *
Martha Skinner **
Hasan Yazici +
Hulya Dede +
Alan S. Cohen **
Aubrey Milunsky #
James C. Skare #

From the * Department of Medicine, Cukurova University, Adana, Turkey, + the Division of Rheumatology, Cerrahpasa Medical Faculty, Istanbul, Turkey, and the ** Arthritis Center and Department of Medicine,the # Center for Human Genetics and Departments of Pediatrics and Microbiology, Boston University School of Medicine, Boston, MA 02118 USA.

ABSTRACT

The first family of Turkish origin with typical familial amyloidotic polyneuropathy type I was studied. Two symptomatic brothers were found to be homozygous for the met 30 mutation of transthyretin (TTR) by examination of their TTR genes using polymerase chain reaction. Both brothers developed symptoms in the sixth decade of life and no family history of FAP was present.

INTRODUCTION

Familial amyloidotic polyneuropathy (FAP) has been reported in families of many ethnic origins and has been shown to be caused by a number of specific point mutations in the transthyretin (TTR) molecule. The disease is inherited in an autosomal dominant manner with symptoms occuring during adulthood and fairly consistent patterns within kinships.

We examined the first family of Turkish origin with symptoms of FAP and found them to be homozygous for the most common FAP TTR mutation, met 30 (Skare, et al 1990).

MATERIALS AND METHODS

Clinical Material

The pedigree of the Turkish family can be seen in Figure 1 and the clinical data of the two affected family members can be seen in Table 1. The rectal biopsies on these individuals were positive for amyloid by Congo red staining. The amyloid deposits reacted with antibody to TTR on immunohistochemical staining.

Blood was obtained and DNA extracted from the two affected brothers II-3 and II-7, another brother II-1, and two sons of one of the affected III-10, III-11.

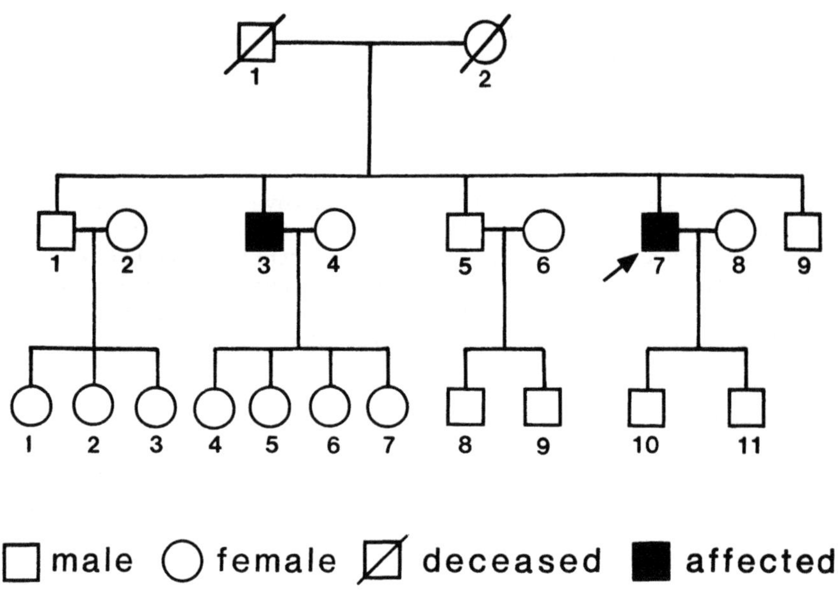

Figure 1 Pedigree of a Turkish family with FAP

Exon 2 of the TTR DNA was amplified by polymerase chain rection (PCR) as previously described (2). After amplification the DNA was digested with Nsi I and the products electrophoresed on 6% polyacrylamide and stained with ethidium bromide.

Table I Turkish Family with Familial Amyloidotic Polyneuropathy

Pedigree	Onset Age	Symptoms	Biopsy	Duration
II-3	51	neuropathy, cardiomyopathy	rectal	alive at age 61
II-7	51	vitreous opacities, sensory neuropathy, cardiomyopathy	rectal vitreous	alive at age 55

RESULTS

Nsi I did not cut the DNA from II-1, but gave only a 219 bp product as expected with normal TTR. In contrast, Nsi I completely cut the DNA from II-3 and II-7 giving fragments of 101 bp and 114 bp plus 4 base tails. Both FAP patients (II-3 and II-7) are therefore homozygous for the met 30 mutation. That is, neither of their two TTR genes are normal. As expected, both sons of II-7 are heterozygous with one normal TTR gene and one met 30 TTR gene.

The same conclusions were obtained when the family was examined using blot hybridization. Equivalent amounts of DNA from the individuals resulted in equivalent hybridization signals, so the PCR data cannot be the result of deletion of the TTR gene from one of the patient's chromosomes 18. Two copies of the met 30 TTR gene are present in each cell.

DISCUSSION

This is the first report of Turkish individuals with FAP, and the second report of individuals who are homozygous for met 30 transthyretin. Holmgren et al reported a Swedish brother and sister homozygous for the met 30 mutation (3). One developed symptoms in the sixth decade, the other was in the seventh decade and still asymptomatic. Some Swedish individuals with met 30 TTR have lived to be 80 years old without developing symptoms. The later age of onset explains why a large percentage of Swedish FAP patients had no family history of disease (4,5).

It is interesting that the first FAP patients to be identified in Turkey are homozygotes. The parents of the two affected brothers died at ages 75 and 84 years old. Although they must have been heterozygotes to have a child with two normal TTR genes and children with two met 30 TTR genes, they showed no symptoms of FAP. All four of the patient's grandparents lived in excess of 75 years and showed no symptoms.

It has been estimated that about 3% of the population in a region of Sweden are met 30 heterozygotes (Holmgren 1988). Given the fact that two heterozygotes married in this family, a high frequency of nonpathogenic met 30 mutations might also exist in regions of Turkey.

Acknowledgements

Supported by grants from NIH CA-49629, AM-07014, AM-20613, RR533 and the Arthritis Foundation.

REFERENCES

1. Skare JC, Yazici H, Erken E, Dede H, Cohen AS, Milunsky A, Skinner M: Homozygosity for the met 30 transthyretin gene in a Turkish kindred with familial amyloidotic polyneuropathy. Human Genetics (in press) 1990.
2. Skare JC, Milunsky JM, Milunsky A, Skare IB, Cohen AS, Skinner M: A new transthyretin variant from a patient with familial amyloidotic polyneuropathy has asparagine substituted for histidine at position 90. Clinical Genetics (in press) 1990.
3. Holmgren G, Haettner E, Nordenson I, Sandgren O, Steen L, Lundgren E: Homozygosity for the transthyretin-met30-gene in two Swedish sibs with familial amyloidtic polyneuropathy. Clin Genet 34:333-338, 1988.
4. Holmgren G, Lindstrom A, Nordenson I, Sandgren O, Steen L, Svensson B, Lundgen E: Familial amyloidotic polyneuropathy in Sweden--RFLP analysis in patients and in healthy controls. In Amyloid and Amyloidosis. T. Isobe (ed), N.Y. Plenum Press 387-392, 1988.
5. Sandgren O, Holmgren G, Lundgren E, Steen L: RFLP analysis of mutated transthyretin in vitreous amyloidosis. In Amyloid and Amyloidosis. T. Isobe (ed), N.Y. Plenum Press 383-386, 1988.

A NEW TRANSTHYRETIN VARIANT ASSOCIATED WITH FAMILIAL AMYLOIDOTIC POLYNEUROPATHY IN AN ITALIAN KINDRED

Maria do Rosário Almeida[1,2], MaryAnn Gawinowicz[3], Pedro P. Costa[1], Fabrizio Salvi[4], Alessandra Ferlini[4], Rosaria Plasmati[4], Carlo Tassinari[4], Maria João Saraiva[1,2]

[1]Centro de Estudos de Paramiloidose, [2]Instituto de Ciências Biomédicas 4000 Porto, Portugal; [3]Dep. of Med., College of Physicians and Surgeons of Columbia University, New York; [4]Instituto di Clinica Neurologica, University of Bologna, Bologna, Italy.

ABSTRACT. A TTR neutral variant was described in an Italian kindred studied by isoelectric foccusing. Clinically, the affected individuals presented cardiomiopathy in addition to neuropathy. Peptide mapping and sequencing of plasma TTR revealed an alanine for threonine substitution at position 49. This substitution explained by a G for A change was detected by hybridization with ASO probes. From the eleven individuals of the kindred studied six were carriers of the mutation, all of them heterozygous.

INTRODUCTION

Different TTR variants have been associated with the hereditary amyloidoses. In most of them polyneuropathy is the main clinical feature but differences in clinical expression and age of onset is found among them.

The characterization of these variants will be very important to elucidate the structure of mutant proteins and other possible factors involved in amyloidogenesis.

In this context, we studied a neutral TTR variant previously detected by isoelectric foccusing (IEF) (Saraiva et al. 1988) in an Italian kindred with familial amyloidotic polyneuropathy (FAP) and cardiomyopathy with onset in the 5th decade.

The genetic defect was determined by analysis of the primary structure of the protein by tryptic peptide mapping of the isolated plasma TTR and the predicted mutation at DNA level was confirmed by allele specific oligonucleotides (ASO) hybridization.

MATERIAL AND METHODS

SUBJECTS: Plasma was obtained from a patient with FAP onset on the 5th decade. Clinically he had amyloid deposition in the vitreous, preceeding by several years the clinical manifestations of neuropathy and by a more pronounced cardiac involvement leading to death by heart failure. His sister presented a similar clinical picture. Blood was also available from 9 asymptomatic offspring from these two patients.

PEPTIDE MAPPING AND SEQUENCE ANALYSIS: comparative tryptic peptide mapping of the patient's plasma TTR and normal TTR was performed by HPLC under similar conditions described previously (Saraiva et al., 1984). Abnormal peptides were collected and sequenced on an Applied Biosystems model 470A gas-phase sequencer.

DNA AMPLIFICATION: exon 3 of the TTR gene was amplified by the polymerase chain reaction (PCR) using the method of Saiki et al. (1985) with appropriate flanking primers for the region of interest. This resulted in the amplification of a piece of DNA of 247 bp. The conditions of amplification were as previously described (Almeida et al. 1990).

ASO HYBRIDIZATION: one third of the amplification mixture was denatured with NaOH, neutralized and dotted onto a Zeta probe membrane (Bio-Rad). The ASO probes employed were: normal (Thr 49) - 5'TATAGGAAAACCAGTGAGT3' and mutant (Ala 49) - 5'ACTCACTGGCTTTCCTATA3'. The probes were labeled by the T4 kinase reaction for 30 min at 37ºC. Hybridization with ASO probes was carried out at 30ºC, followed by washes under highly stringent conditions at 55ºC The blots were then exposed to X-ray film 2-4 h.

RESULTS

TTR was isolated from plasma of a patient with a TTR neutral variant (by IEF) and studied by tryptic peptide mapping. Comparison of peptide mapping of isolated plasma TTR from the propositus and normal plasma TTR revealed an abnormal peptide peak eluting in a posiion close to the normal peptide 7 (residues 49-70). Sequencing of this peptide showed an alanine for threonine substitution at position 49 (fig.1). This substitution could be explained by a G for A change in the codon of threonine (Thr(ACC) - Ala(GCC)) (fig. 1).

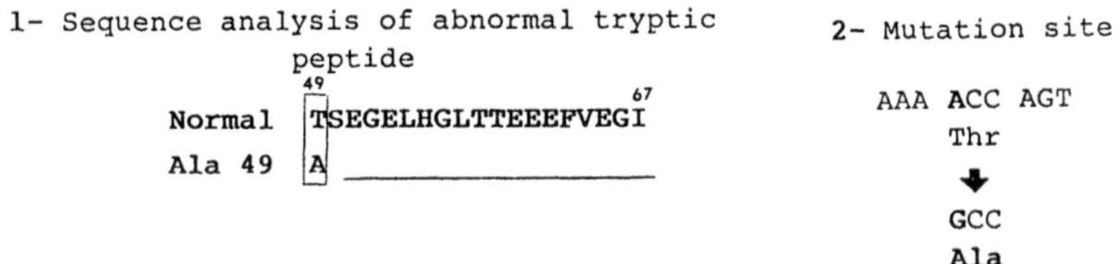

Fig. 1 - Schematic representation of TTR Ala 49 mutation at protein and DNA level.

Since this mutation does not create or abolish any restriction site for endonucleases, we amplified exon 3 of the TTR gene followed by hybridization with ASO probes. We analysed eleven individuals from the same kindred including the propositus. Only two of these individuals were symptomatic. The temperature of washing found to be selective for normal and mutant ASO probes was 55ºC. Six individuals were found to be carriers of the mutation since their amplified DNA hybridized with the normal and mutant ASO probes. Therefore these individuals were all heterozygous for this mutation. As controls we used amplified DNA from a normal individual and amplified cDNA, that hybridized only with the normal ASO probe as expected (fig. 2).

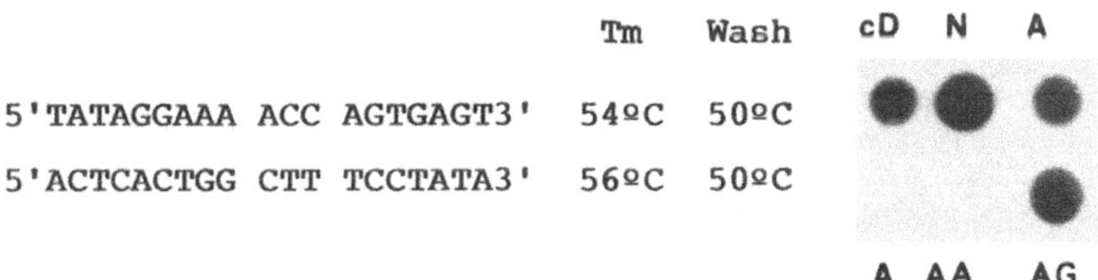

Fig. 2 - Hybridization with allele specific oligonucleotides (ASO) probes. cD means normal TTR cDNA, N DNA from a normal individual and Ala DNA from a carrier of Ala 49 mutation.

CONCLUSIONS

A new TTR variant (TTR Ala 49) was described associated with FAP in an Italian kindred. The deposition of amyloid began in the vitreous and preceeded several years the manifestations of neuropathy. There is also cardiomyopathy leading to death by heart failure.

Another mutation at position 49 and latter assessed to be Ile 33 has been described (Nakazato et al. 1984).

As there were some clinical similarities with Ile 33 we searched for this mutation in the Italian individuals where it was absent (data not shown). Furthermore there are also some clinical differences namely the late age of onset.

It is also interesting to note that position 49 on TTR seems to be related to sites of proteolysis suggesting this position can be important on amyloidogenesis.

Since the substitution originating TTR Ala 49 is explained by a point mutation we performed its detection by ASO hybridization making possible the screening of TTR Ala 49 in other FAP Italian families.

ACKNOWLEDGEMENTS

This work was supported by grant RO1NS25190 from U.S. National Institutes of Health.

REFERENCES

Almeida MR, Alves IL, Sakaki Y, Costa PP, Saraiva MJM. (1990)Prenatal diagnosis of familial amyloidotic polyneuropathy: evidence for an early expression of the associated transthyretin methionine 30. Hum Gen. In press.

Nakazato M, Kangawa K, Minamino N, Tawara S, Matsuo H, Araki S. (1984) Revised analysis of aminoacid replacement in a prealbumin variant (Sko-III) associated familial amyloidotic polyneuropathy of Jewish origin. Biochem Biophys Res Commun 123:921-928.

Saiki RK, Scharf S, Faloona F, Mullis KB, Horn GT, Erlich HA, Arnheim N. (1985) Enzymatic amplification of b-globin genomic sequences and restriction site analysis for diagnosis of sikle cell anemia. Science 230:1350-1354.

Saraiva MJM, Birken S, Costa PP, Goodman DS. (1984). Amyloid fibril protein in familial amyloidotic polyneuropathy, Portuguese type. Definition of molecular abnormality in transthyretin (prealbumin). J Clin Invest 74:104-119.

Saraiva MJM, Costa PP, Almeida MR, Banzhoff A, Altland K, Ferlini A, Rubboli G, Plasmati R, Tassinari CA, Romeo G, Salvi F. (1988) Familial amyloidotic polyneuropathy: transthyretin (prealbumin) variants in kindreds of Italian origin. Hum Genet 80:341-343.

CLINICAL CHARACTERIZATION OF A NEW TTR VARIANT IN AN ITALIAN FAMILY: TTR ALA 49

F. SALVI , R. PLASMATI , R. MICHELUCCI , P. ZONARI,
A. FERLINI*, MR. ALMEIDA**, P.P. COSTA**, M.J. M. SARAIVA**,
C. RAPEZZI°, R. MENCUCCI °°, C.A.TASSINARI.

Institute of Neurology , University of Bologna, Italy
*Istituto di Istologia e Anatomia Umana Normale, University of Modena ,Italy.
**Centro de Estudos de Paramiloidose ,Porto , Portugal .
°Department of Cardiology , S. Orsola Hospital , Bologna , Italy.
°°Institute of Ophthalmology , University of Florence, Italy.

ABSTRACT. We describe the peculiar association among eye ,heart, peripheral nervous system involvement in an Italian late onset FAP family with 49 substitution (THR → ALA) in TTR molecule .
Footplates attached to the posterior surface of the lens are the first clinical signs of the disease appearing many years before the onset of the polyneuropathy .
Polyneuropathy is clinically and electrophysiologically undistinguishable from that occurring in TTR MET 30 patients.
Chronical heart failure due to heavy amyloid deposits within the cardiac walls is responsible for death .

INTRODUCTION. In a collaborative research among the University of Bologna and Modena , the Centro de Estudos de Paramiloidose , and the University of Giessen (Federal Republic of Germany) 2 TTR mutations have been found in Italy through the HIEF tecnique planned by Klaus Altland (Institute of Human Genetics, University of Giessen).(Saraiva et al. 1988) One of this TTR variants has been related to an abnormal transthyretin with a single aminoacid substitution at position 49(ALA for THR).(Almeida et al.,this issue).

In order to correlate clinical and biological findings we studied three patients and six carriers of this abnormal protein. Strict criteria were adopted for the clinical characterization of this FAP variant, thus avoiding any possibility of error : common clinical features in at least three patients , a long clinical follow-up ,and the absence of the same disturbances in other members of the family not TTR ALA 49 carrier.

CASE REPORT.

CASE 1. male, dead at the age of 49 in 1987. At 40 visual acuity was decreased in both eyes without benefit with lens correction.

At 41 cold sensation and intermittent paresthesiae were present in the lower limbs with mild weakness in the legs and both diurnal and nocturnal cramp pain . At 44 the clinical features were that of a mixed polyneuropathy with autonomic disorders. An EKG revealed diffuse T waves inversion with abnormal Q-T prolongation . At 46 considerable worsening of the polyneuropathy. Chest X-ray showed enlarged heart size; echocardiography was compatible with the diagnosis of cardiac amyloidosis. Fundus examination revealed an unclear vitreous with "possible membranes" in the posterior pole of both eyes.At 48 he had several episodes of orthostatic hypotension with dizziness and syncope when standing . A pretibial edema appeared bilaterally . Vision was poor in both eyes . At 49 he was bedridden ,blind , anorexic with dyspnea and widespread edema . On november 1987 he died of intractable heart failure.

CASE 2. Female , 54 yrs. At 48 black specks floating before the left eye were the first visual complains. They increased in size over the time till vitrectomy was performed at 49; visual acuity was very poor in that eye due to vitreous opacities . At 49 a diagnosis of restless legs sindrome was made . After a few months paresthesiae in the feet were the onset symptoms of the polyneuropathy . At 51 an echocardiography revealed enlarged walls with increased refractile pattern;an EKG showed T waves inversion . At 52 she had a sensory-motor polyneuropathy affecting upper and lower limbs with dysautonomic disturbances. At 53 a pretibial edema was evident .

CASE 3. Female ,55yrs. At 47 she complained a slow progressive decrease of vision in both eyes. Slit-lamp examination showed numerous small white dots attached to the posterior surface of the lens. She was submitted to vitrectomy in the left eye . During the surgery it was possible to localize two main areas of deposit :retrolenticular and in front. of the retina of the posterior pole . At 50 she had insomnia caused by restless legs syndrome . At 52 paresthesiae and dysesthesiae appeared in the lower limbs. Neurological examination revealed sensory deficits mainly in the lower limbs. At 53 an echocardiography showed an abnormal increased in the left and right ventricular wall thickness.

CARDIAC EVALUATION OF THE THREE PATIENTS.

EKG: anteroseptal pseudoinfarctional pattern with diffuse T waves inversion with abnormal Q-T prolongation . Echocardiography: abnormal increase in the left and right ventricular wall thickness with " granular sparkling" of ventricular myocardium and normal systolic function. No obvious signs of restrictive physiopathology . Final cardiologic diagnosis: myocardial disease with normal systolic function and absence or mild diastolic dysfunction.

OCULAR FINDINGS.

Slit -lamp examination ; "star sky" appearance of the vitreous body due to small white dots attached to the posterior lens surface(pseudopodia lentis). The amyloid meshwork is visible in periphery. Ocular echography: irregular strand-like echoes in the vitreus, forming a sheet-like membranes extending from the posterior pole towards the lens.

NEUROLOGICAL EXAMINATION.

In all the patients a pseudosyringomyelic dissociated sensory loss appeared in the lower limbs. The progression of the polyneuropathy is clinically undistinguishable from the TTR MET 30 one.

DISCUSSION.

In order to fill the gap sometimes present among biochemical, molecular and clinical findings we tried to delineate the major clinical aspects present in patients affected by TTR ALA 49 Familial Amyloidotic Polyneuropathy. A peculiar triad of symptoms is present in all the patients with a full clinical picture .

According to the litterature vitreous opacities are heterogeneus clinical entities in Familial Amyloidosis. Ocular findings in TTR ALA 49 FAP resemble previous descriptions of vitreous opacities made by IRVINE A.R. (1976), KAUFFMAN H.E. (1959),HITCHING R.A. (1976).

Altough cardiac symptoms appear in the final stage of the disease, amyloidotic depositsare evident in myocardic walls as proved earli er by echocardiography and EKG.

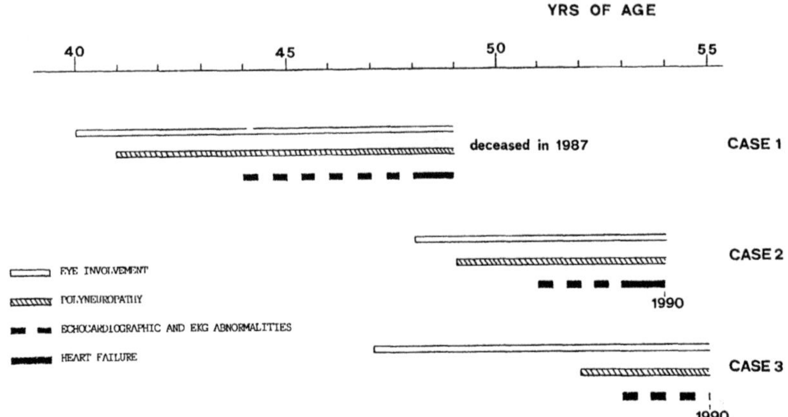

Fig. 1: summary of the major clinical features and their progression.

Acknowledge The authors thank E. Diozzi for her assistance in the preparation of the manuscript.

REFERENCES.

Salvi F., Ferlini A. , Plasmati R. , Rubboli G., Saraiva M.J.M., Costa P.P. , Tassinari C.A. (1989). Familial Amyloidotic Polyneuropathy in Italy; Neurology 39 (Suppl. 1), 408.

Saraiva M.J.M., Costa P.P., Almeida M.R., Banzhoff A., Altland K., Ferlini A. , Rubboli G. , Plasmati R., Tassinari C.A., Romeo G., Salvi F. , (1988) . Familial Amyloidotic Polyneuropathy : Transthyretin (prealbumin) Variants in kindreds of Italian origins. Hum. Genet. 80 : 341- 343.

Almeida M.R., Gawinowicz M. ,Costa P.P., Salvi F. , Ferlini A., Plasma ti R., Tassinari C.A., Saraiva M.J.M. (1990).A new Transthyretin va riant associated with Familial Amyloidotic Polyneuropathy in an Ita lian kindred. This issue .

Kauffman H.E. , Thomas L.B. , (1959). Vitreous opacities diagnostic of Familial Primary Amyloidosis. N. Engl. J . Med. 261: 1267-1271.

Irvine A.R., Char D.H. ,(1976). Recurrent amyloid involvement in the vitreous body after vitrectomy. Am. J. Ophth. 82: 705-708.

Hitching R.A., Tripathi R.C. , (1976). Vitreous opacities in Primary Amyloid disease. Brit. J. Ophth. 60 : 41-54.

A TTR ACIDIC VARIANT DNA ANALYSIS OF HOMOZYGOUS AND HETEROZYGOUS INDIVIDUALS

Maria do Rosário Almeida[1,2], Pedro Pinho Costa[1], Maria João Saraiva[1,2]

[1] Centro de Estudos de Paramiloidose, Hospital de Santo António 4000 Porto, Portugal.

[2] Departamento de Bioquimica, Instituto de Ciências Biomédicas Abel Salazar 4000 Porto, Portugal

ABSTRACT. A TTR acidic variant was previously described in a screening study of the population by isoelectric focusing in immobilized pH gradient. We describe an homozygous individual for this variant and an heterozygous individual showing also the TTR Met 30 monomer. Peptide mapping and sequencing studies revealed a substitution of asparagine for histidine at position 90. We present DNA analysis of these individuals.

INTRODUCTION

A TTR acidic variant was previously described in the Portuguese and German populations in a screening study by isoelectric focusing (IEF) in immobilized pH gradients (Altland et al. 1987). Investigation of this apparently non pathogenic variant can be very interesting since we detected an homozygous individual for the acidic variant and an individual with both the TTR Met 30 and acidic monomers. The study of TTR from these individuals may elucidate modifications in structure originated by these substitutions and how subunit assembly in the tetrameric TTR molecules is affected.

Peptide mapping and sequencing studies of the isolated TTR were performed and the predicted mutation was confirmed by RFLP analysis of PCR amplified material. We further confirmed the mutation by DNA sequencing of this region.

MATERIAL AND METHODS

SUBJECTS: Blood was obtained from a woman homozygous for the TTR acidic variant detected by IEF (Alves et al. 1989), her daughter and her brother both heterozygous. Blood was also collected from an heterozygous individual with acidic variant and TTR Met 30.

PEPTIDE MAPPING AND SEQUENCE ANALYSIS: Comparative tryptic peptide mapping of plasma TTR from the heterozygous individual with the two mutant monomers and normal TTR individuals was performed by HPLC as described previously (Saraiva et al 1984). Some of the peptides were collected and subjected to sequence analysis on an Applied Biosystems model 470A gas-phase sequencer equipped with a 120A PTH analyser.

RFLP ANALYSIS OF AMPLIFIED DNA: TTR gene exons 2 or 3 were amplified with the appropriate flanking primers by the polymerase chain reaction (PCR). The amplification conditions were as described previously (Almeida et al. 1990). Digestion with restriction enzymes was performed in one tenth of the mixture. The enzymes employed included Sph I (BRL), Bsm I and Nsi I (Biolabs). The products were analysed on a 4% Nusieve agarose gel.

DNA SEQUENCE ANALYSIS: Direct asymetric amplification was performed using a ratio of 100:1 pmol of the oligonucleotides primers. The conditions of amplification were the the same as above. The amplified DNA was purified by centrifugation on Centricon 30. Sequencing reactions with Sequenase version 2.0 (USB) were done according to the protocol of the supplier. α-^{32}P-dATP was used. The sequencing gel was 8% polyacrylamide (Gel mix-8 from BRL). Electrophoresis was run at 40 W. The gel was dried and subjected to autoradiography.

RESULTS

The different pI of the TTR acidic variant should result from a change in the primary structure of TTR. In order to elucidate this change we performed structural studies namely tryptic peptide mapping.

Comparison of TTR peptide maps from the acidic carrier and a normal individual showed a distinct abnormal peptide peak eluting close to peptide 10,not observed in the normal TTR. Sequence analysis of this peptide revealed a substitution of asparagine for histidine at position 90. TTR peptide mapping from the acidic and Met 30 heterozygote showed the abnormal peptide 10 and the abnormal peptide 4 due to the Met 30 mutation (data not shown).

The Asn 90 substitution can be explained by a A for C point mutation creating a new restriction site for Bsm I and abolishing one for Sph I.

This was confirmed by RFLP analysis of amplified exon 3 TTR gene. Figure 1 shows the results obtained for three acidic carriers belonging to the same kindred - mother, daughter and brother.

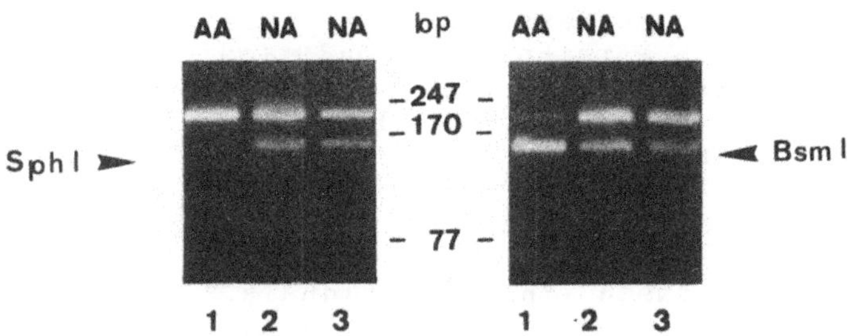

FIG. 1 - RFLP analysis of amplified exon 3 TTR gene from three individuals of the same kindred (1- mother, 2- daughter, 3- brother). A - acidic; N - normal.

As detected by IEF the mother was found homozygous since the amplified DNA is not cut by Sph I (247 bp fragment) but is completly digested with Bsm I presenting only 170 bp and 77 bp fragments. The heterozygous individuals present the 3 fragments 247 bp, 170 bp and 77 bp. These results were further confirmed by DNA sequencing.

For the analysis of the acidic and Met 30 heterozygous individual we made RFLP analysis with Nsi I of amplified exon 2 TTR gene and in parallel with Sph I (fig. 2). We found that this individual (labelled FA) carried the two polymorphisms originating Met 30 and Asn 90 TTR variants.

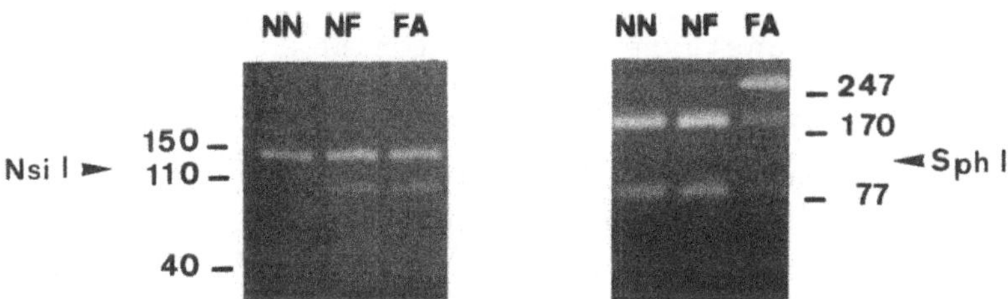

FIG. 2 - RFLP analysis of amplified exons 2 and 3 of the TTR gene. Amplified fragment of exon 2 was digested with NsiI and exon 3 with SphI.

CONCLUSIONS

The acidic variant TTR detected by IEF was characterized and found to have a substitution of asparagine for histidine at position 90. This result obtained by tryptic peptide mapping and sequence analysis was confirmed by RFLP analysis and DNA sequencing.

The individuals studied are very interesting since there is an acidic homozygous, acidic heterozygous and acidic and Met 30 heterozygous individuals.

All the carriers of the acidic variant regardless of their age were healthy, never presented a particular symptomatology, suggesting that this variant is not associated with a pathogenic condition.

The possible structural effects produced by Asn 90 will be distinct in the different carriers of the mutation, that is, in normal and Asn 90 heterozygotes, in Met 30 and Asn 90 heterozygotes and in Asn 90 homozygotes; different molecular tetrameric species will be present and the ratios of normal to variant subunits might vary between the individuals. These variations might affect also the physiological functions of TTR, that is, the binding of thyroxine and retinol binding protein.

Recent studies by Skare et al. (1989) identified the same polymorphism in an American FAP patient. The patient TTR analysed by IEF didn't present the same migration as our TTR Asn 90. Further studies are needed to investigate if the Sph I polymorphisms in the American patient result in the Asn 90 substitution or, whether, an additional post-translational modification occurs.

ACKNOWLEDGEMENTS
This work was supported by grant RO1NS25190 from U.S. National Institutes of Health.

REFERENCES

Almeida MR, Alves IL, Sakaki Y, Costa PP, Saraiva MJM. (1990)Prenatal diagnosis of familial amyloidotic polyneuropathy: evidence for an early expression of the associated transthyretin methionine 30. Hum Gen. In press.

Altland K, Becher P, Banzhoff A. (1987) Paraffin oil protected high resolution hybrid isoelectric focusing for the demonstration of substitutions of neutral aminoacids in denatured proteins: The case of four human transthyretin (prealbumin) variants associated with familial amyloidotic polyneuropathy. Electrophoresis 8: 293-297.

Alves IL, Altland K, Costa PP, Saraiva MJM. (1989) Detection of TTR variants in a Portuguese population by isoelectric focusing in immobilized pH gradients. Arq Med 3: 196- A 38.

Saraiva MJM, Birken S, Costa PP, Goodman DS. (1984). Amyloid fibril protein in familial amyloidotic polyneuropathy, Portuguese type. Definition of molecular abnormality in transthyretin (prealbumin). J Clin Invest 74:104-119.

Skare JC, Saraiva MJM, Alves IL, Skare IL, Milunsky A, Cohen AS, Skinner MA. (1989) A new mutation causing familial amyloidotic polyneuropathy. Biochem Biophys Res Commun 164: 1240-1246.

ASN 90 IS THE VARIANT TTR IN AN ITALIAN FAP KINSHIP

JC Skare *
LA Jones #
J Harding #
JM Milunsky *
A Milunsky *
IB Skare +
AS Cohen #
M Skinner #

* Center for Human Genetics and Departments of Pediatrics and Microbiology, and # Arthritis Center, Boston University School of Medicine; + Department of Biological Sciences, University of Lowell

SUMMARY
A new transthyretin variant which lost an Sph I cleavage site within exon 3 has been characterized. A 260bp sequence containing exon 3 was amplified using the polymerase chain rection, and the variant was found to possess a Bsm I cleavage site not present in normal transthyretin. This led to the conclusion that the histidine at position 90 was replaced by asparagine, and amino acid analysis supported the conclusion.

INTRODUCTION
We studied the DNA from a patient of Italian descent with familial amyloidotic polyneuropathy (Skare et al, 1989). It did not possess any of the mutations which have previously been associated with FAP. However, a novel 7.0kb Sph I restriction fragment was discovered, and the mutation creating it was localized to exon 3 of the transthyretin gene. This mutation was inherited from a parent, and could have resulted in an amino acid substitution at position 89, 90, or 91.

METHODS
PCR reactions contained 10ug/ml human DNA, 2ug/ml of each primer, 25U/ml Taq polymerase, 10mM trisCl, 50mM KCl, 1.5mM Mg Cl_2, 0.1 g/l gelatin and 200uM of each dNTP. There were 30 cycles of amplification, each consisting of 30sec. at 94C, 2min. at 45C and 30sec. at 70C. At the end of amplification, approximately 20ug/ml of PCR product was present . 200ng of product was incubated

with 2U of restriction endonuclease, and the digests were applied to a 6% polyacrylamide gel. The 15cm gel was electrophoresed at 160 volts for 2.5 hours.

RESULTS

There are 18 possible base substitutions that would result in the loss of an Sph I site in exon 2. Of these, 9 would create a recognition site for a commercially available restriction endonuclease. An asp 89 substitution would create a Bcl I recognition site, pro90 would create a Pst I site, asn90 and ser91 would both create Bsm I sites, asp90 and pro91 would both create Fok I sites, leu90 would create an Alu I site, his 90 would create a Bsp 1286 site, and glu91 would create an Mbo II site. Thus, there was a reasonable chance that the mutation could be characterized without sequencing exon 3 or the tryptic peptide or TTR which contains the amino acid substitution. The sequence of exon 3 and flanking intron was reported by Sasaki et al, 1985. Based on this information, two 20 base oligonucleotides were synthesized and used as primers in polymerase chain reactions to amplify a 260 bp sequence (table 1). Figure 1a shows that the product derived from the patient's DNA was homogeneous, which indicates that the Sph I site (at bases 182-187) was missing as a result of a base substitution rather than a deletion.

TABLE 1: The amplified region of normal TTR. Exon 3 is in upper case, and the Sph I recognition sequence is underlined.

ccatgccatt tgtttcctcc atgcgtaact taatccagac tttcacacct
tatagGAAAA CCAGTGAGTC TGGAGAGCTG CATGGGCTCA CAACTGAGGA
GGAATTTGTA GAAGGGATAT ACAAAGTGGA AATAGACACC AAATCTTACT
GGAAGGCACT TGGCATCTCC CCATTCCATG AGCATGCAGA Ggtgagtata
cagaccttcg agggttgttt tggttttggt ttttgctttt ggcattccag
gaaatgcaca

When the patients's PCR product was incubated with Sph 1, over half of the product remained 260bp, while the remainder was converted into fragments of about 184bp and 76bp (figure 1c). We expected only half of the 260bp product would be digested, since we knew that half of the patient's TTR genes lacked Sph I sites in exon 3. In fact, less than half of the product can be cut because part of the 260bp product consists of heteroduplexes

between normal and mutant exon 3.
Incubation of our patient's PCR product with Bsm I cleaved the product into fragments of approximately 240bp, 187bp, 53bp and 20bp (figure 1d). Incubation of 260bp product from a normal individual with Bsm I yielded fragments of about 240 and 20bp (figure 1f). Our patient has an additional Bsm I site in half of her TTR genes that creates fragments of 187bp and 53bp instead of 240bp. We conclude that the same single base substitution which destroyed an Sph I site created a Bsm I site.

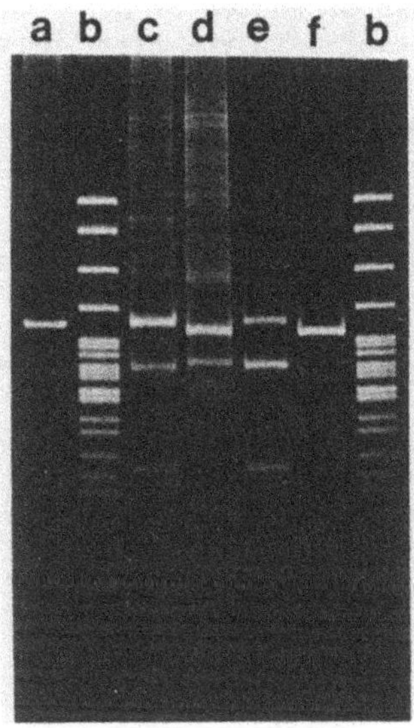

Figure 1: Lane a is the 260bp PCR product from our patient. Lane b is molecular weight markers generated by cleavage of pBR322 DNA with Msp I. In lane c is the product cut with Sph I and in lane d it is cut with Bsm I. Lane e is 260bp PCR product from a normal individual partially digested with Sph I. Lane f shows a Bsm I digest of normal 260bp product.

Therefore, the patient's substitution must be either asn90 or ser91. Fortunately, the size of the Bsm I fragment provides further information. The Bsm I recognition site, GAATGCN, is nonpalindromic and the cleavage is asymmetric. If the mutation were ser91, then the large Bsm I fragment would be 180bp with a 2-base tail. If the mutation were asn90, then the large Bsm I fragment would be 186bp with a 2-base tail. Sph I produces a 182bp fragment with a 4-base tail when it cleaves normal 260bp product. Therefore, the large Bsm I fragment from ser91 DNA should migrate more quickly than the Sph I fragment, but the large Bsm I fragment from asn90 DNA should migrate more slowly than the Sph I fragment. Figure 1d shows that the Bsm I fragment migrates more slowly than the Sph I fragments in lanes c and e, so the histidine at position 90 must have been replaced by an asparagine. This is caused by a substitution of adenine for cytosine in the first base of codon 90.

Amino acid analysis of mutant TTR showed a decrease in histidine and an increase in asparagine-aspartate relative to normal TTR. This provides additional support for the conclusion that asparagine has been substituted for histidine at position 90.

DISCUSSION

This is the first time an FAP mutation has been characterized without protein or DNA sequencing. Recently, exons 2,3, and 4 of the TTR from this patient have been sequenced (data not shown). Other than the asn90 substitution, no mutations were found. Since we have shown that the amyloid fibrils are composed of TTR and that asn90 is the only mutation, it follows that asn90 causes FAP in the patient.

ACKNOWLEDGEMNTS

We wish to thank G. Crombie for assistance with amino acid analysis. This work was supported by N.I.H. grants CA-49629, AM-07014 and AM-20613, and Division of Research Resources GCRC RR-553, and the Arthritis Foundation.

REFERENCES

1. Skare JC, Saraiva MJM, Alves I, Milunsky A, Cohen AS, Skinner M: (1989) A new mutation causing familial amyloidotic polyneuropathy. Biochem Biophys Res Comm 164:1240-1246.
2. Sasaki H, Yoshioka N, Takagi Y, Sakaki Y: (1985) Structure of the chromosomal gene for human serum prealbumin. Gene 37:191-197.

FREQUENCY OF THE POSITION 122 (VAL→ILE) VARIANT TRANSTHYRETIN GENE IN BLACKS WITHOUT AMYLOIDOSIS

D.R. Jacobson*, J.D. Reveille#, and J.N. Buxbaum*, New York University School of Medicine and Department of Veterans Affairs Medical Center, New York, NY*, and University of Texas Medical School, Houston, TX, USA#.

ABSTRACT. Transthyretin (TTR) (122 Val→Ile), caused by a point mutation which destroys a Mae III restriction site, is associated with cardiac TTR-amyloid deposition, causing congestive heart failure, in Blacks. To determine the frequency of the Mae III (-) gene in the Black population, DNA from 177 Black individuals without amyloidosis was amplified by the polymerase chain reaction (PCR) around TTR codon 122 and digested with Mae III. The Mae III (-) gene frequency was 1.1%, suggesting that this variant is relatively common in Blacks.

1. Introduction

The TTR mutation, TTR (122 Val→Ile), caused by a G to A transition which destroys a Mae III restriction site, was found originally in the amyloid fibrils of a 68-year-old Black patient with cardiac amyloidosis. In contrast to the heterozygous pattern typically seen for the TTR variants associated with FAP, the position 122 variant was homozygous in this patient, i.e., PCR-amplified DNA around codon 122 was Mae III (-,-) (1). Two other Blacks with cardiac TTR-amyloidosis have been found with the same TTR variant, one of whom was homozygous (2,3). To address the question of the gene frequency of the TTR position 122 variant in the Black population, we tested DNA from 177 unaffected Blacks for the Mae III (-) genotype.

2. Materials and methods

DNA samples were obtained from 177 unrelated Blacks without amyloidosis or a known family history of amyloidosis. Fourteen samples were from African patients with Burkitt's lymphoma; 14 were from African sickle cell anemia patients; 7 were from American Blacks with sickle cell anemia or sickle trait; 4 were from American Blacks with adenosine deaminase deficiency; 2 were from American Blacks with colon carcinoma; 136 were from healthy volunteer donors (131 from the continental United States, 1 from Ethiopia, 1 from Puerto Rico, and 3 from the West Indies). DNA was also obtained from

86 White controls without overt amyloidosis or cardiomyopathy.

DNA samples were PCR-amplified around TTR codon 122, digested with Mae III, electrophoresed on agarose gels and stained with ethidium bromide as previously described (1), except that cycling times were shortened (94°C x 45 sec and 55-60°C x 30 sec, for 30 cycles) and that different primers were used for some samples.

3. Results and Discussion

Four of 177 samples were heterozygous for the variant, i.e. Mae III (+,-). The other 173 samples showed the "normal", Mae III (+,+) genotype (figure 1). One of the heterozygotes

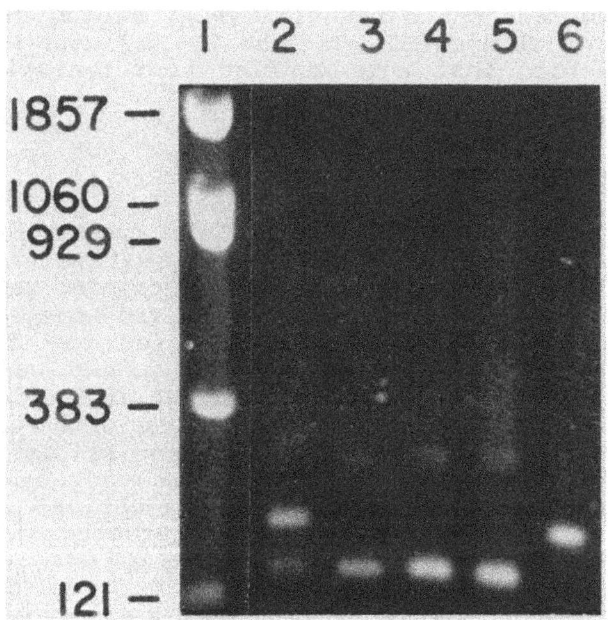

Figure 1. Mae III digests of PCR-amplified DNA around TTR codon 122. Lane 1: DNA size markers, showing sizes in base pairs. Lane 2: DNA sample heterozygous for the codon 122 Mae III site. Lanes 3-5: normal controls, showing complete digestion with Mae III. Lane 6: DNA which is homozygous for the Mae III (-) variant, from the patient with cardiac amyloidosis. Three other samples demonstrated the heterozygous pattern (two bands) seen in lane 2; 172 other samples demonstrated the pattern seen in lanes 3-5.

was from a sickle globin gene carrier (AS at the ß globin locus) who had donated blood during a sickle cell screening program. The other three Mae III (+,-) samples were from normal volunteer donors. The Mae III (-) gene frequency was thus 4/354 (1.1%, 95% confidence interval 0.32-2.7%). 86/86 DNA samples from whites were Mae III (+,+).

In this study the Mae III (-) genotype, originally reported as a homozygous variant in association with SSA, was found as a heterozygous variant in 2.2% of 177 Black individuals without overt heart disease, neuropathy, or amyloidosis. It is not yet known what percentage of TTR (122 Val→Ile) homozygotes develop cardiac amyloidosis, or the degree to which heterozygotes may be at risk for disease. These data indicate that TTR (122 Val→Ile) is a common variant in Blacks, and suggest that cardiac amyloidosis resulting from TTR Ile-122 may be an unrecognized, relatively common cause of heart failure in Blacks.

4. Acknowledgements

We would like to thank Drs. Stephanie Tzall, Rochelle Hirschorn, Ricardo Dalla-Favera, Ronald Nagel, Agathe Pachnis, Sergio Piomelli, and Kishor Bhatia for contributing DNA samples. We thank Immaculata Kane for technical assistance.

5. References

1) Jacobson DR, Gorevic PD, and Buxbaum JN. (1990) A homozygous transthyretin variant associated with senile systemic amyloidosis: evidence for a late-onset disease of genetic etiology. Am. J. Hum. Genet. 47:127-136.

2) Nichols WC, Snyder EL, Liepnieks JJ, Benson MD. (1990) Senile cardiac amyloidosis is a hereditary disease. Proceedings of the 1st International Symposium on Familial Amyloidotic Polyneuropathy 3:190(Abstract).

3) Saraiva MJM, Sherman W, Kyle R, Gertz MA, Costa PP, Figueira A, Gawinowicz MA. (1990) Studies on TTR associated cardiac amyloidosis. Proceedings of the 1st International Symposium on Familial Amyloidotic Polyneuropathy 3:191(Abstract).

VARIANT TRANSTHYRETINS IN FAMILIAL AMYLOIDOTIC POLYNEURO-PATHY (FAP)

M. Miyazato, M. Nakazato, Y. Yamamura, K. Kangawa*, H. Matsuo#, and S. Matsukura
Third Department of Medicine, Department of Biochemistry*, Miyazaki Medical College, Kiyotake, Miyazaki 889-16, and National Cardiovascular Center Research Institute#, Suita, Osaka 565, Japan.

ABSTRACT. We determined amino acid sequences of transthyretins of FAP patients from 10 countries. Serum transthyretin was isolated by using immunoaffinity chromatography and reverse-phase high-performance liquid chromatography (RP-HPLC). Six kinds of variant transthyretins with one amino acid substitution, $Val^{30} \rightarrow Met$, $Phe^{33} \rightarrow Ile$, $Glu^{42} \rightarrow Gly$, $Ser^{50} \rightarrow Arg$, $Thr^{60} \rightarrow Ala$, and $Ser^{77} \rightarrow Tyr$, were identified. Serum level of Met^{30} transthyretin in 29 Swedish, 4 Dutch, and 114 Japanese patients with type I FAP was 9.55 mg/dl, 11.31 mg/dl, and 9.86 mg/dl, respectively. A quantitative method for Met^{30} transthyretin deposited in tissues was developed by using radioimmunoassay (RIA) and extraction of the protein with formic acid. Met^{30} transthyretin occupied 0.8-1.8% of wet tissue weight in the heart, thyroid gland, and kidney, whereas, it comprised only 0.03% of wet tissue weight in the liver. A novel immunohistochemical technique using cyanogen bromide cleavage and an antiserum for subsequence[26-30] in Met^{30} transthyretin was useful for specific staining of amyloid Met^{30} transthyretin in tissue specimen.

Introduction

FAP is a molecular disorder of transthyretin (also called prealbumin). Four kinds of variant transthyretins with one amino acid substitution, $Val^{30} \rightarrow Met$, $Phe^{33} \rightarrow Ile$, $Thr^{60} \rightarrow Ala$, and $Ser^{77} \rightarrow Tyr$, have been known to form amyloid fibrils in the disease. To clarify biochemical etiology of FAP in which variant transthyretin has not been identified, we determined amino acid sequence of serum transthyretin of FAP patients in 10 countries. Serum levels of Met^{30} transthyretin were studied in three different ethnic groups of type I FAP cases; i.e. Swedish, Dutch and Japanese origins. Correlation was investigated between serum level of Met^{30} transthyretin and ages of onset as well as progression of illness in these type I FAP.

Amyloid fibrils accumulate in systemic organs of FAP; however, the amount of amyloid deposition varies according to different organs. To determine tissue distribution and predominance of amyloid deposits in FAP, we developed a method for quantifying Met^{30} variant transthyretin in amyloid-laden tissues by using extraction with formic acid followed by RIA. Furthermore, a novel immunohistochemical method which specifically stains amyloid Met^{30} transthyretin in tissue section was developed.

Materials and Methods

PURIFICATION AND SEQUENCE ANALYSIS OF TRANSTHYRETIN IN SERUM AND URINE: Serum transthyretin was isolated from 1 ml of the serum of FAP patients residing in European countries and Japan using Affi- Gel Blue affinity chromatography, anti- human transthyretin IgG Affi- Gel 10 chromatography, and finally RP- HPLC on a TSK phenyl- 5PW RP column. Urine transthyretin was purified from one litter of the urine of a Japanese FAP case using the same method as described above. Fractions containing transthyretin in chromatographies were detected by RIA for transthyretin. Purified transthyretin was treated with trypsin or Lysyl C endopeptidase in 0.1M Tris-HCl buffer (pH 8.0) at 37 °C for 2 hr. Resulting digests were separated by RP- HPLC on a TSK ODS SIL 120A column. Abnormal peptides detected in patient's peptide maps were subjected to sequence analysis using a gas- phase sequencer linked with RP-HPLC for identifying PTH- amino acids.

DETERMINATION OF TISSUE CONTENT OF MET^{30} TRANSTHYRETIN IN FAP: Tissues listed in Table 1 were obtained at autopsy from a Japanese FAP patient. Three different sites from each of these organs were examined. Tissues were homogenized in 70% formic acid solution and centrifuged. An aliquot of the supernatant was treated with cyanogen bromide in 70% formic acid. The sample was lyophilized twice, incubated in 0.1M Tris- HCl buffer (pH 8.0), and then digested with trypsin. The sample was measured by RIA for Met^{30} transthyretin (1).

IMMUNOHISTOCHEMICAL METHOD FOR MET^{30} TRANSTHYRETIN: Tissue sections fixed on glasses were treated with cyanogen bromide. Samples were successively reacted with antiserum specific for subsequence[26 - 30] in Met^{30} transthyretin, biotinylated antirabbit γ- globulin, avidin- bound peroxidase, and 3,3'-diaminobenzidine according to the manufacturer's instructions (VECTASTAIN ABC kit, Funakoshi Co. Ltd., Japan). The antibody specific for subsequence[26- 30] of Met^{30} transthyretin was isolated from a polyclonal antibody raised against subsequence[22- 30] of Met^{30} transthyretin by using Affi - Gel 10 resin which was coupled with a pentapeptide corresponding to subsequence[26 - 30] with a homoserine residue at position 30.

Results

SEQUENCE DETERMINATION OF VARIANT TRANSTHYRETIN: Transthyretins in the serum and urine were purified by three steps of chromatography coupled with the RIA. An extra peptide which was detected only in a map from patient's transthyretin was subjected to sequence analysis. Six kinds of variant transthyretin with one amino acid substitution, Val^{30} → Met, Phe^{33} → Ile, Glu^{42} → Gly, Ser^{50} → Arg, Thr^{60} → Ala, and Ser^{77} → Tyr, were identified (unpublished observations). Analyses on transthyretin gene causing Glu^{42} → Gly and Ser^{50} → Arg substitutions were reported elsewhere (2).

TISSUE CONTENT OF MET^{30} TRANSTHYRETIN: Met^{30} transthyretin was detected in all organs studied, while its quantity was different in various organs as shown in Table 1. A large amount of the variant transthyretin was deposited in the heart, thyroid gland and kidney. However, the quantity of the variant transthyretin was very low in the liver. These results were compatible with those of semi- quantitative studies of amyloid deposits in organs by Congo red staining and immunohistochemical observations.

TABLE 1. Tissue content of Met^{30} transthyretin amyloid in FAP

Tissues	μg/wet mg	Tissues	μg/wet mg
cardiac atrium	17.8	gall bladder	2.8
ventricle	7.0	spleen	1.0
thyroid gland	12.9	vena cava	1.0
choroid plexus	10.8	tongue	0.7
kidney	7.6	aorta	0.7
lung	4.0	liver	0.3

IMMUNOHISTOCHEMISTRY: Cyanogen bromide cleavage on tissue sections was confirmed by RIA for homoserine at position 30 produced by cyanogen bromide cleavage (2). Amyloid in type I FAP was positively stained with the antiserum specific for subsequence[26-30] of Met^{30} transthyretin. The antiserum did not stain other types of amyloid protein or specimens without amyloid deposition.

Discussion

We reported that FAP of Japanese, Swedish and Dutch origins had a variant transthyretin with $Val^{30} \rightarrow Met$ substitution (3, 4) and FAP of Jewish origin had a variant transthyretin with $Phe^{33} \rightarrow Ile$ substitution (5). In the present study, we found additional four other variant transthyretins from FAP patients from European countries and Japan. Their clinical manifestations were somewhat different from that of type I FAP, which will be reported elsewhere.

The variant transthyretin was verified to be excreted in the urine of FAP patient. Amyloid deposits were marked in the glomerulus, which caused excretion of the variant transthyretin into the urine. Concentration of the variant transthyretin in the urine was correlated to amount of proteinuria. Urinary excretion of the variant transthyretin might be in part responsible for the decrease of its serum level in FAP cases who suffer from renal failure.

Tissue content of Met^{30} transthyretin deposited as amyloid was determined by RIA coupled with extraction of the protein with formic acid. The quantity of Met^{30} transthyretin in the wet tissue weight of liver accounted for 2-4% of that of the heart, thyroid gland and kidney. In the liver of FAP, amyloid deposits were present only in the vessel walls and scarcely present in the interstitial tissue. This is why very little variant transthyretin was detected in the liver. The quantitative method used in this study is promising in elucidating the relationship between the amount of amyloid deposits and the severity of the clinical impairment of various organs in FAP. Furthermore, this method will be also helpful in clarifying the time relationship between amyloid deposition in various organs and the appearance of clinical symptoms in FAP.

The antiserum for transthyretin molecule occasionally cross-reacts various proteins other than transthyretin. To establish an immunohistochemical method specifically staining Met^{30} transthyretin, we prepared the antiserum for its subsequence[26-30]. A methionine residue was changed into a homoserine by cyanogen bromide cleavage followed by incubation in weakly basic solution. Since the antiserum specifically recognized homoserine at position 30 of Met^{30} transthyretin, tissues were treated with cyanogen bromide to yield homoserine, then subjected to immunohistochemical staining. Met^{30} transthyretin in sections from type I FAP patients was positively stained and no cross-reactivity was observed. The method developed in this study, which utilized specific antiserum and chemical treatment to disclose the epitope for the antiserum, can be widely applied to immunohistochemical studies.

References

1. Nakazato, M., Kangawa, K., Minamino, N., Tawara, S., Matsuo, H., and Araki, S. (1984) 'Radioimmunoassay for detecting abnormal prealbumin in the serum for diagnosis of familial amyloidotic polyneuropathy (Japanese type)', Biochem. Biophys. Res. Commun., 122, 719-725.
2. Ueno, S., Uemichi, T., Takahashi, N., Soga, F., Yorifuji, S., and Tarui, S. (1990) 'Two novel variants of transthyretin identified in Japanese cases with familial amyloidotic polyneuropathy', Biochem. Biophys. Res. Commun., 169, 1117-1121.
3. Tawara, S., Nakazato, M., Kangawa, K., Matsuo, H., and Araki, S. (1983) 'Identification of amyloid prealbumin variant in familial amyloidotic polyneuropathy (Japanese type)', Biochem. Biophys. Res. Commun., 116, 880-888.
4. Nakazato, M., Steen, L., Holmgren, G., Kurihara, T., Matsukura, S., Kangawa, K., and Matsuo, H. (1987) 'Structurally abnormal transthyretin causing familial amyloidotic polyneuropathy in Sweden', Clin. Chem. Acta., 167, 341-342.
5. Nakazato, M., Kangawa, K., Minamino, N., Tawara, S., Matsuo, H., and Araki, S. (1984) 'Revised analysis of amino acid replacement in a prealbumin variant (SKO-Ⅲ) associated with familial amyloidotic polyneuropathy of Jewish origin', Biochem. Biophys. Res. Commun., 123, 921-928.

THREE NOVEL VARIANTS OF TRANSTHYRETIN IDENTIFIED IN THREE JAPANESE KINDREDS WITH FAMILIAL AMYLOIDOTIC POLYNEUROPATHY

S. UENO, T. Uemichi, N.Takahashi, F.Soga, S.Yorifuji, and S.Tarui

Second Department of Internal Medicine and Department of Neurology, Osaka University Medical School, Fukushima, Osaka 553, JAPAN

SUMMARY. We identified three novel variants of transthyretin (TTR), TTR-Cys 114, TTR-Gly 42, and TTR-Arg 50, in three Japanese kindreds with familial amyloidotic polyneuropathy. Amyloid deposits reacted with anti-TTR serum. Amino acid mutations were deduced from TTR gene sequences determined. Every four exons were amplified by PCR, cloned into M13 vectors and randomly sequenced by Sanger's method. Base change detected was confirmed by restriction site analysis and ASO differential hybridization analysis. Two genetically different kindreds may originate in rather small area, one was our kindred associated with TTR-Cys 114 in Kunimi and other was already reported FAP type I with TTR-Met 30 in Arao. No cases of FAP as identified by us have been reported outside of Japan and the possibility that the gene mutations occurred originally within Japan can not be excluded. Our discovery of the three new variants adds to the substantial evidence supporting that TTR related FAP are far more varied and prevalent than previously thought.

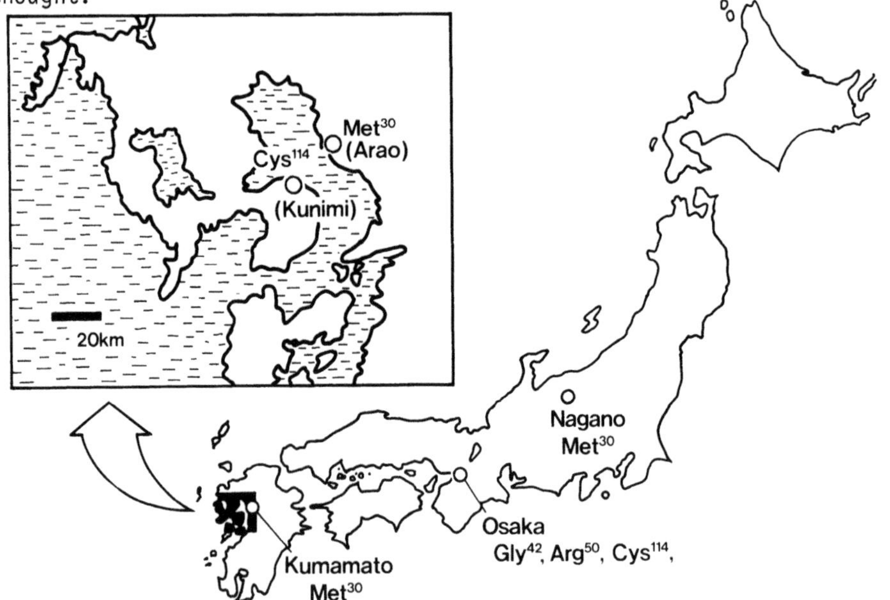

Familial amyloidotic polyneuropathy (FAP) is a dominantly inherited disease, most cases were associated with the genetic variants of plasma transthyretin (TTR). We report three new FAP kindreds from the Osaka area, possessing different three variants of TTR.

MATERIALS and METHODS

PCR amplification and sequencing of TTR gene fragments. Genomic DNA was extracted from the peripheral-blood leukocytes or the autopsied organ tissues of patients and controls. Based on the published sequence of normal human TTR gene, the oligonucleotide primers flanking exons of TTR genes were prepared (Table 1). The four exons of the TTR gene were amplified from the genomic DNA using Gene Ampkit. PCR run consisted of 30 cycles of denaturation at 94° C, annealing at 55° C, and extension at 74° C for 60 sec for each step. PCR products were electrophoretically separated on 3.7 % NuSieve GTG agarose. The gene fragments containing the entire length of each exon were cloned into M13 vectors and sequenced by the dideoxy-chain termination method.

Table 1 Summary of TTR gene amplification primer sets

Exon and size	Primer sequence #	amplified ##
Exon 1 95 bp	5'-AGAATCAGCAGGTTTGCAGTCAGAT-3' 5'-AGCTCAGTAAGCTCAGTGGAACTT-3'	-91-275
Exon 2 131 bp	5'-TGTCGACACTTACGTTCCTGATAAT-3' 5'-ATGCTCAGGTTCCTGGTCACTT-3'	885-1347
Exon 3 136 bp	5'-ATCTACAGTGAGCTTTTCAAAA-3' 5'-TCGAAGGTCTGTATACTCAC-3'	3034-3398
Exon 4 253 bp	5'-GAAATGGATCTGTCTGTCTTC-3' 5'-CAGCGAATTCCTTTGATTCTTTGTAA-3' ###	6659-7035

The primer sequences and the numbering of TTR gene are based on the published data (1). ## The amplified region of TTR gene with each primer set. ### Extra bases (CAGC) are added 5' to the EcoRI recognition sequence to ensure that the efficiency of restriction enzyme cleavage is maintained.

Allele-specific oligonucleotide (ASO) hybridization. Exons of the TTR gene were amplified from genomic DNA of the patients and controls with oligonucleotide primers. Amplified products were denatured after dot-blotting onto nylon membranes. The filters were subsequently hybridized with endlabeled oligonucleotides: 19 bases of normal and mutant ASOs. Filters were washed in 5 X SSC (1 X SSC: 0.15M NaCl, 0.015M sodium citrate) at 54 C for 10 min.

Restriction site analysis. Exon amplifified from genomic DNA of patient was digsted with approprite restriction enzyme and electrophoresed on acrylamide gel.

RESULTS

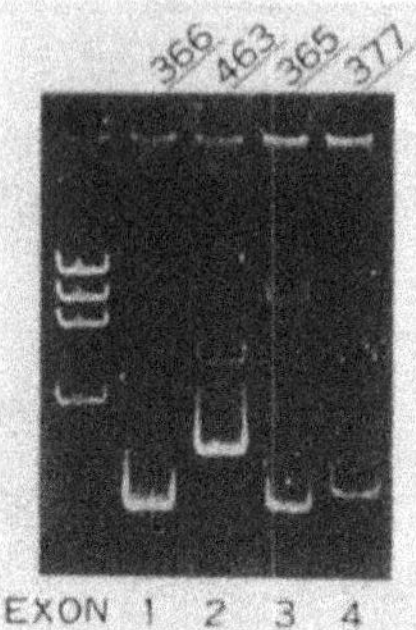

Fig. 1

FAMILY-TK. A 35-year-old man visited us with the complaints of numbness and cold sensation in the under-knee portion of the bilateral lower limbs. Vitreous opacities were present. The gene fragments containing entire length of each exon were effectively amplified (Fig. 1). The sequence data on the exons 1, 2, and 3 were compatible with the published data of normal human TTR gene. Clones containing entire length of exon 4 had the sequence with a single base change from A to G at position 6752 in the TTR gene. This mutation was responsible for the change from codon TAC coding for tyrosine to TGC coding for cysteine at position 114 of the 127-residue TTR molecule. The other clones contained gene fragments with the normal sequence. The identical base change at the same position was established in his affected cousin. ASO test repeatedly confirmed the base change and endorsed that the patients were heterozygous for the TTR gene mutant.

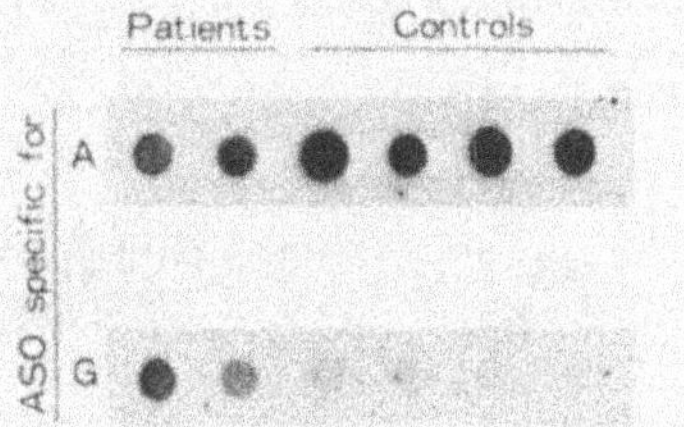

Fig. 2. ASO hybridization of PCR-amplified exon 4 from the two patients and four controls. The two cases hybridize with both the normal (specific for A) and the mutant (specific for G) ASOs, while the controls hybridize only with the normal ASO.

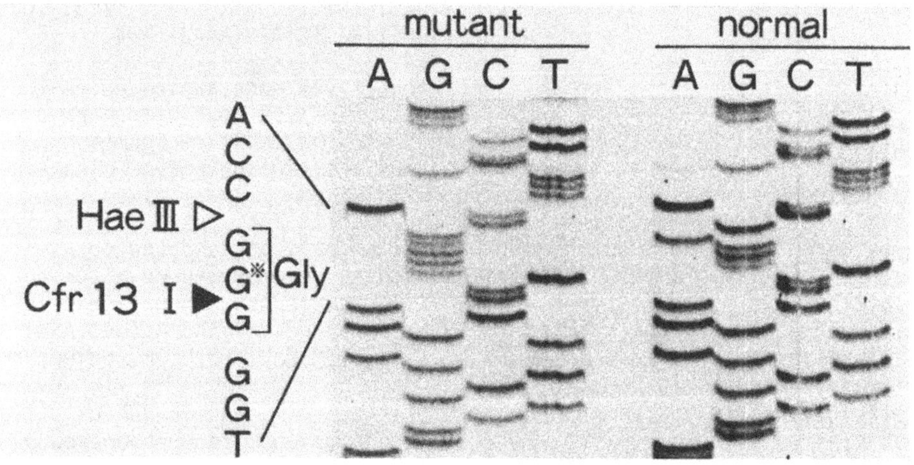

Fig. 3 Nucleotide sequence of exon 2 (FAMILY-KA)

FAMILY-KA. A 42 year-old male proband had lower limb neuropathy and chronic diarrhea. A single base change from A to G at position 1135 was identified in TTR gene. Other clones had normal sequences (Fig.3). This mutation resulted in amino acid change from Glu (GAG) to Gly (GGG) at position 42. The identical mutation was detected in his brother. This base change predicts the generation of new sites of the enzyme Hae III (GG/CC) and Cfr 13 I (G/GGCC) within exon 2. Cfr 13 I digestion of amplified exon 2 (463 bp:885-1347) yielded two extra fragments (250 and 213 bp) in addition to normal fragment. The restriction patterns were explained by the single base change detected by sequence analysis. ASO hybridization confirmed the presence of base change in the patients.

FAMILY-HY.
Two different allelic sequence coding for exon 3 were detected in a 45 year old man. One was normal and the other showed a single base change from T to G at position 3252. This base change resulted in replacement of Ser by Arg at position 50 and predicted new restriction site of enzyme Mva I (CC/AGG) within exon 3. The digestion of amplified exon 3 (365 bp, 3034-3398) with Mva I resulted in the appearance of the two extra bands (216 and 149 bp) in addition to normal band (Fig. 4). ASO hybridization showed that patient's DNA bound both to normal and variant ASO probes.

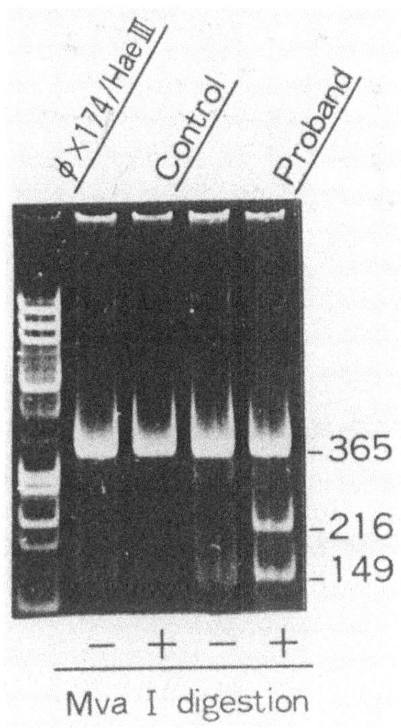

Fig. 4

REFERENCES

1. Tsuzuki, T., Mita, S., Maeda, S., Araki, S., and Shimada, K. (1985) Structure of the human prealbumin gene. J. Biol Chem. 22, 12224-12227.
2. Ueno, S., Uemichi, T., Yorifuji, S., and Tarui, S. (1990) A novel variant of transthyretin (Tyr114 to Cys) deduced from the nucleotide sequences of gene fragments from familial amyloidotic polyneuropathy in Japanese sibling cases. Biochem Biophys Res Commun 169, 143-147
3. Ueno, S., Uemichi, T., Takahashi, N., Soga, F., Yorifuji,S., and Tarui, S. (1990) Two novel variants of transthyretin identified in Japanese cases with familial amyloidotic polyneuropathy: Transthyretin (Glu 42 to Gly) and Transthyretin (Ser 50 to Arg). Biochem Biophys Res Commun 169, 1117-1121

A POSSIBLE NEW TRANSTHYRETIN GENETIC VARIANT IN A FAMILY WITH CARDIAC AMYLOIDOSIS

A. Hesse, K. Altland*, R.P. Linke, A. Steinmetz, B. Maisch**
Zentrum Innere Medizin, Philipps-Universität, D-3550 Marburg
*** Institut für Humangenetik der Universität, D-6300 Giessen**
**** Institut für Immunologie der Universität, D-8000 München, F.R.G.**

ABSTRACT. Several amino acid substitutions in the plasma transthyretin (TTR) molecule have been found to be associated with familial cardiac amyloidosis. We describe a patient and his family with cardiac amyloidosis. The index patient, 63 years old, was seen for chest sensations resembling angina pectoris and arrhythmia. Holter ECG recording revealed severe arrhythmia of the Lown class IVa. In echocardiography hypertrophic non obstructive cardiomyopathy (HNOCM) was diagnosed. Amyloid of the TTR type (AF) was identified in a cardiac biopsy by immunohistochemistry. No amyloid was found in rectum biopsies. Two different forms of TTR varying in their electrophoretic properties, one normal form and an apparently altered one, were identified by hybrid isoelectric focusing suggesting that the patient's plasma was heterogenous for the TTR proteins. Electrophoretic analysis of the plasma from the patient's first degree relatives (son, daughter, brother, mother) identified the son as a carrier of the mutant TTR protein. The variant TTR appears to be different from many others found in described families with amyloidotic individuals.

INTRODUCTION. Amyloidosis characterized by deposition in various organs of fibrillar pathologic proteins is diagnosed by the Congo red binding and their green color in polarized light [1]. Despite the similar morphology the deposited proteins are different. This difference can be used for classification. Immunohistochemistry is the method of choice [2]. Chemically different amyloid-types correlate with the symptomatology. So amyloid AF is often linked to the dominantly inherited familial amyloid polyneuropathy (FAP), sometimes combined with cardiac involvement [3]. FAP is based on point mutations of the plasma protein prealbumin (transthyretin, TTR). Various amino acid substitutions have been identified [4,5,6].

Here we report the data of a 63 year old man and his family. He suffered from a hypertrophic non obstructive cardiomyopathy (HNOCM) due to AF-amyloidosis with signs of polyneuropathy in history. A complete examination failed because of his sudden death by accident. The family investigation revealed the son as a carrier of a mutant TTR protein which has not been reported so far.

METHODS. Besides history taking and physical examination, echocardiography, Holter ECG recording, chest roentgenography and laboratory tests were made with the propositus, his son and his daughter. Gastroscopy, rectoscopy and cardiac catheterization with biopsy from the left ventricle were made in addition with the index patient.

Paraffinembedded sections of the heart muscle and rectum were histochemically examined with a panel of anti-amyloid antibodies directed against various amyloid fibril proteins (AA, A-kappa, A-lambda, AF, AB).

Plasma of the patient and his relatives was submitted to double one-dimensional electrophoresis with polyacrylamide gel electrophoresis followed by hybrid isoelectric focusing as described by Altland et al. [7] with modifications designed for the study of the folding-unfolding properties of TTR in the presence of urea [8].

RESULTS

Patient:
In 1988 the 61 year old patient, W.W., was admitted to the hospital because of arrhythmia and dyspnoea following a bronchitis two months ago. For several years he had suffered from exercise-induced retrosternal pain. In addition he complained about stomach pain, cramps in the calf and dysaesthesia in both hands, especially when working with elevated hands in his profession as a dentist. There was a pan-systolic murmur at the left sternal edge. Electrocardiography demonstrated a left anterior bundle block with an R-reduction in V1 to V4. Holter ECG recording revealed arrhythmias of Lown class IVa. Gastroscopy showed no pathological finding.

One year later the propositus came to hospital for cardiac catheterization because of exercise-induced dyspnoea and mild pretibial oedema as the only signs of congestive heart failure. The chest roentgenogram now demonstrated general heart enlargement. Echocardiography revealed besides small pericardial effusion significant left ventricular hypertrophy with normal left ventricular diameter (enddiastolic diameter 46mm), a dilated left atrium (diameter 50mm, normal <40mm) and a thickened interventricular septum of 21mm (normal <11mm), compatible with hypertrophic non obstructive cardiomyopathy (HNOCM). Doppler echocardiography found mitral valve incompetence. Cardiac catheterization excluded coronary heart disease and demonstrated elevation of right ventricular end-diastolic pressure. Rectum mucosal biopsy did not show any amyloid deposits. Abdominal ultrasound was normal, and no proteinuria was found. The diagnosis polyneuropathy was derived from the complaints of dysaesthesia, whereas neurological examination did not reveal any objective pathological findings. Extensive further studies were not possible and the patient died suddenly abroad.

Biopsy:
Endomyocardial biopsy at the left ventricle showed Congo red positive amyloid with green fluorescence in polarized light. Immunoperoxidase staining revealed amyloid of the TTR type.

Electrophoresis:
Electrophoretic analysis demonstrated the normal and a variant TTR monomer in the plasma of both the propositus and his son, while all other tested relatives were found normal. The isoelectric point of the variant was indistinguishable from that of the normal TTR monomer indicating an electrically neutral amino acid substitution in the variant. Other data to be published elsewhere indicated differences in the molecular properties of the variant from those TTR variants already described to be associated with amyloidosis of the heart and from many others associated with FAP.

Family investigation:

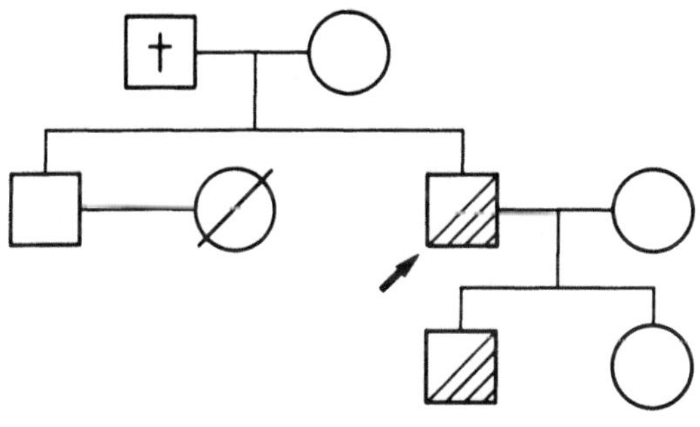

Fig. 1
Variants found in the propositus (arrow) and his son.

The index patient's father had died at the age of 56 of an accident. Serum electrophoresis of the propositus' mother, of his brother, wife and daughter showed normal TTR patterns, whereas the 22 year old son showed normal as well as an altered TTR protein. The prealbumin level in the serum ranged from 0,28 (wife) to 0,37 g/l (mother) as a normal parameter.

History, electrocardiography under rest and exercise, chest roentgenography, echocardiography, laboratory tests, opthalmological and neurological examination with electromyo- and -neurography were completely negative concerning the son, and in addition with regard to the patient's daughter as a control person also. Only the son showed a slightly diminished sensory nerve conductance velocity.

DISCUSSION. A TTR variant in a German family causing cardiac amyloidosis with polyneuropathy is described. The propositus reported revealed typical signs of hypertrophic non obstructive cardiomyopathy combined with arrhythmia and exercise-induced dyspnoea as the most striking features. After exclusion of chronic infection and hematologic disorder by bone marrow aspirate a form of idiopathic amyloidosis was most likely. Because of the lack of amyloid deposits in other organs (rectum biopsies), a senile heart amyloidosis, characterized by ASc1 had to be excluded. Despite immunohistochemical cross reactions with amyloid AF [2], typical for familial amyloid polyneuropathy, biographic data such as dysaesthesia and gastric pain led to the possible diagnosis of FAP. To establish this diagnosis prealbumin/ TTR was examined for a possible variant. The heredity was proven on serum taken from the son who was shown to be a carrier of TTR mutant form as well. Remarkably this mutant has not yet been reported. We expect a new amino acid substitution to be the underlying cause. Although clinically inapparent, the son already demonstrated a slightly diminished sensory nerve conductance velocity. He should be followed up prospectively.

REFERENCES

1. Goffin, Y.A. (1989) 'Amyloid proteins and amyloidoses: complexity updated', Acta Clinica Belgica 44, 37-51
2. Linke, R.P. (1982) 'Immunohistochemical identification and cross reactions of amyloid fibril protein in senile heart and amyloid in familial polyneuropathy', Clinical Neuropathology 1, 172-182
3. Anzai, N.; Akiyama, K.; Tsuchida, K.; Yamada, M.; Kito, S.; and Yamamura, Y. (1989) 'Treatment by pacemaker in familial amyloid polyneuropathy', Chest 96, 80-84
4. Harada, T.; Kito, S.; Shimoyama, M.; Katayama, S.; Sasaki, H.; Furuya, H.; Yoshioka, K.; and Sakaki, Y. (1989) 'Genetic and clinical studies of Japanese patients with familial amyloid polyneuropathy', European Neurology 29, 48-52
5. Jacobson, D.R.; Santiago-Schwarz, F.; and Buxbaum, J.N. (1988) 'Restriction fragment analysis confirms the position 33 mutation in transthyretin from an Israeli patient (SKO) with familial amyloidotic polyneuropathy', Biochemical and Biophysical Research Communications, 153, 198-202
6. Nordlie, M.; Sletten, K.; Husby, G.; and Ranlov, P.J. (1988) 'A new prealbumin variant in familial amyloid cardiomyopathy of Danish origin', Scandinavian Journal of Immunology, 27, 119-122
7. Altland, K.; Becher, P.; and Banzhoff, A. (1987) 'Paraffin oil protected high resolution hybrid isoelectric focusing for the demonstration of substitutions of neutral amino acids in denatured proteins: The case of four human transthyretin (prealbumin) variants associated with familial amyloidotic polyneuropathy', Electrophoresis, 8, 293-297
8. Altland (in preparation)

STRUCTURAL STUDIES OF TRANSTHYRETIN AND RELATED FRAGMENTS OBTAINED FROM A SWEDISH PATIENT (V-ÅS 280) WITH SENILE SYSTEMIC AMYLODOSIS.

TOBIASSEN, R.*, GUSTAFSSON, Å.**, SLETTEN, K.*, JOHANSSON, B.**, WESTERMARK, P.**

* *Department of Biochemistry, University of Oslo, Norway*
** *Department of Pathology, University of Linkøping, Sweden*

ABSTRACT. In the present study, primary structure determination was performed of the TTR-like molecule and of the derived fragments, isolated from amyloid fibrils of the heart of a 83 year old Swedish patient (V-Ås 280) with senile systemic amyloidosis (SSA). The TTR derived fragments started in position 46, 49, 52 and 53, and revealed an amino acid sequence identical to that of normal TTR. Sequence data obtained supports our earlier data that the TTR-like molecule are of the normal type.

1. Introduction

A common feature with amyloid fibrils in senile systemic amyloidosis (SSA), in familial amyloid cardiomyopathy (FAC) and in familial polyneuropathy (FAP) is the involvment of transthyretin (TTR) derived proteins (1).
A point mutation in the TTR gene, leading to an amino acid substitution, is shown to be the hereditary factor in the familial amyloidosis (2).
Several such mutations, each linked to a specific type of amyloid disease, have now been demonstrated (2).
Senile systemic amyloidosis (SSA), earlier called senile cardiac amyloidosis is the most common systemic amyloidosis. About 25 % of the population over 80 years of age, are supposed to have deposits of amyloid fibrils containing TTR in various organs (3).
In most cases SSA does not produce symptoms, but some individuals, mostly men, are more severly affected. Serious deposits in the heart can give rise to cardiomegaly and heart failure (3).
The present study involves characterization of TTR derived proteins from amyloid fibrils of the heart of a patient with typical SSA.

2. Materials and methods

Amyloid fibrils were extracted from the heart of a 83 year old Swedish patient. Gel-filtration of degraded amyloid fibrils gave a TTR fraction A and a cystein-lacking fragment fraction B (4).

2.1 PURIFICATION OF TTR-FRACTIONS

The protein fraction A was dissolved in 6M guanidine hydrocloride (Gu-HCl) containing 0.1 M dithiothreitol (DTT) at pH 8.0. The excess of DTT was removed by gel filtration through a Sephadex G-25 column.
The protein fraction was then applied to a Thiopropyl Sepharose CL-6B column, equilibrated with 4.5 M Gu-HCl at pH 8.0, under which condition the cysteine-containing TTR is being bound. The column was washed with Gu-solution and the TTR was eluted with 25 mM L-cysteine. The eluted TTR-containing fraction was finally gel-filtered in a Sephacryl S-200 HR column equilibrated and eluted with 5 M Gu-HCl.
Fraction B, containing the cysteine-lacking proteins, was taken for purification on reverse phase HPLC (Vydac 214 TP5) using a linear gradient from 0-70 % of acetonitrile in 0.1 % trifluoroacetic acid (TFA). This resulted in several closely eluted peaks.

2.2. STRUCTURAL STUDIES

The TTR-derived polypeptides were hydrolyzed in 6 M HCl and quantitated by amino acid analysis using a Biotronic LC 5000 Amino Acid Analyzer.
N-terminal analysis was performed with an automatic sequence analyzer from Applied Biosystems (Model 477A). The PTH amino acid derivatives were determined with an on line 120A PTH amino acid analyser (Applied Biosystems). The polypeptides were obtained after cleavage with cyanogen bromide and 3'-bromo-3-metyl-2(nitrophenyl-sulphenyl)indolamine (BNPS-skatole) (4). The polypeptides were enzymatically degradated with trypsin and S.Aureus V8 protease (5).
The tryptic peptides, TTR-fragments and BNPS-fragments were purified by reverse phase HPLC (Vydac 218 TP54 and Vydac 214 TP5) using linear gradients from 0-70 %, 0-80 % and 0-90 %, respectively, of solvent B at a rate of 1.0 ml/min. Solvent A was 0.1 % TFA in wather, and solvent B was 30 % of solvent A in acetonitrile (4).

3. Results

3.1. AMINO ACID SEQUENCE ANALYSIS OF A TTR-LIKE MOLECULE

N-terminal sequence analysis of the TTR-like protein showed a ragged N-terminal region starting in position 3, 5, 6, 8 and 11. The sequence from positions 5 to 18 was established, except for positions 6 and 10 (Fig.1).
Cyanogen bromide cleavage of the protein, resulted in a free N-terminus, starting in position 14 of TTR. Twenty six degradation cycles confirmed positions 15-39. Positions 14, 21, 31, 34, 36 and 38 could not be fully established (Fig.1).

The protein was also cleaved with BNPS-skatole, and applied directly to the protein sequencer without purification. Positions 43-64 and 82-102 were confirmed with the exeption for positions 54, 56, 59-61, 63, 83, 88, 90, 92 and 94-95 (Fig.1).
The protein was finally digested with S.Aureus V8 protease. Only positions 105-109 were confirmed (Fig1). In this case the whole sample was applied with no previous HPLC separation.

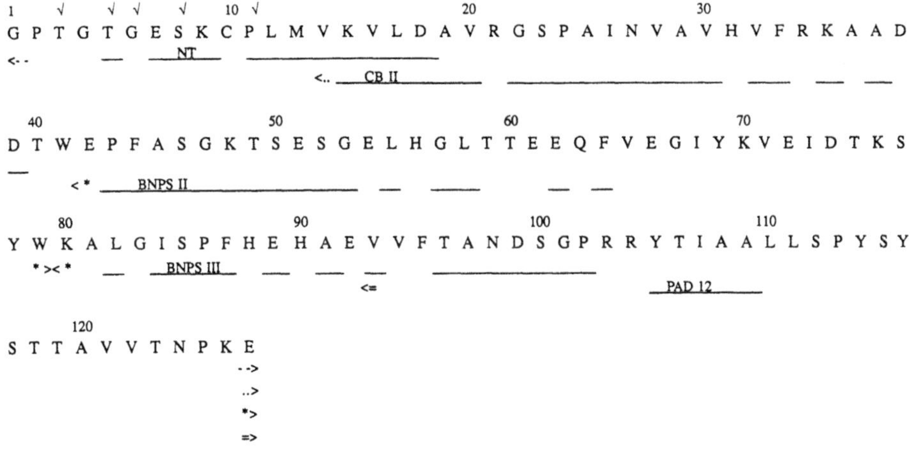

FIG.1. AMINO ACID SEQUENCE OF THE TTR-LIKE MOLECULE

The abbreviations used:

- .. CB , Cyanogenbromide fragment
- * BNPS , BNPS-skatole fragment
- = PAD , S.Aureus V8 protease peptides
- -- NT , N-terminal amino acid sequence of the protein
- √ , Characterised N-terminal residues of the ragged TTR

3.2. ANALYSIS OF TTR-DERIVED FRAGMENTS

The amyloid fibrils were found to contain TTR-derived fragments starting in positions 46, 49, 52 and 53. The N-terminal analyses of different HPLC fractions confirmed positions 47-81 with that of the normal TTR molecule, except for positions 56, 62, 63, 65, 72, 78 and 79, which were not fully established (Fig.2). Some of the fragments, which revealed a blocked N-terminal residue, were cleaved with BNPS-skatole. N-terminal analyses established the amino acid sequence of positions 82-85 (Fig.2).
Tryptic peptides, TD-7, TD-9, TD-10, TD-11+12 and TD-12, were isolated and characterised from a pool of TTR-derived fragments (Fig.2). The amino acid residues in positions 51-64, 78-79 and 83-126 were established. A small amount of tryptic peptides TD-3 (positions 16-21) and TD-4 (positions 22-34) were also identified, which would indicate that some of the TTR-derived fragments even started between position 11 and 16.

4. Discussion

The structural studies of the TTR-like molecule of SSA, as well as of the derived fragments, suggest a degradation of the molecule from the N-terminal region. TTR-derived fragments starting in positions 3, 5, 6, 8, 11, somewhere between 11 and 16, 46, 49, 52 and 53 were shown to exist. Similar fragmentation patterns have also been observed in other forms of amyloid where TTR-like molecules are involved (4).
The data so far supports our earlier data that the TTR-like molecule in SSA has no amino acid substitution, and that differences in the primary structure seems to be of minor importance for the fibrillogenesis.
In that case, it seems likely that the TTR monomer itself or the formation of the tetrameric form of TTR are factors involved in fibrillogenesis, and perhaps that the deposition site is more due to the availability of different proteases within the actual cell.

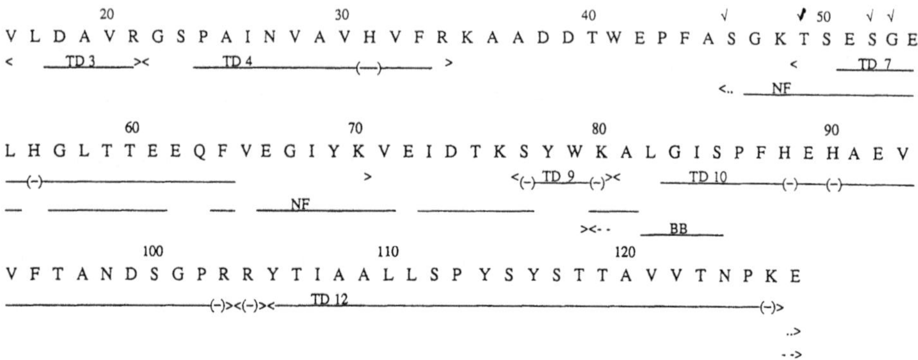

FIG.2. RESULTS FROM SEQUENCING OF TTR FRAGMENTS

The abbreviations used:

TD , Tryptic peptide
-- BB , Blocked fragment cleaved with BNPS-skatole
.. NF , N-terminal amino acid sequence of the fragments
√ , Characterised N-terminal residues of different fragments

5. References

1. Cornwell,G.G., Sletten,K., Olofsson,B.O., Johansson,B., and Westermark,P. (1987) 'Prealbumin:its association with amyloid', J.Clin.Pathol.**40**, 226-231.
2. Benson,M.D. (1989) 'Familial amyloidotic polyneuropathy',TINS.**12**,No.3.
3. Cornwell,G.G., Murdoch,W.L., Kyle,R.A., Westermark,P., and Pitkanen,P. (1983) 'Frequency and Distribution of Senile Cardiovascular Amyloid', Am.J.Med.**75**, 618-623.
4. Westermark,P., Sletten,K., Johansson,B., and Cornwell,G.G. (1990) 'Fibril in senile systemic amyloidosis is derived from normal transthyretin', PNAS.**87**, 2843-2845.
5. Sletten,K., Husebekk,A., and Husby,G. (1987) 'The amino acid sequence of an amyloid fibril protein AA isolated from the horse', Scand.J.Immunol.**26**, 79-84.

The transthyretin cDNA sequence is normal in transthyretin-derived senile systemic amyloidosis

Lars Christmanson[1], Christer Betsholtz[1], Björn Johansson[1] and Per Westermark[2]

[1]*Department of Pathology, University Hospital, S-751 85 Uppsala, Sweden and* [2]*Department of Pathology, University Hospital, S-581-85 Linköping, Sweden.*

A variety of mutations leading to amino acid substitutions have been described in the transthyretin (TTR) gene in association with different familial amyloidoses and have been implicated as the cause of amyloid formation. However, there has been disagreement whether or not a mutation in TTR is present in conjunction with the most common form of transthyretin-derived amyloidosis, the senile systemic amyloidosis (SSA). Therefore, the cDNA sequence of liver TTR was determined in a 91-year-old patient with typical SSA. The sequence was normal. We conclude that other factors than the presence of a mutant TTR must determine amyloid fibril formation in conjunction with this disease.

INTRODUCTION

There are two groups of amyloid syndromes in which the main fibril protein is transthyretin (TTR). These comprise most forms of familial amyloidoses (1-4) and the age-related senile systemic amyloidosis (SSA) (5,6). In the TTR-derived familial amyloidoses, point mutations in the TTR gene, leading to single amino acid substitutions have invariably been found. Several different substitutions spread over the TTR molecule have been described to-date (2-4,7-9). How these lead to fibril formation has, however, not yet been explained.

The familial amyloidoses are comparably rare. SSA, on the other hand, is a very common disorder, affecting about 25% of individuals over 90 years old, although very few of these have more than mild disease (10,11). In spite of this frequency, it has been claimed that SSA, like other TTR-derived amyloidoses, might be a hereditary disorder linked to an amino acid substitution in the TTR molecule (12). However, SSA amyloid protein sequencing studies by us have failed to reveal TTR mutations (5,6,13). We have now determined the cDNA sequence of TTR in a patient with advanced SSA and show that this is identical with previously published normal TTR genomic DNA and cDNA sequences.

MATERIALS AND METHODS

Liver and myocardial tissues were taken from a 91-year-old man at autopsy and frozen at -70 C. Congo red staining revealed massive amyloid infiltrations in the myocardium. Immunohistochemistry showed reaction with an antiserum against TTR. Total cellular RNA was extracted from the liver tissue using the LiCl/urea method (14), poly(A)-selected and used for oligo(dT) primed cDNA synthesis using an Amersham cDNA synthesis kit (Amersham, UK). Approximately 10 ng of cDNA was used for a polymerase chain reaction (PCR) using a sense primer corresponding to the 5' untranslated sequence of the human TTR cDNA sequence (15) immediately upstream of the translation initiation site (5'AATCGAGAATTCAGTCCACTCATTCTTGG CAGG) and an antisense primer complementary to the 3' untranslated sequence immediately downstream of the translation stop codon (5'ATTCGAGGATCCCACTGGAGGAGAAGTC CCTCA). The primers included EcoRI and BamHI sites respectively flanked by six "stuffer" nucleotides in their 5' ends to facilitate restriction enzyme cleavage and subcloning of the amplification product in M13 vectors. Thermostable DNA polymerase was purchased from Perkin Elmer Cetus (Norwalk, CT) and used as recommended by the manufacturer. The following PCR cycle temperature profiles were used: 94°C, 1min; 54°C, 10 min; 72°C, 30 min for two cycles followed by 94°C 1 min; 54°C, 2 min; 72°C, 4 min for 28 cycles. Ten percent of the amplification reaction mixture (10 ml) was analysed on a 1.5% agarose/TBE gel and showed only one amplified DNA fragment of the expected sixe, 507 base pairs. The reaction product was purified by isotachophoresis, cleaved by EcoRI and BamHI and subcloned in M13mp18/19 vectors The complete sequences of ten M13 clones were determined using dideoxynucleotide sequencing methodology (16).

RESULTS

An outline of the strategy to amplify TTR cDNA sequences from the liver of a patient with SSA is shown in Figure 1. A single DNA fragment of the expected size was amplified. The fragment was excised from the agarose gel, subcloned in M13 vectors and sequenced. Ten randomly picked TTR-positive clones were fully sequenced. All clones had a DNA sequence identical to that expected of normal TTR (15,17).

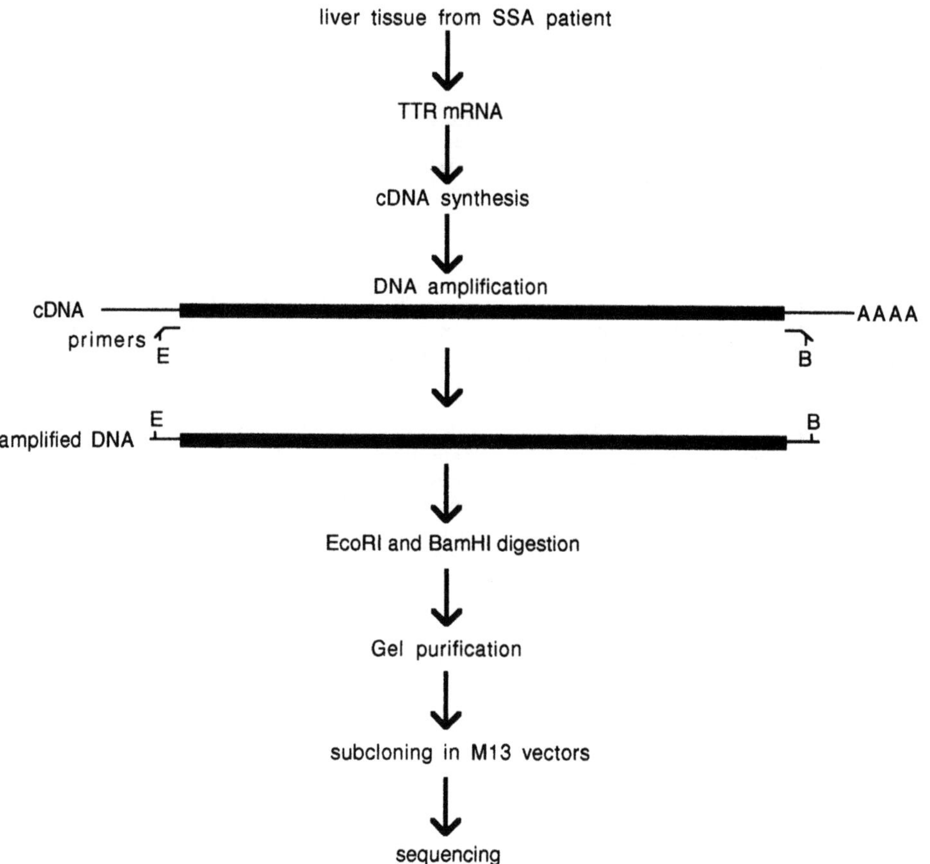

Figure 1. An outline of the strategy to amplify TTR sequences from a patient with advanced SSA.

DISCUSSION

In familial amyloidoses, mutant TTRs have invariably been found (2-4,7-9), but the fibrils have usually been found to contain normal TTR as well (18,19). This raises the question whether normal TTR by itself can give rise to amyloid fibrils. One such instance could be SSA which, since it is a very common disorder, is unlikely to involve specific TTR mutations. In a recent study, we resolved the complete primary structure of TTR in the amyloid of a patient with typical SSA and found it to have a normal amino acid sequence. However, since most of the amyloid was composed of TTR fragments of varying length, a TTR-variant with an amino acid substitution could, theoretically, have escaped detection. Therefore, we found it important to determine the structure of the TTR cDNA from a patient with typical SSA. If one of the TTR alleles is mutant in this disease, we would expect to find a mixture of normal and mutant TTR mRNA molecules. A simple way to study this question is to use PCR to amplify TTR cDNA sequences. Following subcloning and sequencing of the amplified TTR fragment, a fraction of the sequences would be mutant and the rest would be normal. The proportion of each would ideally reflect the transcriptional activity of each TTR allele. We sequenced ten such clones from a SSA patient and found that all of them were normal. Due to the absence of a polymorphic sequence within the TTR coding sequence analysed, we cannot completely exclude the possibility that a putative mutant allele is present and expressed at a very low level. However, we regard this possibility as unlikely.

In combination with the previous reports on normal amino acid sequences of TTR purified from SSA patients (5,6,13), the present result suggest that TTR with a normal primary structure is the sole constituent of amyloid fibrils in SSA. This is an important finding since it suggests that (a) mechanism(s) other than variations in the primary structure of TTR could be involved in the amyloid fibril formation by TTR. This mechanism may also be important in the pathogenesis of hereditary amyloidoses involving mutant TTR:s.

Recently, several investigations have reported an isoleucine for valine substitution in patients with an amyloid disorder resembling SSA (12,20,21). However, several facts indicate that these patients, rather than having proper SSA, suffer from a new form of hereditary amyloidosis with cardiomyopathy. Thus, all affected individuals were black and the onset of the disease appears to have occured at a much younger age than what is normally seen with SSA.

REFERENCES

1. Costa, P.P., Figueira, A.S., & Bravo, F.R. (1978) Amyloid fibril protein related to prealbumin in familial amyloidotic polyneuropathy. *Proc.Natl.Acad.Sci USA* **75**:4499-4503.

2. Nakazato, M., Kangawa, K., Minamino, N., Tawara, S., Matsuo, H. & Araki, S. (1984) Rivised analysis of amino acid replacement in aprealbumin variant (SKO-III) assoviated with familial amyloidotic polyneuropathy of Jewish origin. *Biochem.Biophys.Res.Commun.* **123**:921-928

3. Dwulet, F.E., & Benson, M.D. (1986) Characterization of a transthyretin (prealbumin) variant associated with familial amyloidotic polyneuropathy type II (Indiana/Swiss). *J.Clin:Invest.* **78**:880-886.

4. Nordlie, M., Sletten, K., Husby, G. and Ranlöv, P.J. (1988) A new prealbumin variant in familial amyloid cardiomyopathy of Danish origin. *Scand.J.Immunol.* **27**:119-122.

5. Sletten, K., Westermark, P. and Natvig, J.B. (1980) Senile cardiac amyloid is related to prealbumin. *Scand J Immunol.* **12**:503-506.

6. Cornwell, G.G. III, Sletten, K., Johansson, B. and Westermark, P. (1988) Evidence that the amyloid fibril protein in senile systemic amyloidosis is derived from normal prealbumin. *Biochem.Biophys.Res.Commun.* **154**:648-653.

7. Tawara, S., Nakazato, M., Kangawa, K., Matsuo, H. & Araki, S. (1983) Identification of amyloid prealbumin variant in familial amyloidotic polyneuropathy (Japanese type). *Biochem.Biophys.Res.Commun.* **116**:880-888

8. Wallace, M.R., Dwulet, F.E., Conneally, P.M. & Benson, M.D. (1986) Biochemical and molecular genetic characterization of a new variant prealbumin associated with hereditary amyloidosis. *J.Clin.Invest.* **78**:6-12.

9. Wallace, M.R., Dwulet, F.E., Williams, E.C., Conneally, P.M. & Benson, M.D. (1988) Identification of a new hereditary amyloidosis prealbumin variant, Tyr-77, and detection of the gene by DNA analysis. *J.Clin.Invest.* **81**:189-193.

10. Wright, J.R. & Calcins, E. (1975) Amyloid in the aged heart: frequency and clinical significance. *J.Am.Geriatr.Soc.* **23**:97-103.

11. Pitkänen, P., Westermark, P.& Cornwell, G.G. III. (1984) Senile systemic amyloidosis. *Am.J. Pathol.* **117**:391-399.

12. Gorevic, P.D., Prelli, F.C., Wright, J., Pras, M. & Frangione, B. (1989) Systemic senile amyloidosis. Identification of a new prealbumin (transthyretin) variant in cardiac tissue: Immunologic and biochemical similaroty to one form of familial amyloidotic polyneuropathy. *J Clin Invest* **83**:836-843.

13. Westermark, P., Sletten, K., Johansson, B. and Cornwell, G.G. III. (1990) Fibril in senile systemic

amyloidosis is derived from normal transthyretin. *Proc Natl Acad Sci USA* **87**:2843-2845.

14. Auffrey, C., & Rougeon, F. (1980) Purification of mouse immunoglobulin heavy-chain messenger RNAs from total myeloma tumor RNA. *Eur.J.Biochem.* **107**:303-314.

15. Mita, S., Maeda, S., Shimada, K. & Araki, S. (1984) Cloning and sequence analysis of cDNA for human prealbumin. *Biochem.Biophys.Res.Commun.* **124**:558-564.

16. Sanger, F., Nicklen, S. & Coulson, A.R. (1977) DNA sequencing with chain-terminating inhibitors. *Proc.Natl.Acad.Sci USA* **74**:5463-5467.

17. Sasaki, H., Yoshioka, N., Tagaki, Y. & Sakaki, Y. (1985) Structure of the chromosomal gene for human serum prealbumin. *Gene* **37**:191-197.

18. Dwulet, F.E., & Benson, M.D. (1984) Primary structure of an amyloid prealbumin and its plasma precursor in a heredo-familial polyneuropathy of Swedish origin. *Proc.Natl.Acad.Sci. USA* **81**:694-698.

19. Westermark, P., Sletten, K. and Olofsson, B.-O. (1987) Prealbumin variants in the amyloid fibrils of Swedish familial amyloidotic polyneuropathy. *Clin.Exp.Immunol.* **69**:695-701.

20. Nichols, W.C., Snyder, E.L., Liepnieks, J.J. & Benson, M.D. (1990) Senile cardiac amyloidosis is a hereditary disease. In: *Familial amyloidotic polyneuropathy and other transthyretin-related disorders.* (Costa, P.P, Falcüao de Freitas, A. & Saraiva, M.J.M. eds.) In press.

21. Saraiva, M.J.M., Sherman, W., Kyle, R., Gertz, M., Costa, P.P., Figueira, A. & Gawinowicz, M. (1990) In: *Familial amyloidotic polyneuropathy and other transthyretin-related disorders.* (Costa, P.P., Falcüao de Freitas, A. & Saraiva, M.J.M. eds.) In press.

A RECOMBINANTS SYSTEM FOR PRODUCTION OF VARIANT TYPE HUMAN TRANSTHYRETIN(TTR)

H. Furuya [1,2], M. J. M. Saraiva[3,4], M. A. Gawinowicz [5], I. L. Alves[3,4], P. P. Costa[4], H. Sasaki[1], I. Goto[2] and Y. Sakaki[1]
[1]Research Laboratory for Genetic Information and [2]Department of Neurology, Neurological Institute, Kyushu University 18, Fukuoka 812, Japan
[3]Institute of Biomedical Sciences, University of Porto and [4]Centro de Estudos de Paramiloidose, Hospital de Santo Antonio, 4000 Porto, Portugal
[5]Department of Medicine, Columbia University, New York, USA

ABSTRACT. We used an *Escherichia coli Omp*A secretion vector and achieved an effective production of the recombinant variant TTRs including Ser-10, Met-30, Ile-33, Ala-60, Tyr-77, Ser-84, Met-111 and Ile-122 types. The variant TTRs produced in this system were efficiently secreted to the culture media. The secreted TTR(Met-30 type) was shown to have the same N-termini as the native one, to form tetrameric structure and also to have the thyroxin(T4) binding activity.

1. Introduction

Some variant forms of transthyretin (TTR, prealbumin) have been known as a major component of amyloid fibrils found in familial amyloidotic polyneuropathy(FAP). Furthermore, the variants with different amino acid substitutions cause different clinical features of FAP. These observations indicated that the comparative analysis of the molecular nature of wild and variant TTRs is crucial for understanding the amyloidogenesis in FAP, but little has been known mainly because no pure preparation of the variants has been available. So, we have attempted to establish the system for production of the variant TTRs by recombinant DNA technology.

2. Materials and Methods

2.1. *Site-Specific Mutagenesis*:

Site-specific mutagenesis was performed according to the conventional method by Morinaga *et al*. (1984) and the method using the polymerase chain reaction(PCR) by Higuchi *et al*. (1988). The mutation was confirmed by a dideoxyribonucleic acid sequencing method. As for the construction of pUTR-30, 33, 60 and 77, the conventional method was applied and pUTR-OH, 84, 111 and 122, were constructed by the method of Higuchi *et al*. (1988).

2.2. *Preparation of cell extracts and SDS polyacrylamide gel electrophoresis*:

Bacteria carrying the recombinant plasmid were grown containing 50mg/ml of ampicillin with vigorous shaking. When the density of the culture reached 50-100 Klett units, isopropyl-β-D-thiogalactoside (IPTG) was added to a final concentration of 0.1mM to induce the production of recombinant TTR. The bacterial culture was centrifugated and cell pellets were resuspended in distilled water. Cells were disrupted by sonication and subjected to SDS polyacrylamide gel electrophoresis (SDS-PAGE). On the other hand, the supernatant of the culture medium was dialyzed and concentrated with lyophilization.

2.3. *Immunological analysis and N-terminal sequence determination:*

After SDS-PAGE, the proteins were electrophoretically transferred onto a polyvinylidene difluoride (PVDF) membrane and TTR was visualized by anti-human TTR antibody and second antibody alkaline phosphatase conjugate (ProtoBlot‰). The protein secreted in the media were also electroblotted onto a PVDF membrane and the protein band of 16kDa("M") was then excised in order to be sequenced. Sequencing was carried out on an Applied Biosystems 470A gas-phase peptide sequencer.

2.4. *Thyroxine binding assay*:

The recombinant Met-30 TTR was partially purified and T4 binding assay was carried out essentially as described previously (Saraiva *et al.*, 1984). A parallel assay mixture containing an excess of unlabeled T4 was investigated in order to examine displacement of labeled T4 from specific binding sites. After incubation, protein-bound [^{125}I] T4 was isolated from unbound hormone by gel filtration on minicolumns of Sephadex G-25.

3. Results

3.1. *Construction and expression of the Met-30 TTR expression plasmids:*

We previously constructed plasmid (pINTR-5)(Furuya *et al.*, 1989) for production of Met-30 TTR using pIN III-113-*Omp*A1 vector(Ghrayeb *et al.*, 1984). We then constructed the complete form of Met-30 TTR cDNA and introduced into pIN III-113-*Omp*A1 vector to generate pINTR-

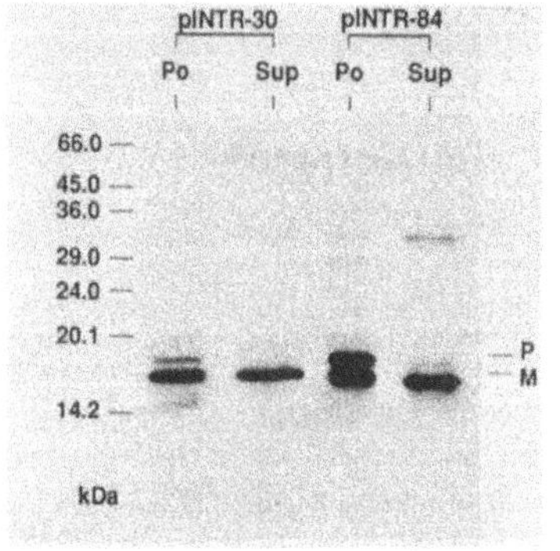

Pr:bacterial lysate (pre IPTG induction)
Po:bacterial lysate (after IPTG induction)
Sup:supernatant (after IPTG induction)

Figure 1. Immunoblot analysis of recombinant variant TTRs(Met-30 and Ser-84). Proteins were treated by anti-human TTR antibody and second antibody alkaline phosphatase conjugate. For each lane, 'Po' means bacterial lysate(after IPTG induction) and 'Sup' means supernatant of culture medium(after IPTG induction). The protein bands corresponding to the molecular weights of monomer TTR(16kDa) and *Omp*A-TTR fusion protein(18kDa) are indicated by 'M'and 'P'.

30(Furuya, H., *et al.*, submitted). *E. coli* carrying the plasmid was grown at 30°C and induced by IPTG. The protein bands of the molecular weight of 18kDa and 16kDa(named "P" and "M", respectively) were inducibly increased in the cell extracts but only the band of "M" was observed in the culture media, which is blotted by anti human TTR antibody(Fig. 1).

3.2. *N-terminus of the secreted TTR*:

To confirm that the 16kDa protein is the TTR monomer, the N-terminal amino acid sequence of the protein(pINTR-30) was determined by gas-phase peptide sequencer. From the profiles, the first nine amino acid sequence of the protein was determined to be Gly-Pro-Thy-Gly-Thr-Gly-Glu-Ser-Lys, which is identical to that of native human plasma TTR (Kanda *et al.*, 1974).

3.3. *Thyroxine binding activity*:

The recombinant TTR in the culture medium was partially purified, incubated with ^{121}I-labeled T4, and then subjected to the gel filtration. A peak of radioactivity was observed at the position corresponding to that of the protein-hormone complex. When the assay was carried out in the presence of an excess amount of cold T4, the protein-bound radioactivity was completely disappeared. This result indicated that the recombinant Met-30 TTR is able to bind T4.

3.4. *Construction of the expression vectors for other variant TTRs*:

The plasmid pUTR-RM having the wild type TTR cDNA was mutagenized to prepare pUTR-HO(Ser-10), 33(Ile-33), 60(Ala-60), 77(Tyr-77), 84(Ser-84), 111(Met-111) and pUTR-122(Ile-122). These mutagenized cDNAs were introduced into pIN III-113-*Omp*A1 vector and the final TTR expression/secretion plasmids(pINTR-HO, 33, 60, 77, 84, 111 and 122) were obtained(Furuya, H., *et al.*, submitted). When cells carrying these plasmids were grown in the presence of IPTG, two types of proteins were inducibly produced. For "P" and "M" proteins were immunologically stained with anti-human TTR antibody by Western blotting(Fig. 1) and the difference of molecular weights between "P" and "M" roughly corresponded to the size of signal leader peptide, it was considered that the larger protein "P" is the *Omp*A signal peptide-TTR fusion protein, and the protein "M" is the processed recombinant TTR itself. Thus, the TTR variants other than Met-30 type were also efficiently synthesized and secreted into the culture media by the *E. coli Omp*A vector system. It is interesting to note that the efficiency of the processing/secretion significantly differed from variant to variant (Table 1.), which may reflect the molecular nature of each TTR variants.

mutation site	10	30	33	60	77	84	111	122	wild type
amino acid substitution	Cys ↓ Ser	Val ↓ Met	Phe ↓ Ile	Thr ↓ Ala	Ser ↓ Tyr	Ile ↓ Ser	Ile ↓ Met	Val ↓ Ile	-
expression of 18kDa protein ("P")	-	-	±	+	+	+	+	+	+
16kDa protein("M")	+	++	++	+	+	+	±	±	-
secretion of "M"	+	+	+	+	+	+	±	±	-

TABLE 1. Comparisons of recombinant TTR secretion ability. The efficiency of ability was estimated after SDS-PAGE following coomassie brilliant blue staining.(+: positive, -: negative)

4. Discussion

In the present work, an expression system using *E. coli* secretion vector was constructed for the efficient production of human TTR variants related to FAP. The presented data suggested that the recombinant TTR(Met-30 type) produced in this system was functionally very similar to the native one.

To date, seven distinct variants of TTR have been identified as the major component of the amyloid fibrils in FAP and the tight linkage between FAP and the variants has been genetically established(Sakaki *et al.*, 1989). These findings indicate that the molecular nature of the variants is a crucial point to be analyzed for understanding the amyloidogenesis in FAP. However, little has been known about the characteristics of these variants mainly because almost all the FAP patients are heterozygous for the mutation and their plasma contains almost equal amount of normal and variant TTRs. The TTR production system developed in the present work enable us to produce any types of pure variants in a large amount.(Furuya *et al.*, submitted).

Native TTR forms tetramer in plasma and this structure is a prerequisite for the T4 binding activity (Blake *et al.*, 1978). Thus, the result indicated that the recombinant(Met-30) TTR forms tetrameric structure as native one. This system would be valuable for studying the effects of the FAP-related amino acid substitutions on the higher order structure as well as for verifying the structure and function relationship of TTR molecule by introducing appropriate amino acid substitutions with the technique of site-specific mutagenesis.

In conclusion, the TTR production system developed in this work opened a new way to study the molecular basis of amyloid formation in FAP and also the structure-function relationship of TTR molecule.

5. References

Blake, C.C.F., Geisow, M.J., Oatley, S.J., Rérat, B. and Rérat, C. (1978) 'Structure of prealbumin: Secondary, tertiary and quaternary interactions determined by Fourier refinement at 1.8Å' *J. Mol. Biol.*, **121**, 339-356.

Furuya, H., Nakazato, M., Saraiva, M.J.M., Costa, P.P., Sasaki, H., Matsuo, H., Goto, I. and Sakaki, Y. (1989) 'Tetramer formation of a variant type human transthyretin(prealbumin) produced by *Escherichia coli* expression system' *Biochem. Biophys. Res. Commun.*, **163**, 851-859.

Furuya, H., Saraiva, M.J.M, Gawinowicz, M.A., Alves, I.L., Costa, P.P., Sasaki, H., Goto, I. and Sakaki, Y. 'Production of recombinant human transthyretin with biological activities toward the understanding of the molecular basis of familial amyloidotic polyneuropathy (FAP)', submitted

Ghrayeb, J., Kimura, H., Takahara, M., Hsiung, H., Masui, Y. and Inouye, M. (1984) 'Secretion cloning vectors in Escherichia coli' *EMBO J.*, **3**,2437-2442.

Higuchi, R., Krummel, B., Saiki, R.K. (1988) 'A general method of in vitro preparation and specific mutagenesis of DNA fragments: Study of protein and DNA interactions' *Nucl, Acids Res.*, **16**, 7451-7367.

Kanda, Y., Goodman, D.S., Canfield, R.E., Morgan, F.J. (1974) 'The amino acid sequence of human plasma prealbumin.' *J. Biol. Chem.*, **249**, 6796-6805

Morinaga, Y., Franceschini, T., Inouye, S., and Inouye, M. (1984) 'Improvement of oligonucleotide-directed site specific mutagenesis using double-stranded plasmid DNA' *Bio/Technology* **2**, 636-639.

Sakaki, Y., Yoshioka, K., Tanahashi, H. Furuya, H. and Sasaki, H. (1989) 'Human transthyretin (prealbumin) gene and molecular genetics of familial amyloidotic polyneuropathy' *Mol. Biol. Med.*, **6**, 161-168.

Saraiva, M.J.M., Birken, S., Costa, P.P. and Goodman, D.S. (1984) 'Amyloid fibril protein in familial amyloidotic polyneuropathy. Portuguese type' *J. Clin. Invest.*, **74**, 104-119.

ASSESSEMENT OF STRUCTURE AND BINDING CAPACITIES OF SECRETED MUTANT TRANSTHYRETINS BY AN E.Coli SYSTEM

I. L. Alves[1,2], H. Furuya[3], H. Sasaki[3], H. Sakaki[3], P.P. Costa[1], M.J.M. Saraiva[1,2]

[1]Centro de Estudos de Paramiloidose and [2]Bioquímica, Instituto de Ciências Biomédicas Abel Salazar, Porto, Portugal; [3]Research Laboratory for Genetic Information, Kyushu University, Fukuoka, Japan

ABSTRACT

Recently, an E. coli expression system was used for the production of several TTR variants. In this work, some properties of the secreted proteins were studied in order to see if they could be used in future structural and functional studies. We concluded that the isolated TTRs were correctly processed to the normal size, could form a stable tetramer and were able to bind T4 and RBP.

INTRODUCTION

Comparative studies of wild and variant types of TTR are necessary for the understanding of the mechanisms of amyloid fibril formation. Recently, Furuya et al (1989) used an E.coli expression system where the recombinant TTR was first synthesized as a fusion protein with E. coli outer membrane protein A (omp A) signal peptide, processed to eliminate the signal peptide and finally secreted to the culture medium. Using site directed mutagenesis several bacterial strains, coding for different TTR molecules, namely wild type, Ser 10, Met 30, Ala 60, Tyr 77, Ser 84, Met 111 and Ile 122, were obtained.

The aim of this work was the study of the characteristics of the products secreted by these E. coli strains, that is, whether the polypeptide chain is correctly processed and has binding capacities to the normal physiological ligands, thyroxine (T4) and retinol-binding protein (RBP), before using these variants in structural and functional studies.

MATERIALS AND METHODS

CELL CULTURE

Bacteria carrying the recombinant plasmid were grown essencially as described (Furuya et al,1989), centrifuged and the supernatant was collected.

TTR PURIFICATION

Purification of supernatant TTR was carried out by a two step procedure. First, the protein was semipurified by chromatography in DEAE-cellulose equilibrated in glycine buffer. The protein was eluted by lowering the pH.

The major peak was collected, applied on a DEAE-cellulose column in Tris/HCl buffer and TTR was eluted by applying a NaCl gradient.

IEF

Isoelectric focusing was performed essentially as described (Altland et al, 1981), to analyse purified TTRs.

RBP BINDING ASSAY

The RBP binding capacity of mutant TTR was analysed by ligand blotting. After electrophoresis on a SDS-polyacrylamide gel, the proteins were transferred to a nitrocellulose membrane. The filter was blocked with bovine serum albumin (BSA) and incubated with human serum RBP at a concentration of 200 µg/ml.

Detection of RBP bound to TTR was made by incubation with anti-human RBP antibody and second biotinylated antibodies.

THYROXINE BINDING ASSAYS

To investigate thyroxine binding to the different TTRs, these proteins were incubated with L-(^{125}I)T4 (Amersham) for 30 minutes and then applied to a native polyacrylamide gel in glycine-acetate buffer (Saraiva et al, 1988). A serum control was run in parallel. The gel was then autoradiographed.

RESULTS

Secreted TTR was purified by a two step procedure. Figure 1 shows the SDS-PAGE analysis of the two major protein peaks from these steps obtained for TTR Met30. Pure TTR Met30 has the correct size for the normal monomer, i.e., approximately 15,000 da.

IEF analysis revealed that the mutant monomers focused at the same pH as the normal serum TTR monomer, indicating that the polypeptide chains are correctly processed. Furthermore, an oxidation product was observed for all proteins except for Ser10. This result strongly confirms the hypothesis of the involvement of Cys10 in the formation of the oxidation product.

Thyroxine and RBP binding capacities of the secreted TTRs were assessed only at a qualitative level. The presence of TTR radioactive bands after autoradiography, in the first case, and stained bands after immunoblotting, in the second, indicates that these TTRs are able to bind T4 and RBP.

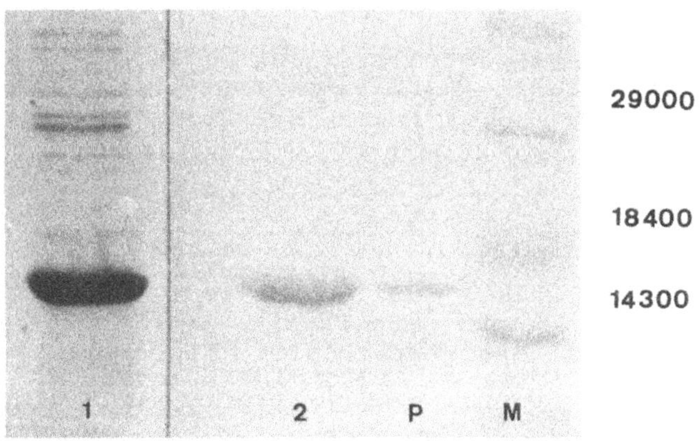

Figure 1: TTR purification. SDS-PAGE analysis of the major protein fractions obtained in each step.
1- Semipurified TTR
2- Purified TTR
P- Purified human TTR
M- Molecular weight markers

CONCLUSIONS

From these studies we can conclude that TTR secreted by the E. coli strains has the following characteristics:

- can be easily purified by ion exchange chromatography
- is properly processed to the correct size and can form a stable tetramer
- is able to bind thyroxine and RBP, the normal physiological ligands of human TTR. Future studies involving determination of binding constants for T4 and RBP will evaluate its affinities to these ligands.

These recombinant TTRs will also serve in studies of the amyloidogenesis process "in vitro"; the Ser10 mutant will be important for studies concerning the role of disulfide bonds in the polymerization process.

ACKNOWLEDGMENTS

This work was supported by grant 87440 from JNICT (Portugal) and grant RO1NS25190 from U.S. National Institutes of Health.

REFERENCES

Altland, K., Rauh, S., Haeckler, R. (1981). Demonstration of human prealbumin by double one-dimensional slab gel electrophoresis. Electrophoresis,2: 148-155.

Furuya, H., Nakazato, N., Saraiva, M.J.M., Costa, P.P., Sasaki, H., Goto, I., Sakaki, Y. (1989). Tetramer formation of a variant type human transthyretin (prealbumin) produced by an E. coli. expression system. Biochem. Biophys. Res. Commun. 163: 851-859.

Saraiva, M.J.M., Costa, P.P., Goodman, D.S. (1988). Advances in Neurology: 189-200.

STRUCTURE AND FUNCTION OF RECOMBINANT HUMAN TRANSTHYRETIN

[1]Murrell, J., [3]Schoner, R., [4]Moses, A., [4]Rosen, H., and [1,2]Benson, M.D.

[1] Indiana University School of Medicine, Department of Medicine, Rheumatology Division, Clinical Building 492, 541 Clinical Drive, Indianapolis, IN 46223, USA

[2] Veterans Affairs Medical Center (583/111RH), 1481 West 10th Street, Room #A772, Indianapolis, IN 46202, USA

[3] Eli Lilly Co., Indpls., IN, USA

[4] Harvard Medical School, Boston, MA, USA

ABSTRACT. In order to gain more insight into the metabolism, structure and function of transthyretin (TR) and its variants, recombinant human TR (r-TR) was synthesized _in vitro_ using a thermoinducible expression vector, pCZ11. Normal TR cDNA was ligated into the NdeI-BamHI sites of pCZ11 and then transformed into E. coli JM103 cells. The r-TR showed the correct size (14kD) on PAGE and Western analysis and self associated into tetramers as seen by size exclusion chromatography. To determine proper function, iodothyronine equilibrium competitive binding assays were performed by incubating $^{125}I\text{-}T_4$ with purified r-TR in the presence of increasing concentration of unlabeled iodothyronines. Affinity constants of r-TR for T_4 were determined by the method of Scatchard. r-TR had the same affinity for T_4 and other iodothyronine analogs (Ka=$1.9 \pm .16 \times 10^{7} M^{-1}$) as normal human TR purified from serum (Ka= $1.06 \pm .36 \times 10^{7} M^{-1}$). Variants of TR were also studied. The rank order of affinity of the TR variants for T_4 was Thr^{109}>normal=Ala^{60}=Ile^{122}(heterozygous)>His^{58}=Tyr^{77}=Ser^{84}=Ile^{122}(homozygous)=Met^{30}(heterozygous)>>Met^{30}(homozygous). These studies demonstrate that _in vitro_ expression of human TR can provide large amounts of pure protein (normal and variant) for the study of structure/function relationships and amyloid forming capabilities.

INTRODUCTION

Familial amyloidotic polyneuropathy (FAP) is a late-onset autosomal dominant disease characterized by extracellular deposition of variant forms of protein. Most FAP cases involve serum transthyretin variants which are due to single base changes. Transthyretin functions as a 55,000 dalton tetramer transporting 20-25% of serum thyroxine and retinol-saturated retinol binding protein. In order to learn more about the structure and function of transthyretin (TR), recombinant human TR was synthesized _in vitro_ utilizing a thermoinducible runaway expression vector, pCZ11 [1]. In addition, the function of native variant transthyretins was studied by performing thyroxine binding analyses.

MATERIAL AND METHODS

pCZ11 Cloning. The 470 base pair (bp) TR cDNA was first subcloned into the PstI/StyI sites of pUC18 along with a StyI/BamHI 3' linker in order to facilitate the final ligation into pCZ11. The resultant pUC18 clones were screened and then cut with BglI and BamHI. This 370 bp fragment was ligated into the NdeI/BamHI sites of pCZ11 along with an NdeI/BglI 5' linker. JM103 cells were transformed and plated on kanamycin (50ug/ ml) TY plates [2]. Colonies were screened and positive clones sequenced using the M13 dideoxynucleotide method [3].

Analysis of Protein. Positive JM103 pCZ11 clones were grown overnight at 25°C and then diluted 1:4 and grown at 37°C for six hours. One milliliter of the cells was centrifuged, and the cell pellet resuspended in buffer (10% SDS, 10% glycerol, 6M urea, .1% bromphenol blue and β mercaptoethanol) and boiled for three minutes. The cell lysate was electrophoresed on a 12.5% SDS-polyacrylamide gel which was stained with Fairbanks A and B. The protein gels were then transferred to nitrocellulose, and Western blots were done with TR antisera.

Isolation of Protein. Protein was isolated by lysing the cells with lysozyme. After centrifuging, the supernate was fractionated on DEAE Sephadex A. TR containing peaks were then subjected to sieve chromatography on Ultra-gel ACA-34 [4]. Molecular weight of the recombinant TR (r-TR) was determined on an Ultra-gel ACA34 column using BSA and OVA as standards. Native variant TRs were isolated from 100 ml of plasma using the same techniques as above except for an additional fractionation on Affigel Blue.

Thyroxine (T_4) Binding. Thyroxine binding was determined by immunoprecipitation assays. For these assays, 1 ug/100ul of protein diluted 1:25 in PBS were incubated with ^{125}I-T_4($6x10^{-12}$M) in 100 ul of PBS containing 1mg/ml of bovine serum albumin for three hours at 37°C. One hundred ul of a 1:20 dilution of anti-TR IgG was added before incubation at 4°C and centrifuged. The pellet was counted in a gamma spectrometer [5]. TR affinity was determined with a competitive binding assay using purified TR [.5ug] as described above except that replicate samples of purified TR were incudbated with ^{125}I-T_4($6x10^{-12}$M) in the presence of varying concentrations of unlabelled T_4. TR bound ^{125}I-T_4 was separated as described above and counted in a gamma spectrometer. Affinity constants were calculated by the method of Scatchard.

RESULTS

Dideoxynucleotide sequencing of the positive kanamycin resistant clones showed the correct cDNA sequence and linker orientation. Protein extracts of cultured cells run on polyacrylamide-SDS gels showed a band of approximately 14,000 molecular weight which was specific for TR on Western blot analysis. Chromatography on ACA-34 of r-TR isolated by ion-exchange and size-exclusion chromatography exhibited a molecular weight between 50,000 and 60,000, consistant with the tetrameric size of TR. Competitive binding assays showed r-TR had the same affinity for T_4 as normal human TR purified from serum; Ka=$1.9\pm.36x10^7M^{-1}$ (Figure 1). Affinity for T_4 of other TR variants was also determined. The Thr 109 variant had the highest affinity for T_4 followed by normal TR. Next were Ala 60 and Ile 122, both heterozygous. Slightly lower

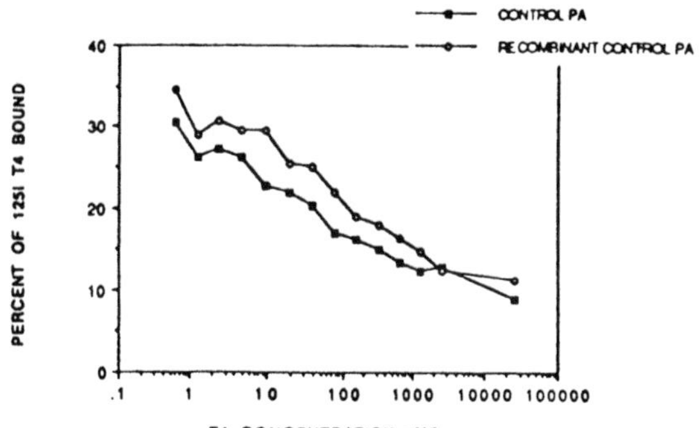

Figure 1. Comparison of T_4 binding by TR and r-TR.

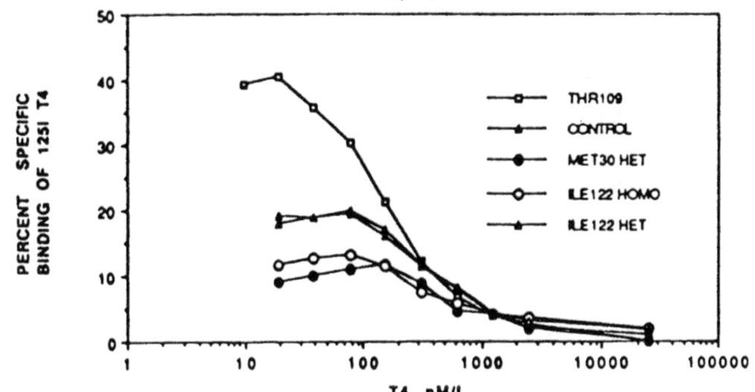

Figure 2. Competitive binding assay with TR variants Thr 109, Met 30, and Ile 122 purified from human serum.

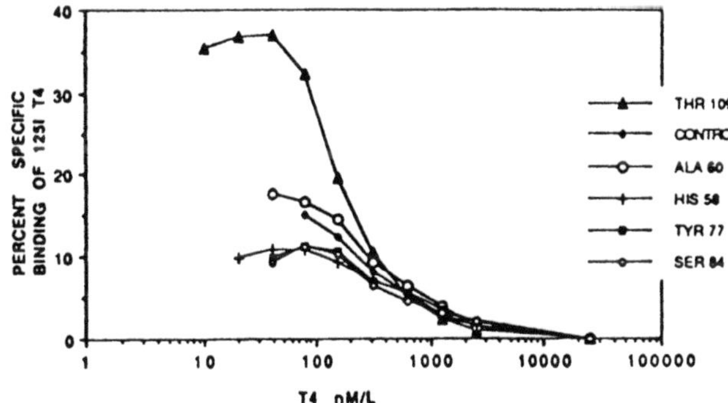

Figure 3. Competitive binding assay with variants Ala 60, His 58, Tyr 77, and Ser 84. The Met 30 homozygous protein was also done but had virtually no specific binding.

affinity constants were found for His 58, Tyr 77, Ser 84 and Ile 122 (homozygous) and Met 30 (heterozygous) (Figures 2 and 3). Homozygous Met 30 [6] had the lowest affinity for T_4.

DISCUSSION

r-TR produced by the pCZ11 vector was found to form tetramers and bind thyroxine the same as native TR. However, T_4 binding by TR variants was altered according to specific amino acid changes. Thr 109, described by Moses et al. in a family with dysprealbuminemic hyperthyroxinemia showed increased affinity compared to normal. This variant to date has not been associated with amyloidosis. The rest of the variants had lower affinity for T_4 than normal TR. This data suggests that the affinity for T_4 is determined by the location of the amino acid change. For example the Thr 109 change is within the thyroxine binding pocket. The Ala 60 amino acid is located on the surface of the molecule, thus affecting T_4 binding much less than the Thr 109 mutation. Another consideration is that the amino acid changes may affect association of the monomers to form tetramers and, therefore, affect the T_4 binding site within the central channel. In the homozygous state, Met 30 binds T_4 with less affinity than heterozygous Met 30. The same is seen with Ile 122. Studies such as these will help determined the effect of single amino acid changes on TR function. In vitro expression and site-directed mutagenesis of human TR can provide large amounts of protein (variant and normal) for the study of structure and function.

ACKNOWLEDGEMENTS

This work was supported by VA Medical Research, the United States Public Health Service (RR-00750, NIDDK-34881, NIAMS-AR20582, AR7448), The Arthritis Foundation, The Grace M. Showalter Trust and The Marion E. Jacobson Fund.

REFERENCES

1. Schoner, B.E., Belagaje, R.M., and Schoner, R.G. (1986) 'Translation of a synthetic 2-cistron mRNA in Excherichia coli', Proc. Natl. Acad. Sci. USA 83, 8506-8510.
2. Maniatis, T., Fritsch, E.F., and Sambrook, J. (1982) Molecular cloning: A laboratory manual, Cold Spring Harbor, NY.
3. Sanger, F., Nicklen, S., and Coulson, A. (1977) 'DNA sequencing with chain termination inhibitors', Proc. Natl. Acad. Sci. USA 74, 5462-5467.
4. Dwulet, F.E. and Benson, M.D. (1983) 'Polymorphism of human plasma thyroxine binding prealbumin', Biochem. Biophys. Res. Commun. 114, 657-662.
5. Moses, A.C., Rosen, H.N., et al., 'The molecular basis of dysprealbuminemic hyperthyroxinemia: identification of a point mutation in transthyretin that increases affinity for thyroxine', JCI in press.
6. Holmgren, G., Haettner, E., Nordenson, I., Sandgren, O., Steen, L., and Lundgren, E. (1988), 'Homozygosity for the transthyretin Met 30 gene in two Swedish sibs with familial amyloidotic polyneuropathy', Clin. Genet. 34, 333-338.

DETECTION OF VARIANT TRANSTHYRETIN GENES BY RESTRICTION ANALYSIS OF PCR-AMPLIFIED GENOMIC DNA.

D.R. Jacobson and J.N. Buxbaum, New York University School of Medicine and Department of Veterans Affairs Medical Center, New York, NY, USA

ABSTRACT. Many of the DNA point mutations causing TTR variants lead to the formation or destruction of a restriction site; the new restriction pattern can be used to detect DNA variants after amplification of TTR coding regions by the polymerase chain reaction (PCR). We have PCR-amplified genomic DNA in order to detect 5 different TTR mutations associated with amyloidosis. These techniques are useful for genetic testing for TTR variants associated with disease.

1. Introduction.

Several transthyretin (TTR) variants are associated with TTR-amyloid deposition in cardiac tissue and along peripheral nerves (1). These TTR variants are encoded by genes containing point mutations, many of which lead to the formation or destruction of a restriction site. The polymerase chain reaction (PCR) represents a powerful tool for the investigation of genetic TTR variants. We have used the new restriction patterns which result from PCR-amplification and restriction enzyme digestion to detect 5 DNA variants associated with amyloidosis.

2. Materials and Methods

HAR was a Black male who died of amyloid cardiomyopathy, whose TTR was homozygous for the variant (122 Val→Ile) (2). DNA samples heterozygous for TTR (122 Val→Ile) were obtained from healthy Black volunteer blood donors. SKO is an Israeli patient with Familial Amyloidotic Polyneuropathy (FAP) and the variant TTR (33 Phe→Ile) (3). DNA coding for TTR (30 Val→Met) was provided by Drs. Merrill Benson and Maria Saraiva. HER and SMA are FAP kindreds with other TTR variants in exon 2 and exon 3, respectively.

Oligonucleotide primers were complementary to genomic sequences flanking TTR exons 2, 3, and 4. The polymerase chain reaction (PCR) was performed as previously described (2), except that cycling times were shortened (94°C x 45 sec and 55-60°C x 30 sec).

To demonstrate the exon 2 and exon 3 TTR variants, aliquots from the PCR reactions were digested with the appropriate enzyme (Nsi I, Bcl I, Fnu4H I, Alu I, or Mae III), electrophoresed through an agarose gel, and stained with ethidium bromide. For the position 122 variant, in some cases an aliquot of the PCR product was subjected to a second round of PCR, using nested primers, prior to Mae III digestion.

3. Results and Discussion

Restriction enzyme analysis of PCR-amplified DNA around TTR exons 2, 3, and 4 permitted demonstration of genes coding for TTR variants associated with amyloidosis: exon 4 PCR and Mae III digestion allowed identification of carriers of the gene coding for TTR (122 Val→Ile), associated with SSA in Blacks (figure 1). Mae III digests the normal DNA cuts completely, whereas the variant gene is resistant to Mae III cleavage.

Similarly, exon 2 PCR permitted identification of the genes coding for TTR (33 Phe→Ile) after Bcl I digestion (figure 2A) and for TTR (30 Val→Met) after Nsi I digestion (figure 2B). In each case, only the abnormal gene is recognized by the restriction enzyme. We have also used this technique to identify new TTR gene mutations in exons 2 and 3 (figure 2B); in each of these cases, the normal gene is completely digested, whereas the variant allele is resistant.

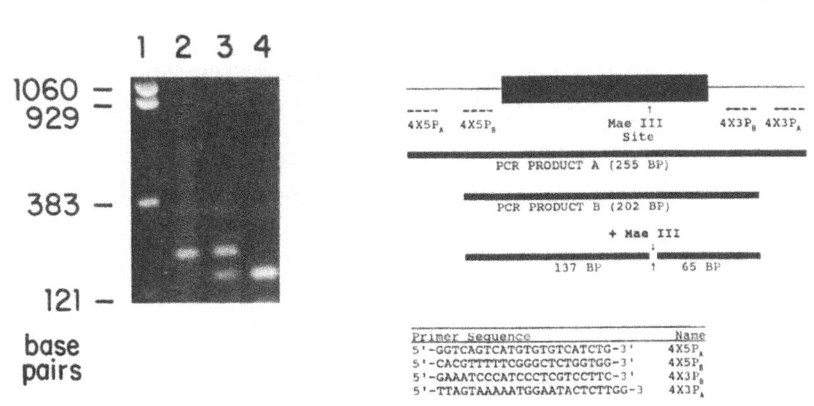

Figure 1. A. Mae III digests of PCR-amplified exon 4 DNA. Lane 1: DNA size markers. Lane 2: DNA homozygous for the codon 122 mutation (Mae III(-)) coding for TTR (Val→Ile). Lane 3: DNA heterozygous for the Mae III (-) variant, showing both the variant (top) and normal (bottom) bands. Lane 4: normal control, showing complete digestion with Mae III. **B.** Schematic diagram illustrating the experimental protocol for demonstrating the Mae III (-) variant.

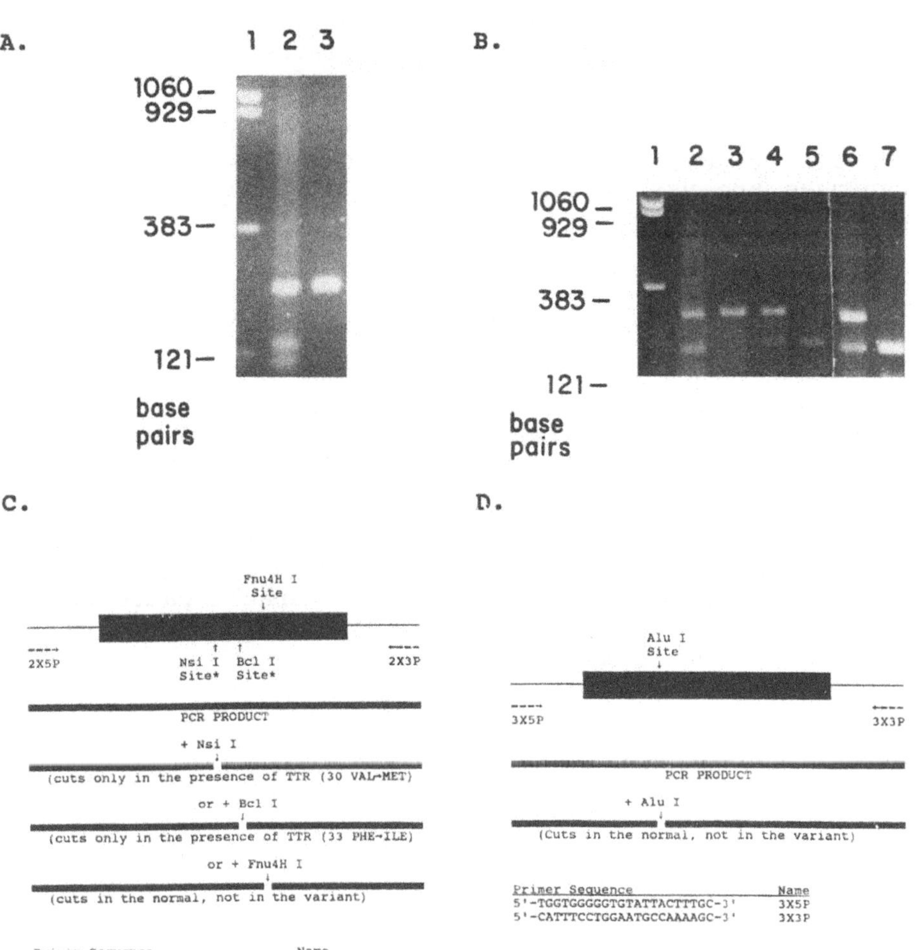

Figure 2. Exon 2 and 3 TTR variants. **A.** Lanes 2-3: exon 2 PCR product digested with Bcl I; lane 2: DNA from an FAP patient heterozygous for TTR (33 Phe→Ile); lane 3: control. **B.** Lanes 2-3: Exon 2 PCR product digested with Nsi I; lane 2: DNA from a patient with TTR (30 Val→Met); lane 3: control. Lanes 4-5: exon 2 PCR product digested with Fnu4H I; lane 4: DNA from a patient with a position 36/37 mutation; lane 5: control. Lanes 6-7: Exon 3 PCR product digested with Alu I; lane 6: a patient from a kindred with a position 54/55 variant; lane 7: control. **C.** Schematic diagram illustrating the experimental protocol for demonstrating exon 2 TTR variants. Asterisks denote restriction sites accompanying TTR variants. **D.** Schematic diagram illustrating the experimental protocol for demonstrating the exon 3 TTR variant.

These tests facilitate identification of DNA variants more easily than Southern analysis, because of the speed and economy of PCR. PCR is particularly useful for detection of the position 122 variant; because of the small size of the genomic Mae III restriction fragments, this variant is difficult to demonstrate by Southern analysis (2). These techniques are useful for genetic testing for TTR variants associated with disease.

4. References.

1) Benson, M.D. (1989) Familial amyloidotic polyneuropathy. Trends Neurosci. 12:88-92.

2) Jacobson DR, Gorevic PD, and Buxbaum JN. (1990) A homozygous transthyretin variant associated with senile systemic amyloidosis: evidence for a late-onset disease of genetic etiology. Am. J. Hum. Genet. 47:127-136.

3) Jacobson DR, Santiago-Schwarz F, and Buxbaum, JN. (1988) Restriction fragment analysis confirms the position 33 mutation in transthyretin from an Israeli patient (SKO) with familial amyloidotic polyneuropathy. Biochem. Biophys. Res. Comm. 153:198-202.

MYELIN P2 PROTEIN IN TRANSTHYRETIN (SER-84) VITREOUS AMYLOID.

R.L. MARTONE, M.D. BENSON and J. HERBERT
Columbia University and Helen Hayes Hospital,
Depts. of Neurology, 630 West 168th Street
New York, NY 10032
and Indiana University and Roudebush VA Medical Center,
Indianapolis, IN 46202, U.S.A.

ABSTRACT.

In familial amyloidotic polyneuropathy, transthyretin (TTR)-amyloid is deposited in peripheral nerve (PN) and frequently in ocular vitreous. We explored the possiblity that a common factor may be implicated in amyloidogenesis in these two tissues. We studied the PN myelin protein, P2, which shares conformational homology with serum retinol-binding protein (RBP), a known ligand of TTR. We performed immunoblot analysis using a polyclonal antiserum to purified bovine P2 (a gift of S.W. Brostoff) and detected an immunoreactive band co-migrating with P2 (apparent M.W. 15 kDa) in bovine vitreous. A prominent P2 band was also detected in 3 of 4 samples of vitreous amyloid fibrils from patients carrying the Serine-84 TTR mutation, but not in supernatant fractions. RBP, a component of the normal mammalian vitreous, was not present in amyloid fibril or supernatant fractions. Our findings raise the possibility that TTR-amyloidogenesis may involve a specific interaction between mutant TTR and P2 protein.

1. INTRODUCTION

It is now well established that FAP is caused by mutations in serum transthyretin (TTR), and numerous point mutations in the TTR monomer have been characterized. However, the mechanism of amyloid fibrillogenesis and the factors determining the tissue distribution of TTR-amyloid are unknown.

In this study we have investigated the possibility that amyloid fibril formation in the vitreous may involve an interaction between TTR and specific tissue determinants.

2. MATERIALS AND METHODS

Purified bovine myelin P2 protein and antiserum to bovine P2 were generous gifts of S.W. Brostoff [1]. Antisera to human TTR and to human RBP were from Boehringer-Mannheim (Indianapolis, IN); purified human RBP was from Calbiochem (San Diego, CA). Acrylamide, bis-acrylamide, TEMED, ammonium persulfate and low molecular weight markers were from Bio-Rad (Richmond, CA). All other reagents were from Sigma Chemical Co. (St. Louis, MO).

Patients were all members of the Indiana/Swiss kindred [2] in which a serine for isoleucine substitution occurs at amino acid residue no. 84 of the TTR monomer [3]. Four vitrectomy specimens were obtained from 3 patients and aspirated into sterile saline. Amyloid fibrils were prepared by centrifugation, resuspension in citrate saline (twice) and extensive dialysis against water. Vitreous supernatant fractions were saved.

Bovine vitreous was prepared by dissecting the vitreous body from whole bovine eyes less than 4 hours post-enucleation. Vitreous contents were homogenized and centrifuged to remove insoluble material.

Total protein concentration was determined by the method of Lowry et al. [4]. When necessary, samples were concentrated in vacuo.

Protein electrophoresis [5] and immunoblotting [6] were performed as follows: All samples were boiled in sample buffer containing SDS and beta-mercaptoethanol before electrophoresis on SDS-15% polyacrylamide gels. Separated proteins were transferred to nitrocellulose and incubated for 1 hour in phosphate buffered saline containing 0.05% Tween-20 (TPBS) and 3% BSA. Filters were incubated overnight with a 1:1000 dilution of primary antibody in 3% BSA-TPBS, washed with TPBS and then incubated for 1 hour in 3% BSA-TPBS containing a 1:1000 dilution of peroxidase-conjugated secondary antibody. After further washes, filters were developed in 1 mg/ml each of diaminobenzidine and imidazole with 0.024% hydrogen peroxide.

3. RESULTS

When purified TTR, P2 and RBP were reacted with the non-homologous antisera, no cross-reactivity was detected.

Western blot analysis of fresh peripheral nerve with antiserum to P2 revealed a single immunoreactive band with an apparent molecular weight of 15 kDa co-migrating with purified P2. Western blot analysis of normal bovine vitreous revealed the presence of both RBP and P2 immunoreactivity.

TTR immunoreactivity was detected in fibril and supernatant fractions of all four samples. On the other hand, no RBP immunoreactivity was detected in either fraction from any sample. P2 immunoreactivity was detected in 3 of 4 fibril preparations; one such immunoblot is illustrated in Figure 1. Supernatant fractions from the same preparations, containing threefold higher concentration of total protein than the fibril fractions, were not immunoreactive for P2.

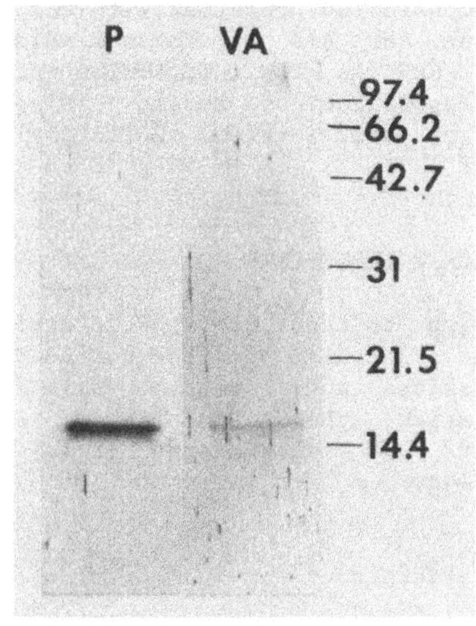

Figure 1. Western blot analysis demonstrating P2 immunoreactivity in vitreous amyloid, patient no. 3.

Lane P: 100 ng. purified bovine P2
Lane VA: 0.7 ug vitreous amyloid fibril

4. DISCUSSION

To address the question of amyloid fibrillogenesis, we have chosen to study the ocular vitreous because it is a relatively acellular structure of simple chemical composition, and because it is a frequent site of amyloidosis in FAP. Vitreous opacities secondary to amyloid deposition are features of FAP Types I and II, the Ashkenazi Jewish variant and familial oculoleptomeningeal amyloidosis. Transthyretin is a major protein component of the normal vitreous [7] and of vitreous amyloid [8,9].

In searching for tissue determinants which may be involved in amyloidogenesis, we concentrated on proteins which may mimic serum RBP in its interaction with TTR. RBP belongs to a family of extracellular lipid-binding proteins which share sequence homology [10]. This family is distinct from a second family of lipid-binding proteins which also share sequence homology, and which includes the cytosolic retinoid-binding proteins and the myelin membrane protein P2 [11]. Despite the absence of primary sequence homology, however, recent crystallographic data indicate that P2 shares significant conformational homology with RBP [12]. This suggested to us the possibility that P2 might also interact with TTR.

Our data demonstrate that P2 is a component of mammalian vitreous and that P2 is present in vitreous amyloid fibrils from 3 of 4 samples from patients with ser-84 TTR mutation. The presence of P2 in amyloid fibrils appears to be specific because P2 was not detected in supernatants from the same fibril preparations and because RBP, a component of normal vitreous, was not detected in amyloid fibrils.

These findings demonstrate that P2 is present in two widely divergent tissues - peripheral nerve and ocular vitreous - which are frequent sites of TTR amyloidosis. Furthermore, P2 is specifically associated with vitreous amyloid fibrils from patients with FAP Type

II. Considered together with the evidence for conformational homology between RBP and P2, these findings raise the possibility that P2 may mimic RBP in its interaction with TTR. Such an interaction may favor the deposition of mutant TTR as amyloid fibrils and thereby account for the distribution of TTR-amyloid in peripheral nerve and vitreous in FAP.

5. ACKNOWLEDGEMENTS

We wish to thank Steven W. Brostoff for his kind gift of antiserum to bovine P2 and of purified bovine P2, and Eric A. Schon for stimulating discussions and comments. This work was supported by the Irving Foundation, the Aaron Diamond Foundation and NIH grants NS01155 and NS26892. JH is Florence Irving Assistant Professor of Neurology and Pathology.

6. REFERENCES

[1] Greenfield, S., Weise, M.J., Gantt, G., Hogan, E.L., and Brostoff, S.W. (1982) J. Neurochem. 39, 1278-1282.
[2] Rukavina, J.G., Block, W.D., Jackson, C.E., Falls, H.F., Carey, J.H., and Curtis, A.C. (1956) Medicine 35, 239-334.
[3] Dwulet, F.E. and Benson, M.D. (1986) J. Clin. Invest. 78, 880-886.
[4] Lowry, O.H., Rosebrough, N.J., Farr, A.L., and Randall, R. (1951) J. Biol. Chem. 193, 265-275.
[5] Laemmli, U.K. (1970) Nature 227, 680-685.
[6] Towbin, H., Staehelin, T., and Gordon, J. (1979) Proc. Natl. Acad. Sci. (U.S.A.) 76, 4350-4354.
[7] Ishizaki, T. (1985) Acta Soc. Ophthalmol. Jpn. 88, 1487-1491.
[8] Sandgren, O., Westermark, P., and Stenkula, S. (1986) Ophthalmic Res. 18, 98-103.
[9] Gorevic, P.D., Rodrigues, M.M., Spencer, W.H., Munoz, P.C., Allen, A.W., and Verne, A.Z. (1987) Ophthalmology 94, 792-798.
10] Sawyer, L. (1987) Nature 327, 659.
11] Sundelin, J., Das, S.R., Eriksson, U., Rask, L., and Peterson, P.A. (1985) J. Biol. Chem. 260, 6494-6499.
12] Alwyn Jones, T., Bergfors, T., Sedzik, J., and Unge, T. (1988) EMBO J. 7, 1597-1604.

CLONING AND TRIMMING OF THE TTR-cDNA GENE BY PCR.

Nordvåg, B.Y.*, El-Gewely, M.R.**, Husby, G.*
*Dep. of Rheumatology, University Hospital of Tromsø, University of Tromsø. **Institute of Medical Biology, Dep. of Biotechnology, University of Tromsø, Norway.

Abstract: To study the molecular basis for hereditary amyloidosis, a human adult liver cDNA was screened using PCR to isolate the normal human TTR-cDNA. Simultaneously trimming of the cDNA in both 5'- and 3'-ends was made. The PCR-product was digested with SphI and XbaI, and resulting fragments indicated successful amplification of modified TTR-cDNA, which was later cloned into vectors M13mp19 and pUC18. Positive hybridization signals were obtained in Southern blots. DNA-sequencing of the cDNA cloned in M13, revealed the successful cloning of the trimmed TTR-cDNA. A mutant TTR-cDNA with a A for G_{76} was observed.

Introduction:

Hereditary amyloidosis was first found to be closely related to the transthyretin (TTR) protein in the Portuguese kindred (1). Recent studies have revealed several different point mutations in the TTR protein (2), each associated to various clinical syndromes of hereditary amyloidosis. Our group has previously reported a Met for Leu substitution at position 111 in the TTR protein in a familial amyloid cardiomyopathy (FAC) of Danish origin (3). Also, normal TTR has been isolated from amyloid fibrils in senile systemic amyloidosis (4). We wanted to clone the normal TTR-cDNA gene, previously cloned and described (5), for further studies related to the molecular basis of hereditary amyloidosis. In addition, a trimming of the gene was designed, making it fit for studies by site directed mutagenesis for heterologuos gene expression.

Materials and methods:

A human adult liver cDNA library was screened using the PCR-reaction. 0,1 - 1μg template DNA was used, prepared by a miniplasmid preparation, using alkaline lysis method of a culture of the E. coli containing the library in PstI site of plasmid vector pKT218 (6). PCR-primers contained nucleotides complementary to some bases of the vector, included PstI-site, and some of the bases in each end of the TTR-cDNA (Fig.1). Annealing temperatures in the PCR-reaction were 45° and 54° C. The PCR-product was restriction enzyme analyzed, using SphI and XbaI. PstI-digested PCR-product was ligated into phage M13mp19 and plasmid pUC18 and subcloned in DHα_5F, respectively RR1 competent cells. Recombinant phages and plasmids were selected by abscense of β-galactosidase activity, isolated and examined for presence of inserts by 0,8% agarose gel electrophoresis after PstI-digestion. Southern blots of vector-DNA and inserts were hybridized with a 5'-end labelled 22 bp oligo (P3) complementary to the middle region of the TTR-cDNA. DNA-sequencing using the dideoxy method, was made on DNA of recombinant M13 from several colonies.

Results:

According to the design, the PCR-product gave a band of 496 bp, and the restriction fragments had the expected sizes. Different annealing temperatures did not have any significant influence on the result. However, the highest annealing temperature gave a more distinct band (result not shown). Inserts of equal size, representing ligated cDNA, were observed

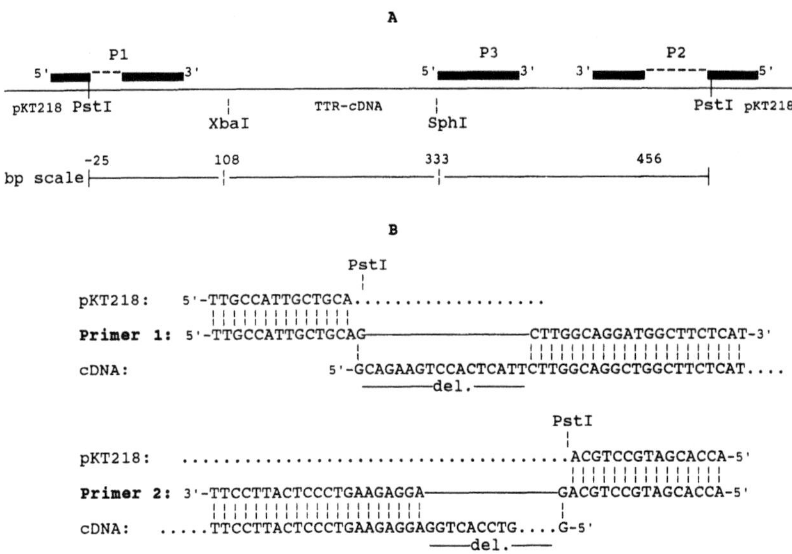

Figure 1 A: A diagrammatic presentation of the normal TTR-cDNA and the flanking regions in vector pKT218. The positions of primers P1 and P2 for the PCR are indicated, and also that for the oligo P3 used in hybridization. Directions of the oligos are indicated. Digestion points for restriction enzymes SphI and XbaI used are indicated in the diagram. The restriction sites are shown on the approximate scale below. Truncated regions of P1 and P2 represent sequences of the cDNA that were trimmed out in the PCR strategy, resulting in the PCR product shown in Fig. 3.
B: Sequences of primers and parts of plasmid pKT218 vector and cDNA-TTR-gene, demonstrating the design of primers regarding complementarity to vector and cDNA sequences and deleted parts of the cDNA. Primer 2 is complementary to the DNA-strand opposite of that shown for primer 1. 16 bp are deleted in the 5'-end by primer 1, while primer 2 deletes 133 bp in the 3'-end of the TTR-cDNA.

as bands in examined, PstI-digested recombinant plasmids and phages (Fig. 2). Strong hybridization signals were obtained in blots of insert-DNA from the examined plasmids and from four of seven phages (Fig. 2B). DNA-sequencing of the cDNA cloned in M13, revealed the sequence of the TTR-gene, as modified by the designed trimming (Fig. 3). A mutation of G to A_{76} was found in three out of four sequenced clones (Fig. 3).

Discussion:

The polymerase chain reaction (PCR) has simplified the process of amplifying specific regions of DNA (7). We succeeded in cloning and trimming of the TTR-cDNA from a human adult liver cDNA-library, using the PCR-reaction. This cDNA is suitable for further study by site directed mutagenesis for heterologuos gene expression.
Our developed technique (8) is a simple and quick tool in the screening of a DNA-library, and reduces the need for use of radioactive isotopes. This method could be utilized in the search also for unknown genes of interest.
A cDNA-variant with a mutation of A for G_{76} was observed, and should give rise to a GS6 substitution in the resulting TTR protein. This mutation is previously described (9), and associated with an increased thyroxine-binding affinity of the TTR protein.

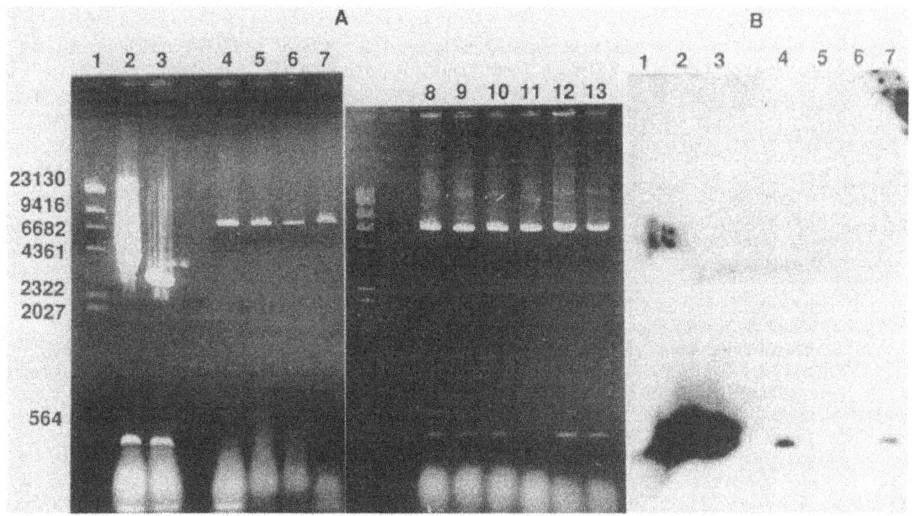

Figure 2: A. Agarose gel electrophoresis of DNA of pUC18 (lanes 2 and 3) and M13mp19 (lanes 4 to 13), examined for the presence of insert after subcloning and digestion with PstI. Lane 1 is a HindIII digest of λ DNA. A significant band representing insert is visible in lanes 2-4,8-10, 12 and 13. (A band in lane 7 is not visible in the picture.)
B. Southern blot of the DNA in A (lanes 1 -7), hybridized to the labelled oligo (P3). Strong signals were obtained from the inserts, and also from inserts in lanes 11 and 12 (not shown), indicating a successfull cloning of trimmed TTR-cDNA.

```
                    PstI
                    |          Met
TCCTCTAGAG TCGACCTGCA GCTTGGCAGG ATGGCTTCTC ATCGTCTGCT CCTCCTCTGC
                    -10                                        30

CTTGCTGGAC TGGTATTTGT GTCTGAGGCT GGCCCTACGG GCACCGGTGA ATCCAAGTGT
                  XbaI                           A             90
                    |
CCTCTGATGG TCAAAGTTCT AGATGCTGTC CGAGGCAGTC CTGCCATCAA TGTGGCCGTG
                  108                                         150

CATGTGTTCA GAAAGGCTGC TGATGACACC TGGGAGCCAT TTGCCTCTGG GAAAACCAGT
                                                              210
GAGTCTGGAG AGCTGCATGG GCTCACAACT GAGGAGGAAT TTGTAGAAGG GATATACAAA
                                                              270
GTGGAAATAG ACACCAAATC TTACTGGAAG GCACTTGGCA TCTCCCCATT CCATGAGCAT
 SphI                                                         330
 |
GCAGAGGTGG TATTCACAGC CAACGACTCC GGCCCCCGCC GCTACACCAT TGCCGCCCTG
 333                                                          390
                                                 Glu
CTGAGCCCCT ACTCCTATTC CACCACGGCT GTCGTCACCA ATCCCAAGGA ATGAGGGACT
          PstI                                                450
          |
TCTCCTCTGC AGGCATGCAA....
          461
```

Figure 3: DNA sequence of the PCR-product after subcloning into M13mp19, using the PstI restriction site (position shown). The flanking regions of the vector are shown in italics. A mutation of G to A in bp # 76 of the cDNA is indicated. This mutation was found in three out of four sequenced colonies. Met and Glu indicate first and last amino acids in the coding region of the cDNA-gene. Restriction sites of enzymes SphI and XbaI are indicated by ¦; bp numbers at the sites are given. Sequences complementary to, or in the primers/oligos, are indicated in bold types.

References:

1. Costa,P.P., Figueira,A.S., Bravo,F.R. (1975) "Amyloid fibril protein related to prealbumin in familial amyloidotic polyneuropathy." Proc. Natl. Acad. Sci. USA, 75:4499-503.
2. Costa,P.P., Falcâo de Freitas,A., Saraiva,M.J.M. (1990) "Proceedings of the First International Symposium on Familial Amyloidosis." Arquivos Medicos, Porto, Portugal. Suppl. 3 in press.
3. Nordlie,M., Sletten,K., Husby,G., Ranløv,P.J. (1988) "A New Prealbumin Variant in Familial Amyloid Cardiomyopathy of Danish Origin." Scand. J. Immunol., 27:119-121.
4: Westermark,P., Sletten,K. Johansson,B., Cornwell,G.G. (1990) "Fibril in senile systemic amyloidosis is derived from normal transthyretin." Proc. Natl. Acad. Sci. USA, 87:2843-2845.
5. Mita,S., Maeda,S., Shimada,K., Araki,S. (1984) "Cloning and sequence analysis of cDNA for human prealbumin." Biochem. Biophys. Res. Commun. 125:558-564.
6. Recombinant DNA Technical Bulletin, NIH (1978)
7. Saiki,R.K., Gelfand,D.H., Stoffel,S., Scharf,S.J., Higuchi,R., Horn,G.T., Mullis,K.B., Erlich,H.A. (1988) "Primer-directed enzymatic amplification of DNA with a thermostable DNA polymerase." Science, 239:487-491.
8. Nordvåg,B.Y., Husby,G., El-Gewely,M.R. (1990) "Library screening and gene reconstruction by PCR." Manuscript in preparation.
9. Fitch,N.J.S., Akbari,M.T., Sheppard,M.C., Ramsden,D.B. (1990) "Serine for Glycine substitution at position 6 in an inherited, non-lethal transthyretin variant with increased thyroxin-binding affinity." Proceedings of the First International Symposium on Familial Amyloidosis, eds. Costa,P.P., Falcâo de Freitas,A., Saraiva,M.J.M. (Arquivos Medicos, Porto, Portugal.) Suppl. 3 in press.

PATHOLOGICAL SIMILARITY OF TRANSGENIC MICE CARRYING THE HUMAN MUTANT TRANSTHYRETIN GENE TO HUMAN FAMILIAL AMYLOIDOTIC POLYNEUROPATHY (FAP) TYPE I

S. YI, K. TAKAHASHI, F. TASHIRO, S. WAKASUGI, K. YAMAMURA and S. ARAKI
The 1st Department of Internal Medicine, 2nd Department of Pathology, and Institute for Medical Genetics, Kumamoto University Medical School, Honjo 1-1-1, Kumamoto 860, JAPAN

ABSTRACT. To analyze pathological processes of amyloid deposition in type I FAP, we produced transgenic mice carrying the human mutant transthyretin (TTR) gene. In these transgenic mice, amyloid deposition started in the gastrointestinal tract, cardiovascular system, and kidneys at 6 months old. At the age of 24 months, the pattern of amyloid deposition was similar to that observed in human autopsy cases of FAP except for the absence of amyloid deposition in the peripheral nervous system. Amyloid deposition was shown to be composed of human mutant TTR. These results indicate that human variant TTR produced in transgenic mice deposits as a major component of amyloid fibrils in their various tissues similar to those of human FAP cases except for the peripheral nervous tissues.

1. INTRODUCTION

Type I FAP is an inherited systemic amyloidosis characterized by the extracellular deposition of fibrilar amyloid protein and by prominent peripheral and autonomic nerve involvement [1]. The amyloid deposits derived from the Japanese type of FAP were found to consist of a variant TTR with a single amino acid substitution of valine in position 30 of normal TTR a methionine [2]. Moreover, genetic studies revealed that there was only one base change (GTG-ATG) in the DNA for TTR [3]. Current techniques of molecular biology enabled to create the transgenic mice of FAP, in which amyloid deposition was induced [4]. This paper describes the pattern of amyloid deposition in the transgenic mice pathologically and discusses their similarity to human FAP.

2. MATERIALS AND METHODS

2.1. Transgenic mice

The recombinant plasmids were isolated from the library of genomic DNA of liver taken from a patient with FAP type I. This gene has a substitution of methionine for valine at amino acid position 30. In order to produce large quantities of variant TTR in transgenic mice, we constructed a 7.8kb StuI-EcoRI fragment in which the promoter region of the mouse methallothionein I (MT-I) gene was ligated to the structural gene of human TTR (MT-hMet30). About 1 pg of DNA solution was microinjected into fertilized eggs of C57BL/6 mice according to the methods described elsewhere [5]. In four out of 12 mice derived from eggs microinjected with the MT-hMet30 gene, gene integration was confirmed by southern blot analysis.

2.2. Morphologic studies

Transgenic mice were sacrificed at 3, 6, 9, 12, 15, 18, and 24 months after birth. The following tissues were excised from the mice, fixed in 10% neutral buffered formalin at the time of autopsy, and embedded in paraffin: brain, heart, kidney, spleen, liver, lung, pancreas, skin, stomach, intestine, thyroid, lymph node, sciatic nerve, urinary bladder, muscle, and reproductive organs. Sections were cut 3-4 μm thick and stained with Congo red. Immunostaining was performed by the avidin-biotin-peroxidase complex (ABC) method. For electron microscopy, small tissues blocks of principal organs were fixed in 2.5% glutaraldehyde in 0.1M cacodylate buffer, followed by fixation with 2% osmium tetroxide, and embedded Epon. Ultrathin sections were cut, stained with uranyl acetate and lead citrate, and observed with an electron microscope.

3. RESULTS

3.1. Light-microscopic changes

In the early stage (6 month-old), amyloid deposited in the mucosa and around the wall of small vessels of the small intestine, particularly the terminal ileum. These deposits appeared more remarkably with age. In the kidneys, glomerular deposits were seen at the age of 6 months and, amyloid deposition was prominent in glomeruli, around the tubules, and in the interstitium of the medulla thereafter. Nodular deposits around the mesangial cells were most frequently observed at 12 months late. In the 24 month-old mice, all of the glomeruli were destroyed by replacement with massive amyloid deposits. At the same time, amyloid deposition began to appear in the myocardium, particularly markedly around the myocardial fibers. Amyloid deposits were more marked in the subendocardial layer of the myocardium than in the deep layer. But small and medium-sized arteries in the myocardium were slightly affected. In the thyroid, amyloid deposition was prominent in the interfollicular area. There were no amyloid deposits in the liver, spleen, pancreas, and lungs except around the blood vessels. In the sciatic nerves, amyloid deposits were not found, and nerve fibers and Schwann cells were normal.

Amyloid substance in the transgenic mice was stained moderately positive by Congo red staining. The staining intensity of amyloid substance in the transgenic mice by the Congo red method was weaker than that in patients with FAP or other types of systemic amyloidosis, though emitting an apple-green birefringence under polarized light. Immunohistochemically, amyloid deposits in the heart, kidneys, and ileum showed a positive staining with anti-human TTR and anti-mouse SAP antisera by ABC method. However, they were not stained with anti-mouse SAA, anti-human SAA, and anti-human SAP antisera.

3.2. Electron-microscopic changes

In the intestines, amyloid deposits were observed to consist of clusters of amyloid fibrils, approximately 7 to 10 nm thick and variable in length, a finding which is consistent with human FAP or other types of amyloidosis. In the initial stage, amyloid deposits were observed in the propria mucosa at the top of the intestinal villi, particularly beneath the epithelial cells. Also, they were found in the basal area of the lamina propria, in the muscularis mucosae, and in the submucosa. In the submucosa, amyloid deposition occurred in the connective tissue and around small blood vessels. In the advanced stage, diffuse amyloid deposition was found in the mucosa, muscularis mucosae, submucosa, and subserosa.

In the kidneys, amyloid fibrils were first detected in the matrix around the mesangial cells or beneath the endothelial cells of glomerular capillaries. With age, the amount of amyloid fibrils increased, and their clusters were observed in the lamina rara interna between the basal lamina and endothelial cells. At the advanced stage, clusters of amyloid fibrils were massively deposited in almost all parts of the glomerular mesangial matrix; the mesangial cells were swollen, and the glomerular epithelial cells showed fusion of their foot processes with each other.

In the myocardium, clusters of amyloid fibrils in the superficial myocardium were observed initially around small blood vessels. Myocardial cells showed atrophy and degenerative changes due to massive amyloid deposition.

4. DISCUSSION

In this paper, some subjects will be discussed in relation to the pathological similarity between the transgenic mice and human FAP autopsy cases.

The pathological changes of the transgenic mice are in good agreement with those reported in previous pathological studies of FAP [6]. Some of the present authors recently reported in nine autopsy cases of type I FAP that amyloid deposition occurred predominantly in the cardiovascular system, peripheral and autonomic nervous system, choroid plexus, kidneys, thyroid, and gastrointestinal tract [7]. However, it was slight or minimal in the pancreas, bone marrow, spleen, lymph nodes, or liver, and absent in the brain parenchyma. The major sites and pattern of amyloid deposition in the transgenic mice are similar to these human autopsy cases except for the peripheral nervous tissues. In the mice, our pathological study revealed that cardiac amyloid deposition initially occurs in the subendocardial layer and in the superficial areas of the myocardium. In the kidneys of the mice, amyloid deposition first occurred in the mesangial areas of glomerular involvement and increased with age. These findings are almost consistent with those reported in autopsy cases of type I FAP. Amyloid deposition in the thyroid gland of the transgenic mice is prominent, and its pattern closely resembles that of human cases of FAP.

Although the most striking pathological feature of FAP is amyloid deposition in the peripheral nervous tissues, no amyloid deposition was observed in the nervous tissues of the transgenic mice examined up to age 24 months. To explain the reasons why no amyloid deposition occurs in the peripheral nervous tissues of the transgenic mice, the following possibilities are pointed out. In the transgenic mice, we demonstrated little or no production of human TTR in the choroid plexus unlike human autopsy cases. This could imply a relationship in amyloid deposition between the choroid plexus and peripheral nervous system. A second possibility is a low level expression of hMet30 gene in these transgenic mice. A third possibility may be responsible for characteristic metabolic features of the mice themselves. Interestingly, degenerative changes in the peripheral nerve tissues prior to amyloid deposition have been reported in FAP patients [7]. This suggests implication of another intrinsic factor(s) for inducing in amyloid deposition in the nervous tissues of FAP. To produce amyloid deposition in the peripheral nerve tissue of transgenic mice, further approaches are in progress.

5. REFERENCES

1) Araki, S. (1984) 'Type I familial amyloidotic polyneuropathy (Japanese type)', Brain Dev 6, 128-133.
2) Tawara, S., Nakazato, M., Kangawa, K., et al. (1983) 'Identification of amyloid prealbumin variant in familial amyloidotic polyneuropathy (Japanese type)', Biochem Biophys Res Commun 116, 880-888.
3) Mita, S., Maeda, S., Ide M. et al. 'Familial amyloidotic polyneuropathy diagnosed by cloned human prealbumin cDNA', Neurology (N.Y.) 1986, 298-301.
4) Wakasugi, S., Inomoto, T., Yi, S., et al. (1987) 'A transgenic mouse model of familial amyloidotic polyneuropathy', Proc Japan Acad 63(B), 344-347.
5) Yamamura, K., Kikutani, H., Takahashi, N., et al. (1984) 'Introduction of human γ1 immunoglobulin genes into fertilized mouse eggs', J Biochem (Tokyo) 96, 357-365.
6) Ikeda, S., Hanyu, N., Hongo, M., et al. (1987) 'Hereditary generalized amyloidosis with polyneuropathy. Clinicopathological study of 65 Japanese patients', Brain 110, 315-337.
7) Takahashi, K., Kimura, Y., Yi, S., et al. (1988) 'Pathology of familial amyloidotic polyneuropathy occurring in Kumamoto', in T. Isobe, S. Araki, F. Uchino, S. Kito and E. Tsubura (eds.), Amyloid and Amyloidosis, Plenum Press, New York, pp. 505-510.

Prealbumin type cerebral amyloid angiopathy in familial amyloid polyneuropathy

Masao Ushiyama*, Shu-ichi Ikeda**, Nobuo Yanagisawa**
*Kenwakai Hospital, Department of Neurology, 1936 Kanae Iida, Nagano 395, Japan
**Shinshu University School of Medicine, Department of Medicine (Neurology), Matsumoto 390, Japan

ABSTRACT. Immunocytochemical and electron-microscopic studies were performed on the central nervous system(CNS) in 10 cases with type I familial amyloid polyneuropathy. All cases showed CNS amyloid deposits, mainly on the leptomeningeal vessels and pia-arachnoid membranes, with arteries and arterioles in subarachnoidal space being the predominant site of cerebral amyloid accumulation. All of these amyloid deposits were specifically immunolabeled by an anti-human prealbumin antibody. However, there were no prealbumin deposits in the brain parenchyma. It is concluded that CNS prealbumin-type amyloid deposition with cerebral amyloid angiopathy is a common pathological finding in this disease.

INTRODUCTION. Cerebral amyloid angiopathy(CAA) is characterized by amyloid deposition on the walls of leptomeningeal and cortical blood vessels[1]. This pathological condition is observed in several different brain disorders including Alzheimer's disease, adult Down's syndrome and Icelandic-type or Dutch-type hereditary cerebral hemorrhage with amyloidosis[2], but rarely occurs in the brains with generalized amyloidosis. In this study, we carried out histological, immunocytochemical and electron-microscopic observations of amyloid deposits seen in the CNS in type I familial amyloid polyneuropathy(FAP) with special attention to cerebrovascular amyloidosis.

MATERIALS AND METHODS. We examined 10 autopsied cases with type I FAP that originated from two foci of this disease, Ogawa and Miyata village in Nagano prefecture, Japan. All cases showed various autonomic dysfunctions and a progressive polyneuropathy starting in the legs. However, with the exception of case 2, they did not suffer from any clinical manifestations suggestive of CNS involvement: case 2 had a late onset and slow course of this disease and at the age of 65 he suddenly died from subarachnoid hemorrhage possibly caused by autopsy proven arteriovenous malformation in the thoracic spinal cord[3].

Tissue samples including cerebrum, cerebellum, brain stem and spinal cord were routinely taken from all cases. Serial sections from formalin-fixed and paraffin-embedded blocks were stained by hematoxylin and eosin, alkaline Congo red and Klüver-Barrera, and by immunocytochemical methods using the following primary reagents: rabbit antisera to human prealbumin (DAKO, Denmark), human cystacin C (AG 8206) and GFAP(DAKO, Denmark), and monoclonal antibody 4D12/2/6 raised against a synthetic peptide consisting of residues 8-17 of amyloid beta-protein. The specimens for electron microscopy were prepared from the formalin-fixed neocortex of case 9. They were postfixed in 1% osmium tetroxide, dehydraded through graded alcohols into propylene oxide, and embedded in an epoxy-resin mixture. Ultrathin sections after staining with uranyl acetate and lead citrate were examined under a Hitachi HS-9 electron microscope.

RESULTS. Gross examination of the brain and spinal cord was unremarkable in all cases, and their brain weights ranged from 1100 to 1400g. General neuropathological examinations revealed localized degeneration of the spinal posterior columns in some cases but no hemorrhages or infarcts in the brains.

Congo red staining commonly showed a variable degree of amyloid deposition in an extensive area of the CNS including vascular walls, leptomeninges, subependymal parenchyma and choroid plexus. Cerebrovascular amyloid deposits were seen mainly in the leptomeningeal vessels: many small vessels in cerebral subarachnoid space were heavily laden with amyloid deposits on the entire vascular walls, frequently showing thickened walls with prominent perivascular accumulation of amyloid, while amyloid deposits on large vessels were confined to the media or adventitia (Fig. 1). These involved vessels were observed to be free of amyloid shortly after entering into the cerebral cortex. The leptomeninges and choroid plexus were also affected by amyloid deposition and the thickened pia-arachnoid showed an irregular meshwork of strands and trabeculae composed of amyloid. These leptomeninges with heavy deposits of amyloid often contained amyloid-laden small vessels, and the subpial amyloid deposits were occasionally surrounded by proliferated GFAP-immunoreactive astrocytes. However, in less involved areas, Congophilic angiopathy was seen without any significant deposits of amyloid on the pia-arachnoid membranes, and except a few subependymal amyloid deposits no senile plaque-like amyloid lesions were found in the brain parenchyma. A similar pattern of amyloid deposition was observed in the brain stem, cerebellum and spinal cord, and among them a marked accumulation of amyloid on the leptomeninges and vessels was noted in the dorsal part of the spinal cord(Table 1).

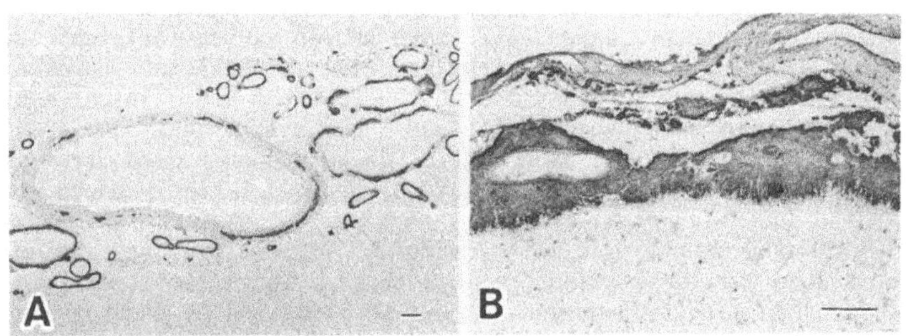

Figure 1. Amyloid deposits in the leptomeningeal vessels from Case 7 oc-

cipital lobe(A) and subpial deposits from Case 9 frontal lobe(B). Immunostaining with anti-human prealbumin antibody. (bars=100μm).

TABLE 1. Severity of amyloid deposition in the CNS in 10 patients with type I FAP

	CASE	1	2	3	4	5	6	7	8	9	10
	AGE, SEX	40F	65M	62M	43M	45M	45F	43F	70M	45F	51F
	DURATION OF ILLNESS(Y)	6	7	8	9	11	15	16	17	25	33
	BRAIN WEIGHT(g)			1320	1300	1400	1100	1200		1260	1300
CEREBRUM	Subarachnoid vessel	+++	+	++	++	+++	+++	+++	++	+++	+++
	Leptomeninx	+++	-	+	-	++	++	+++	+	+++	+++
	Cortical vessel	+	-	+	+	+	+	+	+	+	+
CEREBELLUM	Subarachnoid vessel		+	+	++		+++	+++	+++	+++	+++
	Leptomeninx		-	-	-		-	+	-	+	++
	Cortical vessel		-	-	-		+	+	+	+	+
BRAIN STEM	Subarachnoid vessel		+	++			+++	+++	+++		+++
	Leptomeninx		+	+			++	+++	+		+++
	Parenchymal vessel		-	+			+	+	+		+
SPINAL CORD	Subarachnoid vessel	+++	++		++		+++	+++	+++	+++	+++
	Leptomeninx	+++	++		++		+++	+++	++	++	+++
	Parenchymal vessel	+	+		-		+	+	+	-	+

- negative + slight ++ moderate +++ marked

In electron microscopic examinations these amyloid deposits were identified as aggregations of straight nonbranching fibrils with a diameter of about 10 nm. All amyloid deposits with Congophilic angiopathy seen in the CNS in these patients with type I FAP were invariably immunoreactive to anti-human prealbumin antibody but showed no significant immunocytochemical reactions for anti-human cystacin C antiserum or anti-beta protein antibody.

DISCUSSION. Type I FAP is a genetically determined systemic amyloidosis and amyloid fibril protein in this disorder consist of a variant of prealbumin(also called transthyretin) with a single substitution of a methionine residue for valine at position 30[4]. It is well established that type I FAP patients show severe amyloid deposition in the peripheral somatic and autonomic nerves. However, there has been few detailed report concerning the CNS in this disease[5,6.7].

The present study has revealed that amyloid deposits on the subarachnoid vessels and leptomeninges are a cardinal neuropathological finding in patients with type I FAP, and in some cases CAA was a predominant pattern of amyloid deposition in the CNS. The amyloid fibril protein comprising these deposits was demonstrated by immunohistochemical methods to be prealbumin. This form of CAA with prealbumin immunoreactivity has not been described by previously. Furthermore, prealbumin-type amyloid is the only well characterized example of a systemic amyloidosis with chemically similar amyloid deposits in the cerebrovascular walls and meninges. CAA infrequently occurs in patients with AL or AA-type generalized amyloidosis, but immunocytochemical analysis of these cerebrovascular amyloid deposits has shown that they consists of beta-protein[8].

Cerebrovascular amyloidosis is observed in a variety of brain degenerative diseases, of which beta protein-type CAA is the most common form seen in the aged individuals[9]. However, the pathologic mechanism of amyloid deposition on the cerebral vessels remains unclear. In the CNS of patients with type I FAP the leptomeningeal vessels are the principal site of amyloid deposition. The prealbumin variant noted above was detected in the serum of patients whose sera were available for testing[10]. On the basis of these findings, we concluded that prealbumin-type CAA seen in patients with type I FAP is a further example of cerebrovascular amyloid deposits derived from serum precursor. However, it was noted that this prealbumin-related amyloid did not affect the brain parenchyma as seen in patients with Alzheimer's disease showing CAA and many intracerebral senile plaques with amyloid deposition. This would seem to explain the lack of any CNS symptoms in these patients with type I FAP. Accordingly, it is likely that the etiologic and pathologic processes involved in the formation of senile plaques might be different from those that result in CAA. Further studies are necessary to explain the great variability of pattern of amyloid deposition in the CNS seen in different disorders.

REFERENCES

1. Vinters, H. V. (1987) 'Cerebral amyloid angiopathy. A critical review', Stroke 18, 311-324.
2. Castaño, E. M. and Frangione, B. (1988) 'Biology of disease. Human amyloidosis, Alzheimer disease and related disorders' Lab. Invest. 58, 122-132.
3. Ikeda, S., Hanyu, N. et al. (1987) 'Hereditary generalized amyloidosis with polyneuropathy. Clinicopathological study of 65 Japanese patients' Brain 110, 315-337.
4. Tawara, S., Nakazato, M. et al. (1983) 'Identification of amyloid prealbumin variant in familial amyloidotic polyneuropathy (Japanese type)' Biochem. Biophys. Res. Commun. 116, 880-888.
5. Sumino, S., Nagashima, K. et al. (1983) 'Familial amyloid polyneuropathy with marked hypertrophy of the peripheral nerves' Acta Pathol. Jpn. 33, 629-643.
6. Horta, J. D. S., Filipe, I. et al. (1964) 'Portuguese polyneuritic familial type of amyloidosis' Pathol. Microbiol. 27,809-825.
7. Julião, O. F., Queiroz, L. S. et al. (1974) 'Portuguese type of familial amyloid polyneuropathy. Anatomo-clinical study of a Brazilian family' Europ. Neurol. 11, 180-195.
8. Ishihara, T., Nagasawa, T. et al. (1989) 'Amyloid protein of vessels in leptomeninges, cortices, choroid plexuses, and pituitary glands from patients with systemic amyloidosis' Human Patho. 20, 891-895.
9. Glenner, G. G. and Wong, C. W. (1984) 'Alzheimer's disease: Initial report of the purification and characterization of a novel cerebrovascular amyloid protein' Biochem. Biophys. Res. Commun. 120, 885-890.
10. Nakazato, M., Kangawa, K. et al. (1984) 'Identification of a prealbumin variant in the serum of a Japanese patient with familial amyloidotic polyneuropathy' Biochem. Biophys. Res. Commun. 122, 712-718.

AMYLOID LOCALIZED TO THE TENOSYNOVIUM AT CARPAL TUNNEL RELEASE: IMMUNOHISTOCHEMICAL IDENTIFICATION OF AMYLOID TYPE

Kyle RA*, Linke RP**, and Gertz MA*; *Mayo Clinic, Rochester, Minnesota 55905 USA; **Institüt für Immunologie der Universität, München, West Germany

ABSTRACT. We identified 35 patients seen at the Mayo Clinic from 1968 to 1977 with carpal tunnel syndrome and local deposition of amyloid without evidence of systemic amyloidosis. The unlabeled immunoperoxidase method was used with antisera against purified amyloid proteins of the AA, Aκ, Aλ, AF-AS_{C1} [transthyretin (prealbumin)], and AB (β_2-microglobulin) types. The amyloid stained with antisera to transthyretin in 33 of the 35 patients. Amyloid deposits did not stain with any antisera in two pateints. Nine of the 35 patients had an M-protein in the serum and two others had a monoclonal light chain in the urine. None of these 11 patients developed systemic amyloidosis or multiple myeloma. Only 2 of the 35 patients developed systemic amyloidosis during follow-up. The initial carpal tunnel tissue in both of these cases stained with antisera to transthyretin. Neither had an M-protein in the serum or urine. One patient subsequently developed congestive heart failure and an endomyocardial biopsy stained with antisera to transthyretin. This is consistent with senile systemic amyloidosis. Tissue in the second patient was inadequate for immunohistochemical staining. We conclude that amyloid localized to the tenosynovium consists of transthyretin and systemic amyloidosis rarely develops.

1. MATERIAL AND METHODS

We reviewed the records of all patients with a carpal tunnel release performed at the Mayo Clinic from 1968 to 1977. Sections from tissue blocks embedded in paraffin were stained with Congo red and viewed with a polarizing light source. The unlabeled immunoperoxidase method was used with antisera against purified amyloid proteins of the AA, Aκ, Aλ, AF/AS_{C1}, and AB (β_2-microglobulin) types. All antisera were shown to be able to discriminate the different amyloid types on a larger panel of patients. The antisera to AS_{C1} and AF cross-reacted to an extent that they were interchangeable and recognized transthyretin (prealbumin) type of amyloid fibrils. Conventional positive and negative controls were prepared. Each specimen that was Congo-red positive was tested with each of the above mentioned antibodies.

Evidence of systemic amyloidosis was searched for in historical and physical findings as well as additional biopsies in some cases. Sera and urines were examined for the presence of a monoclonal protein (M-protein). Appropriate biopsy and autopsy evidence of amyloidosis was sought. Follow-up letters were written to all patients and their physicians when we had not seen or heard from them during the previous year. Death certificates were requested when appropriate. The patients, their relatives, or their physicians were contacted by telephone when all other contacts by letter had produced no information.

2. RESULTS

We identified 35 patients seen at the Mayo Clinic from January 1, 1968 to December 31, 1977 with carpal tunnel syndrome and local deposition of amyloid without evidence of systemic amyloidosis. None of the patients were on hemodialysis. The median duration from the onset of symptoms of carpal tunnel syndrome until histologic diagnosis ranged from <1 to 124 months. The median duration was 13.7 months.

The age at diagnosis ranged from 53 to 93 years with a median of 71 years. Sixty-six percent were males. Anemia, thrombocytosis, hypercalcemia, and renal insufficiency were rarely present and were not related to the amyloid deposition in any case.

Nine of the 35 patients had a monoclonal protein in the serum (IgGκ, 4; IgGλ, 3; IgAλ, 1; and IgMκ, 1). Two of these also had a small amount of monoclonal light chain in the urine. Two additional patients had a transient monoclonal light chain in the urine which disappeared without therapeutic intervention. Eight of the 11 patients with an M-protein in the serum or urine have died. The cause of death was cardiac disease in 3, cerebrovascular accident in 2, pneumonia in 2, and a ruptured abdominal aortic aneurysm in 1. None of the patients died of systemic amyloidosis or multiple myeloma. The duration of follow-up ranged from 1 to 15 years. The median survival (Kaplan-Meier) of the 11 patients following histologic diagnosis of amyloid was 11 years.

The median survival of the 24 patients with localized amyloidosis and no M-protein was 10 years. Eleven (46%) of the patients died. The cause of death was cardiac disease in 8 patients and metastatic carcinoma in 3.

Only 2 of the 35 patients showed evidence of systemic amyloidosis during follow-up. The first patient developed symptoms of bilateral carpal tunnel syndrome and 1.5 years later had right carpal ligament decompression performed, and amyloid staining with AS_{C1} antisera was found. Nine years after the symptoms of carpal tunnel syndrome, he developed congestive heart failure. An echocardiogram showed thickening of the left ventricular wall (16 mm) and septum (16 mm). The findings were classic for amyloid heart disease. A rectal biopsy was positive for amyloid. No monoclonal protein was found in the serum or urine with immunoelectrophoresis and immunofixation on multiple occasions. He died of congestive heart failure and cardiac arrest 3 months after the recognition of systemic amyloidosis.

The second patient was a 66-year-old man who had bilateral carpal tunnel decompression for symptoms of 5-year's duration. Amyloid staining with AS_{C1} was found, but there was no clinical evidence of systemic amyloidosis. Ten years later, he returned because of dyspnea, fatigue, and weight loss. He had congestive heart failure. An echocardiogram revealed thickening of the interventricular septum (20 mm) and the posterior wall of the left ventricle (20 mm). The ejection fraction was reduced at 36%. An endomyocardial biopsy (positive for AS_{C1} antisera) and an abdominal fat aspirate were positive for amyloid. Immunoelectrophoresis and immunofixation showed no evidence of an M-protein in the serum or urine on repeated determinations. He died of congestive heart failure 17 years after the onset of symptoms of his carpal tunnel syndrome.

Two of the 35 patients with amyloid localized to the carpal ligament subsequently developed systemic amyloidosis. Neither had a monoclonal protein in the serum or urine. The initial carpal tunnel tissue stained for AS_{C1}, but the subsequent rectal biopsy was inadequate for special staining. The carpal tunnel tissue and the endomyocardial biopsy in the second patient both stained with AS_{C1}. There was no staining with κ or λ antisera. Both of these patients most likely had senile systemic amyloidosis.

Thirty-five patients with amyloid localized to the carpal ligament or synovium were studied with a battery of amyloid antisera. Thirty-three stained for AS_{C1}. Thirty-three stained for AS_{C1}. The amyloid in the carpal ligament tissue did not stain with any of the amyloid antisera in two patients. One of these two patients presented with a 1-year history of carpal tunnel symptoms in July 1977. Surgery was performed and amyloid was identified. The patient had an IgGλ monoclonal protein of 1.2 g/dL which did not increase in size during follow-up. The patient did well clinically and died suddenly of an acute myocardial infarction 9 years later. Her physician said that the patient had developed no features of amyloidosis. Her urine was negative for light chains. The second patient presented with a 10-year history of carpal tunnel syndrome in September 1974. Decompression was performed and amyloid was found. Immunoelectrophoresis and immunofixation of the serum and urine showed no evidence of a monoclonal protein. The patient, aged 84 years, was alive and asymptomatic 25 years after the onset of carpal tunnel syndrome.

3. DISCUSSION

Although all amyloid appears homogeneous with light microscopy and fibrillar with electron microscopy, it is composed of a variety of proteins. In AL and in amyloid localized to the lung or bladder, the fibrils consist of the variable portion of a monoclonal light chain (Glenner, et al., 1971).

We have described a group of patients who had carpal tunnel syndrome from local deposition of amyloid but who had no clinical evidence of systemic amyloidosis (Kyle, et al., 1989). Approximately one-fourth of patients with AL present with a carpal tunnel syndrome (Kyle and Gertz, 1990). In the current study, AL was suspected initially in 11 of the 35 patients because they had an M-protein in the serum or urine. It is important to determine whether the carpal tunnel symptoms are a manifestation of AL or whether the amyloid is localized to the tenosynovium. It is imperative from the standpoint of the patient and his physician to know whether the carpal tunnel syndrome represents AL with a survival of approximately 2 years or is from amyloid localized to the tenosynovium with no effect upon survival. Histologically, the amyloid from both types appears identical with light and electron microscopy and can be differentiated only on the basis of histochemical staining.

The presence of a monoclonal light chain in the serum or urine usually indicates AL, but the M-protein may be unrelated. None of the 11 patients with an associated M-protein in the serum or urine in this study developed symptomatic systemic amyloidosis.

Almost all (33 of 35) cases stained for AS_{C1}. This is different than the expected results from amyloid involving the carpal ligament, because the clinician usually expects the presence of AL. The presence of an M-protein always suggests the possibility of AL amyloidosis. None of our 11 patients with amyloid involving the carpal ligament and an M-protein in the serum or urine had AL. Approximately 3% of patients above the age of 70 years have a monoclonal gammopathy of undetermined significance (Kyle and Lust, 1989). In the current series, the M-protein and the presence of amyloid were unrelated. Immunohistochemical staining of the amyloid tissue is essential in order to determine whether the amyloid fibrils consist of a monoclonal light chain or of transthyretin.

It is important to determine the type of amyloid found in carpal ligament tissue because the patient may have a serious systemic disease with a short survival or localized amyloidosis of no prognostic importance to the patient.

4. REFERENCES

Glenner, G.G., Ein, D., Eanes, E.D., et al. (1971) Creation of "amyloid" fibrils from Bence Jones proteins in vitro, Science, 174:712.

Kyle, R.A., Eilers, S.G., Linscheid, R.L., Gaffey, T.A. (1989) Amyloid localized to tenosynovium at carpal tunnel release. Natural history of 124 cases, Am J Clin Pathol, 91:393.

Kyle, R.A., Gertz, M.A. (1990) Systemic amyloidosis, CRC Crit Rev Clin Oncol Hematol, 10:49.

Kyle, R.A., Lust, J.A. (1989) Monoclonal gammopathies of undetermined significance, Semin Hematol, 26:176.

REEVALUATION OF 134 PATIENTS WITH FAMILIAL AMYLOIDOTIC POLYNEUROPATHY (FAP) IN JAPAN, KUMAMOTO FOCUS

Shinichi Ikegawa, Shigehiro Yi, Shukuro Araki, Yukio Ando and Akira Miyazaki
The First Department of Internal Medicine, Kumamoto University Medical School, 1-1-1 Honjo, Kumamoto 860, JAPAN

ABSTRACTS. Clinical data on FAP in Kumamoto area, Japan from 1967 to 1990, were reevaluated in March 1990. One hundred, thirty four patients in 8 pedigrees, male 70 and female 64 were studied. The initial symptoms occured at 18-69 years of age (mean 34.2) with sensory disturbance at lower extremities (50%), or constipation / diarrhea (33.9%). The duration of illness was 5-19 years (mean 12.5 years). Female patients had a tendency of late onset (36.9 years old) and a long duration of illness (12.5 years). Main clinical symptoms were polyneuropathy, autonomic dysfunction and general manifestations such as edema, arrhythmia and visual disturbances. The diagnosis was made by biopsy, DNA and serum diagnosis. Owing to the recent diagnostic advances, seven late onset cases who had initial symptoms later than 45 years old have been found. Symptomatic treatment such as L-DOPS, DMSO, pace-maker implantation, opthalmological operations, hemodialysis, and other, were not only useful to eliminate subjective symptoms of the disease but also extended the survival from 8.8 years to 9.4 years, compared with those observed in an epidemiological study done in 1982 [1].

1. INTRODUCTION

A large family focus of type I FAP was discoverd by Araki in Kumamoto, Japan in 1967 [2]. Since then, various other FAP foci have been reported from all over Japan, owing to recent DNA diagnostic techniques. They were confirmed type I FAP by DNA diagnosis and have no relation to Kumamoto or Nagano foci. In this paper, we reexamined clinical and genetic features of FAP in Kumamoto from 1967 to 1990.

2. EPIDEMIOLOGY AND CLINICAL MANIFESTATIONS

2.1. Epidemiology

To confirm clinical data, we reviewed all the clinical data of FAP patients and their families in Kumamoto from 1967 to 1990. There were 134 FAP patients (male 70, female 64) in 8 pedigrees 62 cases were examined completely. The inheritance pattern was autosomal dominant. The mean age of onset was 34.3 years old, and the mean duration of the illness was 9.4 years. The causes of death was cardiac or renal failure and infections.

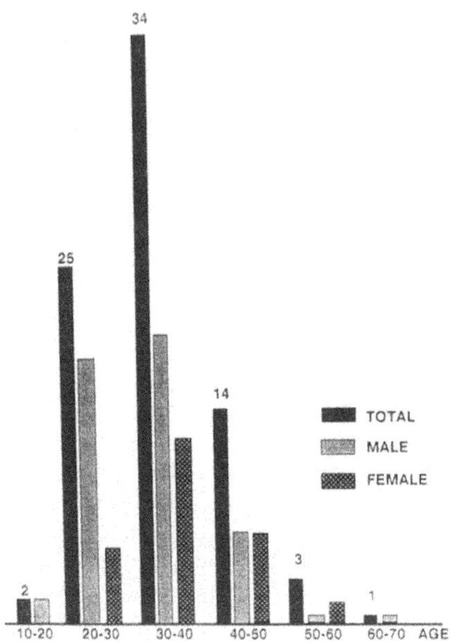

Fig. 1: The distribution of the age of onset. Black bars indicate total number of the patients and shadowed bars shows male and female.

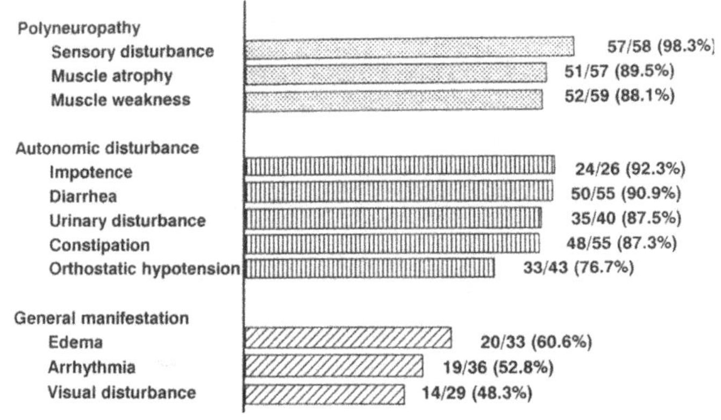

Fig. 2: Clinical manifestations of FAP in Kumamoto (1967-1990)

2.2. Initial symptoms

The distribution of the age of onset is shown in Figure 1. The age of initial symptoms appear from 18 to 69 years. The mean age of onset for male is 32.9 years old and for female patients is 36.2 years. Seven late onset cases who had initial symptoms later than 45 years of age were found.

The initial symptoms of 62 examined cases showed as follows. Sensory disturbance in lower legs was the most common initial symptoms (31/62), and diarrhea or constipation follows (21/62). Other initial symptoms were impotence in male (3/26), nausea (2/62), abdominal pain (2/62), syncope on standing (2/62) and weakness of the lower legs (1/62). Many patients initiate the symptoms with sensory or autonomic neuropathy.

2.3. Clinical manifestations

Clinical manifestations of FAP during the course of the disease are seen in Figure 2. Major clinical symptoms consist of: 1) polyneuropathy, 2) autonomic neuropathy, 3) general manifestations. The clinical stage of FAP were divided by Araki into 4 stages (Table 1). According to the stage, clinical manifestations were analyzed for each. In stage I, dissociated sensory disturbances, with pain and temperature sensation dominantly affected, started in lower limbs. Autonomic nervous system involvement such as impotence, diarrhea, orthostatic hypotension and constipation were also seen in the early stage of the disease. Motor neuropathy followed in stage II and III. General manifestations such as edema and arrhythmia were observed in the late stage.

Table 1. Clinical stages of FAP (by S. Araki)

STAGE	sensory disturbance	autonomic dysfunction*	ADL
I	mild, distal part of lower extremities	+ ~ ++	almost normal or slight disturbance
II	moderate and dissociated in lower extremities	++ ~ +++	difficulty in working moderate disturbance
III	lower and upper extremities	+++	difficulty in walking, stay home, marked disturbance and need help in ADL
IV	severe & generalized	+++	bed ridden (heart & renal failure)

+ : slight, — : moderate, +++ : marked

* autonomic dysfunction: Bowel dysfunction, orthostatic hypotension, urinary disturbances Syncope attack, impotence (male)

2.4. Prognosis

The mean age of death was 45.9 years (32-72 years old). The mean duration of illness was 9.4 years (5 to 19 years). Female patients had tendency toward later onset than males (36.9 vs 32.9) and longer duration of illness (11.5 vs 8.5).

3. TREATMENT

Although there is no specific therapy for amyloidosis, symptomatic treatment such as L-DOPS, DMSO, pacemaker implantation, ophthalmologic surgery, hemodialysis and so on, improve activity of daily life of FAP patients. These therapies were useful to improve the subjective symptoms of the patients, and also extended mean survival from 8.8 years to 9.4 years compared with those observed in epidemiological study in 8 years ago [1]. Monthly plasma exchange have been performed to one patient for three years and progression of the disease seemed to be slow down, evaluated by neurological score [3]. The usefullness and practicability of this treatment requires future study.

4. DNA AND SERUM DIAGNOSIS

DNA [4] and serum [5] diagnosis were performed in 87 members (control 18, FAP patient 25, family members 44). All FAP patients and 13 of familial members are positive by this test. Molecular genetics cannot explain how a biochemical abnormality causes the symptoms of the disease. We must deal with the ethical problems of presymptomatic diagnosis of FAP for which there is no effective treatment.

5. REFERENCES

1) Ikegawa S, Araki S, and Nagata J. (1984) "Review of clinical records and therapeutic trials in familial amyloidotic polyneuropathy (type 1) in Japan. in Amyloid and Amyloidosis, ed by Glenner GG, Osserman EF et al. Plenum, New York, 441-445.
2) Araki S, Mawatari S, Ohta M, Nakajima A and Kuroiwa Y. (1968) "Polyneuritis amyloidosis in a Japanese family", Arch Neurol 18, 593-602.
3) Ikegawa S, Araki S, Yi S, et al. "Plasma exchange therapy to FAP patients", Proceedings of the First International Symposium on FAP and TTR related disease (in press).
4) Mita S, Maeda S, Ide M, Tsuzuki T, Shimada K, Araki S. (1986) "Familial amyloidotic polyneuropathy diagnosed by cloned human prealbumin cDNA", Neurology (NY) 36, 298-301.
5) Ikegawa S, Tanase S, Araki S, and Morino Y. (1987) "Quantitative detection of a variant prealbumin associated with type I familial amyloidotic polyneuroapthy (Japanese type) by high performance liquid chromatography", Clinica Chimica Acta 167, 165-172.

SYMPATHETIC SKIN RESPONSE IN FAMILIAL AMYLOID POLYNEUROPATHY

P. Montagna, MD; F. Salvi, MD; L Monari, MD; R. Plasmati, MD.
Institute of Clinical Neurology, University of Bologna, Via U.Foscolo 7, 40123 Bologna, Italy.

ABSTRACT. In 39 relatives belonging to 6 Italian families affected with Familial Amyloid Polyneuropathy (FAP) we blindly performed Sympathetic Skin Responses (SSR) and EMG/CV studies. Palma SSR were reduced or absent in patients with clinically evident FAP. SSR amplitude was low also in relatives carrying transthyretin (TTR) mutations but without clinical or EMG evidence of polyneuropathy. SSR is useful in assessing autonomic involvement in FAP, even in preclinical stages.

INTRODUCTION

Sympathetic skin response (SSR) is a change in sudomotor skin function and electric resistance induced by exteroceptive arousing stimuli or by deep inspiration. It provides a non-invasive way to test unmyelinated axon function in peripheral neuropathy (Shahani et al, 1984).

Familial amyloid polyneuropathy (FAP) is a genetically determined polyneuropathy characterized by early and prominent autonomic nervous system involvement (Cohen, Rubinow, 1984).

We evaluated the usefulness of SSR in detecting autonomic impairment in patients affected with and in relatives carriers of the TTR mutations responsible for FAP but still asymptomatic. SSR data were then related to clinical staging and EMG/CV findings of involvement of the sensory-motor peripheral nervous system.

MATERIAL

Six Italian families with FAP were studied. Three were characterized by an abnormal TTR with a Met for Val substitution at position 30 (TTR Met 30). One had a Thre-Ala substitution at position 49 and another a

basic variant. In family 6, the genetic defect was still unknown.
In all, 39 subjects were studied. Twelve patients had clinically evident FAP; 8 were carriers of abnormal TTR but without symptoms or signs of FAP; 19 relatives were completely normal.

METHODS
SSRs were obtained by electric stimulation and surface recording from the palma and planta pedis ipsilaterally. Shocks were delivered randomly to avoid habituation. Electric stimulation was performed at the wrist and glabella (Montagna et al, 1985) and, when negative, deep inspiration was tried. The maximal amplitude of palma SSR was considered.
Normal SSR values were from 20 volunteers without signs of neurological involvement.
EMG and CV by near-nerve needle electrodes were performed according to Buchthal's method (Buchthal, Rosenfalck, 1966) on the deep peroneal (motor CV), superficial peroneal and sural (sensory CV) nerves.
All SSR, EMG and CV studies were performed blindly, without prior knowledge of the patient's TTR status.
For the purpose of clinical staging, patients were staged according to Coutinho et al, 1980.

RESULTS
SSR latencies and CV did not change appreciably among clinically affected relatives, asymptomatic carriers, normal relatives and controls.
Mean SSR amplitudes (palma) were lower in patients with clinically evident FAP than in normal relatives not carrying any TTR mutations (0.43 mV ± 0.5 SD versus 1.44 mV ± 0.9 SD). Asymptomatic carriers of TTR mutations also had lower SSR amplitudes (0.88 mV ± 0.4 SD) than completely normal relatives. In patients with severe FAP, SSR were usually absent.
There was a progressive reduction of SSR amplitude with increasing clinical disability as measured by a more advanced clinical stage of FAP (figure).

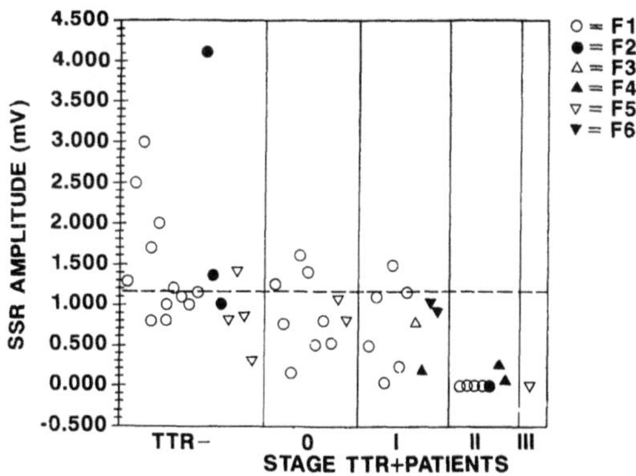

FIGURE: Correlation between TTR status/clinical stage and SSR amplitude. TTR- are normal relatives; TTR+ are carriers of TTR mutations (stage 0= asymptomatic).

On follow-up studies of single patients, SSR amplitude decreased with time, often dramatically, sometimes disappearing in a few months. Planta responses disappeared before palma SSRs.

Compared to EMG/CV studies, SSR were more often abnormal in both asymptomatic and symptomatic FAP patients. SSR amplitude seemed to correlate better with the amplitude of evoked response in extensor digitorum brevis muscle than with sural sensory CV.

DISCUSSION

SSRs are abnormal in clinically developed FAP; abnormalities increase with progression of the disease, leading to a complete disappearance of the responses in late stages.

SSR are also low in amplitude in carriers of TTR mutations without clinical or EMG/CV evidence of polyneuropathy. This confirms our earlier finding on a single FAP family (Montagna et al, 1988) and probably indicates that unmyelinated autonomic fibres are the first to become impaired by the pathogenic mechanisms responsible for FAP. Precise preclinical identification of carriers is however precluded by the wide scatter of

normal SSR values.
SSR are more sensitive than conventional EMG/CV studies. They provide a useful non-invasive method for the detection of autonomic involvement in FAP. It would be interesting to know whether other tests of autonomic function show similar or even better sensitivity in FAP, also in the preclinical stages.

REFERENCES

Buchthal, F. and Rosenfalck, A. (1966) 'Evoked action potentials and conduction velocity in human sensory nerves, Brain Res. 3, 1-122.

Cohen, A.S., and Rubinow, A. (1984) 'Amyloid neuropathy', in P.J. Dyck, P.K. Thomas, E.H. Lambert, R. Bunge (eds), Peripheral Neuropathy, Vol. II, Philadelphia, W.B. Saunders, pp. 1866-1898.

Coutinho, P., Martins da Silva, A., Lopes Lima, J., Resende Barbosa, A. (1980) 'Forty years of experience with Type I Amyloid Neuropathy. Review of 483 cases', Excerpta Medica ICS 497, 88-98.

Montagna, P., Liguori, R., Zappia, M. (1985) 'Sympathetic skin response', J. Neurol. Neurosurg. Psychiatry 48:489-490.

Montagna, P., Salvi, F., Liguori, R. (1988) 'Sympathetic skin response in familial amyloid polyneuropathy', Muscle & Nerve 11, 183-184.

Shahani, B.T., Halperin, J.J., Boulu, P., Cohen, J. (1984) 'Sympathetic skin response: a method of assessing unmyelinated axon dysfunction in peripheral neuropathies', J. Neurol. Neurosurg. Psychiatry 47, 536-542.

EXTRINSIC AND INTRINSIC NERVE LESIONS OF THE INTESTINE IN TYPE I FAMILIAL AMYLOID POLYNEUROPATHY

M. YAZAWA, S. IKEDA, N. YANAGISAWA
Department of Medicine (Neurology), Shinshu University School of Medicine, Matsumoto 390, Japan

ABSTRACT

To demonstrate the severity of the extrinsic and intrinsic nerve lesions in the intestine of type I familial amyloid polyneuropathy(FAP), we studied the rectum of 14 FAP patients (10 biopsy and 4 autopsy cases), using histochemistry and immunohistochemistry. Noradrenaline fluorescent nerve fibers in the rectal mucosae and silver impregnated axons in the nerve bundles in the outer space of the rectum were markedly depleted in FAP. However, s-100 protein, VIP and PHM immunoreactive nerves were normally distributed in the rectum of FAP patients. Severe degeneration of the intestinal extrinsic nerves may occur from an early stage of this disease, whereas the intrinsic nerves are relatively well preserved even in the advanced case. This selectivity of the intestinal nerve damage is presumed to produce the characteristic bowel dysfunction in FAP.

INTRODUCTION

In FAP, uncontrollable diarrhea and constipation develop at its early clinical stage[1,2]. These bowel symptoms are considered to be caused by abnormal neural control of the intestine[2,3], but the details of the pathological mechanisms remain unclear. To clarify the severity of damage in the intestinal nerves consisting of the extrinsic and intrinsic nerves[4], we examined the rectum of FAP patients with histochemistry and immunocytochemistry.

MATERIALS AND METHODS

We examined 14 patients with FAP(32 to 64y. o.), originating from Nagano prefecture, Japan(table 1). All patients suffered from a variable degree of polyneuropathy with autonomic symptoms and their clinical severity was divided into 3 stages(table 1). Rectal mucosae were biopsied from the 10 patients endoscopically, and additionally the rectum and lumbar sympathetic ganglia were obtained from the autopsy cases. The rectums of 12 controls(9 biopsy and 3 autopsy cases, 38 to 72y. o.) were also studied.

Noradrenaline fluorescent histochemistry was performed on the biopsied specimens with the glyoxylic acid method[3]. Nerve bundles in the outer side of

TABLE 1. Autonomic symptoms of 14 FAP patients

Case No.	1	2	3	4	5	6	7	8	9	10	11*	12*	13*	14*
Age	64	40	43	60	33	37	32	40	62	62	65	44	45	51
Sex	F	M	F	M	M	M	M	M	F	M	M	M	F	F
Duration(year)	2	2	3	5	6	7	6	8	11	5	12	16	19	33
Clinical stage	I	I	I	I	I	I	I	I	II	II	III	III	III	III
Orthostatic hypotension	-	-	+	+	+	+	+	2+	+	+	+	3+	3+	3+
Anhidrosis	-	+	-	-	+	-	+	+	+	+	+	3+	3+	3+
Dysuria	-	-	-	-	-	+	+	+	-	2+	+	3+	3+	3+
Bowel symptoms	+	+	+	+	+	+	2+	2+	2+	+	+	3+	3+	3+
Impotence	/	-	/	+	+	+	+	+	/	+	+	+	/	/

Clinical stage; I :can walk unaided; II :can move with help; III :bedridden
Severity of symptoms (except for impotence); -:none; +:mild; 2+:moderate; 3+:severe
(Impotence; -:none; +:involved; /:female) *:autopsied case, M:male, F:female

the rectal wall were stained by silver impregnation to demonstrate axonal loss. The lumbar ganglia were examined by conventional staining methods.

Using avidin-biotin-peroxidase complex, the rectum was immunostained with rabbit antisera(at a dilution of 1:1,000) to s-100 protein[5], vasoactive intestinal polypeptide:VIP(r-501)[6] and peptide histidine methionine:PHM(r-8502)[7], a precursor protein of VIP. The immunoreaction was abolished by preabsorption with the corresponding antigen. An electron microscopic study was carried out after embedding the immunostained specimen into epoxy-resin.

After observation of 10 optic fields(x100) of each layer of the rectum, the density of nerve fibers was graded as shown in table 2. The amyloid deposition was evaluated into 4 degrees(table 2) by the Congo red reaction.

RESULTS

Amyloid deposition was seen in the rectal wall of all FAP patients, but control specimens did not show any Congophilic reactivity.

Control rectal mucosae exhibited several noradrenaline fluorescent nerve fibers(fig. 1a&b). However, in the biopsied rectum of FAP cases, moderate to marked depletion of the noradrenergic fibers was observed(fig. 1c & table 2).

Silver impregnation revealed many axons in the thick nerve bundles in the outer side of the control rectum(fig. 2a). In contrast, autopsy cases of FAP had only a few thin nerve bundles in those spaces, showing a significant axonal

TABLE 2. Amyloid deposition and nerve distributions in the rectum

No.	Amyloid deposition					NA nerve			Axon of ExNB	S-100 nerve					VIP/PHM nerve				
	Lp	Mm	Sm	Cm	Lm	Lp	Mm	Sm		Lp	Mm	Sm	Cm	Lm	Lp	Mm	Sm	Cm	Lm
1	-	+	+			±	±	+		3+	3+	2+			3+	3+	2+		
2	-	2+	+			+	±	+		3+	2+	2+			2+	2+	2+		
3	-	2+	+			+	+	+		3+	3+	2+			3+	3+	2+		
4	-	+	+			+	+	+		3+	3+	2+			3+	3+	2+		
5	-	+	+			±	±	±		2+	3+	2+			2+	2+	2+		
6	-	+	+			±	+	+		3+	3+	2+			3+	3+	2+		
7	-	2+	+			±	+	+		2+	2+	2+			2+	2+	2+		
8	-	2+	+			±	±	+		3+	3+	2+			3+	3+	2+		
9	-	2+	+			±	+	+		3+	2+	2+			3+	2+	2+		
10	-	+	+			+	+	+		2+	3+	2+			2+	3+	2+		
11*	-	2+	2+	2+	+				+	2+	3+	2+	3+	2+					
12*	-	2+	3+	+	2+				±	+	2+	2+	3+	+	+	2+	+	2+	2+
13*	-	+	2+	2+	2+				±	+	2+	2+	3+	2+					
14*	-	2+	2+	+	+				+	+	2+	2+	2+	2+					
N	-	-	-			2+	3+	3+		3+	3+	2+			3+	3+	2+		
N*	-	-	-	-	-				3+	2+	3+	2+	3+	2+	2+	3+	2+	3+	2+

Degree of amyloid deposition; -:none, +:a little, 2+:moderate, 3+:severe
Rectal nerve density; -:none, ±:very few, +:a few, 2+:several, 3+:many
Lp:lamina propria, Mm:muscularis mucosae, Sm:submucosa, Cm:circular muscle, Lm:longitudinal muscle, *:autopsied case, N:normal control
NA:noradrenergic, ExNB:extrinsic nerve bundle

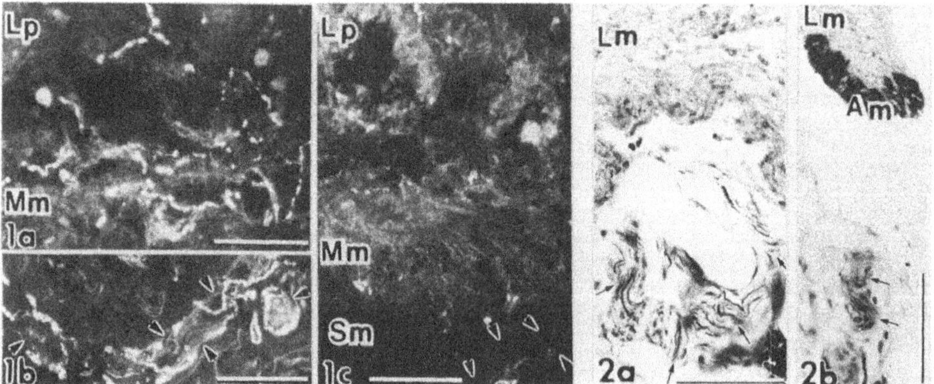

Fig. 1. Noradrenaline fluorescence in the biopsied rectal mucosae. a&b:Control c: FAP. Arrow heads=an arteriole. Fig. 2. Nerve bundles (arrows) in the external side of the rectum. a:Control. b:FAP. Am is amyloid deposit. Bar=100μm.

loss(fig. 2b & table 2).

The lumbar sympathetic ganglia, taken from 3 FAP cases showed a marked decrease of the nerve cells and heavy accumulation of amyloid(fig. 3a&b). Most of the remaining nerve cells were found to be severely degenerated(fig. 3c).

Immunostaining revealed many anti-s-100 protein immunoreactive nerve fasciculi in both the biopsied and autopsied rectal tissues of FAP patients as well as those in the control rectum(fig. 4a-c & table 2). The densities of VIP and PHM immunostained nerve fibers in the rectum biopsied from FAP patients were also similar to those of control rectal mucosae(fig. 5a & table2). Submucosal ganglia were not affected by amyloid deposition and the nerve cell

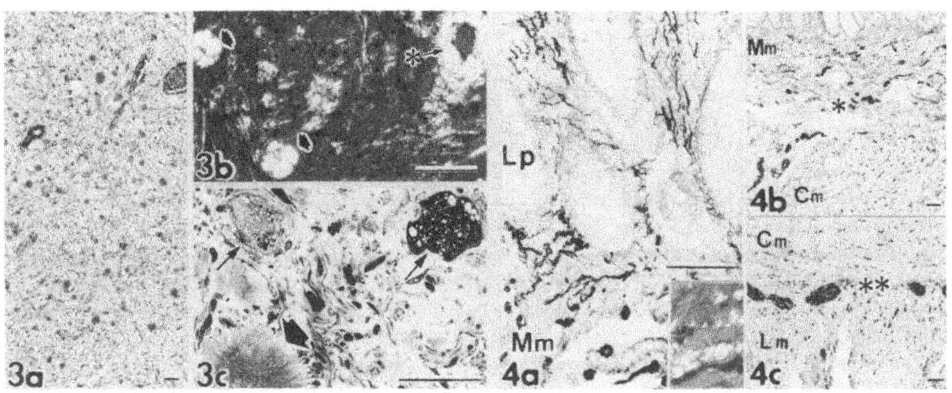

Fig. 3. Lumbar ganglion of FAP. a:Congo red and hematoxylin stain. b:Cross polarized light. *=arteriole, thick arrow=amyloid core. c:Toluidine blue stain Arrow=nerve cell body. Fig. 4. Rectal s-100 protein positive nerves of FAP. a:Biopsied rectal mucosa. Insert=Congo red stain with polarized microsope. b&c: Autopsied rectum. *&**=submucosal and myenteric plexus. Bar=100μm.

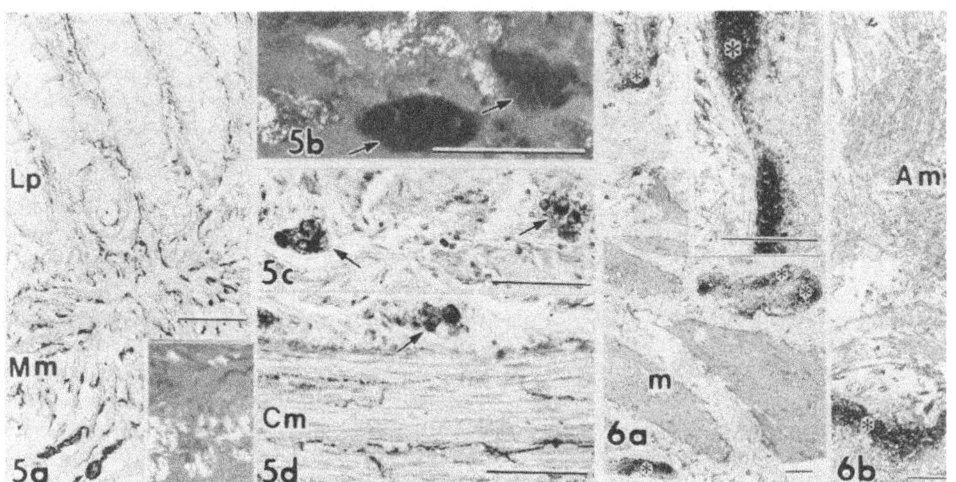

Fig. 5. Rectal VIP neurons of FAP. Arrow=submucosal ganglion. a&b:Biopsied rectal mucosa. Insert(a) & b=Crossed polar view of Congo red stain. c&d: Autopsied rectum. Bar=100μm. Fig. 6a&b. Electron microscopic findings of rectal PHM positive nerve fibers(*) of FAP. m=smooth muscle fiber. Bar=2.0μm.

bodies showed strong immunoreactivity in all biopsy cases and an autopsy one(No. 12) of FAP(fig. 5b-d). Several nerve fibers with either VIP or PHM immunoreactivity were seen in the muscular coats of a FAP autopsy case (fig. 5d). Electron microscopic observation of the rectal mucosa of FAP patients demonstrated unmyelinated nerve fibers with VIP and PHM immunoreactivity(fig. 6a), surrounded by the deposition of amyloid fibrils(fig. 6b).

DISCUSSION

Rectal noradrenergic nerve fibers are the processes of nerves in the lumbar sympathetic ganglia, innervating the rectum extrinsically[8]. The depletion of these nerve fibers in the biopsied rectum of FAP patients indicates that significant damage of the sympathetic nerves, possibly caused by the amyloid laden lumbar ganglia, may occur even in an early stage of this disease. We did not study another extrinsic nerves of the intestine including the parasympathetic nerves. However, our previous report on the vagus nerve [8] provided evidence of the severe parasympathetic nerve lesions in the intestine of FAP patients.

S-100 protein is localized in the enteric glial cells of the nerve fasciculi and ganglia[9], and its immunoreactivity demonstrates the distribution of many nerves in the rectum of FAP patients. On the other hand, the nerves of the alimentary tracts contain many kinds of peptides[10, 11], and in the intestine both VIP and PHM are shown to be present only in the intrinsic nerves[12]. Therefore, well preserved VIP and PHM immunoreactive nerves observed in the rectum of FAP patients elucidate that the intestinal intrinsic nerves are not markedly affected by amyloid accumulation in this disease.

This selectivity of the autonomic nerve lesions in the intestine (severe disturbance of the extrinsic innervation without significant involvement of the intrinsic nerves) may produce the characteristic bowel dysfunction in FAP.

[ACKNOWLEGDEMENTS. We thank Dr. T. Endo and Dr. N. Yanaihara for kindly supplying antisera of s-100 protein, VIP(r-501) and PHM(r-8502).]

REFERENCES

1. Andrade, C. (1952) 'A peculiar form of peripheral neuropathy, familial atypical generalized amyloidosis with special involvement of the peripheral nerves', Brain 75, 408-428. 2. Ikeda, S., et al (1987) 'Hereditary generalized amyloidosis with polyneuropathy. Clinicopathological study of 65 Japanese patients', Brain 110, 315-337. 3. Ikeda, S., et al (1983) 'Histochemical study of rectal aminergic nerves in type I familial amyloid polyneuropathy', Neurology (Cleveland) 33, 1055-1058. 4. Cooke, H. J. (1986) 'Neurobiology of the intestinal mucosa', Gastroenterology 90, 1057-1081. 5. Endo, T., et al (1981) 'Calcium-dependent affinity chromatography of s-100 and calmodulin on calmodulin antagonist-coupled sepharose', J. Biol. Chem. 256, 12485-12489. 6. Yanaihara, N., et al (1977) 'Immunological aspects of secretin, substance P, and VIP', Gastroenterology 72, 803-810. 7. Yanaihara, N., et al (1984) 'Immunochemical study on PHI/PHM with use of synthetic peptides', Peptides 5, 247-254. 8. Ikeda, S., et al (1987) 'Vagus nerve and celiac ganglion lesions in generalized amyloidosis', J. Neurol. Sci. 79, 129-139. 9. Ferri, G. L., et al (1982) 'Evidence for the presence of s-100 protein in the glial component of the human enteric nervous system', Nature 297, 409-410. 10. Furness, J. B., et al (1980) 'Types of nerves in the enteric nervous system', Neuroscience 5, 1-20. 11. Keast, J. R., et al (1985) 'Distribution of certain peptide-containing nerve fibers and endocrine cells in the gastrointestinal mucosa in five mammalian species', J. Comp. Neurol. 236, 403-422. 12. Larsson, L-I., et al (1980) 'Localization of vasoactive intestinal polypeptide (VIP) to central and peripheral neurons', Proc. Natl. Acad. Sci. USA 73, 391-393.

SEX DIFFERENCES AND AGE-DEPENDENT PENETRANCE IN FAP-TYPE I.

J. SEQUEIROS[1,2,3], A. SOUSA[1,3] and T. COELHO[2,3]
[1]Dept. Population Studies, ICBAS; [2]Hosp. Geral de Santo António and [3]Centro de Estudos da Paramiloidose (CEP);
Lg. Abel Salazar, 2
4000 Porto, Portugal.

ABSTRACT. Women are known to be less often affected with FAP-I, and to have later onset. There were 625 men and 447 women affected - a sex ratio of 1.45:1. Among all asymptomatic carriers of TTR^{Met30}, 334 were women and 272 were men (0.81:1). The sex ratio for all (manifesting and non-manifesting) carriers (1678) was 1.15:1. Mean age-of-onset was 34.8 in women and 31.7 years in men. The sex ratio was close to one in patients with intermediate onset; however, both in classic and late-onset patients there was a lack of women. This reflects different age-of-onset distributions, with overall later onset and less affected women. Thus, women and men are not alike in the expression of FAP-I, showing different age-dependent penetrances. We discuss a multifactorial model of inheritance of genetic modifiers, with a different threshold for each sex, and a hypothetical heterozygote's advantage (greater in males?), as possibly explaining all the sex differences found.

1. Introduction

Despite its autosomal dominant mode of inheritance, women are known to be less often affected with FAP-I, and to have later onset than men [1,2,3]. Presumably just due to insufficient sample sizes, sex differences were not statistically significative in some of the previous studies.

2. Subjects and methods

We have now studied sex ratios and age-of-onset distributions in 1072 Portuguese patients, 606 additional proven carriers (TTR ^{Met30}), not yet symptomatic, and 1201 relatives "at risk" who proved to carry the "wild type" gene, all registered at CEP (Porto, September 1989).

3. Results

Taking the whole population that has ever come to CEP (Table 1), there is no difference in proportion between men and women. Among those known to be affected, there were 625 men and only 447 women - a ratio of 1.45:1.

On the other hand, among all proven (asymptomatic) carriers of TTR^{Met30}, 334 were women and only 272 were men - a sex ratio of 0.81:1. The sex ratio for all 1678 (manifesting and non-manifesting) carriers was 1.15:1. The proportion of carriers (patients plus TTR^{Met30} asymptomatic carriers) is significantly greater than that of non-carriers (Table 2). But, most interestingly, the proportion of males among the carriers is greater than expected, whereas the proportion of female carriers is smaller than expected (in other words, the proportion of female non-carriers is greater than that of males) - $X^2{}_1=25.88$, P=0.

Although both curves have similar shapes, the women's distribution shows a definite shift to the right, meaning an overall later onset in women (Table 3). Mean age-of-onset was 34.8 years in 429 women (SD=8.6, SEM=0.418) and 31.7 in 613 men (SD=9.4, SEM=0.379).

The sex ratio was close to one in patients with intermediate onset (40 to 51 years); however, both in patients with classic (before age 40) and late-onset (after age 52 years) there is a lack of women (Table 4). This reflects different sex distributions of age-of-onset, with overall later onset in women, as well as the excess of male patients.

TABLE 1. Sex distribution of persons registered at CEP

	females	males	total
Patients (alive or dead)	447	625	1072
Asymptomatic TTR^{Met30} carriers	170	114	284
Not observed TTR^{Met30} carriers	164	158	322
'Wild type' relatives (TTR^{Val30})	664	537	1201
Relatives still at risk	255	201	456
Other diagnoses	19	24	43
Total	1659	1719	3378

TABLE 2. Total number of carriers and non-carriers

	females	males	total
Carriers (TTR^{Met30})	781	897	1678
Non-carriers (TTR^{Val30})	664	537	1201
Total	1445	1434	2879

TABLE 3. Global and sex distributions of age-of-onset

	Global	Women	Men
Sample size (patients)	1042	429	613
Mean age-of-onset (years)	32.95	34.77	31.68
S.D.	9.1	8.6	9.4
Range	17-73		
Mode	30		

TABLE 4. Groups of age-of-onset (o.) and sex ratios

SEX	Classic (o.<40)	Intermediate (39<o.<52)	Late (o.>51)	Total
Men	515	61	37	613
Women	344	63	22	429
Total	859	124	59	1042
%	82.4	11.9	5.7	100.0
Sex ratios	1.50	0.97	1.76	1.42

4. Discussion

Women and men are not alike in the expression of FAP-I, showing different age-dependent penetrance, as manifested by different sex distributions of age-of-onset and different overall penetrance (more asymptomatic women aged 52 or older) [3].

We have previously proposed that other familial factors, probably genetic modifiers, influenced the phenotypic variation in Portuguese patients with FAP [3,4,5]. These factors, however, seem to affect men and women at a different extent. Men seem to have a lower threshold for the expression of the Portuguese FAP gene: (1) there are more male than female patients; and (2) the age of onset is significantly later, on average, in women than in men.

The study of the parental transmission of the Portuguese FAP gene [6] has suggested a model of multifactorial inheritance of these genetic modifiers (with different thresholds for each sex). Women, having a higher threshold, are more "protected" from the effects of the FAP gene. So, in order for a woman to be affected, she needs to carry more "detrimental factors" (or less "favorable" ones) than a male. This implies that women who have become affected have, on average, more of those "detrimental factors" (or less "favorable" ones) to pass on to their children, who will be then at a greater risk of manifesting FAP earlier in life (and perhaps of having a more severe disease), than the offspring of affected fathers, particularly if they are of the male sex.

A sex-ratio of 1.5 among the classic-onset patients, may be explained by the women's later onset, whereas the predominance of men in the late-onset group may reflect the greater proportion of life-term asymptomatic women (the similar sex-ratios in the intermediate-onset group may be due to a partial overlapping of the classic and late-onset distributions).

It is possible that the FAP gene may confer some (still unknown) advantage to the heterozygote (as opposed to both the "wild type" and TTR^{Met30} homozygotes), explaining the wide diffusion of the FAP mutation (Portuguese type) in Portugal and other countries. It is possible that this advantage (if it does exist) is greater for the male than the female heterozygote: if the gametal segregation is the same (i.e., there is no meiotic drive), the excess of males could be explained by a positive selection of the FAP gene predominantly, or exclusively, in males.

Therefore, it will be of paramount importance to study the segregation of the FAP gene in sibships (proportion of carriers and non-carriers), as well as the proportion of males and females in those families.

5. Acknowledgements

The authors wish to express their gratitude to Profs. Drs. P.P. Costa and M.J. Saraiva, at whose laboratories the biochemical tests were performed, as well as Dr. P. Coutinho and all the other neurologists involved with patient examination. This work was supported in part by a grant from Fundação Luso-Americana para o Desenvolvimento.

6. References

1. Andrade, C., Canijo, M., Klein, D. and Kaelin, A. (1969) 'The genetic aspects of the familial amyloidotic polyneuropathy', Humangenetik 7, 163-175.
2. Coutinho, P., Silva, A.M. and Barbosa, A.R. (1980) 'Forty years of experience with type I amyloidotic polyneuropathy - Review of 483 cases', in G.G. Glenner, P.P. Costa and A. Freitas (eds.), Amyloid and Amyloidosis, Excerpta Medica, Amsterdam, pp. 88-98.
3. Sousa, A., Lobato, L. and Sequeiros, J. (1988) 'Início tardio na neuropatia amiloidótica hereditária - tipo I: Variação familiar e modelos genéticos', Boletim do Hospital (HGSA) 3, 63-69.
4. Sequeiros, J. and Saraiva, M.J. (1987) 'Onset in the seventh decade and lack of symptoms in heterozygotes for the TTR^{Met30} mutation in hereditary amyloid neuropathy - type I (Portuguese, Andrade)', Am. J. Med. Genet. 27, 345-357.
5. Lobato, L., Teixeira, F., Sousa, A. and Sequeiros, J. (1988) 'Genetic Study of Late-onset in Hereditary Amyloid Neuropathy (HAN) - Type I (Portuguese, Andrade)', in T. Isobe et al. (eds.), Amyloid and Amyloidosis, Plenum Press, New York, pp. 413-418.
6. Sousa, A., Coelho, T. and Sequeiros, J. 'Parental transmission and age-of-onset in familial amyloidotic polineuropathy (Portuguese type)' in Natvig, J.B. et al. (eds.), Amyloidosis, Proceedings of the VIth International Symposium on Amyloidosis (in press).

PARENTAL TRANSMISSION AND AGE-OF-ONSET IN FAMILIAL AMYLOIDOTIC POLINEUROPATHY (PORTUGUESE TYPE)

A. Sousa[1,3], T. Coelho[2,3] and J. Sequeiros[1,2,3]
[1]Instituto de Ciencias Biomedicas Abel Salazar, [2]Hospital Santo Antonio and [3]Centro de Estudos da Paramiloidose
Department of Population Studies
ICBAS, Largo Abel Salazar,2
4000 Porto, Portugal

ABSTRACT. We studied the consequences on age-of-onset of both the sex of the patient and that of the transmitting parent in portuguese patients: 505 inherited the FAP gene from the mother, and 429 from the father.
Classic onset (before age 40) was more often inherited from the mother, while patients with intermediate (ages 40-51) or late-onset (52 or after) have more frequently inherited FAP from their fathers. When onset was after age 40 years (last two groups), the father was 1.5 times more likely to be the transmitting parent. Men affected with FAP had, on average, earlier onset than women. Mean age-of-onset was higher for children of transmitting fathers than of transmitting mothers; in any case, daughters have a higher mean age-of-onset. Thus, sons of affected mothers had the earliest onset (29.3), while daughters of affected fathers seemed to be the most "protected" (35.1 yrs) from the effects of the FAP gene. We discuss the possible role of multifactorial inheritance of genetic modifiers, with a different threshold for each sex.

1. INTRODUCTION

In other autosomal dominant diseases, such as Huntington's disease [1,2,3] or Myotonica dystrophy [4], the study of the effect of parental transmission on age-of-onset has been of major importance in the discussion of a genetic model for the phenotypic variation. We studied the consequences on age-of-onset of the sex of the transmitting parent (who, in some cases, may not have shown symptoms).

2. SUBJECTS AND METHODS

We studied parental transmission among portuguese FAP patients with diagnosis established on at least two of the following criteria: typical clinical picture, positive family history, positive biopsy and presence of TTR^{Met30} in the plasma. Among 1072 patients, 505 (224 women, 281 men) inherited the gene from the mother, and 429 (180 women, 249 men) from thefather; 9 had both maternal and paternal family history of FAP; in 74 cases the disease was unknown in their parents' generation and in the 55 remaining no information was available.

3. RESULTS

The proportion of patients who inherited the FAP gene from their mothers is greater than those who inherited it from the father (Z=2.5, P=0.012). They distribute, however,equally in both sexes.

Table 1. Sex of patients and their transmitting parent

Transmitting Parent	Patient Women	Men	Total
Mother	224	281	505
Father	180	249	429
Total	404	530	934

(X^2_1=0.543,P=0.54).

Classic onset (before age 40) was more often inherited from the mother, while patients with intermediate (ages 40-51) or late-onset (52 or after) had more frequently inherited FAP from their fathers (Table 2.). When the onset was after age 40 years (last two groups), the father was 1.5 times more likely to be the transmitting parent.

Table 2. Sex of the transmitting parent and the offspring age-of-onset group

Offspring age-of-onset group	Transmitting Parent		
	Mother	Father	Total
Classic	446	347	793
Intermediate	38	55	93
Late	9	15	24
Total	493	417	910

(X^2_2=10.7,P=0.0046)

Offspring of transmitting mothers have, on average, earlier onset (30.9 yrs) than those who inherited FAP from their fathers (32.9) (Z=-2.99, P=0.0056).
There is an additive effect of the sex of the patient and that of the transmitting parent, with no interaction (ANOVA not shown), with sons of transmitting mothers and daughters of transmiting fathers showing the extreme means (Table 3.).

Table 3. Mean age of onset according to the sex of patient and the sex of the transmitting parent

Sex of Patient	Transmitting parent		
	Mother	Father	Global
Men	29.29 (278)	30.64 (244)	29.92
Women	33.08 (215)	35.10 (173)	33.98
	30.94	32.49	31.65

4. DISCUSSION

In Portuguese FAP patients, men had, on average, earlier onset (32.9) than women (34.8 yrs). However, mean age-of-onset was higher for those who inherited the FAP gene from their fathers (32.6) than for those who inherited it from their mothers (30.9 yrs); in both cases, however, daughters had a higher mean age-of-onset than sons.
Thus, sons of affected mothers had the earliest onset (29.3), while daughters of affected fathers seemed to be the most "protected" (35.1 yrs) from the effect of the FAP gene.
These results toghether with those on anticipation (Sousa et al., 1990) seem to argue in favour of a multifactorial model of inheritance of genetic modifiers, modifying the expression of the FAP gene, showing different thresholds for each sex.

5. Aknowledgements

The authors wish to express their gratitude to Dr. Paula Coutinho and all the other neurologists involved in patient examination. This work was partly supported by the Fundacao Luso-Americana para o Desenvolvimento.

6. References

1. Merritt,A.D., Conneally,P.M., Rahman,N.F. and Drew, A. L. (1969) 'Juvenile Huntington's chorea' in Andre Barbeau and Jean Real Brunette (eds), Progress in Neurogenetics, Excerpta Medica Foundation, Amsterdam, pp. 645-650.
2. Conneally,P.M. (1984) 'Huntington's disease:genetics and epidemiology', Am. J. Hum. Genet. 36, 506-526.
3. Farrer,L.A. and Conneally,P.M. (1985) 'A Genetic Model for Age at Onset in Huntington Disease', Am. J. Hum. Genet. 37, 350-357.
4. Harper,P.S. and Dyken,P.R. (1972) 'Early-onset dystrophia myotonica: evidence supporting a maternal environmental factor', Lancet II, 53-55.

ANTICIPATION OF AGE-OF-ONSET IN FAMILIAL AMYLOIDOTIC POLINEUROPATHY (PORTUGUESE TYPE)

A. Sousa[1,3], T. Coelho[2,3], L. Lobato[2,3] and J. Sequeiros[1,2,3]
[1]Instituto de Ciencias Biomedicas Abel Salazar, [2]Hospital Santo Antonio and [3]Centro de Estudos da Paramiloidose
Department of Population Studies
ICBAS, Largo Abel Salazar,2
4000 Porto, Portugal

ABSTRACT. Among portuguese FAP patients, no late-onset FAP offspring has been found to descend from a classic-onset parent, while late-onset patients often have classic-onset children. Offspring of late-onset patients, though having a higher mean age-of-onset, usually have earlier onset than their parents. Age-of-onset was studied in 147 parent-offspring pairs and so was the mean difference between them. Both the sex of the affected parent and that of the offspring were significant factors with no interaction. Sons of affected mothers (who, on average, started FAP 10.9 yrs earlier than their mothers), and daughters of affected fathers (who had onset 1.3 yrs later than their fathers) showed the extreme means. Anticipation may be the result of sampling and ascertainment biases (less late-onset children and less children of early onset parents) but also of sex differences.

1. INTRODUCTION

No late-onset child (onset at or after age 52 yrs) has ever been found to descend from a classic-onset parent (onset before age 40). Late-onset patients, however, often have classic-onset children (Lobato et al. (1988)). Offspring of late-onset patients, though having a higher mean age-of-onset (36.8) than the overall population (32.9), usually have onset earlier than their own parents.

We have now looked at the transmission of age-of-onset (from affected parents to their offspring), through pedigree analysis and the effect of the sex of the offspring and of his/her affected parent on anticipation.

2. SUBJECTS AND METHODS

Age-of-onset (AO), the age at beginning of first symptoms of the sensory or autonomic neuropathy) was known for 147 parent-offspring pairs examined at Centro de Estudos da Paramiloidose (CEP), Porto: 91 patients (52 men and 39 women) had an affected father and 56 (32 men and 24 women) descended from an affected mother. The male and female offspring were equally distributed within

both groups.
Anticipation was defined as the parent's AO minus the offspring's AO. Three groups were defined: patients showing (1.) anticipation (earlier onset than the affected parent); (2.) no anticipation (same age of onset as the affected parent); (3.) negative anticipation (onset later than the affected parent).

3. RESULTS

Mean AO for all offspring was 30.0 yrs, (range of 19-48), whereas parents' mean AO was 35.9 yrs (range: 22-68).
The proportion of patients showing anticipation is significantly greater than those not showing it; negative anticipation is more often inherited from the father (Table 1).

Table 1. Anticipation according to the sex of the affected parent

Anticipation	Negative	Zero	Positive	Total
Fathers	31	5	55	91
Mothers	9	2	45	56
Total	40	7	100	147
%	27.2	4.8	68.0	100

(X^2_1=6.41, P=0.04)

There are very few children of affected mothers who do not anticipate; however, there are no significant sex differences among them (Table 2).

Table 2. Anticipation in offspring of affected mothers

Anticipation	Negative	Positive	Total
Sons	3	29	32
Daugthers	6	16	22
Total	9	45	54
%	16.7	83.3	100

(X^2_1=2.914, P=0.08)

Among the descendants of affected fathers, there is an association between the sex of the offspring and anticipation: more daughters than expected who do not anticipate (Table 3).
The absence of late-onset offspring (Table 4) may be due to the fact that some late-onset offspring have not yet manifested FAP, but also to the impossibility to establish age of onset for the affected parent of our late-onset cases. Nevertheless, it remains true that no late-onset case has been found descending from a classic or even from an intermediate onset-parent.

Table 3. Anticipation in offspring of affected fathers

Anticipation	Negative	Positive	Total
Sons	8	41	49
Daugthers	23	14	37
Total	31	55	86
%	36.0	64.0	100

(X^2_1=19.3, P=0)

Table 4. Groups of age of onset for parents and their offpring

Parent / Offspring	Classic (0.<40)	Intermediate (39<0.<52)	Late (0.>51)	Total
Classic	106	16	11	133
Intermediate	7	2	5	14
Late	-	-	-	-
Total	113	18	16	147

A two-way ANOVA showed that both the sex of the affected parent and that of the offspring were significant factors with no interaction. Sons of affected mothers (who, on average, started FAP 10.9 yrs earlier than their mothers), and daughters of affected fathers (who had onset 1.3 yrs later than their fathers) showed the extreme means (Table 5):

Table 5. The effect of the sex of the offspring and of his/her affected parent on mean anticipation

Sex of patient	Affected Parent		
	Mother	Father	Global
Sons	10.91 (32)	7.77 (52)	8.96
Daughters	7.0 (24)	-1.33 (39)	1.84
Global	9.23	3.87	5.9

() is the n. of patients.

4. DISCUSSION

Anticipation has been studied in other autosomal dominant diseases as Myotonic Dystrophy (Penrose, 1948), Machado-Joseph disease (Sequeiros and Coutinho, 1981) and Huntingtons' disease (Ridley et al., 1988). It has been explained as the result of sampling and ascertainnment biases (Penrose,1948) though others (Murphy, 1975), however, believe that other factors may be implicated. Anticipation is common in FAP patients and may be found in all parent-offspring classes except, on the overall, in daugthers of affected fathers. Sons anticipate more than daughters, particularly when their mother was the transmitting parent. We have shown (Sousa et al., 1990) that there are important sex differences and these may well account for at least part of the anticipation encountered in this families (less late-onset children and less children of early onset parents). Further studies, either in other populations with the same variant (Swedish, Japanese or Maiorquin), or using other methods can be useful in distinguishing between possible sampling biases and genetic or environmental factors. The study of the possible role of the sex of the affected great-parent is also recommanded.

5. Aknowledgements

The authors wish to express their gratutide to Dr. Paula Coutinho and all the other neurologists involved in patient examination. This work was partly supported by the Fundacao Luso-Americana para o Desenvolvimento.

6. References

Lobato,L., Teixeira,F., Sousa,A. and Sequeiros,J. (1988) "Genetic Study of Late-onset in Hereditary Amyloid Neuropathy (HAN)-Type I (Portuguese,Andrade)" in Takashi Isobe et al (eds.), Amyloid and Amyloidosis, Plenum Press, New York, pp. 413-418.

Murphy, E. A. and Chase, G. A. (1975) Principles of Genetic Counselling, Year Book Medical Publishers, Chicago.

Penrose,L.S. (1948) 'The problem of anticipation in pedigrees of dystrophia myotonica', Ann. Eug. (London) 14, 125-132.

Ridley, R. M., Frith,C.D., Crow, T. J. and Conneally, P. M. (1988) "Anticipation in Huntington's disease is inherited through the male line but may originate in the female", J. Med. Genet. 25, 589-595.

Sequeiros, J and Coutinho, P. (1981) "Genetic Aspects of Machado-Joseph disease", Broteria Genetica (Lisboa) II,137-147.

Sousa, A., Coelho, T. and Sequeiros, J. "Parental transmission and age-of-onset in Familial Amyloidotic Polineuropathy (Portuguese Type)" in Natvig,J.B. et al. (eds.) Amyloidosis, Proceedings of the VIth International Symposium on Amyloidosis.

SPORADIC, LATE-ONSET CASE OF FAMILIAL AMYLOID POLYNEUROPATHY TYPE I (ANDRADE) - A CLINICOPATHOLOGICAL STUDY

Y. Yamamura[1], S. Kito[1], T. Harada[1]
S. Katayama[1], M. Shimoyama[1]
T. Takeshima[2], Y. Inai[2], T. Nakano[3]
1) Third Dep. Int. Med., 2) Second Dep. Pathol.
Hiroshima Univ. School of Med., Hiroshima 734
3) Dep. Int. Med., Nagano Chuo Hosp., Nagano 380

ABSTRACT A solitary, late-onset case of FAP type I originated from Hiroshima Prefecture, Japan, was reported, which had polyneuropathy complicated by mild cardiac changes but was lacking in nephrotic syndrome. Postmortem examination revealed the almost total saving of the kidney from amyloid deposition. The clinical and pathological features of this case were documented in comparison with those of FAP cases from Nagano Prefecture in which renal involvement is usually severe.

1. PREFACE

Familial amyloid polyneuropathy (FAP) type I is an autosomal dominant disease affecting young adults aged 20-45 years. Since the discovery of transthyretin (TTR) with Val-Met substitution at position 30 as the biochemical marker and with advances of DNA analysis an increasing number of late-onset cases have been found. Some pedigrees have only late-onset forms and others have both classical and late-onset forms, and there are small numbers of solitary cases of late onset. According to Ribeiro and Coutinho (1988) the clinical picture of late-onset forms seems more benign than that of classical forms, but the duration of the disease of the late-onset forms is shorter than that of the classical. No significant pathological differences have been observed between the two conditions. In this paper we report a solitary, late-onset case presenting atypical clinical and pathological manifestations.

2. REPORT OF CASE

The patient was healthy until 1979 (the age 63) when she noticed abnormal gustation, tingling dysesthesia and pain in her feet. Next year she visited our clinic. She had a slight sensory and motor disturbances in distal portions of the extremities. Her neurological deficits became progressively worsened. A sural nerve biopsy showed marked loss of myelinated fibers with amyloid deposit. She was admitted in Jan. 1983.

Physical examination revealed slight anemia, early cataract, and functional systolic murmur at the apex. She had a misshapened pupil on the right side, dysgeusia and perioral sensory loss. Weakness of muscle strength of the extremities was slight in the proximal and moderate in the distal portions. Amyotrophy of lower limbs with drop foot was noted. Deep reflexes were totally lost. Superficial sensations was disturbed with distal dominancy in all extremities. She had difficulty of gait due to muscle weakness, impaired deep sensations and neuralgic pain. There were no autonomic symptoms but for constipation. She became bedridden in Mar. 1985. Autonomic failures including orthostatic hypotension, dysuria, hyperhidrosis, decreased salivary secretion became manifested around 1986. She had no decubital ulcers, no episodes of alternating diarrhea and constipation.

Repeated laboratory studies showed iron deficiency anemia, and normal or slightly lower level of serum albumin and cholesterol. Except for during bouts of urinary tract infection there was no albuminuria. ECGs showed right axis deviation, QS pattern, changing ST-T figures, grade I A-V block with occasional ventricular extrasystoles. There were, however, no sick sinus syndrome or severe conduction disorders. Echo cardiograms showed concentric left ventricular hypertrophy, but the wall movement was not so bradykinetic. Motor nerve conduction velocity was decreased in the median nerve and was not detected from the lower limbs.

In the last one and a half years of her life ataxic respiration with paroxysmal respiratory arrest occurred repeatedly. She became akinetic mutism and finally demented. The patient died in Jun. 1989 due to respiratory arrest, 10 years after the onset of the disease.

2.1. FAMILY HISTORY, DNA DIAGNOSIS AND VARIANT TRANSTHYRETIN ASSAY

Details of these studies were reported in the previous paper (Harada et al., 1988). The patient (proband) and her families were inborn inhabitants of Hiroshima Prefecture. DNA analysis to detect the variant TTR ($Val-Met^{30}$) gene gave positive tests in the proband and one of 5 family members examined: her 47 year-old niece with positive DNA test exhibited no clinical features of FAP. Radioimmunoassay of the plasma variant TTR of the proband case was 11.3 mg/dl, comprising 55 % of total plasma TTR.

2.2. PATHOLOGICAL STUDY

The heart was 390 g in weight. Heavy amyloid deposition was noted in the endocardium and valves. The spleen had amyloid deposit in the vascular walls and trabeculae, and in the liver it was limited to the Glisson's sheaths. In the pancreas amyloid deposition was remarkable in the connective tissue with atrophy of exocrine glands, while the islets were relatively well preserved. The thyroid gland showed heavy amyloid deposits in the connective tissue but the follicular epitheial lining and colloidal content were well preserved. In the adrenal amyloid was in the medullary blood vessel wall. The kidney had multiple scars due to pyelonephritis and arteriosclerosis (Fig.1a). There was substantially no amyloid deposit in the glomeruli and peritubular vascular networks, and only a little amount was found in the medullary interstitium (Fig.1b,c).

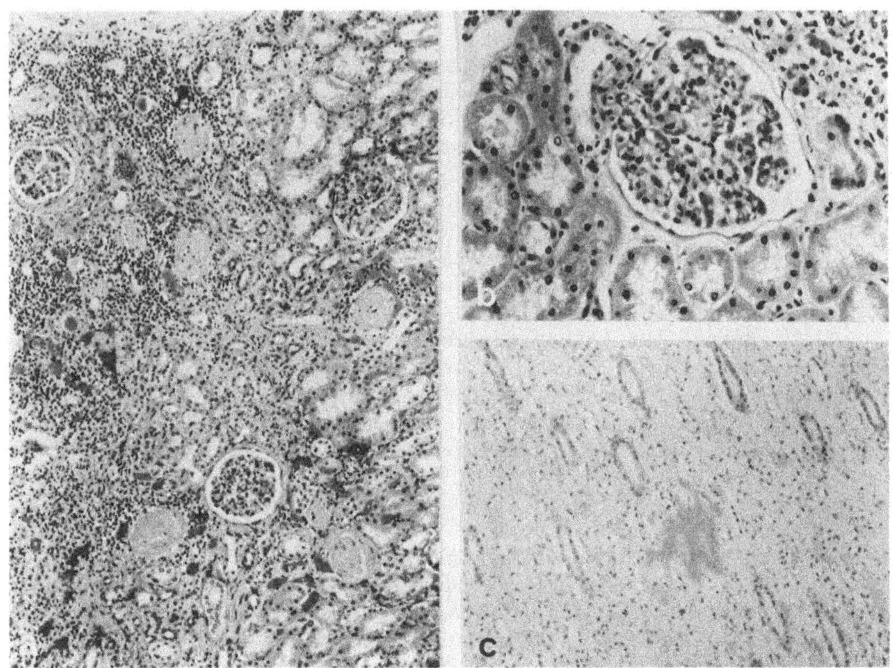

Fig.1 (a) Scars with hyalinized glomeruli. H.E., (b) A glomerulus without amyloid deposits. H.E. (c) Amyloid deposits in the renal medulla.

In the peripheral nerve amyloid deposition was remarkable with a reduced number of myelinated fibers. The posterior root ganglia and sympathetic ganglia showed heavy amyloid deposition and atrophy of ganglion cells. The spinal cord had degeneation of the posterior funiculi. Blood vessels of the pia mater had amyloid deposits but those within the central nervous system tissue did not. Myelin sheath staining revealed diffuse but perivascularly accentuated pallor of the cerebral white matter with minimal gliosis.

3. DISCUSSION

Clusters of late-onset cases or FAP type I have been reported from many countries including Sweden, Portugal, and Japan. Of the Swedish cluster comprising 33 families and 60 patients, of which 68% of patients had the first symptoms after 50 years. Thirteen percent was solitary cases. In the cluster of Nagano average age of onset was 35.1, and 5.2 % of them had the first symptoms after 60 years (Shimoyama et al., 1988). The present case was confirmed to be suffering from FAP by the recombinant DNA technique and the plasma variant TTR assay. Although with an asymptomatic carrier the family history was apparently negative. In the present case, in addition to polyneuropathy same as those of the cases from Nagano, there are some characteristic features. First, autonomic failures were relatively mild: she did not have ducubital ulcers, nor alternative diarrhea and constipation. Second, severe cardiac complications including complete A-V block or sick sinus syndrome were not observed throughout her course. Third, there were no nephrotic syndrome. Postmortem study revealed amyloid deposit in the peripheral nerve, heart, pancreas, thyroid gland, and, to a lesser extent, in the spleen. Conspicuous was the almost total saving of the kidney from amyloid deposition.

In cases of FAP type I from Nagano the important factors leading to death are cardiopathy with arrhythmias and conduction defects, infectious diseases and renal failure. Renal involvement was severe in all cases of classical form (Yamamura et al., 1988), and also in one solitary, late-onset case of Nagano we observed intense histological changes of amyloidotic nephropathy. Although renal involvement varies considerably among different families and even among individuals of the same family, renal dysfunction is a serious complication in Japanese cases (Shimoyama et al., 1988; Itoh et al., 1988). In this respect the clinicopathological features of Japanese cases are different from those of type I FAP from Portugal. The present case is unique for the lack of amyloidotic nephropathy, and is similar to the Portuguese cases. The different organ selectivity suggests the existence of unknown factors, other than the molecular characteristics of TTR, contributing to the development of amyloid deposition in particular organs.

REFERENCES

Ribeiro, I., and Coutinho, P. (1988) 'Late-onset forms of familial amyloid polyneuropathy (Portuguese type), A reappraisal', T. Isobe, S, Araki, F. Uchino, S. Kito, E. Tsubura (eds.), Amyloid and Amyloidosis, Plenum, New York & London, pp.435-439

Harada, T., Kito, S., Shimoyama, M., Katayama, S., Sasaki, H., Furuya, H., Yoshioka, K., Sakaki, Y. (1988) 'Diagnosis of familial amyloid polyneuropathy by recombinanat DNA techniques in relation with clinical features', Ibid, pp365-370

Shimoyama,M. Kito, S., Katayama, T., Togo, M., Yamamura, Y., Nakano, T. (1988) 'Natural history of Ogawa Village typefamilial amyloid polyneuropathy in Japan', Ibid. pp827-832

Yamamura, Y., Kito, S., Shimoyama, M., Katayama, S., Miyoshi, R., Nakano, T., Anzai, N., (1988) 'Pathological studies on familial amyloidosis', Ibid., pp. 511-516.

Itoh, N., Shigematsu H., Ikeda, S., Oguchi, H. (1988) 'Clinicopathological studies on nephropathy of familial amyloid polyneuropathy in Japan', Ibid. 499-504.

FAMILIAL AMYLOIDOSIS WITHOUT TRANSTHYRETIN (TTR) INVOLVEMENT: AN UNUSUAL PRESENTATION

N.J.S. FITCH, A.M. ZALIN* & D.B. RAMSDEN

Department of Medicine,
University of Birmingham,
Queen Elizabeth Hospital,
Birmingham B15 2TH, UK.

*Corbett Hospital,
Stourbridge,
West Midlands, UK.

ABSTRACT. Six members of a family shared the trait of developing petechiae with minimal skin abrasion. All are now dead. Three of them had histologically proven amyloid deposits, and a fourth died of renal failure. There was no clinical evidence of peripheral neuropathy in any of the above, but amyloid was found in the peripheral nerves of one of the cases. The possibility that the amyloid deposits arose from a variant TTR was investigated by sequencing the exonic sections of the TTR gene. No mutations were observed, and it is concluded that the amyloid deposits were not formed from a variant TTR.

1. Clinical Presentation

1.1 HISTORY OF PROBAND (FAMILY MEMBER 8, FIGURE 1)

A 50 year old man underwent a laparotomy for abdominal pain and epigastric mass. He had a large spleen, pale liver and nodular small bowel mesentery. Histology of the spleen, liver, jejunum and mesentery showed amyloid infiltrate.

Since childhood he had been liable to develop skin petechiae after mild abrasion, a propensity he shared with other members of the family. He had proteinuria (up to 1g/L) but normal renal function. Serum immunoglobulins were normal. ECG showed first degree heart block (PR 0.22sec.) Three months later he died of Staph. aureus septicaemia and endocarditis. Amyloid was found in the kidney, lymph node and peripheral nerve.

1.2 CASE HISTORIES OF FAMILY MEMBERS

There was no known foreign ancestry. We have no clinical information regarding family members 1 and 4, except that they both had petechiae and they died aged 60+ and 30 years respectively. Family member 3 (proband's mother) had proteinuria at age 51y. Urea was 20mmol/L. ECG showed a PR interval = 0.22sec. Within a year her urine protein excretion was 9g/L, and her serum albumin was 20g/L. She died of renal failure.

Family member 9 (proband's sister) presented at age 20y with folic acid deficiency. Four years later her creatinine clearance was 28ml/min. Renal and jejunal biopsies showed amyloid. At 34 years of age her renal function deteriorated sharply and she died of a retroperitoneal bleed. Liver, spleen and abdominal nodes were enlarged with amyloid infiltrates. Family member 11 (maternal first cousin of proband) had an enlarged amyloid-bearing spleen removed when 27 years old. Chest X-rays showed widespread mottling. At age 47y he had moderate hepatomegaly but no proteinuria. He died aged 50 of carcinoma of the stomach. The suture line of the anastomosis site failed to hold because the tissue was so heavily infiltrated with amyloid.

Family members 5,6 & 7 died of well documented conditions unrelated to amyloid. Nothing is known of family member 2.

Previous investigations, using antibody staining of histological sections, failed to identify TTR or any other the known amyloidogenic proteins as the major component of the amyloid deposits (Pepys et al. 1983).

2. Aim

In view of :-

i) the clear hereditary character (autosomal dominant) of the amyloidosis,
ii) the fact that antibody staining for TTR amyloidosis is known to give false negative results on occasions (Koeppen et al. 1985), and
iii) familial amyloidosis is frequently associated with mutations in the TTR gene (Costa et a. 1978; Saraiva et al. 1988),

it was decided to elucidate the structure of the TTR gene in one of the affected subjects to ascertain whether this unusual form of amyloidosis was associated with the presence of a TTR variant.

3. Methods

3.1 EXTRACTION OF DNA FROM SPLEEN HISTOLOGY BLOCKS

The only remaining tissue samples from this family were two small histological paraffin wax blocks of material from family members 8 & 11. Sections were cut from the larger of these (proband - spleen). The paraffin wax was removed with toluene (2x1ml) and ethanol (2x1ml), and the tissue dried in vacuo, suspended in 300ul TEK buffer (50mM Tris-Cl, pH 8; 10mM EDTA; 300ug/ml proteinase K) and digested for 72h at 37°C, with a further 300ug of proteinase K added after 24h. After digestion the remaining insoluble material was spun down, the supernatant extracted with phenol/chloroform and the DNA precipitated with ethanol.

3.2 PCR AMPLIFICATION OF TTR EXONS AND BLUNT-ENDING OF PRODUCTS

PCR Amplification of each exon (Saiki et al. 1988) was carried out using spleen DNA and primers complementary to intron sequences on either side of the exon of interest. Amplification was performed for 30 cycles (91°C for 30s, 55°C for 1 min, 72° for 1 min), in 50ul reaction mixtures comprising 50mM KCl, 10mM Tris-HCl (pH 8.3), 1.5mM $MgCl_2$, 0.01% gelatin, 400uM each dNTP, 4uM each primer and 2.5 Units AmpliTaq recombinant Taq DNA polymerase (Perkin Elmer) overlayed with 50ul liquid paraffin. Samples (20-100ng) of the PCR products were rendered blunt-ended with Klenow DNA polymerase. Blunt-ended products were phenol/chloroform extracted and ethanol precipitated overnight at -70°C.

3.3 M13 SUBCLONING

The blunt-ended PCR products were ligated with recombinant-selective M13 RV vector (a gift from Dr. John Bell) linearised with Eco RV, using T4 DNA ligase. The mixture was used to transform E. Coli JM101 rendered competent by the high efficiency method of Hanaham (1985). The recombinant M13 plaques were screened using a full-length TTR cDNA probe (Docherty et al. 1989) according to Maniatis et al.(1982). Single-stranded templates were prepared from TTR exon-containing plaques and sequencing was carried out by the method of Sanger (Sanger 1981;Sanger et al. 1977) using a Sequenase version 2 sequencing kit (United States Biochemical).

4. Results

Six to eight clones were sequenced for each of the four exons. There were no conserved mutations, and the only deviations from the published sequence of Tsuzuki et al. (1985) were random Taq misincorporations. These were far more numerous than we have previously observed with leukocyte DNA as the PCR template and may reflect damage to the cellular DNA caused by formalin fixation and/or paraffin embedding.

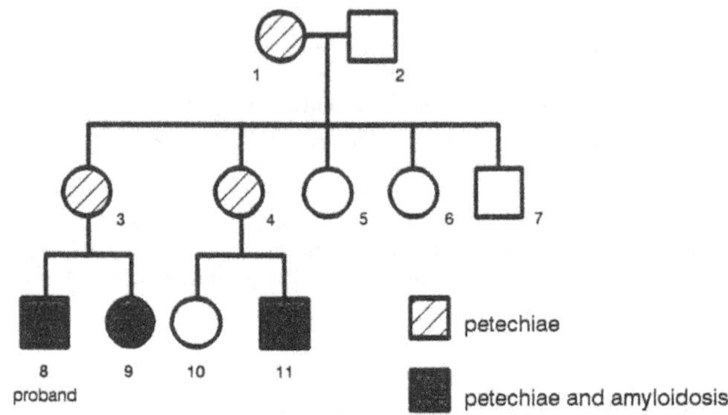

Fig 1: Inheritance of petechiae and amyloidosis in an English family

5. Conclusions

The clinical features of the family presented here are similar to those describe by Ostertag (1950) in that there was familial amyloidosis without peripheral neuropathy. However, in one of our cases there was amyloid deposition in a peripheral nerve. This deposition of amyloid plus the fact that not all TTR amyloid deposits are easily identified by antibody staining techniques, led us to investigate the possibility that a variant TTR may be the major component of the amyloid. Sequencing of all four exons of the TTR gene in the genomic DNA of one of the affected subjects showed that no mutations were present. Therefore the identity of the protein forming the amyloid still awaits elucidation. The clinical symptoms are also similar to those of a Massachusetts family with amyloidosis formed by a variant apolipoprotein A1 described by Jones et al. elsewhere in these Proceedings.

ACKNOWLEDGEMENTS. We wish to acknowledge the financial support of the Central Birmingham Health District Endowment Fund and the Wellcome Trust.

6. References

Costa P.P., Figueira A.S. and Bravo F.R. (1978) Amyloid Fibril Protein Related to Prealbumin in Familial Amyloidotic Polyneuropathy. **Proc Nat Acad Sci USA 75; 4499-4503.**

Docherty K., Shennan K.I.J., Marsden R. and Ramsden D.B.(1989) Subunit assembly and secretion of transthyretin: studies in a cell free translation system and microinjected Xenopus oocytes. **J Molecular Endocrinology 3, 191-197.**

Hanaham D. (1985) Techniques for transformation of E. Coli. in **DNA Cloning; a practical approach vol 1., ed. Glover D.M., IRL Press (Oxford)**

Koeppen A.H., Mitzen E.J., Hans M.B., Peng S-K and Bailey R.O. (1985) Familial Amyloid Neuropathy. **Muscle & Nerve 8;733-749.**

Jones L.A.., Harding J.A., Cohen A.S. and Skinner M. (1990) New USA family has Apolipoprotein A1 (Arg 26) variant. **Proceedings VIth International Symposium on Amyloidosis.** Abstract 4/4.

Maniatis T., Fritsch E.F. and Sambrook J. (1982) in **Molecular Cloning; a laboratory manual,pp312-328, Cold Spring Harbor Laboratory, New York.**

Ostertag B. (1950) Familiare amyloid-erkrankung. **Z.Menschl. Vererbungs Konstit. lehre 30;105-115.**

Pepys M.B., Breathnach, S.M., Black, M.M., Tennent, G., De Beer, F.C., Lanham, J., Zalin, A.M., Tribe, C.R. & Evans, D.J. (1983) Diagnosis and characterisation of amyloid deposits by immunohistochemical staining. **Amyloidosis E.A.R.S. pp189-191 (ed. Tribe, C.R.& Bacon P.A.) Reed Books, Bristol.**

Saiki R.K., Gelfand D.H., Stoffel S., Scharf S.J., Higuchi R., Horn G.T., Mullis K.B. and Erlich H.A. (1988) Primer-directed enzymatic amplification of DNA with a thermostable DNA polymerase. **Science 239; 487-491.**

Sanger F. (1981) Determination of nucleotide sequences in DNA. **Science 214; 1205-1210.**

Sanger F., Nicklen S. and Coulson A.R. (1977) DNA sequencing with chain terminating inhibitors. **Proc Nat Acad Sci USA 74; 5463-5467.**

Saraiva M.J.M., Costa P.P. and Goodman DW.S. (1988) Transthyretin (Prealbumin) in Familial Amyloidotic Polyneuropathy: Genetic and functional aspects. in **Advances in Neurology vol. 48, ed. S. Didonato et al, Raven Press (New York).**

Tsuzuki T.,Mita S., Maeda S.,Araki S. and Shimada K. (1985) Structure of the Human Prealbumin Gene. **J Biol Chem 260; 12224-12227.**

MECHANISMS OF AMYLOID FIBRIL FORMATION IN ALZHEIMER'S DISEASE AND OTHER DEMENTIAS

G.G. GLENNER, P.M. MEHLHAFF AND H. KAWANO
University of California, San Diego
Department of Pathology - 0612
9500 Gilman Drive
La Jolla, California, USA 92093

ABSTRACT Alzheimer's disease is one of several dementing conditions in which amyloid deposits represent a major, if not causative lesion. The characteristics of these deposits and their chemical nature may lead to an understanding of the pathogeneses of these disorders.

INTRODUCTION

Alzheimer's disease is the most common form of amyloidosis (1) affecting over 4 million individuals in the United States and the cost to care for the ravages of the disease totals $90 billion per year. Deposits of amyloid fibrils as visualized in the core of "senile" (neuritic) plaques and cerebrovascular walls have the "classic" fibrillary appearance and crystallographically defined ß-pleated sheet structure (2), while the intracellular neurofibrillary tangles composed of paired helical filaments of 12 nm width with an 80 nm periodicity also have a ß-pleated sheet X-ray diffraction pattern (3), consistent with the definition of amyloid fibrils. Identical lesions have been reported in Down's syndrome individuals over the age of 40. Our initial specific focus in investigating the nature of Alzheimer's disease was on the isolation, purification and characterization of fibrils composing the amyloid-laden vessels found in over 92% of cases.

Isolation of the amyloid fibril protein of the cerebral vessels in Alzheimer's disease revealed a novel polypeptide of 28 amino acids designated the ßP (4). A similar polypeptide differing only by having a Glu instead of a Gln at residue 11 was isolated from the amyloid-laden cerebrovasculature of Down's individuals. (5). The gene encoding for the ßP was as a result assigned to chromosome 21. Three years following the discovery of the ßP, four groups, using oligonucleotide probes based on the ßP amino acid sequence, obtained the nucleotide sequence of the gene product and assigned the gene to chromosome 21. The gene product was suggested to be a glycosylated cell-surface receptor composed of 695 amino acids (6). The deduced amino acid sequence of the ßP domain was identical to that of the Down's syndrome polypeptide (having a Glu at residue 11).

Antibodies raised to the cerebrovascular ßP localized also to senile plaques indicating these amyloid deposits were also composed of ßP fibrils (7). In addition, immunohistochemical localization was found in the cortex in granular (Type 4) and plaque-like (Type 3, "pre-amyloid") structures without evidence of neuritic change or amyloid deposition (8). Not infrequently cerebellar localization primarily to the molecular layer could be seen (9).

COMPARATIVE PATHOLOGY

Sporadic Congophilic Angiopathy: This is a condition in which amyloid deposition occurs predominantly in the walls of leptomeningeal vessels with an apparent paucity of plaques and tangles. Its most common pathologic manifestation is vessel rupture with subarachnoid or intracortical hemorrhage. Immunohistochemical studies reveal the fibrillar protein is ßP.

Hereditary Icelandic Cerebrovascular Amyloidosis (HCHWA-I): This process affects individuals in their 20-30's as an autosomal dominant disease with severe cerebrovascular amyloidosis leading to vessel rupture, hemorrhage and stroke. Atypical plaques but no neurofibrillary tangles are noted. The amyloid fibril protein from this condition was sequenced and shown by Frangione and coworkers to be composed of a segment of cystatin C (gamma trace), a serine protease inhibitor derived from the serum. No sequence homology exists between this protein and ßP.

Hereditary Dutch Cerebrovascular Amyloidosis (HCHWA-D): This is also an autosomal dominant cerebrovascular amyloidosis affecting individuals averaging 25 years of age with evidence of atypical plaques but no tangles. Death or morbidity is caused by rupture of amyloid-laden vessels in the leptomeninges or grey matter. Frangione and coworkers found that a variant ßP having a Gln substitution at residue 22, comprised the protein of the amyloid fibers.

Spongioform Encephalopathies: This group of diseases caused by slow-acting transmissible agents includes in humans Creutzfeld-Jacob disease, kuru and the autosomal dominant process Gerstmann-Sträussler syndrome (GSS) while its most noted animal manifestation is scrapie in sheep. The sole and predominant amyloid lesions in kuru and GSS are numerous often large cortical amyloid-laden plaques while such lesions are rare or absent in Creutzfeld-Jacob. In "natural" scrapie amyloid plaques and often adjacent cerebrovascular amyloidosis can be defined. Prusiner and co-workers have found the amyloid fibrils to be composed of a protein of 27-30 kilodaltons designated the "prion". Recombinant DNA techniques have shown the gene product to be a cell membrane protein. The 27-30 kd prion protein is derived from a 30-35 kd precursor by proteolytic treatment. Thus far the prion protein associated with scrapie has not been chemically distinguished from the normally occurring protein. Recently the nature of the protein forming the plaques in GSS has been shown to be a prion variant having a Leu for a Pro substitution at residue 102 of the gene product.

CAUSE, SIGNIFICANCE AND NATURE OF CEREBRAL AMYLOIDOSIS

1. Overproduction or Increased Concentration of Protein Precursor:
The most relevant example of increased concentration of an amyloid fibril precursor to induce formation of fibrils is found in hemodialysis amyloidosis with the relative concentration in serum of ß2 microglobulin being greatly increased by its failure to pass the dialysis membrane.

Since the gene encoding ßP is on chromosome 21 in Down's syndrome, this results in a 50% increase in the amount of all proteins synthesized on this chromosome. Overproduction of the ß protein precursor (ßPP), overwhelming proteolytic systems, has been suggested as an amyloidogenic mechanism. However, initial evidence for such a ßPP increase, although found in Down's syndrome, could not be demonstrated in Alzheimer's disease. It is also possible that the formation of AIAPP in type 2 diabetic pancreatic islets may represent an example of local overproduction of this hormonal protein.

2. Amino Acid Substitutions (Point Mutations):
In a variety of amyloidoses protein variants have been demonstrated in autosomal dominant conditions as for example in familial amyloidotic polyneuropathy (transthyretin variants), GSS (prion variant), HCHWA-Icelandic (cystatin C variant) and HCHWA - Dutch (ßP variant). The exact effect of these variant ("amyloid-ogenic") proteins in producing amyloid fibril deposits is not known and may vary for each condition.

Possibilities are 1) the induction of a protein conformational change leading to fibril deposition, 2) inhibition of normal proteolytic cleavage or 3) abnormal proteolysis.

3. Post-translational Modifications:
In those cases where a variant protein cannot be demonstrated, an enzyme defect (inherited or acquired) may lead to amyloid deposition e.g. by glycosylation, phosphorylation or sulfation defects. To date no examples of this as a cause of amyloidogenesis are known. Of greater likelihood is abnormalities in proteolysis.

4. Incomplete Proteolytic Processing:
A possible example of this amyloidogenic mechanism may be in medullary carcinoma of the thyroid where the amyloid fibrils are formed from a pre-calcitonin molecule apparently as the result of failure to proteolytically cleave the signal polypeptide. This failure may also be due to overproduction of pre-calcitonin in this condition. Alzheimer's disease may also be an example of this mechanism.

A PATHOGENETIC MECHANISM IN ALZHEIMER'S DISEASE

The frequent presence of ßP reactive plaque-like structures in the cerebellum (9) (where compact amyloid plaques are rarely seen) may indicate that these structures may represent potential precursors to compact plaques only if proteolytic enzymes, e.g. from microglia, are present to cleave the ßPP to release the ßP to produce amyloid fibers (2). In sites where such cleavage does not occur (e.g. in the absence of microglia) the ßPP is digested by non-amyloidogenic proteolysis e.g. by carboxypeptidases.

-2 ↓ 1 5 ↓
VAL - LYS - MET - [ASP - ALA - GLU - PHE - ARG - HIS - ASP - SER-

16 ↓
GLY - TYR - GLU - VAL - HIS - HIS - GLN - LYS - LEU - VAL - PHE-

28 ↓
PHE - ALA - GLU - ASP - VAL - GLY - SER - ASN - LYS] - GLY - ALA-

40
ILE - ILE - GLY - LEU - MET - VAL - GLY - GLY - VAL - VAL - ILE-

Figure 1: Potential proteolytic cleavage sites (arrows) of the ßPP to form ßP amyloid fibrils.

Since a ßP variant, overproduction or a concentration increase of the ßP precursor or evidence of abnormal post-translational modifications have not been demonstrated for the amyloid deposition of Alzheimer's disease, the most likely mechanism is an abnormality in proteolytic processing of the ßP precursor (ßPP) (10). Four sites of the ßPP containing or proximal to the ßP domain which have serine protease-susceptible amino acids (see Figure 1) are at residue: -2 at the Lys-Met bond, residue 5 at the Arg-His bond, residue 16 at the Lys-Leu bond, and residue 28 at the Lys-Gly bond. Based on precedent cleavage at position 5 will not occur if the enzyme is a Lys protease. Cleavage first at the Lys 28 would allow release ("secretion") of the ßPP at the plasma membrane. Cleavage at Lys 16 would approximately halve the ßP domain and prevent amyloid fibril formation. However, if this enzyme is absent, as for example in familial Alzheimer's disease, or inhibited as for example in acquired Alzheimer's disease, cleavage at Lys-2 would release a 1-28 ßP (after aminopeptidase cleavage of Met-1) to afford amyloid fibrils. Recently, normal cleavage of the ßPP at residue Lys 16 has been demonstrated (11) and evidence of abnormal proteolysis of the ßPP in Alzheimer's disease has been suggested (12).

Assuming this mechanism to be correct and absence of inhibition of proteolytic cleavage at Lys 16 is the cause of ßP amyloid formation in Alzheimer's disease, an approach to treatment would be the inhibition of proteolysis at Lys-2 to prevent ßP release and amyloid deposition.

REFERENCES

1. Glenner, G. (1983) 'Alzheimer's disease: multiple cerebral amyloidosis' in R. Katzman (ed.), Banbury Report 15: Biological Aspects of Alzheimer's Disease, Cold Spring Harbor Symposium, pp. 137-144.

2. Glenner, G. (1980) 'Amyloid deposits and amyloidosis: the ß-fibrilloses (Medical Progress Report)', N. Engl. J. Med. 302, 1283-1292, 1333-1343.

3. Kirschner, D., Abraham, C., and Selkoe, D. (1985) 'X-ray diffraction from intraneuronal paired helical filaments and extraneuronal amyloid fibers in Alzheimer disease indicates cross-ß conformation', Proc. Natl. Acad. Sci. USA 82, 1-5.

4. Glenner, G. and Wong, C. (1984) 'Alzheimer's disease: initial report of the purification and characterization of a novel cerebrovascular amyloid protein, Biochem. Biophys. Res. Commun. 120, 885-890.

5. Glenner, G. and Wong, C. (1984) 'Alzheimer's disease and Down's syndrome: sharing of a unique cerebrovascular amyloid fibril protein', Biochem. Biophys. Res. Commun. 122, 1131-1135.

6. Kang, J., Lamaire, H., Unterbeck, A., Salbaum, J., Masters, C., Gryeschik, K., Multhaup, G., Beyreuther, K., and Muller-Hill, B. (1985) 'The precursor of Alzheimer's disease amyloid A4 protein resembles a cell-surface receptor', Proc. Natl. Acad. Sci. USA 82, 8729-8732.

7. Wong, C., Quaranta, W., and Glenner, G. (1985) 'Neuritic plaques and cerebrovascular amyloid in Alzheimer's disease are antigenically related', Proc. Natl. Acad. Sci. USA 82, 8729-8732.

8. Ikeda, S., Yanagisawa, N., Allsop, D., and Glenner, G. (1989) Evidence of amyloid ß-protein immunoreactive early plaque lesions in Down's syndrome brains', Lab. Invest. 61, 133-137.

9. Bugiani, O., Giaccone, G., Frangione, B., Ghetti, B., and Tagliavini, F. (1989) 'Alzheimer's patients: preamyloid deposits are more widely distributed than senile plaques throughout the central nervous system', Neuroscience Letters 103, 263-268.

10. Glenner, G. (1988) 'The proteins and genes of Alzheimer's disease', Biomed. Pharmacother. 42, 579-584.

11. Esch, F., Keim, P., Beattie, E., Blacher, R., Culwell, A., Oltersdorf, T., McClure, D., and Ward, P. (1990) 'Cleavage of amyloid ß peptide during constitutive processing of its precursor', Science 248, 1122-1124.

12. Sisodia, S., Koo, E., Beyreuther, K., Unterbeck, A., and Price, D. (1990) 'Evidence that ß-amyloid protein in Alzheimer's disease is not derived by normal processing', Science 248, 492-495.

AMYLOID β-PROTEIN DEPOSITION AS A SEMINAL PATHOGENETIC EVENT IN ALZHEIMER'S DISEASE

DENNIS J. SELKOE
Center for Neurologic Diseases
Harvard Medical School
Brigham & Women's Hospital
Boston, MA 02115

ABSTRACT. Since the original description of the clinicopathological syndrome of Alzheimer's disease (AD), there has been lively debate about the primacy of amyloid deposition, neuritic/neuronal dystrophy or glial dystrophy in the pathogenesis of the disease. The isolation of the subunit protein [amyloid β-protein (AβP)] from meningovascular [1] and senile plaque core [2,3] amyloid and the production of relevant antibodies has shown that amorphous, largely non-fibrillar deposits of AβP occur in much larger numbers than "classical" compacted plaque cores in AD and Down's syndrome. The precursor polypeptide of AβP (βAPP) is encoded by a gene on chromosome 21 [4-7]. This finding suggests that the premature development of numerous AβP deposits in patients with trisomy 21 as early as the second decade of life is due to the increased dosage of βAPP in such patients. The localization of the βAPP gene to chromosome 21 and the identification of amorphous AβP deposits ("diffuse" or "preamyloid" plaques) in both Down's syndrome and AD strengthens the use of Down's syndrome as a natural model of the pathogenesis of AD. In this chapter, we review the current evidence that deposition of AβP is a seminal event in the pathogenesis of AD which may precede the development of neuritic plaques, neurofibrillary tangles, astrocytosis, microgliosis and other neuropathological changes of the disease.

Distinctions Between AβP From Meningeal and Senile Plaque Deposits

AβP is a ~40-amino acid proteolytic fragment of βAPP. We previously reported βAPP to occur in brain, non-neural tissues, and cultured cells as a heterogeneous group of 110-135 kD membrane-associated glycoproteins [8]. Although it is clear that AβP in meningovascular deposits and AβP in plaque cores have a common protein precursor (βAPP), these two principal forms of AβP deposits differ to some extent in their chemical properties. AβP isolated from meningeal blood vessels is soluble in guanidine HCl (6M), whereas AβP in purified senile plaque cores is insoluble in this reagent [2,3]. Besides this differential solubility, AβP isolated from meningeal blood vessels can readily be sequenced by Edman degradation, whereas there is considerable controversy about the ability to sequence AβP isolated from purified amyloid plaque cores. In our studies, we have consistently found that purified senile plaque cores (prepared by fluorescence-activated cell sorting to achieve maximal purity) cannot be sequenced by Edman degradation, despite loading up to 2 nanomoles of the subunit protein [3]. We have interpreted these results as indicating that AβP present in amyloid plaque cores has a blocked or buried N-terminus [3]. This observation

observation has been confirmed in other laboratories [9,10]. In contrast, one laboratory has reported the straight-forward sequencing of AβP in isolated senile plaque cores [2]; however, the vascular AβP deposits present in these fractions could be the source of the AβP sequences obtained. To date, the identity of a modifying group that might cause the apparent blockage of the N-terminus of AβP from amyloid cores has not been reported. The current evidence that AβP in plaque cores cannot be sequenced from its N-terminus and is insoluble in guanidine HCl suggests that the AβP in such cores is more modified than the AβP which is the subunit of meningovascular-derived amyloid. It could be that the plaque core AβP is a further derivation of the vascular AβP. On the other hand, these two forms of amyloid deposits may arise by separate and parallel routes from βAPP.

Origin and Molecular Pathogenesis of AβP Deposits in Alzheimer's Disease and Down's Syndrome

In the case of Down's syndrome, it has been possible to obtain evidence about the temporal sequence of AβP deposits versus other cytopathological alterations. Patients with Down's syndrome prior to the age of 30 have been found to have diffuse or preamyloid AβP deposits with little or no surrounding neuritic dystrophy or glial alteration and with very few or no neurofibrillary tangles. Since all patients with Down's syndrome develop the full-blown pathologic lesions of AD if they survive below 40-50 years, it appears that diffuse AβP deposits lacking morphologically surrounding neuronal/glial abnormality can precede the classical lesions of AD. Such a conclusion is supported by studies of AβP deposition in regions of AD brain that are usually clinically asymptomatic. We have described abundant diffuse AβP deposits in the cerebellar molecular layer of AD brains [11]. Antibodies to neurofilaments, tau protein and glial fibrillary acidic protein as well as certain markers for microglial cells fail to demonstrate neuronal or glial abnormality in the immediate vicinity of such cerebellar deposits. Our results indicate that AβP deposition occurs in a variety of brain regions, but that the response to its presence varies greatly as a function of the local milieu [11]. The absence of significant neuronal and glial structural abnormality in AD cerebellum even at the end of the disease may be the reason for the lack of significant cerebellar symptoms in most AD patients.

Since we last reviewed the issue of the origin of AβP deposits in AD [12], further data has accumulated that supports a vascular or blood origin of at least some AβP deposits in Alzheimer's disease and Down's syndrome. Potentially the most persuasive new evidence is the discovery of small numbers of AβP-immunoreactive deposits in and around microvessels in the skin, subcutaneous tissue, small and large intestine and adrenal gland of most patients with AD and a minority of aged non-AD subjects [13]. Further studies we have performed since this initial report support the notion that most AD subjects demonstrate some systemic AβP-immunoreactive deposits [14]. In addition, we have observed that antibodies to the native AβP subunit protein purified from brain amyloid deposits are more sensitive and specific in detecting these extracerebral deposits than are antibodies to synthetic AβP

[13,14]. The latter results suggest that there are certain conformational epitopes in native AβP that are not mimicked by synthetic AβP and that these epitopes are present in extracerebral deposits. However, much further work is needed to clarify the similarities and differences between systemic AβP-immunoreactive deposits and the much more abundant and well-characterized AβP deposits in the brain. It is important to emphasize that the AβP deposits we have detected in extracerebral sites are highly selective; many microvessels are unaffected by AβP deposition while a few react positively. It seems unlikely that an irrelevant cross-reactive antigen related to aging of microvessels would have this kind of highly selective distribution. Instead, the selectivity of involvement mimics that seen in microvessels of the brain and meninges in AD. The fact that four different AβP antisera (three native and one synthetic) can label the same immunoreactive deposits in a particular microvessel wall in a section of AD intestine supports the notion that such AβP immunoreactivity, while of low abundance in peripheral tissues, is chemically related to the AβP deposition process in the brain.

Further studies are currently under way to try to determine whether the detection of AβP in peripheral tissues (particularly fresh skin biopsies) has any diagnostic utility in cases of clinically-suspected Alzheimer's disease. It may turn out that the amount and detectability of AβP deposits in the skin may be insufficient to serve as a reliable diagnostic marker. In any event, the reason that we searched for extracerebral AβP deposits and the significance of these findings relate to the hypothesis that AβP might arise from a circulating source. The principal conclusion from our non-neural studies is that AβP-immunoreactive deposits can occur in the absence of preceding neuronal and/or glial alteration (indeed, in the absence of local neurons and glia) in and around vessels of the skin, intestine and adrenal gland and perhaps other tissues. Although this data suggests that a vessel-derived or blood-borne source of AβP could give rise to amyloid deposits in AD, it does not address the critical question of why there is much more abundant AβP deposition in cerebral than extracerebral tissues.

A Hypothesis about the Seminal Role of Altered APP Expression and Catabolism in Familial Alzheimer's Disease

Based on the evidence summarized above and numerous other observations, we derive the following hypothesis about the mechanism of familial Alzheimer's disease. The model begins with a description of the processing of APP into AβP during normal aging and in Down's syndrome.

In Normal Aging: An alternate pathway for the proteolytic processing of some APP molecules exists. While most molecules are processed by the primary pathway, a variable minority are cleaved by an alternative mechanism, resulting in fragments that contain the intact AβP region and are potentially amyloidogenic. This occurs over years, even decades.

The relatively modest number of "mature" neuritic/glial plaques that develop in normal limbic and association cortices apparently produce limited neuronal dysfunction and thus few symptoms.

<u>In Trisomy 21</u>: The increased gene dosage of APP (and other genes on ch. 21) results in increased transcription of APP. This presents an excess number of precursor molecules for proteoytic processing, resulting in more molecules being diverted into the alternate, minor pathway.

The result is an augmented and accelerated deposition of AβP, first in non-fibrillar form and then (in selected brain regions only) in a fibrillar, compacted form that gradually becomes associated with dystrophic neurites and glia.

<u>In familial AD</u>: Genetic rearrangement(s) or mutation(s) (occurring on ch. 21 in some kindreds) lead to a disregulation of APP biosynthesis that results in enhanced production of precursor molecules and thus increased usage of the alternate proteolytic pathway.

Allelic heterogeneity in the FAD locus (or loci) could result in varying degrees of APP up-regulation, producing either milder or more malignant amyloidogenic cascades and, thus, delayed or accelerated disease.

<u>Origin of AβP Deposits</u>: Forms of APP containing the intact AβP region exist in blood cells and/or plasma and can reach the microvasculature of both brain and peripheral tissues via this route.

In considering this hypothesis, one need not conclude that AβP deposition per se is the direct cause of clinical dementia in AD. Rather, it is more likely that early AβP deposition can initiate a regionally-selective cascade of complex molecular and cellular alterations that, over time (many years or decades) lead to selective neuronal degeneration and aberrant regeneration and hence to the cortical dysfunction which characterizes AD. Thus, AβP deposition may not be the proximate cause of clinical dementia but may well be the critical underlying event that ultimately leads to the tragic symptoms of Alzheimer's disease.

<u>References</u>

1. Glenner, G.G. and Wong, C.W. (1984) 'Alzheimer's disease: initial report of the purification and characteristics of a novel cerebrovascular amyloid protein', <u>Biochem</u>. <u>Biophys</u>. <u>Res</u>. <u>Commun</u>. 120, 885-890.

2. Masters, C.L., Simms, G., Weinman, A., Multhaup, G., McDonald, B.L., and Beyreuther, K. (1985) 'Amyloid plaque protein in Alzheimer's disease and Down's syndrome', Proc. Natl. Acad. Sci. USA 82, 4245-4269.
3. Selkoe, D.J., Abraham, C.R., Podlisny, M.B., and Duffy, L.K. (1986) 'Isolation of low-molecular-weight proteins from amyloid plaque fibers in Alzheimer's disease', J. Neurochem. 146, 1820-1834.
4. Kang, J., Lemaire, H.-G., Unterbeck, A., Salbaum, J.M., Masters, C.L., Grzeschik, K.-H., Multhaup, G., Beyreuther, K., and Muller-Hill, B. (1987) 'The precursor of Alzheimer's disease amyloid A4 protein resembles a cell-surface receptor', Nature 325, 733-736.
5. Goldgaber, D., Lerman, M.I., McBride, O.W., Saffiotti, U., and Gajdusek, D.C. (1987) 'Characterization and chromosomal localization of a cDNA encoding brain amyloid of Alzheimer's disease', Science 235, 877-880.
6. Tanzi, R.E., Gusella, J.F., Watkins, P.C., Bruns, G.A.P., St. George-Hyslop, P.H., Van Keuren, M.L., Patterson, D., Pagan, S., Kurnit, D.M., and Neve, R.L. (1987) 'Amyloid β protein gene: cDNA, mRNA distribution, and genetic linkage near the Alzheimer locus', Science 235, 880-884.
7. Robakis, N.K., Ramakrishna, N., Wolfe, G., and Wisniewski, H.M. (1987) 'Molecular cloning and characterization of a cDNA encoding the cerebrovascular and the neuritic plaque amyloid peptides', Proc. Natl Acad. Sci. USA 84, 4190-4194.
8. Selkoe, D.J., Podlisny, M.B., Joachim, C.L., Vickers, E.A., Lee, G., Fritz, C., and Oltersdorf, T. (1988) 'β-Amyloid precursor protein of Alzheimer disease occurs as 110- to 135-kilodalton membrane-associated proteins in neural and nonneural tissues', Proc. Natl. Acad. Sci. USA 85, 7341-7345.
9. Bobin, S.A., Currie, J.R., Chem, M.-C., Iqbal, K., Miller, D.L., et al. (1987) 'Comparisons between the structures of cerebral vascular amyloid (CVA) and senile plaque core amyloid (SPCA) peptides found in Alzheimer's disease. Fed. Proc. Am. Soc. Exp. Biol. 46, 2137.
10. Frangione, B. Personal Communication.
11. Joachim, C.L., Morris, J.H., and Selkoe, D.J. (1989) 'Diffuse amyloid plaques occur commonly in the cerebellum in Alzheimer's disease', Am. J. Pathol. 5, 309-319.
12. Selkoe, D.J. (1986) 'Altered structural proteins in plaques and tangles: what do they tell us about the biology of Alzheimer's disease?', Neurobiol. Aging 7, 425-432.
13. Joachim, C.L., Mori, H., and Selkoe, D.J. (1989) 'Amyloid β-protein deposition in tissues other than brain in Alzheimer's disease', Nature 341, 226-230.
14. Selkoe, D.J., Lemere C., and Joachim, C. (1990) 'Analysis of non-neural deposition of amyloid β protein in Alzheimer's disease (AD) and Aging', Neuroscience Abstract, in press.

PROTEOLYTIC PROCESSING OF ß-AMYLOID PROTEIN-RELATED SYNTHETIC PEPTIDES AND THE ß-PROTEIN PRECURSOR BY A PROTEASE PURIFIED FROM ALZHEIMER'S DISEASE BRAIN

C. R. Abraham, B. L. Razzaboni, A. Ben-Meir and G. Papastoitsis
The Arthritis Center,
Boston University School of Medicine,
Boston, MA 02118
U.S.A.

ABSTRACT

In Alzheimer's disease, Down's syndrome, Hereditary Cerebral Hemorrhage with Ayloidosis of Dutch origin and normal aging, amyloid accumulates in the brain parenchyma and blood vessels. The major protein in the deposits is the ß-protein, a 4Kd peptide possibly generated by an abnormal degradation of its precursor, the ß-protein precursor (ß-PP). We found, as a second component of the brain amyloid, the serine protease inhibitor alpha 1-antichymotrypsin (ACT). Since ACT is tightly associated with the ß-protein and is never found in other amyloidoses, we hypothesize a role for ACT in the degradation of the ß-PP. We used synthetic peptides made according to the sequence flanking the N-terminus of the ß-protein to screen brain fractions for protease activity. Following several purification steps, a protease fraction was found that can cleave the peptide between methionine and aspartic acid, aspartic acid being the N-terminus of the ß-protein. The protease is activated by calcium and inhibited by ACT, ß-PP containing the Kunitz-type inhibitory domain and diisofluorophosphate, all three inhibitors being serine protease inhibitors. The protease fraction is also able to degrade the ß-PP in vitro.

INTRODUCTION

In normal aging of humans and, to a much greater extent, in Alzheimer's disease and Down's syndrome, three major neuropathological changes can be seen: neurofibrillary tangles, neuritic plaques and congophilic angiopathy Tangles are made of fibrous intraneuronal proteinaceous material believed to accumulate as a result of inadequate posttranslational processing of cytoskeletal proteins. In the center of the plaques and in the blood vessel walls extracellular deposits, termed amyloid, are found. In 1984, Glenner and Wong purified the amyloid fibrils from the meninges of Alzheimer's disease (AD) and Down's syndrome (DS) and sequenced the first 28 amino acids of the 4Kd peptide they named the ß-protein (Glenner and Wong, 1984). A similar, but not identical, peptide was also purified from the amyloid cores of senile plaques (Masters et al., 1985; Selkoe et al., 1986). The ß-protein is a 39-42 amino acid fragment derived from a larger precursor protein (ß-PP) whose gene has been cloned and sequenced. The finding of multiple transcripts indicates alternative splicing of the ßPP. In addition to the ß-protein, the brain amyloid contains a tightly associated serine protease inhibitor, a1-antichymotrypsin (ACT) (Abraham et al., 1988). Interestingly, two of the ßPP transcripts were shown to contain a domain homologous to the Kunitz-type of protease inhibitors. Today we know that the secreted forms of ß-PP bearing the inhibitor domain is identical to the previously described inhibitor—protease nexin 2 (PN2)(Van Nostrand et al., 1989). We described a protease inhibitor actually in the AD brain amyloid, i.e., ACT (Abraham et al., 1988). ACT was also detected in the amyloid of aged humans and monkeys (Abraham et al., 1989) and in all brain amyloidoses that have the ß-protein as their major component (Abraham et al., 1990). It is not known whether ACT, which is a serum protein, gets into the amyloid from the circulation or from the local synthesizing cells—the astrocytes (Pasternak et al., 1989). There seems to be a very strong association between the ß-protein and ACT in the amyloid filaments since harsh SDS/ß-ME extraction cannot separate these two molecules (Abraham et al., 1988).

Studying the enzymes involved in the pathway of proteolytic processing of the ß-PP is fundamental to understanding the formation of amyloid deposits, which in turn are believed to be trophic/toxic to their surroundings. We searched for a brain protease which could make the N-terminal of the two cleavages necessary to generate the ß-protein from its precursor. It is not yet clear where exactly the physiologic cleavage that releases the soluble form of the ßPP occurs in brain, but recent findings suggest that it may occur inside the ß-protein, and outside the putative membrane domain (Palmert et al., 1989, Sisodia et al., 1990, Esch et al., 1990). Such a cleavage would never generate an amyloidogenic peptide. Alternatively, we may have a mixture of soluble ßPP molecules, some containing the entire ß-protein, some containing part of it, and some containing none.

METHODS

In order to find a protease which cleaves in the vicinity of the N-terminus of the ß-protein, we synthesized two peptides according to the ß-PP sequence. One peptide is ten amino acids long, peptide 1 (P1: HSEVKMDAEF), and the second is eighteen amino acids long (P2: HSEVKMDAEFRHDSGYEV). The histidine was added at the N-terminus of the peptides for the purpose of radio-iodination. Iodinated peptides were used to follow the protease in two ways. First, the labelled peptide was incubated with the various brain fractions and then the resulting cleaved peptides separated on thin layer chromatography (TLC). The TLCs were exposed to film overnight. Second, a novel technique was applied to follow the specific cleavage enzymes. Brain fractions were incubated with the iodinated peptide and then treated with disuccinimidyl suberate (DSS), an agent which can cross-link amino groups that are 11.4 Angstroms apart. Only proteins that were in intimate contact with the peptide, i.e., a protease-substrate complex, will be cross-linked by DSS and thus radioactively labeled. This method has been successfully used to bind labeled ligands to receptors, and is here shown to be useful for identifying and following the enzymes through purification procedures. Homogenates of

Alzheimer's brain were spun at 10,000g and the supernatant subjected to DEAE and CMC columns, ammonium sulfate precipitation and finally a gel filtration column. At each step the ability of the protease to cleave the 125I-P1 was checked by autoradiography after separating the cleaved products on TLC. The brain fractions were also reacted with both iodinated peptides (P1 and P2), cross-linked with DSS, subjected to SDS-PAGE, and then then the gel was dried and exposed to X-ray film.

RESULTS

Specific inhibitors were used on our cleanest fractions to characterize the type of protease that we have purified: EGTA, a specific inhibitor of calcium-activated proteases; DFP, a specific inhibitor of serine proteases; and two serine protease inhibitory proteins potentially involved in the proteolytic degradation of the ß-PP, a1-antichymotrypsin and the purified Protease Nexin 2 from human brain (PN2 or ß-PP) which includes two secreted forms, one with and one without the Kunitz inhibitory domain. All above inhibitors prevented the cleavage of the 125I-P1, indicating that the fraction is enriched in a calcium-activated, serine protease. Protease nexin 1 and albumin did not influence the enzymatic activity. Finally, since we suspected that a chymotrypsin-like or a cathepsin G-like enzyme would cleave between the methionine and the aspartic acid at the N-terminus of the ß-protein (corresponding to the middle of P1), we compared the sequence of the cleaved products generated by cathepsin G to the ones generated by our protease fraction and other known serine proteases. The peptide was cleaved between methionine and aspartic acid, and lysine and methionine, aspartic acid being the first amino acid in the ß-protein. Both cathepsin G and our protease fraction cleaved after the methionine, and are thus capable, in principle, of generating the first cleavage required to release the ß-protein from its precursor. Very preliminary studies suggest that our protease is also able to degrade ßPP770 into a lower molecular form as detected on a western blot using antibodies to total ßPP.

DISCUSSION

It is believed today that an abnormal post-translational proteolytic processing of the ß-PP results in the ß-protein fragment which can adopt a ß-pleated sheet conformation and precipitate as amyloid. Our finding of a serine protease from brain that degrades ß-PP related synthetic peptides, and is inhibited by both PN2 and ACT may shed light on this abnormal processing event. The finding that this protease cleaves after lysine suggests that it may also be able to cleave at amino acids 15-17 (QKL) of the ß-protein, the normal physiologic site of ß-PP processing. Minor changes in the ß-PP structure could then account for one cleavage site being favored over the other. This however remains to be proven. Finally, in addition to having an effect on abnormal processing of ß-PP, an imbalance in proteases and inhibitors may influence many normal brain processes, for instance, neurite extension. Taken together then, the data suggest that an aberrant proteolytic degradation of the ß-PP can contribute to amyloid deposition, which in turn may be trophic or toxic to neurons and astrocytes, causing the neuritic response, neuronal cell death and cognitive deficits. The identification of proteases and/or inhibitors which may be responsible for amyloid formation and deposition may be the first step leading to the design of therapeutic agents for Alzheimer's disease.

Acknowledgements

This work was supported by ADRDA grant IIRG-89-125 and NIH grant AR-20613 to C.R.A.

REFERENCES

1) Abraham, C.R., Selkoe, D.J. and Potter. H., 1988, Immunochemical identification of the serine protease inhibitor a1-antichymotrypsin in the brain amyloid deposits of Alzheimer's disease. Cell 52: 487-501.
2) Abraham, C.R., Selkoe, D.J., Potter, H., Price, D.L. and Cork, L.C., 1989, a1-antichymotrypsin is present together with the ß-protein in monkey brain amyloid deposits. Neuroscience, 32:715-720
3) Abraham, C.R., Shirahama, T., and Potter, H., 1990, a1-antichymotrypsin is associated solely with amyloid deposits containing the ß-protein. Neurobiol. Aging 11:123-129.
4) Abraham, C.R., 1989, Potential roles of protease inhibitors in Alzheimer's disease. Neurobiol. Aging 10:463-465.
5) Esch, F.S., Keim, P.S., Beattie, E.C., Blacher, R.W., Culwell, A.R., Oltersdorf, T., Mclure, D., Ward, P.J., 1990, Cleavage of amyloid ß peptide during constitutive processing of its precursor. Science 248:1122-1124.
6) Glenner, G.G. and Wong, C.W., 1984, Alzheimer's disease and Down's syndrome: sharing of a unique cerebrovascular amyloid fibril protein. Biochem. Biophys. Res. Commun. 122:1131-1135.
7) Masters, C.L., Simms, G., Weinmann, N.A., Multhaup, G., McDonald, B.L., and Beyreuther, K., 1985, Amyloid plaque core protein in Alzheimer's disease and Down's syndrome. Proc. Natl. Acad. Sci. 82:4245-4249.
8) Palmert, M.R., Siedlak, S.L., Podlisny, M.B., Greenberg, B., Shelton, E.R., Chan, H.W., Usiak, M., Selkoe, D.J., Perry, G., Younkin, S.G., 1989, Soluble derivatives of the ß amyloid protein precursor of Alzheimer's disease are labeled by antisera to the ß amyloid protein. Biochem. Biophys. Res. Commun. 165:182-188.
9) Pasternak, J.M., Abraham, C.R., Van Dyke, B., Potter, H. and Younkin, S.G., 1989, Astrocytes in Alzheimer's disease gray matter express a1-antichymotrypsin mRNA. Am. J. Pathol., 135: 827-834
10) Selkoe, D.J., Abraham, C.R., Podlisny, M.B., and Duffy, L.K., 1986, Isolation of low-molecular weight proteins from amyloid plaque fibers in Alzheimer's disease. J. Neurochem. 46:1820-1834.
11) Van Nostrand, W.E., Wagner, S.L., Suzuki, M., Choi, B.H., Farrow, J.S., Geddes, J.W., Cotman, C.W. and Cunningham, D.D., 1989, Protease nexin-II, a potent antichymotrypsin, shows identity to amyloid ß-protein precursor. Nature 341:546-549.

IMMUNOREACTIVITY OF ALZHEIMER AMYLOID PRECURSOR PROTEIN (APP) SPECIFIC ANTISERA WITH PLATELET GRANULE CONSTITUENTS

J. E. Gardella [1], J. Ghiso [2], G. A. Gorgone [3], D. Marratta [3], A. P. Kaplan [3], B. Frangione [2], P. D. Gorevic [1,3].

Departments of [1]Pathology and [3]Medicine,
State University of New York at Stony Brook, and,
[2]Pathology, New York University Medical Center, USA.

ABSTRACT. Utilizing polyclonal antisera directed against APP amino-terminal and carboxyl-terminal epitopes, we have found the presence of APP species in the membrane and saline soluble fractions of unstimulated platelets, and in the conditioned medium of thrombin-stimulated platelets. Five signals ranging in molecular weight from 105 kD to 140 kD were detected. The largest species detected was isolated solely from platelet membranes and reacted with both amino-terminal and carboxyl-terminal specific antiseras. Thrombin stimulation of platelets abrogated this reactivity. None of the non-membrane associated forms reacted with the carboxyl-terminal specific antisera. The existence of a membrane bound form of APP in platelets suggests that APP may be produced by cells of megakaryocyte lineage and/or sequestered from the plasma. Processing of APP for release may then occur via successive carboxyl-terminal truncations, as well as by the release of an intact form. Our results also suggest that proteolysis of these molecules may precede, as well as be a result of, degranulation. Elucidation of APP-specific proteases in thrombocytes may provide insight into the pathogenesis of AD and beta amyloid diseases.

Introduction

The amyloid beta protein (A_B) comprises the bulk of fibrillar material in senile plaques and cerebrovascular amyloid in Alzheimer's Disease (AD), Down's Syndrome, Hereditary Cerebral Hemorrhage with Amyloidosis - Dutch Type (HCHWA-D), and Sporadic Cerebral Amyloid Angiopathy [1,2,3,4,5]. This protein is a proteolytically derived degradation product of one or more species of precursor molecules, five differentially spliced versions of which have been described to date [6,7,8,9,10,11,12,13]. Amyloid precursor proteins (APPs) have been identified in the membrane fraction of brain cortex, as extracellular secreted forms, as soluble proteins in cerebrospinal fluid, and in blood [14,15,16,17,18]. Only four of the five known mRNAs ($APP_{695,\ 751,\ 770,\ 714}$) encoding products of the APP gene contain a region specifying the 39-42 residue [19] hydrophobic A_B sequence, the carboxyl 11-14 residues of which extend into the proposed transmembrane domain of the intact molecule [20]. This polymerized fragment constitutes the amyloid material deposited in the senile plaques and cerebrovasculature of AD patients, and patients with the related beta-fibrilloses [1,2,3,4,5,21]. However, it has been shown that only 14 residues of the A_B sequence are necessary for amyloid fibril formation [22]. Two of the transcripts ($APP_{751,770}$) encoding A_B also possess an insert sequence which is homologous to the active site of Kunitz-type protease inhibitors [9,10,11]. Substantial evidence indicates that APP_{751} is a protease inhibitor initially isolated from cultured human fibroblasts, designated protease nexin II (PN II) [15,16]. Purified APP and recombinant APP deletion mutants expressing the Kunitz insert domain have been demonstrated to inhibit a number of proteases including; trypsin, epidermal growth factor-binding protein, alpha-chymotrypsin, gamma-nerve growth factor, plasmin, and, mGK-22 [23,24]. Amino terminal sequence analysis indicates that a hepatoma cell line, HepG2, also secretes PN II, and immunologic, kinetic, and biochemical evidence supports identity of this molecule with a coagulation factor XIa inhibitor (XIaI) contained in platelets [25]. With the exception of XIa, no physiologic substrate for PN II has been described in humans [24].

Our inquiry ultimately concerns proteases which may be responsible for cleaving A_B from APP. With the exception of a single nonfibrillar report [26], the A_B of AD is seen in the central nervous system (CNS) and associated cerebrovasculature, suggesting the action of CNS specific proteases. However, the general scheme of the amyloidoses as systemic disorders [21], and the primarily vascular deposition of A_B in HCHWA-D [4], indicate that non-neuronal tissues should also be carefully considered as possible sources of APP and beta amyloidergic proteases. We feel that the most logical origin of a search for these putative proteases should be an examination of those cells which express the APP. Although current studies indicate that expression of APP transcripts with the A_B sequence are fairly ubiquitous [13], we examined blood platelets in this report due to their obvious role as vehicles for PN II transport and delivery.

Materials and Methods

PLATELETS

Platelet units were diluted 1:1 with 20 mM phosphate buffered saline, pH 7.4, 5 mM ethylene diamine tetraacetic acid (EDTA), and 10 mM glucose (PBS-EG), and centrifuged at 200 g to pellet non-platelet cellular elements. Platelet rich supernatants were then removed and recentrifuged at 2000 g. Platelet pellets were resuspended in RPMI-1640 (Gibco). Thrombin (1 U/ml) was used for stimulation studies. Both stimulated and unstimulated platelet pellets were extracted of saline soluble proteins by resuspension of pellets into 2 volumes of Tris saline buffer with inhibitors (50 mM Tris, pH 7.4, 150 mM NaCl, 5 mM EDTA, 5 mM EGTA, 2 mM PMSF, 5 ug/ml Soybean Trypsin Inhibitor, 10 ug/ml Aprotinin, 0.1 ug/ml Pepstatin, 1 ug/ml TLCK, 1 ug/ml TPCK, 5 ug/ml Leupeptin, all inhibitors purchased from Sigma) and performing 2 successive cycles of freezing in dry ice and thawing at 4°C. Saline insoluble material from the lysed cells was centrifuged out of the saline extract at 100000 g for 60 minutes at 4°C. Saline insoluble pellets were extracted by sonication with a Heat Systems Sonicator for 15 seconds on 90% duty cycle, setting 6, continuous emission with a micro tip probe, in Tris saline buffer with inhibitors plus 2% Triton X-100. Clarification of the final homogenate was performed by centrifugation at 100000 g for 60 minutes at 4°C.

All extracts for immunoblotting, and chromatography, were stored at minus 70°C.

ELECTROPHORESIS and IMMUNOBLOTTING

Performed essentially as described [27].

ANTISERA PRODUCTION

Anti-SP18 was raised against a KLH conjugated synthetic peptide as described [14]. Anti-C7 was raised against a synthetic peptide as described [28].

Results

Although thrombin is itself a serine protease, published reports indicate that thrombin is not inhibited by PN II [23,25]. We examined the immunoreactivity of saline soluble APP from unstimulated platelets to characterize the prestimulus nature of platelet APP. The saline soluble extract of unstimulated platelets revealed two anti-SP18 (an APP amino-terminal specific antiserum) reactive species with molecular weights of approximately 110 and 130 Kd. In contrast to this result, thrombin-stimulated platelet-conditioned media possessed four anti-SP18 reactive signals with molecular weights of approximately 105, 110, 125, and 130 Kd. None of the soluble species were reactive to anti-C7 (an APP carboxyl-terminal specific antiserum) before or following thrombin stimulation.

Similarly, we made a comparison of the immunoreactivities of unstimulated platelet membranes vs. an identical preparation which had first been stimulated by thrombin prior to homogenization. The membranes of unstimulated platelets possess at least one species of APP with an approximate molecular weight of 140 kD. This molecule is reactive to anti-SP18, and to anti-C7 (Figure 1). This unstimulated membrane form of platelet APP is therefore an intact, non-truncated molecule. The membranes of platelets which had been stimulated with thrombin prior to membrane isolation were non-reactive to both of these antisera at this molecular weight.

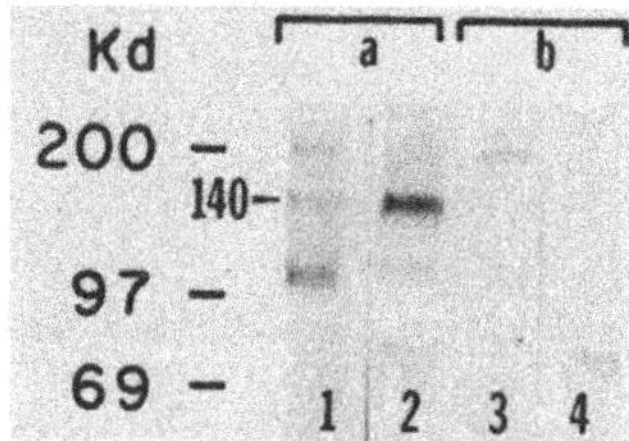

Figure 1. Western blot of Triton X-100 extracts (60 ug of protein per lane) of saline insoluble (membrane) fractions from (a) unstimulated platelets, and, (b) thrombin-stimulated platelets. Lanes: 1 and 3, anti-SP18 (1:1000); 2 and 4, anti-C7 (1:1000). Only the 140 Kd signals are specific, as indicated by peptide absorbtion studies (data not shown).

Discussion

The neuronal origin of A_B has not been established to date. Our interest in the localization of APP within platelets has been to examine the possibility that A_B, or a molecule capable of giving rise to A_B, might originate from these blood borne cellular elements. Our findings are supported by the recent report of PN II existing as an alpha granule constituent [29], as well as a report citing immunologic, kinetic, and substrate relatedness between a platelet-released coagulation factor XIaI and a form of APP produced by the hepatoma cell line HepG2 [25]. It therefore seems reasonable that one or more of the immunoreactive species detected in thrombin-stimulated platelet-conditioned media in this report is PN II or a carboxyl terminal truncation thereof. Similarly, this assumption suggests that one of the saline soluble anti-SP18 reactive species detected in unstimulated platelets is PN II. Confirmation of coidentity of PN II with any of the soluble platelet derived molecules we have described will require further immunologic (anti-kunitz) and enzymologic study.

The role of platelet APP in the pathogenesis of AD remains speculative. Presumably, the physiologic processing of PN II involves truncation after either residue 15 (Gln), or 16 (Lys), of the A_B sequence upon release from a membrane bound state into the soluble phase [30]. This would prevent PN II from playing a direct role in the formation of A_B. Possibly the antiprotease functionality of one or more platelet form of PN II imparts an indirect role upon these molecules in amyloid deposition within cerebral cortex and/or leptomenigial vessels in AD. However, our data clearly shows that unstimulated platelets also possess a membrane bound form of APP which is not carboxyl-terminal truncated. The unstimulated membrane preparation is reactive to both the amino-terminal specific antiserum and the carboxyl-terminal specific antiserum, at a single molecular weight. The stimulated membrane preparation is negative to both antisera. Therefore, we have demonstrated that physiologic (thrombin) stimulation of platelets results in a release of the 140 kD species from platelet membranes. Whether this molecule or its derivatives contribute to the antiprotease capacity of the soluble forms or not, *it could serve as a source of A_B.*

The presence of an intact form of APP in platelets is significant in that it provides a circulating substrate upon which proteases from a multitude of tissues (vascular and extraneuronal) may act.

Acknowledgements

We are grateful to Dr. Dennis Selkoe (Center for Neurologic Diseases, Brigham and Women's Hospital) for his gift of C7 antiserum. Peptide SP18 was synthesized in the Center for the Analysis and Synthesis of Macromolecules (CASM) at the State University of New York at Stony Brook by Ms. Karen Springer. This work was supported by grants from the American Heart Association, and the Center for Biotechnology at Stony Brook.

References

1. Glenner, G. G., et al. (1984). *Biochem. Biophys. Res. Comm., Vol. 120, No. 3, pp. 885-890.*
2. Masters, C. L., et al. (1985). *EMBO, Vol. 4, No. 11, pp. 2757-2763.*
3. Masters, C. L., et al. (1985). *Proc. Natl. Acad. Sci. USA, Vol. 82, pp. 4245-4249.*
4. van Duinen, et al. (1987). *Proc. Natl. Acad. Sci. USA, Vol. 84, pp. 5991-5994.*
5. Coria, F., et al. (1987). *Amer. Jour. Path., Vol. 129, No. 3, pp.422-428.*
6. Goldgaber, D., et al. (1987). *Science, Vol. 235, pp. 877-880.*
7. Robakis, N. K., et al. (1987). *Proc. Natl. Acad. Sci. USA, Vol. 84, pp. 4190-4194.*
8. Tanzi, R. E. et al. (1987). *Science, Vol. 235, pp. 880-884.*
9. Ponte, P., et al. (1988). *Nature, Vol. 331, pp. 525-527.*
10. Tanzi, R.E., et al. (1988). *Nature, Vol. 331, pp. 528-530.*
11. Kitaguchi, N., et al. (1988). *Nature, Vol. 331, pp.530-532.*
12. de Sauvage, F., et al. (1989). *Science, Vol. 245, pp. 651-653.*
13. Golde, T. E., et al. (1990). *Neuron, Vol. 4, pp. 253-267.*
14. Ghiso, J., et al. (1989). *Biochem. Biophy. Res. Comm., Vol. 163, No. 1, pp. 430-437.*
15. Van Nostrand, W.E., et al. (1987). *J. Biol. Chem., Vol. 262, No. 18, pp. 8508-8514.*
16. Oltersdorf, T., et al. (1988). *Nature, Vol. 341, pp. 144-147.*
17. Palmert, M. R., et al. (1989). *Proc. Natl. Acad. Sci. USA, Vol. 86, pp. 6338-6342.*
18. Rumble, B., et al. (1989). *New England Journal of Medicine, Vol. 320, No. 22, pp. 1446-1452.*
19. Prelli, F., et al. (1988). *Biochem. Biophys. Res. Comm., Vol. 151, No. 3, pp. 1150-1155.*
20. Kang, J., et al. (1987). *Nature, vol. 325, pp. 733-736.*
21. Castano, E.M., et al. (1988). *Journal of Laboratory Investigation, Vol. 58, No. 2, pp. 122-132.*
22. Gorevic, P. D., et al. (1987). *Biochem. Biophys. Res. Comm., Vol. 147, No. 2, pp. 854-862.*
23. Van Nostrand, W. E., et al. (1990). *J. Biol. Chem., Vol. 265, No. 17, pp. 9591-9594.*
24. Sinha, S., et al. (1990). *J. Biol. Chem., Vol. 265, No. 16, pp. 8983-8985.*
25. Smith, R. P., et al. (1990). *Science, Vol. 248, pp. 1126-1128.*
26. Joachim, C. L., et al. (1989). *Nature, Vol. 341, pp. 226-230.*
27. Harlow, E., Lane, D. (1988). In, Antibodies: A Laboratory Manual. Cold Spring Harbor Laboratory Press, USA, pp.174-195, 471-505, 635-657.
28. Selkoe, D.J., et al. (1988). *Proc. Natl. Acad. Sci. USA, Vol. 85, pp. 7341-7345.*
29. Van Nostrand, W. E., et al. (1990). *Science, Vol. 248, pp. 745-748.*
30. Esch, F. S., et al. (1990). *Science, Vol. 248, pp. 1122-1124.*

SITE OF FORMATION OF BETA-PROTEIN AMYLOID FIBRILS

H. M. WISNIEWSKI, J. WEGIEL, E. KIDA*, T. BURRAGE, and J. CURRIE

NYS Institute for Basic Research in Developmental Disabilities
Department of Pathological Neurobiology
1050 Forest Hill Road, Staten Island, NY 10314

Abstract: Ultrastructural, three-dimensional reconstruction of cells surrounding the amyloid star in classical plaques in Alzheimer's disease (AD) were carried out to determine the cells associated with the deposits of beta-protein amyloid fibrils. These studies showed that the amyloid fibrils appear first within the altered cisternae of endoplasmic reticulum (ER) and infoldings of plasma membranes of microglia/macrophages further supporting our conclusion that the microglia/macrophages are the site of formation of amyloid fibrils.

1. Introduction

Amyloid is deposited in the brain during normal aging and Alzheimer disease (AD) as well as during unconventional viral diseases (e.g., Gerstmann-Straussler syndrome, kuru, Creutzfeldt-Jakob disease and scrapie). In AD, one of the most prominent lesions is the classical plaque, which is composed of amyloid star, microglial cells, abnormal neuritic processes and reactive astrocytes (Wisniewski and Terry, 1973; Wisniewski et al., 1981). Immunohistochemical and in situ hybridization procedures have shown that many cell types both within and outside the central nervous system could generate the beta protein precursor of AD or the protease resistant protein (PrP) that accompanies the unconventional viral diseases. In both cases, brain microglia/ macrophages appear closely associated with amyloid formation and/or deposition. However, because this cell type is also phagocytic, it has been unclear whether the microglia/macrophages operate to remove amyloid or whether they actively produce the amyloid fibrils. Recent morphological studies indicate a primarily manufacturing relationship between the cytoplasmic membrane compartments of microglial cells and the amyloid fibrils (Wisniewski et al., 1989; Wisniewski et al., 1990; Wegiel and Wisniewski, 1990).

This study uses morphometric methods and three-dimensional reconstruction techniques to examine the spatial relationships between the cytoplasmic components of the microglia/macrophages and the cell membrane and the spatial organization of the amyloid star-microglial complex in the context of fibril formation.

2. Materials and Methods

Four cortical biopsies (kindly provided by Dr. B. Lach and Dr. A. P. Anzil) from patients with Alzheimer disease were examined. The tissue was fixed with 3% glutaraldehyde and 1% osmium tetroxide and embedded in Epon. A biopsy from a 72-year old woman was used for the reconstruction of the plaques. The reconstruction was accomplished using serial semithin (0.3μm) and ultrathin (0.06μm) sections alternately. Three complexes were reconstructed. Ultrathin sections were stained by immunogold technique using a monoclonal antibody (mAb) raised against the synthetic peptide corresponding to the first 24 amino acids of the beta amyloid protein (4G8, IgG_{2b}, Kim et al., 1988).

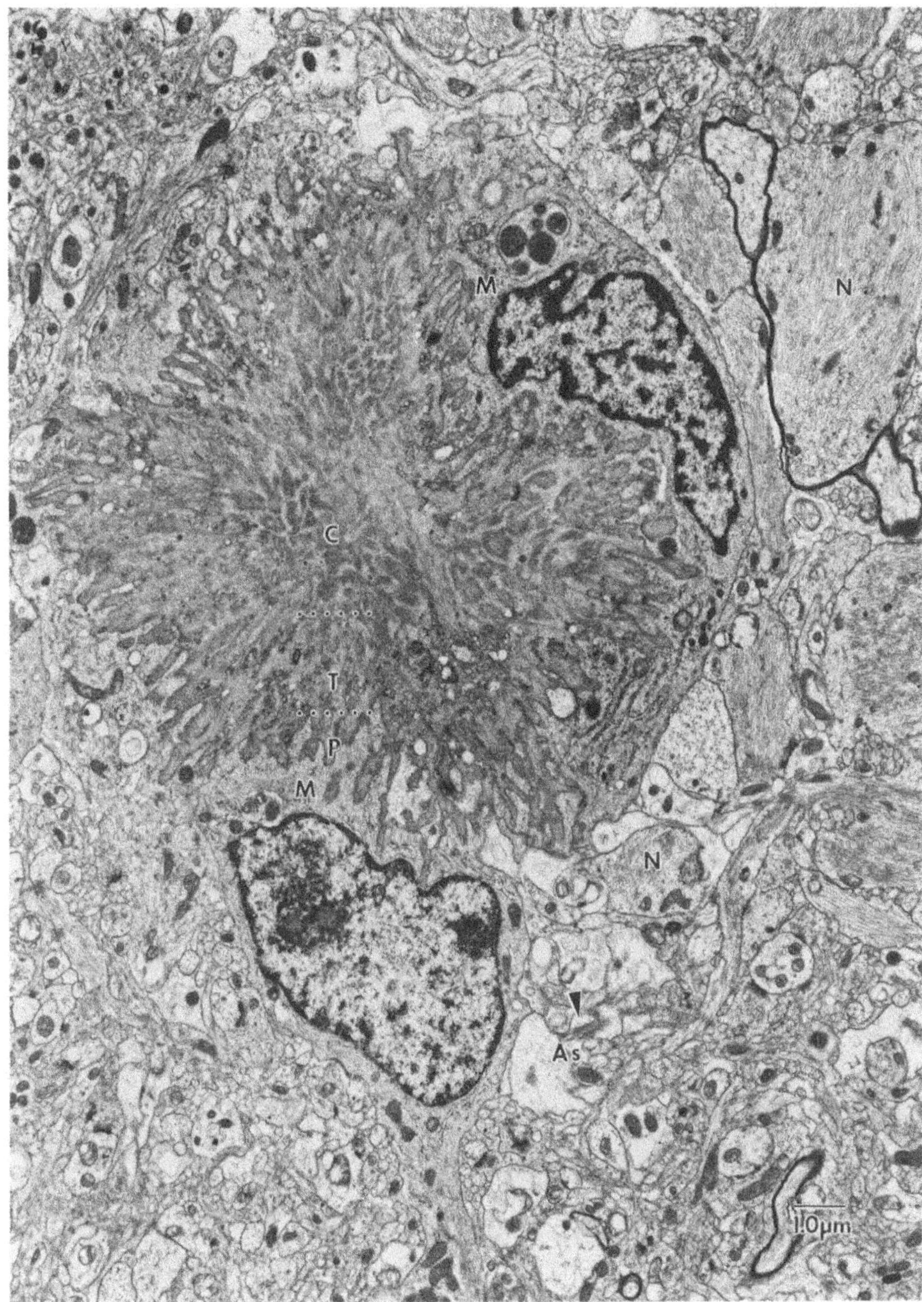

Figure 1. A classical plaque with two microglial cells (M) surrounding the amyloid star. The star has a peripheral (P), a transitional (T) and a central (C) zone. Also present are abnormal neuritic processes (N) and proliferating astrocytic processes (As), which isolate the amyloid wisps (arrowhead) from neuropil.

3. Results

3.1 ORGANIZATION OF CLASSICAL PLAQUES

The general features of classical plaques shown by ultrathin sections include the topography of the amyloid star, the spatial arrangement of the 4 to 5 associated microglial cells and the presence of abnormal neurites and proliferating astrocytic processes. Ultrastructural reconstruction of these plaque components revealed that the star was surrounded by a mantle of cytoplasm of several microglial cells (Fig. 1). The cytoplasm contained a well-developed system of rough and smooth endoplasmic reticulum (RER and SER), mitochondria and polymorphic dense bodies. Some segments of the RER were in continuity with distended SER membranes and deep infoldings of the plasma membrane. The plasma membrane facing the star consisted of a labyrinth of hundreds of such channels filled with newly formed amyloid fibrils. These amyloid fibrils were decorated with gold label after incubation with amyloid specific monoclonal antibody (Fig. 2). The transitional zone of the amyloid star contained degenerated microglial cytoplasmic fragments trapped between aggregates of amyloid fibrils arranged in parallel bundles. The central zone of the amyloid star contained only amyloid fibril bundles, which were more densely packed than at the amyloid star periphery.

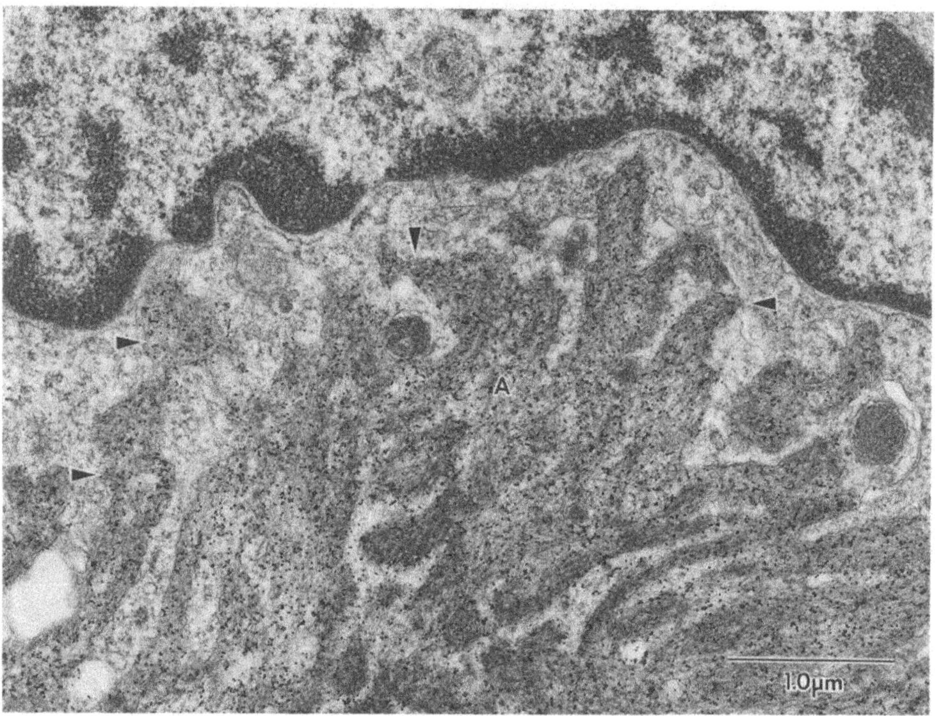

Figure 2. Well-ordered bundles of amyloid fibrils (A) labelled with colloidal gold reside in channels formed by cytoplasmic and plasma membranes of microglial cells (arrowheads).

3.2 THREE-DIMENSIONAL RECONSTRUCTION OF CLASSICAL PLAQUES

The three-dimensional reconstruction of three amyloid star-microglial complexes reveals their spatial organization. The bulk of the amyloid occurs as the star in the center of the plaque and is almost completely isolated from the neuropil by surrounding microglial cells. Amyloid wisps, on the other hand, are present at the periphery of the plaque and are also surrounded by astrocytic processes. Five microglial cells surround stars in two of the classical plaques, whereas six were involved in the third. The microglial cells had three distinctive morphologies depending upon their topographical relationship to plaque, extent of contact with star, overall size and shape. The most numerous morphological type (2 or 3/complex) was a cap-like microglial cell, which had the greatest contact with the amyloid star (Fig. 3a). The perikarya were closely applied to the star; only a few short cytoplasmic processes radiated into the neuropil. Each plaque had one or two macrophage-like cells (Fig. 3b). The macrophage-like cells were large and extended from the amyloid star to the plaque periphery, but the area of contact with amyloid was quite small. Numerous polymorphic, osmiophilic bodies could sometimes be found throughout cytoplasm (occupying up to 44% of cytoplasmic volume in one cell), and occasionally, phagocytic vacuoles could be observed containing components of degenerating synapses and neuronal processes. However, the vast majority of the microglial cells associated with the amyloid star demonstrated very little phagocytic activity. A third microglial cell, an octopus microglia, was present at the outside of plaque. The octopus-microglial cell had scanty cytoplasm about the nucleus and cytoplasmic projections extended in all directions from the soma (Fig. 3c). Usually, a small area of one of these projections would reach the amyloid star after traversing the degenerating neuropil. The identity of these microglial cells was deduced only after three-dimensional reconstruction. All microglial cells involved in the complex had an organized interface with the amyloid star such that they formed a border zone consisting of a system of channels 2-3 μm deep, filled with amyloid fibrils.

Discussion

Three-dimensional reconstruction of the cells surrounding the amyloid star in Alzheimer disease reveal that the microglia/macrophage cells are engaged in the formation of the amyloid fibrils. The complex morphology of the microglial cells around the star identifies them as reactive microglia cells, as opposed to the resting population also found in mature brain (Ferrer and Sarmiento, 1980). Microglial cells that stain intensely with a mAb AD11/8 have also been implicated by others in amyloid fibril formation (Haga et al., 1989). The polarized orientation of the microglial cell with its protein synthetic machinery (RER, SER and Golgi) complex directed towards the star and the site of formation of the amyloid fibrils, makes the mission of the AD microglial cell manifest. The polarized configuration of microglial membranous compartments also occurs in association with amyloid deposits in aged dogs and scrapie-infected mice (Vorbrodt et al., 1988; Wisniewski et al., 1981; Wisniewski et al., 1982). A similar polarization of the Kupffer cells in the liver, the reticular cells of the spleen, and the mesangial cells in the kidney has been observed in murine experimental amyloidosis (Cohen, 1965; Cohen et al., 1965; Bari et al., 1969; Shirahama and Cohen, 1973; Uchino et al., 1985). In systemic amyloidosis, amyloid precursor protein is first produced and then processed, either locally or at distant sites, to

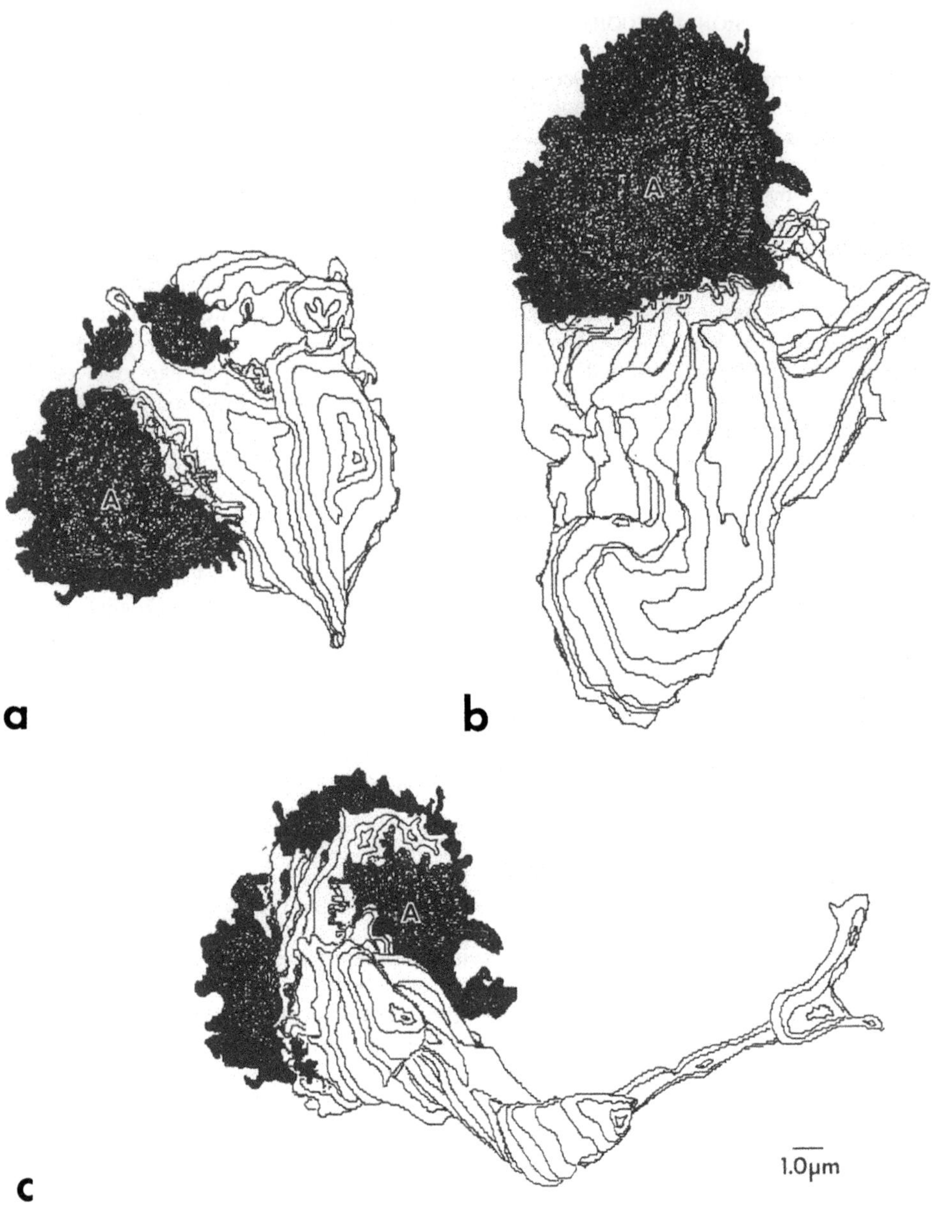

Figure 3. Three dimensional reconstruction of cap-like (a), macrophage-like (b) and octopus-like microglial cells (c). Amyloid star (A).

yield amyloid fibrils (Wegelius, 1976; Wisniewski and Wrzolek, 1988). Our approach at present is to focus our studies of amyloidogenesis, both in the brain and in other organs, on this microglia/macrophage population of cells, in order to determine whether these cells are only the processor of the amyloid protein or both the producer and processor cells.

*Acknowledgements. Dr. Kida is a visiting scientist from Polish Academy of Sciences, Medical Research Center, Warsaw, Poland

Supported in part by funds from the New York State Institute for Basic Research in Developmental Disabilities and a grant from the National Institute on Aging NIH, #AGO-4220-06.

References

Bari, W. A., Pettengill, O. S., and Sorenson, G.D. (1969) Lab. Invest. 20, 234-242.
Cohen, A. S. (1965) Int. Rev. Exp. Pathol. 4, 159-243.
Cohen, A. S., Gross, E., and Shirahama, T. (1965) Am. J. Pathol. 47, 1079-1111.
Ferrer, I. and Sarmiento, J. (1980) Acta Neuropathol. (Berl) 50, 69-76.
Haga, S., Akai, K., and Ishii, T. (1989) Acta Neuropathol. (Berl) 77, 569-575.
Kim, K. S., Miller D. L., Sapienza, V. J., Chen, C. M. J., Bai, C., Grundke-Iqbal,I., Currie, J. R., and Wisniewski, H. M. (1988) Neurosci. Res. Com. 2, 121-130.
Shirahama, T. and Cohen, A. S. (1973) Am. J. Pathol. 73, 97-114.
Uchino, F., Takahashi, M., Yokota, T., and Ishihara, T. (1985) Appl. Pathol. 3, 78-87.
Vorbrodt, A. W., Dobrogowska, D. H., Kim, K. S., Lossinsky, A. S., and Wisniewski, H. M. (1988) Acta Neuropathol. (Berl) 75, 277-287.
Wegelius, O. (1976) in O. Wegelius and A. Pasternak (eds.) Amyloidosis, Academic Press, London, pp. 1-13.
Wegiel, J., and Wisniewski, H. M. (1990) Acta Neuropathol. (Berl.) In press.
Wisniewski, H. M., and Terry, R. D. (1973) in H. M. Zimmerman (ed.) Progress in Neuropathology, Volume 11, 1-26.
Wisniewski, H. M., Moretz, R. C., and Lossinsky, A. S. (1981) Ann. Neurol. 10, 517- 522.
Wisniewski, H. M., Vorbrodt, A. W., Moretz, R. C., Lossinsky, A. S., and Grundke-Iqbal, I. (1982) in S. Hoyer (ed.) The Aging Brain-Physiological and Pathophysiological Aspects, Exp. Brain Res (Suppl 5) Springer, Heidelberg, pp. 3-9.
Wisniewski, H. M., and Wrzolek, M. (1988) in Novel Infectious Agents and the Central Nervous System Ciba Foundation Symposium 135 John Wiley and Sons, Chichester, pp. 224-238.
Wisniewski, H. M., Wegiel, J., Wang, K. C., Kujawa, M., and Lach, B. (1989) Can. J. Neurol. Sci. 16, 535-542.
Wisniewski, H. M., Vorbordt, A., Wegiel, J., Morys, J., and Lossinsky, A.S. (1990) Am. J. Medical Genetics (in press).

A SEARCH FOR VASCULAR AMYLOID USING A4 AMYLOID ANTIBODY IMMUNOSTAIN IN CAA (CLASSIC METHODS) NEGATIVE ALZHEIMER'S CASES

T.I. MANDYBUR, M.D., PH.D.
Department of Pathology and Laboratory Medicine
University of Cincinnati Medical Center
Cincinnati, Ohio 45267-0529

ABSTRACT: It has been postulated that CAA is an important morphological feature of Alzheimer disease, although it is not present in all classic cases. It was uncertain, however, if the negative cases, showing numerous plaques and tangles only but no CAA are indeed negative or rather, the stains used were not sensitive enough to detect small amounts of vascular amyloid. Recently, it has been demonstrated that A4 amyloid immunostain (with formic acid) is capable of discovering much more amyloid than any of the previously used techniques (Thio S, Congo red, crystal violet). It seemed appropriate, therefore, to examine 15 of such CAA negative Alzheimer cases from our collection using the mentioned stain. From each case a section of hippocampus with temp. neocortex and a section of visual cortex were stained. The results were as follows: In all sections examined of all cases numerous amyloid positive interstitial cortical plaques were present. Thirteen cases showed occasional positive vessels in leptomeninges and/or in the cortex, and two revealed no CAA. Present results indicate that in majority of classic methods CAA-negative AD cases, A4 amyloid stain is capable of detecting traces or small amounts of vascular amyloid. In rare AD cases, however, even this stain shows no vascular amyloid.

Introduction

Three main pathomorphological features characterize Alzheimer's disease (AD) as well as so-called "normal" brain aging (NBA). These are the Alzheimer's tangles (AT), senile plaques (SP), and cerebrovascular amyloidosis (CAA).

It is well known, however, that there can be substantial differences as to how these features mix and in what proportion in a particular instance. Many cases show predominance of tangles and others of plaques. Although plaques and tangles tend to appear together in a given case, CAA is known to be the most variable component as to its intensity, only about 10-20% of AD cases displaying severe changes of this nature. The previous statistics agreed that not all AD cases show CAA when stained with classic amyloid detecting histological techniques like Congo red with green polarization, Thioflavine S and crystal violet. The percentages of positive cases are quoted as about 90%.[1-3] It was uncertain, however, if the negative cases showing numerous plaques and tangles only but no CAA are indeed negative or if the stains used were not sensitive enough to detect small amounts of vascular amyloid. Recently, it has been demonstrated that A4 amyloid immunostain, especially after formic acid pretreatment, detects more cerebral amyloid than any of the previously used techniques (Thio S, Congo red, crystal violet). It seem appropriate, therefore, to examine 15 of such CAA negative classic Alzheimer cases from our collection using the mentioned stain.

Materials and Methods

From each classic method CAA negative Alzheimer's case, a section of hippocampus with adjacent temporal neocortex and a section of visual cortex were stained with Congo red, A4-amyloid immunostain after formic acid pretreatment, in addition to H&E, Bodian and Bielschowsky stain. (The A4 antibody was kindly donated by Dr. C. Masters, Melbourne, Australia.)

Results

Of 15 cases, two were completely free of any trace of CAA, although they revealed massive, densely distributed A4 positive plaques, including perivascular globoid SP as well as encircling perivascular SP. Twelve other cases showed minimal A4 positive vascular amyloid component. There were distinct differences in distribution of vascular amyloid in these particular cases:

A) occasional positive small intracortical vessels only were seen in two cases

B) occasional small positive vessels in the leptomeninges only in four cases

C) A and B together in four cases

D) the large leptomeningeal vessels displaying a biphasic mild intensity positive stain were observed in all eight previous cases (of groups A, B and C) and an additional two cases as the only A4 positive finding

<u>Note</u>: All cases showed some degree of uniform (uniphasic) A4 positive stain of the adventitia. At the present time, we believe this to be an artifact because similar findings were observed in nondemented age-matched controls. The biphasic adventitia-stain means that its inner perimuscularis layer is considerably darker in A4 stain than in its outer layer.

E) in one case, A4 stain detected widespread CAA in the leptomeninges and some cortical positive vessels

<u>Note</u>: Positive changes, if any, prevailed in the visual cortex vs. hippocampus. Also, the choroid plexus perivascular connective tissue revealed a mild intensity uniphasic stain (also present in age-matched controls). Most likely, this finding is a staining artifact.

Discussion

Present results indicate that in many classic methods CAA-negative AD cases A4 amyloid stain is capable of detecting traces or small amounts of unpolymerized vascular amyloid. It was observed previously (similarly as for senile plaques) that in CAA (congophilic angiopathy), A4 stain usually shows more amyloid-positive vessels than the classic amyloid detecting histopathological methods.[4]

An interesting observation was that the minimal A4 positive could affect different vessels. In most cases, the change was observed in the leptomeningeal vessels. In some cases, the stain affected only the larger leptomeningeal arteries, all other vessels being negative. This could point to CSF as the source of amyloidgenic material. The visual cortex region proved more likely to show traces of CAA than the hippocampus.

The one Congo red (CAA) negative case that showed conspicuous infiltration of leptomeningeal vessels by A4 positive material suggest that sometimes even substantial amounts of such material may not necessarily convert into Congo red positive amyloid. This parallel cases (areas) showing many amorphous A4 positive SP but few, if any, Congo red positive SP (especially of the neuritic type).

The present study indicates also that in rare AD cases even A4 stain is incapable of brining out any vascular amyloid. This suggests that CAA is not a constant pathological feature of AD. In previous studies,[4-6] we have pointed out that in AD, CAA is often out of phase with the intensity of SP and NT; that with massive SP and NT it might be weak and spotty only. On the other hand, in other cases with few SP and NT, it might be extremely severe. Moreover, we also studied cases with minimal or no NT, minimal SP, and extensive CAA. Recently, we examined a case of severe granulomatous cerebral vasculitis with A4 positive CAA associated with only a few amorphous SP. AT are known to appear in masses in SSPE without any traces of any associated A4-positive changes.[7,8]

Perhaps the fluctuation and dissociation of the three phases of AD (NT, SP, CAAO is a phenomenon which requires more attention.

References

1. Mandybur, T.I. (1975) 'The incidence of cerebral amyloid angiopathy in Alzheimer's disease', Neurology 25, 120-126.

2. Vinters H.V., et al. (1988) 'Brain amyloid and Alzheimer's disease', Annals of Internal Medicine 109, 41-54.

3. Glenner, G.G., Henry, J.H., Fujihara, S. (1981) 'Congophilic angiopathy in the pathogenesis of Alzheimer's degeneration', Annals of Pathology 1, 120-129.

4. Vinters, H.V., Pardridge, W.M., Yang, J. (1988) 'Immunohistochemical study of cerebral amyloid angiopathy: use of an antiserum to a synthetic 28-amino-acid peptide fragment of the Alzheimer's disease amyloid angiopathy', Human Pathology 19, 214-222.

5. Mandybur, T.I. (1986) 'Cerebral amyloid angiopathy: the vascular pathology and complications', Journal of Neuropathology and Experimental Neurology 45, 79-90.

6. Mandybur, T.I. (1986) 'The tole of cerebral amyloid angiopathy in dementia of Alzheimer's type (preliminary results). Amyloidosis 783-788.

7. Mandybur, T.I., et al. (1977) 'Alzheimer neurofibrillary change in subacute sclerosing panencephalitis', Annals of Neurology 1, 103-107.

8. Tabaton, M., Mandybur, T.I., et al. (1989) 'The widespread alteration of neurites in Alzheimer's disease may be unrelated to amyloid deposition. Annals of Neurology 26, 771-777.

A variant of Gerstmann-Sträussler-Scheinker disease with β-protein epitopes and dystrophic neurites in the peripheral regions of PrP-immunoreactive amyloid plaques

S. Ikeda[1], N. Yanagisawa[1], D. Allsop[2], G.G. Glenner[3]
1) Shinshu University School of Medicine, Matsumoto 390, Japan
2) Queen's University of Belfast, Belfast BT9 7BL, 156, Northern Ireland, UK
3) University of California at San Diego, CA 92093, U.S.A.

(Abstract)

We report immunohistochemical and electron microscopic findings of the brains obtained from two siblings aged 67 and 79 possessing pathological features of both Gerstmann-Sträussler-Scheinker disease (GSS) and Alzheimer's disease: they showed a large number of PrP immunoreactive amyloid plaques in an extensive area of the brain, and around these plaques a "crown-like" appearance of β-protein immunoreactivity was also seen in sections pretreated with formic acid. Electron microscopic examinations revealed that these β-protein immunoreactive structures consisted of sparse aggregations of amyloid fibrils. Additionally, tau-immunoreactive abnormal neurites were observed in the peripheral regions of many cerebral plaques with neurofibrillary tangle formation in some neurons. These two cases seemed to be atypical GSS cases with hibrid plaques containing both PrP- and β-protein amyloid deposits. As such, they may provide a link between the transmissible prion dementias and Alzheimer's disease.

(Introduction)

Gerstmann-Sträussler-Scheinker disease (GSS) is a familial but transmissible degenerative brain disease characterized pathologically by the presence of PrP-immunoreactive amyloid plaques throughout the cerebrum and cerebellum.

In this study we report unique pathological findings of atypical GSS cases, showing the coexistence of both PrP-and β-protein immunoreactivity in their brain amyloid plaques, with tau-immunoreactive abnormal neurites.

(Subjects and Methods)

i) Case reports:

Case 1 was a 67 year-old female who developed difficulty in walking and changing position, and her condition rapidly deteriorated. Finally she showed dysphagia, incontinence and confusion, and she died in the same year. Case 2 was her 79 year-old her brother with a history of progressive intellectural failure that started at the age of 74. We were unable to obtain any additional informations concerning other family members.

ii) Staining methods:

Serial sections from formalin-fixed and paraffin-embedded brain blocks were stained with hematoxylin-eosin, alkaline Congo red, modified Bielshowsky's silver impregnation, and immunocytochemical methods using the avidin-biotin-peroxidase technique. The primary reagents were rabbit antisera to PrP 27-30[1] or denaturated scrapie-associated fibrils (SAF) from Sinc ^{s7} mice with ME7 scrapie[2], a monoclonal antibody (4D12/2/6) for β-protein[3] and anti-tau antiserum[4], and in the staining with anti-β-protein antibody some sections were pretreated with 98 % formic acid. An electron microscopic study was performed on the brain tissues of case 2: in addition to conventional ultrastructural examination, dewaxed sections were stained with immunoperoxidase methods, and then embedded in epoxy resin. Thin sections without further electron-dense stainings were observed.

(Results)

i) Light microscopic findings:

There were numerous amyloid plaques of varying size and form throughout the cerebral and cerebellar cortices in both cases. These plaques were most dense in the cerebellar molecular layer where they lacked neuritic components. In the cerebrum multicentric plaques were abundant, and the vast majority of these plaques were accompanied by argyrophilic abnormal neurites. The amyloid cores in both the cerebral and cerebellar plaques were strongly immunoreactive with the

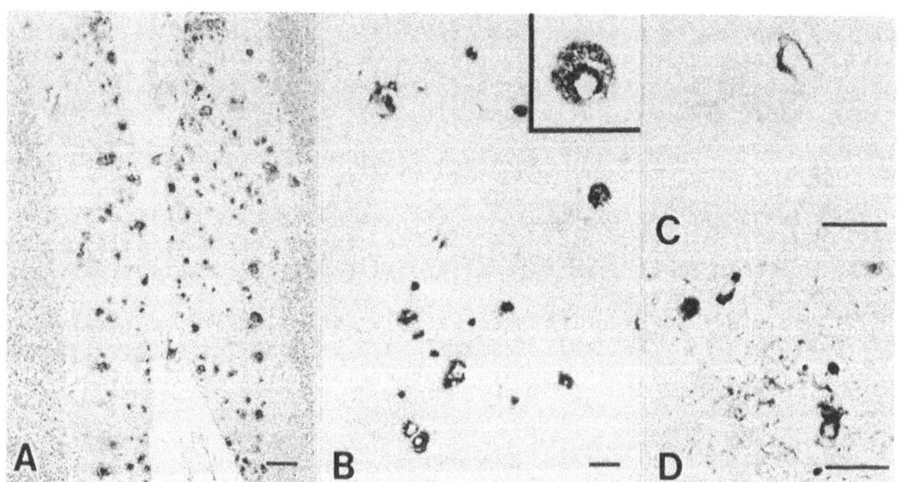

Figure 1. A: PrP-immunoreactive cerebellar plaques, B: β-protein immunoreactive cerebral deposits in the periphery of PrP-immunoreactive plaque. C: β-protein type cerebrovascular amyloid, D: tau-immunoreactive abnormal neurites and tangles. (Bars=50 μm)

anti-PrP antiserum (Fig 1-A) but showed no reaction with the antibody to β-protein even after the formic acid pretreatment. The immunohistochemical reaction to β-protein did, however, produce faintly stained granular or small nodular areas which surrounded many of the non-reactive amyloid deposits; this was greatly enhanced by the formic acid pretreatment (Fig 1-B), and β-protein immunoreactive cerebrovascular amyloid deposits were very occasionally seen (Fig 1-C). Neurofibrillary tangles and dystrophic neurites around amyloid cores were invariably immunoreactive to the anti-tau antibody (Fig 1-D).

ii) Electron microscopic findings:

A routine examination showed that in the periphery of discrete amyloid cores there were loose bundles of amyloid fibrils that were closely adjacent to degenerating neurites. In immunoelectron microscopy dense core deposits of amyloid fibrils were diffusely immunolabeled by anti-PrP antiserum, and the β-protein immunoreactive structures located in the peripheral regions of the cerebral plaques were shown to be composed of sparse aggregations of amyloid fibrils (Fig 2).

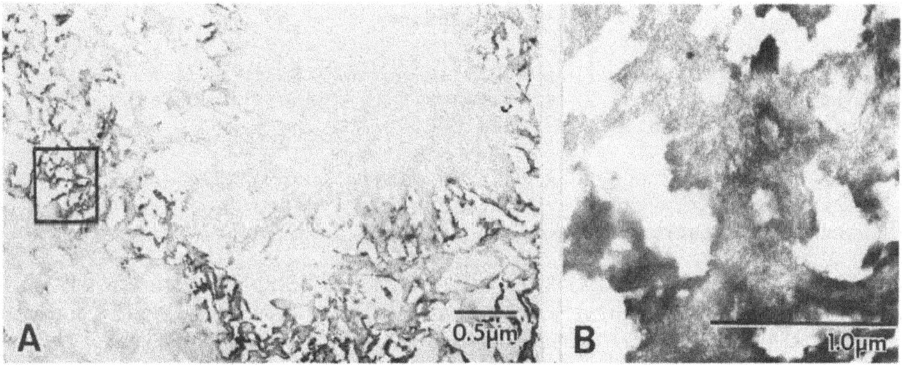

Figure 2. Electron micrographs of a cerebral plaque stained by anti-β protein antibody. B is higher magnification of the framed area in A. Note that an amyloid core is not immunolabeled and immunoreactive areas in the periphery consist of amyloid fibrils.

(Discussion)

The present two cases both showed some pathological features of Alzheimer's disease, including neurofibrillary tangles and β-protein type cerebrovascular amyloid deposition. However, the morphology and distribution of the amyloid plaques seen in these cases were consistent with the categorized pathology of GSS[5], and the amyloid fibril protein comprising the central cores of these plaques was immunohistochemically demonstrated to be PrP. These were, therefore, considered to be atypical GSS cases.

The pathological hallmark of GSS is the presence of numerous kuru-type amyloid plaques throughout the brain showing PrP-immunoreactivity without any dystrophic neurites[6]. Recently a variant of GSS with PrP-immunoreactive amyloid plaques and numerous Alzheimer's neurofibrillary tangles has been described[7], suggesting clinical and pathological heterogeneity of this disease. The present atypical GSS cases revealed a previously unknown type of amyloid plaques apparently containing two chemical classes of amyloid fibril protein: PrP in the core and β-protein in the periphery. Moreover, these plaques were also accompanied by neuritic components with tau-immunoreactivity that is a characteristic finding of senile plaques seen in Alzheimer's disease. A search for further examples of this unusual variant of GSS and analysis of the probable gene defect would be worth-while, since these patients seemed to provide a heuristic link between the transmissible prion dementias and Alzheimer's disease. The present study also suggests the β-protein amyloid fibril accumulation and the development of tau-immunoreactive abnormal neurites share some common pathological mechanism.

(Aknowledgments)

We express our appreciation to Drs. S. Prusiner and M. Bruce for providing anti-PrP antisera, and Dr. Y. Ihara for anti-tau antiserum.

(References)

1. Wiley, CA., Burrola, PG., Buchmeier, MJ., et al. (1987) 'Immunogold localization of prion filaments in scrapie-infected hamster brains', Lab. Invest. 57, 646-656.

2. Bruce, M.E., McBride, P.A. and Farquhar, C.F. (1989)'Precise targeting of the pathology of the sialoglycoprotein, PrP, and vacuolar degeneration in mouse scrapie', Neurosci. Lett. 102, 1-6.

3. Allsop, D., Landon, M., Kidd, M., et al. (1986)'Monoclonal antibodies against a subsequence of senile plaque core protein react with plaque core, plaque periphery and cerebrovascular amyloid in Alzheimer's disease', Neurosci. Lett. 68, 252-256.

4. Ihara, Y. (1988) 'Massive somatodendritic sprouting of cortical neurons in Alzheimer's disease', Brain Res. 459, 138-144.

5. Masters, CL., Gajdusek, DC. and Gibbs, CJ.(1981)' Creutzfeldt-Jakob disease virus isolations from the Gerstmann-Straussler syndrome', Brain 104, 559-588.

6. Kitamoto, T., Tateishi, J. and Sato, Y. (1988) 'Immunohistochemical verification of senile and kuru plaques in Creutzfeldt-Jakob disease and the allied disease', Ann. Neurol. 24, 537-542.

7. Ghetti, B., Tagliavini, F., Masters, CL., et al. (1989) 'Gerstmann-Sträussler-Scheinker disease. II. Neurofibrillary tangles and plaques with PrP-amyloid coexist in affected family', Neurology 39, 1453-1461.

ANTIGENIC HETEROGENEITY OF CEREBRAL AMYLOID DEPOSITS IN ALZHEIMER'S DISEASE

R.P. Linke, R. Schifferegger, H. Kretzschmar*, L. Gerhard&,

Institute of Immunology, Goethestr. 31 and *Institute of Neuropathology, Thalkirchnerstr. 36, D-8000 München 2/FRG, &Institute of Neuropathology, Huflandstr. 55, 4500 Essen/FRG

ABSTRACT. Amyloid plaques and cerebrovascular amyloid in Alzheimer's disease and Down's syndrome are shown to be composed of β-protein fibrils, designed Aβ. To investigate, whether Aβ deposits could also bind antibodies directed against non-Aβ amyloid fibril proteins, sections of cerebral tissues of eight patients with Alzheimer's disease were examined with a panel of antibodies directed against the major known amyloid-types, i.e. anti-AA, -Aλ, -Aκ, -AF(TTR), -AB (β_2m), and -Aβ. Anti-Aβ was prepared by us against β-protein purified from a patient's leptomeningeal vessels.
The immunohistochemical results show, that anti-Aβ reacted most consistently with cerebral amyloid deposits of all examined tissues, confirming the diagnosis. In addition, also non-β protein antisera (in particular Anti-Aλ) reacted to various extent also with some Aβ-amyloid deposits, indicating that plasma proteins or fragments thereof are associated with amyloid plaques and cerebrovascular amyloid. The demonstration of the presence of serum proteins in Aβ-amyloid strongly indicates a disturbance of the blood-brain barrier in Alzheimer's disease.

1. INTRODUCTION

Alzheimer's disease (AD) is characterized clinically by progressive dementia and morphologically by cerebral storage of the 4.2 kD β-protein (1), which is deposited within plaques either in amyloid conformation (Aβ) or in unstructured β-deposits (βD) and in addition in vascular leptomeningeal and cortical vessels (2). Aβ is the product of limited proteolysis from larger precursor membrane proteins (3) which are present throughout the organism, including the brain. Antibodies directed against the β-protein are able to lable immunohistochemically Aβ-deposits and βD, confirming the diagnosis. These antibodies are also useful in assisting the evaluation of the extent of the past cerebral damage (2). Since also other proteins have been found in Aβ-deposits, e.g. enzymes (4), we have investigasted cerebral tissue sections for the presence of amyloidogenic proteins different from Aβ. The immunohistochemical results show further antigenic heterogeneity of amyloid deposits in Alzheimer's disease.

2. MATERIAL AND METHODS

a. **Postmortem specimens and immunohistochemistry** of brain tissue from 8 patients with clinical diagnosis of typical Alzheimer's disease were obtained after fixation in 10% of buffered formalin in form of paraffin blocks. Unstained paraffin sections (approximately 4µm) were available for immunohistochemistry using the unlabelled immunoperoxidase technique of Sternberger as decribed (5).

b. **Antibodies** directed against purified amyloid fibril proteins were prepared in form of murine monoclonal (5) or rabbit polyclonal antibodies (6). The following antibodies were used: murine monoclonal anti-AA antibody mc29 (directed against the conserved segment of the AA/SAA protein; see Frankenberger et al. in this issue. This antibody is able to inhibit the inhibitory action of SAA on neutrophile function and thus may bind to a funtional important segment of the SAA-molecule; mc29 is reacting very similarly to mc1 (Dakopatts) on tissue sections). Both monoclonal antibodies have so far stained all tissue sections with AA-amyloid tested, without any false negative or false positive reactions which could give rise to confusion. Anti-Aλ (HAR) covers almost all Aλ-amyloid deposits (6). Whether the few not reacting amyloid syndromes are indeed of the Aλ-type is still under investigation. Anti-Aκ (SIN) has so far stained all Aκ-amyloids. Anti-AF (TIE) was prepared against a purified TTR-amyloid isolated from a vitreous of patient TIE (7) and was shown to identify amyloid of both groups of TTR-amyloids, the idiopathic senile systemic amyloidosis and the variant types of hereditary TTR-amyloids. Anti-AB (WOE) is directed against the isolated amyloid fibril protein of patient WOE treated with long-term hemodialysis; it covers all β_2m-derived AB-amyloids. Anti-Aβ (RAP) was induced against a purified and chemically characterized Aβ protein from a patient (RAP) with congophilic angiopathy (in progress). All employed antibodies have met the test on a large panel of tissue sections obtained from different amyloid types (8, in part unpublished).

3. RESULTS AND DISCUSSION

A summary of all immunohistochemical data is shown in Table 1. All eight cases, including a familial case (No. 8) showed strong reaction with the anti-Aβ antibody as the most consistent feature. However, also reactions with non-Aβ antisera have been documented. How could these rather unexpected reactions be explained and what do they mean?
Cerebral amyloids in different clinical syndromes are reported to be chemically of different nature. Aβ is found in the idiopathic and heretitary Alzheimer's disease, in the Dutch-type of hereditary cerebral hemorrhage and in Down's syndrome, cystatin C is found in amyloid in Islandic hereditary hemorrhage and prion protein in transmissible amyloid encephalopathies such as Kuru, Creutzfeld-Jacob disease, Gerstmann-Stäußler-Schenkein syndrome, and animal diseases of the scrapie group (9). These syndromes can be distinguished in various laboratories on tissues section with suitable antibodies. Nevertheless, the amyloid deposits are not composed of a single substance, but represent a complex of different proteins and other constituents, including amyloidogenic proteins which are not present in amyloid conformation but which are merely adsorbed in different amounts. These adsorbed proteins can confuse the correct

immunochemical typing, in particular when an antibody to the amyloidogenic core protein is not available or unsuitable. The results presented here document the presence of adsorbed proteins which are recognized by anti-amyloid antibodies of non-Aβ specificity. In two out of 8 patients a moderate reaction with anti-AF was seen, indicating the presence of transthyretin, which was formerly confused with the correct amyloid fibril protein Aβ. In one patient a borderline reaction was seen with anti-AB indicating small amounts of β_2m. This weak reaction, however, could hardly confuse the identification of the correct amyloid type, because other stronger reactions were present. The most abundant adsorbed proteins detected here in seven out of eight examined cases, however, are immunoglobulin light chains. In case, the anti-Aβ antibody would not have been appropriate for immunohistochemical typing, these reactions with anti-Aλ could have resulted in the incorrect amyloid-type. Cerebral tissue section of another patient (not in Table 1) reacted only with anti-Aλ and indicating a light chain amyloid (in progress). For obtaining the correct immunochemical diagnosis it seems essential, to employ anti-amyloid antibodies that detect a given amyloid class entirely and at the same time does not react with another amyloid type. Only when anti-amyloid antibodies meet these criteria, can they be used for typing of amyloid. These tests have been done with all anti-amyloid antibodies used here (8). These data are important also for another reason. Serum proteins are usually not present in easily detectable amounts within the cerebral substance. Yet, when they are found, as has been demonstrated here in Alzheimer's disease within amyloid plaques and cerebrovascular amyloid deposits, it stronly indicates the presence of these proteins in diffusible form within the brain, and demonstrates a disturbance of the blood-brain barriers. In addition, the Aβ-precursor proteins could enter the brain from plasma by this route and the impaired blood-brain barrier could play a role during the development of Alzheimer's disease.

Fig. 1a: Analysis of Aβ-deposits in Alzheimer's disease using a panel of anti-amyloid antibodies, including anti-Aβ

Pat.	Sex m/f	age (y)	Immunohistochemical reaction against anti- AA (mcl)	Aλ (HAR)	Aκ (SIN)	AF (TIE)	AB (WOE)	Aβ (RAP)
1	m	69	o	+	o	+	o	+++
2	m	63	o	++	o	+	(+)	+++
3	nd	nd	o	++	o	o	o	++
4	m	81	o	++++	++	o	o	++++
5	m	76	o	++	(+)	o	o	++
6	m	77	o	+	(+)	o	o	+++
7	m	89	o	o	o	o	o	++
8	f	39	o	++	o	o	o	++

nd, no data available; strength of reaction: o, negative; (+) borderline reaction; + moderate reaction; ++ strong reaction; +++ very strong reaction; ++++ extremely strong reaction.

disease by increasing the Aβ-deposits and the βD. Whether the severity of the dementia can be related to the amount of serum proteins present within the amyloid deposits is a matter of further investigation.

4. REFERENCES

1. Glenner, G.G., Wong, C.W.: Alzheimer's disease: initial report of the purification and characterization of a novel cerebrovascular amyloid protein. Biochem. Biophys. Res. Commun. 120, 885-890 (1984)

2. Selkoe, D.J., Podlisny, M.B., Gronbeck, A., Mammen, A., Kosik, K.S.: Molecular relation of amyloid filaments amd paired helical filaments in Alzheimer's disease. Adv. Neurol. 51, 171-179 (1990)

3. Kang, J., Lemaire, H.G., Unterbeck, K.A., Salbaum, J.M., Masters, C.L., Grzeschik, K.H., Multhaupt, G., Beyreuther, K., Müller-Hill, B.: The precursor of Alzheimer's disease amyloid A4 protein resembles a cell surface receptor. Nature 325, 733-736 (1987)

4. Cataldo, A.M., Nixon, R.A.: Enzymatically active lysosomal proteases are associated with amyloid deposits in Alzheimer brain. Proc. Natl. Acad. Sci. USA 87, 3861-3865 (1990)

5. Linke, R.P.: Monoclonal antibodies against amyloid fibril protein AA. Production, specificty and use of immunohistochemical localization and classification of AA-type amyloidosis. J. Histochem. Cytochem. 32, 322-328 (1984)

6. Linke, R.P.: Immunochemical typing of amyloid deposits after microextraction from biopsies. Appl. Path. 3, 18-28 (1985)

7. Linke, R.P.: Immunohistochemical identification and cross reactions of amyloid fibril proteins in senile heart and amyloid in familial polyneuropathy. Lack of reactivity with cerebral amyloid in Alzheimer's disease. Clin. Neuropathol. 1, 172-182 (1982)

8. Linke, R.P., Nathrath, W.P.J., Eulitz, M.: Classification of amyloid syndromes from tissue sections using antibodies against various amyloid fibril proteins: report of 142 cases. In: Amyloidosis, Glenner, G.G. et al. (eds.), pp. 599-605, Plenum Press, New York and London 1986

9. Glenner, G.G., Murphy, M.A.: Amyloidosis of the nervous system. J. Neurol. Scie. 94, 1-28 (1989).

6. ACKNOWLEDGMENTS

Supported by the Deutsche Forschungsgemeinschaft, Bonn, Grant Li 247/7-2, Sonderforschungsgemeinschaft 207, Grant G8, and Sandersstiftung, Grant 89.036.1. For technical assistance we thank Ms. A. Rail and A. Kerling.

Systemic Vascular Amyloidosis Associated with Alzheimer's Disease.

Lathi D; Cathcart E.S.; Sipe J.D.
Department of Research and Department of Pathology;
E.N.R.M. V.A. Hospital, Bedford, Massachusettes, U.S.A.

Abstract: Vascular amyloidosis, with minimal parenchymal or interstitial involvement, is extremely rare. This is a report of a case of dementia of Alzheimer's type, confirmed at autopsy, by the presence of senile plaques, neurofibrillary tangles, and congophilic angiopathy. In addition, amyloid was seen in parenchymal arteries of various organs. Extracerebral vsacular Amyloid was negative for AA protein.

Introduction.

Amyloid deposits other than AL are reported infrequently, in the coronary arteries and systemic paranchymal arteries.[Ref 1]. Cerebral Congophilic angiopathy has been considered as one of the morphologic changes frequently seen in the brain of Alzheimer's disease.[Ref 2].

To our knowledge, co-existence of systemic vascular amyloidosis and cerebral vascular amyloidosis has been reported 0nly in three cases, [Ref 3].

We report a case of systemic vascular amyloidosis in a patient with clinical history compatible with the diagnosis of senile dementia, and who, at autopsy, showed cerebral congophilic angoipathy, neuro fibrillary tangles, and neuritic plaques, consistent with Alzheimer's disease.

Amyloid in the coronary arteries, was analysed for the presence of AA, by Potassium permanganate digestion method.

Case history

The patient, an 88 year old caucasian man with the family history of dementia in the mother and one brother, was committed to a psychiatric hospital in 1975 for one year history of increasing forgetfulness, confusion and aggressive, assaultive behaviour.

Physical examination showed no gross abnormalities. BP 120/80; Pulse 78/min, Regular. Neurological examination showed ++ deep tendon reflexes, steady gait and down going plantar reflexes.

Evaluation of mental status revealed lack of orientation to time, place and person. He showed no understanding of his predicament and could not perform simple mathemetical calculations.

Serum B12 level, thyroid function, and heavy metal screen were normal.

The patient's symptoms progressed rapidly. Within six years patient became obtunded, mute and developed flexion contracture deformities in all four extremities. He suffered from multiple urinary tract, and respiratory infections. Terminally, he became suddenly unresponsive, hypotensive bradycardic; and died inspite of supportive therapy.

Pathological Findings.

The autopsy study revealed a pulmonary embolus,multifocal myocardial necrosis with acute inflammation, and pneumonia as immediate causes of death. The heart was flabby with four chamber dilation and a mural thrombus in the right auricular process. There was diffuse scarring in the apical portion of the left ventricle. Atherosclerosis was minimal and the major coronary arteries were patent. The most unusual finding was the presence of congophilic material in the parenchymal arteries of all the organs (Fig 1) including the lungs. Coronary arteries were most severely affected and many showed marked narrowing and occlusion of the lumina.(Fig 2) In contrast to typical cases of primary, and secondary amyloidosis, parenchyma was spared, apart from smal foci in the myocardium. The congophilic material showed only foci of apple green birefringence described as characteristic of amyloid. with large portions showing only white birefringence or no refringence at all.

Postmortem serum electrophoresis did not show any protein abnormalities. Urine was not available to rule out presence of light chains.

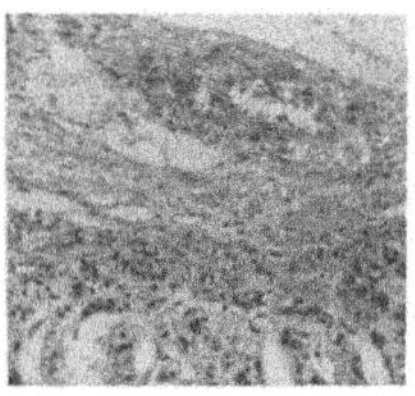

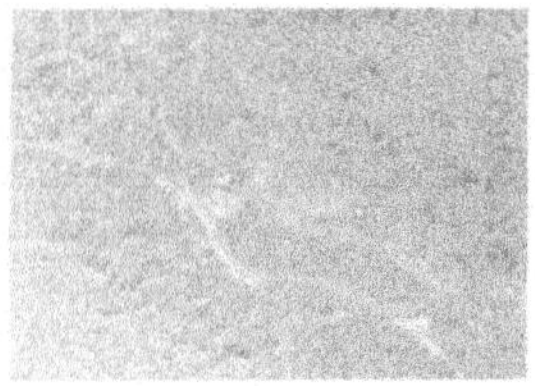

Fig 1. Amyloid in parenchymal arteries.
Congored stain; polarised light.
A. Periadrenal tissue B. Pancreas

Fig 2. Coronary artery:
Congored stain

Method and materials

Paraffin blocks from the formalin fixed tissues were stained with alkaline congo red stain,and differentiated by 80% ethanol to elicit amyloid birefringence.

Since collagen and fibrin are also congophilic [Ref 4], sections from the myocardial block used for the study were also stained with trichrome and PAS stains to identify collagen and fibrin respectively.

Positive and negative control tissue paraffin blocks for detection of AA protein, using potassium permanganate digestion method were kindly provided by Dr Wright, from Departments of Pathology and Medicine, State University Of New York in Buffalo. Potassium permanganate digestion study was performed on one block of left ventricle of the heart, according to the method described before [ref 5].

Results.

The congophilic material in the arteries stained bright pink with PAS stain suggesting presence of fibrin, but did not stain for collagen.

Congophilia and green birefringence in the coronary arteries persisted after potassium permanganate digestion. (Fig 3)

Fig 3. Coronary artery. Congored stain; Polarised light
A. Before and B. After potassiun permanganate digestion

Discussion.

In the case presented, the amyloid deposits were found predominantly in the small arteries of various organs, without parenchymal involvement, except in the heart. The cardiac changes were secondary to acute and chronic ischemia, due to coronary vascular amyloid deposits. Amyloid was also seen in the cerebral vessels, plaques and neurofibrillary tangles

"Senile systemic amyloidosis" and "Small artery Amyloidosis" have been described as subgroups of "Peripheral Amyloid Angiopathies". The former group shows small, mostly vascular amyloid deposits with focal parenchymal deposits in various organs, and connective tissue. In the second group, the amyloid depsits are vascular, and occasionally may be severe enough to cause visceral ischemia. In a series of fifty cases studied from this group, cerebral plaques tangles and angiopathy were either absent or not mentioned [Ref 6].

The non-birefringent congophilic material in the vessels was probably fibrin. The vascular hayaline and fibrinoid degenerative changes associated with amyloid deposits have been described. Thus far, this phenomenon is identified only in cerebral vessels. [Ref 7].

Although the staining and optical properties of all amyloids are uniform, diversity in it's chemical composition under different clinical settings has been demonstrated by using immunohistopathologic techniques, amino acid sequencing, autoclaving and digestion by alkaline guadine and potassium permanganate [Ref 5, 8, 9].

Inspite of recurrent infections over a long period of time, AA protein was not seen in the systemic vascular deposits in the case reported here. Presence of AL protein was ruled out because of the normal serum protein electrophoresis and lack of clinical evidence of Myeloma.

ASc1 proteins, homologus to Prealbumin have been identified in Senile cardiac and senile systemic amyloid [ref 10]. Prealbumin has also been demonstrated in the senile plaques, neurofibrillary tangles, and cerebral congophilic vessels of Alzheimer's disease, and senile non-demented patients [Ref 8]. Association between senile systemic and senile cerebral amyloid has not been very clear.

Recently, several investigators have identified beta peptide as part of the amyloid in Alzheimer's disease, senile (age-related) changes, as well as in familial and sporadic cerebral congophilic angiopathies [Ref 11]. It has been postulated that precursor protein to Beta peptide is present on cell membranes of neurons, and parenchymal cells of other organs [Ref 12]. In a recent study, Beta protein has been demonstrated in extracerebral tissues of non -demented senile patients, and patients with Alzheimer's disease, indicating extacerebral expression of the disease. [Ref 13].

Isolation, biochemical analysis and immunohistochemical analysis of the amyloid from cerebral lesions has not yet been performed and compared with systemic vascular amyloid in the case reported here. However, concurrent presence of non-AA amyloid in cerebral and extacerebral vessels in a non-myeloma patient indicates that the pathological process resulting in the senile and Alzheimer's lesions, may be widespread in the body, and the systemic vascular amyloid deposits, as seen in our case, may be a rare manifestation of such a process. The mechanism of selective vascular involvement with the amyloid is unknown. Presence of yet unidentified component with vascular affinity or different processing of the precursor in the vessel walls has been suggested.[Ref 1, 12].

Acknowledgements.

Authors wish to thank Dr. Wright for providing positive and negative controls for potassium premanganate digestion study; Dr. Rosalis for interpreting the brain sections from the patient; Carol Kubilus, Jean Thomson and Robert Landrigan for technical assistance.

Bibliography

1. Jennette Charles J., M.D.; Sheps David S., M.D.; McNeil Donald D., M.D., Exclusively Vascular Systemic Amyloidosis with Visceral Ischemia. Arch. Pathol. Lab. Med. 1982. Vol 106 (p.323 - 327).

2. Bergeron C; Ranalli P.J.; Miceli. Amyloid Angiopathy In Alzheimer's Disease. Canadian Journal of Neurological Sciences. 1987. Vol. 14 (p.564-569)

3. Haberland C. Primary Systemic Amyloidosis; Cerebral Involvement and Senile Plaque Formation. J. Neuropath Exp. Neurology. 1964 Vol. 23 (p.135-150)

4. Elghetany Tarek M.; Saleem Abdus. Methods For Staining Amyloid in Tissues. Stain Technology 1988. Vol. 63, No. 4. (p.201-212)

5. Wright JR; Calkins E; Humphrey RL. Potassium Permanganate Reaction in Amyloidosis. Lab. Investigation 1977. Vol.36 No 3 (p.274-281)

6. Muckle TJ. Peripheral Angiopathy, in "Amyloidosis". Marrink J; VanRijswijkm. (Edit) Martinus Nijhoff Publishers 1986 (p.271-282)

7. Mandybur T. I. Cerebral Amyloid Angiopathy. Journal of Neuropathology and Experimental Neurology 1986. Vol. 45, No.1. (p.79-90)

8. Shirahama T.; Skinner M.; Westermark P.; Rubinow A; Cohen A; Brun A; Kemper T. Prealbumin As a Common Constituent in the Neuritic Plaque, in the Neurofibrillary Tangle, and in the Microangiopathic Lesion. Am. J. Pathol. 1982. Vol. 107 (p.41-50)

9. Tetsuyuki Kitamoto; Takatoshi Tashima; Jun Tateishi ; Novel Histochemical Approaches To The Prealbumin-Related Senile And Familial Forms OF Systemic Amyloidosis. American Journal Of Pathology 1986. Vol 123 No.3 (p 407-412)

10. Westermark P.; Johansson B.; Natvig J.B. Senile Cardiac Amyloidosis: Evidence of Two Different Amyloid Substances in the Aging Heart. Scand. J. Immunology 1979. Vol.10 (p.303-308)

11. Coria F.; Prelli F.; Castano E.M.; Lorrondo-Lillo M.; Fernandez-Gonzalez J.; vanDuinen S.G.; Bots G.T.A.M.; Luyendijk W.; Shelanski M.L.; Frangione B. Beta-protein Deposition: A Pathologic Link Between Alzheimer's Disease And Cerebral Amyliod Angiopathies. Brain Research 1988. Vol 463.(p187-191).

12. Prelli F.; Castano E.M.; vanDuinen S.G.; Bots G.; Luyendijk W.; Blas F.; Diferent Processing Of Alzheimer's Beta protein In the Vessel wall O Patints With Hereditary Cerebral Hemorrhage With Amyloidosis - Dutch Type. Biochem. and Biophysical Research Comm. 1988. Vol.151, No 3,(p 1150-1155)

13. Joachim C.L.; Mori Hiroshi; Selkoe D.J. Amyloid Beta Protein Deposition in Tissue Other than Brain in Alzheimer's Disease. Nature 1989. Vol. 341, (p.226-230)

PATHOLOGICAL CHANGES IN HEREDITARY CEREBRAL HEMORRHAGE WITH AMYLOIDOSIS - DUTCH TYPE

R.A.C. ROOS[1], J. HAAN[1], M.L.C. MAAT-SCHIEMAN[1],
S.G. VAN DUINEN[1] AND G.T.A.M. BOTS[2]
Department of Neurology[1] and Pathology[2]
Academic Hospital Leiden
P.O. Box 9600
2300 RC Leiden
The Netherlands

ABSTRACT. Neuropathological findings in hereditary cerebral hemorrhage with amyloidosis - Dutch type are described.

Pathological findings

The main pathological findings in patients with hereditary amyloidosis are a normal or slightly elevated brain weight (1300 - 1400 grams), no cortical atrophy and in some patients cerebral edema. Recent large cerebral hemorrhages and remnants of older ones are mainly located in the subcortical white matter. Recently developed and old hemorrhagic infarcts are present in cortex and subcortical white matter. Amyloid deposits are found in cortical arterioles and small leptomeningeal arteries (green birefringence in polarized light after staining with Congo-red), with typical irregularly arranged non-branching filaments with a diameter of 7.5 to 10 nm when studied by electron microscope. No senile plaques or neurofibrillary tangles in Bielschowsky block staining could be demonstrated. Outside the brain, in the skin, fascia, muscle, eye, no amyloidosis is found. [1]

In further studies it was shown that almost all hemorrhages appeared to be surrounded by or related to a zone of infarction, suggesting hemorrhagic infarction rather than primary hemorrhage.

In a large series the most remarkable finding was the presence of large numbers of so-called 'senile plaques of the amorphous type'. Neurofibrillary tangles were not found. With the aid of a polyclonal antibody to a 28-residue synthetic peptide (anti-SP 28) homologous to the N-terminal region of the ß-protein of Alzheimer's disease and Down's syndrome intensive staining of the arterioles and the plaque like lesions appeared. [2] Neurofibrillary tangles did not stain with antibodies against prealbumin, amyloid A protein, kappa and lambda immunoglobulin light chains, or against monomeric amyloid protein of hereditary cerebral hemorrhage with amyloidosis - Icelandic type (HCHWA-I). The presence of amyloid P-component in the amyloid deposits in the vessel walls and in the plaque like structures of two patients with HCHWA-D was shown. [3]

Further studies revealed that the complete sequence of the amyloid protein in the arachnoidal blood vessels in HCHWA-D was three residues shorter (39 in stead of 42) than that reported of plaque amyloid of Alzheimer's disease patients. [4] This finding may reflect a difference in degradation of the amyloid precursor that occurs in the vessel wall compared with the degradation in the brain parenchyma. A relation between the cerebral amyloid deposits and α_1-anti-chymotrypsin was found in HCHWA-D. [5] This appears to indicate deranged proteolysis as a cause for the cerebral amyloid deposits. P-component (see above) is a common component of virtually all types of amyloidosis [6] and not specific for ß-protein deposition, but $\alpha 1$-antichymotrypsin seems to have an unique association with ß-protein. [5, 7]

In HCHWA-D and in Alzheimer's disease coexistence of ß-protein and its precursor was proven in the cerebral vessel-walls. [8] This strongly suggests that the vascular system is a source of the precursor.

Pathological examination of two patients with periventricular lesions also showed circumscript cortical areas in which axons and myelin sheaths had disappeared, but glia cells and neuropil were preserved. In the white matter sparing of the 'U-fibers' with prominent demyelination of axons was seen. These lesions (called 'incomplete infarctions'), probably reflect focal hypoxic brain damage and resemble the 'incomplete infarctions' described in Alzheimer's disease and multi-infarct dementia as well as the 'hemorrhagic leukoencephalopathy' described in sporadic amyloid angiopathy. [9] Amyloid induced stenosis and loss of compliance of cortical and long perforating arterioles with chronic hypoperfusion of the deep white matter was presented as a possible pathogenetic mechanism for the diffuse white matter involvement in sporadic amyloid angiopathy and in HCHWA-D.

In conclusion, the pathological changes described in HCHWA-D reflect a whole spectrum of damage to the brain probably all caused by amyloid angiopathy. Although difficult to demonstrate rupture of affected blood vessels and obliteration occurs in amyloid angiopathy. [10] And also chronic damage is represented by accumulation of residual lesions of previous strokes, by cortical infarcts, and by diffuse white matter involvement, probably caused by chronic ischemia. The occurrence of senile plaques only of the amorphous type possibly suggests an effect of amyloid angiopathy on brain parenchyma. This is contrary to Alzheimer's disease, Down's syndrome and normal aging, where cortical atrophy, all categories of plaques, neurofibrillary tangles and a minor degree of amyloid angiopathy occur. The amyloid deposits in HCHWA-D have a relation with protease-inhibitors, and the source of the precursor seems to be the vessel walls. A comparison between patients who died as a result of their first cerebral stroke and patients who survived their first attack more than a decade revealed a higher number of amorphous plaques in the latter.

References.

1 Wattendorf A.R., Bots G.T.A.M., Went L.N., Endtz L.J. (1982) Familial cerebral amyloid angiopathy presenting as recurrent cerebral hemorrhage. J. Neurol. Sci. 55:121-135.

2 Van Duinen S.G., Castaño E.M., Prelli F., Bots G.T.A.M., Luyendijk W.,

Frangione B. (1987) Hereditary cerebral hemorrhage with amyloidosis in patients of Dutch origin is related to Alzheimer's disease. Proc. Natl. Acad. Sci. USA 84:5991-5994.

3 Coria F., Castaño E., Prelli F., Larrondo-Lillo M., Van Duinen S.G., Shelanski M.L., Frangione B. (1988) Isolation and characterization of amyloid P component from Alzheimer's disease and other types of cerebral amyloidosis. Lab. Invest. 58:454-458.

4 Prelli F., Castaño E.M., Van Duinen S.G., Bots G.T.A.M., Luyendijk W., Frangione B. (1988) Different processing of Alzheimer's ß-protein precursor in the vessel wall of patients with hereditary cerebral hemorrhage with amyloidosis-Dutch type. Biochem. Biophys. Res. Comm. 151:1150-1155.

5 Picken M.M., Larrondo-Lillo M., Coria F., Gallo G.R., Shelanski M.L., Frangione B. (1990) Distribution of the protease inhibitor α_1-antichymotrypsin in cerebral and systemic amyloid. J. Neuropathol. Exp. Neurol. 49:41-48.

6 Coria F., Castaño E.M., Frangione B. (1987) Brain amyloid in normal aging and cerebral amyloid angiopathy is antigenically related to Alzheimer's disease ß-protein. Am. J. Pathol. 129:422-428.

7 Abraham C.R., Selkoe D.J., Potter H. (1988) Immunochemical identification of the serine protease inhibitor α_1-Antichymotrypsin in the brain amyloid deposits of Alzheimer's disease. Cell 52:487-501.

8 Tagliavini F., Ghiso J., Timmers W.F., Giaccone G., Bugiani O., Frangione B. (1990) Alzheimer's disease and hereditary (Dutch type) cerebral hemorrhage: Coexistence of amyloid precursor protein and amyloid protein in cerebral vessel walls. J. Neuropathol. Exp. Neurol. 49:332.

9 Englund E., Brun A., Alling C. (1988) White matter changes in dementia of Alzheimer's type. Biochemical and neuro-pathological correlates. Brain 111:1425-1439.

10 Vinters H.V., Miller B.L., Pardridge W.M. (1988) Brain amyloid and Alzheimer's disease. Ann. Int. Med. 109:41-54.

HEREDITARY CEREBRAL HEMORRHAGE WITH AMYLOIDOSIS - DUTCH TYPE

J. HAAN and R.A.C. ROOS
Department of Neurology
University Hospital
P.O. Box 9600
2300 RC Leiden
The Netherlands

ABSTRACT. Hereditary cerebral hemorrhage with amyloidosis - Dutch type (HCHWA-D) is an autosomal dominant disease, characterized by recurrent cerebral hemorrhages and dementia, occurring at a relatively young age. The symptoms are caused by extensive deposition of amyloid in cerebral arterioles and leptomeningeal arteries. A point-mutation in the β-protein precursor gene on chromosome 21 is the underlying cause of the disease. In this chapter the clinical, radiological, pathological and genetic features of this disease will be summarized, with special attention for the relation between HCHWA-D and Alzheimer's disease, which is also characterized by β-protein deposition.

Introduction

Hereditary cerebral hemorrhage with amyloidosis - Dutch type (HCHWA-D) is an autosomal dominant disease, occurring in several large families in two coastal villages in the Netherlands [1-3]. The disease is characterized by recurrent strokes and affects normotensive middle-aged patients. About 50% of the patients die as a result of their first stroke, whereas the remaining half suffers from recurrent strokes [1]. Extensive cerebral amyloid angiopathy has been identified as the cause of the strokes [1,2].

The amyloid, present in cortical arterioles and small leptomeningeal arteries, is biochemically homologous with the β-protein found in Alzheimer's disease (AD) [4], and therefore, HCHWA-D is categorized as one of the cerebral β-amyloid diseases [5].

In this chapter, the present knowledge about HCHWA-D will be summarized, with special attention to the differences and similarities between HCHWA-D and AD. The pathological findings will be presented in another chapter in this volume.

History

In the early sixties, the familial occurrence of cerebral hemorrhages in a small Dutch coastal village, called Katwijk, was recognized [6]. The transmission of the disease appeared to be autosomal dominant. The discovery of amyloid angiopathy as the cause of cerebral hemorrhages in another autosomal dominant disease, occurring in Iceland [7], led to a specific search for amyloid angiopathy in the Dutch cases. Indeed, amyloid angiopathy was found, and consequently it was presumed that the Dutch and Icelandic patients were genealogically related [1]. One important difference between the patients from both countries, however, was that the Icelandic patients suffered from their first hemorrhage around the age of 25 [7], whereas the Dutch patients had the first stroke approximately 20 years later [1]. At first, different expression of one single disease process was used as explanation.

In 1983 it was discovered that the amyloid fibrils in hereditary cerebral hemorrhage with amyloidosis - Icelandic type (HCHWA-I) are related to cystatin C (gamma-trace) [8]. The subsequent discovery of β-protein in the amyloid deposits of patients with HCHWA-D [4] made clear that HCHWA-I and HCHWA-D are different diseases. Furthermore, it showed a biochemical relation with AD and Down's syndrome, two other examples of β-protein deposition diseases [5].

Clinical features

HCHWA-D is characterized by recurrent strokes, occurring between 45 and 60 years of age, resulting in death or persistent focal neurological deficits [1,2]. Recently, we reviewed the neuropsychological investigations of 16 patients surviving one or more strokes [9]. All patients showed cognitive dysfunction and in 12 patients moderate to severe dementia was present. The dementia was correlated with the number of focal lesions on CT-scans of the brain [9]. This suggests 'multi-infarct (hemorrhage) dementia. However, many patients also had a history of progressive cognitive decline, apparently unrelated to the strokes. In three patients with such a history, repeated neuropsychological investigations documented progression of the mental deterioration [9]. Apparently, amyloid angiopathy leads (next to focal cerebral damage) to chronic, diffuse damage.

Radiological findings

CT and MRI studies of HCHWA-D patients have revealed recent cerebral hemorrhages, infarcts or remnants of them [3,10]. Remarkably, also diffuse white matter damage seems to be present, visible on CT scans as hypodensity of the white matter and on MRI as hyperintensity in T2-weighted images of the same structure [3,9,10].

These white matter lesions resemble the lesions seen in patients with sporadic cerebral amyloid angiopathy [11] and AD [12]. The lesions are most likely caused by amyloid induced stenosis of arterioles to the white matter [11,13].

Genetics

HCHWA-D is an autosomal dominant disease [1]. As the gene for the precursor of β-protein has been located (on the long arm of chromosome 21), we were able to perform linkage studies in HCHWA-D aimed at this gene. Close linkage was found [14]. In a small number of HCHWA-D patients a point-mutation in the region of the β-amyloid gene coding for β-protein was found subsequently [15].

Conclusion

The main importance of HCHWA-D lies in the biochemical resemblance of the amyloid fibrils with those found in AD.

Clinically, both AD and HCHWA-D are characterized by the development of dementia. In HCHWA-D, however, this has the features of multi-infarct (hemorrhage) dementia. Only the slowly progressive dementia, additionally occurring in HCHWA-D, may point at a pathogenetic process which also plays a role in AD (e.g. chronic ischemic or metabolic damage of the brain due to amyloid angiopathy).

Radiologically, the occurence of white matter damage in HCHWA-D shows a striking resemblance with AD. This also may point at a similar pathogenetic mechanism: chronic ischemia of the cerebral structures that are most vulnerable to ischemia [10,11,13].

Genetically, the linkage to the β-amyloid gene on chromosome 21 and the point-mutation in this gene suggests a different etiology for HCHWA-D and AD, because (familial) AD is not linked with the same gene [16]. The process leading to amyloid formation in HCHWA-D probably is the inability of the proteolytic system to degradate an abnormal β-protein precursor, whereas in AD it is most likely that the degradation system itself is defective.

1. Luyendijk W., Bots G.T.A.M., Vegter-van der Vlis M., Went L.N., Frangione B. (1988) Hereditary cerebral hemorrhage caused by cortical amyloid angiopathy. J. Neurol. Sci. 85, 267-280.
2. Haan J., Roos R.A.C., Briet P.E., Herpers M.J.H.M., Luyendijk W., Bots G.T.A.M. (1989) Hereditary cerebral hemorrhage with amyloidosis - Dutch type. Clin. Neurol. Neurosurg. 81, 285-290.
3. Haan J., Algra P.R., Roos R.A.C. (1990) Hereditary cerebral hemorrhage with amyloidosis - Dutch type: clinical and CT analysis of 24 cases. Arch. Neurol. 47, 649-653.
4. Van Duinen S.G., Castaño E.M., Prelli F., Bots G.T.A.M., Luyendijk W., Frangione B. (1987) Hereditary cerebral hemorrhage with amyloidosis in patients of Dutch origin is related to Alzheimer's disease. Proc. Natl. Acad. Sci. USA 84, 5991-5994.
5. Castaño E.M., Frangione B. (1988) Human amyloidosis, Alzheimer's disease and related disorders. Lab. Invest. 58, 122-132.
6. Luyendijk W., Schoen J.H.R. (1964) Intracerebral haemetomas. A clinical study of 40 surgical cases. Psych. Neurol. Neurosurg. 67, 445-468.
7. Gudmundsson G., Hallgrimsson J., Jonasson T., Bjarnason O. (1974) Hereditary cerebral haemorrhage with amyloidosis. Brain 95, 387-404.
8. Cohen D.H., Feiner H., Jensson O., Frangione B. (1983) Amyloid fibril in hereditary cerebral hemorrhage with amyloidosis (HCHWA) is related to the gastroentero-pancreatic neuroendocrine protein, gamma trace. J. Exp. Med. 158, 623-628.
9. Haan J., Lanser J.B.K., Zijderveld I., Does I.G.F. van der, Roos R.A.C. (in press) Dementia in hereditary cerebral hemorrhage with amyloidosis - Dutch type. Arch. Neurol.
10. Haan J., Roos R.A.C., Algra P.R., Lanser J.B.K., Bots G.T.A.M., Vegter-van der Vlis M. (in press) Hereditary cerebral hemorrhage with amyloidosis - Dutch type: Magnetic resonance imaging of seven cases. Brain.
11. Gray F., Dubas F., Roullet E., Escourolle R. (1985) Leukoencephalopathy in diffuse hemorrhagic cerebral amyloid angiopathy. Ann. Neurol. 18, 54-59.
12. Erkinjuntti T., Ketonen L., Sulkava R., Sipponen J., Vuorialho M., Iivanainen M. (1987) Do white matter changes on MRI and CT differentiate vascular dementia from Alzheimer's disease? J. Neurol. Neurosurg. Psychiat. 50, 37-42.
13. Janota I., Mirsen T.R., Hachinski V.C., Lee D.H., Merksey H. (1989) Neuropathological correlates of leuko-araiosis. Arch. Neurol. 46, 1124-1128.
14. Broeckhoven C. van, Haan J., Bakker E., Hardy J.A., Hul W. van, Wehnert A., Vegter-van der Vlis M., Roos R.A.C. (1990) Amyloid β-protein precursor gene and hereditary cerebral hemorrhage with amyloidosis (Dutch). Science 248, 1120-1122.
15. Levy E., Carman M.D., Fernandez-Madrid I.J., et al. (1990) Mutation of the Alzheimer's disease amyloid gene in hereditary cerebral hemorrhage, Dutch type. Science 248, 1124-1126.
16. Broeckhoven C. van, Genthe A.M., Vandenberghe A., et al. (1987) Failure of familial Alzheimer's disease to segregate with the A4-amyloid gene in several European families. Nature 329, 153-155.

PERIPHERAL DISTRIBUTION OF A DERMATAN SULFATE PROTEOGLYCAN (DECORIN) IN AMYLOID PLAQUES AND THEIR PRESENCE IN NEUROFIBRILLARY TANGLES OF ALZHEIMER'S DISEASE

ALAN D. SNOW
University of Washington,
Department of Pathology SM-30,
Seattle, WA U.S.A. 98195

ABSTRACT: A polyclonal antibody recognizing the protein core of the small dermatan sulfate proteoglycan (DSPG)(known as decorin) derived from human skin fibroblasts was used to immunolocalize decorin in Alzheimer's (AD) brain at the light and electron microscopic levels. Decorin was identified as a component of both the amyloid deposits of neuritic plaques (NPs) and the filamentous structures within neurofibrillary tangles (NFTs). Unlike heparan sulfate proteoglycans (HSPGs) which tend to be evenly distributed throughout NPs containing amyloid fibrils, decorin was primarily localized to the periphery of the spherically-shaped amyloid plaques, and to the edges of amyloid fibril bundles within the plaque periphery. Decorin was also immunolocalized to the paired helical and straight filaments within NFTs, and to collagen fibrils surrounding blood vessels. The unique distribution of decorin to the periphery of amyloid plaques in AD brain suggests that this particular PG may play an important role in containing the size and/or shape of the forming plaque.

INTRODUCTION

Previous studies have identified a specific group of complex, anionic macromolecules known as proteoglycans (PGs), specifically localized to the amyloid deposits in both NPs and in the wall of blood vessels (1-3). The particular class of PG present in the amyloid deposits of these lesions have been identified by immunocytochemistry as a basement membrane derived heparan sulfate proteoglycan (HSPG) (3). Although HSPG core protein was not immunolocalized to NFTs, histochemical studies (1,2) suggested that PGs were also associated with the paired helical and straight filaments of NFTs. However, the major types of PGs/GAGs within NFTs have not been identified. In the present investigation, a polyclonal antibody primarily recognizing the small dermatan sulfate proteoglycan (DSPG), known as decorin (4-6), was identified as a new component uniquely associated with the amyloid deposits of NPs and the filamentous structures within NFTs.

MATERIALS AND METHODS

An affinity-purified polyclonal antibody to the protein core of the DSPG (decorin) of human fibroblasts (4) was used to determine the localization of this molecule in 8 cases of AD. Congo red staining was used on adjacent serial sections to detect NPs, NFTs and congophilic angiopathy in each of the cases. Additionally, antibodies raised to the beta-amyloid protein (BAP)(7) or against residues 1-42 of the BAP identified amyloid deposits in NPs and congophilic angiopathy. Detection of the core protein of decorin in 1 micron deplasticized sections of AD brain tissue was accomplished according to the avidin-biotin-immunoperoxidase method (8). Immunogold labelling employing the DSPG core protein antibody enabled its localization in NPs and NFTs at the ultrastructural level.

RESULTS

Decorin immunostaining was demonstrated in 1 micron deplasticized sections and at the ultrastructural level in AD hippocampus, specifically localized to amyloid plaques, NFTs and collagen fibrils in blood vessels. At the ultrastructural level, immunogold labelling for decorin was only evident after removal of epon from ultrathin sections prior to colloidal gold immunostaining (9) indicating that interference due to the presence of resin occurred. Non-neuritic star-shaped amyloid plaques contained both a central core region and periphery. Decorin was primarily localized to the periphery of the amyloid plaque as a whole, and to the edges of amyloid bundles in the periphery region (Fig. 1A). Less positive immunogold labelling for decorin was found in the center of amyloid plaques, in comparison to the periphery. As a negative control, the adjacent serial thin section from Fig. 1A was immunostained with a polyclonal antibody to the AA amyloid protein. Little immunogold labelling was observed in both the periphery and center of the identical amyloid plaque. Collagen fibrils present in the adventitia of arterioles in the brain parenchyma also demonstrated positive immunogold labelling of decorin. The localization of decorin to collagen fibrils served as a positive internal control since previous studies demonstrated a close association of decorin with collagen fibrils (10).

Decorin was also immunolocalized to extraneuronal and intraneuronal NFTs in AD brain at the ultrastructural level. Immunogold labelling for decorin was primarily associated with bundles of both paired helical and straight filaments in NFTs (Fig. 1B), correlating with decorin immunostaining of NFTs in 1 u deplasticized sections. Little to no immunogold labelling of paired helical and straight filaments of NFTs was found when the adjacent serial section from Fig. 1B was immunolabelled with a polyclonal antibody against the AA amyloid protein.

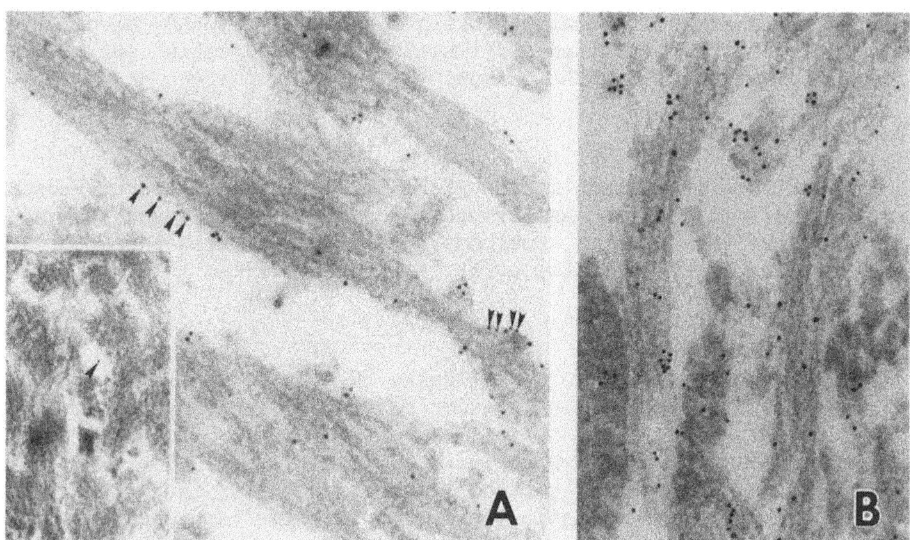

Fig. 1A: Immunogold labelling of decorin in the periphery of an amyloid plaque primary localized to the edges of amyloid bundles (arrowheads). Inset shows lack of immunogold labelling (arrowhead) of plaque periphery with a polyclonal antibody to the AA amyloid protein
Fig. 1B: Immunogold localization of decorin to paired helical and straight filaments in a NFT in AD brain.

DISCUSSION

The major finding of the present study was the immunolocalization of the small DSPG core protein (known as decorin) as a newly identified component within the amyloid plaques and NFTs in AD brain. Unlike HSPG core protein, previously shown to be evenly distributed throughout NPs containing amyloid fibrils (3), decorin was primarily localized to the periphery of the amyloid plaque, as a whole, and to the edges of amyloid fibril bundles within this plaque periphery. The lack of decorin immunostaining in the centre of amyloid plaques may be due to masking of the antigen by other components. However, this seems unlikely since no particular protein or macromolecule has been found preferentially localized to the centre of amyloid plaques.

Currently, it is not known why amyloid plaques are generally spherically shaped and are confined to a certain size (generally 15 microns in diameter) within the AD (Down's syndrome and normal aging) brain. The unique and specific localization of decorin to the periphery of the amyloid plaque suggests that these molecules may contribute to containing the size of amyloid accumulation within the cores of NPs and/or in maintaining their spherical shape. A somewhat analogous situation has been described in collagen, where decorin has been implicated in influencing collagen fibril formation and the ultimate diameter of collagen fibrils formed (11). In AD, decorin may similarly play a role by controlling the size and extent of amyloid fibril formation within the plaque.

Acknowledgements

This work was supported by the Alzheimer's Disease Research Program of the American Health Assistance Foundation. We thank Dr. Hans Kresse for the decorin antibody, Dr. Dennis Selkoe for the BAP antibody and Dr. Robert Kisilevsky for the AA amyloid antibody.

References

1. Snow, A.D., Willmer, J., Kisilevsky, R. (1987) 'Sulfated glycosaminoglycans in Alzheimer's disease', Lab Invest, 18, 506-510.
2. Snow, A.D., Lara, S., Nochlin, D., Wight, T.N. (1989) 'Cationic dyes reveal proteoglycans structurally integrated within the characteristic lesions of Alzheimer's disease', Acta Neuropath, 78, 113-123.
3. Snow, A.D., Mar, H., Nochlin, D., Kimata, K., Kato, M., Suzuki, S., Hassell, J., Wight, T.N. (1988) 'The presence of heparan sulfate proteoglycans in the neuritic plaques and congophilic angiopathy in Alzheimer's disease', Am J Path, 133, 456-463.
4. Glossl, J., Beck, M., Kresse, H. (1984) 'Biosynthesis of proteodermatan sulfate in cultured human fibroblasts', J Biol Chem, 259, 14144-14150.
5. Fisher, L.W., Termine, J.D., Dejter, S.W. Jr., Whitson, S.W., Yanagishita, M., Kumura, J.H., Hascall, V.C., Kleinman, H.K., Hassell, J.R., Nilsson, B. (1983) 'Proteoglycans of developing bone', J Biol Chem, 258, 6588-6594.
6. Day, A.A., McQuillan, C.I., Termine, J.D., Young, M.R. (1987) 'Molecular cloning and sequence analysis of the cDNA for small proteoglycan II of bovine bone', Biochem J, 248, 801-805.
7. Selkoe, D.J., Abraham, C.R., Podlisny, M.B., Duffy, L.K. (1986) 'Isolation of low-molecular-weight proteins from amyloid plaque fibers in alzheimer's disease', J Neurochem, 46, 1820-1834.
8. Snow, A.D., Mar, H., Nochlin, D., Wight, T.N. (1990) 'Congo red staining on 1 micron de-plasticized sections for the detection of lesions in alzheimer's disease and related orders', in K. Iqbal, H. Wisniewski and B. Winblad (eds.), Alzheimer's Disease and Related Disorders, Alan R. Liss Inc., New York, pp. 383-391.
9. Mar, H., Wight, T.N. (1988) 'Colloidal gold immunostaining on deplasticized ultra-thin sections', J Histochem Cytochem, 36, 1387-1395.
10. Scott, J.E., Orford, C.R. (1981) 'Dermatan sulphate-rich proteoglycan associates with rat tail-tendon collagen at the d band in the gap region', Biochem J, 197, 213-216.
11. Scott, J.E. (1988) 'Proteoglycan-fibrillar collagen interactions', Biochem J, 252, 313-323.

CHOROID PLEXUS AMYLOID

L. Eriksson and P. Westermark
Department of Pathology, University of Uppsala and
Department of Pathology, University of Linköping, Sweden

ABSTRACT. Intracellular inclusions with staining properties of amyloid have long been known to occur in the choroid plexus epithelial cells. These inclusions are very common in choroid plexus of aging persons. Morphologically the inclusions show some similarities with the neurofibrillary tangles found in cortical neurons from patients with Alzheimer type of dementia. However, immunochemical characterization of the inclusions reveals that they are different from the neurofibrillary tangles and represent an unique form of intracellular amyloid.

INTRODUCTION

Threadlike structures, demonstrable by silver impregnation, have long been observed in the choroid plexus epithelial cells. These structures occur in two different forms, one that is needle-shaped or crystal-like and one ring-form called the Biondi-ring (1).

These inclusions have been shown to bind to Congo red with green birefringence in polarized light (2) and to have a fine fibrillar ultrastructure (3,4). The inclusions may therefore be regarded as a form of amyloid although a cross ß-pleated conformation has not yet been shown.

We present here purification and morphological characterization of the choroid plexus amyloid (CPA) (5,6).

MATERIAL AND METHODS

The choroid plexus material was obtained at autopsy. For light microscopy, material was immediately fixed in 4% formaldehyde solution. Electron microscopy was performed on material fixed in 2% glutaraldehyde. For immunocytochemistry at the EM-level, material was fixed in 4% paraformaldehyde/0.5% glutaraldehyde and embeded in Lowicryl K4M (7).

The amyloid was purified by homogenizing the choroid plexuses in a Tris-Triton buffer and treatment with collagenase A from Clostridium histiolyticum, 1M acetic acid, and pepsin (6).

A rabbit antiserum to CPA was obtained by subcutaneous injections bimonthly of purified CPA. The preparation was solubilized in 100% formic acid and mixed with Freund's adjuvant. Antisera to other amyloid proteins were also used. Antisera to microtubule-associated protein Tau and SDS-isolated paired helical filaments were a kind gift from Dr DJ Selkoe, Boston.

RESULTS

Morphology: In light microscopy, two different forms of congophilic inclusions were identified. The most common form was needle-shaped, but in some cases, ring-formed inclusions occurred in large amounts.

In material from 250 patients, intracellular choroid plexus amyloid was found in all patients over 60 years of age, and there was a tendency for more pronounced amyloid deposits with increasing age (Table 1).

TABLE 1 Occurence of amyloid inclusions in Tris-Triton smear from choroid plexus in different age-groups.

	GRADE				
AGE	0	1	2	3	N
- 9	2				2
10-19	4				4
20-29	11				11
30-39	12	2			14
40-49	6	4	3		13
50-59	2	3	8	2	15
60-69		5	20	14	39
70-79		1	47	25	73
80-89		4	41	23	68
90 -		1	8	2	11
Total	37	20	127	66	250

Grade 0 - No amyloid inclusions found
Grade 1 - Amyloid inclusions represent less than 1% of the material
Grade 2 - Amyloid inclusions represent 1-50% of the material
Grade 3 - Amyloid inclusions represent more than 50% of the material

Ultrastructurally, the inclusions consist of bundles of parallel fibrils of about 20 nm thickness. Apparently they were built up by two filaments twisted around one another. Often, the bundles were limited by a membrane and intermingled with lipid droplets. Scanning EM and transmission EM of sectioned material of the ring-form showed that in reality they are imperfect spherical bodies with a thin rim of fine fibrils and a large central core, probably consisting of lipid.

Immunology: Rabbit antiserum to CPA showed a specific reaction with the amyloid fibrils. This antiserum also labelled the choroid plexus inclusions specifically in immunogold preparations of EM sections. It did not react with amyloid of other types.

This antiserum did not react with neurofibrillary tangles, amyloid core of senile plaques or amyloid in congophilic angiopathy from patients with Alzheimer-type of dementia. It did not react with intracellular amyloid inclusions in the adrenal cortex.

No reaction in the choroid plexus amyloid could be seen when antisera or antibodies against ATTR, AA, AL, Cystatin-C (a kind gift from Dr. A Grubb, Lund, Sweden), microtubule-associated protein Tau, or SDS-isolated paired helical filaments were used. Antiserum against TTR gave a reaction with all choroid plexus epithelial cells irrespective of the occurrence of amyloid.

Biochemistry: Biochemical analysis was performed on purified CPA. The purification method resulted in a preparation rich in amyloid. SDS-PAGE revealed two zones corresponding to about 40-50 kDa and less than 10 kDa. In western blot analysis the antiserum to CPA reacted only with material between 40-50 kDa.

DISCUSSION

Intracellular inclusions with properties of amyloid have been described in nerve cells (8-9), adrenal cortical cells (10) and choroid plexus epithelial cells (11). Our study indicates that CPA is not identical with the other intracellular amyloids since its morphological appearance is unique. It is also immunologically different, as no immunological cross-reactivity were demonstrated between our antiserum to CPA and antisera or antibodies to different epitopes in neurofibrillary tangles.

A unique feature was the close contact between fibrils and large structures resembling residual bodies. Such structures seem to be the explanation of the ring-forms (Biondi rings). Ringforms of neurofibrillary tangles in cortical neurons occur but are rare.

Neurofibrillary tangles are one of the main pathological findings in Alzheimer dementia and are thought to indicate cell injury (12). Whether the CPA is associated with any specific neurological disease or with cellular dysfunction is not known.

ACKNOWLEDGEMENTS

Supported by the Swedish Medical Research Council and the Research Fund of King Gustaf V.

REFERENCES

1. Biondi, G. (1934) 'Zur Histopathologie des menschlichen Plexus choroideus und des Ependyms', Arch. Psychiatr. Nervekrankn. 101,666-728.

2. Divry, P. (1955) 'De la nature des formations argentophiles des plexus choroideus', Acta Neurol. Psychiatr. Belgica 55,282-293.
3. Dohrmann, GJ., Bucy, PC. (1970) 'Human choroid plexus: a light and electron microscopic study', J. Neurosurg. 33,506-516.
4. Bargmann, W., Katrisis, E. (1966) 'Über die sog. Filamente und das Pigment im Plexus choroideus des Menschen', Z. Zellforsch. Mikrosk. Anat. 75,366-370.
5. Eriksson, L., Westermark, P. (1986) 'Intracellular neurofibrillary tangle-like aggregations . A constantly present amyloid alteration in the aging choroid plexus', Am. J. Pathol. 125,124-129.
6. Eriksson, L., Westermark, P. (In press) 'Characterization of intracellular amyloid fibrils in the human choroid plexus epithelial cells', Acta Neuropathol.
7. Carlemalm, E., Villiger, W., Hobot, JA., Acetarin, JD., and Kallenberger, E. (1985) 'Low temperature embedding with Lowicryl resin: two new formulations and some applications', J. Microsc. 140,55-63.
8. Kawasaki, H., Murayama, S., Tomonaga, M., Izumiyama, N., and Shimada, H. (1987) 'Neurofibrillary tangles in human upper cervical ganglia'. Acta Neuropathol. 75:156-159.
9. Kirschner, DA., Abraham, C., Selkoe, DJ. (1986) 'X-ray diffraction from intraneuronal paired helical filaments extraneuronal amyloid fibers in Alzheimer disease indicate cross-ß conformation' Proc. Natl. Acad. Sci. USA 83:503-507.
10. Eriksson, L., Westermark, P. (1990) 'Age-related accumulation of amyloid inclusions in adrenal cortical cells' Am J Pathol136:461-466
11. Kidd, M. (1963) 'Paired helical filaments in electron microscopy in Alzheimer's disease', Nature 197,192-193.

NEW IMAGES OF CLINICAL AMYLOIDOSIS

M.B. PEPYS
Immunological Medicine Unit, Department of Medicine
Royal Postgraduate Medical School, Hammersmith Hospital
London W12 0NN
U.K.

ABSTRACT. Serum amyloid P component (SAP) is a normal plasma protein which is the precursor of amyloid P component (AP), present in all known forms of systemic and local amyloidosis. We have devised procedures for use of radiolabelled SAP as a specific tracer for amyloid deposits in man. These approaches have elucidated the normal metabolism of SAP and its pathophysiology in amyloidosis, demonstrating in particular the rapid normal catabolism of SAP in the plasma and the remarkable persistence of SAP molecules which have localised in amyloid deposits. We have investigated 111 patients with histologically confirmed amyloid, 30 more with amyloid identified by SAP tracer studies, 65 patient controls with diseases predisposing to amyloidosis, 8 patients with other diseases, and 14 healthy normal controls; 19 amyloid patients have undergone 1-3 repeat studies. The results show conclusively that labelled SAP is a safe, non-invasive and effective tool for *in vivo* diagnosis, localisation, quantification and monitoring of amyloidosis. It provides clinically important information which is not otherwise available, makes a valuable contribution to patient management and should assist in the assessment of existing and novel treatments for amyloidosis.

1. DIAGNOSIS OF AMYLOIDOSIS

Amyloidosis is a histological diagnosis which depends on the pathognomonic green birefringence of amyloid-containing tissue stained with Congo red and viewed under polarised light. When amyloid is suspected the classical approach is to biopsy an accessible site, such as the rectum or subcutaneous fat. If amyloid is not detected these biopsies may be repeated or biopsies taken from clinically affected sites such as kidney, liver, heart, peripheral nerve, salivary glands, etc. A positive specimen will eventually be found in nearly all patients with systemic amyloidosis. However, there is also a classical clinical situation in which amyloidosis is not suspected and biopsy is not performed. Amyloid may then be missed completely or it may be discovered incidentally when biopsy or resection is performed in the course of other investigative or therapeutic procedures. Often, amyloid is discovered only at autopsy.

Successful biopsy diagnosis of amyloidosis depends on sufficient clinical awareness to initiate the procedure, on an adequate tissue sample, and on correct staining and interpretation. Although subcutaneous fat biopsy is safe, biopsies of other sites carry varying but not insignificant risks, especially of haemorrhage. Biopsy specimens are extremely small and sample only a minute proportion of the tissue or organ involved; they cannot provide quantitative assessment of amyloid deposition even in the biopsied organ, let alone other sites.

Referral centres with experience of amyloidosis are aware of these problems and overcome many of them. However, this is often not the case elsewhere. Among the last 87 consecutive referrals with systemic amyloidosis from other hospitals to the Royal Postgraduate Medical School, Hammersmith Hospital, which is a tertiary referral centre, rectal biopsies had already been performed in 47 cases but 50% had been reported as negative. In 5 other cases there were false positive reports, whilst among 31 patients who had undergone renal biopsy elsewhere 2 had suffered life-threatening complications. Of 5 patients with suspected cardiac amyloidosis there were false positive reports on endomyocardial biopsies in 2 cases and equivocal or false negative reports in 3.

The prompt and safe diagnosis or exclusion of amyloidosis in thus not, in practice, a straightforward matter. Furthermore, the limited information available from biopsies means that most of the central questions about the natural history of amyloidosis in man remain unanswered. We do not know why amyloid fibrils persist, what is their rate of deposition, whether amyloid deposits turn over or whether in general they can regress, and most importantly whether treatments are effective in promoting regression of amyloid *per se* rather than affecting organ function. Apart from their academic interest these questions are of practical importance. Cytotoxic anti-inflammatory treatment of rheumatoid arthritis and juvenile chronic arthritis can halt progression of AA amyloid occurring as a complication of those disorders and greatly improve life expectancy. Cytotoxic therapy of AL amyloidosis may also be beneficial in a minority of cases, whilst renal transplantation alleviates the symptoms of haemodialysis-associated amyloidosis. Heart transplantation for cardiac amyloidosis has been successful in the few cases attempted so far, and liver transplantation in familial amyloid polyneuropathy has recently been attempted. Availability of a safe and effective method for rapidly diagnosing or excluding the presence of amyloid, and for localising, quantifying and monitoring it, should thus make an important contribution to basic knowledge and clinical management.

2. SERUM AMYLOID P COMPONENT AS A SPECIFIC TRACER IN AMYLOIDOSIS

2.1. Introduction

AP is present in all the different forms of amyloid. Although there was controversy about the intracortical senile plaques of Alzheimer's disease, failure to demonstrate AP there immunohistochemically was apparently due to loss of antigenicity in fixation [1].

In 1977 we discovered that SAP had the capacity for calcium-dependent binding to specific ligands and in 1979 showed that it bound to amyloid fibrils *in vitro* in this way. In 1984 we reported that circulating SAP was indeed the precursor of AP in amyloid deposits, and suggested that labelled SAP could be used as a specific targeting agent for amyloid deposits *in vivo* [2,3]. In mice with AA amyloidosis, radiolabelled SAP was demonstrated to localise specifically to amyloid deposits, to persist there and to permit gamma camera imaging *in vivo* [4,5].

Since 1987 we have developed this approach in man. SAP is isolated in sterile, pure form from the plasma of single accredited donors to the British National Blood Transfusion Service. This plasma is the most rigorously screened and safest material available and is heated at 56°C for 30 min before isolating the SAP. Each patient receives only about 100 μg compared to the 5-10 mg of SAP contained in a single unit of normal blood transfusion. For all these reasons, and the fact that no adverse effects have been seen in some 250 individuals studied over the past 3 years, we do not believe that there is any "risk" [6] associated with administration of this product.

SAP is oxidatively labelled with radioiodine: ^{123}I (T½ 13 hr) for gamma camera imaging, single photon emission computed tomography and short term metabolic studies; ^{124}I (T½ 4 days) for positron emission tomography; ^{125}I (T½ 6 weeks) and ^{131}I (T½ 1 week) for metabolic studies. The radiation dose involved in metabolic studies with 5 μCi of ^{125}I is minute whilst that from an imaging procedure with 5 mCi of ^{123}I, 4 mSv, is the same as a barium series or intravenous urogram. Detailed reports of the results of our studies are included in this volume and are published elsewhere [7-9].

2.2. Specificity

The specificity of deposition of labelled SAP in amyloid, established in mice, has been confirmed in man. In individuals without amyloid, SAP which has been injected intravenously is rapidly distributed in the blood volume and a small extravascular space, compatible with the high M_r of SAP, and is then cleared with T½ of about 24 hr. The SAP is catabolised and the iodinated products are promptly and completely excreted in the urine; there is no detectable retention within the body. In marked contrast, labelled SAP localises rapidly to amyloid deposits if they are present and is retained there for prolonged periods. The distribution of SAP to different sites occurs in proportion to the amount of amyloid present determined at autopsy.

2.3. Diagnostic information

Imaging and metabolic procedures with labelled SAP are particularly useful in patients in whom biopsies have been negative or have failed to yield suitable tissue. We have diagnosed amyloid before biopsy in 19 individuals and confirmed it in all 11 subjects subsequently biopsied. Imaging results in patients with histologically confirmed systemic amyloid are summarised in the Table. The extreme variability of severity and distribution of AL deposits at the time of diagnosis, which has long been recognised clinically, is elegantly confirmed by SAP-imaging. In some cases presenting with carpal tunnel syndrome only deposits in the carpal region were identified, whilst in 5 of the 7 AL patients with negative scans the only clinical abnormality was in the heart. The demonstration of cardiac amyloid is discussed below.

SAP imaging in biopsy proven amyloidosis

Type of amyloid	No of patients	Positive scans	Negative scans
AA	44	44	-
AL	41	37 (4 in carpal region only)	7 (5 with cardiac amyloid)
Familial amyloid polyneuropathy	5	4 (kidney, adrenal, spleen, liver, nerve)	1
Ostertag-type hereditary systemic amyloidosis	7	7	-
Cystatin C: Icelandic HCHWA	4	4 (speen, liver)	-

2.4. Distribution of amyloidosis

The relatively constant distribution of AA amyloidosis contrasts with the variability of AL amyloidosis [8, and this volume]. We have demonstrated, for the first time *in vivo*, major visceral deposits in cystatin C amyloidosis (hereditary cerebral haemorrhage with amyloidosis, Icelandic type) and confirmed their presence in familial amyloid polyneuropathy, type I. Amyloid has also been detected in otherwise inaccessible sites, such as adrenal and bone, when all other imaging procedures were normal. Half our patients with adrenal amyloid had impaired adrenal reserve function. No visceral deposits of amyloid were seen in 29 cases of haemodialysis-associated amyloid, although 1 individual studied serially over 2 years developed SAP uptake in the spleen. No redistribution of amyloid between different anatomical sites has been observed and there is a variable and poor correlation between the extent of amyloid deposition and the presence and severity of organ dysfunction. The liver and spleen may contain enormous quantities of amyloid without any sign of liver dysfunction or hyposplenism. This highlights the difficulty in monitoring progression of amyloidosis or its response to therapy by measuring the function of affected organs.

2.5. Quantification of amyloidosis

Whole body and regional amyloid deposits can be quantified by scintigraphy using ^{123}I-SAP and by PET using ^{124}I-SAP. Measurements of plasma clearance, whole body retention and the extrapolated extravascular compartment give precise and highly reproducible quantitative information. This approach, using an extremely small dose of ^{125}I-SAP is simple, does not require an expensive scanner, and is ideal for serial monitoring.

2.6. Natural history of amyloidosis

Over the past 3 years we have been able to study *in vivo* in man for the first time, the natural history of amyloidosis *per se*, rather than its effects on organs and tissues. In most cases there has been inexorable progression but in a few patients, most encouragingly some rheumatoids treated with cytotoxic drugs, the deposits have apparently remained unchanged. Even more exciting is the evidence that in some individuals with juvenile chronic arthritis and AA amyloidosis treated over 10 years ago with chlorambucil, the amyloid deposits have resolved completely.

2.7. Disadvantages of SAP tracer studies

There are both theoretical and practical problems associated with material of human origin as an *in vivo* tracer, although there is no ethical or health risk associated with the present use of SAP. Radioiodine, especially ^{123}I, is expensive and not always universally available. Its short half-life is ideal for the present purpose but is a disadvantage for a routine product. Gamma cameras are widely available but PET scanners are not and ^{124}I is a rare and expensive isotope. The procedure for radioiodination of SAP is simple in expert hands but is an aspect of a sophisticated new test which may be unfamiliar in nuclear medicine departments.

^{123}I-SAP imaging has relatively low sensitivity for cardiac amyloid deposits and has failed so far to identify intracerebral amyloid. Problems with the heart are that it is motile and that it includes the blood pool with high activity from tracer which has not yet localised. Once unlocalised SAP has been eliminated most of the ^{123}I activity has decayed and low levels in cardiac deposits may not be imaged because of tissue attenuation effects. These difficulties have now been overcome by the use of ^{124}I-SAP and PET scanning, which gave convincing images in a patient with cardiac biopsy proven amyloidosis but no evidence of amyloid elsewhere in the body, in whom ^{123}I-SAP scanning had been negative. In patients with extensive visceral deposits as well as cardiac amyloid the labelled SAP distributes *pro rata* to the deposits. When the heart contains, for example, only 5% of the total amyloid and 5% of the total AP, it also attracts just 5% of the labelled tracer. This may not be detected by the gamma camera, although it is visible using ^{124}I-SAP and PET. In any event this is of little practical importance since diagnosis of systemic amyloidosis by SAP imaging effectively establishes the cause of the patient's cardiomyopathy.

Our studies on brain amyloid are preliminary and still in progress. The presence of AP, presumably derived from circulating SAP, in cerebral amyloid deposits suggests that with suitable labels and detecting technology our approach should also succeed here. However, there are limits of sensitivity, and microscopic deposits, to which only minute amounts of SAP can localise, may not be detectable by this method.

2.8. Advantages and future prospects

Labelled SAP as a specific tracer in amyloidosis is a safe, non-invasive, rapid and quantitative diagnostic tool which reveals clinically significant deposits throughout the body, including those in otherwise inaccessible sites and allows monitoring of progression and response to therapy. In the future more convenient radionuclides for labelling SAP should help to promote wider availability of the imaging procedures, although ^{125}I is ideal as a tracer label for metabolic studies. Elucidation of the three dimensional structure of SAP, currently in progress, should identify the ligand-binding region and may lead to superior synthetic or engineered tracer molecules. Finally our 1984 prediction of the possible use of SAP as a means to target to amyloid deposits molecules with therapeutic effects, remains valid and is strengthened by the specificity of SAP localisation and its remarkable persistence in the deposits.

REFERENCES

1. Kalaria, R.N. and Grahovac, I. (1990) Serum amyloid P immunoreactivity in hippocampal tangles, plaques and vessels: implications for leakage across the blood-brain barrier in Alzheimer's disease. *Brain Res.,* **516:** 349-353.
2. Baltz, M.L., Caspi, D., Rowe, I.F., Hind, C.R.K., Evans, D.J. and Pepys, M.B. (1986) Pathogenetic mechanisms and precursor product relationships in murine amyloidosis. ***In:*** *Amyloidosis* (Glenner, G.G., ed.), Plenum Publishing Corporation, New York, pp. 101-113.
3. Baltz, M.L., Caspi, D., Evans, D.J., Rowe, I.F., Hind, C.R.K. and Pepys, M.B. (1986) Circulating serum amyloid P component is the precursor of amyloid P component in tissue amyloid deposits. *Clin. Exp. Immunol.,* **66:** 691-700.
4. Caspi, D., Zalzman, S., Baratz, M., Teitelbaum, Z., Yaron, M., Pras, M., Baltz, M.L. and Pepys, M.B. (1987) Imaging of experimental amyloidosis with ^{131}I-labeled serum amyloid P component. *Arth. Rheum.,* **30:** 1303-1306.
5. Hawkins, P.N., Myers, M.J., Epenetos, A.A., Caspi, D. and Pepys, M.B. (1988) Specific localization and imaging of amyloid deposits *in vivo* using ^{123}I-labeled serum amyloid P component. *J. Exp. Med.,* **167:** 903-913.
6. Cohen, A.S. and Skinner, M. (1990) New frontiers in the study of amyloidosis (Editorial). *New Engl. J. Med.,* **323:** 542-543.
7. Hawkins, P.N., Myers, M.J., Lavender, J.P. and Pepys, M.B. (1988) Diagnostic radionuclide imaging of amyloid: biological targeting by circulating human serum amyloid P component. *Lancet* **i:** 1413-1418.
8. Hawkins, P.N., Lavender, P.J. and Pepys, M.B. (1990) Evaluation of systemic amyloidosis by scintigraphy with ^{123}I-labeled serum amyloid P component. *New Engl. J. Med.,* **323:** 508-513.
9. Hawkins, P.N., Wootton, R. and Pepys, M.B. (1990) Metabolic studies of radioiodinated serum amyloid P component in normal subjects and patients with systemic amyloidosis. *J. Clin. Invest.* (in press).

SCINTIGRAPHIC IMAGING OF AMYLOIDOSIS WITH ^{123}IODINE SERUM AMYLOID P COMPONENT

P.N. HAWKINS, J.P. LAVENDER & M.B. PEPYS
Immunological Medicine Unit, Department of Medicine
Royal Postgraduate Medical School, Hammersmith Hospital
London W12 0NN
U.K.

ABSTRACT. Purified human serum amyloid P component labelled with ^{123}I, given intravenously, localised rapidly, specifically and quantitatively to amyloid deposits. In contrast any ^{123}I-SAP which had not localised to amyloid was promptly eliminated from the body. This permitted characteristic scintigraphic images to be obtained in the gamma camera identifying the presence, distribution and extent of amyloid deposits in 50 patients with systemic amyloidosis (25 AA type, 25 AL type), compared to 26 disease controls and 10 normal healthy subjects. In AA amyloidosis the spleen was always involved whilst amyloid in the heart, skin, carpal region and bone marrow was seen only in the AL type; clinically silent adrenal amyloidosis occurred in both types. Positive images were seen in 6 patients in whom biopsies had either been negative or had failed, and the presence of amyloid was subsequently confirmed histologically in all cases either by further biopsy or at autopsy. Progressive amyloid deposition was observed in 9 out of 11 patients studied serially over 6-12 months. Scintigraphy after injection of ^{123}I-SAP allows specific diagnosis, localisation and monitoring of systemic amyloidosis, and can provide clinically important information which is not otherwise available.

1. INTRODUCTION

Knowledge of the distribution, progression and natural history of systemic amyloidosis has been limited by the fact it is a histological diagnosis. Serum amyloid P component (SAP) is a normal plasma protein which is deposited in all known types of amyloid [1,2], suggesting that it could be used as a specific targeting agent for amyloid deposits.

SAP binds specifically to amyloid fibrils *in vitro* [3] and also *in vivo* [4-7], where it is then retained in the tissue amyloid deposits for prolonged periods, apparently protected from the normal rapid catabolism to which it is subject in the plasma. The results of the present study of 50 patients with systemic AA and AL amyloidosis suggest that scintigraphy using ^{123}I-SAP can be used for the diagnosis, localisation and monitoring of systemic amyloidosis, and are reported in full elsewhere [8].

2. METHODS [8]

2.1. Preparation of Radiolabelled SAP

Sterile, 99% pure SAP was isolated from heated (56°C, 30 min) serum of a single accredited donor (UK National Blood Transfusion Service) and labelled with ^{123}I. Each lot was sterile, non-pyrogenic and retained full ligand binding reactivity.

2.2. Patients and Controls

The following individuals were studied: 1) 50 patients with systemic amyloid, 25 AA type, 25 AL; 2) 26 patient controls, 18 with chronic inflammatory diseases, 6 with monoclonal gammopathy and 2 patients with cardiomyopathy; 3) 10 healthy volunteers. Amyloid was not confirmed in 3 AA and 3 AL patients until after the scan. It was excluded in all controls. All subjects gave informed consent.

2.3. Imaging and Analysis of ^{123}I-SAP Clearance

Following thyroid blockade subjects received ^{123}I-SAP (200 MBq, 200 μg) by bolus i.v. injection. Whole body scans were obtained 30 min and 6, 24 and 48 hr later, and interpreted "blind". Radioactivity was counted in venous blood taken at intervals for 6 hr and in all urine passed for 48 hr after injection.

2.4. Autopsy Studies

The distribution of amyloid was established at autopsy by Congo red staining in 5 patients who died 2-52 weeks after ^{123}I-SAP study. In a further AL patient who died suddenly, shortly after 6 hr images had been obtained, the precise organ distribution of both ^{123}I-SAP and amyloid was determined, and the microscopic localisation of ^{123}I-SAP was determined by autoradiography.

3. RESULTS

In the 10 healthy volunteers and 26 disease controls ^{123}I-SAP remained confined to the blood pool and underwent rapid metabolism. The mean (SD) quantity of ^{123}I-SAP remaining in the plasma of normals at 6 hr was 74.5 (4.9)% and at 48 hr around 47% of the tracer had been excreted into the urine. In all amyloid patients, including 6 individuals in whom previous biopsies had been negative or not performed, there was rapid uptake of ^{123}I-SAP into one or more sites including the viscera, bone marrow and carpal regions producing characteristic scintigraphic images. Most amyloid patients showed significantly increased 6 hr plasma clearance and whole body retention of tracer corresponding to the proportion of injected SAP (up to 95%) which had localised to the amyloid. This correlated closely with clinical and/or subsequent pathological estimates of the quantity of amyloid present. The persistence of tracer sequestrated in the amyloid deposits indicated that ^{123}I-SAP in this site was degraded at a very much slower rate than that remaining in the circulation.

The specificity of localisation of ^{123}I-SAP to amyloid deposits was demonstrated at autopsy in 6 patients in whom the histological distribution of amyloid, and the previous *in vivo* images corresponded precisely. In the patient who died suddenly 8 hr after injection, the density of amyloid demonstrated histologically in different tissues corresponded exactly with the quantity of tracer present, and with the *in vivo* images. Autoradiography confirmed the microscopic co-distribution of radioactivity and amyloid.

Tracer localisation frequently occurred in sites for which there had been no previous clinical suspicion of amyloid deposition (Table 1), and for which no suggestive clinical or laboratory features could be detected following scintigraphy and in some sites was non-homogenous which may reflect patchy amyloid deposition.

Serial studies were performed at intervals of 6-12 months. In 3 normals, SAP turnover values were within 1% of the original results. In 2 AA and 3 AL patients with clinical evidence of increased amyloid deposition, the images in the second study were more intense with a higher target:background ratio (Fig. 1).

Table 1. Organ distribution of ^{123}I-SAP in patients with systemic AA and AL amyloidosis

	AA		AL	
Spleen	25	(100%)	18	(72%)
Liver	8	(32%)	15	(60%)
Kidneys	19	(76%)	5	(20%)
Adrenals	6	(24%)	1	(4%)
Carpal region	0/7		4/18	(22%)
Bone marrow	0		5	(20%)
Skin	0		2	(8%)
Patients studied	25		25	

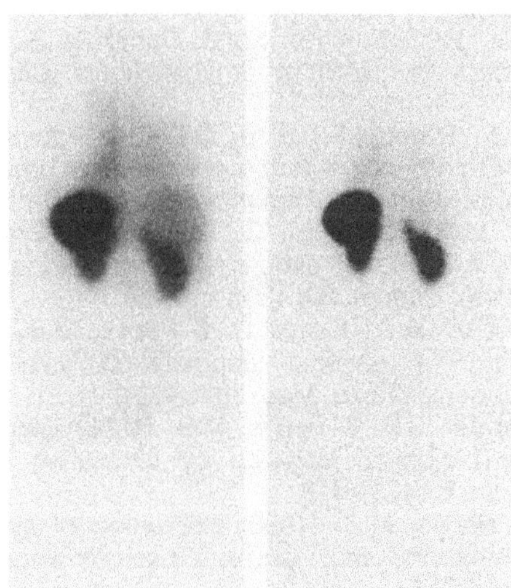

Figure 1. Serial ^{123}I-SAP scans in systemic AA amyloidosis. Posterior whole body images at 24 hr at presentation (left) and 12 months later (right). The proportion of tracer taken up into the splenic, renal and adrenal amyloid deposits is greater in the second study resulting in a greater target:background ratio.

In each case early plasma clearance and whole body retention of ^{123}I-SAP were significantly increased. Among a further 3 AA and 3 AL patients showing no measurable clinical change, scanning and turnover results indicated increased SAP deposition in 1 AA and 3 AL cases, and no change in the remainder.

4. DISCUSSION

These studies demonstrate that the uptake and retention of ^{123}I-labelled SAP in amyloid deposits provides a highly specific targeting mechanism permitting high quality scintigraphic images of amyloid to be obtained *in vivo*. The quantity of labelled SAP in each tissue correlated with the amount of amyloid present.

In most amyloid patients, early plasma clearance and whole body retention of ^{123}I-SAP were significantly greater than in controls. Serial SAP turnover studies in normals were notably stable, but 9 of 11 amyloid patients re-tested after 6-12 months showed significantly increased clearance and retention, and had correspondingly enhanced scintigraphic images, even though 4 of them had not deteriorated clinically. A gratifying absence of progression was observed in 2 patients with AA amyloid and rheumatic disease treated with cytotoxic drugs. The present method can thus be used to quantify amyloid deposition *per se* rather than the function of amyloid-laden organs. The use of labelled SAP as a targeting agent is non-invasive, safe and, on the basis of our present findings, it can confirm or exclude significant amyloidosis rapidly and easily.

REFERENCES

1. Pepys, M.B. (1988) Amyloidosis. ***In*** *Immunological Diseases, 4th ed.* (M. Samter, D.W. Talmage, M.M. Frank, K.F. Austen, & H.N. Claman, editors), Little Brown & Co., Boston, p. 631-674.
2. Coria, F., Castano, E., Prelli, F., Larrondo-Lillo, M., Van Duinen, S., Shelanski, M.L. & Frangione, B. (1988) Isolation and characterization of amyloid P component from Alzheimer's disease and other types of cerebral amyloidosis. *Lab. Invest.* **58:** 454-458.
3. Pepys, M.B., Dyck, R.F., de Beer, F.C., Skinner, M. & Cohen, A.S. (1979) Binding of serum amyloid P component (SAP) by amyloid fibrils. *Clin. Exp. Immunol.* **38:** 284-293.
4. Baltz, M.L., Caspi, D., Evans, D.J., Rowe, I.F., Hind, C.R.K. & Pepys, M.B. (1986) Circulating serum amyloid P component is the precursor of amyloid P component in tissue amyloid deposits. *Clin. Exp. Immunol.* **66:** 691-700.
5. Caspi, D., Zalzman, S., Baratz, M., Teitelbaum, Z., Yaron, M., Pras, M., Baltz, M.L. & Pepys, M.B. (1987) Imaging of experimental amyloidosis with ^{131}I-serum amyloid P component. *Arth. Rheum.* **30:** 1303-1306.
6. Hawkins, P.N., Myers, M.J., Epenetos, A.A., Caspi, D. & Pepys, M.B. (1988) Specific localization and imaging of amyloid deposits *in vivo* using ^{123}I-labeled serum amyloid P component. *J. Exp. Med.* **167:** 903-913.
7. Hawkins, P.N., Myers, M.J., Lavender, J.P. & Pepys, M.B. (1988) Diagnostic radionuclide imaging of amyloid: biological targeting by circulating human serum amyloid P component. *Lancet.* **i:** 1413-1418.
8. Hawkins, P.N., Lavender, P.J. & Pepys, M.B. (1990) Evaluation of systemic AA and AL amyloidosis by scintigraphy with iodine-123-serum amyloid P component. *New Engl. J. Med.* **323:** 508-513.

LONGTIME FOLLOW UP OF PATIENTS WITH AL-AMYLOIDOSIS WITH MRI

Benson L, Thuomas KA, Westermark P. and Wibell L.
Departments of Internal Medicine and Diagnostic Radiology, University Hospital, Uppsala,
Department of Pathology, University Hospital, Linkoping, SWEDEN.

We have previously reported prolonged longitudional relaxations time (T1) in heart, liver and fat in patients with AL-amyloidosis, and suggested magnetic resonance imaging (MRI) as a possible method to evaluate the amount of amyloid deposition (1). After chemotherapy patients have now been followed for 20-60 month.

PATIENTS AND METHODS

Five patients with AL-amyloidosis have undergone regular examinations with MRI every 3-6 month. The diagnosis of systemic amyloidosis was achieved by subcutaneous fine needle biopsy, and the amyloid was classified in all patients from extracts made of subcutaneous fat (2). MRI was carried out with a superconductive 0.5 T equipment (Magnetom, Siemens). Spin echo (SE) sequences with the following repetion time (TR) and echo time were used: TR 500 ms; TE 35/70 ms and TR 1500 ms, TE 120/35 ms. Examination were made in the axial plane with slice thickness of 10 mm. Matrix size was 256 x 256.

PRELIMINARY RESULTS

In all patients T1-relaxation time changed over time after treatment was started, and has returned into normal range in four patients. Two of these patients have been follow for 60 month and are well; one patient survived 20 month, and therapy was just started in one patient observed for 6 month. A change in T1 was seen in a patient surviving 24 month. T2 values were within normal range in liver and fat tissue. In healthy individuals and patients with neurological diseases acting as controls T1 and T2 in liver and fat did not change over time.

DISCUSSION

In physics relaxation is a term used to describe a process which brings a system back to equilibrium after the system has been interfered with. At the site of the nucleus, relaxation is caused by time dependent magnetic fields, which arise from random thermal motion as local magnetic fields, diffusing spins, fields of unpaired electrons, molecular rotation and changes in chemical shielding. The main cause of relaxation of protons is the magnetic coupling between two protons. There is an intramolecular contribution due to rotation of the other protons of the same water molecule and intermolecular contribution caused by to translational motion of neighboring water molecules. In a magnetic field protons will orient themselves in the direction of the magnetic field. A pulse of energy - in this case a radiosignal - will flip the protons out of their orientation and afterwards they will return to their position.

Relaxation of a spin or spin system is characterized by relaxation times T1 and T2. The spin-lattice relaxation time or T1 describes the thermal energy absorbed to the surrounding tissues. The spin-spin relaxation time or T2 gives the redistribution of the absorbed energy among the spins in the spin system. In water and other liquids the main source of relaxation is rotational and diffusional motions, dominated by Browninan motions of molecules. Prolonged T1-relaxation time is found in water, where many protons easily can move. T2 can be used to evaluate oedema.

Tissues are mixtures of a large variety of biological components. A simplified model is mostly accepted for the interpretation of data from biological tissues (3). This model comprises a phase of free (bulk) water in exchange with bound water. In fat T1 is short and in body fluids long T1 relaxation time is observed.

Extra-cellular deposition of protein changes not only the amount of water in the extracellular space but also how watermolecules are bound. Proton movement is influenced by the amount of protein and its structure. A prolonged T1-relaxation time in liver and fat tissue probably reflects rearrangement of watermoleculs indicating the deposition of amyloid fibrils in tissue. A change in T1-value associated with clinical improvement may therefore indicate restructuring or dissolving of amyloid fibrils in the extracellular space. Theoretically very high amount of amyloid fibrils would not allow movement of protons and therefore short T1-value could be anticipated. Further studies are needed to address this problem.

REFERENCES

1. Benson L, Hemmingsson A, Ericsson A, Jung B, Sperber G, Thoumas KA, Westermark P.
Magnetic resonance imagining in primary amyloidosis.
Acta Radiologica, 28:13:1986.

2. Westermark P, Benson L, Olofsson BO.
Fine needle aspiration biopsy of abdominal subcutaneous fat tissue for the diagnosis and typing of amyloidosis. In Amyloidosis, Eds Glenner GC,Osserman EF, Benditt EP et al,
Pergamon Press N.Y., 613-615, 1986.

3. Mansfield P and Morris P.G. NMR imaging in Biomedicine, in Advances in magnetic resonance, Supp 2, Ed J.S. Waugh, Academic Press, N.Y.,1982.

DETECTION OF AUTONOMIC DYSFUNCTIONS IN PATIENTS WITH FAMILIAL AMYLOIDOTIC POLYNEUROPATHY (FAP) BY LASER DOPPLER METHOD

Yukio Ando, M.D., Shukuro Araki, M.D., *Osamu Shimoda, M.D., Shinichi Ikegawa, M.D. and *Tatsuhiko Kano, M.D.
The First Department of Internal Medicine and *Surgical Center, Kumamoto University Medical School, 1-1-1 Honjo, Kumamoto 860, Japan

ABSTRACT. Laser Doppler flowmetry (LDF) examination was conducted in 11 FAP patients, 3 asymptomatic carriers of FAP and 29 normal controls. The vasoconstrictive responses induced by deep inspiration in the 11 FAP patients were markedly depressed, compared with those in healthy volunteers. In the 7 patients advanced to the stages 2 (moderate) to 4 (terminal), the responses were not elicited at all. To our interest, the vasoconstrictive responses following deep inspiration were also depressed in two of the 3 asymptomatic carriers of FAP, who had normal sensory nerve conduction velocity. Some patients with other diseases, such as Shy-Drager disease and pandysautonomia, also failed to exhibit the decrease of blood flow for various stimulations. Thus, these data suggest that the autonomic nervous system, especially the sympathetic vasomotor nerve regulating peripheral circulation, might be affected prior to the somatic polyneuropathy in FAP patients.

INTRODUCTION

Pathologically, amyloid deposition is found in peripheral and autonomic nerves as well as other organs except for central nervous system [1]. In addition to sensory dominant polyneuropathy, very serious complaints of FAP patients reflect disordered autonomic nerve functions, such as alternating diarrhea and constipation, orthostatic hypotension, and urinary retention [1]. The symptoms of FAP started in between 20 and 45 years of age in 69 individuals from 7 pedigrees in Kumamoto district, Japan. However, it is not known as yet when autonomic dysfunctions start in FAP patients. Although there are several tests for autonomic functions, we have had no proper tools to detect and evaluate dysfunctions autonomic nerves noninvasively and quantatively.

Laser Doppler flowmetry (LDF) technique developed recently by Bonner et al [2] has made it possible to monitor regional blood flow noninvasively with real time. Kano et al [3] recognized three different components in the LDF waves recorded from the pulp of the finger or the toe. From the studies used for neural blockade or anesthesia, they have demonstrated that the reflex wave, one of the three components and a transient marked decrease in blood flow following by a deep inspiration or various sensory stimuli, reflected phasic sympathetic activities regulating vasomotion on the skin.

We have applied for the first time this Laser Doppler method for FAP patients to detect the peripheral autonomic nerves dysfunction.

SUBJECTS AND METHODS

Patients

Eleven FAP patients and 3 asymptomatic carriers of FAP included in the study had a definite diagnosis of FAP based upon clinical findings, amyloid deposition in biopsied materials and genetic investigations (11 FAP patients; 4 females and 7 males, 27-59 years of age). Three individuals with asymptomatic FAP, carring a variant TTR (Met30), were a female and 2 males, 18-24 years of age. FAP patients were divided in 4 groups as the progression of the disease. Stage 1 (initial), sensory impairment limited in lower limbs with almost normal life; Stage 2 (moderate), sensory impairments in four limbs with limited daily activity; Stage 3 (marked), home stay life with supports; Stage 4 (terminal), bed ridden [1]. Twenty-nine age matched healthy volunteers were selected as normal controls to monitor their LDF.

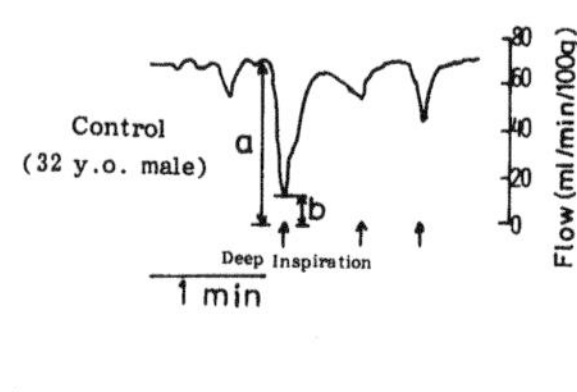

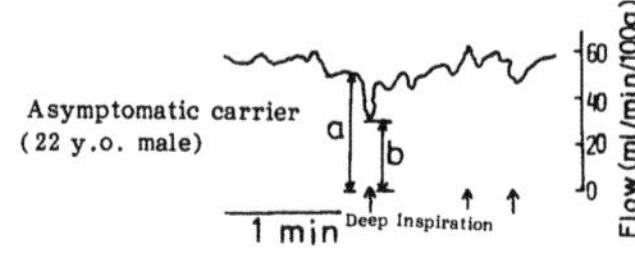

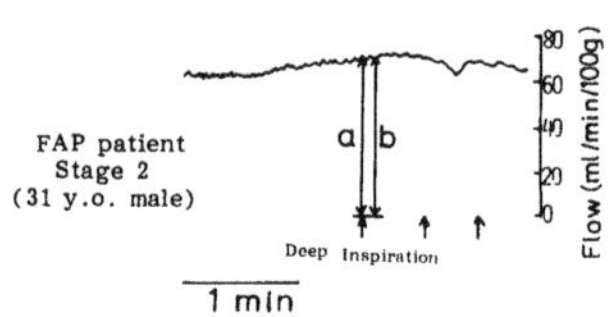

Fig. 1. Changes of peripheral blood flow after deep inspiration.

The arrow indicates the deep inspiration. A: Normal responses in a healthy volunteer (32 y.o., male), B: moderately depressed responses in an asymptomatic carrier without any clinical manifestations (22 y.o., male), C: marked depressed responses in an FAP patient at stage 2 (31 y.o., male). a: Baseline level of the blood flow, b: maximamly reduced level after deep inspiration.

Method to monitor the LDF

The blood flow was measured by using laser Doppler flowmeter (Advance Model ALF2100). A probe for LDF was attached to the pulp of the second finger and the vasoconstrictive response induced by deep inspiration was quantatively evaluated.

RESULTS

To analyze the functional vasoconstrictive changes of autonomic nerves in the peripheral tissues, laser Doppler flowmetry (LDF) examination was conducted in 11 symptomatic patients and 3 asymptomatic carriers of FAP (Fig. 1). The vasoconstrictive responses induced by deep inspiration in the 11 patients manifesting the FAP symptoms were markedly depressed (75.6±6.1% of blood flow), compared with those in 29 healthy volunteers. Three FAP patients without any sensory disturbance of their upper limbs (stage 1) failed to show their normal responses. These vasoconstrictive responses diminished as the progression of FAP. In the 7 patients advanced to the stages 2 to 4, the responses were not induced at all. To our interest, the vasoconstrictive responses following deep inspiration were also depressed in two of the 3 asymptomatic carriers of FAP with normal sensory nerve conduction velocity (Table 1). These depression was also confirmed by other stimulations such as standing, Aschner test and hearing large sound. The patients with spino cerebellar degeneration also failed to exhibit the decrease of blood flow for various stimulations.

Stage	Name	Age	Sex	Variant TTR	Decreased blood Flow (%)	SCV
Normal (n=29)		28.9±6.2		-	75.8±6.1	
Asymptomatic carrier	K.H.	18	F	+	59.4	62.5
	O.H.	22	M	+	54.1	58.3
	T.H.	24	M	+	72.3	62.1
FAP Stage 1	H.F.	35	M	+	17.2	
	U.S.	34	M	+	12.0	48.2
	K.M.	29	F	+	-	44.9
Stage 2	T.T.	34	M	+	9.9	
	M.S.	36	F	+	-	45.1
	H.T.	27	M	+	-	
	H.M.	31	M	+	-	38.1
Stage 3	K.N.	42	M	+	-	34.3
	S.H.	41	M	+	-	
	M.K.	59	F	+	-	
Stage 4	J.S.	41	F	+	-	

Table 1. Percent decrease of peripheral blood flow in FAP patients and asymptomatic carriers after loading deep inspiration.

The response reduction was calculated with the following formula; ((a-b)/a x 100 (a: baseline level of the blood flow, b: maximamly reduced level after deep inspiration)). -: no detectable responses for deep inspiration.

DISCUSSION

The present study has demonstrated that autonomic nervous system, especially the sympathetic vasomotor nerve regulating peripheral circulation, was affected prior to the somatic polyneuropathy in all FAP patients. In addition to their amyloid deposition to the peripheral nerves, other factor(s) has been extensively discussed as the pathogenesis of polyneuropathy of FAP [4]. For example, disorders of the vessels in and around the peripheral nerves might play an important role to induce polyneuropathy of FAP [4]. However, direct evidence has been lacking because there has been no proper method for detecting peripheral autonomic dysfunctions around the vessels. Since laser Doppler flowmetry is non-invasive and sensitive method, minor changes of autonomic dysfunction can be detected and evaluated [3].

Recently, late onset cases of FAP have been focused in the attention. Clinical symptoms of these patients were slowly progressive and most of these cases showed mild autonomic dysfunction [5]. Moreover, it is well konwn that type II FAP patients whose amyloid deposition was also caused by the mutant transthyretin exhibit very mild autonomic disorders and the period from the onset to the

for evaluating autonomic dysfunctions in FAP patients during the progression of illness.

Our preliminary examination by frequency analysis of R-R interval of ECG [6] revealed that one asymptomatic carrier of FAP and all the patients examined in the early stage also showed lower coefficient of variation (CV) levels, indicating dysfunction of cardiac autonomic nerves, than those of control subjects. This disorder increases along with the progression of FAP. Analysis by newly developed capsule polyhydrograph, which can ditect trace amount of sweating, revealed that no responses were ditected in the patients with the early stage of FAP while control subjects showed sweating for various stimulations, such as culculation, thinking and deep inspiration. These findings were consistent with the result obtained by the laser Doppler method.

This might be the first report to have demonstrated that peripheral autonomic nerves dysfuction started prior to the sensory neuropathy in FAP patients. The data obtained from the LDF examination provide a useful tool to elucidate the degree of pathophysiology of FAP.

REFERENCES

1) Araki S, Kurihara T, Tawara S, Kuribayashi T. (1980) "Familial amyloidotic polyneuropathy in Japanese: Clinical, pathophysiological, biochemical and therapeutic studies", In Amyloid and Amyloidosis Eds. by Glenner GG, Costa PP and Freitas F. Excerpta Medica, pp67-77.
2) Bonner RF, Clem TR. (1981) "Laser-Doppler continuous real-time monitor of pulsatile and mean blood flow in tissue microcirculation. In Scattering techniques applied to supramolecular and non-equilibrium systems", Eds by Chen SH, Chu B, Nossal R. New York, Plenum Press, pp 685-701.
3) Kano T, Shimoda O, Yasumoto M, Tsutsumi R. (1987) "Component analysis of Laser Doppler blood flow waves from the skin", Igaku No Ayumi 143, 791-792.
4) Asbury AK, Johnson PC.(1980) "Pathology of peripheral nerve", In: Major problems in pathology. Ed by Bennington JL, W.B. Saunders Co., Philadelphya Vol 9, pp148.
5) Ikeda S, Koh C-S, Miyasaka M, Yanagisawa N, Tsukagoshi H. (1981) "Familial amyloidotic neuropathy with late onset and benign course", Clin Neurol 21, 135-142.
6) Campbell IW, Ewing DJ, Clarke BF. (1980) "Tests of cardiovascular reflex function in diabetic autonomic neuropathy", Horm Metab Res. Suppl 9, 61-67.

NON-INVASIVE IN VIVO DETECTION OF AB-AMYLOIDOSIS USING ITS RADIOLABELLED PRECURSOR PROTEIN*

J. FLOEGE, S. SHALDON**, K.M. KOCH
Department of Nephrology
Medizinische Hochschule Hannover,
3000 Hannover 61, W-Germany
***86, Rue de Grézac*
Montpellier 34080, France.

ABSTRACT. AB-amyloidosis, characterized by the presence of ß2-microglobulin in the amyloid fibrils has become an important complication of long-term renal replacement therapy. Due to the mainly musculoskeletal manifestations of the disease standard approaches to obtain the diagnosis of amyloidosis, such as rectal biopsy or fat aspiration, often yield negative results. Currently the definitive diagnosis relies on biopsies, usually of synovial membranes or bone cystic radiolucencies. Recently two radiopharmaceuticals, namely radiolabelled serum amyloid P component and radiolabelled ß2-microglobulin have been shown to be able to detect amyloid deposits *in vivo* in a non-invasive manner. In the case of labelled ß2-microglobulin we have shown that it allows the detection of clinically and radiologically unrecognizable AB-amyloid deposits and that it is specific. These latter tests therefore may have the potential to alleviate the need for biopsy confirmation in the diagnostic work-up of a suspected AB-amyloidosis. Furthermore, the use of radiolabelled precursor molecules may allow more insight into the processes underlying amyloid formation in man.

1. Introduction

Amyloid deposition is increasingly recognized as an important complication of long-term dialysis therapy [1,2]. In 1985 Geyjo et al identified the main fibrillar protein in the amyloidosis of chronic hemodialysis patients as ß2-microglobulin [3], thereby establishing the existence of a new type of amyloidosis. The prevalence of AB-amyloid deposition in patients on chronic hemodialysis treatment for more than 10 years is estimated to range from 30 to 100% [1,2]. Except for rare cases, the amyloidosis will not manifest clinically before 5-7 years of chronic dialysis therapy [1,2]. Manifestations of AB-amyloid deposition are largely restricted to (peri-) articular sites [1,2] and include the carpal tunnel syndrome, arthralgias, destructive arthropathies, pathological fractures due to amyloid deposition in bones, spondylarthropathies and tenosynovites. In contrast, other systemic manifestations, especially in regard to organs, seem to be exceptional [1,2,4].

In view of the manifestations, the clinical diagnosis of AB-amyloidosis has mainly been based upon the presence of the carpal tunnel syndrome or juxta-articular radiolucent cystic bone lesions in long term dialysis patients [1,2,4]. However, neither these nor any of the other clinical manifestations of AB-amyloidosis can be regarded as

* Synonyms used for AB-amyloidosis amongst others include: dialysis-related amyloidosis, dialysis amyloidosis, Aß2M-amyloidosis.

pathognomonic for this disease. Consequently, specific tests are needed to confirm the clinical diagnosis of AB-amyloidosis. Standard procedures to diagnose amyloid, such as rectal or skin biopsy or fat aspiration, are rarely successful and can therefore not be recommended [1,2]. The only diagnostic *in vivo* approach that has repeatedly been shown to yield positive findings in the majority of affected patients has been the biopsy of synovial membranes or bone radiolucencies [1,2]. On the other hand it seems unrealistic to assume that these procedures have the potential to become routine tools in the work-up of a suspected AB-amyloidosis.

2. Radiodiagnostic Approaches

In the past, several radiopharmaceuticals, such as ^{99m}Tc-tagged phosphates [5] and (^{99m}Tc(V))DMSA [6], have been described for the *in vivo* detection of amyloidoses. However, besides being non-specific and subject to false-positive findings [6], the usefulness of these compounds in the diagnosis of AB-amyloidosis, when evaluated, has yielded conflicting results [1,5].

Recently, two more specific radiodiagnostic tests have been described. Hawkins et al. [7] by injecting ^{123}I-serum amyloid P component, were able to detect *in vivo* the amyloid fibril ligand for this protein. Injection of the radiolabelled molecule allowed the non-invasive detection of amyloid deposits in the carpal tunnel region and metacarpophalangeal joints of long-term hemodialysis patients [7]. An alternative to scanning with radiolabelled serum amyloid P component is offered by the injection of radiolabelled human β_2-microglobulin which we first described in 1989 [8; reported in more detail in 9]:

3. ^{131}I-β_2-Microglobulin Radiodiagnostic Imaging

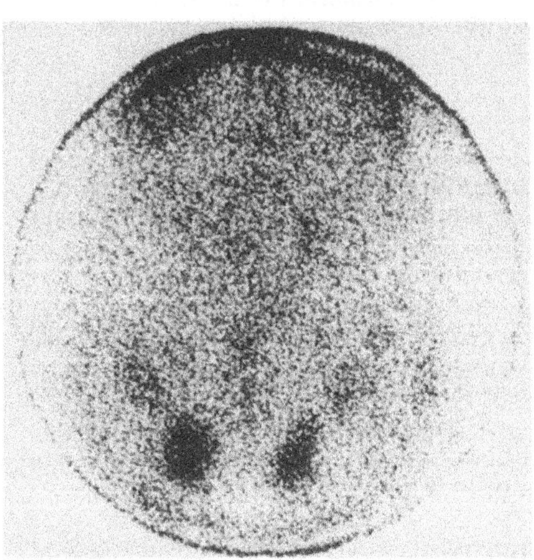

Figure 1. Dorsal pelvic image, 72 hrs after injection of ^{131}I-β_2-microglobulin, of a patient on chronic hemodialysis for 16 years. Subcutaneous nodules, probably representing AB-amyloid tumors [8], could be felt over both ischiac bones.

β_2-microglobulin, purified from uremic plasma ultrafiltrate, was radiolabelled with Na^{131}I. After approval by the local ethics committee, 42 oligo-anuric patients on chronic hemodialysis for between 0.5 to 18 years were studied. All patients were evaluated clinically for AB-amyloid associated symptoms and X-ray images of the hands, shoulders, pelvis and knees were obtained. Each examination was initiated by intravenous injection of radiolabelled β_2-microglobulin, followed after 72-96 hours by gamma-camera imaging of the shoulders, pelvis, knees and hands.

The results showed that localized tracer accumulations occurred in pelvic sites (fig. 1), shoulders, hip regions, vertebral column, knees or hands of 23 of the 42 hemodialysis patients studied (table 1). In contrast, no localized tracer accumulations were detected in patients on hemodialysis for 5 years or less (table 1). Both, the prevalence of scan positivity (table 1) and the number of tracer accumulation sites increased with increasing time of chronic hemodialysis. The number of involved predilection sites as judged by scanning was approximately two-fold higher than as judged by combined clinical and radiological evaluation.

Table 1. Percentage of hemodialysis patients, in whom ^{131}I-ß$_2$-microglobulin accumulations were detected versus percentage of patients, in whom clinical or radiological findings compatible with AB-amyloidosis were present [data modified from 9].

Time on Chronic Hemodialysis (Years)	n	Localized Tracer Accumulation(s)	Clinical/Radiological Findings Compatible with AB-amyloidosis.
0.0 - 5.0	12	0 %	0 %
5.1 - 10.0	16	63 %	44 %
10.1 - 15.0	9	89 %	89 %
15.1 or more	5	100 %	80 %

In four patients tissue was obtained during surgery at 4-10 days after tracer injection. In these samples up to 48-fold tracer enrichment was noted in amyloid-tissue as compared to amyloid-free tissue. When amyloid fibrils were extracted from an amyloid-infiltrated synovial membrane at 4 days after tracer injection 255 counts/g starting material were detected in the isolated fibrils, as compared to 14 counts/g starting material in samples obtained from non-amyloidotic control tissue.

The presence of AB-amyloidosis at prior tracer enrichment sites was confirmed histologically in 12 sites of 8 patients. In a ninth patient on hemodialysis for 6.5 years, five months before death the scan was negative. At autopsy, although the synovial membranes had normal macroscopic appearances, there was moderate microscopic AB-amyloid infiltration in the synovial membrane of the hip and shoulder joints.

Concerning the specificity of the ^{131}I-ß$_2$-microglobulin scan, no local enrichment was seen when free ^{131}I was used for scanning in a patient eight weeks after a positive ß$_2$-microglobulin scan. Furthermore, no local tracer enrichment at the respective site of disease occurred in patients with various inflammatory disorders, including chronic polyarthritis, primary oxalosis or localized bacterial infections. In three additional patients with a biopsy proven AB-amyloidosis, scanning was performed with ^{99m}Tc-labelled nanocolloidal human serum albumin (Nanocoll; Solco Nuclear, Switzerland), which has been shown to accumulate at sites of inflammation and increased phagocytotic activity. No local enrichment of this tracer around large joints or at prior ß$_2$-microglobulin accumulation sites was noted. In two patients with a biopsy-proven AA-amyloidosis, a weak image of the liver only was obtained.

Taken together these data suggest a specific localization of the injected ^{131}I-ß$_2$-microglobulin in or around the amyloid fibrils. The mechanism(s) underlying positive scans remain(s) hypothetical, but could involve three possibilities:

a) Binding or incorporation into amyloid fibrils. This could also explain the low-grade tracer accumulation in the livers of two AA-amyloidosis patients, as it is known that small amounts of other amyloidogenic proteins occur together with the main amyloid protein [9].
b) Binding to altered ground substance within or around the amyloid deposits. This could involve e.g. glycosaminoglycans or collagen [9].

c) Binding to inflammatory cells, especially macrophages, surrounding the AB-amyloid fibrils. However, although these cells have the capacity to bind exogenous ß2-microglobulin via an HLA-related mechanism on their cell surfaces [9], this possibility seems least likely, as negative scans were obtained in hemodialysis patients with non-amyloid inflammatory disorders.

4. Conclusion

Scanning with radiolabelled ß2-microglobulin seems to offer a specific, sensitive and non-invasive way to demonstrate AB-amyloid deposits and it may have the potential to alleviate the need for biopsy confirmation. Also, it offers the possibility to obtain more complete data on the incidence of AB-amyloidosis. This could serve as the basis of prospective studies, in which the influence of dialysis strategies on the *de-novo* appearance or the progression of established sites of AB-amyloid deposits is examined.

From a more general point of view this study for the first time provides direct evidence that uptake of an injected amyloid precursor protein into its derived deposits can occur in man. This technique or similar approaches may thereby become important tools to gain more insight into the mechanisms underlying *in vivo* amyloid formation in man.

5. Acknowledgements

The help of W. Burchert, B. Nonnast-Daniel, P. Gielow, A. Brandis and E. Spindler in performing the studies is gratefully acknowledged.

6. References

1) Kleinman, K.S. and Coburn, J.W. (1989) Amyloid syndromes associated with hemodialysis. Kidney Int. 35: 567-575.
2) Bardin, T., Zingraff, J., Kuntz, D., Drüeke, T. (1986) Dialysis-related Amyloidosis. Nephrol. Dial. Transplant. 1: 151-154.
3) Gejyo, F., Odani, S., Yamada, T., Nakagawa, Y., Arakawa, M., Kunitomo, T., Kataoka, H., Suzuki, M., Hirasawa, Y., Shirahama, T., Cohen, A.S., Schmid, K. (1986) ß2-microglobulin: a new form of amyloid protein associated with chronic hemodialysis. Kidney Int. 30: 385-390.
4) Gejyo, F., Homma, N., Arakawa, M. (1988) Carpal tunnel syndrome and ß2-microglobulin related amyloidosis in chronic hemodialysis patients. Blood Purif. 6: 125-131.
5) Sethi, D., Naunton Morgan, T.C., Brown, E.A., Jewkes, R.F., Gower, P.E. (1990) Technetium-99-labelled methylene diphosphonate uptake scans in patients with dialysis arthropathy. Nephron 54: 202-207.
6) Ohta, H., Endo, K., Kanoh, T.: Technetium-99m (V) DMSA uptake in amyloidosis. J. Nucl. Med. 30: 2049-2052.
7) Hawkins, P.N., Myers, M.J., Lavender, J.P., Pepys, M.B. (1988) Diagnostic radionuclide imaging of amyloid: biological targeting by circulating human serum amyloid P component. Lancet I: 1413-1418.
8) Floege, J., Nonnast-Daniel, B., Gielow, P., Brandis, A., Spindler, E., Hundeshagen, H.H., Koch, K.M., Shaldon, S. (1989) Specific imaging of dialysis-related amyloid deposits using ^{131}I-ß2-microglobulin. Nephron 51: 444-447.
9) Floege, J., Burchert, W., Brandis, A., Gielow, P., Nonnast-Daniel, B., Spindler, E., Hundeshagen, H.H., Shaldon, S., Koch, K.M. On the imaging of dialysis related amyloid (AB-amyloid) deposits with ^{131}I-ß2-microglobulin. Kidney Int. in press.

CARDIAC INVOLVEMENT IN SECONDARY AMYLOIDOSIS

Robert W. Simms
Mary H. Coats[+]
Martha Skinner
Alan S. Cohen
Rodney H. Falk[+]

From the Arthritis Center, and Section of Cardiology[+], Department of Medicine, Boston City Hospital and Boston University School of Medicine, Boston, MA 02118 USA.

Introduction

Cardiac symptoms are reported to occur rarely in patients with secondary (AA) amyloidosis (1), and while autopsy data have indicated that cardiac amyloid deposits occur in up to 25% of patients, the cause of death is not usually felt to be related to cardiac disease (2). Although a number of reports have documented the diagnostic utility of echocardiography in primary amyloidosis, there is little information regarding the echocardiographic and clinical cardiac features of patients with secondary amyloidosis. We sought to better characterize the clinical, electrocardiographic and echocardiographic features of secondary amyloidosis in a retrospective review of consecutive patients evaluated at the Thorndike Memorial Laboratory of Boston City Hospital.

Methods

The clinical, electrocardiographic and 2-dimensional echocardiographic features of consecutive patients with secondary (AA) amyloidosis were reviewed. The diagnosis of secondary amyloidosis was made by typical congophilic staining of tissue biopsy material, the presence of an underlying inflammatory disorder, typical organ involvement (e.g. kidney, gastrointestinal) and the absence of features (clinical or laboratory) suggestive of either primary (AL) or hereditary (FAP) amyloidosis. Patients with known ischemic or congenital cardiac disease were excluded from the study.

All patients underwent a detailed cardiologic evaluation, including evaluation by a cardiologist, routine 12 lead electrocardiography and conventional 2-D echocardiography.

Results

Table 1 shows the clinical features of the 23 patients with secondary amyloidosis. Inflammatory arthropathy, typically juvenile rheumatoid arthritis (JRA) or rheumatoid arthritis (RA) were the most common underlying conditions in the study patients. The mean duration of underlying disease to time of amyloid diagnosis was 16.2 years. Most patients had a substantial time interval between date of amyloid diagnosis and clinical cardiac evaluation (mean 4.2 years).

Table II shows the cardiac evaluation in the study patients. No patients had symptoms indicative of cardiac disease, and no patient had clinically evident heart failure by examination, including three patients with strong electrocardiographic and echocardiographic evidence of cardiac amyloidosis. Low voltage was the most common electrocardiographic abnormality, identified in 5 of the 23 patients. Both first degree heartblock and pathologic Q waves occurred together in a single patient.

TABLE 1. Clinical Features of Patients with Secondary Amyloidosis

Mean Age (years)	45
Mean amyloid disease duration at time of evaluation (years)	4.2
Underlying disease (no. of pts.)	
Inflammatory arthritis	13
Chronic infection	2
Inflammatory Bowel Disease	2
Familial Mediterranean Fever	3
Hodgkin's Disease	1
Unknown	3

TABLE 2. Prevalence of Cardiac Features in Patients with Secondary Amyloidosis

Cardiac Symptoms	0/23
Abnormal Cardiac examination	0/23
Electrocardiographic abnormalities	
1^0 AV Block	1/23
Low voltage	5/23
Pathologic Q waves	1/23
Echocardiographic abnormalities	
Ventricular wall thickening	4/23
Intra-atrial wall thickening	1/23

Echocardiographic abnormalities consisting of ventricular or septal wall thickening were present in 4 patients. Intratrial septal thickening was present in one patient with low voltage on ECG. Classical myocardial scintillation or granular sparkling was not detected in any patient. Correlation of ECG and echocardiography indicated that 4 of 5 patients with wall thickening displayed low voltage. One patient with low voltage had normal ventricular and septal wall thickness, but had intra-atrial thickening.

Conclusion

In summary, these data indicate that: 1) echocardiographic and/or electrocardiographic evidence of cardiac involvement appears to be uncommon in patients with secondary amyloidosis, and 2) when cardiac involvement occurs in secondary amyloidosis, it does not appear to be associated with clinically evident heart disease. This latter finding is in contrast to cardiac involvement in the primary (AL) form, where similar degrees of cardiac involvement by echocardiogram or electrocardiogram may result in important and often life-threatening disease. Studies of myocardial technetium-99 pyrophosphate scanning in AA-amyloid and cardiac involvement have shown no significant uptake (3) compared with primary (AL) amyloidosis which is characterized by diffuse uptake in the presence of cardiac involvement (4), possibly reflecting differences in fibrillar uptake of technetium pyrophosphate. Therefore the absence of congestive heart failure with laboratory evidence of cardiac amyloid in secondary amyloid disease may indicate a different pathogenesis of cardiac deposition than that which occurs in the primary type. Differences in the location or rate of fibrillar deposition may explain this phenomenon, however, confirmation of this hypothesis will await serial prospective studies.

Acknowledgements

Supported by grants from the U.S. Public Health Service, NIAMDD (AM 07014), the General Clinical Research Branch of the Division of Research Resources, National Institutes of Health (RR 533), the Multipurpose Arthritis Center, National Institutes of Health (AM 20613), and the Arthritis Foundation.

REFERENCES

1. Falk RH. (1989) Cardiac amyloidosis. Progress in Cardiology 2:143-155.

2. Brandt K, Cathcart ES and Cohen AS. (1968) A clinical analysis of the course and prognosis of fourty-two patients with amyloidosis. Am J Med 44:955-969.

3. Leinonen H, Totterman KJ, Tammola-Korppi T and Korhola O. (1984) Negative myocardial technetium-99 m pyrophosphate scintigraphy in amyloid heart disease associated with type AA systemic amyloidosis. Am J Cardiol 53:380-381.

4. Falk RH, Lee VW, Rubinow A, Hood WB and Cohen AS. (1983) Sensitivity of technetium-99 m pyrophosphate scintigraphy in diagnosing cardiac amyloidosis. Am J Cardiol 61:826-830.

IMAGING HEREDITARY AMYLOIDOSIS OF OSTERTAG

P.N. HAWKINS, T.G. FEEST & M.B. PEPYS
*Immunological Medicine Unit, Department of Medicine,
RPMS, Hammersmith Hospital, London W12 0NN, and
Royal Devon and Exeter Hospital,
Exeter, Devon, UK*

ABSTRACT. We have used scintigraphy with ^{123}I-labelled serum amyloid P component to investigate members of 4 families with hereditary systemic amyloidosis conforming to the syndrome described by Ostertag. Clinical features included hypertension, proteinuria and renal impairment though one individual presented with keratoconjunctivitis sicca and two others with hepatomegaly. Immunohistochemistry was performed on tissue obtained by biopsy from members of 3 families; amyloid stained positively for SAP in all cases but no reactivity was observed using antibodies to transthyretin, serum amyloid A, β_2-microglobulin or immunoglobulin light chains. Positive images were obtained by ^{123}I-SAP scintigraphy in all individuals with histologically demonstrated amyloid, unsuspected major visceral deposits being identified in each case. Scans of asymptomatic relatives from 2 families were normal in 3 cases, but demonstrated massive hepatic and splenic amyloid deposits in 2 individuals.

Scintigraphy with ^{123}I-SAP appears to be a sensitive, non-invasive method for the diagnosis and screening of familial amyloidosis of Ostertag.

1. INTRODUCTION

A syndrome of hereditary nephropathic amyloidosis was described by Ostertag in 1950 [1], who reported a German kindred in which amyloid was transmitted in an autosomal dominant pattern and was deposited mainly in the kidneys, livers and spleens of affected individuals; lesser amounts were also sometimes found in the lungs and heart. These patients presented in early middle-age with hypertension and rapidly progressive renal failure, neural involvement was conspicuously absent. Only two further kindreds have so far been reported [2,3]. In the present study, members of one of the above [3] and 3 additional families with hereditary systemic amyloid syndromes conforming to that described by Ostertag were investigated with scintigraphy using ^{123}I-labelled serum amyloid P component (SAP), a specific targeting agent for amyloidosis [4-6].

2. METHODS AND RESULTS

SAP, greater than 99% pure, was radiolabelled with ^{123}I and given to subjects as an i.v. bolus. Anterior and posterior whole body gamma camera scans were performed at 24 hr and limited measurement of ^{123}I-SAP turnover was made for

48 hr [6]. Clinical details of individuals studied were as follows (Fig. 1): *Family 1.* A 30 yr old male who presented 7 yr previously with keratoconjunctivitis sicca. Minor proteinuria and renal impairment were noted and amyloid was demonstrated in salivary gland, rectal and renal biopsies. Further details have been described by Lanham *et al.* [3]. *Family 2.* A male aged 42 yr, presented 6 yr previously with hepatomegaly, renal impairment, hypertension, gut disturbances and testicular failure. Biopsies of rectum, duodenum and kidney were positive for amyloid. *Family 3.* A 37 yr old female who presented with hypertension and marked renal impairment. Amyloid was demonstrated in a nephrectomy specimen obtained after an attempted needle biopsy caused severe haemorrhage. Asymptomatic relatives also studied were her brother, aged 40, in whom amyloid had been shown to be present on salivary gland biopsy as a screening procedure, and three siblings, aged 17, 20 and 24, whose mother was a cousin of the proband, and who died aged 35 with systemic amyloid. *Family 4.* A 32 yr old female who presented with hypertension, nephrotic syndrome and renal impairment. Amyloid was demonstrated on renal biopsy. Her father, aged 58, documented to have hepatic amyloid and her asymptomatic sister, aged 28, were also studied. Where possible, tissues were obtained for immunohistochemical studies of the amyloid fibril protein.

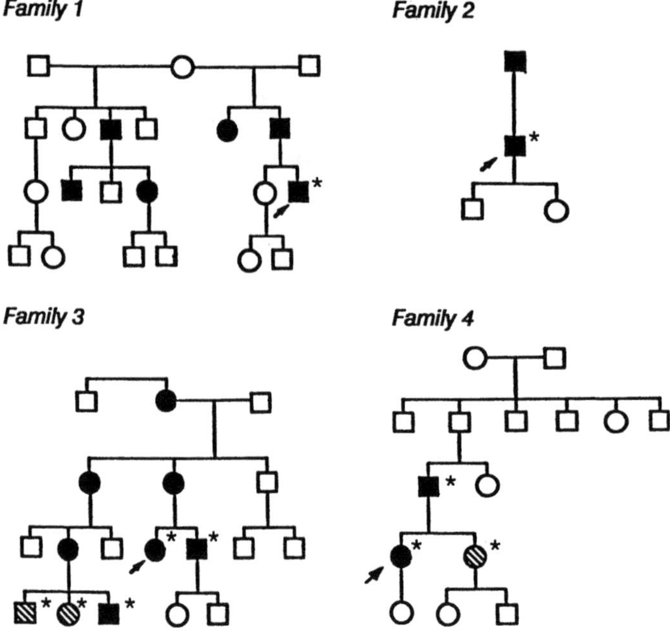

Fig. 1. Details of 4 families with hereditary amyloidosis of Ostertag. The probands are arrowed and individuals who underwent ^{123}I-SAP scintigraphy are marked by an asterisk. □ denotes no history of amyloidosis, ▧ screened for amyloid by ^{123}I-SAP scintigraphy with negative results and ■ tissue or scanning evidence of amyloidosis.

The images obtained 24 hr after ^{123}I-SAP administration in all of the probands from families 1, 2 and 3 were remarkably similar, demonstrating intense localisation of the tracer to the liver and spleen, associated with very rapid clearance of activity from the plasma during the first 6 hr and much increased whole body retention of tracer at 48 hr. Although renal images were also present in the proband of Family 2, visualisation of uptake into the kidneys may have been precluded in other cases by the relatively high intensity of signal arising from adjacent livers and spleens which were sometimes enlarged.

The images of SM, proband of Family 4, showed tracer uptake in the same distribution though this was quantitatively much less; similar observations were made in her father, NC.

Studies of 5 asymptomatic relatives revealed normal results in 3, both with respect to the images and limited measurement of SAP turnover. However, there was major localisation of tracer to the liver and spleen in one individual in whom screening with salivary gland biopsy had been positive for amyloid, and to the liver, spleen and kidneys in a further 24 yr old male (Fig. 2). Despite evidence of major amyloid deposits in both the latter subjects, routine laboratory tests for renal, liver and haemopoetic function were normal.

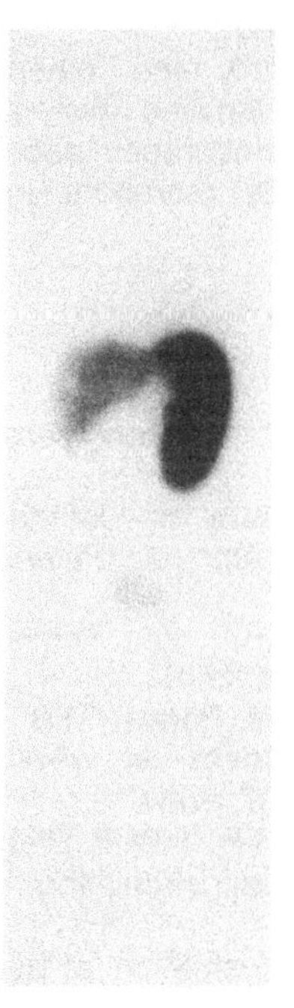

Fig. 2. Anterior whole body scintigraph taken 24 hr after i.v. injection of ^{123}I-labelled SAP. The subject was an apparently fit and healthy 24 yr old male whose mother died with hereditary systemic amyloidosis aged 35. Amyloid is demonstrated by intense uptake of tracer in the liver and spleen which is enlarged. In addition renal uptake was discernable on the posterior view. A small amount of degraded radioactive material can be seen in the bladder.

Small amounts of tissue were available from the probands of Families 1, 2 and 3. The fibril proteins were not identified in immunohistochemical studies using antibodies to transthyretin, serum amyloid A, β_2-microglobulin and immunoglobulin light chains, though SAP/AP was present in the amyloid deposits in each case.

3. CONCLUSIONS

The 4 families described here with familial nephropathic amyloidosis share similar clinical and pathological features with the family described by Ostertag in 1950. An autosomal dominant mode of inheritance was implied in all of the present cases although the phenotypic expression, even within a particular family, varied considerably both with respect to age and mode of presentation.

SAP scintigraphic studies were positive in all subjects in whom there was histological evidence of amyloid identifying major unsuspected visceral involvement in each case. Major deposits were identified in 2 individuals who were entirely without symptoms though a notable feature in the majority of positive studies, including those of the 2 asymptomatic relatives, was that despite relatively large quantities of amyloid being present, particularly in the liver, there were often only very minor functional abnormalities.

Although immunohistochemical studies failed to identify the biochemical nature of the amyloid fibril proteins(s) involved in these families and, as yet, further chemical studies have not been undertaken, SAP scintigraphy appears to have the potential for effective screening of at-risk family members in early adult life.

REFERENCES

1. Ostertag, B. (1950) Familiare amyloid - erkrankung. *Z. Menschl Verebungs Konsit Lehre,* **30**: 105-115.
2. Weiss, S.W. and Page, D.L. (1973) Amyloid nephropathy of Ostertag with special reference to renal glomerula giant cells. *Am. J. Pathol.,* **72**: 447-455.
3. Lanham, J.G., Meltzer, M.L., de Beer, F.C., Hughes, G.R.V. and Pepys, M.B. (1982) Familial amyloidosis of Ostertag. *Quart. J. Med.,* **51**: 25-32.
4. Hawkins, P.N., Myers, M.J., Epenetos, A.A., Caspi, D. & Pepys, M.B. (1988) Specific localization and imaging of amyloid deposits *in vivo* using ^{123}I-labeled serum amyloid P component. *J. Exp. Med.,* **167**: 903-913.
5. Hawkins, P.N., Myers, M.J., Lavender, J.P. & Pepys, M.B. (1988) Diagnostic radionuclide imaging of amyloid: biological targeting by circulating human serum amyloid P component. *Lancet,* **i**: 1413-1418.
6. Hawkins, P.N., Lavender, P.J. & Pepys, M.B. (1990) Evaluation of systemic AA and AL amyloidosis by scintigraphy with iodine-123-serum amyloid P component. *New Engl. J. Med.,* **323**: 508-513.

COMPUTER-AIDED IMMUNOHISTOCHEMICAL QUANTITATION OF AMYLOID IN RENAL BIOPSIES

U. Donini[1), S. Casanova[2)], P Zucchelli[1)], C. Poli[3)], G. Carboni[3)], R.P. Linke[4)]

[1)]Department of Nephrology and [2)]Laboratory of Electron Microscopy, Malphigi Hospital, [3)]ENEA, Bologna, Italy, [4)]Institute of Immunology, University of Munich, Munich, FRG

ABSTRACT
A computer program of image analysis has been designed for the quantitation of glomerular amyloid deposits in renal tissue. Computer digitalized microscopic images were obtained from glomeruli stained histochemically with Congo red (CR) and immunohistochemically by peroxidase anti-peroxidase (PAP) and by immunofluorescence (IF) methods using antibodies against different amyloid fibril proteins: AA, Aλ, Aϰ, AF, AB. Seven patients with renal amyloidosis (4 AA, 3 Aλ) were studied to quantify their glomerular amyloid deposits.

INTRODUCTION
In order to classify amyloid deposits by immunohistochemistry, it is crucial to compare immunohistochemical reactions with a panel of antibodies against different types of amyloid fibril proteins (1). The comparison of these reactions is done microscopically by inspection. The result is qualitative and does not include quantitation of the amyloid present. Therefore, the aim of this study was to apply computer-based techniques to quantitate the amount of amyloid stained histochemically and immunohistochemically in tissue sections.

MATERIALS AND METHODS
Cryostat (C), paraffin (P) and hydroxiethylmethacrylate (GMA) sections from 7 patients (4 with AA, 3 with Aλamyloidosis) were stained with antibodies against AA (monoclonal, mcl), Aλ, Aϰ, AF, AB amyloid fibril proteins, by indirect IF and PAP methods as previously described (1-2). The CR stained sections were observed under polarized light to identify the tissue deposits as amyloid, and by fluorescence microscopy to compare the surface area (SA) of histochemically stained deposits with those stained by IF or PAP methods. In observation and digitalization the following equipment was used: 1) a Photomicroscope II Zeiss equipped for fluorescence microscopy with epicondenser IIIRS and XB0 75 W xenon lamp, 2) a video camera Hamamatsu C3077 (Hamamatsu Photonics K.K., Japan) attached to the microscope and with the video output matched both to the image-aquisition hardware and to a monitor for direct viewing and adjusting of the image, 3) image-acquisition-hardware made up of a ATARI MEGA ST4 computer, a hard disk MEGAFILE 44 (Atari Corporation, Sunnyvale, California) and a video digitizer. For image processing a program was written with he following objectives: 1) to recognise the stained amyloid deposits inside the glomerulus and measure their SA and their mean grey level (GL), that is their brightness, 2) to automize the process as much as possible and minimize operator monitoring. With these objectives in mind, the program consists of two steps: The operator encloses the digitalized glomerulus images in a rectangle (Fig. 1). The computer then automatically analyses the images, identifying and measuring the deposit areas inside the glomerulus (Fig. 2) and stores the data. As a result of the image analysis, the computer gives three values 1) percent (P) of amyloid deposits present inside the glomerulus; 2) mean of the GL of the deposits (DGL); 3) mean of the GL of the total glomerular surface (GGL). For the sections stained with PAP (Fig. 3), the DGL and GGL were considered not valid for quantitation because

too much dependent on microscope light conditions. When there was doubt on glomerulus boundary in IF, bright light was additionaly used to determine the limits of the glomerulus (Fig. 4).

RESULTS

Agreement was found in the qualitative and computer quantitative methods (Table 1). IF proved the best staining method to match this image analysis system. The digitizing of images was most important step, and to obtain valid quantitative results unclear images should be excluded. There was no difference in digitalizing and processing of images in respect to embedding media used. The case AM286 was examined with both IF and PAP methods with similar results. Amyloid quantified on CR stained sections agreed with that measured by IF or PAP staining.

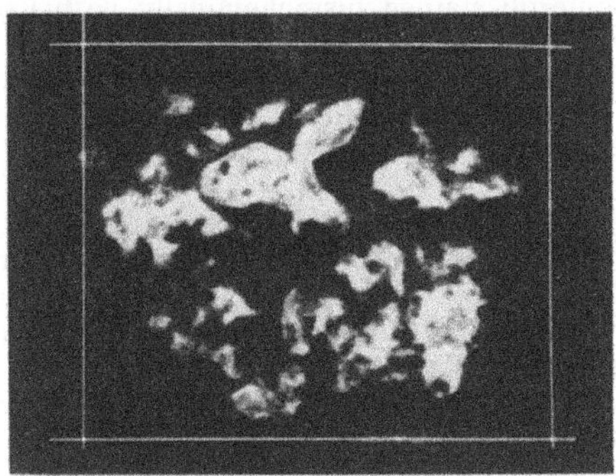

Fig. 1 Case AM286. Digitalized image of glomerulus stained by IF with anti-AA monoclonal antibody (mc1). The glomerulus is limited by 4 lines.

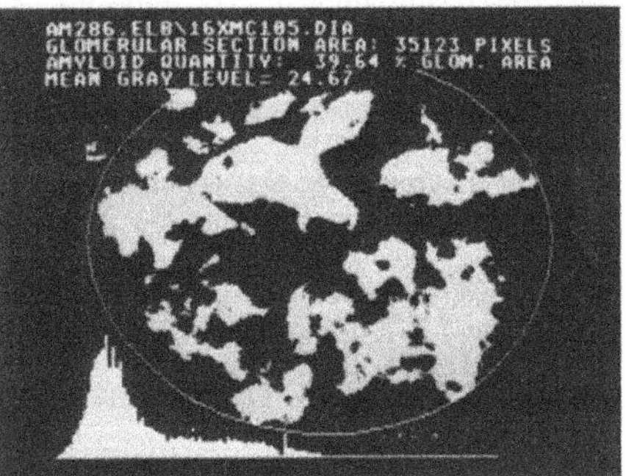

Fig. 2 Case AM286. Results of computer image analysis as they appear on the screen. The histogram of grey level of glomerular area at the bottom.

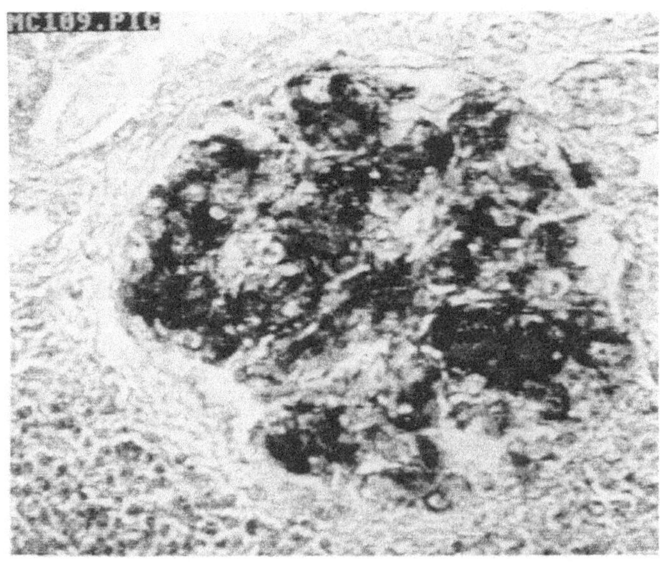

Fig. 3 Case AM286. Digitalized image of glomerulus stained by PAP with anti-AA monoclonal antibody (mc1)

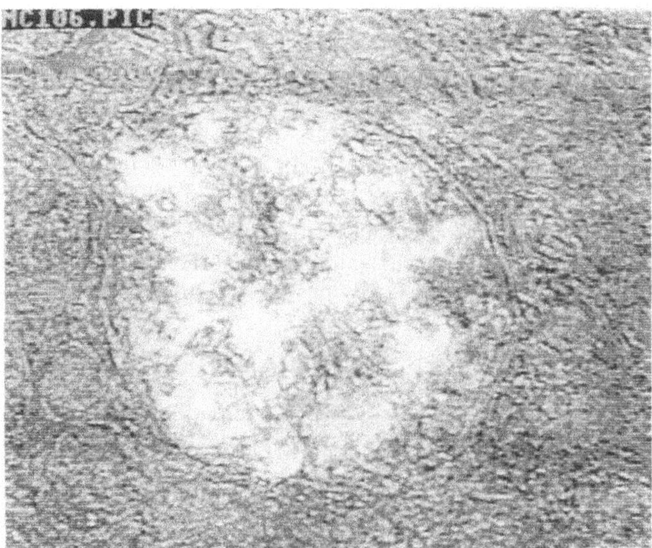

Fig. 4 Case AM1148. Digitalized image of glomerulus stained by IF with monoclonal antibody anti-AA (mc1) and observed both under bright and ultraviolet light.

Only in the case AM1424 the CR staining was significantly less than the PAP staining, meaning that λ-chain deposits other than amyloid were detected (LCDD ?).

Table 1. QUANTITATIVE AND QUALITATIVE RESULTS OBTAINED IN AMYLOID IF AND PAP STAINING AND COMPARISON WITH CR STAINING QUANTIFICATION

CASE	EMB/MET	AMYLOID TYPE	CR (qnt evl)	IMMUNOHISTOCHEMISTRY (qnt evl)	(qlt evl)
AM286	par/IF	AA	35.6/52.4/36*	46.6/48.6/33.3	++++*
AM1148	par/IF	AA	51/47/35.5	23.6/33.1/20.28	++++
CR1924	cry/IF	AA	32.4/54.5/35	48.26/60.2/34.3	++++
AM1345	par/IF	Aλ	0.6/32.2/10.2	2/32.5/6.25	+++
AM286	par/PAP	AA	35.6/52.4/36	40/-/-/	++++
AM1424	par/PAP	Aλ	6.1/30.8/16	25.5/-/-/	+++
AM1350	par/PAP	Aλ	17/38/16	20.7/-/-	++++
AM1150	par/PAP	AA	34/50/32	38.7/-/-	++++

*The values are expressed as P/DGL/GGL (see MATERIALS AND METHODS)
** grading + to ++++
Abbreviations: EMB=embedding; MET=immunostaining method; qnt=quantitative; evl=evaluation; qlt=qualitative; par=paraffin; cry=cryostat.

DISCUSSION

We have applied image analysis to quantitate amyloid in renal tissue sections to compare CR, IF and PAP staining. IF was found the most practical because of its constant light condition and high image contrast. Others have validated quantitative IF using a comparison based on radiolabelled antigens (3). On the other hand PAP may also be used when measuring SA of amyloid deposits. The best results are obtained under optimum, constant staining and digitalizing conditions. Our system is simple and relatively of low cost and permits general use of image analysis in amyloidotic tissue evaluation. It provides precise amyloid quantitation and allows for better amyloid classification when different amyloid types are probed. This technique may be used for documentation of an effective therapy, when sample error can be minimized, as could be done in liver and renal biopsies.

REFERENCES

1. Linke, R.P., Nathrath, W.J.B., Eulitz, M. (1986) Amyloidosis, Plenum Press, London
2. Donini, U., Casanova, S., Dal Bosco, F., Linke, R.P. (1985) Immunhistochemical typing of amyloid on hydroxyethyl-methacrylate-embedded renal biopsies, Appl. Path. 2, 299-307
3. Basgen, J.M., Nevins, T.E., Michael, A.F. (1989) Quantitation of antigen in tissue by immunofluorescence image analysis, J. Immunol. Methods 124, 77-83

ABDOMINAL FAT BIOPSY FOR CHARACTERIZATION OF THE MAJOR AMYLOID FIBRIL PROTEINS BY AMINO ACID SEQUENCE ANALYSIS

A.-H. FORSBERG[1], K. SLETTEN[2], L. BENSON[3] AND P. WESTERMARK[1]

[1]Department of Pathology, University of Linköping, Sweden
[2]Department of Biochemistry, University of Oslo, Norway and
[3]Department of Internal Medicine, University of Uppsala, Sweden

ABSTRACT Needle biopsy of subcutaneous fat is a realiable diagnostic method for most systemic amyloidosis. We describe here a simple method to use surgical subcutaneous fat biopsies for purification of amyloid fibril proteins in patients with AL- and AA-amyloidosis. Using this method we have obtained N-terminal amino acid sequence analysis in six patients with systemic amyloidosis.

INTRODUCTION AL-amyloidosis, AA-amyloidosis and transthyretin derived amyloidoses (familial amyloidoses and senile systemic amyloidosis) are all amyloid diseases where amyloid can be deposited in almost all organs, including subcutaneous fat tissue. Biopsy from this tissue can be used as a method for the diagnosis of amyloidosis (1-6). We have also shown previously that subcutaneous fat biopsies can be utilized for immunological typing of amyloid (7,8). In the present study we show that amyloid fibril proteins can be purified from fat biopsy and the type determined by N-terminal sequence analysis.

MATERIAL AND METHODS

Abdominal subcutaneous fat tissue pieces (about 1 cubic cm) were excised from patients with systemic amyloidosis, (AA- and AL-type). The presence of amyloid was determined by Congo red-stained thick smears of the biopsies. The unfixed biopsy was washed in normal saline over night, rinsed in distilled water, defatted in acetone, air dried and homogenized in 6 M guanidine-HCl containing 0.1 M Tris-HCl/ 0.2 % EDTA/ 0.02 M dithiothreitol, pH 8.0. After centrifugation, the supernatant was dialyzed against deionized water and lyophilized. About half of this material was used for immunological typing (8). The rest of the material was redissolved in guanidine-HCl as above and centrifuged. The supernatant was gel filtered through a Sephacryl S-200 HR column. The small retarded peak was dialyzed, lyophilized, redissolved in guanidine-HCl and applied to a Vydac 214 TPS column for reversed phase HPLC. The main peak materials were applied to a 477A protein Sequencer (Applied Biosystems, Foster City, California).

RESULTS

For this study, only biopsies containing considerable amount of amyloid, determined in Congo-red stained smears, were used (roughly 75 % of the patients with AL- and AA-amyloidosis). In samples from six patients, N-terminal sequence analysis allowed exact typing of the amyloid (see Table). Five of these patients had AL-amyloidosis and only one had AA-amyloidosis. This proportion depends mainly on difficulties in clinical typing of AL-amyloidosis and does not reflect the actual frequency of AL-amyloidosis in Sweden. In materials from three other patients, no free N-terminal was found. No further studies (e.g. after cleavage with cyanogenbromide) were performed with these latter samples. Except for the amyloid fibril proteins, only hemoglobulin α and ß chains were often identified, probably as a result of hemolysis in the samples.

TABLE N-terminal amino acid sequences (one letter code) of amyloid fibril proteins purified from abdominal fat biopsies of six patients with systemic amyloidosis.

Patient 1.	D F M L T Q P H S V S E S P G	Ref.9
AL-AR lambda VI	- - - - - - - - - - - - - - -	
Patient 2.	? E L T Q P P S V S V S P G Q T A S I T	Ref.12
AL-GIL lambda IV	S - - - - D - A - - - A L - - - V R - -	
Patient 3.	D I Q V T Q S P S S L S A S V G D R V T	Ref.10
BJ-AG kappa I	- - - M - - - - - - - - - - - - - - - -	
Patient 4.	S F F S F L	Ref.11
Protein AA	- - - - - -	
Patient 5.	D I Q M T Q S	Ref.10
BJ-AG kappa I	- - - - - - -	
Patient 6.	Y E L T Q P P S V S V S P G	Ref.10
BJ-Kern lambda III	- A - - - - - - - - - - - -	

CASE REPORTS

The following two cases will illustrate the value of this method

Patient 1. 47-year old woman with nephrotic syndrome for 3 years. Renal biopsy exhibited amyloid, by potassium permanganate test determined to be of AA-type. However, amino acid sequence analysis of protein purified from subcutaneous fat tissue showed that the amyloid was of AL-type, lambda VI.

Patient 5. 68-year old woman with myelomatosis and amyloidosis. Immunohistochemical study (performed in another laboratory) revealed reaction both with antisera to kappa immunoglobulin light chain and with protein AA. Sequence analysis showed that the amyloid was of AL-type, kappa I.

DISCUSSION

It is usually possible to determine with reasonable safety the type of systemic amyloidosis from which a patient suffers. Sometimes, however, the nature of an amyloid disease is uncertain. The present study shows that abdominal fat biopsy can be used not only for immunological typing but also for purification and amino acid sequence analysis of the main amyloid fibril protein. Since the proportion of amyloid proteins compared to other proteins is very high, a simple purification method can be used. This technique makes it possible to get exact information on the amyloid fibril protein in many patients during life. When more data on the types of amyloid fibril proteins is available, it is possible that information on the fibril protein will be of value, for treatment or for estimation of prognosis.

ACKNOWLEDGEMENTS

Supported by the Swedish Medical Research Council and the Research Fund of King Gustaf V.

REFERENCES

1. Westermark P., Stenkvist B. 'A new method for the diagnosis of systemic amyloidosis'. Arch Int Med 1973;132:522-3.
2. Stenkvist B., Westermark P., Wibell L. 'Simple method of diagnostic screening for amyloidsis'. Ann Rheum Dis 1974;33:75-76.
3. Libbey C.A., Skinner M., Cohen A.S. 'Use of abdominal fat tissue aspirate in the diagnosis of systemic amyloidosis'. Arch Int Med 1983;143:1549-52.
4. Orfila C., Giraud P., Modesto A., Suc J.-M. 'Abdominal fat tissue aspirate in human amyloidosis: Light ,electron and immunofluorescence microscopic studies'. Human Pathology.1986;17:3669.
5. Marujyma K., Ikeda S., Yanagisawa N., Nakazato M. 'Diagnostic value of abdominal fat tissue aspirate in familial amyloid polyneuropathy'. J Neurol Sci 1987;81:11-18.
6. Gertz M.A., Li C.-Y., Shirahama T., Kyle R.A. 'The subcutaneous fat aspirate: a controlled and blinded evalution of the technique in the diagnosis of primary amyloidosis (AL)'. In Isobe T., Arakis S., Uchino F., et al, eds. Amyloidosis. New York: Plenum, 1988:801-5.
7. Westermark P., Stenkvist B., Natvig J.B., Olding-Stenkvist E. 'Demonstration of protein AA in subcutaneous fat tissue obtained by fine needle biopsy'. Ann Rheum 1979;38:68-71
8. Westermark P., Benson L., Olofsson B.-O. 'Fine needle aspiration biopsy of abdominal subcutaneous fat tissue for the diagnosis and typing of amyloidosis'. Glenner G.G., Osserman E.F., Benditt E.P., Calkins E., Cohen A.S., Zucker-Franklin D., eds. Amyloidosis. New York: Plenum,1986:613-15.
9. Sletten K., Husby G., Natvig J.B. 'N-terminal amino acid sequence of amyloid fibril protein AR, prototype of a new λ-variable subgroup, V λ V'. Scand J Immunol 1974;3:833-836.
10. Benditt E.P., Eriksen N., Hermodson M.A., Ericsson L.H. 'The major proteins of human and monkey amyloid substance: common properties including amino acid sequences'. FEBS Lett. 1971;19:169-73.

11. Kabat E.A., Wu T.T., Bilofsky H., Reid-Miller M., Perry H., Gottesman K.S. 'Sequences of proteins of immunological interest'. Fourth ed. Bethesda, Maryland: National institute of Health, 1987.
12. Fykse E.-M., Sletten K., Husby G, and Gibbons G. Cornwell III. 'The primary structure of the variable region of an immunoglobulin IV light-chain amyloid-fibril protein (AL GIL)'. Biochem J 1988;256:973-980.

BETA-2-MICROGLOBULIN DOES NOT DEPOSIT IN ABDOMINAL FAT TISSUE OF LONG-TERM HEMODIALYSIS PATIENTS

G. MERLINI, D. LIMIDO*, V. BELLOTTI, E. BUCCIARELLI, P. BERRETTA*, P. MARIANI*, V. PERFETTI, E. ASCARI.
*Institute of Clinical Medicine II, University of Pavia, IRCCS Policlinico S. Matteo, 27100 Pavia; and *Div. Nephrology and Hemodialysis, S. Gerardo Hospital, 20052 Monza, Italy*

ABSTRACT. The absence of amyloid deposits in subcutaneous fat tissue has been reported in patients with amyloid deposits composed of beta-2-microglobulin (B2M) undergoing long-term hemodialysis (HD). We considered it of interest to ascertain, by combining abdominal fat aspiration with the immunoblot technique, if B2M is nevertheless deposited in non-amyloid form in the fat tissue. Twenty-seven patients undergoing regular HD for a median time of 11 yr (range 2-21) were evaluated; seventeen patients had demonstrated carpal tunnel amyloidosis (13 cases) or amyloid arthropathy (4 cases). The fat aspirate was divided into two portions: one for Congo red staining and microscopic analysis, the other for immunoblotting with anti-B2M and anti-P component antisera. Microscopic analysis detected definite amyloid deposits in only one patient, who turned out to have a previously undiagnosed AL amyloidosis. The immunoblot revealed trace amounts of B2M in 11 patients and no detectable B2M in 16. The search for P component was negative in all 11 patients investigated. Conclusion: our study confirms the absence of amyloid in abdominal fat aspirate in patients undergoing long-term HD, and demonstrates that B2M does not accumulate in this tissue.

Introduction

In patients on long-term hemodialysis (HD) the appearance of chronic musculoskeletal syndromes (carpal tunnel syndrome, CTS, osteoarthropathies and synovial effusion), related to a unique variety of amyloid deposits composed of beta-2-microglobulin (B2M)[1,2], has been extensively documented. Systemic amyloid deposition in cases undergoing long-term HD has been reported [3-6], in these cases amyloid deposition in visceral organs is usually mostly perivascular and seldom becomes heavy, although cases of extensive systemic amyloidosis associated with clinical disease have been reported [7-9]. The examination of tissues outside the musculoskeletal system, such as abdominal fat aspirates, for amyloid deposition in the cases of HD-associated amyloidosis gives a low positive rate [10], or none at all [11-12] .

Extensive tissular deposits of B2M lacking the characteristic birefringence after Congo red staining has been reported in one patient: the authors suggested that B2M can deposit in tissues without undergoing complete amyloidogenic changes [13]. Recent data indicate that the interaction of the amyloid proteins with collagen and/or collagen-like molecules may play an important role in the supramolecular organization of the amyloid fibrils [14] and in determining the clinical characteristics of HD-associated amyloidosis [15]. Therefore, it may be possible that an amyloid protein, B2M in this case, which does not interact efficiently with fat tissue collagen/collagen-like molecules could be deposited in non-amyloid form. In order to clarify this point we combined abdominal fat aspiration with the biochemical characterization of the tissue components by immunoblotting.

Patients and Methods

The characteristics of patients are reported in Table 1. Informed oral consent was obtained from all patients.

B2M was determined on fresh sera using a competitive immunoassay (Enzygnost β_2-microglobulin, Behringwerke, Marburg, WG). Abdominal fat aspiration was performed in all patients from the periumbilical area using a 19-gauge needle. The fat aspirate was divided into two portions: one for Congo red staining and microscopic analysis under polarized light, the other for immunoblotting with anti-B2M and anti-P component antisera. The fat samples were washed three times with saline and then mixed with the SDS-PAGE sample buffer, boiled for 5 minutes and then applied to 5-20%-gradient SDS-PAGE slabs. Immunoblotting was performed using rabbit anti-B2M and anti-P component as first antibody and peroxidase-labelled goat anti-rabbit immunoglobulins as second antibody (Dako, Copenhagen, DK); 0.1% diaminobenzidine and 0.1% imidazole were used as peroxidase substrate.

Results

Table 1 reports the main characteristics of the patients studied and the findings in fat aspirates.

Only one patient out of the 13 who had surgery for the carpal tunnel syndrome (definite CTS) had been in dialysis for less than 10 years; the others were on HD for a median time of 16 years (range 11-21). The fat aspirate showed a characteristic birefringence in one patient (no 27). The cause of the end-stage renal disease of this patient was unknown; further studies revealed that he had a plasma cell dyscrasia producing free k chains, this protein was also detected by immunoblot in the abdominal fat aspirate. These findings made the diagnosis of AL amyloidosis the most likely explanation. In two other samples, one from a patient with CTS and amyloid arthropathy and the other from an asymptomatic patient, a scant and difficult-to-detect birefringence was noted.

As reported in the Table 1, in 11 samples trace amounts of B2M were detected by immunoblot, with no restriction to samples from patients with definite CTS or amyloid arthropathy. No P-component was found by immunoblot in any of these 11 patients with traces of B2M in the fat aspirate (not shown).

Discussion

The negative outcome of the search for amyloid in the abdominal fat tissue of patients undergoing long-term dialysis reported in several series of patients [11-12] indicates that this form of amyloidosis is prevalently confined to the musculoskeletal system, at least in the early stages [11]. However, in another series, 12 out of 30 patients (40%) with CTS and/or amyloid arthropathy had amyloid deposits which were often scant and difficult to detect [10]. This finding can be accounted for by the systemic deposition of this type of amyloidosis, but to a far lesser degree than in other forms of systemic amyloidosis. Also in our series, a very weak birefringence was noted in two abdominal fat aspirates. Apart from the fact that one of these was apparently a false positive, since the patient did not present CTS or other musculoskeletal symptoms, such dubious positivity cannot be useful in the screening for hemodialysis-associated amyloidosis.

Table 1.Characteristics of patients receiving long-term hemodialysis and findings in fat aspirate.

Pt.no	Sex	Age	Yrs HD	B2M (mg/L)	CTS	MSC	CRS	IB-B2M	IB-PC
1	M	42	9	65	-	-	-	-	nd
2	F	62	6	57	-	-	-	-	nd
3	F	69	5	68	-	-	-	±	-
4	F	59	3	43	-	-	-	-	nd
5	F	55	4	62	-	-	-	-	nd
6	F	55	2	47	-	-	-	-	nd
7	M	62	4	28	-	-	-	-	nd
8	F	68	3	61	-	-	-	-	nd
9	F	59	6	59	-	-	-	-	nd
10	M	56	10	62	-	-	±	-	nd
11	M	59	14	101	-	+	-	±	-
12	M	58	15	63	+	+	-	±	-
13	F	53	10	101	-	+	-	±	-
14	F	70	8	74	+	+	-	±	-
15	M	48	19	53	+	+	-	±	-
16	M	49	18	96	+	+	±	±	-
17	F	51	16	25	+	-	-	-	nd
18	F	58	13	105	+	+	-	±	-
19	M	56	16	78	+	+	-	-	nd
20	F	52	16	105	+	+	-	±	-
21	M	50	21	101	+	+	-	±	-
22	F	59	11	97	+	+	-	-	nd
23	M	58	16	99	+	-	-	-	nd
24	M	62	19	57	-	+	-	-	nd
25	M	40	17	105	+	+	-	±	-
26	F	46	15	103	+	+	-	-	nd
27*	M	53	4	80	-	+	+++	-	nd

HD= Hemodialysis; CTS= Carpal Tunnel Syndrome (definite); MSC= MusculoSkeletal Complaints; CRS= Congo Red Staining; IB-B2M= Immuno Blot for Beta-2-Microglobulin; IB-PC= Immuno Blot for P Component; nd= not done; * Patient with AL amyloidosis.

The report of extensive tissular deposits of B2M lacking the characteristic birefringence of amyloid in one patient suggested that B2M can be deposited in the fat tissue without undergoing complete amyloid supramolecular organization [13]. Our preliminary data obtained by immunoblot of fat aspirates in AL amyloidosis indicate that in certain cases the monoclonal light chain can also be present in minimal amounts in the fat tissue samples which did not show any birefringence after Congo red staining (unpublished observation). This observation combined with other experimental data suggested that the interaction between certain light chains and some tissue components can play a role in the supramolecular organization and deposition of amyloid fibrils [14].

Homma et al. [15] reported that the collagen-binding activity of B2M depends upon the collagen concentration, and suggested that this may explain the deposition of amyloid in collagen-rich tissue such as those of the joints. Subcutaneous abdominal fat biopsy specimen has been used successfully for detailed typing of amyloid fibril protein [16]. The fat is removed *surgically* and the amyloid fibrils extracted: the fibril proteins are then typed by double immunodiffusion or characterized by amino acid sequence analysis [16]. In our experience the immunoblot technique applied *directly to fine needle fat aspirate* proved to be helpful in detecting light chain deposits in AL amyloidosis; therefore, we extended this approach to B2M amyloidosis. We were unable to detect discrete amounts of B2M in the fat biopies, the trace amounts of B2M detected in some samples reflect the very limited deposition of B2M outside the musculoskeletal system.

Acknowledgements

Study supported by the C.N.R. Target Project on Biotechnology and Bioinstrumentation.

References

1. Gejyo, F., Yamada, T., Odani, S.,et al. (1985) 'A new form of amyloid protein associated with chronic hemodialysis was identified as β_2-microglobulin', Biochem. Biophys. Res. Comm. 129, 701-706.
2. Gorevic, P.D., Casey, T.T., Stone, W.J., DiRaimondo, C.R., Prelli, F.C., and Frangione, B. (1985) 'Beta-2 microglobulin is an amyloidogenic protein in man', J. Clin. Invest. 76, 2425-2429.
3. Herve, J.P., Cledes, J., Bourbigot, B., et al (1985)'Systemic amyloidosis in the course of maintenance hemodialysis', Nephron 40, 494.
4. Hillion, D., Villeboeuf, J., Hillion, Y., Nakamura, S., and Bruet, A.(1985) 'Appearance of systemic amyloidosis in a chronic hemodialysis patient', Nephron 41, 127-128.
5. Bardin, T., Zingraff, J., Shirahama, T., et al (1987) 'Hemodialysis-associated amyloidosis and beta-2 microglobulin. Clinical and immunohistochemical study', Am. J. Med. 83, 419-424.
6. Ogawa, H., Saito, A., Hirabayashi, N., Hara, K.(1987) 'Amyloid deposition in systemic organs in long-term hemodialysis patients', Clin. Nephrol. 28, 199-204.
7. Gejyo, F., Homma, N., Maruyama, H., Ohara, K., and Arakawa, M.(1988) 'Coexistence of B2-microglobulin-derived amyloid deposits and hectopic calcification in the heart of a chronic hemodialysis patient', in Isobe T, Araki S, Uchino F, Kito S, Tsubura E (eds) *Amyloid and Amyloidosis*. Plenum, New York, p. 617-622.
8. Theaker, J.M., Raine, A.E.G., Rainey, A.J., Heryet, A., Clark, A., Oliver, D.O.(1987) 'Systemic amyloidosis of b_2-microglobulin type, a complication of long term dialysis', J. Clin. Pathol. 40, 1247-1251.
9. Maher, E.R., Hamilton Dutoit, S., Baillod, R.A., Sweny, P., Moorhead, J.F.(1988) 'Gastrointestinal complications of dialysis related amyloidosis', Br. Med. J. 297, 265-266.
10. Arqués, M.S., Campistol, J.M., and Muñoz-Gòmez, J. (1988) 'Abdominal fat aspiration biopsy in dialysis-related amyloidosis', Arch. Intern. Med. 148, 988, letter.
11. Varga, J., Idelson, B.A., Felson, D., Skinner, M., and Cohen, A.S.(1987) 'Lack of amyloid in abdominal fat aspirates from patients undergoing long-term hemodialysis', Arch. Intern. Med. 147, 1455-1457.
12. Orfila, C., Goffinet, F., Goudable, C., et al (1988) 'Unsuitable value of abdominal fat tissue aspirate examination for the diagnosis of amyloidosis in long-term hemodialysis patients' Am. J. Nephrol. 8, 454-456.
13. Terreros, D.A., Knight, J.A., Peric-Golia, L., and Cheung, A.K.(1989) 'Generalized β_2-microglobulin deposition. A preamyloidosis disorder?', Arch. Pathol. Lab. Med. 113, 31-35.
14. Bellotti, V., Merlini, G., Arbustini, E., Pucci, A., Stoppini, M., and Ferri, G. (1990) 'High molecular weight proteins sensitive to collagenase digestion are intimate consituents of amyloid deposits', VI Int Symp Amyloidosis, Oslo, August 5-8, 1990, Abstract.
15. Homma, N., Gejyo, F., Isemura, M., and Arakawa, M.(1989) 'Collagen-binding affinity of beta-2-microglobulin, a preprotein of hemodialysis-associated amyloidosis', Nephron 53, 37-40.
16. Westermark, P., Benson, L., Juul, J., and Sletten, K.(1989) 'Use of subcutaneous abdominal fat biopsy specimen for detailed typing of amyloid fibril protein-AL by amino acid sequence analysis', J. Clin. Pathol. 42, 817-819.

HISTOPATHOLOGIC CLASSIFICATION, CLINICAL CHARACTERISTICS AND SURVIVAL OF 18 PATIENTS WITH INCONCLUSIVE CLINICAL DATA TO IDENTIFY THE AA OR AL TYPE OF THEIR SYSTEMIC AMYLOIDOSIS

ANTON S.M. DOFFERHOFF[$#], BOUKE P.C. HAZENBERG[$], KORNELIS TE VELDE[#], JORIS GROND[*], JAN MARRINK[$], MARTIN H. VAN RIJSWIJK[$]
Dpt. Medicine[#], Deventer, The Netherlands and
Dpt. Medicine[$] and Dpt. Pathology[*]
State University Hospital, 59 Oostersingel
9713 EZ Groningen, The Netherlands

ABSTRACT. 189 Patients with non-familial systemic amyloidosis were evaluated from 1960 to november 1988. No precursor producing process like a monoclonal gammopathy or underlying inflammatory disease could be identified in 11 "idiopathic" patients. In 10 other patients the concurrent presence of chronic inflammation as well as a monoclonal gammopathy as the possible precursor producing process made a division into AA or AL difficult. Aim of this study was to classify these 21 patients by histopathology and to look at their symptoms and survival. Three patients of the "idiopathic" group could not be classified; 4 were classified AA and 4 AL. In the "double" precursor producing process group 6 patients were classified AA and 4 AL. All but one of the 10 with the AA-type presented with a nephrotic syndrome, while the 8 with the AL-type had a more diverse presentation. The 1-year survival of these 10 AA patients was 52% and of the 7 AL patients 29%. However, this difference was not significant.

1. INTRODUCTION

AA and AL amyloidosis do not only differ with regard to the precursor protein, but also to the clinical pattern of organ involvement, prognosis, therapy, monitoring of the disease and cause of death. So it is essential to be informed about the type of amyloid protein involved. Classification into the AA- or AL-type can often be suspected from the clinical situation: An associated precursor producing process like a chronic inflammatory disease points at the AA-type and the detection of a monoclonal gammopathy points at the AL-type. However, sometimes this situation is non-conclusive. We looked in our patient population to the clinical presentation and survival of this particular group of 18 patients.

2. MATERIALS AND METHODS

189 Patients with non-familial systemic amyloidosis were evaluated in a

referral-based university hospital from 1960 to november 1988. In 168 patients classification was easy: 116 patients had an associated chronic inflammatory disease and were supposed to have the AA-type, 52 patients had an associated plasma cell dyscrasia and were supposed to have the AL-type. In 9 patients (2 with AL and 7 with AA) a histologic diagnosis was made at the autopsy.

In 11 "idiopathic" patients no associated monoclonal gammopathy or inflammatory disease could be identified. In 10 other patients the concurrent presence of chronic inflammation as well as a monoclonal gammopathy made a clinical division into AA or AL difficult.

No tissue could be retrieved in 3 patients of the "idiopathic" group. Histologic classification was performed in 18 patients by the Congo red stain with $KMnO_4$ pretreatment, and in recent specimens also by immunohistochemistry with a panel of antibodies directed against AA [1], lambda and kappa light chains, transthyretin and β_2-microglobulin.

Actuarial survival curves were made starting at the time of histological diagnosis. The logrank test was used to detect differences in survival. Level of significance was $p<0.05$.

3. RESULTS

The results of classification are shown in table 1. Four patients of the "idiopathic" group were classified AA and the other 4 (1 of them at autopsy) classified AL. Six patients of the "double" group were classified AA and the other 4 classified AL.

Table 1. Clinical classification of 189 patients with systemic amyloidosis

	Chronic Inflam. (C.I.)	Monoclonal Gammopathy (M.G.)	C.I. + M.G.	Idiopath.	total
AA-type	116	-	6	4	126
AL-type	-	52	4	4	60
Unknown	-	-	-	3	3
Total	116	52	10	11	189

Prominent clinical details of the 18 patients are presented in table 2. No carpal tunnel syndrome was observed. Haemorrhagic diathesis was present in patients 4 (vaginal), 5-7 (skin) and 18 (bowel). Diarrhoea was seen in patient 5, 12 and 14 and malabsorption in patient 5 and 10. The thyroid gland appeared to be enlarged in patient 10. All but one of the 10 with the AA-type presented with a nephrotic syndrome, while the 8 with the AL-type had a more diverse presentation, especially with heart failure and macroglossia.

The survival curves are shown in figure 1. The 1-year survival for

Table 2: Patient characteristics and histopathology.

No	Age	Sex M/F	Associated disease	SAA mg/l	M-component Serum	M-component Urine	Bone-marrow	Histopathology CR + $KMnO_4$	K	L	TTR	β_2M	AA	Protein-uria g/day	ECC ml/min	CF/PN/Gl/Hp	Survival (months)	Cause of death
1	69	M	–	1.9	–	–	norm	sens	ND	ND	ND	ND	+	14	4	– –[#] – +[$]	8	Uremic
2	67	F	–	4.2	–	–	norm	sens	ND	ND	ND	ND	+	6	3	– – – –	11	Uremic
3	77	M	–	13	–	–	norm	sens	ND	ND	ND	ND	+	7	85	– – – –	18	Uremic
4	32	F	–	4.6	–	–	norm	sens	–	±	–	–	+	0.5	32	– – – –[$]	133	?
5	58	M	–	ND	–	–	dub	res	ND	ND	ND	ND	ND	1	9	+ + + –	1	Uremic
6	56	M	–	ND	–	–	dub	res	ND	ND	ND	ND	ND	0.5	24	– + + +	-0	Ileus
7	60	M	–	ND	–	–	dub	res	ND	ND	ND	ND	ND	0.5	14	+ – + +[$]	9	CF
8	52	F	–	ND	–	–	norm	res	–	+	–	–	–	8	38	– – – +[$]	65	CVA
9	71	F	RA	69	IgG-K	K	norm	sens	–	–	–	–	+	9.3	29	– – – –	81	Uremic
10	78	F	RA	65	IgM-K	–	norm	sens	–	–	–	–	+	4.1	36	– – – –	4	Bowel
11	66	F	Rec Pulm Inf	10	IgG-K	K	abn[&]	sens	–	–	–	–	+	3.4	64	– – – +[$]	>6	–
12	62	M	TBC (+RA)	191	–	L	norm	sens	–	–	–	–	+	6.0	81	– –[#] – –[$]	51	Sudden
13	44	F	RA	0.5	IgG-K	–	ND	sens	ND	ND	ND	ND	ND	5.2	84	– – – –	0	Uremic
14	61	F	Crohn	1.0	IgG-K	–	norm	sens	–	–	–	–	+	6.5	86	– – – –	71	?
15	32	M	Rec Pulm Inf	ND	–	K	dub	res	ND	ND	ND	ND	ND	2.0	30	+ + + –	1	CF
16	68	M	Rec Pulm Inf	ND	IgG-K	L	dub	res	±	+	–	–	–	14.4	10	–[*] – – –	>22	–
17	71	M	Rec Pulm Inf	ND	spike	K,L	norm	res	–	+	–	–	–	1.3	30	+ + – –	8	CF
18	49	M	RA	ND	spike	–	ND	res	–	+	–	–	±	0.0	2	–[*] – + +[$]	0	Uremic

SAA = serum amyloid A (N ≤2.6 mg/l); ND = not determined; – = absent; ± = weak, non specific; + = positive, present; norm = normal; dub = dubious (5-15% plasma cells); abn = abnormal (>15% plasma cells); & = Multiple Myeloma; CR = Congo red; $KMnO_4$ = potassium permanganate pretreatment; sens = sensitive; res = resistent; K = kappa; L = lambda; TTR = transthyretin; β_2M = β_2-microglobulin; AA = amyloid A; ECC = endogenous creatinine clearance; CF = cardiac failure; * = low voltage ECG; PN = polyneuropathy; # = autonomic neuropathy; Gl = macroglossia; Hp = hepatomegaly; $ = elevated alkaline phosphatase; -0 = autopsy

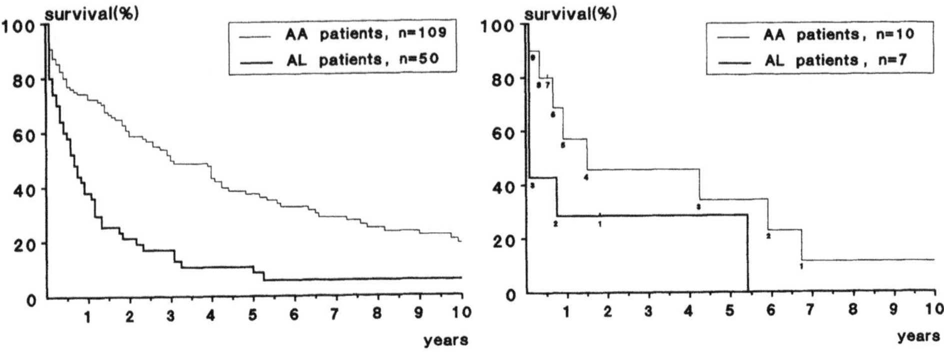

Figure 1. Survival curves of AA and AL patients

these clinically classified amyloid patients appeared to be 72% for those with the AA-type and 36% for those with the AL-type ($p<0.001$); a difference in survival between AA and AL patients could be detected from 3 months ($p<0.05$). The 1-year survival of the 18 patients classified by histology was 52% for those (n=10) having the AA-type and 29% for those (n=7) with the AL-type. No significant difference in survival between AA and AL could be observed in these two small groups.

4. DISCUSSION

The number of "idiopathic" non-hereditary patients in our population was small (6%); in this group AA- and AL-type were seen in the same frequency (each in 4 patients). The monoclonal protein was often of the Kappa-type in the "double" precursor producing process group, especially in the patients with the AA-type.

The concurrent presence of a monoclonal protein in AA patients with an associated inflammatory disease (in 6 out of 122 patients, 5%) could have been expected by chance in this age group. The concurrent presence of a chronic inflammatory disease in AL patients (in 4 out of 56 patients, 7%) is not understood easily, but may be explained by a relative immunodeficiency state due to suppression of normal immunoglobulin production.

5. REFERENCES

1. Janssen, S., Elema, J.D., Van Rijswijk, M.H., Limburg, P.C., Meijer, S. and Mandema, E. (1985) ' Classification of amyloidosis: Immunohistochemistry versus the potassium permanganate method in differentiating AA from AL amyloidosis', Appl. Pathol. 3, 29-38.

IMMUNOHISTOCHEMICAL DETECTION OF AMYLOID AA IN FORMALINE-FIXED PARAFFINE-EMBEDDED RECTAL BIOPSIES WITH THE MONOCLONAL ANTI-HUMAN SAA ANTIBODY REU.86.2

BOUKE P.C. HAZENBERG, JORIS GROND*, DICKY VAN DEN TOP*, JOHAN BIJZET, PIETER C. LIMBURG, MARTIN H. VAN RIJSWIJK
Division of Rheumatology and Department of Pathology*
State University Hospital, 59 Oostersingel
9713 EZ Groningen, The Netherlands

ABSTRACT. The present study addresses the reliability of a monoclonal anti-human SAA antibody (Reu.86.2) to detect amyloid AA in formaline-fixed paraffine-embedded rectal biopsies. A total of 34 rectal biopsies obtained from amyloidotic patients from 1986 until februari 1990 were positive for amyloid in the Congo red (CR) stain. Pretreatment with $KMnO_4$ eliminated CR staining in 30 specimens (AA-amyloid) whereas in 4 biopsies CR staining was resistent to $KMnO_4$ (non-AA). A murine monoclonal antibody (Reu.86.2) was raised against apo-SAA coupled to Helix Pomatia Haemocyanin. After pretreatment with 0.1% protease routine paraffine sections were incubated with Reu.86.2 as the first layer and peroxidase-conjugated Rabbit anti-Mouse antibody as the second. All 30 $KMnO_4$ sensitive specimens showed moderate or strong reactivity in immunostaining with the monoclonal antibody (in these biopsies the intensity of CR staining was moderate or strong in 18 and weak in 12). Twenty CR-negative controls and all 4 $KMnO_4$-resistent biopsies were negative in immunohistochemistry with Reu.86.2. In conclusion, immunohistochemistry with monoclonal anti-SAA antibody Reu.86.2 is an easy and highly reliable method to detect amyloid AA in rectal biopsies.

1. INTRODUCTION

Patients with chronic inflammation (like rheumatoid arthritis) are at risk to develop AA amyloidosis. Proteinuria or loss of renal function are the most frequent presenting symptoms (88%) of this complication [1]. The biopsy of rectal mucosa is the safest and best diagnostic procedure (sensitivity 81%) in cases of suspected amyloidosis [1]. Apple-green birefringence after staining with Congo red and under examination with polarized light is specific. However, amyloid deposits are sometimes small and easily overlooked. Routine immunohistochemistry with anti-AA antibodies could offer advantages.

Aim of the present study was to establish the reliability and ease of a monoclonal anti-human SAA antibody (Reu.86.2) to detect amyloid AA in formaline-fixed paraffine-embedded rectal biopsies.

2. MATERIALS AND METHODS

2.1. Rectal biopsies

From 1986 until februari 1990 in our University Hospital 34 rectal biopsies obtained from different patients were found to be positive for amyloid in the Congo red (CR) stain. Pretreatment with $KMnO_4$ eliminated CR staining in 30 specimens (AA-amyloid) whereas in 4 biopsies CR staining was resistent to $KMnO_4$ (non-AA). Twenty other rectal biopsies were used as negative controls.

2.2. Murine monoclonal antibody Reu.86.2

A murine monoclonal antibody (Reu.86.2) was raised against apo-SAA coupled to Helix Pomatia Haemocyanin. In short: HDL_3 was isolated from pooled sera (150 with CRP level >100 mg/l). SAA was purified by chromatography after HDL_3 delipidation. Monoclonal anti-SAA antibodies were raised to apo-SAA complexed (by glutaraldehyde) to Helix Pomatia Haemocyanin (HPH).

The produced monoclonal antibodies were screened and tested against: 1. Control antigens (HPH, CRP, and other amyloid proteins) in ELISA. 2. Purified SAA and AA from several donors in ELISA. 3. Native serum and purified SAA in immunoblotting techniques (PAGE and IEF). 4. Control and amyloid tissues in immunohistochemistry.

Reu.86.2 was chosen for its specificity and good results to be used in immunohistochemistry.

2.3. AA-immunohistochemistry

Formaline-fixed paraffin-embedded sections were treated as follows:
1. Deparaffination for 2 x 5 min in Xylol and successively in 100%, 96%, 70%, 50% and 30% ethanol/H_2O. 2. Endogenous peroxidase was blocked with 0.3% H_2O_2 for 30 min and subsequent washing in PBS. 3. Pretreatment with 0.1% protease (type XXIV, Sigma) in PBS for 15 min to enhance staining intensity. 4. Incubation with murine monoclonal anti-human apo-SAA antibody Reu.86.2 (culture supernatant diluted 1:100 in PBS) for 60 min. 5. Conjugate incubation: HRPO-Rabbit-anti-Mouse-IgG for 15 min; optional enhancement with HRPO-Swine-anti-Rabbit-IgG. 6. Incubation for 10 min with 20% AEC (3 amino-9-ethylcarbazole, A 5754, Sigma) in acetate buffer pH 5.0; a final concentration of 0.002% H_2O_2 was added before incubation.
NB. Frozen sections can be treated likewise, excluding step 1 and 3.

All specimens were processed and scored under code. Congo red staining as well as immunostaining with anti-SAA were scored for intensity: Negative (0), weak (+), moderate (++), strong (+++).

3. RESULTS

All 30 $KMnO_4$ sensitive specimens showed moderate or strong positivity in immunostaining with Reu.86.2; in these biopsies the intensity of CR staining was moderate or strong in 18 and weak in 12. Twenty CR-negative controls and all 4 $KMnO_4$-resistent biopsies were negative in immunohistochemistry; no background staining was observed. Table 1 summarizes these results. An example of a negative control is shown in figure 1 and an example of a positive biopsy in figure 2.

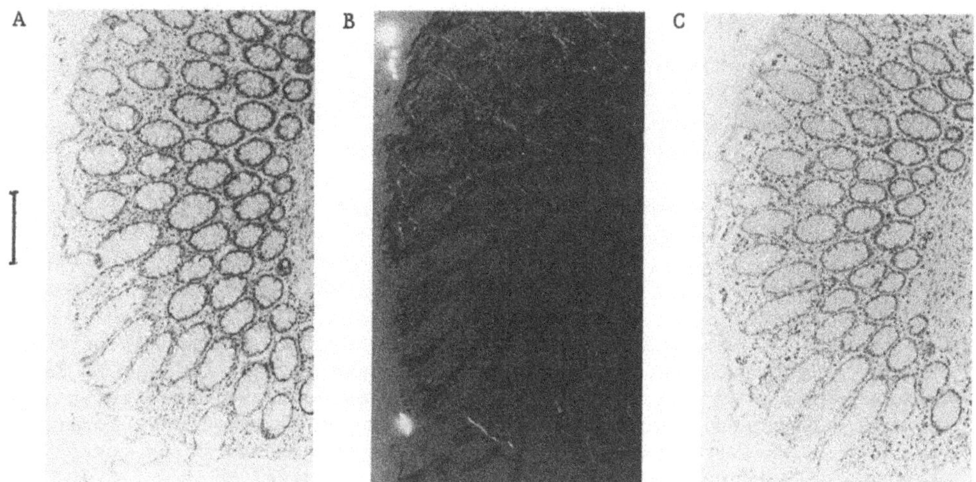

Figure 1. Rectal biopsy, negative control. A) Congo red, B) Congo red, birefringence, C) Reu.86.2 (anti-SAA). Bar length 0.2 mm.

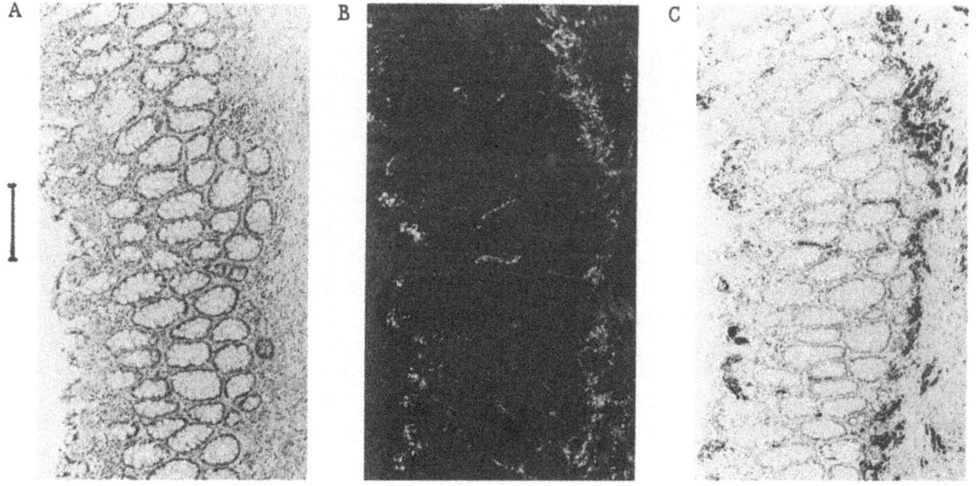

Figure 2. Rectal biopsy with amyloid AA. A) Congo red, B) Congo red, birefringence, C) Reu.86.2 (anti-SAA). Bar length 0.2 mm.

TABLE 1. A comparison of Congo red stain and immunostaining with Reu.86.2 in 54 rectal biopsies.

	Congo red				
Reu.86.2	0	+	++	+++	Total
0	20#	-	1*	3*	24
+	-	-	-	-	-
++	-	5	3	-	8
+++	-	7	6	9	22
Total	20	12	10	12	54

negative controls * $KMnO_4$ resistent specimens

4. DISCUSSION

The results of immunohistochemistry with Reu.86.2 obtained in this limited study material were at least as good as the CR stain. This method may be even better since small deposits could be detected easily whereas background staining was absent. However, it should be realized that the sensitivity and specificity of this method has to be confirmed prospectively in patients at risk for AA amyloidosis.

In conclusion, immunohistochemistry with our monoclonal anti-SAA antibody Reu.86.2 is an easy and highly reliable method to detect amyloid AA in rectal biopsies.

5. ACKNOWLEDGEMENTS

This study was supported by the Dutch Kidney Foundation.

We are grateful to our collegue L.de Leij for his assistance in monoclonal antibody production.

6. REFERENCES

1. Janssen, S., Van Rijswijk, M.H., Meijer, S., Ruinen, L. and Van der Hem, G.K. (1986) 'Systemic amyloidosis: a clinical survey of 144 cases', Neth. J. Med. 29, 376-395.

LONG SURVIVAL IN PATIENTS WITH AL AMYLOIDOSIS

N Ferrante
AS Cohen
JJ Anderson
M Skinner

From the Arthritis Center and Department of Medicine, Boston University School of Medicine, Boston

ABSTRACT

Eighteen of 127 patients with AL amyloidosis seen before October 1984 were found to have survived 60 months or longer. For this study, a control patient matched for the nearest date of diagnosis was analyzed with each long survivor. Six male and 12 female patients comprised the long survivor group, compared to 10 males and 8 females in the control group. Median survival from diagnosis was 93.3 months (range 60.9-205.3) for the long survivors and 12.3 months (2.3-56.5) for the controls. The marked difference in survival could not be predicted by organ system involvement.

INTRODUCTION

Primary (AL) amyloidosis is a non-malignant plasma cell dyscrasia characterized by overproduction of monoclonal immunoglobulin light chains which are the amyloid precursor proteins. The fibrillar protein is arranged in a ß-pleated sheet conformation and is deposited extracellularly in organs and tissues throughout the body. Progressive infiltration of normal tissues by the insoluble protein results in organ failure and ultimately death.

The average survival from the time of amyloid diagnosis is approximately one year with studies reporting 4.9 to 17.0 months (Kyle and Bayrd 1975, Kyle, et al 1986, Cohen, et al 1987). In spite of this generally poor prognosis, there are anecdotal reports of remarkably long survival with AL amyloidosis (Fritz, et al 1989). The scarcity of analyses of prognostic factors and the great disparity in survival time of small numbers of patients with AL amyloidosis prompted us to undertake this study.

MATERIALS AND METHODS

Patient population

Dates of diagnosis and death for all patients with AL amyloidosis seen at our Clinical Research Center (CRC) prior to Oct. 1984 were reviewed. Patients with amyloidosis and multiple myeloma were excluded. Survival was calculated from the date of histologic diagnosis to the date of death. Of 127 patients diagnosed between Apr. 1960 and Oct. 1984, 18 survived 60 mos. or longer, and were considered long survivors for this study. Each long survivor was paired with a control patient matched for the nearest date of diagnosis. The interval between dates of diagnosis of long survivors and paired controls was 5 mos. or less for all 18 pairs, with a mean of 1.3 mos.

Statistical Analysis

Medical records from CRC evaluations and referring physicians were reviewed for measurable parameters defining organ system involvement and laboratory results. For comparison of survival of long survivor and control groups after organ involvement the log-rank test was used, with adjustment for censored data (i.e. 5 long survivors are still living, and 1 was lost to follow-up at 78 months after diagnosis).

RESULTS

Six males and 12 females comprised the long survivor group, compared to 10 males and 8 females in the control group. Mean age at the time of diagnosis was 57.6 years for long survivors and 54.6 for controls. All patients were diagnosed between April 1971 and October 1984. Median survival from the date of diagnosis until death was 93.3 months for the long survivor group and 12.3 months for the control group. No discernible differences were noted in treatments of amyloid, and presence of plasmacytosis or serum M-component (Table 1).

The mean number of organ systems involved at the time of diagnosis was 2.4 for long survivors and 3.0 for controls. The mean number of organ systems involved over the entire course of disease was 5.1 for long survivors and 5.7 for controls. This difference was not significant.

The number of patients with involvement of a particular organ system and the median survival after organ involvement was examined. For controls median survival after specific organs were involved ranged from 5.1 mos. after onset of neuropathy (other than carpal tunnel syndrome) to 29.9 mos. after onset of arrhythmia or abnormal conduction. For long survivors median survival ranged from 41.6 months after onset of abnormalities in cardiac ECHO to 98.3 mos. after onset of carpal tunnel syndrome. Differences in median survival after organ involvement between long survivors and controls was highly significant for all organ involvement except echocardiographic abnormalities.

TABLE 1 LONG SURVIVOR STUDY GROUP

	Long Survivors	Controls
Median Survival		
(months)	93.3	12.3
(range)	(60.9-205.3)	(2.3-56.5)
Sex: male	6	10
female	12	8
Age at diagnosis	57.6	54.6
(range)	(37-72)	(28-73)
Alive: female	4	0
male	1	0
Plasmacytosis	9	12
M-Component	6	8
Treatment:		
Colchicine	18	15
Melphalan	8	6

DISCUSSION

No apparent organ system involvement (or lack thereof) distinguishes long survivors from controls in this study. Different organ systems were involved with comparable frequency in both groups. It does not appear that long survivors merely were diagnosed earlier in the course of their disease, since the mean number of organ systems involved at the time of diagnosis was similar for both groups.

Median survival from diagnosis of 12.3 mos. for the controls is similar to survival reported in other studies (Cohen, et al 1987, Kyle, et al 1975, 1983, 1986). Median survival of 6.5 mos. after onset of CHF in the control group is comparable to survival of 4 and 6 months. Peripheral neuropathy has been associated with relatively longer survival (Duston, et al 1989,

Kyle, et al 1983), but this was not found among controls in our study, with median survival of only 5.1 mos. after onset of symptoms being the shortest survival for any organ involvement in the control group.

A study of prognostic factors in AL amyloidosis cited CHF and hepatomegaly among factors that had adverse effects on survival, at least in the first year after diagnosis (Kyle, et al 1986). Neither factors were good predictors of clinical outcome for long survivors in our study with median survival after onset of symptoms of 65.9 mos. in these subsets.

Perhaps, most surprising, is the relatively mild influence of cardiac arrhythmias on survival. Studies cite cardiac involvement as a cause of death in roughly 40% of patients with primary amyloidosis, and sudden cardiac death due to arrhythmias is felt to be a relatively frequent event. Yet in our study both long survivors (89.3 mos.) and controls (29.9 mos.) had good median survival after the onset of arrhythmias.

ACKNOWLEDGEMENTS

Supported by grants from the U.S. Public Health Service, NIAMDD (AM 07014), the General Clinical Research Centers Branch of the Division of Research Resources, National Institutes of Health (RR 533), the Multipurpose Arthritis Center, National Institutes of Health (AM 20613), and the Arthritis Foundation.

REFERENCES

1. Cohen AS, Rubinow A, Anderson JJ, Skinner M, Mason JH, Libbey C, Kayne H: (1987) survival of patients with primary (AL) amyloidosis. Amer J Med 82:1182-1190.
2. Duston MA, Skinner M, Anderson JJ, Cohen AS: (1989) Peripheral neuropathy as an early marker of AL amyloidosis. Arch Int Med 149:358-360.
3. Fritz DA, Luggen ME, Hess EV: (1989) Unusual longevity in primary systemic amyloidosis, a 19-year survivor. Amer J Med 86:245-248.
4. Kyle RA, Bayrd ED: (1975) Amyloidosis: review of 236 cases. Medicine 54:271-299.
5. Kyle RA, Greipp PR: (1983) Amyloidosis (AL) clinical and laboratory features in 229 cases. Mayo Clin Proc 58:665-683.
6. Kyle RA, Greipp PR, O'Fallon WM: (1986) Primary systemic amyloidosis: multivariate analysis for prognostic factors in 168 cases. Blood 68:220-224.

SECONDARY SYSTEMIC AMYLOIDOSIS (AA): RESPONSE AND SURVIVAL IN 64 PATIENTS

M. A. GERTZ, M.D.
R. A. KYLE, M.D.
Dysproteinemia Clinic
Mayo Clinic and Mayo Foundation
200 First Street Southwest
Rochester, Minnesota 55905
United States

ABSTRACT. From 1956 through 1989, 38 men and 26 women were seen at the Mayo Clinic with biopsy-proven secondary amyloidosis (AA). The underlying disease was rheumatic in 42, infectious in 11, inflammatory bowel disease in 6, and other causes in 5. Of the 64 patients, 58 had proteinuria or renal insufficiency at diagnosis. Symptoms of gastro-intestinal amyloid were seen in 14 and 6 had amyloid goiter. None of the patients had symptomatic cardiac involvement, and only three had palpable hepatomegaly. Renal, gastric, rectal, fat, and marrow biopsies were positive for amyloid in 100, 94, 82, 58, and 46 percent of tested patients, respectively. The median survival of the entire group was 24.5 months. Of the 47 deceased patients, 35 died as a direct result of their amyloidosis, primarily complications of renal failure. Nine were successfully treated and had regression of the disease. Two with bronchiectasis responded to antibiotic therapy as did one patient with osteomyelitis. One patient with inflammatory bowel disease responded to surgical resection and one with familial Mediterranean fever responded to colchicine. Four patients with rheumatic disease were treated with cyclophosphamide (2) and methotrexate (2) with resolution of their renal disease. All nine patients are alive with a median follow-up of 58 months. Multivariate analysis revealed that creatinine ≥ 2.0 mg/dl ($p < 0.003$) and serum albumin <2.5 g/dl ($p < 0.02$) had an adverse impact on survival. The strongest variable predicting survival was serum creatinine >2 mg/dl with a median survival of 11.2 months compared to patients with a creatinine <2.0 mg/dl where median survival was 56.9 months.

Introduction

Secondary amyloidosis (AA) represents the first recognized form of amyloidosis. It was also the first form of amyloid to be isolated, sequenced, and recognized as unique in its derivation (1). In view of the changing spectrum of the disease and the absence of information on survival, we undertook a retrospective review of the Mayo Clinic experience in this disorder.

Materials and Methods

All patients with the diagnosis of secondary amyloidosis seen at the Mayo Clinic between 1956 and 1989 were included in this study. The diagnosis of AA required biopsy or autopsy confirmation. Patients with a monoclonal immunoglobulin protein in the serum or in the urine were excluded. All patients in the series were required to have a compatible clinical syndrome (long-standing inflammatory process) or positive immunochemical stains for amyloid A protein (2) in order to be eligible. No patient was lost to follow-up.

Results

The median age of males and females was 51 (n = 38) and 64 years (n = 26), respectively. When examining only patients with an underlying rheumatic disorder, the male to female ratio was 1:1 and the median age of men and women was 63 and 66 years, respectively. There were 31 patients who had rheumatoid arthritis, 5 ankylosing spondylitis, 3 psoriatic arthritis, and 3 other rheumatic diseases. Five patients had osteomyelitis, five had bronchiectasis, six had inflammatory bowel disease, and two had familial Mediterranean fever. The median time between first symptoms of the underlying disorder and a tissue diagnosis of AA was 19 years (range, 0.2 months to 42.5 years). Only 15 patients had their disease less than 10 years prior to the diagnosis of AA.

Clinical Presentation

The clinical target organ was the kidney in 90 percent of patients. At diagnosis, 62 percent of the patients had $\geq$3 grams protein/day. A serum creatinine >2 mg/dl was present at diagnosis in 31 of the 64 patients. Only three patients had palpable hepatomegaly. The serum alkaline phosphatase was elevated in 8 of the 56 patients in whom the test was performed. The median sedimentation rate for the group was 84 mm/hour. Six of the patients had thyromegaly, but none were hypothyroid. Clinical gastrointestinal symptomatology was present in 23 percent (3,4). The most common symptoms were those of malabsorption or pseudo-obstruction. There were 14 patients who underwent 2-D echocardiography, but none had an echo diagnostic of amyloid.

Biopsy Verification of Amyloid

The incidence of positive biopsies in AA is quite similar to AL with renal, gastric, rectal, fat, and marrow biopsies showing amyloid deposits in 100, 94, 82, 58, and 46 percent of patients tested, respectively (5). There were 14 patients whose amyloid was reconfirmed at autopsy. Widespread vascular deposits were seen in virtually all organs examined, but the dominant deposits were limited to the intestinal tract and kidneys. Liver amyloid was not considered contributory to death in any patients.

Survival

At this time, 47 of the 64 patients have died (73 percent). Of the surviving 17, 6 are on dialysis. The median survival of the entire group was 24.5 months. Of the deaths, 35 were directly due to amyloidosis, with 32 dying of renal failure and 3 dying of intestinal dysfunction resulting in cachexia and malnutrition. Of the entire group, 21 patients received dialysis. At this time, 15 have died with a median survival of one year from the start of dialysis. Multivariate analysis showed that serum alkaline phosphatase, ESR, 24-hour urine total protein loss, age, and gender were found to have no predictive survival value. A serum creatinine level $\geq$2.0 mg/dl ($p < 0.003$) and serum albumin level <2.5 g/dl ($p < 0.02$) had significant predictive value toward survival. The median survival of patients with both the creatinine $\geq$2.0 mg/dl and albumin <2.5 g/dl was 7.0 months ($n = 20$).

Treatment Response

Following the diagnosis of amyloidosis, 44 patients received therapy. Nine of the patients showed a clear-cut response to treatment. All nine patients are alive with a median follow-up of 58 months; one of the patients is on dialysis. Two patients were treated with cytoxan and two were treated with methotrexate with regression of proteinuria (all four had rheumatic diseases). Two patients with bronchiectasis responded to cyclic antibiotics, one patient with familial Mediterranean fever responded to colchicine, one patient with inflammatory bowel disease responded to total colectomy, and one patient with osteomyelitis responded to debridement, surgery, and antibiotics.

Discussion

Secondary amyloidosis is rare. The ratio of AA to AL seen at Mayo Clinic currently is approximately 1:17. In the past, most cases of secondary amyloidosis were associated with tuberculosis and syphilis (6). In a study conducted by the AFIP (7), 63 percent of the patients had an infectious process underlying the amyloidosis. Only 15 percent were rheumatic in origin. In the current study, two-thirds of the patients had rheumatic diseases underlying their amyloid. The optimal method for diagnosing AA remains controversial. Our study did reveal a large number of positive endoscopic biopsies of gastric and small intestinal mucosa which proved to be valuable in the diagnosis of AA (8). Amyloid goiter was seen in 10 percent of our patients. Of patients with rheumatic disease, half were rheumatoid factor negative (9). Whether effective treatment exists for AA remains controversial. Since this study was retrospective and patients were not treated uniformly, it is impossible to comment on whether specific therapies are warranted. It was clear nonetheless that there was a subset of patients who had significant regression of clinical manifestations of AA. Resolution of AA amyloidosis following resection of diseased bowel in inflammatory bowel disease has been well reported (10). Antibiotic use has drastically reduced the incidence of amyloidosis complicating osteomyelitis and tuberculosis (11). Colchicine has clearly been shown to be useful in the treatment of amyloid associated with familial Mediterranean fever, as well as Muckle-Wells syndrome and Behcet's disease. In the current study, there were four patients with rheumatic disease with resolution of organ dysfunction associated with their amyloid. Immunosuppressive therapy has previously been reported to be useful in the treatment of AA, as has chlorambucil therapy. In conclusion, the majority of patients with symptomatic renal amyloidosis have an underlying rheumatic disorder. In virtually all patients, the kidney is the affected organ followed by the GI tract. Endoscopic biopsy of the upper intestinal tract was positive in 94 percent. The liver and myocardium do not appear to be clinically significant target organs in this disease. The median survival in this series was 24.5 months with three-fourths of the deaths a direct result of amyloidosis. Serum creatinine and albumin values are useful survival predictors. Aggressive immunosuppressive therapy may produce disease remissions that can be durable and dramatic.

References

1. Benditt, EP, Eriksen, M, Hermodsen, MA, Ericsson, LH. (1971) FEBS Lett 19, 169.
2. Linke, RP, Huhn, D, Nathrath, WBJ. Isobe, T, Araki, S, Uchino, F, Kito, S, Tsubura, E, eds. (1988) New York, Plenum, 247.
3. Dey, C, Duvoisin, B. (1989) J Comput Assist Tomgr 13, 1094-1095.
4. Legge, DA, Carlson, HC, Wollaegen, EE. (1970) Am J Roentgenol, Radium Ther Nucl Med 110, 406-412.
5. Gulati, PD, Aurora, AL, Mathur, GP, Vaishnaud, H. (1970) Postgrad Med J 46, 137-141.
6. Dahlin, DC. (1949) Ann Intern Med 31, 105-119.
7. Brownstein, MH, Helwig, EB. (1971) South Med J 64, 491-496.
8. Tada, S, Iida, M, Iwashita, A, Matsui, T, Fuchigami, Yamamoto, T, Yao, T, Fujishima, M. (1990) Gastintest Endosc 33, 10-14.
9. Maury, CPJ. (1984) Rheumatol Int 5, 1-7.
10. Edwards, P, Cooper, DA, Turner, J, O'Connor, TJ, Byrnes, DJ. (1988) Gastroenterology 95, 810-815.
11. Sunga, MN Jr, Reyes, CV, Zvetina, J, Kim, TW. (1989) South Med J 82, 92-93.

RENAL MANIFESTATIONS OF AMYLOIDOSIS COMPLICATED WITH RHEUMATOID ARTHRITIS

Yasuo Matsuoka, Mitsuo Obana, Shoichiro Irimajiri.
Kawasaki Municipal Hospital
P.O. 210
12-1, Shinkawa-dori, Kawasaki city, Kanagawa
Japan

ABSTRACT. Renal manifestations of 25 cases with amyloidosis complicated with rheumatoid arthritis (RA) were investigated. The duration of RA prior to the diagnosis of amyloidosis was 16.1±12.0 years. Urinary protein was positive in 18 cases (72%). The degree of proteinuria varied in each case. Nephrotic syndrome was observed in 7 cases. Azotemia (Cr>1.5mg/dl) was present in 20 cases (80%). Among them, 3 cases did not show proteinuria in their clinical courses. Azotemia preceded to proteinuria in 2 cases. The duration of proteinuria prior to the emergence of azotemia was 0.2 to 6 years (2.6±1.3 years). Hemodialysis was done in 7 cases. The duration from the emergence of azotemia to the start of hemodialysis was 0.5 to 6 years (2.4±2.0 years). The duration of azotemia prior to death was 0.1 to 6.5 years (2.8±2.3 years). These data suggested that although renal manifestations were frequently observed in amyloidosis, their courses were varied.

Although nephropathy was frequent in the patients of amyloidosis complicated wiht RA, the detailed clinical course was not reported. We intensively investigated the clinical course of nephropathy in amyloidosis complicated with RA.

Patients and method

Twenty-five patients with RA who were diagnosed as amyloidosis by biopsy or autopsy at Kawasaki municipal hospital in the 21 years from 1969 to 1989 were selected. Among them, 4 cases were confirmed as amyloidosis for the first time at autopsy. Five cases were alive and the remaining 20 cases were dead.

The diagnosis of amyloidosis was confirmed by the presence of greenish birefrigence under polarized microscope in the sections stained with Congo-red and by the indirect immunofluorescent technique using anti-AA antibody. The sites of biopsy to make the initial diagnosis of amyloidosis were stomach in 17 cases, rectum in 3 cases and kidney in 1 case.

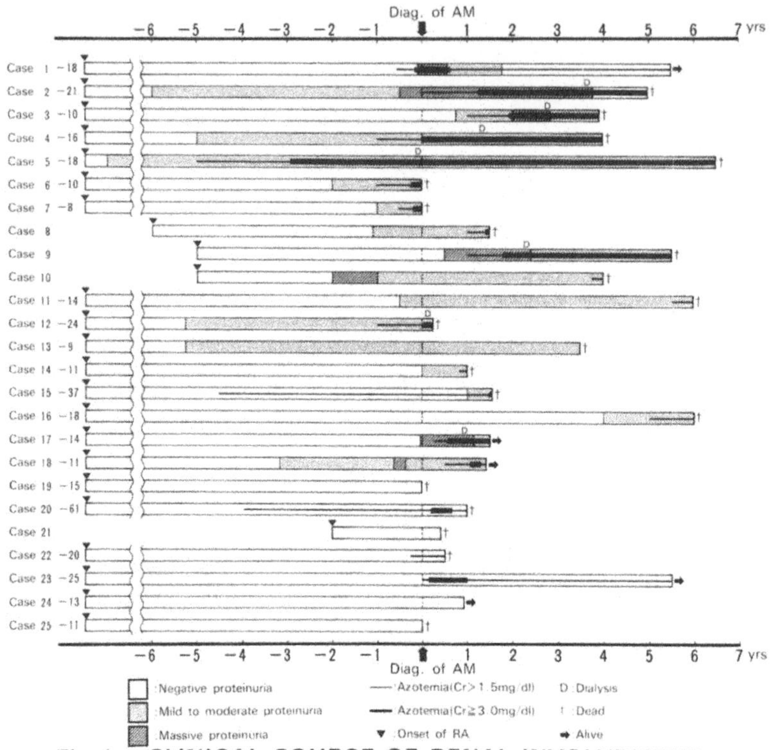

Fig.1. CLINICAL COURSE OF RENAL INVOLVEMENT

Results

The clinical course of amyloid nephropathy starting from the onset of RA in each case is shown in Fig. 1. The duration of RA prior to the diagnosis of amyloidosis was 16.1 years on the average (less than 5 years in one case, from 5 to 9 years in 5 cases and 10 or more years in 19 cases).

Urinary protein was positive in 18 cases (72%). The duration of RA prior to the emergence of proteinuria was 12.9 years on the average, ranging from 3 to 38 years. Most cases showed persistent proteinuria. Intermittent proteinuria was found only in one case. The degree of proteinuria varied between cases. Nephrotic syndrome was observed in 7 cases (28%). In some cases, nephrotic syndrome occured abruptly and in the other cases, it occured after several years of mild proteinuria.

Hematuria was observed in 13 out of 18 cases with proteinuria, but was not seen in any patients without proteinuria. Hematuria was intermittent in 6 cases, continuous in 4 cases and transient in 3 cases.

Hypertension was present in 14 out of 18 cases with proteinuria (77.8%), and in 4 out of 7 without proteinuria (57.1%).

Table 1 CASES TREATED WITH DIALYSIS

	Duration from onset of proteinuria to dialysis (yrs)	Duration from onset of azotemia to dialysis (yrs)	Duration from dialysis to death (yrs)
Case 2	10 (HD)	4	1.5
Case 3	2.5 (HD)	2	1.5
Case 4	6.5 (CAPD)	2.5	3
Case 5	10 (HD)	6	6.5
Case 9	2 (CAPD)	1	4
Case 12	5 (CAPD)	0.5	0.1
Case 17	0.9 (HD)	0.7	Alive
	5.3±3.7	2.4±2.0	2.8±2.3

Azotemia (Cr>1.5mg/dl) was present in 20 cases (80%). Among these cases, proteinuria was absent in 3 patients. Therefore, both azotemia and proteinuria were observed in 17 cases. The duration of RA prior to the emergence of azotemia was 18.2 years on the average, ranging from 6 to 57 years. The duration from the emergence of proteinuria to that of azotemia was ranging from 0.2 to 6 years (2.6 years on the average) in 15 cases, excluding 2 cases in which azotemia preceded proteinuria (case 1 and 15).

Hemodialysis or continuous ambulatory peritoneal dialysis was implemented in 7 cases (Table 1). The period from occurence of proteinuria and that of azotemia to start of dialysis was ranging from 0.9 to 10 years (mean 5.3 years) and from 0.7 to 6 years (mean 2.4 years), respectively. The duration from the start of dialysis to the death was ranging from 0.1 to 6.5 years in 6 dead cases.

Twenty out of 25 cases were dead. All of them died within 7 years after the initial diagnosis of amyloidosis. The mean survival period was 3.2 years (0.1 to 6.5 years) after the diagnosis was made in 16 cases, excluding 4 cases in which the diagnosis of amyloidosis was made at autopsy. The cardinal causes of death were uremia in 11 cases, heart failure, sepsis and malignancy in 2 cases, respectively.

Discussion and conclusion

Some investigators reported that male rheumatoid patients appear to be more susceptible to secondary amyloidosis than female patients in western countries. Cohen [1] reported that the ratio of males to females with amyloidosis complicated with RA was 1.1 : 1.0. In the present study the ratio was 1 : 24. We cannot precisely explain this discrepancy, but there might be differences due to the race in the susceptibility to amyloidosis.

The usefulness of rectal biopsy has been emphasized for the diagnosis of secondary amyloidosis. In our present study, we were able to make the diagnosis of amyloidosis by gastric biopsy in 17 out of 21 cases [2]. Gastroscopy is not only easy but also is safe in comparison with colonoscopy. Moreover gastroscopy is useful to confirm the existence of gastric lesions such as gastric ulcer induced by nonsteroidal anti-inflammatory drugs. Therefore, we consider that gastric biopsy is sufficient to determine the diagnosis of amyloidosis rather than employing rectal biopsy. In this study proteinuria was observed in 18 out of 25 cases and the frequency of hematuria was 52%. Although nephrotic syndrome is said to be characteristic of amyloidosis complicated with RA, in our cases proteinuria greatly varied both in degree and course. Nephrotic syndrome was observed only in 7 cases. There were 3 cases in which renal manifestations were clinically absent. However deposition of amyloid fibril in the kidney was observed in these cases at autopsy. These results suggested that it is impossible to deny the existence of renal amyloidosis even if renal manifestations were clinically absent.

Azotemia was found in 20 cases. The periods from the occurence of proteinuria to those of azotemia were quite different from case by case. We elucidated that there were some cases which presented azotemia without proteinuria during the clinical course, as Falck et al. [3] have reported.

Although it has been reported that hypertension is comparatively rare in secondary amyloidosis even when renal function is deteriorated [4], our data suggested hypertension was rather common in secondary amyloidosis complicated with RA.

In conclusion, although renal manifestations were frequently observed in secondary amyloidosis complicated with RA, their clinical courses were varied in case by case.

References

1. Cohen, AS. (1968) 'Amyloidosis associated with rheumatoid arthritis', Med. Clin. North. Am. 52, 643-653.
2. Obana, M., Matsuoka, Y,. Irimajiri, S. (1990) 'Clinical studies on amyloidosis complicated with rheumatoid arthritis', Jap. J. Med. in press.
3. Falck, HM., Tornroth, T., Wegelius, O. (1983) 'Predominantly vascular amyloid deposition in the kidney in patients with minimal or no proteinuria', Clin. Nephrol. 19, 137-142.
4. Husby, G. (1985) 'Amyloidosis and rheumatoid arthritis', Clin. Exp. Rheumatol. 3, 173-180.

CRP AND SAA SERUM LEVELS IN CHRONIC ACTIVE HEPATITIS

BOUKE P.C. HAZENBERG, BART VAN HOEK*, PIETER C. LIMBURG, JOHAN BIJZET, J. REINT HUIZENGA*, JORIS GROND#, MARTIN H. VAN RIJSWIJK, CHRIS H. GIPS*
Div. Rheumatology, Div. Hepatology* and Dpt. Pathology#
State University Hospital, 59 Oostersingel
9713 EZ Groningen, The Netherlands

1. INTRODUCTION

C-reactive protein (CRP) and serum amyloid A (SAA) were studied in chronic active hepatitis (CAH), a disease of the principal site of CRP and SAA production. CRP and SAA levels were compared with histological severity and levels of cholinesterase (CHE), a representative of liver synthesis capacity.

2. MATERIALS AND METHODS

2.1. Patients

Sera were studied in 81 untreated patients with CAH (male-female ratio 1:1.5, median age 49 years). Thirty-six had "autoimmune" (AI) CAH. Liver biopsies and sera were studied in 29 untreated AI-CAH patients.

2.2. Liver histology

Liver biopsies (examined under code) were assigned a Histologic Activity Score (HAS). This HAS is a numerical score (0-18), and the summation of portal (0-4), periportal (0-10) and lobular (0-4) inflammation and necrosis.

2.3. Serology

Sera were immediately frozen and stored (-20°C) until analysis.

CRP and SAA were quantified by a sandwich ELISA. Basal control values: CRP ≤2.0 mg/l, SAA ≤2.6 mg/l.

Cholinesterase was measured by its activity: Lower reference 1600 U/l (women) and 1800 U/l (men).

2.4. Statistical analysis

Mann Whitney U and Spearman's rank correlation were used. $P<0.05$ was significant.

3. RESULTS

In 81 untreated CAH patients, elevated CRP levels were found in 54 (68%, $p<0.0001$ vs. controls) and elevated SAA levels in 12 (15%, n.s.). Median CRP was 6.6 mg/l in AI-CAH patients and 2.9 mg/l in the others with CAH; no difference was found between both CAH groups. Median SAA in these groups were 0.7 resp. 0.5 mg/l.

In 29 untreated patients with AI-CAH the CRP levels correlated with HAS ($R=0.40$, $p<0.05$) and especially with periportal inflammation ($R=0.48$, $p<0.05$). No correlation was seen between CRP and CHE ($R=-0.06$, $p=0.75$). SAA correlated with CHE levels ($R=0.61$, $p<0.005$). However, neither inflammation ($R=0.06$, $p=0.76$) nor CRP levels ($R=0.22$, $p=0.24$) correlated with SAA. No correlation was found between inflammation and CHE levels ($R=-0.10$, $p=0.62$).

4. DISCUSSION

In CAH of all aetiologies, the acute-phase response is depressed with regard to CRP and especially to SAA. SAA levels are usually not elevated in CAH, whereas CRP is elevated, but not to levels reflecting the high degree of inflammation in such a voluminous organ. SAA correlates with cholinesterase, while CRP does not. CRP modestly reflected the degree of histological (periportal) inflammation, while SAA did not. Impairment of the hepatic capacity to synthesize proteins probably affected SAA more severely than CRP, resulting in this different behaviour of both proteins.

5. ACKNOWLEDGEMENTS

This study was supported by the Dutch Kidney Foundation.

SERUM AMYLOID A AND C-REACTIVE PROTEIN IN THE FIRST 4 WEEKS AFTER LIVER TRANSPLANTATION

BOUKE P.C. HAZENBERG, PIETER C. LIMBURG, J. REINT HUIZENGA*, JOHAN BIJZET, ANNET S.H. GOUW#, MARTIN H. VAN RIJSWIJK, CHRIS H. GIPS*
Div. Rheumatology, Div. Hepatology* and Dpt. Pathology#
State University Hospital, 59 Oostersingel
9713 EZ Groningen, The Netherlands

ABSTRACT. SAA and CRP serum levels were monitored for 4 weeks after liver transplantation (Tx) in 10 patients. Median age of these 6 women and 4 men was 41 years (range 17-55). Therapy consisted of high dose glucocorticoids with azathioprine. One week after Tx a biopsy was taken to detect acute rejection. SAA and CRP were measured by ELISA. Median SAA level before Tx was 2.5 mg/l and median CRP 9.4 mg/l. Top SAA and CRP levels were seen after 1 to 3 days. The severity of acute rejection did not correlate with SAA and CRP levels 2, 3, 7 and 14 days after Tx. Basal reference values for "healthy" (N=19) patients 1-3 years after Tx were calculated: Median SAA 2.1 mg/l, 95% upper limit 6.2 mg/l. Median CRP 0.35 mg/l, 95% upper limit 3.7 mg/l. SAA values were higher than basal values of 50 healthy controls ($p<0.0001$), while CRP values did not differ. In conclusion, the diseased liver was deficient in the production of CRP and especially SAA. CRP and SAA levels did not correlate with the acute rejection found one week after Tx. Basal reference values of "healthy" patients years after Tx showed a modest elevation of SAA levels compared to healthy controls. This elevation of SAA in combination with normal CRP might be caused by maintenance therapy with glucocorticoids, although subclinical rejection cannot be excluded.

1. INTRODUCTION

Serum amyloid A (SAA) is claimed to be a sensitive marker of rejection in renal transplantation (Tx) and to be more sensitive than C-reactive protein (CRP) [1]. However, liver graft rejection is more complex while the principal production site of SAA and CRP is involved. The clinical diagnosis of rejection is made by exclusion of other causes of graft dysfunction. Serial biopsy monitoring of the graft is a safe and accurate diagnostic aid to detect rejection. Recently SAA appeared to be a sensitive marker of acute rejection in all 11 episodes of liver graft rejection [2], while CRP levels were elevated in only 5 out of 9 rejection episodes [3].

Aim of this study was to investigate in 10 patients the clinical usefulness of SAA and CRP serum levels to detect acute rejection 1 week after liver Tx. Basal reference values for this group of patients were obtained from 19 other "healthy" patients 1, 2 and 3 years after Tx.

2. MATERIALS AND METHODS

2.1. Patients

A group of 10 patients was selected from a total of 53 patients receiving a liver allograft. These 10 patients were without graft pathology other than acute rejection: no viral infections (like CMV, HSV and HBV) and no biliary and vascular complications. SAA and CRP levels were monitored daily for 4 weeks after Tx. The median age of these 6 women and 4 men was 41 years (range 17-55). Immunosuppressive therapy consisted of high dose glucocorticoids with azathioprine.

In 19 other patients SAA and CRP were measured 1, 2 and 3 years after Tx. All were without serious infection, surgery or rejection and with low dose prednisolone and azathioprine as maintenance therapy.

SAA and CRP levels were monitored in one particular patient from the detection of her primary biliary cirrhosis (PBC) 9 years before Tx until 8 years after Tx.

2.2. Liver histology

Needle biopsies from the liver graft were taken at the end of the first week after Tx. All biopsies were examined under code for the presence and severity (numerical score ranging from 0-3) of acute rejection [4].

2.3. Serology

All serum samples were immediately frozen and stored (-20°C) until analysis. CRP and SAA were quantified by a sandwich ELISA. Basal control values (N=50) are for CRP ≤2.0 mg/l and for SAA ≤2.6 mg/l with a median level of 0.5 mg/l for CRP and 0.7 mg/l for SAA [5].

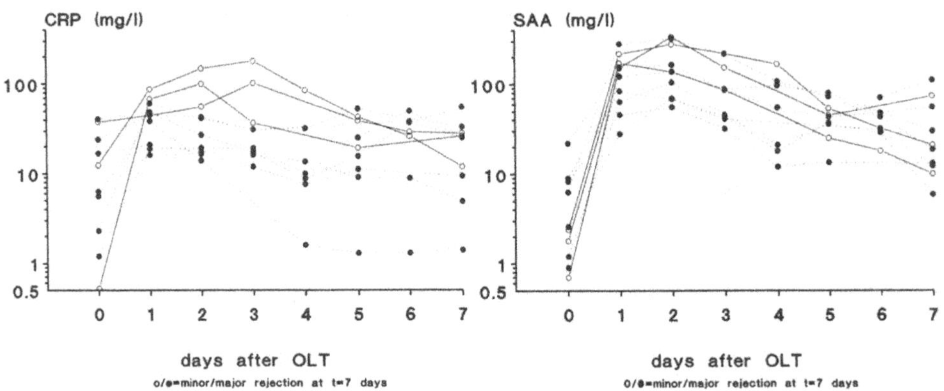

Figure 1. a) CRP and b) SAA serum levels for 7 days after liver Tx.

2.4. Statistical analysis

The Mann Whitney U test and Spearman's rank correlation were used where appropriate, with $p<0.05$ as the level of significance.

3. RESULTS

Before Tx median SAA level was 2.5 mg/l (range 0.7-22), median CRP level 9.4 mg/l (range 0.2-41) and median SAA/CRP ratio 0.65 (range 0.05-3.9). Top levels of SAA and CRP were seen 1 to 3 days after Tx, as shown in figure 1. One week after Tx median SAA level was 22 mg/l (range 5.9-111), median CRP 26 mg/l (range 1.4-55) and median SAA/CRP 1.6 (range 0.2-39). Median values for CRP gradually fell down: 12.8, 7.9 and 5.2 mg/l after 2, 3 and 4 weeks respectively. However, concurrent values for SAA fluctuated: resp. 8.4, 17.3 and 15.0 mg/l.

Rejection after one week: score 0 (N=1), score 1 (N=2), score 2 (N=6) and score 3 (N=1). No correlation was detected between the score of rejection and SAA and CRP levels at 2, 3, 7 and 14 days after Tx. In figure 1 the 3 patients with score 0 or 1 are presented with open dots.

Basal reference values for SAA and CRP in 19 "healthy" patients 1, 2 and 3 years after Tx were calculated by taking the lowest couple of values for each patient. After log-transformation this resulted in a median value for SAA of 2.1 mg/l (mean 2.0 mg/l) with a 95% upper limit of 6.2 mg/l. The median CRP was 0.35 mg/l (mean 0.4 mg/l) with a 95% upper limit of 3.7 mg/l. SAA values were higher than basal values of healthy controls ($p<0.0001$), while CRP values did not differ.

Figure 2 shows SAA and CRP serum levels in the patient with PBC. A small rise of CRP can be observed during disease progression, while SAA levels remain low. After Tx the SAA/CRP ratio inverts and the effects of surgery, cytomegalovirus (CMV) infection and a humerus fracture can be seen clearly. No distinct effects are visible on SAA and CRP levels induced by the acute rejection. However, this may be masked by the concurrent acute-phase reaction caused by CMV. Five months after Tx the CRP levels have fallen into the reference range, while the SAA levels fluctuate around the upper limit; both CRP and SAA remain so for years.

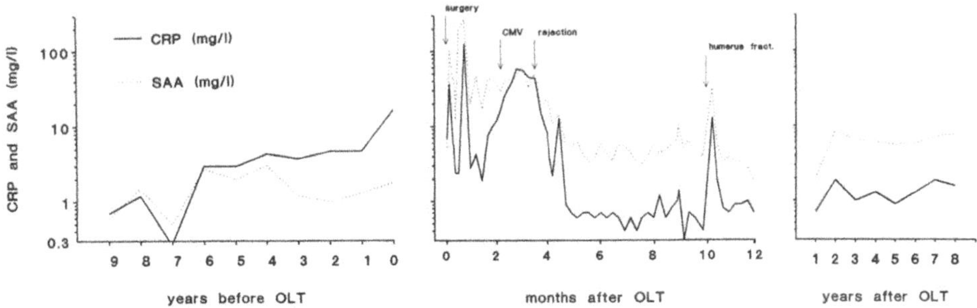

Figure 2. A patient with PBC.

4. DISCUSSION

The diseased liver just before Tx was deficient in the production of CRP and especially SAA. We have observed this in chronic inflammatory diseases of the liver, especially in chronic active hepatitis [5].

SAA and CRP values were still elevated one week after Tx without a relation with rejection. The most likely explanation of the lack of correlation between SAA (and CRP) levels and acute rejection is that we were too early after Tx to detect an additional effect on SAA (and CRP) levels while the new liver was recovering from major surgery (maybe even from the events leading to the death of the donor). Acute and chronic rejections have to be studied on various moments after Tx to establish the value of SAA (and CRP) for the detection of rejection.

The basal SAA reference values of "healthy" patients years after Tx are higher than the basal values of healthy controls, while those of CRP do not differ. Subclinical rejection might be a theoretical cause of this moderate SAA elevation, but a relationship with glucocorticoid therapy is a more likely explanation as has been observed in rheumatoid arthritis and polymyalgia rheumatica [6].

5. ACKNOWLEDGEMENTS

Part of this study was supported by the Dutch Kidney Foundation.

6. REFERENCES

1. Maury, C.P.J. and Teppo, A.-M. (1984) 'Comparative study of serum amyloid related protein SAA, C-reactive protein and β_2-microglobulin as markers of renal allograft rejection', Clin. Nephrol. 22, 284-292.
2. Maury, C.P.J., Höckerstedt, K., Lautenschlager, I. and Scheinin, T.M. (1987) 'Monitoring of high-density lipoprotein-associated amyloid A protein after liver transplantation', Transplant. Proc. 19, 3825-3826.
3. Maury, C.P.J., Teppo, A.-M. and Höckerstedt, K. (1988) 'Acute phase proteins and liver allograft rejection', Liver 8, 75-79.
4. Snover, D.C. (1986) 'The pathology of acute rejection', Transplant. Proc. 18, 123-127.
5. Hazenberg, B.P.C., Limburg, P.C., Bijzet, J. and Van Rijswijk, M.H. (1988) 'SAA versus CRP serum levels in different inflammatory conditions, studied by ELISA using polyclonal anti-AA and monoclonal anti-SAA antibodies', in T. Isobe, S. Araki, F. Uchino, S. Kito and E. Tsubura (eds.), Amyloid and Amyloidosis, Plenum Press, New York, pp. 229-233.
6. Hazenberg, B.P.C., Van Leeuwen, M.A., Bijzet, J., Van Rijswijk, M.H., Limburg, P.C. (1990) 'Differential influence of glucocorticoids on CRP and SAA serum levels in rheumatoid arthritis and polymyalgia rheumatica', Proceedings of the VIth Internat. Symposium on Amyloidosis, Kluwer, Dordrecht, (in press).

DIFFERENTIAL INFLUENCE OF GLUCOCORTICOIDS ON CRP AND SAA SERUM LEVELS IN RHEUMATOID ARTHRITIS AND POLYMYALGIA RHEUMATICA

BOUKE P.C. HAZENBERG, MIEK A. VAN LEEUWEN, JOHAN BIJZET, MARTIN H. VAN RIJSWIJK, PIETER C. LIMBURG
Division of Rheumatology, Department of Medicine
State University Hospital, 59 Oostersingel
9713 EZ Groningen
The Netherlands

ABSTRACT. Aim of this study in patients with rheumatoid arthritis (RA) and polymyalgia rheumatica (PMR) was to investigate the differential effects of immunosuppressive therapy on the serum levels of C-reactive protein (CRP) and serum amyloid A (SAA), two acute-phase proteins. CRP and SAA were both quantified by ELISA. In a cross sectional study of RA patients, prednisolone therapy (median 7.5 mg daily) was associated with a higher SAA/CRP ratio compared to untreated patients (median value 1.67 vs. 0.63, $p<0.005$). Azathioprine did not show a similar effect on this SAA/CRP ratio. A longitudinal study in RA patients showed also a rise of the SAA/CRP ratio after the initiation of low dose (median 7.5 mg) prednisolone therapy ($p<0.05$). In a cross sectional study of PMR patients a positive correlation was observed between the daily dose of prednisolone and the SAA/CRP ratio ($r=0.65$, $p<0.001$). A longitudinal study in PMR patients showed a rise of the SAA/CRP ratio after the start of high dose (median 40 mg) prednisolone ($p<0.05$). Conclusion: Although glucocorticoid treatment suppresses both CRP and SAA synthesis, this effect is more pronounced for CRP than for SAA. This may have consequences for the choice of drug treatment and for the evaluation of its effect in diseases complicated by AA amyloidosis.

1. INTRODUCTION

Amyloidosis of the AA-type is a well-known complication of chronic inflammatory conditions, particularly rheumatoid arthritis. The acute-phase protein serum amyloid A (SAA) is thought to be the precursor of this type of amyloid. Both C-reactive protein (CRP) and SAA are useful tools to monitor the course of inflammatory diseases. The progression to renal insufficiency in patients with AA amyloidosis is correlated with persistent elevation of CRP and SAA serum levels [1]. However, considerable differences in the altitude of CRP and SAA serum levels have been observed among diseases [2,3].

Aim of this study was to investigate the influence of immunosuppressive therapy with prednisolone and azathioprine on the absolute and relative serum levels of CRP and SAA in patients with rheumatoid arthritis (RA) and polymyalgia rheumatica (PMR).

2. MATERIALS AND METHODS

2.1. Patients

Consecutive patients with RA and with PMR were evaluated both in cross-sectional and longitudinal studies. Patients with giant-cell arteritis were included in the group of PMR patients.

Thirty-five patients with RA receiving no immunosuppressive therapy were compared with three therapy groups: 21 patients treated with azathioprine (median 100 mg daily), 37 with prednisolone (median 7.5 mg) and 34 with the combination (median doses 150 mg resp. 6.5 mg).

SAA and CRP levels were correlated with the prednisolone dosage (median 7.5 mg daily) in 29 patients with PMR.

Other patients, 17 with RA and 13 with PMR, were evaluated before therapy and at various time intervals after the start of prednisolone. The mean value of three samples was chosen as the value before therapy. Random samples were taken in the first 4 days ("days"), the first 4 weeks ("weeks") and the first 4 months ("months") after start of therapy. Median daily dose of prednisolone was 7.5 mg in RA (days, weeks and months). Median dose in the PMR group was 40 mg (days), 20 mg (weeks) and 25 mg (months).

2.2. Serology

CRP and SAA were quantified by a sandwich ELISA. Basal healthy control values: CRP ≤ 2.0 mg/l, SAA ≤ 2.6 mg/l [3].

2.3. Statistics

Mann Whitney U, Wilcoxon matched pairs and Spearman's rank correlation were used. Level of significance: $p<0.05$.

3. RESULTS

In the cross sectional study of the 127 RA patients, therapy with prednisolone was associated with a higher SAA/CRP ratio (median value 1.67 vs. 0.63, $p<0.0001$) compared to patients not treated with glucocorticoids. This effect was not observed for azathioprine alone, but the combination of azathioprine with prednisolone yielded also a higher SAA/CRP ratio (median value 2.02 vs. 0.58, $p<0.005$).

The cross sectional study of the 29 PMR patients showed a positive correlation between the daily dose of prednisolone and the SAA/CRP ratio ($r=0.65$, $p<0.001$).

In the longitudinal study of 17 RA patients median CRP level fell from 83 mg/l (range 15-303 mg/l) before start of prednisolone therapy to 21 mg/l (days, range 6.4-130 mg/l; $p=0.005$), 32 mg/l (weeks, range

7.0-119 mg/l; p<0.001) and 33 mg/l (months, range 2.0-110 mg/l; p<0.005). However, SAA showed a different response: the median level of 201 mg/l (range 7.5-613 mg/l) before start of therapy was followed by 53 mg/l (days, range 12-540 mg/l; n.s.), 62 mg/l (weeks, range 5.0-380 mg/l; p<0.01) and 79 mg/l (months, range 6.0-325 mg/l; n.s.).

In the longitudinal study of 13 PMR patients median CRP level fell from 83 mg/l (range 34-213 mg/l) before therapy to 8.4 mg/l (days, range 0.7-53 mg/l; p<0.01), 2.6 mg/l (weeks, range 0.6-172 mg/l; p=0.01) and 9.8 mg/l (months, range 1.6-159 mg/l; p<0.05). Also in these patients the SAA response was less distinct: the median level of 112 mg/l (range 43-530 mg/l) before therapy was followed by 23 mg/l (days, range 7.3-205 mg/l; p=0.01), 31 mg/l (weeks, range 4.5-900 mg/l; p<0.05) and 19 mg/l (months, range 3.4-610 mg/l; n.s.).

In the RA patients (fig. 1A) the median SAA/CRP ratio before therapy was 1.3 and rose to 3.2 (days, p<0.05), to 2.3 (weeks, n.s.) and to 2.6 (months, p<0.05), all compared with pretreatment values. No difference in this ratio was observed among days, weeks and months after start of therapy.

In the PMR patients (fig. 1B) the median SAA/CRP ratio before therapy was 1.3 and rose to 2.8 (days, p<0.05), to 5.0 (weeks, p<0.005) and to 2.6 (months, p<0.05), all compared with pretreatment values. The SAA/CRP ratio after weeks was higher than after days (p<0.05) and months (p<0.05); no difference was seen between days and months.

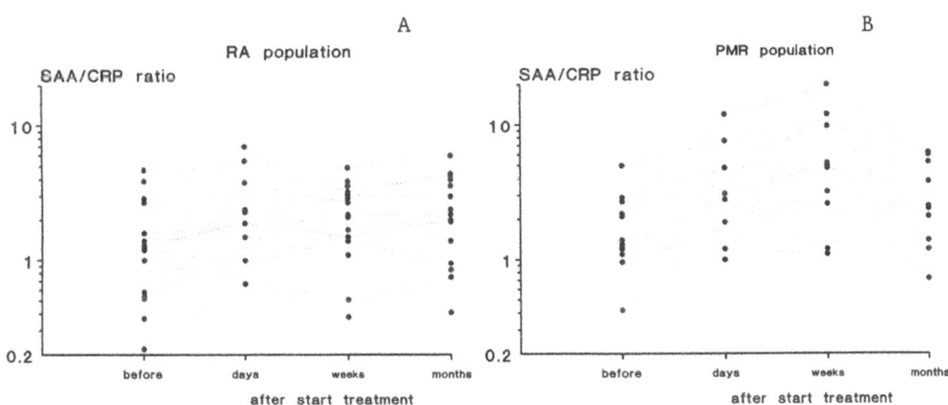

Fig. 1. Prednisolone therapy and SAA/CRP ratio in longitudinal studies: A) RA and B) PMR patients.

4. DISCUSSION

CRP and SAA levels fell after prednisolone therapy. However, this decline was more distinct for CRP than for SAA. Both in RA and in PMR the SAA/CRP ratio increased during prednisolone therapy. The actual values of this ratio differed between both studies in RA, probably explained by differences between the two groups related to the inclusion criteria of both kind of studies.

In hepatocyte cultures a stimulatory effect of glucocorticoids was seen on SAA but not on CRP production [4]. This (amongst others) might offer an explanation of the increased SAA/CRP ratio during prednisolone therapy.

In conclusion glucocorticoids suppress both CRP and SAA levels, but CRP is affected more than SAA. This may influence the choice of drug therapy in diseases complicated by AA amyloidosis. It is advisable in AA amyloidosis to monitor SAA instead of CRP levels, particularly if glucocorticoids are used for therapy.

5. ACKNOWLEDGEMENTS

This study was supported by the Dutch Kidney Foundation.

6. REFERENCES

1. Falck, H.M., Maury, C.P.J., Teppo, A.-M. and Wegelius, O. (1983) 'Correlation of persistently high serum amyloid A protein and C-reactive protein concentrations with rapid progression of secondary amyloidosis', Br. Med. J. 286, 1391-1393.
2. Maury, C.P.J. (1985) 'Comparative study of serum amyloid A protein and C-reactive protein in disease', Clin. Sci. 68, 233-238.
3. Hazenberg, B.P.C., Limburg, P.C., Bijzet, J. and Van Rijswijk, M.H. (1988) 'SAA versus CRP serum levels in different inflammatory conditions, studied by ELISA using polyclonal anti-AA and monoclonal anti-SAA antibodies', in T. Isobe, S. Araki, F. Uchino, S. Kito and E. Tsubura (eds.), Amyloid and Amyloidosis, Plenum Press, New York, pp. 229-233.
4. Castell, J.V., Gómez-Léchon, M.J., David, M., Hirano, T., Kishimoto, T. and Heinrich, P.C. (1988) 'Recombinant human interleukin-6 (IL-6/BSF-2/HSF) regulates the synthesis of acute phase proteins in human hepatocytes', FEBS. Lett. 232, 347-350.

OCULAR MICROANGIOPATHY IN FAMILIAL AMYLOIDOTIC POLYNEUROAPTHY (FAP) TYPE I

Eiko Ando, *Yukio Ando, Shoko Maruoka, Yumiko Sakai, *Susumu Watanabe, Riichiro Yamashita, *Shinichi Ikegawa, Ryoichi Okamura and *Shukuro Araki
The Department of Ophthalmology and *the First Department of Internal Medicine, Kumamoto University Medical School, Kumamoto 860, JAPAN

ABSTRACT. We performed ophthalmological and histopathological studies for 23 FAP patients and 6 asymptomatic individuals with a mutant transthyretin (TTR) gene. The vascular abnormalities of the conjunctiva and the retina were more frequently found in FAP patients than those in control subjects. Conjunctival abnormal vessels (CAV) were found mainly in the limbal area of FAP patients while they were not seen in asymptomatic individuals. Conjunctival biopsy of 5 FAP patients and autopsy of 2 other FAP patients revealed that significant amount of amyloid deposition was recognized in the superficial substantia propria of the conjunctiva and around the conjunctival vessels in all cases, which gets diagnostic value. In regard to retinal vessels, abnormal arteriovenous ratio (A/V ratio), tortuosity of retinal vessels, cotton wool exudates and retinal hemorrhages were found in 10 FAP patients and also one asymptomatic individual. Ophthalmological examination of 3 patients with pandysautonomia revealed that abnormalities of conjunctival and retinal vessels of these patients were quite similar to those of FAP patients. From these results, the ocular amyloid microangiopathy may be related to autonomic dysfunction in FAP patients as well as amyloid deposition.

INTRODUCTION

Various types of ocular complications occur in FAP patients in addition to the systemic disorders [1-3]. Significant amyloid deposition was detected around the vessels as well as stroma of ocular tissues of the patients with FAP. However, little is known especially about the vascular involvements in the ocular tissues, such as the conjunctiva and the retina. Recently, production of transthyretin (TTR) in the retina, has been focused in the attention [4-6]. Thus, precise examination of ocular vessels might give an important clue to understand the pathogenesis of FAP.

One of the most serious complaints of FAP patients are disorders of autonomic nervous systems. These autonomic dysfunctions might influence on the microcirculation. There has been the report that patients with orthostatic hypotension on pandysautonomia showed abnormalities of retinal vessels [7]. Thus, it is possible that FAP patients with disordered autonomic function might show abnormal ocular pathology.

We took ophthalmological examinations of conjunctival and retinal vessels in 23 patients and 6 asymptomatic individuals with a variant TTR gene. Moreover, biopsy and autopsy of the conjunctiva for 7 FAP patients were also carried out.

PATIENTS AND METHODS

Sujbects

We examined 23 patients with FAP (46 eyes) (male; 15, female; 8, age; 28-62 years, average; 38.3 ± 8.3 years), 6 asymptomatic individuals with a mutant TTR gene (12 eyes) (male; 2, female; 4, age; 18-29 years, average; 22.7 ± 3.7 years), 3 patients with pandysautonomia (3 females, 23-33 years, average; 29.7 ± 5.8 years) and 101 normal, healthy volunteers (202 eyes) (male; 85, female; 16, 23-46 years, average; 25.4 ± 3.5 years).

Observation of the conjunctival vessels

All the subjects underwent slitlamp examination on existence of conjunctival abnormal vessels (CAV). CAV were divided in three types, such as red spot, spindle and spider by the method of Sakai et al [8].

Measurement of the diameter of the retinal vessels

In all subjects, 14 patients with FAP (27 eyes), 2 asymptomatic individuals with a mutant TTR gene (4 eyes), 2 patients with pandysuautonomia (4 eyes) and 41 control subjects (41 eyes) underwent funduscopic examination at 30 min after the instillation of one drop of tropicamide. Photographs of the fundus were taken by the fundus camera and each diameter of retinal arterioles and veins was measured at one diameter from the center of the optic disc on the printing papers. A/V ratio out of the mean ± SD range in control subjects was defined as abnormal A/V ratio.

RESULTS

1. Incidence of the conjunctival abmormal vessels (CAV) in FAP patients

Thirty three eyes of 46 eyes (71.7%) showed CAV in FAP patients. On the contrary, only 35 eyes of 202 eyes (17.3%) exhibited CAV in control subjects. The incidence of CAV in FAP patients was significantly higher than those of control subjects ($P < 0.01$). This abnormal findings were not recognized in asymptomatic individuals with a mutant TTR gene. All the patients with pandysautonomia also exhibited CAV.

2. Histopathological findings of the conjunctiva in FAP patients

Biopsy and autopsy were performed in 5 and 2 FAP patients, respectively. Analysis by Congo red staining revealed that significant amount of amyloid deposit was recognized around the conjunctival vessels in all cases.

3. Disorders of the fundus vessels in FAP patients

In 27 eyes of the patients with FAP, tortuosity of the retinal vessels was recognized in 6 eyes (22.2%) and 2 eyes of one individual with a mutant TTR gene. Moreover, tortuosity of the retinal vessels found in 2 patients with pandysautonomia were quite similar to those of some FAP patients described above. To our interest, abnormal A/V ratio in FAP patients (55.6%) is divided in two groups such as low A/V ratio group (44.4%) and high A/V ratio group (11.1%) (Fig. 1). In other groups, one in asymptomatic individuals with a mutant TTR gene and one in patients with pandysautonomia showed low A/V ratio. In control subjects, only 7 subjects exhibited abnormal A/V ratio (17.1%). The incidence was significantly higher than those of control subjects ($P < 0.05$).

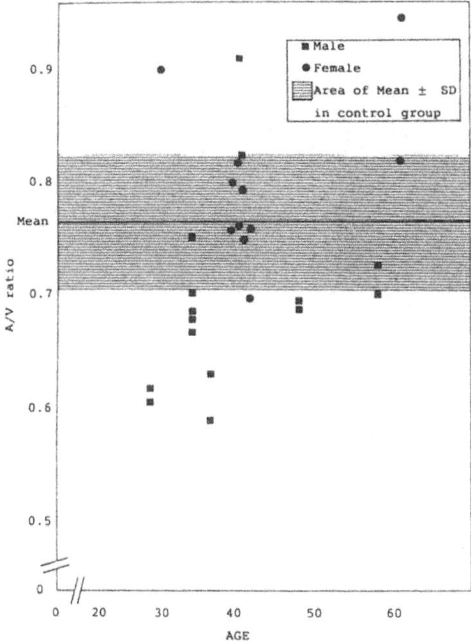

Fig. 1 Distribution of A/V ratio in FAP patients
In 27 eyes of the patients with FAP, more than a half of FAP patients showed abnormal A/V ratio (high A/V ratio; 11.1%, low A/V ratio; 44.4%).

DISCUSSION

The present study demonstrated that ocular microangiopathy in the conjunctiva and the retina was observed in FAP patients. Although those findings were not specific in FAP patients, the incidence of these abnormalities was surprisingly higher than that of control subjects. Evaluation of these abnormal microcirculatory changes in FAP patients might give the diagnostic value of FAP.

We carried out histopathological study for the conjunctiva in 5 biopsy and 2 autopsy cases of FAP patients. Surprisingly, all the cases showed significant amyloid deposition around the vessels we examined.

The same study for diabetic patients in our laboratory revealed that about 50% of these patients showed CAV (data no shown). However, this incidence was significantly lower than that found in the patients with FAP (71.7%) while it is higher than that of the control subjects (17.3%). Recently, microangiopathy in diabetic patients has been considered to be induced some complicated factors, such as the metabolic dysfunction, the rupture of hemostatic balance and the changes of blood fibrinolytic activity [9]. Thus, much higher incidence of CAV found in the patients with FAP might also be induced by additional other factor(s) as well as amyloid deposition.

We also examined retinal microangiopathy in FAP patients. Significant abnormal vessels were also found in the patients with FAP. Histopathological analysis for the autopsied eye revealed that although a cotton wool exudate was seen in the retina by fundus examiantion, only a trace amount of amyloid deposition was detected around retinal vessels. Thus, other factor(s) might take part in the pathogenesis of these disorderd veseels. We also examined three patients with pandysautonomia, who showed various dysautonomic complications. Interestingly, all of these patients had multiple CAV and two patients showed retinal disorders, such as tortuosity of retinal vessels and abnormality of A/V ratio, which was quite similar to those of FAP patients.

These results suggest that combination of the examination of the vessels of the conjunctiva and the retina of FAP-suspected patients might be regarded as the diagnostic value.

REFERENCES

1. Fall, H.F., Jackson J., Caray J.H., Rukavina J.G., and Block W.D. (1982). "Ocular manifestation of hereditary primary systemic amyloidosis." Arch Ophthalmol 54, 660-664.
2. Kaufman H.E. (1958). "Primary familial amyloidosis." Arch Ophthalmol 60, 1036-1043.
3. Savage D.J., Mango C.A. and Streeten B.W. (1982). "Amyloidosis of the vitreous: fluorescein angiographic findings and association with neovascularization." Arch Ophthalmol 100, 1776-1779.
4. Martone R.L., Herbert J., Dwork A. and Schon E.A. (1988). "Transthyretin is synthesized in the mammalian eye." Biochem Biophs Res Commun 151, 905-912.
5. Murakami T., Yasuda Y., Mita S., Maeda S., Shimada K., Fujimoto T., and Araki S. (1990). "Prealbumin gene expression during mouse development studies by in situ hybrization." Cell Differe (in press)
6. Inada K. and Okamura R. (1988). "Localization of human prealbumin in ciliary epithelium and retina." Acta Soc Ophthalmol Jpn 92, 741-745.
7. Goldberg M.F., Payne J.W. and Brunt P.W. (1968). "Ophthalmologic study of familial dysautonomia." Arch Ophthalmol 80, 732-743.
8. Sakai Y., Maruoka S., Ando E., and Okamura R. (1990) "Vascular abnormalities of the bulbar conjunctiva. Study on ophthalmological in-patients and medical students." Ther Res (in press).
9. Lazarow A. and Speidel E. (1964) "Small blood vessel involvement in diabetes mellitus". in Siperstein, M.D., Colawell, A.K.Jr. and Meyer, K. eds., American Institute of Biological Science, Washigton, D.C., pp127-131.

SPECTRAL ANALYSIS OF R-R VARIABILITY IN FAMILIAL AMYLOIDOTIC POLYNEUROPATY, Andrade type

M.Carvalho,J.Freitas,J.Puig,T.Coelho,P.Fernandes,
O.Costa and Falcão de Freitas.
Terapeutica Medica,Faculdade Medicina Porto,Porto.
Instituto Gulbenkian de Ciencias, Lisboa.
Centro de Estudos de Paramiloidose,Porto,Portugal.

ABSTRACT. Spectral analysis of R-R variability has been done in twenty subjects with Familial Amyloidotic Polyneuropathy in order to define intensity, chronology and discriminative capacity of this method in parasympathetic and sympathetic disturbances. The subjects were subdivided in 3 groups. Group I with far advanced disease, group II in early stages of the disease and group III with asymptomatic carriers. The R-R spectral analysis was calculated after fast Fourier transform in supine and after 60 tilt. Valsalva manoeuvre, deep breathing and standing were performed in groups II and III. The results showed a very severe autonomic disturbance in group I.The parasympathetic system seems to be early affected even in some asymptomatic carriers. Heart rate spectral analysis seems to be more sensitive for detection of autonomic disturbances than other autonomic tests

INTRODUCTION

Familial Amyloidotic Polyneuropathy (FAP) is a hereditary disease of the peripheral nervous system with a very high prevalence in Portugal (Andrade,1952). The biochemical basis of the disease is a point mutation in the gene responsible for the synthesis of transthyretin (TTR), the major component of the deposited amyloid, with a methionine for valine substitution at position 30 (Saraiva et al,1983). Deposition of amyloid in many organs and tissues, including typically the peripheral nerves, is a constant feature of FAP (Guedes,1976). A mixed polyneuropathy (motor, sensory and autonomic) appears concomitantly with autonomic involvement taking a preponderant role in the course of the disease because it is responsible for the majority of the most incapacitating symptoms such as impotence, orthostatic hypotension, bladder dysfunction and gastrointestinal symptoms (Freitas,1976).

In the last phases of the disease severe parasympathetic and sympathetic dysfunctions are observed.

The spectral analysis of R-R variability has been used to assess parasympathetic and sympathetic activity in different diseases and experimental studies (Appel et al,1989, Paganini et al,1986).In the present study spectral analysis has been done in order to define intensity, chronology and its discriminative capacity for parasympathetic and sympathetic disturbances in FAP.

MATERIAL AND METHODS

Twenty seven subjects were studied. Seven of them were withdrawn from the study by sinus node disease or conduction disturbances. The remaining twenty were subdivided in three groups. Group I (9 patients) with far advanced disease, group II (6 patients) in an early stage of the disease and group III (5 subjects) with asymptomatic TTR met30 carriers. The subjects were allocated within the different groups according to a clinical scale (15). The mean age was 34.8 +- 5.8. An age matched group (35.4 +- 5.6)has been used as a control.

After 30 minutes of supine rest, a simultaneous record of ECG, breathing and finger blood pressure (Finapress) was performed with an analog digital rate sample of 300 Hz. The spectral analysis of R-R variability was calculated by a fast Fourier transform of 512 consecutive beats with breathing controlled at 15 cycles/minute. This procedure was repeated after 10 min of 60º head up tilt. The power spectra of both low frequency component (LF:0.01-0.15 Hz) and high frequency component (HF:0.15-0.50 Hz) were calculated. The mean R-R and their standard deviation (SD) were determined. Valsalva manoeuvre and deep breathing were performed in all subjects. In group II, III a standing test was still done.

RESULTS

Group I had extremely low values of LF and HF components in supine position. There wasn't any significant change after tilt (Fig 1). Valsalva manoeuvre and deep breathing were abnormal. Postural hypotension was present with tilt in all patients.The R-R standard deviation was very low (0.007 +- 0.003 s).

In group II there was a decrease of both LF and HF components, at rest, with a higher decrease of HF. After tilt there was a decrease of both LF and HF components.In two patients Valsalva manoeuvre, deep breathing and standing were still in the normal range.

In group III, three subjects had normal LF and HF components and the HF component was decreased at rest in the other two. There was apparently a qualitative normal variation after tilt. Valsalva manoeuvre, deep breathing and standing test were normal (fig.2).

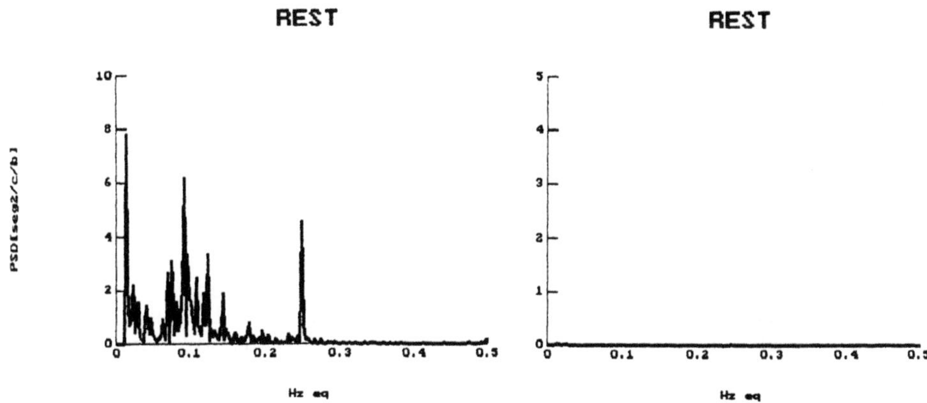

Fig 1. Power spectra from a control (left) and from a patient with advanced disease (right), at rest.

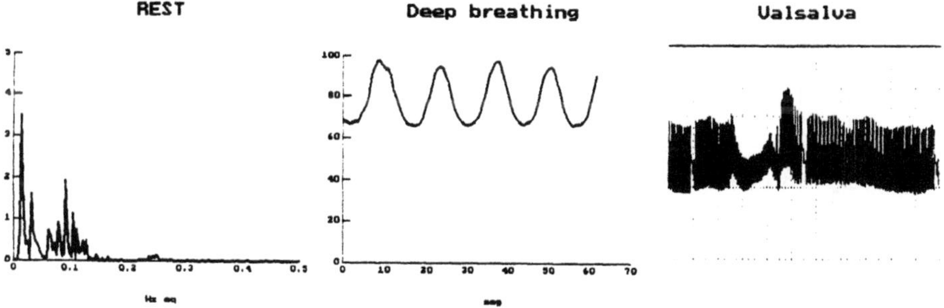

Fig 2. Power spectra from an asymptomatic carrier with low HF component (left) and normal deep breathing (center) and Valsalva manoeuvre (right).

DISCUSSION

In FAP patients with far advanced disease it was observed a severe disturbance of sinus node regulation by the autonomic nervous system with an almost absence of power spectra. The results observed in patients with few symptoms and in asymptomatic carriers suggest a progressive deterioration of the autonomic nervous system. The parasympathetic system was very early affected even in some asymptomatic carriers. Spectral analysis of R-R variability seems to be a more sensitive method to detect vagal and sympathetic impairment in FAP when compared with more classical tests. It is necessary to extend this preliminary observation,increasing the number of subjects and making a longitudinal study to get more definitive conclusions about the fiability of this method to detect early parasympathetic and sympathetic disturbances. FAP, a disease with progressive autonomic impairment, seems to be a very good model to asses precocity, sensitivity and discriminative capacity of spectral analysis of R-R variability in the study of autonomic disturbances.

References

Andrade C. (1952) A peculiar form of peripheral neuropathy: familial atypical generalized amyloidosis with special involvement of peripheral nerves.Brain, 75, 408-427.

Appel M L,Berger R D,Saul P,Smith J M,Cohen R J.(1989) Beat to beat variabity in cardiovascular variables: Noise or music? JAAC, 14, 1139-1146.

Guedes P.(1976) Anatomia patologica da polineuropatia amiloidotica familiar (tipo portugues). Bol.Hosp. 1, 51-59.

Freitas A F.(1976) Aspectos clinicos da polineuropatia amiloidotica familiar (tipo Andrade). Bol. Hosp. 1, 17-25.

Paganini M, Lombardi F, Guzzti S, et al. (1986) Power spectral analysis of heart rate and pressure variabilities as a marker of sympatho-vagal interaction in man and conscious dog. Circ Res,59, 178-193.

Saraiva M J M, Costa P P, Goodman D S.(1985) Biochemical marker in Familial Amyloidotic Polyneuropathy, Portuguese type. Family studies on the transthyretin (prealbumin)-methionine-30 variant. J.Clin. Invest., 76, 2171-2177.

MICROALBUMINURIA IN PATIENTS WITH FAMILIAL MEDITERRANEAN FEVER

S. Oren, J.R. Viskoper, S. Ilan, M. Schlesinger[1]
Department of Medicine B and [1]Clinical Immunology
Barzilai Medical Center, Ashkelon, ISRAEL. Affiliated to the Ben-Gurion University of Negev, Beer-Sheva.

Abstract

Amyloidosis of the kidney is the most threatening complication in FMF. Colchicine has been shown to reduce its occurrence. In the preclinical stage of kidney amyloidosis no proteinuria is observed using the standard Albustix method. However, it is not known whether these patients have normal or increased urinary albumin excretion. The purpose of this study was to evaluate albumin excretion in FMF patients treated with colchicine and to compare these values to those of a normal control group. Twenty-two subjects with FMF were compared with 16 normal subjects matched for age and body surface area. The two groups did not differ with regard to female/male ratio and arterial pressure. Urine samples were collected overnight while recumbent and in the daytime while ambulant. Albumin concentration (Ua) was evaluated using radioimmunoassay, and creatinine concentration was measured using the standard method. Urinary albumin excretion rate (UaV) and urinary albumin creatinine ratio (Ua/c) were calculated. Microalbuminuria was defined as albumin excretion rate higher than 20 µg/min. In the FMF group, three patients had microalbuminuria, two of them only in the early morning collection. These patients were characterized by a longer duration of symptoms (18 vs. 9 years). No patient in the control group had microalbuminuria. The mean urinary albumin excretion rate in the FMF group did not differ significantly from the control group. However, whereas in the control group the albumin excretion in the early morning was only slightly greater than in the night samples, in the FMF group the three indices of albumin excretion Ua, UaV and Ua/c were significantly greater ($p<0.01$) in the morning than at night. This exaggerated pattern of response to orthostatic changes in albumin excretion might indicate a subtle glomerular damage in these patients.

Introduction.

Familial Mediterranean fever occurs most commonly in Sephardic Jews and Armenians (1). Its most threatening complication is amyloidosis of the kidney. Recently,

colchicine has been found to prevent **amyloidosis** in these patients. The preclinical stage of **amyloidosis** is characterized by a positive biopsy and the absence of proteinuria, using the standard albustix method.
As has been shown with diabetic nephropathy (2,3), **microalbuminuria** in patients with **FMF** may precede the stage of persistent proteinuria and may predict, in the preclinical stage, the damage to the kidney caused by **amyloidosis**. The purpose of this study is to evaluate the urinary albumin excretion in **FMF** patients treated with colchicine who did not have proteinuria and to compare this value to that in a healthy matched control group.

Patients and methods

Twenty two patients with **FMF** were included in the study. All the patients were treated for various periods with colchicine and none of them had 1+ proteinuria (Albustix;detection threshold ≥300 mg/L). Patients with arterial hypertension, diabetes mellitus and cardiac, liver or kidney disease were excluded from the study. Sixteen healthy subjects matched for age and body surface area served as a control group. Arterial pressure was measured in the supine position after 5 minutes of rest. Urine was collected over night while lying down and during the early morning after 3 hours of walking around. We did not perform 24-h collection, as these are cumbersome for out-patients and prone to errors (4). It has been shown previously that albumin excretion is significantly higher in daytime ambulant samples than in overnight recumbent samples, and that the albumin/creatinine ratio determined from an early morning urine sample is a useful screening test to detect microalbuminuria making timed urine collection unnecessary (4). Therefore, urine albumin (Ua) and creatinine concentration were assessed from the two collections, and two indices were calculated; Urinary albumin excretion rate (UaV) and ratio of albumin to creatinine excretion (Ua/c). **Microalbuminuria** was assessed using a commercial kit (DPC-Diagnostic Products Co, Los Angeles, CA, USA), based on competitive radioimmunoassay with ^{125}I. Values are expressed as mean ± s.e.

Results.

The **FMF** patients did not differ significantly from the controls in arterial pressure and female/male ratio. The mean duration of the **FMF** symptoms was 12 years (8-30 y). All the patients were treated with colchicine (1 to 2 mg/day). The results of urinary albumin excretion are summarized in table 1.

Table 1. Urinary Albumin Excretion.

time of collection	Albumin Ecretion	Controls (mean ± s.e)	FMF (mean ± s.e)
OR	Ua(mg/L)	4.9 ± 0.8	5.4 ± 1.4
OR	Ua/c(mg/mmol)	0.5 ± 0.1	0.4 ± 0.1
OR	UaV (μg/min)	2.1 ± 0.4	2.7 ± 0.7
DA	Ua	5.7 ± 1.0	10.3 ± 2.6*
DA	Ua/c	0.5 ± 0.07+	1.0 ± 0.2**
DA	UaV	3.0 ± 0.5*	5.6 ± 1.4**

OR=overnight, recumbent urine collection;
DA=daytime ambulant urine collection.
Ua=urinary albumin concentration; Ua/c=urinary albumin creatinine ratio. UaV=albumin excretion rate.
*=$p<0.05$ (day vs. night); **=$p<0.01$ (day vs. night);
+=$p<0.05$ (vs. FMF).

In the **FMF** group three patients had **microalbuminuria**, defined as UaV higher than 20 mcg/ml, two of them only in the early morning collection. These patients were characterized by a longer duration of **FMF** symptoms (18 vs. 9 years). No subject from the control group had **microalbuminuria** during the night or early morning.
The mean urinary albumin concentration and albumin excretion rate were higher in the **FMF** group than in the control group in both urine collections. However, these differences reached statistical significance only when considering the ratio of albumin to creatinine in the early morning collection (1.0±0.2 in the **FMF** group vs. 0.5±0.07 in the control group, $p<0.05$). The albumin excretion rate was slightly higher in the daytime ambulant sample than in the overnight recumbent sample in the control group (3.0±0.5 vs. 2.1±0.4 μg/min, $p<0.05$), whereas the other two indices of albumin concentration and albumin-to-creatinine ratio were not altered by the time or posture of urine collection. On the contrary, the **FMF** group (Table 1) was characterized by a significantly higher albumin excretion rate ($p<0.01$), as well as albumin concentration ($p<0.05$) and albumin to creatinine ratio ($p<0.01$) of the early morning urine. The magnitude of increment was double in these three indices of albumin excretion.

Discussion.

The present study demonstrated that, out of 22 **FMF** patients treated with colchicine, 3 had **microalbuminuria**, in 2 of them it was found in the morning samples only. These three patients were characterized by a longer duration of

symptoms, and their **microalbuminuria** might be attributed to glomerular damage that occurred before colchicine treatment was started. Although no subject in the control group had **microalbuminuria** the urinary albumin concentration and the albumin excretion rate were not higher in the **FMF** group than in the control group, only the urinary albumin-to-creatinine ratio in the early morning samples was significantly higher in the **FMF** patients.
It has previously been shown (4) that normal subjects have higher albuminuria during the day and when upright than at night when recumbent. Watts et al (4) found an increase in the magnitude of the three measured indices of **microalbuminuria**; Ua,UaV,Ua/c being 1.3, 1.4 and 1.5, respectively.
In the present study, the subjects in the control group had no higher increase than a 1.4-fold of all the indices of albumin excretion in the morning sample, whereas in the **FMF** patients all three indices of Ua,UaV and Ua/c were double in the daytime ambulant sample.
In conclusion the urinary albumin excretion in **FMF** patients treated with colchicine is within normal range and does not differ significantly from that of a control group. However, the greater increase in albumin excretion in the morning samples in the **FMF** patients might indicate a subtle glomerular damage, and only further longitudinal studies may clarify its significance.

References

1. Sohar, E., Gafni, J., Pras, M. and Heller, H. (1967) 'Familial Mediterranean Fever;a survey of 470 cases and review of the literature', Am. J. Med. 43,227-53.

2. Viberti, G.C., Jarrett, R.J., Mahmud, U., et al. (1982) 'microalbuminuria as a predictor of clinical nephropathy in insulin-dependent diabetes mellitus', Lancet 1,1430-2.

3. Mogensen C.E. and Christensen, C.K. (1984) 'Predicting diabetic nephropathy in insulin-dependent patients', N. Engl. J. Med. 311,89-93.

4. Watts, GF., Morris, R.W., Khan, K. and Polak, A. (1988) 'Urinary albumin excretion in healthy adult subjects;reference values and some factors affecting their interpretation', Clinica Chimica Acta 172,191-8.

DOPAMINE-ß-HYDROXYLASE IN FAMILIAL MEDITERRANEAN FEVER.

Anis M.[1], Broadbent P.[2], McAdam K.P.W.J.[2], and Raynes J.G.[2]

1. Harpur Memorial Hospital,
Menouf,
Egypt.
2. Department of Clinical Sciences,
London School of Hygiene and Tropical Medicine,
Keppel St.,
London WC1E 7HT

Abstract

A recent report that Dopamine ß-hydroxylase (DßH) was increased in the serum of individuals with FMF and could be used as a diagnostic test, prompted us to examine the activities of this enzyme in sera from Egypt which had been collected from five groups of patients. FMF patients were subdivided into three groups, those in acute attack, those on colchicine, and those with FMF and not on colchicine for 10 days. Two groups of controls (surgical patients for acute abdominal conditions and healthy individuals) were analysed for DßH. We could demonstrate no significant difference between the DßH activities in any of the groups. Acute FMF and surgical control groups were shown to be in the acute phase by assay of SAA and CRP. We can see no diagnostic potential for this enzyme assay.

Introduction

Familial Mediterranean Fever (FMF) or Recurrent Hereditary Polyserositis has no specific laboratory test and diagnosis has been based on exclusion [1]. FMF is characterised by brief, recurrent painful attacks of peritonitis, synovitis or pleuritis and is most common in Jews, Arabs, Turks, and Armenians. The metaraminol test was described in which FMF patients could be diagnosed by provocation of attacks with this alpha adrenergic agonist [1]. Barakat et al. [2] measured plasma dopamine-ß-hydroxylase (DßH) on the hypothesis that the disorder is related to an abnormality in catecholamine metabolism. They reported a greatly elevated DßH concentration in patients not recieving treatment compared with patients on continuous colchicine or healthy controls [2]. More recently this result has been questioned [5] in a study which could find no differences in DßH in another group of FMF patients. DßH is released simultaneously with catecholamines, and catalyses the conversion of dopamine to the neurotransmitter and hormone norepinephrine within the catecholamine-secreting vesicles (chromaffin granules) of the adrenal medulla and the large dense cored synaptic vesicles of the sympathetic nervous system [3].

Materials and Methods

Sera were collected and stored at -20 C until assay.

DßH activity was determined using a previously described method [5]. Repeat assay of the same sample was performed and gave a mean coefficient of variation of 9%. It was important to use the same dilution of sample since higher dilutions often gave higher enzyme activities. The sample volume used during these assays was 10ul as it was found that results were reproducible using the same sample volume. Results are expressed in umoles/min/l of serum at 37° C.

Serum SAA and CRP concentrations were determined using competitive inhibition ELISAs. The ELISA for SAA is described elsewhere [6]. The ELISA for CRP uses a similar method with antibody to CRP coated to the solid phase and an alkaline phosphatase conjugate of CRP competed with sample and standards.

Results

Sera was collected from 3 groups of FMF patients and 2 control groups (table I) and the DßH activity was measured as previously described. We could detect no significant differences between any groups. Since we wished to confirm that the patients were indeed in the acute phase of the attack we also measured serum amyloid A (SAA) and C-reactive protein (CRP) using ELISA methods developed in this laboratory as indicators of an inflammatory response [4]. Raised levels were found in the acute FMF goup, and the control group with a medical abdominal condition (Table II). This confirmed that the FMF group were in an active phase of the disease. There was no correlation between the acute phase response to inflammation and DßH concentrations.

The activity of the DßH was similar to that that reported by Ben-Chetrit [4]. Our results were lower than those of Barakat but approximately similar to those of Ben Chetrit et al. Our results suggest that there was no diagnostic value in DßH.

Table I DßH activities in FMF.

Group	No	DßH (umoles/min/l) Mean ± S.D.	Range
FMF (acute)	13	15.9 ± 8.0	1.7-26.7
FMF (colchicine)	23	17.7 ± 8.9	7.3-49.7
FMF (no colchicine)	15	16.0 ± 7.9	9.3-33.0
Control	12	15.6 ± 6.9	2.9-28.3
Healthy volunteers	16	15.5 ± 6.0	5.0-30.0

Table II Acute phase protein response in FMF patients and controls.

Group	No	SAA	CRP
FMF (acute)	5	354 ± 225	108 ± 75
FMF (colchicine)	13	46 ± 96	10 ± 11
FMF (no colchicine)	11	67 ± 120	25 ± 44
Control	5	257 ± 247	63 ± 47
Healthy volunteers	12	14 ± 9	6 ± 2

Discussion

We have been unable to confirm the results obtained by Barakat et al and thus we agree with ben Chetrit et al [4] that there is no diagnostic value of DßH values. Our results confirm that there is no correlation between DßH levels and inflammation as found previously. We find that the DßH values are very variable over a range of 2 - 30 units between patients. There is no obvious explanation for the differences between the results in Barakat's initial report and those of Ben-Chetri and this report.

Acknowledgements

We would like to thank the Wellcome Trust, the Medical Research Council and the Arthritis Research Council for their support.

References

1. Barakat M.H., Gumaa K.A., Malhas L.N. El-Sobki N.I., Moussa M.A., Fenech F.F. (1988). Plasma dopamine-ß-hydroxylase: a specific diagnostic test for recurrent hereditary polyserositis. Lancet,ii, 1280-1283.

2. Barakat M.H., Karnik K.M., Majeed H.W. El Sobki M.I. Fenech F.F. (1984) Lancet i, 656-657. Metaraminol provocative test: a specific diagnostic test for familial Mediterranean fever.

3. Stewart L.C. Klinman J.P. (1988) Dopamine-ß-hydroxylase of adrenal chromaffin granules: structure and function. Ann Rev. Biochem. 57, 551-592.

4. Ben-Chetrit E., Gutman A., Levy M. (1990) Dopamine-ß-hydroxylase activity in familial Mediterranean fever Lancet,i, 176.

5. Nagatsu T and Udenfriend S (1972) Photometric assay of Dopamine-ß-hydroxylase activity in human blood. Clin. Chem.,18, 980-983.

6. Raynes J.G. and McAdam K.P.W.J. (1988) Purification of serum amyloid A and other high density lipoproteins by hydrophobic interaction chromatography. Anal Biochem,173, 116-124.

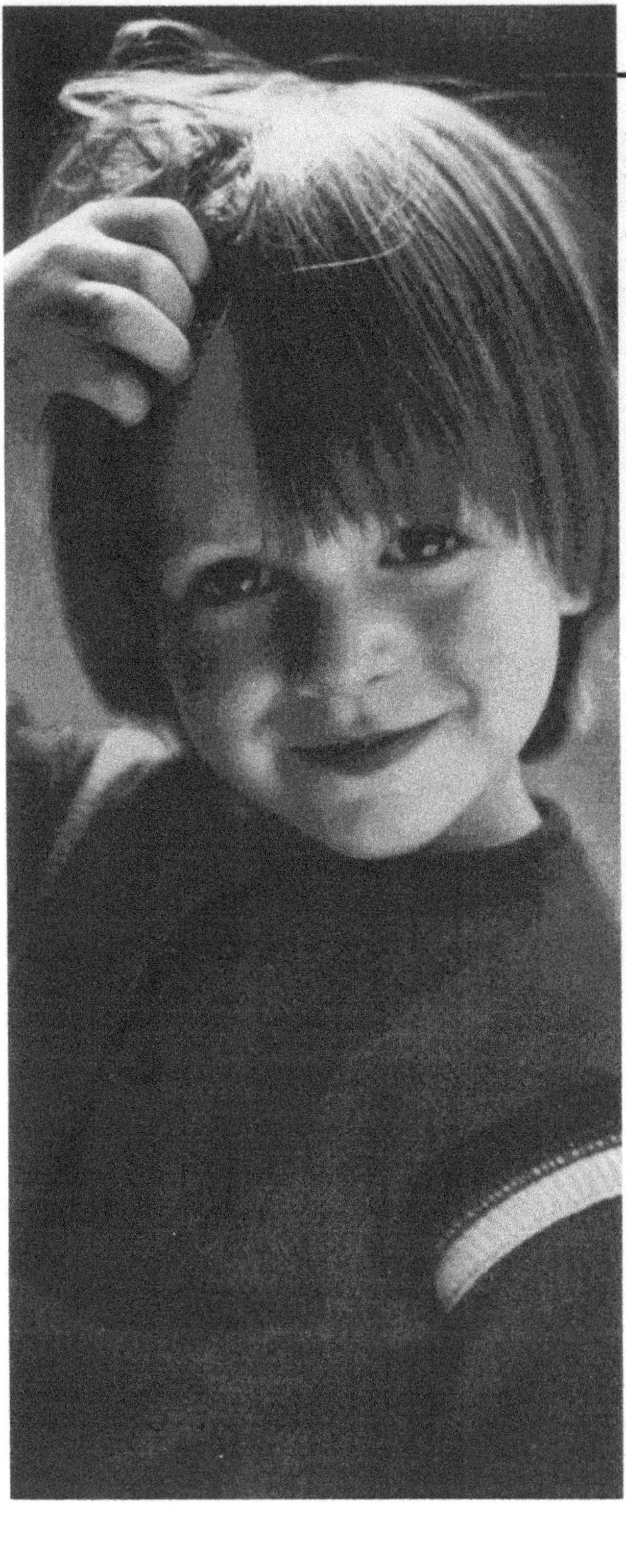

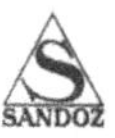
SANDOZ

A MULTICENTRIC STUDY ON HEMODIALYSIS AMYLOID OSTEOARTHOROPATHY IN 747 DIALYSIS PATIENTS

Shiro Maruyama, Fumitake Gejyo, Hiroki Maruyama,
Ryuji Aoyagi, Yasushi Suzuki, E. Hoque,
and Masaaki Arakawa
Department of Medicine(II),
Niigata University School of Medicine,
Niigata 951, Japan.

ABSTRACT. In order to clarify the clinical profile of dialysis amyloid osteoarthropathy, we studied 747 patients. The patients were divided into 5 groups according to the duration of dialysis(HD): group I: 0-5years, group II: 6-10 years, group III: 11-15 years, group IV: 16-20 years, and group V : over 21 years. Osteoarticular symptoms were observed 28.9% in group I, 41.1% in group II, 49.2% in group III, 73.6% in group IV and 80.0% in group V. The patients, treated by HD for more than 10 years, had osteoarticular symptoms in more than 50% cases. The longer the HD duration, the more the cystic radio-lucency (CRL) became frequent and clear by radiological examination. Carpal tunnel syndrome (CTS) and destructive spondyloarthropathy (DSA) had the same tendency. Among the older age patients (above 40 years), 60% revealed CRL in carpal bones. These patients recieved HD for more than 10 years. In the patients without osteoarticuar symptoms, the frequency of CRL was 26.7% in carpal bones, 26.2% in shoulder joints and 17.3% in hip joints respectively. The serum β_2-microglobulin (β_2MG), C-PTH and aluminum levels were not significantly different between patients with or without CRL and DSA. These results revealed that HD duration and age are important factors in the pathogenesis of dialysis amyloid osteoarthoropathy.

1. INTRODUCTION

It has been known that long-term hemodialysis patients have osteoarticular complications related to β_2MG amyloid deposion(1). Such deposits may be responsible for radiological abnormalities of the bone and joints, which are very similar to those observed in primary amyloidosis and can be included in the spectrum of renal osteodystrophy(2). In order to clarify the clinical features and dialysis amyloid osteoarthropathy, we studied 747 patients with long-term HD.

2. MATERIALS AND METHODS

The subjects were 747 patients (455 males and 292 females, mean age:

52.6±15.5 years old), who were dialyzed for 1 month to 273 months (mean HD duration: 6.8±5.4 years). We performed the questionnaire studies including 12 questions, and gain one point to each positive answer. We also analyzed clinical factors such as age, HD duration, underlying disorder of chronic renal insufficiency, hematologic parameters, and CRL of bone. The patients were divided into 5 groups according to the duration of hemodialysis. Group I (HD duration: 0-5 years) were 352 patients, group II(HD duration: 6-10 years) 196, group III (HD duration: 11-15 years) 112, group IV (HD duration: 16-20 years) 82, group V (HD duration: above 21 years) 5. CRL of bone was evaluated by modified Homma's classification(3). It was classified into 4 grades: (-); no findings, (±); single or multiple cyst with unclear cyst margin, (+); single cyst with clear cyst margin and over 2mm diameter and (++); single cyst with clear cyst margin and over 10mm diameter except in carpal bone, or multiple cyst with clear cyst margin and over 2mm diameter in carpal bone. In the profiles of 747 patients, the ages according to the decade were indicated as follows: 11-20 years aged patient was 1, 21-30 years aged patients 43, 31-40 years aged patients 120, 41-50 years aged patients 156, 51-60 years aged patients 204, 61-70 years aged patients 148, 71-80 years aged patients 70, and 81-90 years aged patients 5. Regarding the primary disease, 498 patients (66.5%) were chronic glomerulonephritis, diabetes mellitus 76 patients (10.2%), nephrosclerosis 61 patients (8.4%), polycystic kidney 33 patients (4.4%) and others. We analyzed and evaluated the radiological findings of systemic bone X-rays such as carpal bone (621 patients), shoulder joint (248), hip joint (268), pelvic bone (198), knee joint (76), elbow joint (77), skull (86), cervical vertebra (112) and lumbar vertebra (109).

3.RESULTS AND DISCUSSIONS

The result of questionnaire studies of osteoarticular symptoms are summerised as follows. Three hundred nineteen out of 747 patients (42.4%) showed positive answers for osteoarticular symptoms. Among the patients with positive answers had at least one or two osteoarticular symptoms. We studied the relationship between HD duration and osteoarticular symptoms.

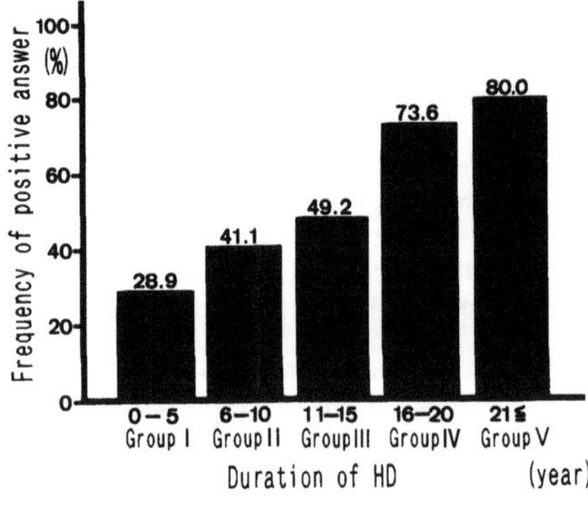

Fig.1: Relationship between HD duration and osteoarticular symptom.

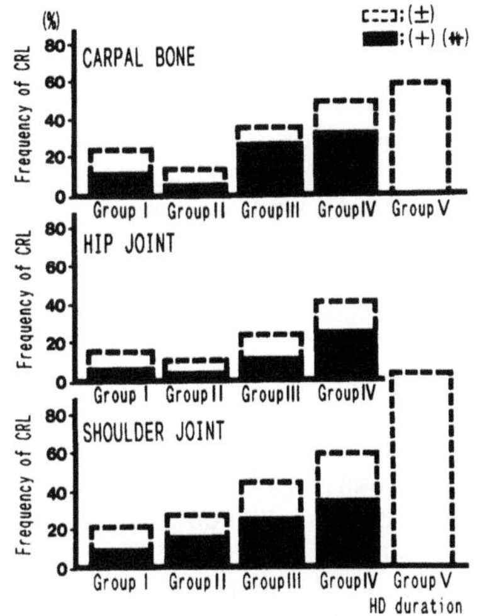

Fig.2: Relationship between HD duration and cystic radio-lucency.

Fig. 2 shows the relationship between HD duration and CRL of carpal bones or hip and shoulder joints. The frequency of CRL of these bones and joints were closely related to HD duration. The longer the HD duration, the higher the frequency of CRL. Mean HD duration in each grade of CRL at carpal bones and hip joints was described in Fig.3. The HD duration became longer according to the grade of CRL. The same tendency could be observed in other joints. On the other hand, the patients without osteoarticular symptoms demonstrated CRL in carpal bones (88/329, 26.7%), shoulder joint (34/130, 26.2%) and hip joint (22/127, 17.3%).

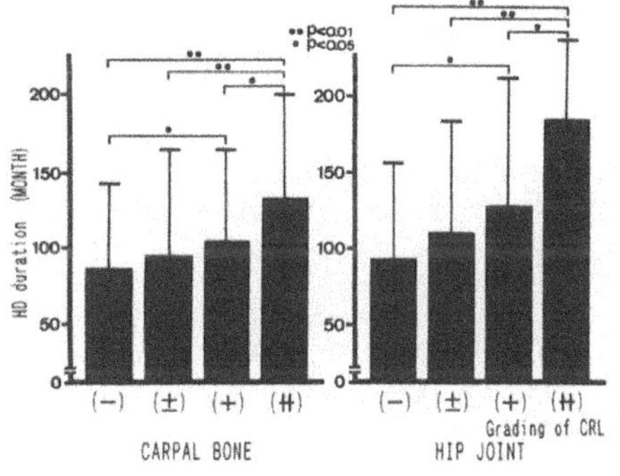

Fig.3: Relationship between cystic radio-lucency (CRL) and HD duration.

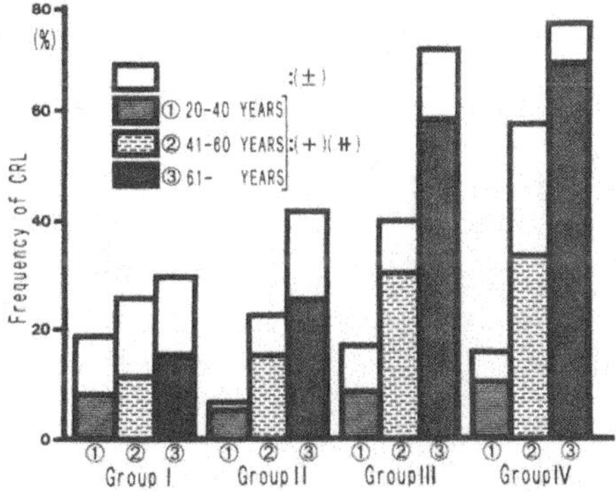

Fig.4: Relationship between frequencyof CRL (carpal bone cyst) and HD duration in different age groups.

Fig.4 shows the relationship between the frequency of CRL and duration of HD in the different age groups. It was found that the high age group (at the age of 41 years old or more) showed significantry higher frequency of CRL of carpal bones than the younger age group (at the age of 40 years old or less). This confirmed that the presence of CRL was related not only to HD duration but also to the age of patients.

CTS was noticed 2.0% in group I, 0.5% in group II, 8.5% in group III, 34.8% in group IV and 20.0% in group V. The number of cases with CTS and DSA was significantly higher in patients with longer HD duration as well as in older patients. The serum β_2MG, C-PTH and aluminum levels were not significantry different between patients with or without CRL and DSA.
The mechanism of β_2MG deposition and amyloid formation leading to osteoarticular symptoms has been unknown, although it may be due to cytokines (IL-2, TNF, etc), ultrafiltrating membrane, endotoxin and pyrogens, which activate macrophage to increase secretion of β_2MG. Increased β_2MG deposition followed by amyloid formation in joints and synovia may produce CRL and DSA, the unique clinical features of HD amyloidosis.

4.CONCLUSION

From these results, we could summarize as follows. [1]. CRL increased more frequently and became more clear accordirg to HD duration. [2]. Among the older age patients (above 40 years), 60% revealed CRL in carpal bones. They received HD for more than 10 years.[3]. More than 50% of these patients had osteoarticular symptoms.[4]. Some of the patients without osteoarticular symptoms also revealed CRL.

5.ACKNOWLEDGEMENT

We wish to thank Drs. Katagiri M., Ei K., Oda M., Oomori T.,Kawada K.,Shimizu M., Kobayashi K., Nagao M., Miyamura S., Suzuki K., Obata N., Satou H., Homma N., Fukagawa M., Kainuma T., Ogino S. and Morita Y. for their corporation to this multi-centric study.

6.REFERENCE

(1)Gejyo, F., Odani, T., Yamada, T., et al.(1986) β_2-Microglobu lin: A new form of amyloid protein associated with chronic hemodialysis, kidney Int.30, 385-389.

(2)T. Bardin, F. Bellini, J.D. Laredo.(1989) Radiological evaluation of Beta-2 microglobulin amyloidosis, DIALYSIS AMYLOIDOSIS. 91-100

(3)Homma, N., Sato, T., Ohara, K., Ueki, K., Gejyo, F., Masaaki, A., Saito, H.(1989) Relationship between cystic radiolucency of hands and amyloid osteoarthropathy in hemodialysis patients, Kidney Metab Bone Dis.2, 497-503.

RENAL TRANSPLANTATION IN RENAL AMYLOID END-STAGE DISEASE.

ANDERS HARTMANN, HALLVARD HOLDAAS, PER FAUCHALD, KNUT J. BERG, TORE TALSETH, KNUT P. NORDAL, CARL E. STRØMSÆTHER, DAGFINN ALBRECHTSEN and AUDUN FLATMARK.
Medical and Surgical Department B, Rikshospitalet, 0027 Oslo 1, Norway.

ABSTRACT. *Renal amyloid end-stage disease has been treated with renal transplantation (tx.) in 62 cases at our center from 1974 until april 89. 43 cases (74%) of these complicated rheumatoid disease. The average follow-up time is 5.1 years. 42 patients (72%) were transplanted after start of dialysis. 29 of the patients received necro donor grafts, the other half living donor grafts. The actuarial patient survival was 82% at 1 year falling to 65% at 5 years. Graft survival was 76% at 1 year and 60% at 5 years. Most graft-losses were due to deaths with functioning grafts. Septicaemia was the major cause of death usually occuring within 3 months after tx. Recurrent graft amyloid was diagnosed in 6 cases (9.6%), but only 2 graft losses could be ascribed to amyloidosis. Despite a high early mortality these long-term results encourage an active transplant program in renal end-stage amyloidosis.*

1. INTRODUCTION.

Renal involvement in systemic amyloid disease is a common feature, and renal failure has been a major cause of death in these patients. Most cases complicate rheumatoid disease, especially rheumatoid artritis (RA) (1,2). Decades of active illness often precedes amyloid renal failure at which time other organs are often affected (1,2). Renal replacement therapy by transplantation has therefore not traditionally been considered the choice of therapy in these patients (2,3,4).

Belzer et al (5) described the first successful case of renal transplantation in a patient with amyloidosis. Later publications have focused on relatively small number of patients or summarized data from several transplantation units (4,6).

In 1986 a transplantation material of 45 patients was published by Pasternack et al.(7) yielding good results in 45 patients, although the results were not as good as for well-matched glomerulonephritic patients. Our preliminary experience also stimulated an active transplant program in our amyloid patients. We now present long-term follow-up results of 62 renal transplantations in renal amyloid end-stage disease from one center.

2. MATERIALS AND METHODS.

2.1. PATIENT DATA.

From november 1974 until april 1989 62 renal transplantations were performed in 58 patients with end-stage amyloid renal failure, 27 men and 31 women. All these transplantations were performed at Rikshospitalet, Oslo. The outcome was evaluated in august 89, and the observation time after transplantation was on average 5.1 years, ranging from 0.3 to 14.5 years. The mean age at transplantation was 46.2 years, range 18-69 years.

Amyloid renal failure complicated rheumatoid disease in 43 patients (74%), 30 of these suffered from rheumatoid artritis (RA), 7 from psoriatic artropathy and 6 from ancylosing spondylartritis (AS). 7 patients (12%) suffered from

Mb.Crohn which in 2 cases was combined with RA or AS. 8 patients (14%) were considered primary amyloid.
Renal amyloid complicated the primary disease after 20±9 years, estimated at the time of transplantation and was confirmed by biopsy in 44 patients (76%).

2.2. HEMODIALYSIS DATA (HD).

HD was started in 42 patients on average 9.6 months (range 1-32 months). before transplantation, 16 were transplanted predialytically.

2.3. DONOR SOURCE.

Donor was living related in 27 patients, 2 patients received grafts from spouse and 33 patients received necro donor grafts.

2.4. IMMUNOSUPPRESSION.

The immunosuppressive therapy consisted of prednisolone and azathioprine until 1983. Since 1983 most patients have been treated with cyclosporine A superimposed on this regimen. Rejections have usually been treated with repeated boluses of methylprednisolone (1-2 grs.).

3. RESULTS.

The observation time after renal transplantation varies widely but the average of 5.3 years demonstrates a long-term follow-up in this material.

3.1. PATIENT SURVIVAL.

The early mortality is relatively high, the actuarial patient survival is down to 90% at 3 months, 86% at 6 months and 82% at 1 year after tx. Still 68% are alive at 3 years and 65% at 5 years . With 10 years observation time the patient survival is still almost 50%. Not suprisingly the patient survival is influenced by age. Those with a higher age than average (>46 years) had a significantly lower survival rate compared to the younger group ($p<0.01$). Less obvious was the finding that patients with RA had somewhat better survival compared to other diseases ($p<0.03$). No other significant differences were found between groups of patients. Alltogether 18 patients died. 11 died from infections, mostly septicaemia. More than half occurred during the first 3 months after tx. 3 patients died from cardiovascular disease, 1 from gastrointestinal bleeding and 1 from pancreatitis. 2 died from uncertain reasons more than 1 year after transplantation.

3.2. GRAFT SURVIVAL.

The graft survival rates are highly influenced by the fact that 16 graft losses were due to patient deaths with functioning grafts. The actuarial graft survival was 76% at 1 year and 60% at 5 years. 42% were functioning after 10 years. Only 9 graft losses occurred in the surviving patients. 4 of these were lost during the 1st year due to rejection and another one after 2 years. 2 patients lost their grafts due to recurrent amyloid 3.5 and 7 years after tx. Finally, 2 grafts were

lost after more than 5 years from uncertain reasons. Recurrence of amyloid in the renal graft was diagnosed in 6 patients (9,6%) but in 4 of these renal function was not compromized. The earliest case of recurrent amyloid was found at autopsy 18 months after tx. in a patient with a functioning graft at the time of death.
2 patients were retransplanted, 1 patient received 3 grafts 6 and 7 years after the first tx.

4. DISCUSSION.

The long-term survival rates in this material with almost 2/3 of the patients alive after 5 years, support the use of renal transplantation as a major mode of therapy in renal end-stage amyloid disease. However, a high early mortality by infection was seen in these patients. These findings are similar to those reported by Pasternack et. al. (7) but the observation time is longer in our material. To further improve the results, diagnosis and treatment of infections are challenged. These patients may well be immunodeficient both due to the primary disease as well as to the treatment of such disease. Since the amyloid patients received the same immunosuppressive therapy as other renal transplant recipients, they might well have been "overtreated", especially during rejection episodes. However, such a hypothesis remains speculative. Careful diagnostic procedures and aggressive antibiotic treatment may improve the results, especially during the first 3 months and during rejection therapy. Why RA patients seem to do somewhat better than others can not be explained by our data, in any case it gives support to an active treatment of this group of patients.
The primary disease may well be affected by the immunosuppressive regimen given after tx. The development of amyloidosis may therefore be retarded or even prevented in the transplanted kidney. In our patients less than 10% suffered from graft amyloidosis. This is less than previously estimated (7) and only 1/3 of the cases led to graft loss in the time range of this study.
Despite a high early mortality by infection and some recurrence of graft amyloid disease, the long-term survival are suprisingly high. Experience elsewhere with chronic dialysis of patients with amyloidosis have not been too encouraging (2). Treatment of amyloidosis with renal end-stage disease may therefore best be performed with renal transplantation.

5. REFERENCES.

5.1. Cohen, A.S. (1967) 'Amyloidosis'.
N.Engl.J.Med. 277: 628.

5.2. Jones, N.F. (1975) 'Renal amyloidosis.' Clin. Nephr. 6: 459.

5.3. Kennedy, C.L and Castro J.E. (1977) 'Transplantation for renal amyloidosis'. Transplantation 24: 382.

5.4. Heering, P, Kutkuhn, B, Frenzel, H, Linke, R.P and Grabensee, B. (1979) 'Renal transplantation in amyloid nephropathy'. Int. Urol. and Nephrol. 21: 339.

5.5. Belzer, F, Ashby, B, Gulyassy, P, and Powell, M. (1968) 'Successful seventeen-hour preservation and transplantation of human-cadaver kidney'. N. Engl. J. Med. 278: 608.

5.6. Kuhlbäck, B, Falck, H, Törnroth, T, Wallenius, M, Lindström, B.L, and Pasternack A. (1979) 'Renal transplantation in amyloidosis'. Acta. Med.Scand. 205: 169.

5.7. Pasternack, A, Ahonen, J, and Kuhlbäck, B. (1986) 'Renal transplantation in 45 patients with amyloidosis'. Transplantation 42: 598.

EFFECT OF CONTINUOUS COLCHICINE TREATMENT IN FAMILIAL MEDITERRANEAN FEVER (F.M.F)

D. ZEMER, E. SOHAR and M. PRAS
Heller Institute of Medical Research, Tel-Aviv University Medical School
Sheba Medical Center, Tel Hashomer 52621
ISRAEL

ABSTRACT. Two-thousand FMF patients are currently being treated with chronic prophylactic colchicine at our center since 1973. Results are reported here on two population groups considered to be at risk from prolonged use of this drug: young children and pregnant women.

Data on 350 patients who started treatment before age 16 are presented. Treatment had a positive effect on growth and development was normal. Proteinuria did not appear in any of the children during treatment.

In 131 pregnancies conceived among colchicine treated mothers, no deviation in spontaneous abortion rate, birth weight and length of pregnancy were observed. No untoward effects have been observed among the offspring of this group and their development is normal.

Our results show that continuous, long term colchicine treatment, is safe. Development, growth and pregnancies are normal. The prevention of amyloidosis in FMF patients, including those whose attacks are not affected by treatment, makes early diagnosis and initiation of treatment imperative. Treatment must be continued uninterrupted for life.

INTRODUCTION. Chronic, daily colchicine treatment for the prevention of the febrile attacks of FMF, was introduced in our clinic in 1973, in accordance with Goldfinger's suggestion.(1). Statistical analysis of our data after several years demonstrated that, in addition, this treatment modality prevents development of the nephropathic amyloidosis which previously caused death at an early age in untreated patients, 13% of whom died before age 16 (2,3). Chronic colchicine treatment was also found to modify the progression of amyloidotic kidney disease after it had been clinically manifested. Consequently, colchicine treatment in daily doses of 1 - 2 mg is being prescribed as soon as the diagnosis of FMF is made, regardless of age, weight, attack rate or stage of nephropathy. It is prescribed after kidney transplantation as well in order to prevent transplant-amyloidosis.(4).

Since the introduction of the treatment 17 years ago, awareness of the clinical manifestation of FMF and its complications increased considerably and with it our patient population, which includes at present about 2000 colchicine-treated patients. Analysis of our roster by age shows that most of the patients belong to the growing, developing and reproductive age groups who, supposedly, would be endangered if exposed for a long period of time to this anti-mitotic drug.

The results of a 15 year continuous follow up of these patients at risk are being reported here.

MATERIAL AND METHODS. Six hundred and thirty FMF patients were started on colchicine when they were less then 16 years of age. They were being routinely examined twice yearly and assessed for compliance, attack rates, side effects of colchicine, presence of proteinuria and general physical status. A detailed analysis on 350 of these patients was completed 3 years ago.

The influence of continuous colchicine intake on growth was studied by comparing height of pre-treatment birth cohorts with height of treated birth cohorts.

Of 220 women who conceived while on colchicine, 131 were followed up in a special obstetric clinic for FMF patients.

RESULTS. While in the great majority (81%) of the 350 treated children onset of symptoms was recorded before age 6, colchicine treatment was started in only 19% of them before this age. In 32%, treatment initiation was between 6 - 10 years of age and in 49% between 11 - 15. In almost all cases there was a delay of several years between the onset of symptoms and the initiation of treatment, indicating in many instances delay in confirming the diagnosis. Duration of continuous treatment was less than 6 years in 32%, 6-10 years in 50% and between 11 of 13 years in 18% of the patients. At present, only 9% of these treated children are below 10 years of age, while 32% are between 16 to 20 and close to 40% are in their third decade of life.

In most children who were initially started on a daily dose of 0.5 mg colchicine, the dose had to be increased in order to suppress the febrile attacks. Forty percent of this group required 1 mg per day, 25% - 1.5 mg day and 35% required 2 mg daily.

The remission from attacks achieved by these doses in this group is identical to the remission rate of the total treated population: 65% responded with complete remission, an additional 30% achieved partial remission, defined as either a significant decrease in frequency and severity of all forms of attacks, or remission of one form (usually abdominal) but persistence of another (usually arthritic). In 5% of the patients the attack-rate did not decrease even when the daily dose was elevated to 2.5 and to 3 mg. This group of non-responders experienced at least one febrile attack per month or more for many years. They were maintained on 2 mg colchicine daily; none of them developed amyloidosis.

Amyloidotic kidney disease did not develop in any of the children who started treatment without proteinuria as long as they adhered to regular colchicine intake. Among the 23 children in whom proteinuria was present for an unknown period of time prior to the onset of treatment, 7 deteriorated to terminal renal failure within a mean period of 7 years. An additional 7 patients were stable for a mean period of 7 years; in 5 intermittent proteinuria often coincided with episodes of noncompliance and in the remaining 4, proteinuria disappeared completely after 2 - 3 years. Proteinuria appeared in 3 children for the first time after an 18 - 24 month lapse in treatment. in spite of re-institution of colchicine, the kidney disease deteriorated in 2 of these to terminal renal failure and required renal transplantation within one year; the third has remained stable to this day.

There was no deviation from normal development detected in any of the children during the continuous colchicine treatment over many years. The heights of the untreated 91 patients, who reached age 17 before treatment was introduced, were compared to 121 long term treated patients at the age of 17. The later group had been on colchicine for a third of their life. The mean height of 62 untreated male patients was 168.3 cm as compared to 171.8 cm among the 70 treated males. The height of 29 untreated female patients was 158.4 cm as compared to 160.7 cm of 51 treated females. The treated groups showed a tendency to decrease the gap in growth with their matched normal controls. In none of our patients was discontinuation of colchicine necessary because of side effects.

One hundred thirty one pregnancies were followed up in the FMF obstetric clinic in our hospital. No deviation from the norm were observed in the spontaneous abortion rate, length of pregnancy or birth weight. (Table 1). Since 2

TABLE 1. Treated and untreated pregnancies

	Treated (131)	Untreated (94)
Abortion/live birth ratio	12.2	20.2
Gestational age at delivery < 37 w.	88 %	89 %
Birth Weight (grams)	3013	3112
Cases of trisomy 21	2	-

cases of trisomy 21 were found in this series (one live-born and one aborted), amniocentesis is routinely advised in each pregnancy where one of the parents is on colchicine. All 130 offspring born to these patients are developing normally: seventeen are 12 years and older, 16 are now between 8-11 years old and 54 are less then 7 years of age. It is of interest that 31 of the pregnancies were in women who started colchicine before age 16, up to 10 years prior to pregnancy.

DISCUSSION. Our results confirm the safety of chronic, long term preventive colchicine treatment in young FMF-patients. Maturation is normal, mean height increasing, approaching normal and reproductive functions are normal. The two cases of trisomy 21 identified among the 131 pregnancies followed up by our team, are not significantly different than the number expected by chance. Nationwide 430 amniocentesis were performed in FMF-patients and no additional cases of trisomy 21 were found. The most exciting finding is the prevention of amyloidosis in all our "non responders", 100 out of our 2000 patients, whose attacks were not alleviated by colchicine. This is in contrast to the 30% incidence of amyloidosis in the course of 2 - 9 years in untreated patients (2). The fact that the colchicine treated group of FMF patients with frequent attacks was protected from amyloid, supports the hypothesis of the genetic etiology of amyloid in FMF, indicating that amyloidosis is not secondary to the febrile attacks. This is in accordance with the presence of renal amyloidosis in untreated family members of FMF patients with no history of inflammatory attacks (1). The practical implications are of extreme importance: It makes early diagnosis imperative. We have seen that there was a delay, sometimes of close to 10 years, between the onset of symptoms and the institution of treatment. In children, kidney disease may rapidly deteriorate to terminal renal failure - our youngest patient died at age 5. To prevent the amyloidotic kidney disease, diagnostic efforts must be intensive and treatment must be started immediately. Continuous colchicine treatment must be given to all cases of FMF, including those who have sporadic attacks, and the non-responders, and even after kidney transplantation, to prevent graft amyloidosis (4).

REFERENCES.

1. Goldfinger, SE. (1972) Colchicine for Familial Mediterranean Fever. N. Eng. J. Med. 287: 1302.
2. Sohar, E. Gafni, J. Pras, M. and Heller, H. (1967) Familial Mediterranean Fever. A survey of 470 cases and review of the literature. Am. J. Med. 43:227-253.
3. Zemer, D. Pras, M. Sohar, E. Modan, M. Cabili, S. Gafni, J. (1986) Colchicine in the prevention and treatment of the amyloidosis of familial Mediterranean fever. The New Engl. J. Med. 314: 1001-1005.
4. Livneh, A. et al, Submitted for publication.

TREATMENT OF AMYLOIDOSIS ASSOCIATED DIARRHEA WITH A SOMATOSTATIN ANALOGUE.

MORTON A. SCHEINBERG
ELIANE CHAPIRA

FROM THE DEPARTMENT OF RHEUMATOLOGY/IMMUNOLOGY,
CANCER INSTITUTE ARNALDO VIEIRA DE CARVALHO
Rua Dr. Cesario Mota Jr., 112 - São Paulo - Brazil - 01221

ABSTRACT
A Somatostatin analogue (SMS201-995) was used to treat amyloidosis associated diarrhea. Considerable improvement was observed suggesting a beneficial effect of this drug on the diarrhea observed in some patients with amyloid associated neuropathy.

Somatostatin inhibits the release of numerous peptides hormones and has many effects on gastrointestinal function. (1). The effect of the long acting somatostatin analogue SMS 201-995 on the diarrhea associated with familial amyloid polyneuropathy type I was evaluated in two patients that were followed on the outpatient clinic of the Cancer Institute. Each subject received a subcutaneous injection of 25 ug of SMS 201-995 (kindly provided by Sandoz AG, Basel, Switzerland) every eight hours. This dose of somatostatin was chosen as being clinically relevant since it has been suggested as the dose for future long term treatment of patients. The injections of SMS-201-995 were given for periods of seven days. Treatment with SMS 201-995 was started and considerable improvement of the diarrhea in both patients were observed as shown on Fig. 1. During the treatment period the administration of SMS 201-995 was associated with a feeling of abdominal fullness and abdominal cramps.

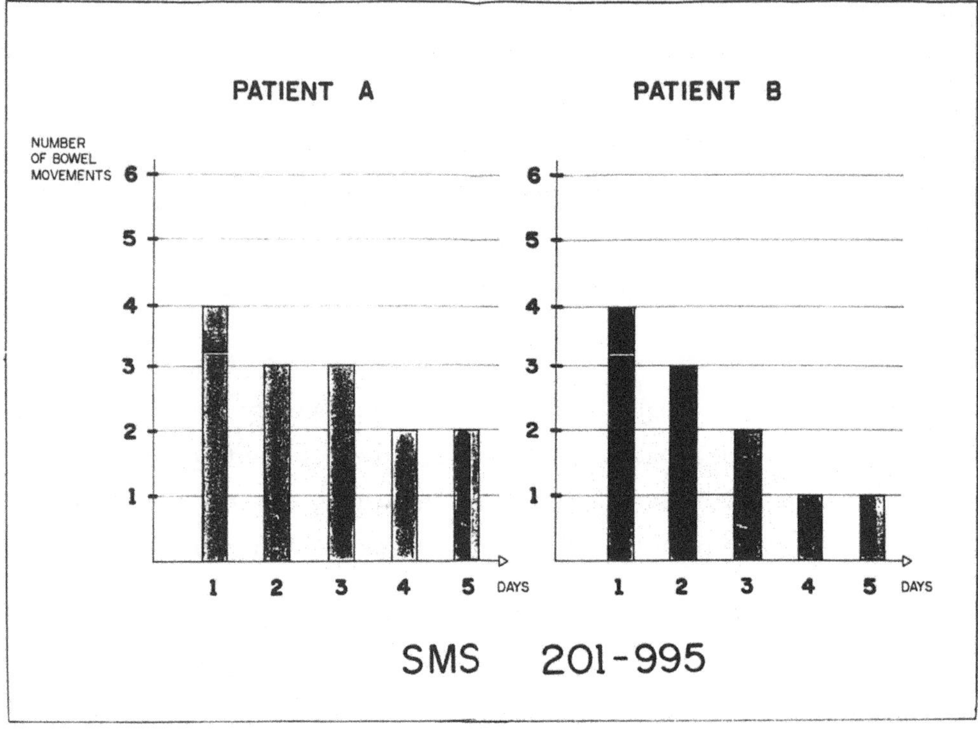

Figure 1 - Reduction on the number of bowel movements observed after SMS 201-995.

Funds for these investigations provided vy CNPq/FAPESP. This is publication nº 104 fron the Department of Immunology.

Somatostatin appears to inhibit intestinal secretion by suppres ing the release of secretagogues. It has also been used on the treatment of diarrhea associated with carcinoid syndrome, chole ra and AIDS patients. These preliminary observations suggests that a trial of somatostatin analogue should be undertaken in patients with diarrhea associated with familial amyloid polineuropathy.

REFERENCES

1) Arnold R, Lankisch P.L.: (1980) Somatostatin and the gastro intestinal tract. Clin. Gastroenterol 9: 733-753.

2) Bauer W, Briner U, Doefner W.: (1982) SMS 201-995: a very potent and selective octapeptide analogue of somatostatin with prolonged action. Life Sci. 31: 1133-1140.

3) Dharmsathaphorn K, Sherwin R.S, Catalano S, Jaffe B, Dobbins J.: (1980) Somatostatin inhibits diarrhea in the carcinoid syndrome. Ann. Int. Med. 92: 68-69.

4) Santagelo W.C, O'Dorisio T.M, Severino G, Kreys G.J.: (1985) Pancreatic cholera syndrome: Effect of a synthetic somatostatin analogue on intestinal water and ion transport. Ann. Int. Med. 103: 363-367.

GASTROINTESTINAL MALABSORPTION IN FAMILIAL AMYLOIDOTIC POLYNEUROPATHY (FAP): URSODEOXYCOLIC ACID ABSORPTION TEST

Yutaka Kawaguchi, Yukio Ando, Isamu Chou, Toru Yamanaka, Shinichi Ikegawa, Shukuro Araki
The First Department of Internal Medicine, Kumamoto University Medical School, 1-1-1 Honjo, Kumamoto 860, JAPAN

ABSTRACT: We applied to use ursodeoxycolic acid (UDCA), which is often used for the evaluation of liver dysfunction, as the useful tool evaluating the grades of gastrointestinal malabsorption in FAP patients. In most of FAP patients, serum levels of total bile acid were not sufficiently elevated after administration of UDCA. Interestingly, oral administration of L-threo-3,4-dihydroxyphenylseline (L-threoDOPS), the artificial precursor of norepinephrine, improved the malabsorption of UDCA when orally administered in FAP patients with mild and moderate diarrhea. This may be because L-threoDOPS suppress the hyperperstarsis of the gastrointestinal tract in FAP patients by elevating serum norepinephrine levels. Moreover, nasal application of L-threoDOPS, the mixture of L-threoDOPS and others, elevated serum levels of total bile acid in FAP patients with severe diarrhea. Procaterol hydrochloride, β_2-stimulant, also showed significant anti-diarrhea effect in mild and moderate diarrhea. These results suggest that malabsorption and diarrhea found in FAP patients may be improved by oral and nasal administration of adrenergic drugs.

INTRODUCTION

One of the most serious complains in FAP patients is disorders of the autonomic nervous systems [1]. In general, diarrhea found in FAP patients seems to be induced by disordered autonomic nervous systems and amyloid deposition of the gastrointestinal tracts [2]. It is also well known that generalized emaciation occurs in many FAP patients even at their early stage predominantly by diarrhea. Thus, it is very important ot control the gastrointestinal function in FAP patients. In most of FAP patients, plasma levels of orally administered drugs may not be so sufficient to express their effect than in normal subjects. We applied to use ursodoxycolic acid (UDCA) as an useful tool for evaluation of absorptional ability of the gastrointestinal tract in FAP patients. The measurement of serum levels of total bile acid is very simple and UDCA itself has no side effect. For the therapeutic purpose, adrenergic drugs, such as L-threoDOPS and procaterol hydrochloride were also orally and nasally administered whether gastrointestinal function improved or not. Nasal administration of L-threoDOPS would be the first trial to FAP patients with severe diarrhea and may be useful in treating gastrointestinal dysfunction.

SUBJECTS AND METHODS

Ten patients with FAP had a definite clinical findings, amyloid deposition of the tissues and a mutant TTR gene (26-58 years old, 8 males and 2 females). We have examined 4 control subjects without diarrhea and 4 with functional diarrhea.

Materials

Ursodeoxycolic acid (UDCA, Tanabe Pharmaceuticals Co.) was used as the tool of evaluation of malabsorption. L-threo-3,4-dihydroxy-phenylserine (L-threoDOPS, Sumitomo Pharmaceuticals Co.) and Procaterol hydrochloride (Ohtsuka Pharmaceuticals Co.) were used for therapeutic purpose of the gastrointestinal function in FAP patients.

Test of UDCA for FAP patients and control subjects

Serum levels of total bile acid were measured at 0, 30, 60 and 120 minutes after oral administration of UDCA (300mg) for FAP patients and control subjects.

Synthesis and administration of nasal application of L-threoDOPS

Nasal L-threoDOPS was synthesized by Sumitomo Pharmaceuticals Co. by mixing of L-threoDOPS and others. Nasal application of this mixture was carried out 30 minutes before administration of UDCA.

RESULTS

1. Absorption of UDCA from the gastrointestinal tract in FAP patients

To evaluate the gastrointestinal function in FAP patients with diarrhea, we measured serum levels of total bile acid after oral administration of UDCA (300mg) in 10 FAP patients and 8 control subjects. As indicated in Fig. 1, serum levels of total bile acid in FAP patients were much lower than in control subjects.

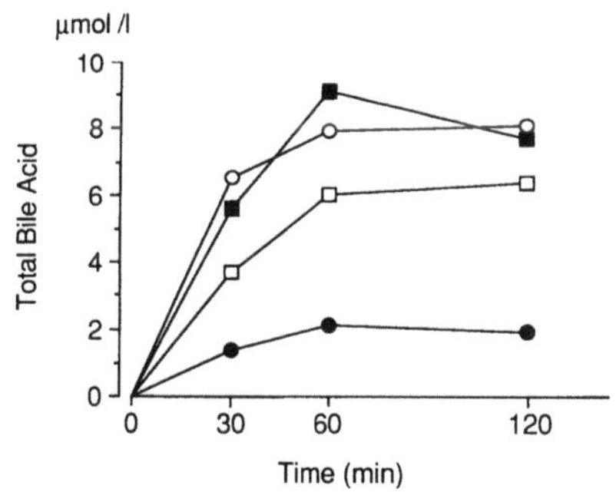

Fig. 1 Absorption test of oral administration of UDCA
○;control without diarrhea
■;control with mild diarrhea
□;control with moderate diarrhea
●;FAP patients with diarrhea

2. Effect of L-threoDOPS on the gastrointestinal function in FAP patients with mild and moderate diarrhea

To know the effect of L-threoDOPS on the

gastrointestinal function in FAP patients with diarrhea, we performed the absorption test using oral administration UDCA (300mg). In case 1 and case 4, absorptional ability of the gastrointestine and symptoms of diarrhea were much improved by L-threoDOPS (Fig. 2). Serum levels of norepinephrine were very low in case 10 even after oral administration of L-threoDOPS (data not shown).

3. Effect of nasal L-threoDOPS on FAP patients with severe diarrhea

To overcome little effect of orally administered L-threoDOPS in FAP patients with severe diarrhea, other drug delivery systems was considered for FAP patients. We synthesized nasal drop type of L-threoDOPS mixture. After administration of nasal L-threoDOPS, serum levels of norepinephrine were extremely elevated biphasically at 30 and 120 min (Fig. 3). With the correlation to serum levels of norepinephrine, malabsorption of UDCA was significantly improved after administration of nasal L-threoDOPS (data not shown).

4. Effect of pocaterol hydrochloride on UDCA absorption

Since sympathetic and parasympathetic denervation of the gastrointestinal tract is considered to be one of the pathogenesis in malabsorption of FAP, we tested the effect of procaterol hydrochloride on FAP patients with mild and moderate diarrhea. The malabsorption of the gastrointestinal tract and symptom of diarrhea were

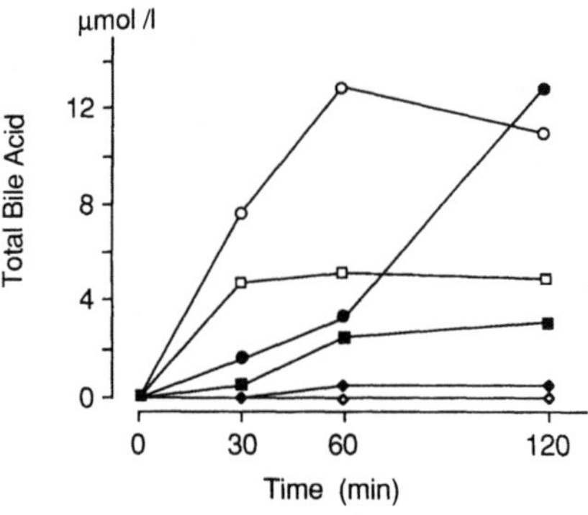

Fig. 2 Effect of L-threoDOPS on FAP patients
One hundred mg of L-threoDOPS was administered to the patients with FAP (case 1, 4 and 10) at 30 min before administration of UDCA.
Group with L-threoDOPS; ○(case 1), □(case 4), ◇(case 10)
Group without L-threoDOPS; ●(case 1), ■(case 4), ◆(case 10)

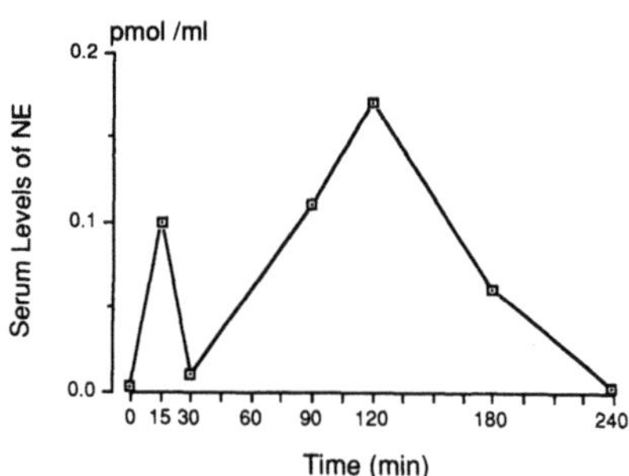

Fig. 3 Effect of nasally administered L-threoDOPS on serum level of NE in FAP patients with severe diarrhea.
Nasal type of L-treoDOPS mixture was administered to FAP patient with severe diarrhea (case 10). Bar represents biphasic serum level of NE.

moderately improved in these patients (data not shown).

DISCUSSION

This work demonstrated that gastrointestinal function in FAP patients could easily be evaluated by UDCA with very little water. It has been reported that L-threoDOPS was effective for gastrointestinal dysfunction as well as orthostatic hypotention [3-5]. However, the effect of oral administration of L-threoDOPS was not recognized in the FAP patients with severe diarrhea. This may be because absorption of L-threoDOPS as well as UDCA was perturbed in these patietns. Analysis of serum norepinephrine levels, converted form of L-threoDOPS, revealed that administered L-threoDOPS was not effectively absorbed the gastrointestinal tract in these FAP patients. Thus, other drug delivery systems should be considered to control severe diarrhea in FAP patients. Administration of nasal L-threo-DOPS improved malabsorption of UDCA in FAP patients with severe diarrhea. Procaterol hydrochloride, β_2-receptor stimulant, also exibited anti-diarrhea effect for FAP patients. These results suggest that adrenergic drugs were effective on gastrointestinal dysfunction via stimulation of the adrenergic receptors, when administered in the effective way.

REFERENCES

1. Araki S., Kurihara T., Tawara S. and Kuribayashi T. (1980) "Familial amyloidotic polyneuropathy in Japanese: clinical, pathophysiological, biochemical and therapeutic studies" In Amyloidosis eds. by Glenner GG, Costa PP and Freitas F. Excerpta Medica, pp67-77.
2. Ikeda S., Oguchi K., Kobayashi S., Tsukahara S., and Yanagisawa N. (1983) "Histochemical study of rectal aminergic nerves in type I familial amyloid polyneuropathy" Neurology 33, 1055-1058.
3. Suzuki T., Azuma T., Araki S., Ikegawa S., Kito S., Matsubayashi H., Yanagisawa N. and Ikeda S. (1987) "Treatment of autonomic dysfunction with L-threo-3,4-dihydroxyphenylserine in patients with familial amyloidotic polyneuropathy: a multicenter study" In Amyloid and Amyloidosis, Isobe T., Araki S., Uchino F., Kito S., and Tsubura E., eds. Plenum New York, pp851-856.
4. Araki S., Ikegawa S., Yi S., Ando Y. and Miyazaki A. (1987). "Treatment of orthostatic hypotention in familial amyloidotic polyneuropathy with L-threo-3,4-dihydroxyphenylserine" In Amyloid and Amyloidosis, Isobe T., Araki S., Uchino F., Kito S. and Tsubura E. eds. Plenum New York, pp863-868.
5. Inagaki C. and Tanaka C. (1982) "Characteristics of enzymic decarboxylation of L-threo-3,4-dihydroxyphenylserine using hog renal L-aromatic acid decarboxylase" Biochem Pharmacol 23, 463-469.

THE PREVALENCE, IMPORTANCE AND SIGNIFICANCE OF AMYLOIDOSIS WITH RHEUMATIC DISEASES IN TURKEY

N.DİLŞEN, M.KONİÇE, O.ARAL, L.ÖCAL
Istanbul Faculty of Medicine, Department of Internal Medicine
Division of Rheumatology, Çapa, Istanbul, Turkey

ABSTRACT. The association of secondary (AA) amyloidosis with rheumatic diseases has been well documented. We reevaluated its prevalence and characteristics in our cases observed during last 25 years. We detected 106 cases of histologically proven renal AA amyloidosis among 2340 cases of rheumatic diseases. The distribution of them were as follows: familial Mediterranean fever (FMF) 51, rheumatoid arthritis (RA) 30, idiopathic ankylosing spondylitis (ASi) 10, Behçet's disease (BD) 8 and the others 7. The diagnosis of AA amyloidosis was proven by renal biopsy in each case.
The main characteristics of our cases of amyloidosis were as follows: male predominance, high prevalence of juvenile onset and long duration of the rheumatic disease.
In conclusion our study reveals that main causes of amyloidosis associated with rheumatic diseases are FMF, RA, ASi and BD in Turkey.

Introduction

The association of secondary (AA) amyloidosis with rheumatic diseases has been well documented[1-7]. We reevaluated the prevalence and characteristics of secondary amyloidosis in 2340 cases of various chronic rheumatic diseases associated with arthritis observed and followed up by us during last 25 years.

Patients and Methods

2340 cases of chronic rheumatic diseases with arthritis diagnosed at the Division of Rheumatology during last 25 years were reevaluated for the presence of amyloidosis and its characteristics. The diagnoses and number of the cases were as follows: rheumatoid arthritis 886, other collagen diseases 553, seronegative arthritides 901 (idiopathic ankylosing spondylitis 320, psoriatic arthritis 76, Reiter's syndrome 15, ulcerative colitis 13, Crohn's disease 2, familial Mediterranean fever 230 and Behçet's disease 245). In patients having either proteinuria or any other findings of nephrotic syndrome or renal dysfunction renal biopsy was performed. Congo red and cresyl violet stainings were done in biopsy specimens of all patients. Light and polarized light microscopy were used in all. Electrone microscopy and potassium permanganate ($KMnO_4$) method were performed in some.

Results

106 out of 500 cases of biopsy proven renal amyloidosis observed at the Department of Internal Medicine belonged to our Division of Rheumatology. All 106 had AA type

amyloidosis. Cases of AL type amyloidosis were not included in this study. The distribution of 106 cases of amyloidosis in 2340 cases of various chronic rheumatic diseases is shown in Table 1. The prevalence of AA amyloidosis ranged from 0.72 to 22.2 % with a mean of 4.53%. The highest prevalence was found in patients with familial Mediterranean fever.
Male preponderance was significantly higher in patients with amyloidosis associated with rheumatoid arthritis and Behçet's disease (Table 2). Although there was no significant difference between the number of juvenile and adult cases of amyloidosis, the number of cases of amyloidosis of juvenile onset of the main disease was found to be significantly higher in cases of familial Mediterranean fever and rheumatoid arthritis (Table 3).
Duration of the main disease in cases of rheumatic diseases associated with amyloidosis was longer than those without amyloidosis (Table 4) particularly in cases of familial Mediterranean fever and Behçet's disease.

TABLE 1. Distribution of our 106 cases of amyloidosis in 2340 cases of various rheumatic diseases

Rheumatic disease	Total	with Amyloidosis	
	n	n	%
Rheumatoid arthritis (RA)	886	30	3.4
Other collagen diseases*	553	4	0.72
Seronegative arthritides	(901)	(72)	(8.0)
Ankylosing spondylitis (idiopathic)(ASi)	320	10	3.12
Psoriatic arthritis (PsA)	76	3	3.95
Reiter's syndrome	15	0	-
Ulcerative colitis	13	0	-
Crohn's disease	2	0	-
Familial Mediterranean fever (FMF)	230	51	22.2
Behçet's disease (BD)	245	8	3.26
Total	2340	106	4.53

TABLE 2. Sex distribution in 1757 cases of various rheumatic diseases with or without amyloidosis

Rheumatic diseases	Male (n=851)			Female (n=906)		
	Amyloidosis			Amyloidosis		
	(+)	(-)	Total	(+)	(-)	Total
FMF (n=230)	32	98	130	19	81	100
RA (n=886)	17[a]	255	272	13	601	614
ASi (n=320)	9	242	251	1	68	69
BD (n=245)	8[b]	152	160	0	85	85
PsA (n=76)	3	35	38	0	38	38

a: $\chi^2 = 8.40$, $p<0.05$= b:$p=0.03$

TABLE 3. Distribution of juvenile and adult onset of the main disease in our cases of various rheumatic diseases with or without amyloidosis

	Amyloidosis present				Amyloidosis absent			
	T	JO	AO	AO/JO	T	JO	AO	AO/JO
FMF (n=230)	51	42*	9	0.2	179	140	39	0.28
RA (n=886)	30	14**	16	1.14	856	186	670	3.6
ASi (n=320)	10	3	7	2.3	310	107	203	1.9
BD (n=245)	8	2	6	3	237	9	228	25.3
PsA (n=76)	3	0	3	all AO	73	7	66	9.4
Total (n=1757)	102	61	41	0.67	1655	449	12.06	2.68

* χ^2= 4.79, p<0.05=; ** χ^2= 8.24, p<0.001
T:total = JO:juvenile onset; AO:adult onset

TABLE 4. Duration of the main disease in our cases of various types of arthritides with or without amyloidosis

Amyloidosis		FMF	RA	ASi	BD	PsA	Total
Present	(No of Cases)	51	30	10	8	3	102
	Duration of Disease(yrs)						
	Mean	15.9*	8.1	9	16*	8	12.4
	Range	2-43	1-25	4-19	7-27	3-16	1-43
Absent	(No of Cases)	179	856	310	237	73	1655
	Duration of Disease(yrs)						
	Mean	11.9	7.48	7.65	9.4	7.4	8.28
	Range	1-50	1.5-79	1-40	1-25	3-17	1-79

*p<0.001 vs others

Discussion

It is established that secondary (AA) amyloidosis accompanies not infrequently with chronic rheumatic diseases particularly with rheumatoid arthritis (juvenile and adult), juvenile chronic arthritis, idiopathic ankylosing spondylitis, psoriatic arthritis and rarely with enteropathic arthropathies, and collagen diseases other than rheumatoid arthritis[1-7]. Familial Mediterranean fever has received the great attention as a source of amyloidosis for many years. Although previously it was accepted as a hereditary amyloidosis, it has recently been proved to be as a secondary AA amylodiosis[7-10]. It was also confirmed and consolidated by us that Behçet's disease is another disease associates commonly with arthritis and infrequently with secondary AA amyloidosis[11]. As we proposed before familial Mediterranean fever and Behçet's disease should be included into the spectrum of seronegative arthritides since they perfectly fulfill its diagnostic criteria(12,13). Our view was also shared by some other workers(14,15). The main characteristics of our cases of amyloidosis associated with chronic rheumatic diseases were as follows: It is quite common (4.53%). Its prevalence is highest in cases of familial Mediterranean fever (22.2%). It is more common in males and this is particularly true in rheumatoid arthritis and Behçet's disease ($p<0.05$, $p=0.03$ respectively). Although the number of the juvenile cases of amyloidosis was not more common than the adult cases, the number of the cases of juvenile onset of the main disease was found to be significantly higher in our cases of familial Mediterranean fever and rheumatoid arthritis associated with amyloidosis ($p<0.05$ and $p<0.001$ respectively) than in cases without it. Duration of the main disease was found to be longer in cases of most rheumatic diseases associated with amyloidosis than those without amyloidosis.

References

1. Missen,G.A.K and Taylor,J.D. (1956) 'Amyloidosis in rheumatoid arthritis', J.Pathol. and Bacteriol. 71, 179-192.
2. Jayson,M.I.V., Salmon,P.R. and Harrison,W. (1971) 'Amyloidosis in ankylosing spondylitis', Ann. Rheum. Dis. 11, 78-82.
3. Schnitzer,T.J. and Ansell,B.M. (1977) 'Amyloidosis in juvenile chronic polyarthritis', Arthritis Rheum. 20, 245-252.
4. Maldykovwa,H. and Krasnowolska,A. (1977) 'Amyloidosis in psoriatic arthritis', Rheumatologia. 15, 37-41.
5. Husby,R.A. (1985) 'Amyloidosis and rheumatoid arthritis', Clin. Exp. Rheumatol. 3, 173-180.
6. Dhillon,V., Woo,P. and Isenberg,D. (1989) 'Amyloidosis in rheumatic diseases', Ann. Rheum. Dis. 48, 696-701.
7. Cathcart,E.S. (1989) 'Amyloidosis' in W.N.Kelley,E.D. Harris, S.Ruddy and C.B.Sledge (eds), Textbook of Rheumatology, W.B.Saunders Company, Philadelphia, pp.1522-1547.
8. Cohen,A.S. (1989) 'Amyloidosis' in D.J.McCarty (ed.), Arthritis and Allied Conditions, Lea and Febiger, Philadelphia, pp.1273-1293.
9. Gafni,J., Sohar,E. and Heller,H. (1964) 'The inherited amyloidoses. Their clinical and theoretical significance', Lancet, 1, 71-74.
10. Eliakim,M., Levy,M. and Ehrenfeld,M. (1981) Recurrent Polyserositis (Familial Mediterranean Fever, Periodic Disease), Elsevier/North-Holland Biomedical Press, Amsterdam.
11. Dilşen,N., Koniçe,M., Aral,O., Erbengi,T., Uysal,V., Koçak,N. and Özdoğan,E. (1988) 'Behçet's disease associated with amyloidosis in Turkey and in the world', Ann. Rheum. Dis. 47, 157-163.
12. Dilşen,N. (1973) 'Ankylosing spondylitis in familial Mediterranean fever (periodic disease)' (Abstract), Proceedings of the XIIth International Congress of Rheumatology, Kyoto, Japan. Exerpta Medica: Abstract No 364. (International congress series No 299).
13. Dilşen,N., Koniçe,M., Aral,O. (1986) 'Why Behçet's disease should be accepted as a seronegative arthritis' in T.Lehner, C.G.Barnes (eds), Recent Advances in Behçet's Disease. Royal Society of Medicine, London, pp.281-284.
14. Moll,J.M.H., Haslock,I., Macrae,I.F. and Wright,V. (1974) 'Association between ankylosing spondylitis, psoriatic arthritis, Reiter's disease, the intestinal arthropathies and Behçet's syndroma', Medicine (Baltimore). 53, 343-364.
15. Hamza,M., Ayed,K., Bardi,R. and Sellami,S. (1989) 'Maladie périodique et spondylarthrite ankylosante', Rev. Rheum. 56, 703-704.

CYCLOSPORIN REDUCES THE INCIDENCE OF AMYLOID DISEASE IN CASEIN TREATED MICE

Morton A. Scheinberg, Vânia Aparecida Bakkenist, Merrill D. Benson, from the Division of Rheumatology/Immunology, Instituto do Cancer Arnaldo Vieira de Carvalho, São Paulo, Brazil - 01221, and University of Indiana - Indianopolis, In., 46223, USA.

ABSTRACT. Evidence is presented that cyclosporin administration reduces the incidence and severity of amyloid disease in casein treated mice. This inhibition occurs at therapeutic levels and raises the possibility that this agent may be helpful in the treatment of secondary amyloid disease.

INTRODUCTION

Experimental (secondary) amyloid deposition is composed of a non immunoglobulin polypeptide with unique amino acid sequence termed amyloid A protein (AA). Tissue AA is believed to be derived from a larger antigenically related precursor, serum amyloid AA protein (SAA), which is an apoprotein of high density lipoprotein (HDL) (1).

Over the past ten years our laboratory has been engaged in studies of amyloid disease by using the murine model. The trend of all these studies have pointed to the concept that disturbances of immune function play a major role in the pathogenesis of this disorder. (2) (3).

The present study was undertaken to determine weather cyclosporin is capable of preventing or reducing the incidence of amyloid disease in Swiss mice exposed to repeated injections of casein.

Cyclosporin is a cyclic undecapeptide metabolite derived from the fungus Tolypocladium inflatum ganus, and represents a new class of immuno regulator (4). There are multiple mechanisms by which cyclosporin A may affect immune function. Unlike most of these agents, it does not cause myelosupression, selectively alters the immune response by directly interfering with T cell function and thereby inhibiting production of interleukin 1 and 2. (5)

MATERIALS AND METHODS

Animals. Swiss mice, 8 to 10 weeks old, maintained in an Animal Division were used in this study.

Casein. Sodium caseinate (Nutritional Biochemical corporation, Cleveland, Ohio) was prepared as a 10% solution in sodium bicarbonate (10%) and given subcutaneously in 0,5 ml doses five times a week for two consecutive weeks.

Cyclosporin. The powder was obtained from Sandoz Laboratories, dissolved in olive oil and adjusted to the concentration of 20 mg/ml at 65ºC for 45 minutes, and stocked for two days in the dark at room temperature.

Cyclosporin Administration. Cyclosporin was given by subcutaneous injection dose in a volume of five times a week for two consecutive weeks. Animals were sacrificed one day after the last injection. The cyclosporin injection was given in the afternoon while the casein injection was given in the morning of each respective day.

Histologic Preparation. Mice were killed by cervical dislocation and their spleens were removed to be fixed in buffered formalin, embebed in paraffin section and stained with Congo Red. All sections were viewed by polarizing light microscopy and considered positive for amyloid when green birefrigent material was observed in characteristic perifollicular location.

Histologic grading of Amyloid. The method used for determining the amount of amyloid in the spleens of casein treated mice was previously described by our laboratory (6) and recorded as follows: grade 1 - a rim of amyloid around one or more splenic follicles: grade 2 - a rim of amyloid in more than 50% of splenic follicles; grade 3 - a rim of amyloid in all splenic follicles; grade 4 - diffuse splenic amyloid with bridging between almost all follicles and some distortion of the splenic architecture.

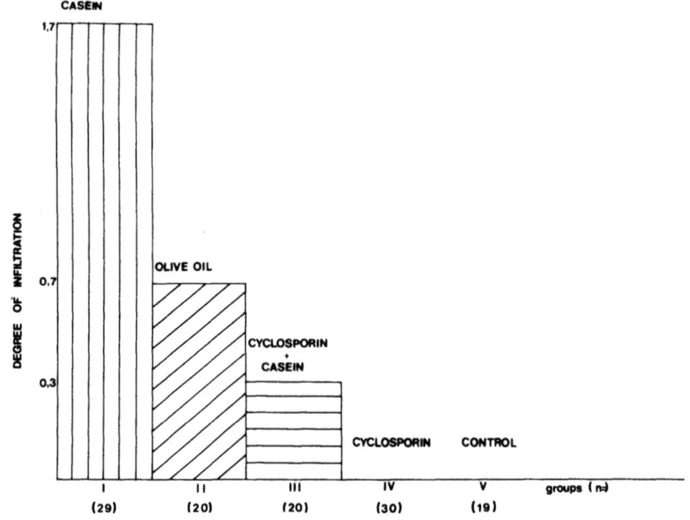

Figure 1. Degree of amyloid infiltration in casein treated mice who also received cyclosporin dissolved in olive oil. Number of mice in each group in parentheses.

T A B L E 1

CYCLOSPORIN SERUM LEVELS IN CASEIN TREATED MICE

CYCLOSPORIN (ONLY)

75% animals > 4,0ug/ml < 8.0 ug/ml

25% animals 1.85 ug/ml

CYCLOSPORIN + CASEIN

70% animals 1.8 ug/ml - 3.4 ug/ml

20% animals less than 0,125 ug/ml

10% > 4.0 ug/ml < 8.0 ug/ml

T A B L E 2

Mouse SAA levels in groups of mice treated with Casein, Cyclosporin A and Mineral Oil.

Casein	Cyclosporin A + Casein	Mineral Oil
2820 ± 550 (1)	4800 ± 1000	880 ± 120
(4)	(4)	(5)

Normal Mouse Sera

< 100 u/ml

P < 0,01 when compared to normal values.

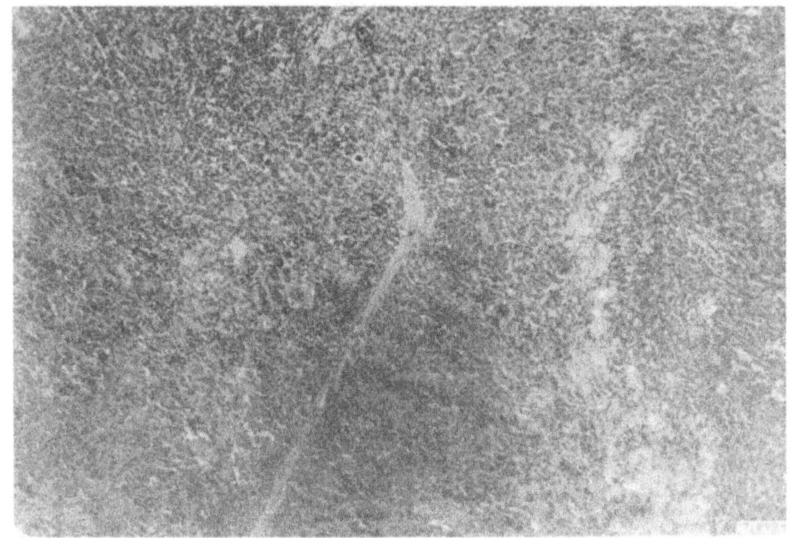

Figure 2. Amyloid infiltration in the spleens of casein treated mice. (HE - Congo Red x 100).

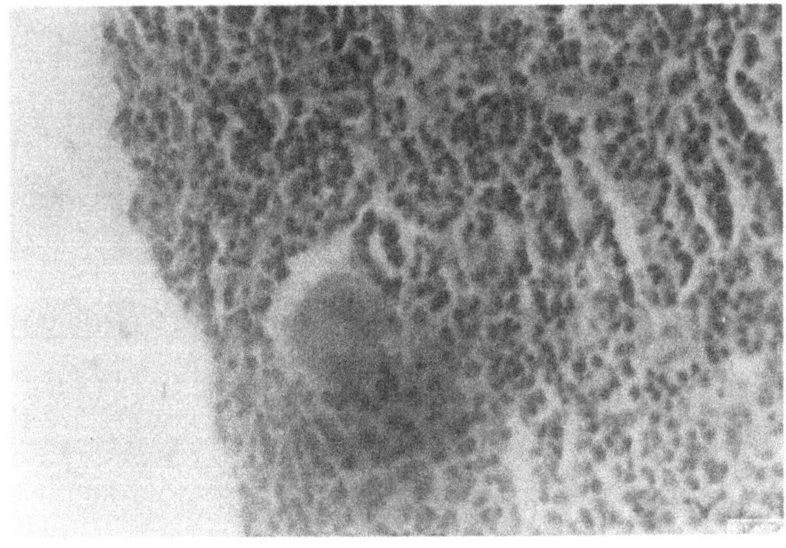

Figure 3. Lack of amyloid infiltration in the spleens of casein treated mice who also received cyclosporin injections (HE - Congo Red x 100).

The microscopic slides were read by two observers without knowledge of the tissue source. Differences between observers ocurred in a small number of slides but never more than one grade. When that ocurred the mean of the two readings were used as a definitive result.

Cyclosporin Serum Levels. A liquid phase radioassay obtained from Sandoz Laboratories and adapted for mouse sera was used to determine the levels in cyclosporin treated mice. Sera from five mice in each group were assayed on the last day of the experiment.

Serum Amyloid Protein Determination. Serum levels of SAA were measured by radioassay as previously described (7). Results expressed as units/ml using AA protein as a reference.

RESULTS

In the first series of experiments we found that olive oil alone (solvent for cyclosporin) was capable of inducing deposition of moderate amount of amyloid in the spleens of casein treated mice. In a second set of experiments a large group of mice receiving only olive oil was also used as controls. On Fig. 1 a representative group of experiments are presented. On the regimen employed in this study more than 95% of the animals receiving casein were shown to have amyloid deposits in the spleen. A marked reduction on the amount and incidence of amyloid deposition was found in casein treated mice that simultaneously received cyclosporine injections. Animals that received saline injections alone as controls showed no amyloid deposits. (Fig. 2 and 3).

Cyclosporin serum levels ranged from below 0,125ug to 4,0 ug/ml. The majority of the mice showed levels between 1.5 and 3.4 ug/ml. - SAA levels in casein treated mice were similar to those observed in cyclosporin plus casein treated mice while animals who received olive oil alone showed values similar to those found in normal mouse sera.(Table 2).

DISCUSSION

Cyclosporin A has been shown to be a potent immunomodulator with apparent benefit in studies of patients with autoimmune diseases including chronic inflammatory arthritis, demyelinating disorders and their correspondent experimental models. (8).

In this study cyclosporin at therapeutic levels was able to reduce substantially the rate and amount of secondary amyloid disease in casein treated mice.

The nature of the mechanism involved in these observations is still unknown. Cyclosporin exerts a number of pharmacologic effects including modulation of a sub population of immune competent cells capable of inhibiting the capacity of T cells to synthesize and release interleukin 2 and impair the secretion of Il 1. (9, 10, 11).

The pathogenesis of casein induced experimental amyloid disease is still unknown although immune mechanisms are believed to play a major role. Evidence has been presented for the participation of T and B lymphocyte, macrophages and neutrophils. (12).

A number of possibilities can be pointed out in relation to the inhibitory activity of cyclosporin in casein induced amyloid disease in mice. Cyclosporin treated animals had elevated SAA levels suggesting that the drug prevents amyloidosis through some other mechanism. It appears to affect amyloid deposition at levels correspondent to its therapeutic use in man.

The results here presented suggest that cyclosporin maybe helpful in the treatment of secondary amyloid disease in man.

Studies are now underway to determine the precise mechanism behind the current observations.

REFERENCES

1. Scheinberg, M.A., (1977) 'Immunology of Amyloid disease. A. Review. Seminars in Arthritis and Rheumatism'. A Review 7: 133-140.
2. Scheinberg, M.A., Wohlgethan, J.R., Cathcart, E.S.(1980) 'Humoral and Cellular Aspects of Amyloid Disease.' Progress in Allergy' 27: 250-70.
3. Herman Hernandez, C.C., Scheinberg, M.A., Benson,M.D., Filkelstein, A.F. (1986) 'The Effect of Gold Salts in Casein Induced Macrophage Activation and Serum Amyloid Protein SAA Levels'. Clin. Exp. Rheumatol. 4: 347-350.
4. Borel, J.F., Feurer, C., Gubler, H.V., Stabelin, H.(1986) 'Biological Effects of Cyclosporin A. A New Lymphocyte Agent'. Agents and Actions 6: 468-475.
5. Burges, D., Hardt,C., Rullinghoff, M., Wagner, H.(1981) 'Cyclosporin A Mediates immunosupression of primary cytotoxic T cell responses by impairing the release of Interleukin 1 and Interleukin 2.' Europ J. of Immunol. 11: 657-661.
6. Scheinberg, M.A., Goldstein, A.L., Cathcart, E.S.(1976) 'Thymosin restores T Cell function and reduces the Incidence of Amyloid Disease in Casein treated mice.' The Journal of Immunology 116: 156-158.
7. Benson, M.S., Scheinberg, M.A., Shirahama , T., Cathcart, E.S., Skinner, M. (1977) 'Kinetics of Serum Amyloid Protein A in Casein Induced Murine Amyloidosis.' The Journal of Clinical Investigation 59: 412-417.
8. Schindler, R.: Editor (1985) 'Cyclosporin in Auto Immune Diseases.'Springer Verlag. Basle.
9. Britton, S., Palacios, R.: (1982) 'Cyclosporin, A. Usefullness, risks and mechanisms of action.' Immunological Review 65: 5-22.
10. Klauss, G.G.B., Kunklc, A.: (1983) 'Dissociation of T helper Cell function and helper cell priming by Cyclosporin A. Transplant Proceedings 2: 321-322.
11. Kahan, B.D.: (1985) 'Cyclosporin. The Agent and its Actions.' Transplant Proceedings 17: 5-18

12. Glenner, G., Osserman, E., Benditt. E.P., Calkins, E., Cohen, A.S., Franklin, D.
Editors Amyloidosis (1986) Plenum Press.

ACKNOWLEDGEMENTS

This is publication nº 81 from the Division of Rheumatology/Immunology. Funds of these investigations provided by CNPq/FAPESP. Address reprint requests to: Morton A. Scheinberg, Rua Dr. Cesario Mota Jr., 112 - Capital - São Paulo - 0121 - Brazil.

REPORT OF SPECIAL SESSION ON BIOASSAYS AND STANDARDIZATION OF AMYLOID PROTEINS AND PRECURSORS

J. D. SIPE, F. C. DE BEER, M. PEPYS, A. HUSEBEKK, B. SKOGEN, R. KISILEVSKY, D. SELKOE, J. BUXBAUM, R. P. LINKE AND M.A. GERTZ.
Boston, MA, USA; Lexington, KY, USA; London, UK; Tromso, Norway; Kingston, Ontario, Canada; New York, NY, USA; Munich, West Germany; and Rochester, MN, USA.

PURPOSE: To identify and resolve technical difficulties and inconsistencies surrounding analysis of amyloid proteins and precursors in tissues and biological fluids, emphasizing work in progress and future studies.

1. SAA: F.C. de Beer

1.1 Identification of isoforms by isoelectric focusing

The unequivocal identification of apo-SAA isoforms can be performed by assigning the major isoforms separated by electrofocusing to published gene sequences. Designating the relative electrofocusing relationship of each apo-SAA moiety within a phenotypic IEF spectrum, a concept introduced by Drs. Strachan, de Beer and colleagues, will facilitate clearer communication of apo-SAA research within the scientific community. In the case of human SAA, it has been possible to identify five mature gene products and three post-translational modifications at the amino termini. The structure of the human SAA gene family has investigated with nonoverlapping genomic clones. Until the entire SAA gene region on human chromosome 11 is sequenced, the total number of genes remains uncertain. Even when all SAA specific bands in restriction maps can be accounted for, the total number of genes may be underestimated because of small structural differences between the genes.

In the case of the mouse SAA gene family, while four closely linked mouse SAA genes have been localized to a 79 kb region of mouse chromosome 7, isoelectric focusing studies of SAA variants within inbred strains have identified a minimum of five loci. Mouse apo-SAA 1 and apo-SAA 2 variants lack charged amino acid residues at the amino termini and are not susceptible to isoform shifts from post-translational modifications caused by aminopeptidase activity.

During the session it was pointed out that isoelectric separation of apo-SAA variants can be influenced by a variety of post-translational protein modifications such as carbamylation and phosphorylation. Although it is a common impression that the technique of isoelectric focusing is fraught with technical difficulties resulting in artefacts, in fact the technique has permitted accurate assignment of apo-SAA proteins and their post-translational modifications to specific gene sequences as documented by several reports in the literature.

1.2 Technical difficulties with apo-SAA assays

Since the discovery of SAA in the early 1970s, SAA determination in plasma and biological fluids has largely remained a research assay because of technical difficulties stemming in large part from the association of SAA with lipids and apolipoproteins, and from the relative ease with which SAA undergoes conformational changes and forms hydrophobic associations with itself. Recent advancements in SAA assay methodology were presented. One is the monoclonal antibody based ELISA for human SAA presented by Dr. Limburg and his colleagues from Groningen. They used two different monoclonal antibodies that recognize different epitopes on SAA. There was no need for sample pretreatment and the problems with underestimation of SAA inherent in competitive immunoassays were eliminated. The other, developed by Dr. Sipe and colleagues, is the direct binding ELISA for SAA in which noncovalent interactions of SAA with other plasma constituents are disrupted, eliminating problems of self-association and self-coating of surfaces by SAA.

2. Antigen and antibody standards for interlaboratory standardization: M. Pepys

At the invitation of the World Health Organization Laboratory at the National Institute for Biological Standards and Control, Professor Pepys´ laboratory is preparing material for an International Reference Standard of the WHO for human SAA. It is planned to establish a large pool of acute phase SAA rich serum that will be lyophilized for a large scale fill to support an international collaborative study including major academic laboratories and commercial companies involved in SAA assays. Based upon the results of this collaborative study, a report will be forwarded to the Expert Committee on Biological Standards in Geneva for approval of the preparation.

Drs. Pepys and Nelson and colleagues have undertaken a large immunoassay study of several hundred normal volunteer blood donors to establish the normal concentration range for SAP. The assays were standardized on a preparation of highly purified SAP, the concentration of which has been determined by spectrophotometry using a precisely determined extinction coefficient. The extinction coefficient was measured using cryodried SAP, obtained by a process which reduces water content to less than a few parts per million and is thus several orders of magnitude better than the usual lyophilization. This new standard will be valuable for interlaboratory standardizations. Dr. Floyd-O´Sullivan described a panel of monoclonal antibodies to human SAP that distinguish between native and denatured SAP. Some of the monoclonal antibodies recognize SAP only in the presence of calcium.

3. Analysis of SAA distribution and clearance: A. Husebekk, B. Skogen

Either pure amyloid protein or monoclonal antibodies are required to establish an accurate quantitation method for SAA or AA proteins. The heterogeneity of SAA complicates the analysis of the protein; there are multiple allotypes of SAA, as well as post-translational modifications at both the amino and carboxyl termini (e.g. AA). Serum might have over a thousand fold variation in apo-SAA content and can contain AA as well as SAA. In addition, labelling of SAA may influence its metabolic rate and its reactivity with antibodies. It was suggested that a suitable assay system for SAA in biological fluids is a double monoclonal antibody system with the capture and detection antibodies recognizing separable epitopes. In addition, the antibodies have to react with all SAA variants with the same affinity.

The complexities of SAA metabolism are summarized in the following scheme:

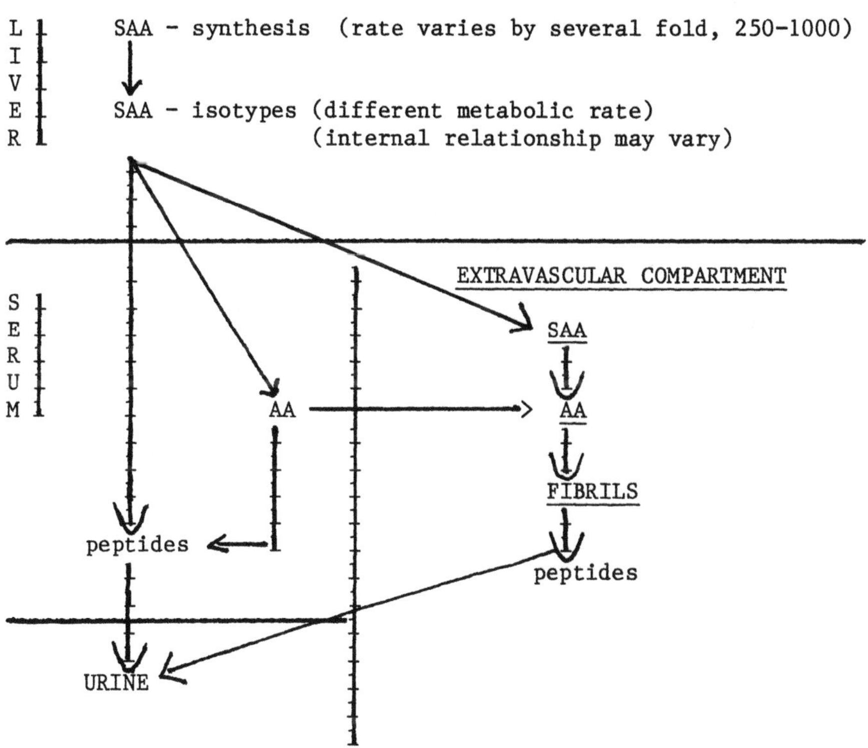

In studying the metabolism of SAA, one has to consider all possible pathways of the protein.

Dr. Shainkin-Kestenbaum and coworkers demonstrated that an apo-SAA fraction isolated and purified from acute phase human plasma modulates growth of transformed cells. Biological effects of SAA may be a function of its metabolic form.

4. Definition of amyloid enhancing factor(s): R. Kisilevsky

As outlined in the introductory talk for scientific session 3 and in other presentations in this symposium, several substances have been implicated as amyloid enhancing factor (AEF). At the moment, AEF is defined strictly in functional terms as a noninflammatory, nonamyloidogenic substance that when coadministered with a single inflammatory stimulus shortens the preamyloid phase to result in splenic amyloid deposition after 36 hours. The issues are to determine the nature, chemistry, potency, kinetics. Intimately connected is how to quantify fibrillar and nonfibrillar AA and SAA in tissues. Morphometric and immunochemical assays have been used. Could the rate of uptake of radiolabeled SAP as described by Pepys and coworkers be used experimentally?

5. Identification of brain amyloid related proteins: D. Selkoe

Amyloid β- fibril proteins isolated from brain vary in length from 39 to 42 amino acids. This size heterogeneity can complicate studies using antisera to synthetic peptides.

The observed heterogeneity in anatomic distribution may be associated with biochemical differences; it has been difficult to sequence the core β-protein from its amino terminus, whereas microvascular derived β-protein can readily be sequenced.

A few antibodies to the β-protein have been reported to recognize neurons containing the neurofibrillary tangles, but this does not mean that the β-protein is the subunit of the abnormal filaments in neurofibrillary tangles.

The β-amyloid precursor protein APP should be designated β-APP to distinguish it from other types of fibril protein precursor. The biochemistry of the intracellular β-APP components needs to be defined. As a result of alternative splicing and processing there is protein heterogeneity of β-APP in extracellular fluids.

Immunochemical studies to develop diagnostic tests must include positive standards. There is a lack of full characterization of antibodies (and epitopes recognized by these antibodies) to synthetic β-protein peptides versus to native purified β-proteins.

Dr. Shinoda and colleagues introduced an ELISA method using a monoclonal antibody and polyclonal antisera to a synthetic peptide corresponding to residues 1-10 of the beta-amyloid protein to measure beta protein cross-reactivity in patients' sera. Higher beta-amyloid protein cross-reactivity values were obtained for senile dementia of the Alzheimer type than for multi-infarct dementia and non-specified senile dementia patients and for members of a non-affected control group. However, the antigen in serum being measured by this ELISA has not yet been defined. Dr. Shinoda stated he was not yet certain whether the assay was detecting true β -protein (or β -protein containing fragments of β-APP) in serum or rather a "cross-reacting protein".

6. Non-SAA amyloid precursors and proteins in tissues and circulation:

J. Buxbaum: AL amyloidosis, Identification of serum precursors

In experienced laboratories, 80-90% of AL patients will have detectable serum M-proteins or urinary monoclonal L-chains when assayed by either conventional immunoelectrophoretic or immunofixation techniques utilizing specific anti-Ig antibodies. In cases in which these proteins are not detectable, immunohistochemical techniques can usually identify a distortion in the usual kappa/lambda ratio in bone marrow cells. The latter may also be revealed by a variety of techniques which may not be generally available. The use of specific light chain immunoglobulin DNA probes may detect clonal rearrangements in cell populations in which only 1-5% of the marrow cells are plasma cells. The latter technique has also revealed the presence of aberrant Ig peptides in marrow samples from patients with both Ig deposition disease. Hence the combination of immunoelectrophoresis or immunofixation of the marrow cell population in conjunction with biosynthetic analysis should be diagnostic in virtually 100% of patients with either AL or non-Congophilic monoclonal Ig deposition.

There is a gap in our knowledge concerning the state of the precursor Igs from the time they are synthesized to the time they are deposited. In those cases in which no fragments can be identified intracellularly, more data are required to define the relationship between the fragments found in the marrow cells and the deposited fibrils and the steps involved in the genesis from intact L-chain to fibril subunit. More precise qualitative analyses of sera of patients with deposition diseases should be performed to define whether there are small amounts of polymerized or process L-chains present in the circulation. Western blotting of serum with appropriate antisera may be the best current appraoch, however more sensitive assays may be necessary.

More information is required concerning the relationship between the fibrillar and non-fibrillar forms of Ig deposition, particularly in the same patient. Whether these represent the products of related, but not identical, clones, differences in tissue processing, differences in Ig-matrix interactions or merely different phases of the same process must be established. The immediate need appears to be a structural analysis of the fibrillar and non-fibrillar material from the same patient. It appears that several forms of amyloid may exhibit deposition of the presursor in similar amorphous and fibrillar states, e.g. the β-protein of Alzheimer's disease, and that knowledge gained from these patients may be broadly applicable.

R.P Linke:

1) Plasma precursor proteins

Identification of amyloid precursor proteins is important in AL-amyloidosis in that the presence and chemical nature of the Bence Jones proteins can give clues as to the chemistry of the amyloid present in a given patient. The diagnosis of plasma precursor variants of TTR by high resolution isoelectric focusing is also indicative of the presence of (familial) TTR-amyloid. Of less value in this respect is the determination of the SAA or β 2-microglobulin concentration in AA- or Aβ2m amyloidosis, respectively.

While the determination of the amyloid precursor proteins is performed in many laboratories, the identification of the preamyloid polypeptide (defined as the soluble polypeptide before aggregation into the enzyme-resistant fibril with the typical tinctorial properties toward Congo red) has been examined only rarely. Whether this is useful in light of the possibility of local processing has to be evaluated. This approach could also lead to preclinical diagnostic tools in some amyloid types.

2) Amyloid fibril proteins in tissues

The identification and the determination of plasma concentration of amyloid precursors can only be indicators for the chemical nature of the amyloidosis present but can never prove it. Proof can only come from direct examination of the amyloid deposits of a patient. This can be done chemically and immunochemically or (more indirect) immunohistochemically. The latter is the most useful, because this procedure can be performed in most laboratories. A precondition for this type of diagnosis is the availability of suitable anti-amyloid antibodies. The production of these antibodies is not an easy task since amyloid fibril proteins express a different epitope repertoire as compared with their precursor proteins. Amyloid deposits adsorb large amounts of plasma proteins which can confuse immunohistochemical classification, and the specimens may be fixed in proteinaceous fluids, adding to the chemical heterogeneity of the amyloid deposits. These pitfalls have been overcome in our laboratory by the production of antibodies against the amyloid fibril protein rather than the precursor, using monoclonal antibodies selected for this purpose, and testing a panel of antibodies against a known amyloid class to demonstrate which of the antibodies is specific for a given class and which covers an entire amyloid class.

By refining our method during the last 14 years, we have come up with monoclonal anti-AA antibodies (mcl, Dako-Patts) which cover the entire class and which have never unspecifically stained a non-AA section in a manner that could give rise to confusion. Our polyclonal anti-Aλ (HAR) and anti-Aλ (ULI) antibodies, and anti-Aκ (SIN) antibodies cover almost the entire spectrum of AL-amyloidoses. Whether the few remaining unreactive cases are of AL-nature is still under investigation. ATTR and Aβ2m amyloidoses can be stained with suitable commercial antibodies, although we prefer the respective antibodies against the purified amyloid fibril proteins, because they stain more intensively. Brain amyloids and endocrine amyloids are best stained with peptide antibodies, as found by several investigators including our own group. Diagnostic identification using immunoelectron microscoscopy is also possible with these antibodies because antigenic epitopes are in part preserved after glutaraldehyde fixation and plastic embedding, so that some monoclonal antibodies may be used together with the protein A gold technique. The preclinical identification of even very small amyloid deposits may be useful for early treatment.

M.A. Gertz:

Detection of a monoclonal light chain is essential to properly classify patients with systemic amyloidosis as AL. Immunoelectrophoresis and immunofixation of the serum and urine will successfully accomplish this in 85 per cent of patients subsequently shown to have AL. Immunostains of amyloid deposits obtained from tissue biopsies may not be helpful since subgroup antisera are not generally abvailable. Antisera may not recognize AL deposits where deletion of the C-terminus of the light chain is common.

One approach to detection of the light chain is to do immunofluorescent microscopy on a Ficoll purified preparation of bone marrow. In 90 per cent of patients with no serum or urine monoclonal protein, immunofluorescence will detect a clonal excess of plasma cells verifying the amyloidosis as AL. Non-AL amyloid invariably reveals a polyclonal population of plasma cells. In vitro culture of plasma cells from patients with AL has shown direct synthesis of immunoglobulin fragments and free light chains which does not occur in the plasma cells of patients without AL.

Identification of apo-SAA isoforms in man and mouse.

F.C. de Beer*, M.C. de Beer* and J.D. Sipe•
*Department of Medicine, University of Kentucky Medical Center, Lexington, Kentucky, USA. •Department of Biochemistry, Boston University School of Medicine, Boston, Massachusetts, USA.

ABSTRACT: Isoelectric identification of apo-SAA isoforms in mouse and human plasma is important in analyzing function and involvement in amyloidogenesis. In this paper we show the influence of altering the pH gradient on the migration of the human isoforms and identify novel minor apo-SAA isoforms. The NH_2-terminals of these isoforms are analyzed by sequencing of the isoforms electroblotted onto polyvinylidene difluoride (PVDF) membranes. Integrity of the COOH-terminal is confirmed by blotting using a rabbit anti-human apo-SAA (aa 95-104) antibody. Isoelectric focusing (IEF) is compared to urea-SDS-acrylamide gel electrophoresis for the analysis of apo-SAA isoforms in haplotype A and B mouse strains [1,2].

INTRODUCTION: Human apo-SAA is a polymorphic protein that can be separated into six major isoforms by electrofocusing of delipidated acute phase high-density lipoprotein (AP-HDL) in the presence of urea [1]. Some individuals display all six isoforms - pI's 6.0; 6.4, 7.0, 7.4, 7.5 and 8.0, whereas others apparently lack the pI 7.4 and 8.0 or the pI 7.0 and 7.5 isoforms. The pI 6.4, 7.5 and 8.0 isoforms are the respective products of the genes corresponding to cDNA pA1, cDNA pSAA82 and genomic DNA clone SAAg9. The 6.0, 7.0 and 7.4 isoforms result from the proteolytic cleavage of the respective NH_2-terminal argenines of the above [3].

Four SAA genes have been described in BALB/c mice [4] of which only 2 yield the protein products designated apo-SAA_1 and apo-SAA_2. Apo-SAA_2 has been identified to be selectively removed from circulating HDL_3 and to give rise to amyloid A protein (AA).

MATERIALS AND METHODS: HDL was isolated from plasma by sequential ultracentrifugation [1]. Delipidated HDL was electrofocused on ultrathin (0.3 mm) polyacrylamide gels containing 7 M urea [1]. To identify basic apo-SAA isoforms, an ampholine ratio of 20% (v/v) pH

3-10, 40% (v/v) pH 4-6.5 and 40% (v/v) pH 7-9 was used. Acidic apo-SAA isoforms were exposed using an ampholine ratio of 20% (v/v) pH 3-10 and 80% (v/v) pH 4-6.5

Immunochemical analysis of apo-SAA isoforms was performed after pressure-blotting apo-SAA isoforms, separated by isoelectric focusing, onto nitrocellulose membranes [1]. The integrity of the COOH-terminal was confirmed with a rabbit anti-human SAA (aa 95-104) (gift from Prof. A.R. Steinmetz, University of Marburg, FRG).

NH_2-terminal sequencing was performed on isoforms electroblotted on to PVDF membrane. Briefly, isoforms were excised from coomassie-stained electrofocused gels. Isoforms of a particular pI were pooled and resolved by electrophoresis in a 5-20% acrylamide SDS-gel, from which the individual isoforms were electroblotted on to PVDF membrane. Electroblotted isoforms were subjected to Edman degradation on an Applied Biosystems 477A pulsed liquid phase peptide sequencer.

Mouse HDL was analyzed by urea-SDS-polyacrylamide gel electrophoresis using 11.5% polyacrylamide and 6.4 M urea [5].

RESULTS: Figure 1: Isoelectric focusing of human acute phase HDL

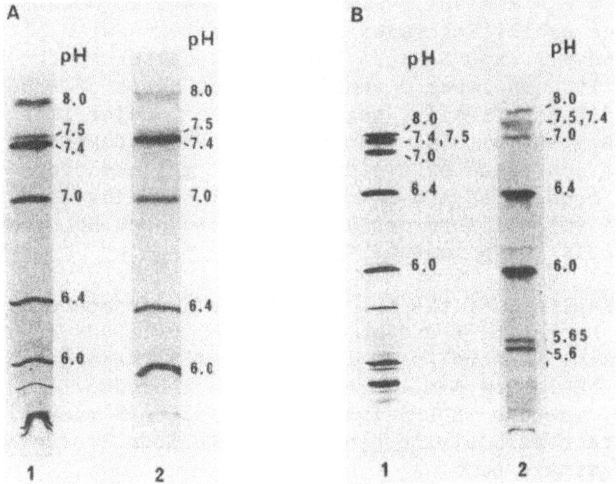

Figure 1: The six major human apo-SAA isoforms, separated by electrofocusing using an ampholine gradient of 20% (v/v) pH 3-10, 40% (v/v) pH 4-6.5 and 40% (v/v) pH 7-9 are depicted in fig. 1A. Lane 1, coomassie-stained gel; lane 2, immunochemical staining of apo-SAA isoforms in lane 1 with rabbit anti-human SAA (aa 95-104). The same isoforms, electrofocused in an ampholine gradient of 20% (v/v) pH 3-10 and 80% (v/v) pH 4-6.5 are shown in fig. 1B. Lane 1, coomassie-stained gel; lane 2, immunochemical staining of apo-SAA isoforms in lane 1 with rabbit anti-human SAA (aa 95-104) identifying acidic apo-SAA isoforms pI 5.65 and pI 5.6 which cannot be resolved by the gradient used in A.

Figure 2A and 2B: Comparative analysis of mouse HDL by IEF and Urea-SDS-acrylamide gel electrophoresis.

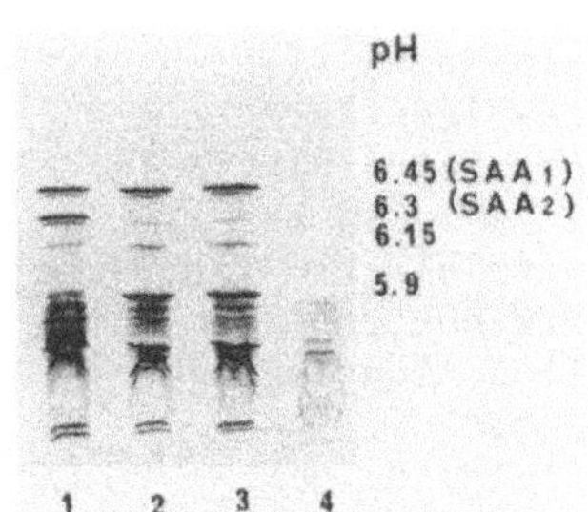

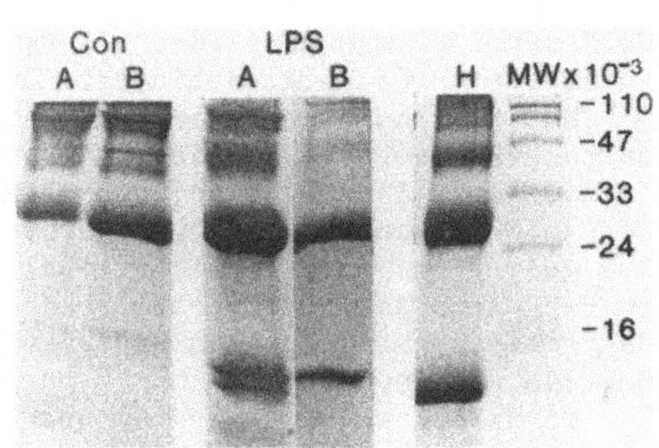

Figure 2A: Coomassie stain of electrofocused HDL from acute and non-acute mice, using an ampholine gradient of 20% (v/v) pH 3-10, 40% (v/v) pH 4-6.5 and 40% (v/v) pH 7-9. Lane 1, HDL from acute C3Heb/FeJ mice exhibiting major apo-SAA isoforms with pI's 6.45 (apo-SAA_1) and 6.3 (apo-SAA_2). These mice belong to the haplotype A SAA gene family. In lanes 2 and 3, the apo-SAA's of P/NCR mice (hapotype B SAA gene family) segregate into 2 major isoforms of pI 6.45 (apo-SAA_1) and pI 5.9. The identity and integrity of these isoforms were confirmed by two-dimensional gel electrophoresis, NH_2-terminal sequencing and immunochemical staining with rabbit anti-mouse AA (unpublished data). Electrofocused HDL from non-acute 3Heb/FeJ mice is shown in lane 4.

Figure 2B: Analysis of the HDL of acute and non-acute mice belonging to haplotype A and haplotype B by urea-SDS-acrylamide gel electrophoresis. Control mice lack apo-SAA. The apo-SAA of LPS-injected haplotype A mice resolve into 2 bands, i.e., apo-SAA_1 and apo-SAA_2, whereas in LPS-injected haplotype B mice all apo-SAA isoforms migrate as a single band. Apo-SAA from Syrian hamsters migrate as a single band.

DISCUSSION: There are precedents for the existence of other molecules related to, but distinct from, "classical" apo-SAA. An SAA-like protein with the capacity for autocrine induction of collagenase has been reported to be produced by PMA-stimulated rabbit synovial fibroblasts [6]. Another human SAA-family member, $GSAA_1$, has been described at the gene level [7]. Our data show the value of using expanded pI ranges during isoelectric focusing to identify the novel apo-SAA gene products pI 5.6 are 5.65. Integrity of these products was confirmed by NH_2-terminal sequencing and blotting with appropriate COOH-terminal directed antibodies in addition to two-dimensional gel electrophoresis.

The difference in migration between mouse apo-SAA_1 and apo-SAA_2 in urea-SDS-acrylamide gels is unlikely due to a difference in molecular weight but is rather due to differential unfolding in 6.4M urea. The limitations of this technique in defining isoforms is apparent in haplotype B mice where all the apo-SAA isoforms migrate as a single band corresponding to apo-SAA_1. This can lead to inaccurate conclusions as to the isoforms present in these mice.

REFERENCES

1. Strachan, A.F.; de Beer, F.C.; Van der Westhuyzen, D.R. and Coetzee, G.A. (1988). Identification of three isoform patterns of human serum amyloid A protein. Biochem. J. 250, 203-207.
2. Taylor, B.A. and Rowe, L. (1984). Genes for serum amyloid A proteins map to chromosome 7 in the mouse. Mol. Gen. Genetics. 195, 491-499.
3.. Strachan, A.F.; Brandt, W.F.; Woo, P.; Van der Westhuyzen, D.R.; Coetzee, G.A.; de Beer, M.C.; Shephard, E.G. and de Beer, F.C. (1989). Human serum amyloid A protein. The assignment of the six major isoforms to three published gene sequences and evidence for two genetic loci. J. Biol. Chem. 264, 18368-18373.
4. Yamamoto, K.; Goto, N.; Kosaka, J.; Shiroo, M.; Yeul, Y.D. and Migita, S. (1987). Structural diversity of murine serum amyloid A genes: evolutionary implications. J. Immunol. 439, 1683-1688.
5. Goldsmith, M.R.; Rattner, E.C.; Koehler, M.M.D.; Balikov, S.R. and Bock, S.C. (1979). Two-dimensional electrophoresis of small-molecular-weight proteins. Analyt. Biochem. 99:33-40.
6. Brinckerhoff, C.E.; Mitchell, T.I.; Karmilowicz, M.J.; Kluve-Beckerman, B. and Benson, M.D. (1989). Autocrine induction of collagenase by serum amyloid A-like and β_2-microglobulin-like proteins. Science 243,655-657.
7. Sack, G.H. and Talbot, C.C. (1989). The human serum amyloid A (SAA)-encoding gene $GSAA_1$: nucleotide sequence and possible autocrine-collagenase-inducer-function. Gene 84:509-515.

NORMAL LIPOPROTEINS INHIBIT BINDING OF SAA-RICH LIPOPROTEINS TO POLYVINYLCHLORIDE SURFACES

J. D. SIPE, W. A. GONNERMAN, G. KNAPSCHAEFER AND W-J XIE
Department of Biochemistry
Boston University School of Medicine
80 East Concord Street, Boston, MA 02118

ABSTRACT. A direct binding ELISA for serum amyloid A (SAA) proteins has been developed in which noncovalent interactions of SAA with other plasma constitutents are disrupted with heat, high salt and alkaline pH to permit coating of the wells of polyvinyl chloride microtitration plates with an amount of SAA antigen proportional to its concentration in plasma (J. Immunol. Methods, 125:125, 1989). When standard preparations of SAA-rich high density lipoprotein (HDL) were added to plasma lacking SAA, the ELISA values were lowered by 100-fold. Therefore standard curves were constructed by adding known amounts of SAA-HDL complex to solutions of purified human IgG and albumin of the same concentration as the diluted plasma samples. In the present study, it was found that addition of the lipoprotein fraction of normal plasma to the mixture of albumin, IgG and SAA-HDL, inhibited binding of SAA antigens by the polyvinylchloride surface. This suggests a strong affinity between SAA and lipoproteins lacking SAA.

INTRODUCTION. Since the discovery of SAA in the early 1970s, it has been widely noted that SAA measurements would be clinically useful in the diagnosis and management of disease (e.g. detection of active inflammation and prediction of graft survival or rejection) [1,2]. However, until recently, SAA determination has largely remained a research assay because of numerous technical difficulties (Table 1). A major factor contributing to these problems is the capacity of SAA proteins for conformational changes [3]. Apo-SAA proteins contain amphipathic helical regions and form alpha helices upon association with lipid [4]; while upon proteolytic removal of 28 amino acids from the carboxyl portion of the molecule, insoluble beta pleated sheet fibrils are produced from SAA [5]. SAA is "sticky", forming hydrophobic associations with itself and other plasma constituents and, depending upon the epitope specificity of antibody preparations, may or may not require denaturation for maximal stable exposure of the antigenic sites [6].

In order to be useful for quantitative clinical measurements, it is desirable to have an assay which is capable of measuring absolute amounts over the concentration range of 1 to 2000 ug/ml, which can be automated and which is simple and safe.

TABLE 1. TECHNICAL DIFFICULTIES SURROUNDING SAA IMMUNOASSAY

1. Denaturation required, depending upon epitope specificity of antibodies.
2. Multiple dilutions required to measure SAA over 1000 fold range result in high variability.
3. Lack of absolute standard, results first expressed in terms of AA equivalents or relative units.
4. Conformation flexibility and physicochemical changes in SAA result in variable results with prolonged sample storage.

For a number of years, SAA concentrations were reported in relative units or in AA equivalents. Recently, stable SAA-rich high density lipoprotein preparations have been used as quantitative standards for SAA immunoassay [7,8] in purified human albumin and IgG rather than plasma lacking SAA. In the present study, the effect of whole plasma and the lipoprotein fraction of plasma on the binding of SAA-rich HDL to polyvinylchloride wells was investigated.

MATERIALS AND METHODS. SAA was isolated by ultracentrifugation as its complex with high density lipoprotein as described in detail elsewhere along with the procedure for coating wells and ELISA analysis [8]. The total lipoprotein fraction of normal plasma lacking HDL was also obtained by ultracentrifugation of plasma with no detectable SAA adjusted to density 1.21 g/ml. Protein concentration was determined using the BCA kit from Pierce Chemical Co (Rockford, IL) according to manufacturers´ instructions.

RESULTS. When varying amounts of purified SAA-rich HDL were added to normal human plasma lacking SAA, much lower absorbance values were measured by ELISA than when the SAA standards were added to a solution of purified IgG, 13 mg/ml, and purified albumin, 45 mg/ml. Both plasma and the solution of IgG and albumin were diluted 1:900 (Fig. 1). Because inhibition of SAA binding was observed when SAA-rich HDL was added to normal plasma immediately before the 60 C incubation, it seemed possible that diminished SAA binding resulted from an increased affinity for the liquid compartment resulting from strong positive interaction with a plasma constituent rather than degradation by a plasma protease.

The lipoprotein fraction from normal human plasma lacking SAA inhibited binding of apo-SAA from SAA-rich lipoprotein fraction (Fig. 2).

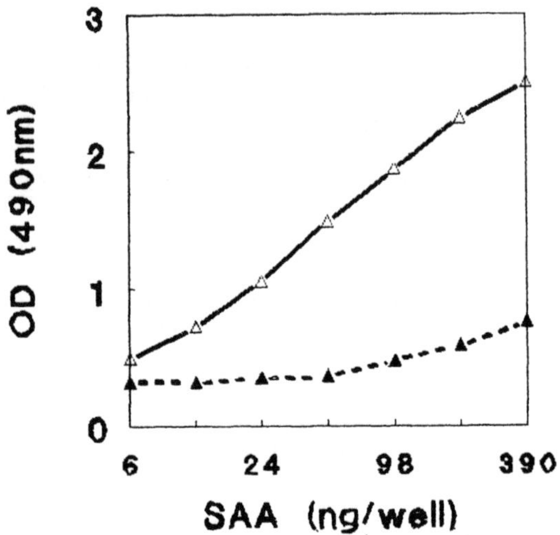

Figure 1. Inhibitory effect of plasma on SAA binding to wells of microtiter plates. SAA-rich HDL was added to a 1:900 dilution in 3M KBr in bicarbonate, pH 9.6, of albumin, 45 mg/ml, and IgG, 13 mg/ml, -△- or plasma lacking SAA, -▲-. Coating was carried out by incubation at 60 C overnight followed by incubation with rabbit anti-human SAA, with peroxidase conjugated anti-IgG and color development in the presence of o-phenylenediamine dihydrochloride substrate and hydrogen peroxide [8].

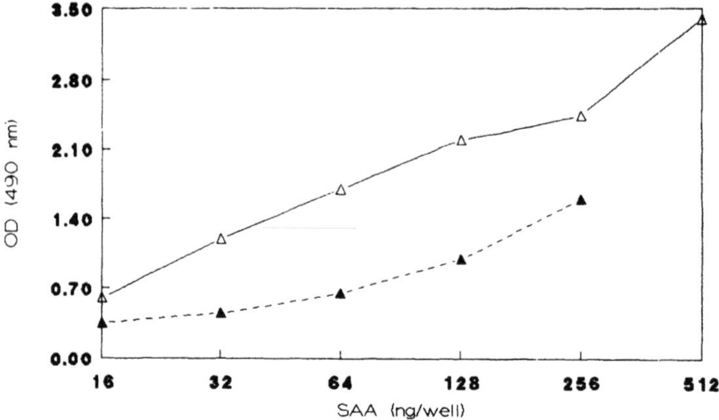

Figure 2. Inhibitory effect of the lipoprotein fraction of normal human plasma lacking SAA, -▲-, on binding of apo-SAA from the lipoprotein fraction from SAA-rich plasma, -△-, in a 1:100 dilution in 3MKBr in bicarbonate, pH 9.6, of purified IgG, 13 mg/ml, and albumin, 45 mg/ml. Coating and color development as described for Figure 1.

DISCUSSION. In the present study we demonstrate that SAA, once isolated as its complex with HDL by ultracentrifugation, cannot be reintroduced into plasma without reduction in its capacity to be bound by plastic surfaces. We show that the interaction of SAA with other lipoproteins may result in diminished binding by polyvinyl chloride wells. The measurement of SAA, like that of other lipophilic plasma proteins has historically been difficult. Conformational changes have been observed when SAA in serum or plasma is analyzed by immunodiffusion or charge shift electrophoresis [9]. Treating with heating, acid, alkali, guanidine hydrochloride and extraction with organic solvents can also induce changes in apo-SAA conformation [1,3,10]. The inherent stickiness of apo-SAA (i.e., tendency to form non-specific hydrophobic interactions with other molecules of similar structure, (self-association) and with the surfaces of laboratory vessels has caused inaccurate measurement of SAA by immunoassays [6]. The direct binding ELISA circumvents these difficulties by dissociation of noncovalent interactions, thus permitting a fraction of SAA to bind to polyvinylchloride surfaces according to its concentration and its relative affinity for the polyvinyl chloride surface relative to that of other constituents.

REFERENCES

1. Pepys, M.B. and Baltz, M.L. (1983) ´Acute phase proteins with special reference to C-reactive protein and related proteins (pentraxins) and serum amyloid A protein´, Adv. Immunol., 34, 141-212.
2. Gorevic, P.D., Rosenthal, C.J. and Franklin, E.C. (1976) ´Amyloid -related serum component (SAA)-Studies in acute infection, medullary thyroid carcinoma and post surger. Behavior as an acute phase reactant, Clin. Immunol. Immunopathol., 6, 83-93.
3. Sipe, J.D., McAdam, K.P.W.J., Torain, B.F. and Glenner, G.G. (1976) ´Conformational flexibility of the serum amyloid precursor SAA´ Br.J. Exp. Pathol. 57, 582-592.
4. Segrest, J.P., Pownall, H.J., Jackson, R.L., Glenner, G.G and Pollock, P.S. (1976) ´Amyloid A: Amphipathic helixes and lipid binding´ Biochemistry, 15, 3187-3191.
5. Benditt, E.P. and Eriksen, N. (1977) ´The major proteins of human and monkey amyloid substance: Common properties including unusual N-terminal amino acid sequences´ Am J. Pathol. 65, 231-252.
6. Marhaug, G. (1983) ´Three assays for the characterization and quantitaation of human serum amyloid A´, Scand J. Immunol., 18, 329-338.
7. Godenir, N.L., Jeenah, M.S., Coetzee, G.A., vanderWesthuyzen, D.R., Strachan, A.F. and De Beer, F.C. (1985) ´Standardization of the quantitation of serum amyloid A protein (SAA) in human serum´ J. Immunol. Methods. 83,217-225.
8. Sipe, J.D., Gonnerman, W.A., Loose, L.D., Knapschaefer, G., Wie, W-J. and Franzblau, C. (1989) ´Direct binding enzyme-linked immunosorbent assay (ELISA) for serum amyloid A (SAA)´ J. Immunol. Methods 125, 125-135.
9. Linke, R.P. (1981)´Amphipathic properties of the low molecular weight component of serum amyloid-A protein shown by charge-shift electrophoresis. Biochim. Biophys. Acta, 668, 388-396.
10. Eriksen, N and Benditt, E.P. (1986) ´Serum amyloid A (apoSAA) and lipoproteins. Methods Enzymol. 128, 311-320.

MONOCLONAL ANTIBODY BASED ELISA FOR HUMAN SAA

BOUKE P.C. HAZENBERG, PIETER C. LIMBURG, JOHAN BIJZET, MARTIN H. VAN RIJSWIJK
Division of Rheumatology, Department of Medicine
State University Hospital, 59 Oostersingel
9713 EZ Groningen, The Netherlands

ABSTRACT. We developed an ELISA for human SAA in which two different monoclonal antibodies (MAb) were used (Reu.86.1 and Reu.86.5) that recognized different epitopes on SAA. These MAb's were raised against purified SAA coupled to Helix pomatia haemocyanin (by glutaraldehyde). The MAb's reacted with isolated AA-proteins and with SAA (all major isotypes), both isolated and after reconstitution in HDL_3. The MAb's could be used in ELISA, in immunohistochemistry, and in immuno-blotting after SDS-PAGE or IEF. In ELISA one of the MAb's was coated to the microtiterplate (Reu.86.5), while the other (Reu.86.1) was coupled to HRPO. The internal standard in the ELISA consisted either of SAA isolated from a serum pool (150 patients with CRP >100 mg/l) reconstituted into normal serum or of a reference serum sample. The lower detection limit of the assay for SAA was 5 μg/l, allowing the use in biological fluids (serum, urine, synovial fluid) and in in-vitro systems (cultured human hepatocytes). In routine serology we found an intra-assay coefficient of variation (CV) and an inter-assay CV both <10% (N=15 res. N=17). In this assay no pretreatment of testsamples was necessary and there was no interference of rheumatoid factors. The basal reference values of healthy controls had a 95% upper limit of 2.6 mg/l. This SAA-ELISA uses well defined MAb's for the detection of SAA, which permits standardization, inter-laboratory comparability and general availability.

1. INTRODUCTION

Serum amyloid A (SAA), an acute-phase protein is supposed to be the precursor of amyloid AA. Quantification of SAA remains a problem. Although about 40 assays (with minor and major modifications) have been developed since the discovery of SAA in 1973 [1], none of them is really satisfactory and what is more, currently available for general use. Apart from standardization and technical differences, the real problem is the lack of general available specific antibodies to human SAA.

Aim of this study was to produce a panel of monoclonal murine anti-human apo-SAA antibodies and to construct an entirely monoclonal (and thereby general available) enzyme-linked immunosorbent assay (ELISA) for the quantification of SAA.

2. MATERIALS AND METHODS

2.1. Murine monoclonal antibodies Reu.86.1 and Reu.86.5

Murine monoclonal antibodies (Reu.86.1 and Reu.86.5) were raised against apo-SAA coupled to Helix Pomatia Haemocyanin (HPH). In short: HDL_3 was isolated from pooled sera (150 with CRP level >100 mg/l). SAA was purified by chromatography after HDL_3 delipidation. Monoclonal anti-SAA antibodies were raised to apo-SAA complexed (by glutaraldehyde) to HPH.

The produced monoclonal antibodies were screened and tested against: 1. Control antigens (HPH, CRP, and other amyloid proteins) in ELISA. 2. Purified SAA and AA from several donors in ELISA. 3. Native serum and purified SAA in immunoblotting techniques (PAGE and IEF). 4. Control and amyloid tissues in immunohistochemistry.

Reu.86.1 and Reu.86.5 were chosen for their specificity and excellent results to be used in the sandwich ELISA for SAA.

2.2. Sandwich ELISA for SAA

Microtiter plates (Labstar Microtest Plates F, Costar, Cambridge, USA.) were coated for 1 h at 37°C with the IgG fraction of Reu.86.5 ("catcher", 1:500, 2.6 mg/l) in 0.01 M PBS, pH 7.4. After being washed (with 0.025 M Tris-HCl, pH 8.0, 0.15 M NaCl and 0.05% Tween-20) the plates were incubated with patient sera and standards for 1 h at 37 °C. Because of the wide range in SAA levels sera were routinely analysed at dilutions 1:250 to 1:16,000. After washing the plates were incubated with the HRPO labeled IgG fraction of the "detector" monoclonal anti-SAA Reu.86.1 (1:400, 2 mg/l) for 1 h at 37°C. Ten mg of the chromogen OPD (O-phenylenediamine dihydrochloride, Kodak Laboratory Chemicals, Rochester, USA) was dissolved in 50 ml 0.05 M phosphate buffer, pH 5.6. After incubation at room temperature for 20 min the reaction was stopped by adding 1 M H_2SO_4, and the absorbance at 492 nm was read in a Titertek Multiskan. All incubations were done in 0.01 M PBS, pH 7.3, 2% BSA and 0.05% Tween-20. The sample and conjugate incubation may be combined in one step.

Reconstitution of an exact amount of the purified apo-SAA into normal plasma (initial SAA concentration 0.6 mg/l), provided the ultimate standard of our ELISA: final SAA concentration 90 mg/l. In every routine assay an aliquot of a well known plasma was used as an internal standard.

2.3. Patients

Plasma samples of fifty apparently healthy members of the medical and nursing hospital staff were taken at three consecutive moments with monthly intervals. The 50 median values served as basal controls for SAA.

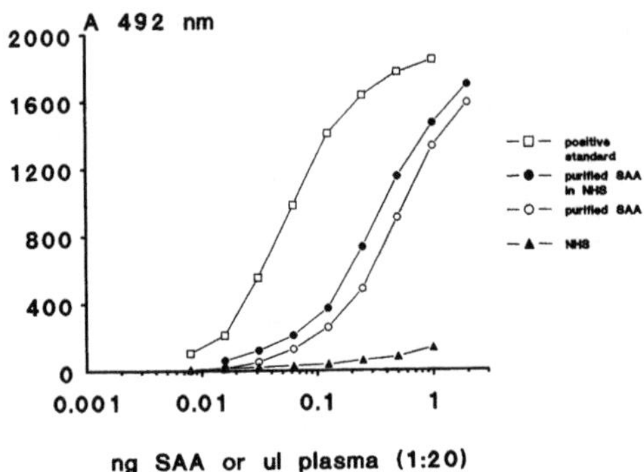

Figure 1. SAA-ELISA: Absorbance at 492 nm.

3. RESULTS

Acute-phase plasma with a concentration of 141 mg/l was used in the SAA-ELISA as the routine standard. ELISA results using apo-SAA in PBS (-O-) and apo-SAA reconstituted in normal (SAA level 0.6 mg/l) plasma (-●-) are presented in figure 1 together with the diluted routine standard plasma (-□-) and plasma from one of our basal controls (-▲-). The absorbance values of apo-SAA reconstituted plasma were slightly higher than those of apo-SAA in PBS.

Denaturation of serum samples with formic acid, alkali, or heating resulted in a decline of SAA reactivity compared to native serum. Repeated (5x) freezing and thawing of serum or plasma did not affect the results. No differences were found between plasma and serum levels. The presence of rheumatoid factors did not affect the results.

The ultimate detection limit of the assay for serum and plasma (using samples diluted 1:50) was 30 μg/l: this value was lower in supernatants of hepatocyte cultures (using samples diluted 1:5) namely 5 μg/l. SAA values >1,000 mg/l were measured; there was no upper limit of this assay. The intra-assay CV (coefficient of variation) and the inter-assay CV were both <10% (N=15 resp. N=17).

The healthy control group had a median basal SAA value of 0.7 mg/l, and a 95% upper confidence limit of 2.6 mg/l.

4. DISCUSSION

Constant quality and general availability make monoclonal antibodies excellent tools for ELISA. Murine monoclonal antibodies were raised against human apo-SAA prepared from acute-phase sera. The monoclonal antibodies Reu.86.1 and Reu.86.5 were selected to construct a sandwich ELISA for SAA.

In routine practice of this SAA-ELISA the intra-assay CV and the inter-assay CV were both <10%. Samples could be quantified from a concentration of 5 μg/l, like in our former assay [2]. No upper limit was observed, values could be measured easily above 1,000 mg/l. No pretreatment of testsamples was necessary and there was no interference of rheumatoid factors. Basal values of healthy controls were ≤2.6 mg/l.

In conclusion: Well defined monoclonal antibodies are used in this assay to detect SAA, which permits standardization, inter-laboratory comparability and most important, a general availability of this SAA-ELISA.

5. ACKNOWLEDGEMENTS

This study was supported by the Dutch Kidney Foundation.

We are grateful to our collegue L.de Leij for his assistance in the monoclonal antibody production.

6. REFERENCES

1. Levin, M., Pras, M., Linke, R. and Franklin, E.C. (1973) 'Immunologic studies of ASF, the major nonimmunoglobulin component of certain amyloid fibrils [Abstract]', Arthritis Rheum. 16, 23-24.
2. Moshage, H.J., Roelofs, H.M.J., Van Pelt, J.F., Hazenberg, B.P.C., Van Leeuwen, M.A., Limburg, P.C., Aarden, L.A. and Yap, S.H. (1988) 'The effect of interleukin-1, interleukin-6 and its interrelationship on the synthesis of serum amyloid A and C-reactive protein in primary cultures of adult human hepatocytes' Biochem. Biophys. Res. Commun. 155, 112-117.

SERUM AMYLOID P COMPONENT IN CHRONIC RENAL FAILURE AND DIALYSIS

S.R. NELSON, G.A. TENNENT, D. SETHI, P.E. GOWER, F.W. BALLARDIE, S. AMATAYAKUL-CHANTLER & M.B. PEPYS
Immunological Medicine Unit, Royal Postgraduate Medical School, London, Renal Unit, Charing Cross Hospital, London, Department of Renal Medicine, Manchester Royal Infirmary, Manchester, and Biochemistry Department, University of Oxford, U.K.

ABSTRACT. A normal reference range for serum amyloid P component (SAP) concentration in the serum was established in 500 healthy adult subjects (274 women, 226 men), by electroimmunoassay calibrated with standards of highly purified, isolated SAP. The mass of SAP in these was determined from the extinction coefficient of SAP at 280 nm measured here precisely for the first time by spectrophotometry and cryogenic drying. The mean (SD, range) SAP concentration was significantly lower ($P < 0.001$) in women: 24 mg/l (8, 8 - 55), compared to 32 mg/l (7, 12 - 50) in men. In 38 patients with chronic renal failure, 79 on haemodialysis and 66 on continuous ambulatory peritoneal dialysis, the mean values for SAP concentration were all significantly higher than normal (range of means, 39-59 mg/l in men and 35-42 mg/l in women), but did not correlate with serum creatinine, duration of dialysis or the presence of an acute phase response. The metabolism of SAP is thus altered in renal failure and is not normalised by dialysis, but it is not clear whether this is relevant to the pathogenesis of dialysis related arthropathy and amyloidosis.

1. INTRODUCTION

High circulating concentrations of β_2-microglobulin (β_2M) are a necessary condition for development of haemodialysis-associated, β_2M-type amyloidosis but may not in themselves be sufficient. The role, if any, of serum amyloid P component (SAP) in amyloidosis is not known but there is a preliminary report of raised SAP levels in dialysis patients [1].

2. METHODS

Venous samples were from 500 normal healthy adult volunteer blood donors, from 38 patients with chronic renal failure (serum creatinines 150-1000 μmol/l), 79 with end stage renal failure on haemodialysis and 66 with end stage renal failure on continuous ambulatory peritoneal dialysis. Serum SAP and CRP were quantitated by electroimmunoassay [2], calibrated with standards of over 99% pure SAP and CRP [3] respectively. The extinction coefficients at 280 nm of these proteins were used to calculate the mass of protein present in primary standard solutions and these in turn were used to calibrate secondary standards of normal human serum spiked with additional pure SAP or CRP. The extinction coefficient of CRP at 280 nm was based on measurement of concentration by interferometry, the refractive index increment for proteins being taken as 0.19 ml/g [4], and was estimated at 17.5 for a 1% solution of CRP and a 1 cm light path. The extinction coefficient of SAP at 280 nm determined by the same method was 17.1. In order to independently check this value a sample of over 99% pure SAP containing 56.2 AU at 280 nm was extensively dialysed against pure water and then cryogenically dried over activated charcoal at -196°C under reduced pressure of < 0.1 Pa for at least 3 days. The mass recovered at complete dryness was 32.81 mg, giving an extinction coefficient of 17.13.

3. RESULTS

The values for SAP were normally distributed and as we have previously reported [2], significantly lower in females than in males (Table). Age was not a significant determinant of SAP levels.

All groups with renal failure had significantly raised SAP values (Table) which were not affected by the level of serum creatinine or duration of dialysis. However, among the male patients on CAPD, the SAP levels were significantly higher than in either the chronic renal failure alone or HD groups. Some patients had acute phase responses, with raised CRP levels. Although modest increases may occur [2] in SAP in patients with chronic disease and raised CRP levels, this did not account for the present findings.

4. DISCUSSION

All the control individuals met stringent conditions for being in good health at the time of sampling and they are by far the largest group in whom serum SAP has been measured. The lower levels than previously reported [2] may reflect the different and larger population sample, and refinements of assay technology. No other published study of serum SAP concentrations adequately documents how assays were standardised for mass units of SAP and it is therefore not possible to ascertain whether different normal ranges reported by others reflect genuine variation between populations. Our values were normally distributed within the range with a slight skewing towards the lower end in females, and we confirmed that SAP concentrations overall are significantly lower in women than in man [2].

The observation of increased serum levels of SAP in patients with chronic renal failure confirms that of Ogawa and Saito [1] and extends it to those not yet on dialysis. The absence of a strong general correlation with CRP values indicates that the modest rise in SAP is not likely to be simply a reflection of the acute phase response. Although there was no correlation with creatinine levels the common factor seems to be impairment of an aspect of renal function which is not replaced by dialysis therapy. Human SAP metabolism is normally extremely closely regulated and increased production or altered breakdown of SAP, reflected even by the relatively minor increases in SAP level seen here, could be related in some way to the pathogenesis of dialysis amyloidosis.

Group	n	Age mean (SD) yrs range	SAP mean (SD) mg/l range	CRP median, mg/l range
Serum SAP concentration in normal healthy subjects				
Males	226	39 (10) 19 - 63	32 (7) 12 - 50	
Females	274	38 (11) 20 - 64	24 (8) 8 - 55	
SAP and CRP levels in male patients with renal insufficiency				
CRF	20	54 (14) 25 - 74	44 (16) 15 - 72	3 2 - 45
CAPD	40	51 (14) 19 - 76	59 (20) 28 - 114	5 2 - 70
HD (all)	49	52 (13) 28 - 74	40 (14) 9 - 72	7 2 - 143
HD + DA	15	57 (11) 33 - 70	39 (11) 24 - 55	13 2 - 37
HD - DA	34	50 (13) 28 - 74	41 (16) 9 - 72	7 2 - 143
SAP and CRP levels in female patients with renal insufficiency				
CRF	17	49 (15) 27 - 77	35 (9) 23 - 51	2 2 - 19
CAPD	26	43 (17) 19 - 72	42 (12) 17 - 64	3 2 - 54
HD (all)	26	52 (18) 14 - 77	35 (12) 20 - 57	5 2 - 89
HD + DA	5	61 (10) 44 - 70	35 (10) 29 - 52	14 2 - 24
HD - DA	21	50 (20) 14 - 77	35 (13) 20 - 57	4 2 - 89

SAP concentration, normal males vs normal females: t statistic, 11.33; $P < 0.001$; difference between means, 8; 95% confidence interval for difference between means, 6-10.
CRF, chronic renal failure patients not on dialysis; HD+DA, haemodialysis patients with dialysis arthropathy; HD-DA, haemodialysis patients without dialysis arthropathy.

Further work on the properties of SAP and the pathogenesis of β_2M amyloid deposition will be required to elucidate this possibility.

REFERENCES

1. Ogawa, H. and Saito, A. (1987) Significance of amyloid P component in dialysis related amyloidosis. *Xth International Congress of Nephrology*, London, p. 163 (abstract).
2. Pepys, M.B., Dash, A.C., Markham, R.E., Thomas, H.C., Williams, B.D. and Petrie, A. (1978) Comparative clinical study of protein SAP (amyloid P component) and C-reactive protein in serum. *Clin. Exp. Immunol.,* **32**: 119-124.
3. de Beer, F.C. and Pepys, M.B. (1982) Isolation of human C-reactive protein and serum amyloid P component. *J. Immunol. Methods,* **50**: 17-31.
4. Dubin, S.B. (1972) Measurement of translational and rotational diffusion coefficients by laser light scattering. *In: Enzyme Structure, Part D, Methods in Enzymology,* Vol. 26 (Hirs, C.H.W. and Timasheff, S.N., eds.), Academic Press Inc., London, pp. 119-174.

MONOCLONAL ANTIBODIES TO HUMAN SERUM AMYLOID P-COMPONENT

G. O'SULLIVAN, K.P.W.J. MCADAM, and J.G. RAYNES
Department of Clinical Sciences
London School of Hygiene and Tropical Medicine
Keppel Street
London WC1E 7HT
U.K.

ABSTRACT. Eighteen mouse hybridomas secreting monoclonal antibodies (mAbs) to human serum amyloid P-component (SAP) were prepared and characterized. The relative avidities of purified mAbs for Human SAP (HuSAP) ranged from 0.05 to 3.3 μg/ml. The mAbs were assigned to three groups on the basis of epitope specificity determined by competitive inhibition. In group I (13 mAbs) nine mAbs bind to native HuSAP only and four bind to native and denatured HuSAP. The four mAbs comprising group II recognize native and denatured HuSAP. One mAb only comprises Group III. Seven mAbs were tested for their ability to precipitate iodinated HuSAP from solution. The mAb from Group III does not precipitate. Eleven out of twelve mAbs, tested by gel immunodiffusion precipitate HuSAP in a calcium independent manner. Calcium is not required for recognition of HuSAP by any of the monoclonals.

1. Introduction

Serum amyloid P-component (SAP) is a 230,000 Da glycoprotein which has 52% amino acid homology with human C-reactive protein (CRP) [1]. It is the major acute phase reactant in the mouse. Although it has been reported to bind to many complex ligands in a calcium dependent manner, the function of SAP, its major physiological ligand(s) and its own binding epitopes are unknown. The aim of this work is to generate a panel of monoclonal antibodies (mAbs) which may be useful in characterizing the binding epitopes on SAP.

2. Methods

Native human SAP was isolated from serum by affinity chromatography on Sepharose 4B, followed by DE52 anion exchange and zinc chelate chromatography on Sepharose 6B. An alkaline extract of zymosan was prepared according to the method of Kubak [2]. SP2/0-Ag 14 myeloma cells were fused to immune mouse spleen cells by the method of Galfre and Milstein [3] with modifications by Lane *et al.* [4]. Hybridomas positive for antibody to HuSAP by screening ELISA were cloned two to four times by limiting dilution. Each hybridoma was screened three times: in the presence of 1mM $CaCl_2$; 10mM EDTA; and a 1/10 dilution of an alkali extract of zymosan. The class and subclass of each mAb in tissue culture supernatant was determined using a red cell agglutination test. MAbs were purified on protein A and concentrated to 1 mg/ml. They were biotinylated. Epitope specificity was studied by measuring the percentage inhibition of binding of biotinylated mAb to HuSAP by unlabelled mAb. The ability of selected mAbs to precipitate HuSAP in the presence of $CaCl_2$ or EDTA was tested using gel immunodiffusion and ^{125}I-SAP in a liquid phase assay. HuSAP was electrophoresed using the method of Laemmli [5], blotted onto Immobilon-P membrane and probed with mAbs.

3. Results

Eighteen mAbs (all IgG1) were produced from three separate fusions. The mAbs were assigned to 3 groups on the basis of epitope specificity (Table 1): Group 1, comprises 13 mAbs of which 8 (3.3D, 5.4A, 7.5C, 6.9F, 8.5P, 13.6G, 7.7F and 1.3) are very cross-reactive (i.e. more than 80% inhibited by unlabelled mAbs) and 5 (4.7D, 6.12C, 9.1H, 2.0A and 1.1O) are moderately cross-reactive (i.e. 50 - 79% inhibited by unlabelled mAbs). Group 2, has 4 members of which 3 (5.3E, 5.4D and 5.4D.3B) are highly cross reactive and one (5.4D.9H) is moderately cross-reactive. Group 3 has one member (9.3F) which does not inhibit binding of other antibodies.

Table 1

% Inhibition of Reactivity of biotinylated mAb by unlabelled mAb

Unlabelled	Biotinylated mAb								
mAb	3.3D	5.4A	7.5C	6.12C	8.5P	13.6G	5.3E	5.4D	1.3
None	0	0	0	0	0	0	0	0	0
Group 1 (examples)									
5.4A	91	100	100	100	100	100	0	0	44
1.3	97	100	100	100	100	100	0	0	99
6.12C	77	32	34	100	15	76	16	0	42
Group 2 (examples)									
5.4D.3B	0	0	0	0	0	0	100	100	0
5.4D.9H	0	17	10	100	53	0	60	74	0
Group 3									
9.3F	26	13	0	0	0	37	0	0	0

100% inhibition is the reactivity inhibited by an excess of homologous unlabelled mAb. 0% inhibition is the reactivity in the absence of unlabelled mAb.

Four mAbs (9.1H, 9.3F, 4.7D and 13.6G) were selected and cloned on the basis of zymosan and/or EDTA inhibition of their reactivity with HuSAP in tissue culture screening ELISA. However, after purification such inhibition could not be demonstrated (Fig.1).

All mAbs react with native HuSAP blotted onto Immobilon P. Group II mAbs react strongly with SDS and DTT denatured HuSAP. MAbs 5.4A, 7.5C, 1.1O and 7.7F from Group I, react weakly with denatured HuSAP.

Three patterns of immunoprecipitation of ^{125}I-HuSAP by selected mAbs were observed (Fig. 2). MAb 7.5C showed increased precipitation of SAP in the presence of EDTA compared with $CaCl_2$, although maximum precipitation was observed at 1 μg for both conditions. MAbs 4.7D, 5.4D.9H, 6.12C, 5.4A and 8.5P all demonstrated calcium independent precipitation. MAb 9.3F did not precipitate ^{125}I-HuSAP.

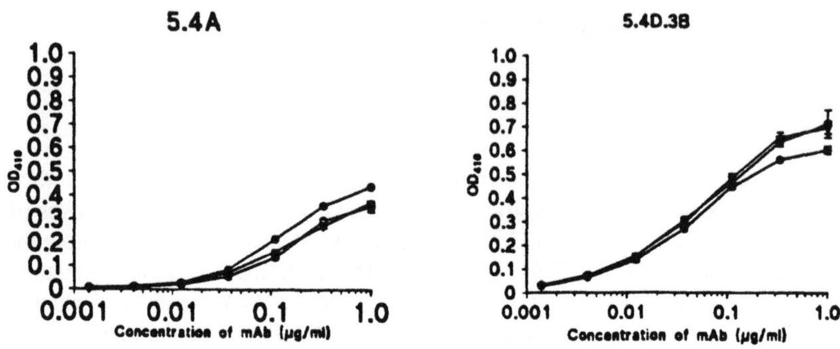

Figure 1. Effect of Ca^{2+}, EDTA and Zymosan on MAb reactivity with 1μg/ml HuSAP

○ = 1mM $CaCl^{2+}$

● = 10mM EDTA

△ = 1/10 dilution of alkaline extract of Zymosan

Results = mean +/− s.d., n = 3

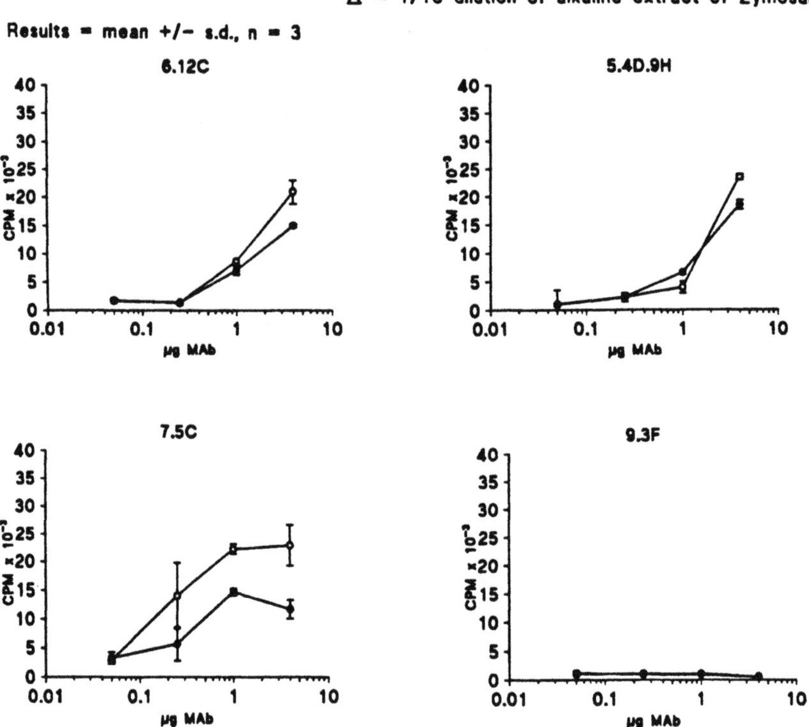

Figure 2. Precipitation of ^{125}I–HuSAP by MAbs.

50ng ^{125}I–HuSAP (sp. act. = 0.74 μCi/ug) were added to 860ng unlabelled HuSAP in 200μl $TBSCa^{2+}$ or TBSEDTA. Pellets were washed, dissolved in 0.1M NaOH and counted.

results = mean +/− s.d. ● = 0.5mM $CaCl^{2+}$ ○ = 5mM EDTA

Immunodiffusion of mAbs and HuSAP in polyacrylamide gels confirmed the results using ^{125}I-SAP (Fig.3). However, mAb 9.3F may precipitate HuSAP weakly by this method and not by the former method. Other mAbs which precipitate HuSAP are 3.3D, 5.3E, 7.7F, 9.1H and 5.4D.3B.

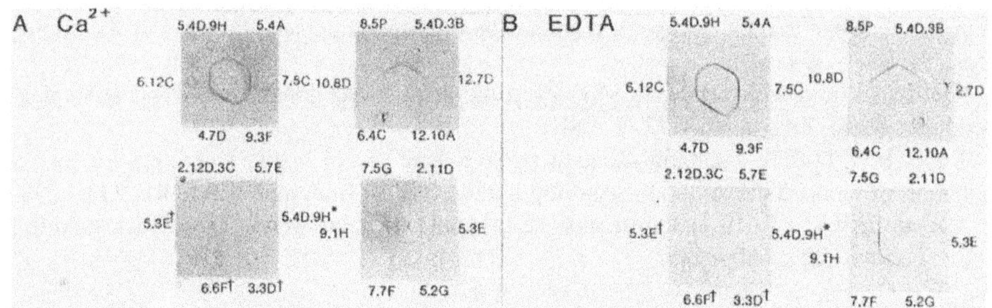

Figure 3. Polyacrylamide gel immunodiffusion of mAbs and HuSAP.
The central wells contain 5µg HuSAP. The outer wells contain 4µg purified mAb. The gel consists of 4% acrylamide (2.7% w/v bis-acrylamide) in 0.125M Tris/HCl, pH8.6. MAbs and SAP were allowed to diffuse in the presence of 0.5mM $CaCl_2$ or 5mM EDTA for 1 week before staining with Coomassie Blue. * = Ascites † = MAb purified on protein A (low [NaCl].

4. Discussion

The results presented here suggest that the region of HuSAP defined as Group I epitopes by reciprocal inhibition patterns (Table 1) are very immunogenic, since 13 of the 18 mAbs generated bind to them. Also clones from this group represent three different fusions. Four members of Group I (5.4A, 7.5C, 7.7F and 1.1O), which have a similar pattern of cross reactivity (Table 1), weakly recognise a linear epitope on denatured and native HuSAP. The others bind to conformational epitopes only.
Group II mAbs, which represent one fusion, react with a linear epitope that is also present on the native protein. They inhibit each other fully and thus are probably different clones of the same antibody.

5. Acknowledgements

We would like to thank the Wellcome Trust and the Arthritis Research Council. We acknowledge very helpful discussions with A.K. Falconer, Dr. A. Hamilton, Dr. G. Holland and Prof. M. Stewart.
G.O'S. would like to thank D.N.O'Sullivan.

6. References

[1] Prelli, F., Pras, M. and Frangione, B. (1985) The primary structure of human tissue amyloid P component from a patient with primary idiopathic amyloidosis, J. Biol. Chem. 260, 12895 - 12898.

[2] Kubak, B.M., Potempa, L.A., Gewurz, A., Slodki, M.E., Venegas, M., Anderson, B. and Gewurz, H. (1986) Binding of serum amyloid P-component (SAP) to soluble saccharomyces cerevisiae zymosan extract, and yeast mannans and phosphomannans, Protides of the Biological Fluids, 34, 391 - 394.

[3] Galfre, G. and Milstein, C. (1981) Preparation of monoclonal antibodies: strategies and procedures, Meth. Enzymology 73, 1 - 46.

[4] Lane, R.D. (1985) A short-duration polyethylene glycol fusion technique for increasing production of monoclonal antibody-secreting hybridomas, J. Immunol. Meth. 81, 223 - 228.

[5] Laemmli, V.K. (1970) Determination of protein molecular weight in polyacrylamide gels, Nature (London) 227, 680 - 685.

SCREENING WITH MONOCLONAL ANTI BETA-PROTEIN ANTIBODY FOR IMMUNO-REACTIVITY IN THE SERA OF PATIENTS WITH ALZHEIMER'S DISEASE

T.SHINODA,[1] Y.KAMETANI,[1] K.MIYANAGA,[2] and K.IINUMA[3]
[1] Department of Cheimistry, Tokyo Metropolitan University, Setagaya-ku, Tokyo; [2] Department of Neuropsychiatry, Gunma University School of Medicine, Maebashi; [3] National Children's Hospital, Setagaya-ku, Tokyo, Japan

ABSTRACT. A monoclonal antibody(aSP01) and a polyclonal antibody was raised against a synthetic peptide corresponding to residues(N:1-10, SP01) of the beta-protein. Using the aSP01 and sandwitch ELISA technique immunoreactivities in sera were determined for four groups, three affected(Alzheimer's disease, senile dementia of Alzheimer's type(AD/SDAT), multi-infarct dementia(MID), dementia of not otherwise satisfied (NOS)), and a non-affected group. Whereas a high value in the cross-reactivity was observed on AD(35.11±7.91), relatively low values were obtained for the latter groups(MID;16.76±2.58, NOS;13.28±2.20, non-demented;14.41±1.94). No difference in the mean value of the CRM was shown between male and female groups(male;16.04±3.51, female; 14.99±2.47). Practically no corroration was observed between the age and CRM of the two affected groups(AD;r=-0.0585, MID;r=0.0353)and non-affected group(r=0.2758).

1. INTRODUCTION

Beta-protein, a 42-residue peptide, has been reported to be a principal constituent of the brain amyloid of patients with Alzheimer's disease and also of adult Down's syndrome brain amyloid[1-3]. Recentry, the base sequence of a cDNA for a much larger precursor amyloid protein[4], consisting of 695 amino acid residues, has been determined. Two additional putative amyloid beta-proteins, consisting of 751 and 770 amino acid residues, have also been reported more recently[5].

Several questions may be raised regarding the nature and the role of these precursor amyloid proteins in relation to the pathogenesis of Alzheimer's disease and related neurological disorders. First, from where do the precursors arise? If primarily from brain, then it may be of value to test cerebrospinal fruid for its preseise; alternatively if it arises from blood, the plasma may be of primary importance for examination. Second, if the precursor(s) and its metabolites exist in the plasma, at what levels? Third, is there any difference in the level of the precursor(s) in the plasmas between patients with Alzheimer's disease and normal individuals? These are all basic problems to be solved.

In order to investigate further the role of the precursor protein(s) in Alzheimer's disease and in some other groups with neurological disorders,we measured the levels of the immunoreactivity in the sera obtained from them using a sandwitch ELISA method employing a monoclonal antibody against a beta-protein subpeptide.

2. MATERIALS AND METHODS

2.1. Preparation of Antigen

A 10-residue peptide corresponding to the first 10 amino acid residues of the amyloid beta-protein(sequence: DAEFRHDSGY; referred to as SP01), which was coupled with an additional cysteine residue at the carboxy terminus was synthesized and purified by reverse-phase HPLC under the reported conditions[6]. The purified peptide was covalently coupled to either KLH(SP01-KLH) or rabbit serum albumin(SP01-RSA).

2.2. Monoclonal Antibody

Four five-week-old female Balb/c mice were immunized subsutaneously with a total of 100ug of SP01-KLH in complete Freund's adjuvant into several parts of the body. Hybridomas were prepared conventionally and selected for monoclonal antibody as reported[7].

2.3. Serum Samples

The sera were collected from three affected and one non-affected groups. (A) Alzheimer's disease and senile dementia of Alzheimer's type; (B) multiinfarct dementia (cerevrovascular involvements); (C) senile dementia not otherwise specified; (D) non-demented group.

2.4. Determination of Immunoreactivity

The immunoreactivity assay of sera was performed by a sandwitch ELISA technique using 40ul of test sera. The microplates were incubated with a peroxydase-conjugated goat anti-rabbit IgG (final dilution;1:2000); and after final washing with 0.01M Tris-HCl 0.2% Tween 20, the presence of the antibody was visualised by incubation of the sample with 0.2mM o-phenylenediamine and 0.44mM hydrogen peroxide in phosphate-citrate buffer.

Table 1. Mean Concentration of the Immunoreactivity in the Sera of Four Different Groups

Group	Number of Samples	Concentration (mean+s.d.)
A (AD/SDAT)	24	35.11±7.91
B (MID)	51	16.76±2.58
C (NOS)	25	13.28±2.20
D (non-demented)	94	14.41±1.91

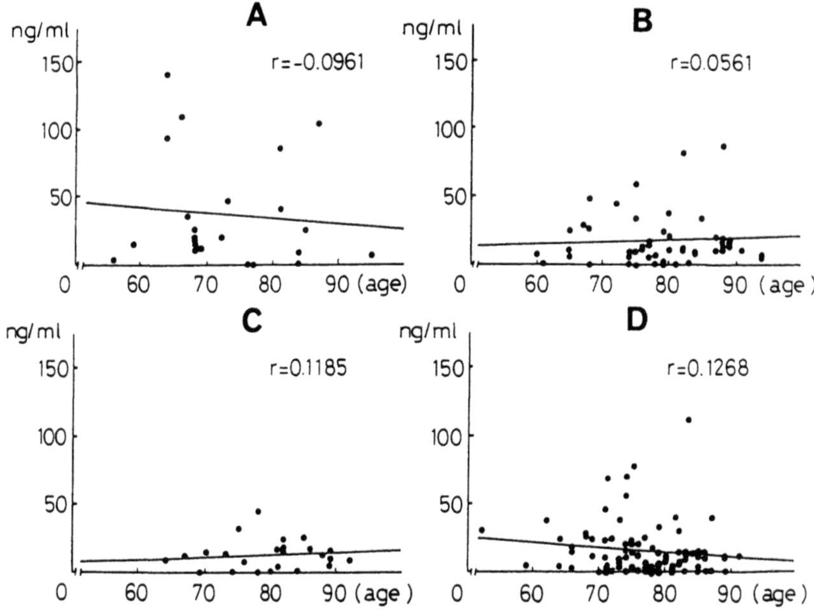

Figuro 1. Distribution of the concentration of SP01-CRM in the sera of patients and non-demented group. Corelation coefficient for each sample group with age was also shown in Fig. 1.

3. RESULTS AND DISCUSSION

Using aSP01 in the sandwitch ELISA technique, we determined cross-reactivities in the sera for four sample groups described above. Practically no significant difference in the mean value of the level of the crossreactivity was seen between male and female groups(male: 16.04±3.51 ng eq/ml, female:14.99±2.47 ng eq/ml). No correlation was seen between the age and the value of immunoreactivity in the sera from either sex. The mean values of the immunoreactivities are summarized in Table 1 for four sample groups.

The monoclonal antibody aSP01 was effective in sandwitch ELISA system for conventional screening. The antibody was also shown to decorate the senile plaques of different stages in the brains of patients with Alzheimer's disease and somewhat less intensely the ones in the brain ofan adult Down's syndrome patient (findings to be published elsewhere).

As indicated in Table 1, when the mean values of the immuno-reactivitywere compared, the highest value was attained with Alzheimer's disease cases. The difference was significant between

AD/SDAT and control($p<0.05$). The increase in the level of the immunoreactivity in the sera of patients with Alzheimer's disease does not necessarily mean that the brain is the principal source of this immunoreactivity, since mRNA for amyloid precursor(s) has recently been found in many other organs. If these mRNAs are indeed translated, the products would more likely be transported into blood circulation. Even if its translation is within the normal level, if there are certain metabolic disturbances in the Alzheimer's disease patients, the level of such immunoreactivity in the serum would be expected to increase with time.

Although our data presented here suggest that there is a significant difference in the level of immunoreactivity between the group with Alzheimer's disease and the control without dementia, further studies are obviously needed in many respects before we can arrive at an overall conclusion.

4. ACKNOWLEDGMENT

This work was supported in part by grants-in-aid from the Primary Amyloidosis Research Committee of the Ministry of Health and Welfare, and by the Human Science Foundation.

5. REFERENCES

[1] Glenner, G.G. and Wong,C.W. (1984) 'Alzheimer's disease and Down's syndrome; sharing of a unique cerebrovascular amyloid protein', Biochem. Biophys. Res. Comm. 122,1131-1136.
[2] Glenner, G.G. and Wong,C.W. (1984) 'Alzheimer's disease: initial report of the purification and characterization of a novel cerebrovascular amyloid protein', Biochem. Biophys. Res. Comm. 120, 885-890.
[3] Masters, C.L., Simms, G., Weinman, N.A., Multihaup, G., MacDonald, B.L., and Beyreuther,K. (1985) 'Amyloid plaque core protein in Alzheimer's disease and Down's syndrome', Proc. Natl. Acad. Sci. USA 82, 4245-4249.
[4] Kang, J., Leaire, H.G., Unterbeck, A., et al., (1987) 'The precursor of Alzheimer's disease amyloid A4 protein resembles a cell-surface receptor', Nature 325, 733-736.
[5] Tanzi, R.E., MacLatchey, A.I., Lamperti, E.D., Komaroff, L.V., Gusella, J.F., and Neve, J.F. (1988) 'Protease inhibitor domain encoded by an amyloid protein precursor mRNA associated with Alzheimer's disease', Nature 331, 528-530.
[6] Shinoda, T., Kametani, F., Tonoike, H., and Kito, S., (1986) 'Sailent structural features of low molecular weight amyloid fibril protein in FAP of Japanese origin', in G.G. Glenner et al. (eds.), Amyloidosis, Plenum, New York, pp.331-336.
[7] Kametani, Y., Hiroi, T. Takenawa, T., Shinoda, T., Okuyama, T., Miyanaga, K., Iinuma, K., 'Preparation of a monoclonal antibody against the beta-protein subpeptide and scleening for an immunoreactivity in serum. submitted to Dementia.

Symposium Day 1: Overview

E.P. Benditt,
Seattle, WA

Having been fortunate to be a member of the original International Symposium group that met in Gröningen, it is a great pleasure for me to be able to participate in this VIth. International Symposium and to comment on the first day's sessions. The questions that were being asked in 1966 were the starting point for the list of questions represented in the VIth. Symposium's first day.

The first question asked was, "What is amyloid composed of?" It was beginning then to be clear that the major constituent of amyloid fibrillar substance is protein. Protein chemistry was very cumbersome in 1966 and our molecular biology was at best primitive. The contrast is dramatic. We know now that there are different chemical classes of amyloid substance based on their major peptide structures. As we see from this first day's proceedings, the questions posed are 1) In any particular case what is its major constituent peptide?; 2) What is the precursor of this peptide?; 3) Where does it come from, i.e. what cells make the precursor?; 4) What does the precursor do physiologically; and finally, 5) What does the peptide do pathologically? While it took some time to recognize that there were a number of different chemical classes of amyloid substance, we presently recognize at least a dozen. In this portion of the Symposium, papers were presented from different laboratories reporting on variants of a given class of amyloid gene products within a single individual and variants among different individuals, the aim being to see if there are amyloidogenic patterns in the amino acid sequences of the peptides. A good deal of effort has gone into investigating the amino acid sequences of peptides from the AL, AA and other amyloidoses in search of particular sequences that might be especially amyloidogenic. This has yielded specific information but not yet any integrating concept.

The genetic features of the SAA family of proteins in several different vertebrate species has become more detailed and elegant with the use of molecular biologic methods. It is now clear that there are several genes that belong to this family in all the species examined so far. This, along with the fact that the gene family and its products are highly conserved among a variety of species of mammals and birds, suggests that it has some important function. The SAA gene family is the most dramatically elevated of the acute phase proteins, and this has led to a number of studies of the gene structure and its responses to various injurious stimuli. Transcriptional control of Serum Amyloid A gene expression by various cytokines turns out to be more complex with several of these signals working in concert and further exploration of this area should be fruitful.

The search for the nature of amyloid substances and the pathogenesis of amyloidosis is leading us to new insights about physiological systems. For example, the serum precursor of the amyloid A protein is a new apolipoprotein family whose functions we are just beginning to appreciate. Similarly, the most recent member of the amyloid peptides family found in pancreatic islets of type II diabetics has a hitherto unknown precursor that seems important for the metabolism of glucose. Clearly the search for the function of the precursors of the amyloid substances, while still elusive in many instances, becomes more and more interesting.

Another feature of the pathogenesis of amyloidosis of the AA type is the apparent role of the enhancing factor (AEF). Although several laboratories have been studying AEF, and it has proved as a substance to be rather elusive, the effects of AEF now appear reproducible and we can expect further clarification of its role.

Some new elements of the pathogenesis of AA and other amyloidoses are being explored including factors such as what localizes the precursor, is it due to selection from the circulation or local formation? Other factors needing study include the fact that amyloid precursors have a tendency to self aggregation, and the amphipathic nature of precursors, suggesting the potential for interactions of the hydrophobic regions of the molecule could be important. Such concerns have become part of the study of amyloidosis and we see some examples of the investigations in this day's sessions. Not much attention has been given to processes of stabilization of the aggregates once they are formed, although the role of the beta conformation of the proteins has been emphasized, there are probably other factors at work.

Unfortunately, the least progress appears to be in developments in therapy. The AL variety shows stubborn resistance to most of the therapies tried so far. The only therapy still that seems to have very much effect is colchicine, and this mainly if not entirely effective in the AA type of amyloid.

A striking feature as one looks over the program for the Symposium is the very extensive collaborative efforts among groups in different parts of the world and in different fields of medicine working on amyloidosis. This is good to see and augers well for future rapid progress in understanding the general features of the disease process and the specific features of each of its varieties.

AMYLOIDOSIS: MOLECULAR INSIGHTS AND CELLULAR BLINDSPOTS

Dorothea Zucker-Franklin, M.D.
Department of Medicine
New York University Medical Center
550 First Avenue
New York, N.Y. 10016

Since the introductory speakers presented very complete overviews of each subject dealt with on the second day of this meeting, mere reiteration of this material seems redundant. Instead, I shall point out what, in my opinion, may be the highlights of the new contributions and where I think we should go from here.

By far the largest number of papers dealt with transthyretin (TTR), a protein which has been fully characterized (1, 2). The normal function of this protein is to carry thyrozine and the retinol-binding protein which is involved in the transport of vitamin A.

A major breakthrough in the field of amyloidosis occurred 6 years ago when the amyloid of the Andrade familial amyloid polyneuropathy (FAP I) was found associated with a mutation in this protein i.e. a substitution of methionine for valine at position 30 of the molecule (3-5). Clinical variants of this condition were soon described in kindreds of Greek, Swiss, Italian and Japanese descent. The genetic polymorphism of TTR became apparent after other mutations in the molecule were reported. Recently, it was found that TTR deposited in the heart in senile amyloidosis has an amino acid substitution at position 122, where isoleucine replace valine (6). The abstracts in the Proceedings of this meeting attest to the fact that a host of other point mutations in the transthyretin molecule may become associated with amyloidosis (e.g. abstracts 07/2, 07/6, P7/9, P7/12, P7/19, P7/24, P7/26, P7/28), and that even perfectly normal TTR is able to polymerize into fibrils (P7/27) whereas the acid variant of the mutated TTR-met 30 may not be pathogenic (P7/7).

The message we take home from this symposium is that in the case of amyloids consisting of TTR, there is enormous biochemical heterogeneity as well as variantion in the clinical syndromes and the ethnic origin of the populations affected.

Technical Advances

There is little doubt that much of the progress made since the last International Amyloid Symposium is attributable to the new biomolecular tools which have become available during the interim. Among these are the polymerase chain reaction (PCR) which has been applied to an assessment of the genotype frequency of the Mae III - TTR in the Black population (see 07/3 an P7/5) or to the DNA extracted from blood cells of individuals who may be carriers of the HCCAA allele, (P4/2). In the former instances, this may lead to the recognition of the etiology of a form of congestive heart failure that was formerly not understood. In the latter case, it may enable us to provide prenatal councilling when this is desirable. In the least, these techniques will permit us to determine, for a relatively small price, the incidence of variant peptide structure or the extent of polymorphism among large populations.

Equally exciting has been the production of hybrid peptides where one or two amino acids in the human peptide sequence has been substituted by rodent residues, which is a boon for studies on fibrillogenesis, the development of a recombinant system for variant type transthyretin (07/1), and the advent of a transgenic mice (07/5) which will facilitate studies on the *in vivo* behavior of variant peptides. These are only few of the techniques which will have a major impact on our knowledge of the amyloid diseases.

Cell Biology

Despite the enormous amount of information gained on the biomolecular level, we have a long way to go. As yet there is no clear understanding of how and why any of the fibrils form in any of the amyloids, how we can intercept the process, or how the polymerized fibrils can be eliminated once they have formed. To elucidate these processes, we must return to studies of intact cells. There have been astoundingly few of these presented at this meeting. The time alotted to this discussion permits only a few suggestions as to the direction future studies might take.

Amyloid is usually deposited in the vicinity of, and sometimes even within the cells responsible for the synthesis of its percursor. This has been amply illustrated in very early publications related to AA and AL (reviewed in ref. 7) and at this Symposium it has been shown to hold true also for islet amyloid polypeptide (IAPP) (05/2) and the β protein (08/5). It is now beyond cavail, that in each of these amyloids it is possible for the fibrils to be located partially intracellularly and partially extracellularly with complete destruction of the intervening plasma membrane. However, this observation alone does not elucidate the process by which fibrils are formed. What could be the mechanism(s) involved?

Within the cellular cortex as well as anchored in the membrane itself, there are numerous proteins which become highly insoluble when they are cross-linked. In addition, the external aspect of the plasma membranes of amy cells bears proteolytic enzymes (e.g. 8, 9), which can be up or down regulated by external stimuli and which are likely to be involved in the processing of secreted molecules. Defective enzymatic degradation has been shown to be a factor in the deposition of AA (10), and we have learned at this meeting that attempts are being made to identify enzyme(s) relevant to the processing of the β-protein (08/2).

Gelsolin

Because of the relatively new discovery by Maury (11, 04/4) and confirmation at this meeting (P4/3, P4/5, P4/6) that a variant form of gelsolin may be responsible for the formation of amyloid in the Finish type of familial amyloidotic polyneuropathy (FAP IV), it seems appropriate to use this protein to illustrate intracellular processes which should be explored in the near future.

Gelsolin was first described in rabbit macrophages and platelets (12, 13) and held responsible for alternating gelation and "solation" of the cytoplasm necessary for contraction and chemotaxis. Gelsolin does not only sever actin molecules, but can also laterally associate or link them to other cytoskeletal proteins depending on ionic conditions and calcium ion concentration (for review see ref. 14) Do patients with FAP IV have aberrant gelsolin all their cells? On the basis of immunohistochemical studies presented at this meeting, this is likely. It has also been established that the aberrant protein circulates in plasma. How is gelsolin normally degraded? The catabolism of circulating proteins generally takes place by lysosomal digestion within the macrophage phagocytic system, whereas non-lysosomal degradation of intracellular proteins is often mediated by ubiquitin. Ubiquitin, when activated by ATP, is covalently linked to its target protein via an isopeptide bond between its carboxy terminal and the ε-amino group of lysine of the target protein. It is conceivable that ubiquitin recognizes the aberrant gelsolin molecule as it would normally occurring, but effete, intracellular proteins. If so, it may accelerate binding and cause an accumulation of cross linked protein which could overwhelm further degradative mechanisms. Ubiquitin has also been reported to possess intrinsic proteolytic activitiy over a broad pH range whereby it specifically modifies proteins intrinsic to membranes (15).

Interestingly, ubiquitin has been found associated with neurofibrillar tangles, senile plaques, Lewy bodies and Pick bodies (16). Therefore, it would not be surprising to find that it cross-links gelsolin and particularly, the molecular variant of this peptide.

Some years ago, we postulated that transglutaminase may play a similar role in the cross-linking of AA, the incomplete degradation product of SAA (10.)

Space does not permit a discussion of these concepts relevant to the "amyloidogenic" isotypes of transthyretin or the endocrine amyloids which were also considered at this meeting. However, the same theories are applicable to them.

We have come a long way towards a biochemical definition of various amyloid fibrils and the molecular genetics of their component proteins. In the next few years new advances my come from studies dealing with processes involving degradative enzymes, their inhibitors, and the physiopathologic turnover of the "amyloidogenic" proteins following their synthesis.

References

1. Kanda Y., Goodman D.S., Canfield R.E., Morgan F.J. (1974) 'The amino acid sequence of human plasma prealbumin', J. Biol. Chem. 249: 6796-6805.

2. Blake CCF, Geisow M.J., Swan IDA (1974) 'Structure of human plasma prealbumin at 2.5 A resolution', A preliminary report of the polypeptide chain conformation, quaternary structure and thyroxine binding. J. Mol. Biol. 88: 1-12.

3. Dwulet F.E., Benson MD (1984) 'Primary structure of an amyloid prealbumin and its plasma precursor in a heredofamilial polyneuropathy of Swedish orgin', Proc. Natl. Acad. Sci. 81: 694-698.

4. Tawara S., Nakazato M., Kangawa K., Matsuo H., and Araki S.(1983) 'Indentification of amyloid prealbumin variant in familial amyloidotic polyneuropathy (Japanese type)', Biochem. Biophys. Res. Commun. 116: 880-888.

5. Saraiva MJM, Birken S., Costa PP, Goodman D.S. (1984) 'Amyloid fibril protein in familial amyloidotic polyneuropathy, Portuguese type', Definition of molecular abnormality in transthyretin (prealbumin), J. Clin. Invest. 74: 104-119.

6. Gorevic P.D., Prelli F.C., Wright J., Pras M., Fangione B. (1989) 'Systemic Senile amyloidosis'. Indentification of a new prealbumin (transthyretin) variant in a cardiac tissue: immunologic and biochemical similarity to one form of familial amyloidotic polyneuropathy. J. Clin. Invest. 83: 836-843.

7. Franklin E.C. and Zucker-Franklin, D. (1972) 'Current concepts of amyloid', Adv. Immunol. 15: 249-304.

8. Lavie G., Zucker-Franklin D., and Franklin E.C. (1978) 'Degradation of serum amyloid A protein by surface-associated enzymes of human blood monocytes', J. Exp. Med. 148: 1020-1031.

9. Zucker-Franklin, D., Lavie G., and Franklin E.C. (1981) 'Demonstration of membrane-bound proteolytic activity on the surface of mononuclear leukocytes', J. Histochem. Cytochem. 29: 451-456.

10. Fuks A., and Zucker-Franklin, D. (1985) 'Impaired Kupffer cell functon precedes development of secondary amyloidosis', J. Exp. Med. 161: 1013-1028.

11. Maury C.P.J., Alli, K., and Baumann M. (1990) 'Finnish hereditary amyloidosis', Amino acid sequence hamology between the amyloid fibril protein and human plasma gelsolin. FEBS 260: 85-87.

12. Yin H.L., and Stossel T.P. (1979) 'Control of Cytoplasmic actin gelsol transformation by gelsolin, a calcium-dependent regulatory protein', Nature 281: 583-586.

13. Yin H.L., Albrecht J., and Fattoum A. (1981) 'Indentification of gelsolin. a Ca++ - dependent regulatory protein of actin gel-sol transformation: its intracellular distribution in a variety of cells and tissues, J. Cell Biol. 91: 901-906.

14. Kwiatkoski D.J., Mehl R., and Yin H.L. (1988) 'Genomic organization and biosynthesis of secreted and cytoplasmic forms of gelsolin', J. Cell Biol. 106: 375-384.

15. Fried, et al. (1987) 'Ubiquitin has intrinsic proteolytic activity', Proc. Natl. Acad. Sci. 84: 3684-3689.

16. Perry G., Friedman R., Shaw G., and Chau V. (1987) 'Ubiquitin is detected in neurofibrillary tangles and senile plaque neurites of Alzheimer disease brains'. Proc. Natl. Acad. Sci. 84: 3033-3036.

SUMMARY OF DAY 3

Martha Skinner, M.D.

Today's scientific session began with the topic of amyloid in Alzheimer's disease. The neurobiologists joined the amyloidologists in 1984 at the Fourth International Amyloid Symposium held in New York and are now an integral part of this group. Today, we have heard 16 papers from 14 different centers with participants from 5 countries.

George Glenner's introductory talk highlighted the remarkable progress in this area of research from the precise identification of the amyloid protein, called beta protein, and its precursor, amyloid beta protein precursor, to the current work on proteolytic processing. He presented evidence suggesting that a serine protease cleaves the beta protein from its precursor at the site where it is embedded in the cell membrane.

Several definitive studies were presented. Dennis Selkoe presented studies which documented the presence of amyloid beta protein immunoreactive deposits in vascular and perivascular tissues of skin and intestine. Carmela Abraham presented data identifying a protease in brain tissue that belongs to the serine protease family. This protease is able to cleave the beta protein precursor at the amino terminus of amyloid beta protein. We look forward to her further characterization and identity of this protease. Marcia Podlisny presented evidence for the remarkable homology of the beta protein precursor in monkey and in man. It is hoped that this will make an excellent animal model. Dr. Erikssen showed his immunohistochemical characterization of choroid plexus amyloid. Dr. Wisniewski presented the finding of amyloid fibrils in an identical location to enzymes in non-amyloid cells.

Eleven more presentations were made in the poster session. Two of these studies were from the Netherlands on the hereditary cerebral hemorrhage with amyloidosis - Dutch type which occurs as an autosomal dominant disorder and in which the amyloid fibril deposit is homologous to beta protein. Others were on vascular amyloid deposits in brain, vascular amyloid in various organs other than brain in Alzheimer's disease, and the distribution of dermatan sulfate proteoglycans in Alzheimer's disease. Several studies further charaterized the immunoreactivity of amyloid deposits in brain.

The scientific sessions continued with the diagnostic, clinical and therapeutic aspects of amyloidosis. In the clinical session 29 abstracts were presented. The large numbers was surpassed only by the AA/SAA session which had 36.

Dr. Pepys in his eloquent introduction and Dr. Hawkins in the the first talk showed us data on an exquisitely sensitive radiolabeled SAP which identifies amyloid deposits in most organ systems. This test promises to be useful in defining and monitoring the "amyloid burden" in tissues before and after therapy.

Other methodologic advances were presented by L. Benson in an assessment of the use of MRI for staging AL amyloid disease followed by Yukio Ando's discussion of an analysis of autonomic dysfunction by laser doppler flowometry. Three large amyloid population studies were presented. A. Dofferhoff reminded us of the clinical dilemma in defining amyloid type and reported to us on the Netherlands experience in a large amyloid population where resolution could be obtained by histopathologic classification. A long term follow up on colchicine treatment in patients with familial Mediterannean fever presented by D. Zemer was very encouraging. And Morie Gertz presented the experience of the Mayo Clinic from 1956 to 1989 with AA amyloidosis. Two-thirds of their 64 patients had AA amyloidosis secondary to a rheumatic disease. All patients had renal involvement and 46 patients had died after a median survival of 30 months.

It was clear in the papers and the posters that as physicians and scientists we still lack an effective treatment for our patients that suffer from these diseases. Sadly, we realize that this will be difficult and will require much more basic research. Although no major advances in therapy have been discovered, a number of supportive measures including the use of organ transplantations, were discussed.

In conclusion, I can say

Day 3, today, has been an interesting day with profitable discussion. We thank our meeting organizers and the presenters.

LIST OF CONTRIBUTORS

SUBJECT INDEX

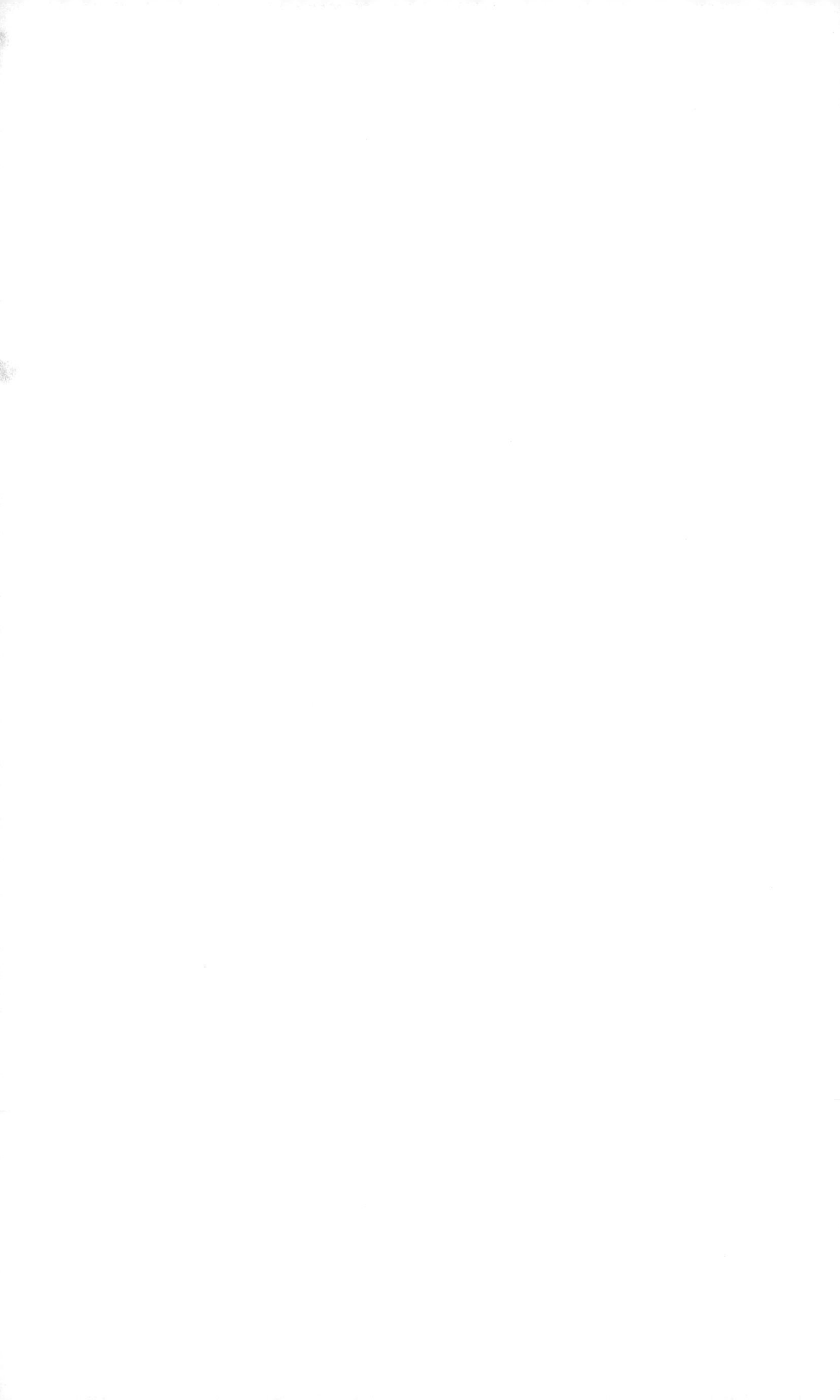

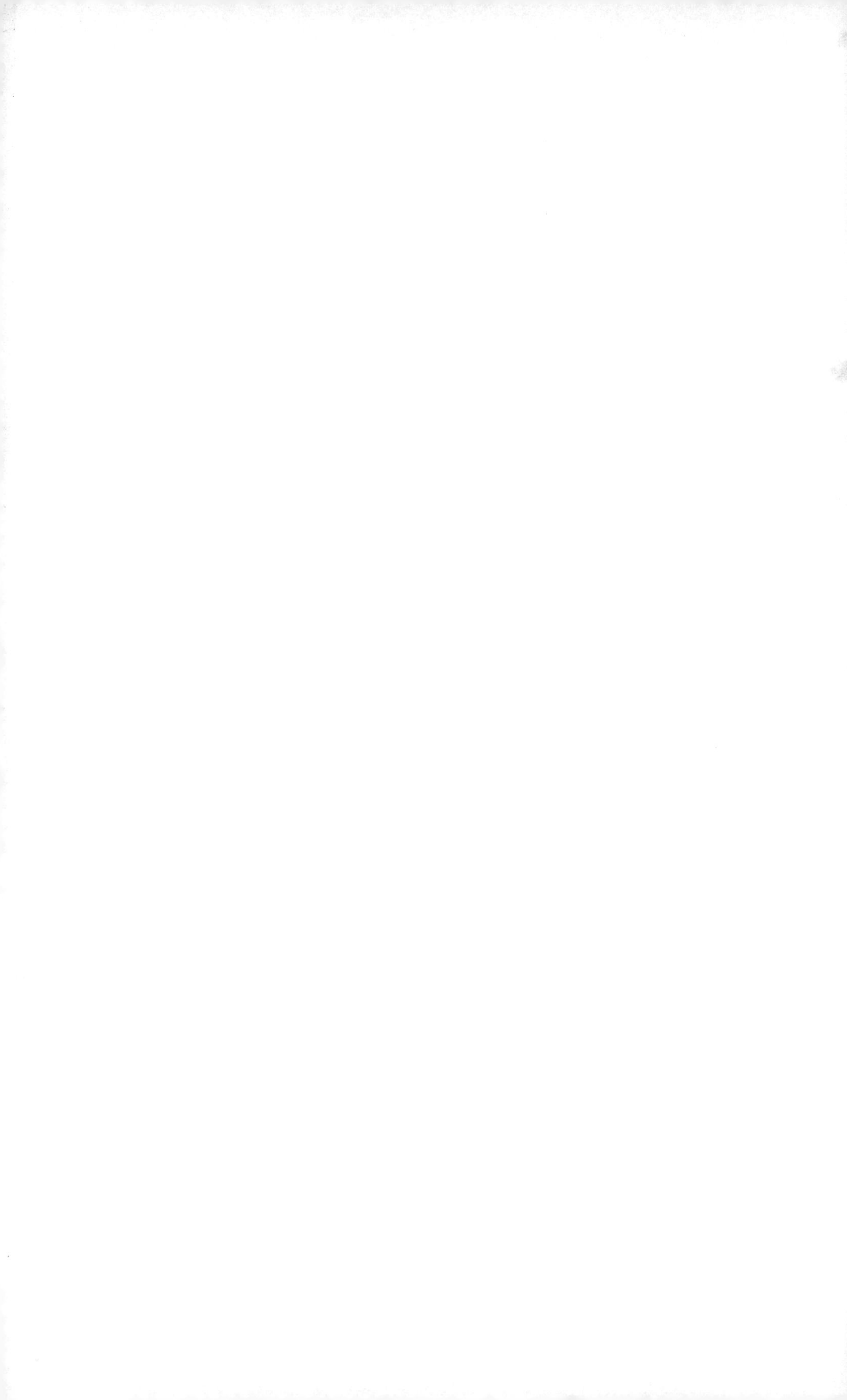

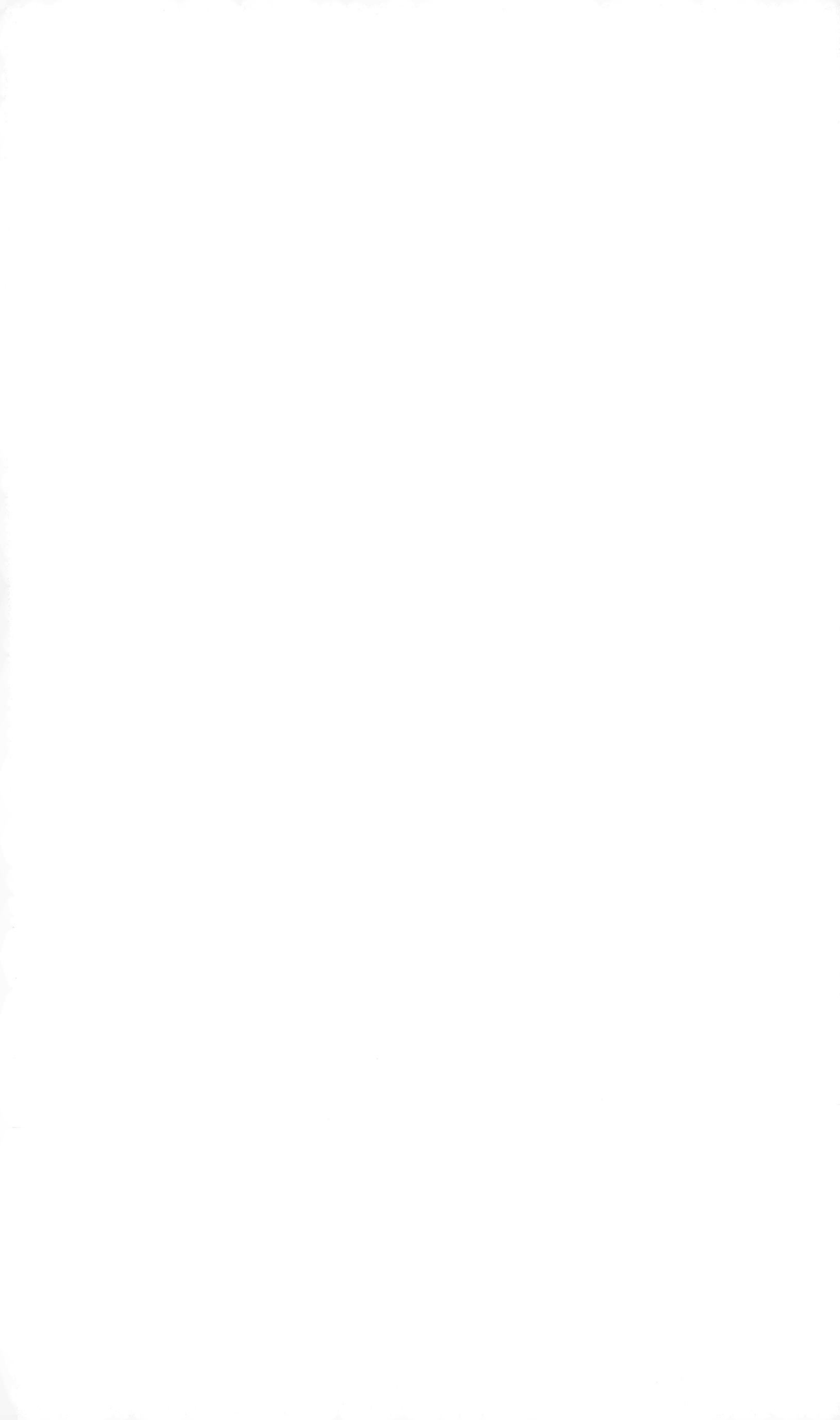

GPSR Compliance
The European Union's (EU) General Product Safety Regulation (GPSR) is a set of rules that requires consumer products to be safe and our obligations to ensure this.

If you have any concerns about our products, you can contact us on

ProductSafety@springernature.com

In case Publisher is established outside the EU, the EU authorized representative is:

Springer Nature Customer Service Center GmbH
Europaplatz 3
69115 Heidelberg, Germany

www.ingramcontent.com/pod-product-compliance
Ingram Content Group UK Ltd.
Pitfield, Milton Keynes, MK11 3LW, UK
UKHW021434280726
14060UKWH00001BA/82